Handbook of Clinical
Neuropsychology

Handbook of Clinical Neuropsychology

SECOND EDITION

Edited by:

Jennifer M. Gurd
University Department of Clinical Neurology,
John Radcliffe Hospital, Oxford, UK

Udo Kischka
Rivermead Research Centre,
Oxford Centre for Enablement,
Oxford, UK

John C. Marshall (deceased †)
Formerly of Neuropsychology Unit,
University Department of Clinical Neurology,
John Radcliffe Hospital, Oxford, UK

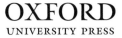
OXFORD
UNIVERSITY PRESS

OXFORD

UNIVERSITY PRESS

Great Clarendon Street, Oxford ox2 6DP

Oxford University Press is a department of the University of Oxford.
It furthers the University's objective of excellence in research, scholarship,
and education by publishing worldwide in

Oxford New York

Auckland Cape Town Dar es Salaam Hong Kong Karachi
Kuala Lumpur Madrid Melbourne Mexico City Nairobi
New Delhi Shanghai Taipei Toronto

With offices in

Argentina Austria Brazil Chile Czech Republic France Greece Guatemala
Hungary Italy Japan Poland Portugal Singapore South
Korea Switzerland Thailand Turkey Ukraine Vietnam

Oxford is a registered trade mark of Oxford University Press
in the UK and in certain other countries

Published in the United States
by Oxford University Press Inc., New York

British Library Cataloguing in Publication Data
Data available

Library of Congress Cataloging in Publication Data
Data available

Typeset in Minion by Glyph International, Bangalore, India
Printed on acid-free paper by
CPI Anthony Rowe

ISBN 978–0–19–923411–0

10 9 8 7 6 5 4 3 2 1

Oxford University Press makes no representation, express or implied, that the drug dosages in this book are
correct. Readers must therefore always check the product information and clinical procedures with the most
up-to-date published product information and data sheets provided by the manufacturers and the most
recent codes of conduct and safety regulations. The authors and the publishers do not accept responsibility
or legal liability for any errors in the text or for the misuse or misapplication of material in this work. Except
where otherwise stated, drug dosages and recommendations are for the non-pregnant adult who is not breast
feeding.

Preface

Sadly, since the publication of the first edition in 2003, John Marshall has passed away, but leaving a hugely inspirational body of consequential neuropsychology research on which to build. Much has changed, and much remains the same since 2003. Technology and philosophical approaches to embracing its fruits have progressed considerably, while patients and their symptomatology remain timeless. We dedicate this second edition to M.C. Gurd, and to Joan Critchley (without whose help and support this volume would not have come to light.) We would also like to extend our gratitude to Carol Maxwell and Martin Baum of Oxford University Press for their generosity and guidance.

As ever, we are aware of the importance of curiosity and imagination in the application of hypothesis-driven (problem solving) approaches to clinical neuropsychology. This plays out over progressively new understanding of human neurophysiology and neuro-anatomy. The future will see further subdivisions of brain regions, vastly outstripping the broad categories initially delineated by Brodmann. Despite this rapidly changing context within the field of neuroscience, task-analytic approaches to testing remain apposite, including the salience of qualitative error analyses to augment quantitative scoring. Other key points emerging from this new edition include: (a) the pre-requisite of baseline measures (e.g. speech rate) in cognitive assessments of motor disorders; (b) the relevance of longitudinal functional imaging, particularly with respect to neurodegenerative conditions such as cortico-basal degeneration; (c) the continued sub-fractionation ('carving the cognitive chicken') of syndromes and conditions (e.g. dementias, MS, MND); (d) sources of bias in clinical research (particularly pharmacologically related ones); (e) the increasing importance of the cross-fertilization between experimental and clinical neuropsychology.

To quote a tongue-in-cheek cherished letter from an esteemed clinical neuropsychology colleague, found in JCM's first edition:

> *I have a problem. My working life is dominated by two groups of people with very different requirements, expectations, and modes of behavior, and yet I am expected, or expect myself, to somehow achieve a reconciliation between them.*
>
> *The first group, with whom I am in contact most weekdays, are people to whom a variety of unpleasant, and in some cases tragic, misfortunes have occurred. It is in the nature of these misfortunes that their origins and consequences are often unclear to those who have suffered them, though undoubtedly in most cases they are aware that some change, usually for the worse, has occurred. In general, the sufferers and their families attempt to deal with their difficulties honestly and realistically, though sometimes the very unfamiliarity of the states in which these people find themselves, coupled with the fact that they have often experienced profound changes in world views lead them to conclusions which others, myself included, would judge to be erroneous, and in some cases, where excessively firmly held and not susceptible to argument or modification, they may even be judged to be deluded. However, such*

delusions where they occur are not propagated widely, though they may cause some distress to friends and relatives.

The second group with whom I am in regular, though less frequent, contact causes me more concern, because delusions are more widely propagated and more powerfully maintained. Superficially, this group has far fewer problems. In general, they are intelligent, well-educated, and healthy. Such misfortunes as do befall them tend to occur in the mental and intellectual sphere, rather than the physical. My meetings with this type of person often occur when they are in large groups, though I also meet with them individually and in small groups. The problem with these people tend to be most noticeable when they are in large groups, and is in the nature of some very strange, but extremely strongly-held beliefs, which they go to great trouble and expense to pursue and substantiate. (This is in contrast to the first group I described, who rarely associate and have few funds or resources available to them.)

There are a number of beliefs of this second group which are so strongly and unshakably held as to merit being called delusions, but for brevity I will just mention two. The first of these is the belief that counting, or in some other sense measuring, external manifestations of behaviour is the same as understanding it. The delusion is marked by a virtually complete inability to empathize with selected other classes of people, who they often refer to as 'subjects'. I believe this term is not used because they consider themselves to have a monarchical relationship to such people, but arises from religious teachings that in this way they are achieving the hallowed state of 'objectivity'. The scriptures relating to these matters are very extensive, but I believe they can be traced back in part to two prophets, 'What's on' and 'Skin hur', who were early proponents of the doctrine of positive science. However, my researches into the origin of this delusion are partial and rudimentary, and other sources and prophets may also be involved.

A second strange belief held by many of these people is that the well-being of the first group of people I have mentioned can be best advanced by the use of large, powerful and complex machinery. Such machinery is said to perform an operation known as 'localizing impairments', and it is considered that the knowledge of where in the body a misfortune, difficulty, or even an intact ability can be said to reside is equivalent to understanding, and indeed treating the problem. I have tried to point out to my associates the error of this belief, and the dangers of placing too much faith in expensive and impressive machinery at the expense of more homely considerations of human purpose, attitudes, and needs, but I fear they pay little attention. The rapt attention which is paid to coloured pictures and diagrams shown by our leaders in the meetings we attend tends to produce a collective excitement which only serves to reinforce the delusion. These days I tend not to raise my arguments overtly a great deal to avoid giving distress to or suffering exclusion by my associates. I merely content myself with the reflection that should any of us have the misfortune to suffer a breakdown in our cars on the way home, it is to be hoped that the repairman has a pragmatic appreciation of the functioning of the systems as a whole, the purpose of the individual components, and a problem-solving approach to diagnosis, and does not lose himself in contemplation of the precise location of the petrol (gas) tank, measurement of the spark plug leads, or other extraneous matters.

JMG
UK
16 March 2009

Contents

Contributors

Anne M. Aimola Davies,
Department of Experimental Psychology,
Faculty of Philosophy and NIHR
Biomedical Research Centre,
University of Oxford, Oxford, UK, and
Department of Psychology,
The Australian National University,
Canberra, Australia

Nicole D. Anderson,
Kunin-Lunenfeld Applied Research Unit,
Baycrest, Toronto, Ontario, Canada

Peter A. Arnett,
Penn State University, Psychology
Department, University Park, PA, USA

Claudius Bartels,
Department of Neurology,
Otto-von-Guericke University,
Magdeburg, Germany

Pelagie M. Beeson,
National Center for Neurogenic
Communication Disorders, The
University of Arizona, Tucson AZ, USA

Vaughan Bell,
Institute of Psychiatry, London, UK

Gerhard Blanken,
Department of Neurology,
Otto-von-Guericke University,
Magdeburg, Germany

Gabriella Bottini,
Psychology Section, Philosophy
Department, University of Pavia, Pavia, Italy

Veronica Bradley,
Hurstwood Park Neurological Centre,
Haywards Heath, West Sussex, UK

Chris M. Bradshaw,
Psychopharmacology Section,
Division of Psychiatry, University of
Nottingham, Nottingham, UK

Paul W. Burgess,
Institute of Cognitive Neuroscience,
University College London, London, UK

Marinella Cappelletti,
Institute of Cognitive Neuroscience,
University College London, London, UK

Lisa Cipolotti,
Department of Neuropsychology,
National Hospital for Neurology &
Neurosurgery, London, UK, and
Dipartimento di Psicologia,
Universita degli Studi di Palermo,
Palermo, Italy

Martin Davies,
Faculty of Philosophy and
Department of Experimental Psychology,
University of Oxford,
Oxford, UK

Jennifer Duncan Davis,
Warren Alpert Medical School of
Brown University, Department of
Psychiatry and Human Behavior,
Providence, Rhode Island, USA

David M. Erlanger,
Department of Neurology,
Albert Einstein College of medicine,
Bronx New York, and Department of
Neuroscience and Education,
Columbia University New York,
NY, USA, and HeadMinder,
incorporated New York, NY, USA

Jonathan J. Evans,
Section of Psychological Medicine,
Division of Community Based Sciences,
University of Glasgow, Glasgow, UK

Jessica Fish,
MRC Cognition & Brain Sciences Unit,
Cambridge, UK

Joaquín M. Fuster,
Neuropsychiatric Institute, University of
California, Los Angeles, CA, USA

Guido Gainotti,
Servizio di Neuropsicologia, Policlinico
Gemelli, Roma, Italy

Martina Gandola,
Psychology Department, University of
Pavia, Pavia, Italy

Georg Goldenberg,
Neuropsychological Department,
Krankenhaus München Bogenhausen,
München, Germany

Laura H. Goldstein,
Department of Psychology, Institute of
Psychiatry, London, UK

C Groh-Bordin,
Clinical Neuropsychology Unit, Dept. of
Psychology, Saarland University,
Saarbrücken, Germany

Jennifer M. Gurd,
University Department of Clinical
Neurology, John Radcliffe Hospital,
Oxford, UK

J. Richard Hanley,
Department of Psychology, University of
Essex, Colchester, UK

Paola Invernizzi,
Psychology Department, University of
Milan-Bicocca, Milan, Italy

Eli J. Jaldow,
Neuropsychiatry and Memory Disorders
Clinic, St Thomas' Hospital, London, UK

Helga Johannsen-Horbach,
School of Speech and Language Therapy,
Freiburg, Germany

Narinder Kapur,
Neurosciences, Addenbrookes Hospital,
Cambridge, UK

Luke Kartsounis,
Essex Neuroscience Centre,
Queen's Hospital, Romford,
Essex, UK

Janice Kay,
Department of Psychology,
University of Exeter, Exeter, UK

Georg Kerkhoff,
Clinical Neuropsychology Research
Group, Neuropsychological Department,
Bogenhausen Hospital, München,
Germany

Nigel King,
Community Head Injury Service, The
Camborne Centre, Aylesbury, UK

Udo Kischka,
Rivermead Research Centre,
Oxford Centre for Enablement,
Oxford, UK

Michael Kopelman,
University Department of Psychiatry,
GKT School of Medicine,
London, UK

Tom Manly,
MRC Cognition and Brain Sciences Unit,
Cambridge, UK

Lilianne Manning,
Laboratoire de Neurosciences
Comportementales et Cognitives,
Université Louis Pasteur, Strasbourg,
France

Hans J. Markowitsch,
Department of Psychology, University of
Bielefeld, Bielefeld, Germany

Jane Marshall,
Department of Language and
Communication Science,
City University,
London, UK

John C. Marshall,
(deceased) formerly of Neuropsychology
Unit, University Department of Clinical
Neurology, John Radcliffe Hospital,
Oxford, UK

Michaela McGowan,
Case Management Services Ltd.,
Edinburgh, UK

William W. McKinlay,
Case Management Services Ltd.,
Edinburgh, UK

Nick Miller,
Institute of Health and Society,
Speech language sciences,
University of Newcastle,
Newcastle, UK

Ronan O'Carroll,
Department of Psychology, University of
Stirling, Stirling, UK

Heather Palmer,
Maximum Capacity,
Toronto, Ontario, Canada

Eraldo Paulesu,
Psychology Department, University of
Milan-Bicocca, Milan, Italy

Martina Piefke,
Physiological Psychology, University of
Bielefeld, Bielefeld Germany

Mervi Pitkanen,
Neuropsychiatry and Memory Disorders
Clinic, St Thomas' Hospital, London, UK

Amanda Rabinowitz,
Penn State University,
Psychology Department,
University Park, PA, USA

Steven Z. Rapcsak,
National Center for Neurogenic
Communication Disorders, The
University of Arizona, Tucson AZ, USA

Bjørn Rishovd Rund,
Institute of Psychology, University of
Oslo, Oslo, Norway

Ian H. Robertson,
Department of Psychology,
Trinity College Dublin, Dublin, Ireland

Jane V. Russell,
Case Management Services Ltd.,
Edinburgh, UK

Carlo Semenza,
Department of Neuroscience,
University of Padova, Padova, Italy

Clive Skilbeck,
School of Psychology, University of
Tasmania, Hobart, Tasmania, Australia

Julie Snowden,
Cerebral Function Unit, Greater
Manchester Neuroscience Centre,
Salford Royal Foundation Trust,
Salford, UK

Joke Spikman,
Department of Neurology, University
Hospital Groningen, Groningen,
The Netherlands

Pamela J. Thompson,
Consultant Clinical Neuropsychologist,
University College, London
Hospital Trust and National Society
for Epilepsy, UK

Geoffrey Tremont,
Warren Alpert Medical School of
Brown University, Department of
Psychiatry and Human Behavior,
Director, Neuropsychology Program,
Rhode Island Hospital, Providence,
Rhode Island, USA

Andrew Tyerman,
Community Head Injury Service,
The Camborne Centre, Jansel Square,
Bedgrove, Aylesbury, UK

Ed van Zomeren,
Department of Neurology, University
Hospital Groningen, Groningen,
The Netherlands

Derick T. Wade,
Neurological Rehabilitation Service,
Oxford Centre for Enablement,
Oxford, UK

Claus-W. Wallesch,
Department of Psycholinguistics,
University of Erfurt, Germany

Rebekah C. White,
Department of Experimental Psychology,
University of Oxford, Oxford, UK

Steven Whitfield,
David Lewis Centre, Warford,
Nr Alderley, Cheshire, UK

Klaus Willmes,
Section of Neuropsychology,
Department of Neurology,
RWTH Aachen University,
Aachen, Germany

Barbara A. Wilson,
MRC Cognition and Brain
Sciences Unit, Cambridge, UK

Gordon Winocur,
Rotman Research Institute,
Baycrest, Toronto Ontario,
Canada

Andrew D. Worthington,
Brain Injury Rehabilitation Trust,
Birmingham, UK

Abbreviations

5-HT	5-hydroxytryptamine (serotonin)	BAER	brainstem auditory evoked responses
AAC	alternative and augmentative communication	BAI	Beck Anxiety Inventory
		BAS	British Ability Scales
AAN	American Academy of Neurology	BBB	blood-brain barrier
AAT	Aachen Aphasia Test	BDAE	Boston diagnostic aphasia examination
ACA	anterior communicating artery		
AChI	acetylcholinesterase inhibitor	BDI	Beck Depression Inventory
ACT	Anagram and copy treatment	BINS	Bayley Infant Neurodevelopmental Screener
ACTH	adrenocorticotrophin hormone		
ACTIVE	Advaned Cognitive Training for Independent and Vital Elderly	BIT	Behavioural Inattention Test
		BORB	Birmingham Object Recognition Battery
AD	Alzheimer's disease		
ADC	(HIV-1)- associated dementia complex	BMIPB	BIRT memory and information processing battery
ADHD	attention deficit hyperactivity disorder	BNT	Boston naming test
		BPRS	Brief Psychiatric Rating Scale
ADL	activities of daily living	BPVS	British Picture Vocabulary Scale
ADT	Auditory Discrimination Test	BRB	Brief Repeatable Battery (of Neuropsychological Tests in Multiple Sclerosis)
AED	antiepileptic drug		
AI	androgen insensitivity		
AIDS	acquired immune deficiency syndrome	BVRT-R	Benton's Visual Retention Test – Revised
ALS	amyotrophic lateral sclerosis	CADASIL	cerebral autosomal dominant arteriopathy with subcortical infarcts and leukoencephalopathy
ALS	articulatory loop system (in working memory)		
AMI	Autobiographical Memory Interview	CAH	congenital adrenal hyperplasia
AMIPB	Adult Memory and Information Processing Battery	CANTAB	Cambridge Neuropsychological Test Automated Battery
AMP	adenosine monophosphate (adenosine 5' –phosphate)	CART	Copy and Recall Treatment
		CBGS	Coronary Bypass Graft Surgery
AMPA	DL-ά–amino-3-hydroxy-5-methyl-isoxazole proprionate	CBT	cognitive behavioural therapy
		CCAP	Centre for Child and Adolescent Psychiatry (Oslo)
ANELT	Amsterdam-Nijmegen Everyday Language Test	CCC	Children's Communication Checklist
APM	Advanced (Raven's) Progressive Matrices		
		CCST	California Card Sorting Test
APT	Attention Processing Training	CDC	Centers for Disease Control (USA)
ATP	adenosine 5' –triphosphate	CELF	Clinical Evaluation of Language Fundamentals
AVM	arteriovenous malformation		
BA	Brodmann area	CES	Central executive system
BADS	Behavioural Assessment of the Dysexecutive Syndrome	CFQ	Cognitive Failures Questionnaire
		CH	congenital hypothyroidism

CICA	Criminal Injuries Compensation Authority (UK)
CJD	Creutzfeldt-Jakob disease
CMDI	Chicago Multiscale Depression Inventory
CMS	Children's Memory Scale
CMV	cytomegalovirus
CN-REP	Children's Test of Non-Word Repetition
CNS	Central nervous system
CNV	contingent negative variation
COWA	Controlled Oral Word Association (test)
CPM	Coloured (Raven's) Progressive Matrices
CPM	Central pontine myelinolysis
CPR	(Lord Woolf's) Civil Procedure Rules (England)
CPT	(Connors) Continuous Performance Test
CRH	corticotrophin-releasing hormone
CS	contrast sensitivity
CSF	cerebrospinal fluid
CT	computerized tomography
CVA	cerebrovascular accident
CVLT	California Verbal Learning Test
CVS	caloric vestibular stimulation
DA	discriminant analysis
DAT	dementia of the Alzheimer's type
DEX	Dysexecutive Questionnaire
DHEA	dehydroepiandrosterone
DHEA-S	dehydroepiandrosterone sulfate
D-KEFS	Delis-Kaplan Executive System (battery)
DLBD	diffuse Lewy body disease
DNET	dysembryoplastic neuroepithelial tumour
DSM-IV	Diagnostic and statistical manual (of mental disorders) (American Psychiatric Association)
DSS	double simultaneous stimulation
DST	dexamethasone suppression test
DTVP	Developmental Test of Visual Perception
EDSS	(Kurtzke's) Expanded Disability Status Scale
EPS	extrapyramidal side-effect

ERPs	event related potentials
ERT	oestrogen replacement therapy
ESES	electrical status epilepticus during slow-wave sleep
FAS	Fluency Controlled Oral Word Association
FEEST	Facial Expressions of Emotion Stimuli Test
FEFs	frontal eye-fields
FIQ	full intelligence quotient
FIRDA	frontal intermittent rhythmic delta activity
FIS	Fatigue Impact Scale
FLD	frontal lobe degeneration of non-Alzheimer type
fMRI	functional MRI
FSH	follicle-stimulating hormone
FSS	Fatigue Severity Scale
FTD	frontotemporal dementia
GABA	y-aminobutyric acid
GAS	Global Assessment Scale
GCS	Glasgow Coma Scale
GDA	Graded Difficulty Arithmetic (test)
GH	growth hormone
GnRF	gonadotrophin-releasing factor
GPI	general paresis of the insane
HAART	highly active antiretroviral therapy
HADS	Hospital Anxiety and Depression Scale
HIV	human immunodeficiency virus
HPT	hypothalamic-pituitary-thyroid (axis)
HRT	hormone replacement therapy
IADLs	instrumental activities of daily living
IAP	intracarotid amytal procedure
ICC	item characteristic curve
ICD-10	(WHO) International Classification of Disease
ICIDH	International Classification of Impairments, Disabilities, and Handicaps (WHO)
IDDM	insulin-dependent diabetes mellitus (type I diabetes)
IES	Impact of Event Scale
IHH	idiopathic hypogonadotrophic hypogonadism
IM	intramuscular

IPT	integrated psychological therapy (for schizophrenia)	NEPSY	Neuropsychological Assessment of Children
IV	intravenous	NFTs	neurofibrillary tangles
K-ABC	Kaufman Assessment Battery for Children	NIDDM	Non-insulin-dependent diabetes (type II diabetes)
KR-20	Kuder Richardson Formula	NIH	National Institute of Health
LBD	left brain damage	NINDS	National Institute of Neurological Disorders and Stroke (USA)
LBL	letter-by-letter (reading)		
L-dopa	laevodopa	NMDA	N-methyl -D-aspartate
LH	luteinizing hormone	NPH	normal pressure hydrocephalus
LICA	Left Internal carotid artery	NV	neck muscle mechanical vibration
LIP	lateral intraparietal (sulcus)	NVLD	nonverbal learning disability
LIPS-R	Leiter International Performance Scale-Revised	OCD	obsessive-compulsive disorder
		OKS	optokinetic stimulation
LGB	Lateral Genicular Body	PALPA	Psycholinguistic Assessment of Language Processing in Aphasia
LPC	lateral prefrontal cortex		
LSD	lysergic acid diethylamide	PASAT	Paced Auditory Serial Addition Task
LTD	long-term depression	PAT	Phonological Abilities Test
LTP	long-term potentiation	PCP	phencyclidine
MAAT	Memory and Attention Adaptation	PCRS	Patient Competency Rating Scale
MAO	monoamine oxidase	PCS	post-concussion symptoms
MAOI	monoamine oxidase inhibitor	PD	Parkinson's disease
MCI	Mild cognitive Impairment	PET	positron emission tomography
MDMA	methylenedioxymeth-amphetamine ('ecstasy')	PFND	progressive focal neuropsychological deficits
MEG	magnetoencephalography	PhAB	Phonological Assessment Battery
MEP	motor evoked potentials	PIQ	performance IQ
MI	Motricity Index for Motor Impairment after Stroke	PML	progressive multifocal leukoencephalopathy
MET	Multiple Errands Test	PMS	peripheral magnetic stimulation
MID	multi-infarct dementia	PMS	premenstrual syndrome
MIT	Melodic Intonation Therapy	PPC	posterior parietal cortex
MMPI	Minnesota Multiphasic Personality Inventory	PPVT	Peabody Picture Vocabulary Test
		PR	percentile rank
MMSE	Mini-Mental State Examination	PROMPT	Prompts for Restructuring Oral Muscular Targets
MND	Motor neuron disease		
MOR	multiple oral re-reading	PSD	poststroke depression
MRC	Medical Research Council	PSP	progressive supranuclear Palsy
MRI	magnetic resonance imaging	PST	Problem Solving Training
MS	multiple sclerosis	PTA	posttraumatic amnesia
NADDs	non-Alzheimer degenerative dementias	PTS	Posttraumatic stress
		PTSD	Posttraumatic stress disorder
NARA	Neale Analysis of Reading	RA	retrograde amnesia
NARI	noradrenaline re-uptake inhibitor	RAVLT	Rey Auditory Verbal Learning Test
NART	National Adult Reading Test	RBD	right brain damage
NEAD	non-epileptic attack disorder	RBMT	Rivermead Behavioural Memory Test

RBMT-C	Rivermead Behavioural Memory Test for Children	TE	toxoplasma encephalitis
RBMT-E	Rivermead Behavioural Memory Test – Extended Version	TEA	Test of Everyday Attention
		TEA-Ch	Test of Everyday Attention for Children
rCBF	regional cerebral blood flow	THC	β –tetrahydrocannabinol
rCMR	regional cerebral metabolic rate	TIA	transient ischaemic attack
RDLS	Reynell Developmental Language Scales	TLE	temporal lobe epilepsy
		TMS	transcranial magnetic stimulation
RFs	receptive fields (of neurons)	TOTs	time-on-task effects
RMI	Rivermead Mobility Index	TOWK	Test of Word Knowledge
RIMA	reversible inhibitor of MAO-A	TPM	Time Pressure Management (training)
RPAB	Rivermead Perceptual Assessment Battery		
		TRH	thyrotrophin-releasing hormone
RPMS	Repetitive peripheral magnetic simulation	TROG	Test for the Reception of Grammar
RR	relapsing-remitting (course type for MS)	TS	Tourette Syndrome
		TSH	thyroid-stimulating hormone
RSAB	Rating Scale of Attentional Behaviour	VER	Visual evoked responses
		VFD	Visual field disorders
RT	reaction time	VIQ	verbal IQ
RTA	road traffic accident	VMI	Visual-Motor Integration (test)
SAH	subarachnoid haemorrhage	VOSP	Visual Object and Space Perception (test)
SART	Sustained Attention for Response Test		
		VSSP	visuospatial scratchpad
SAS	Supervisory attentional system	WAB	Western Aphasia Battery
SCOLP	Speed and Capacity of Language Processing	WAIS	Wechsler Adult Intelligence Scale
		WASI	Wechsler Abbreviated Scale of Intelligence
SET	Six Elements Test		
SMA	supplementary motor area	WCST	Wisconsin Card Sorting Task
SMT	Self-monitoring Training	WIPPSI	Wechsler Preschool and Primary Scale of Intelligence
SNRI	serotonin-noradrenaline re-uptake inhibitors		
		WISC	Wechsler Intelligence Scale for Children
SPECT	single-photon emission computerized tomography		
		WMS	Wechsler Memory Scale
SpLDs	specific learning difficulties	WMTB-C	Working Memory Test Battery for Children
SPM	Standard (Raven's) Progressive Matrices		
		WOND	Wechsler Objective Numerical Dimensions (test)
SSER	somatosensory evoked responses		
SSRI	selective serotonin re-uptake inhibitors	WORD	Wechsler Objective Reading Dimension
		WRAML	Wide Range Assessment of Memory and Learning
SVD	Small Vessel Disease		
T^3	triiodothyronine		
T 4	thyroxine	WRAT3	Wide Range Achievement Test (3rd edn)
TAP	Test for Attentional Performance		
TBI	traumatic brain injury	WRMB	Warrington's Recognition Memory Battery
TCA	tricyclic antidepressant		
		WS	William's syndrome
TCI	transitory cognitive impairments	WTAR	Wechsler Test of Adult Reading

Part 1

Historical context

Chapter 1

Neuropsychology: past, present, and future

John C. Marshall and Jennifer M. Gurd

1 Past

Just how far back one might wish to trace the prehistory of neuropsychology is a moot point. Evidence of trepanning of living 'patients' in the Mesolithic period (Lillie 1998) suggests, although it does not prove, that early modern man had some idea of the importance of that cold grey mass within the skull. But we must wait for the Egyptians before hard evidence becomes available. Egyptian surgeons certainly knew that brain and behaviour are related: The Edwin Smith surgical papyrus, which dates from 1700 BCE, describes language disorder consequent on brain damage after head injury. And over a millennium later the Hippocratic corpus (circa 425 BCE) states unambiguously that *all* mental functions have their seat in the brain:

> It ought to be generally known that the source of our pleasure, merriment, laughter, and amusement, as of our grief, pain, anxiety, and tears, is none other than the brain. It is specially the organ which enables us to think, see, and hear, and to distinguish the ugly and the beautiful, the bad and the good, pleasant and unpleasant… It is the brain too which is the seat of madness and delirium, of the fears and frights which assail us, often by night, but sometimes even by day; it is there where lies the cause of insomnia and sleep-walking, of thoughts that will not come, forgotten duties, and eccentricities.

Aristotle (384–322 BCE), who believed that the brain merely cools the blood, had clearly not been keeping up with the literature.

Nonetheless, it was another two millennia before relatively reliable associations were discovered between the locus of brain damage (established at autopsy) and the nature of the mental impairment (aphasia, agnosia, apraxia, amnesia, etc.) that in life had resulted therefrom. The ground had been prepared by the Viennese physician Franz Joseph Gall (1758–1828) who conjectured that the brain consists of many 'mental organs', each dedicated to a particular cognitive, conative, or affective function. Many of the organs in Gall's classificatory scheme proved to be valid psychobiological modules that could, to a first approximation, be independently impaired by brain damage. The Gallist organs of form, size, weight, colour, arithmetic calculation, locality (topographic learning and memory), eventuality (memory for facts), time, music, and language are still of intense interest to neuropsychologists. In one instance, that of language, Gall even managed to get the (frontal) localization correct.

Inspired by Gall's achievements, the first golden age of neuropsychology, as practised by behavioural neurologists and neuropsychiatrists from 1861 to 1914, was associated with significant advances in the fractionation of the aphasias (Bastian, Broca, Wernicke), the agnosias (Lissauer), the apraxias (Liepmann), and the alexias (Déjerine), along with the relevant autopsy-confirmed anatomoclinical correlations. Jackson (who first suggested that the right hemisphere was 'leading for spatial cognition') and Balint began to elucidate a wide range of spatial disorders, and Bianchi explored the role of the frontal lobes in reasoning and planning. The study of neurodegenerative diseases that could lead to different types of dementia was also inaugurated by Alzheimer, Korsakoff, and Pick. It is of interest that the early aphasiologists made serious attempts to retrain language skills, often deploying many of the same pedagogical techniques that were currently used to teach children. In Paris, Paul Broca himself attempted to remediate language and reading problems, but noted that the time a busy clinician could devote to speech and language therapy was ridiculously brief. Although employing traditional teaching methods, Broca nonetheless thought it probable that 'the adult and the child will follow different procedures to attain the same end' (Howard and Hatfield 1987). He also conjectured that recovery from aphasia involved training the right hemisphere homologue of (what became known as) Broca's area to take over the functions of the damaged frontal language region in the left hemisphere.

For the most part, classical neuropsychology was based upon patients who had suffered cerebrovascular accidents (and patients with progressive or degenerative conditions, including neurosyphilis). But the period from 1914 to 1956 saw two world wars and the Korean war (and their medical aftermaths). In contrast to previous patients who had typically been elderly and sick, neurologists were now also dealing with the behavioural sequelae of focal lesions caused by high-velocity projectile injury to the brains of young, previously healthy men (and, more rarely, women). Many of the seminal contributions of Gordon Holmes to the understanding of visual and visuospatial deficits were made while he was on active service as a consultant neurologist in France during World War I. Likewise, the neurologist Pierre Marie spent the war studying 'les aphasies de guerre' after gun-shot and shrapnel injuries. Such wounds are often self-sterilizing consequent upon the heat generated by the transit of the missile: As a result there were often fewer medical complications than might initially have been anticipated. Accordingly, the necessity of cognitive rehabilitation became far more pressing as patients who recovered medically from their injuries could often look forward to another 30, 40, or even 50 years of life. This period also saw the development of more formal testing procedures (to ensure the comparability of observations made on different patients). The desirability of using standardized tests and test-batteries (with appropriate norms) for the assessment of language, memory, praxis, and visuospatial skill was reinforced by the earlier success of Alfred Binet in devising intelligence tests for Parisian children (cf. Weisenburg and McBride 1935). When, in Cologne, Poppelreuter (1917/1990) was studying impairments of visual attention in brain-injured soldiers, he noted that 'only a result that lies below the normal range should be judged to be definitely pathological'. Poppelreuter's (1917/1990) monograph, *Disturbances of lower and higher visual capacities caused by occipital damage,* is subtitled 'with special reference to the psychopathological, pedagogical, industrial, and social implications', which reflects the concerns of the time. Poppelreuter, a neurologist who had also trained in psychology (with Carl Stumpf in Berlin), was well placed to address these concerns. Rehabilitation was also stressed in the Berlin clinic of Hermann Gutzmann where psychologists and speech therapists treated both organic and functional disorders of language, speech, and voice in the casualties of trench warfare on the Western Front.

Classical neuropsychology had also taken an interest in affective disorders as well as cognitive impairments. The Hippocratic corpus incorporated a humoural theory of the emotions with different temperaments being associated with a preponderance of black bile, phlegm, blood, or yellow bile. Much later, Otto Loewi discovered (in 1924) that synaptic transmission from the vagus nerve to the heart muscle was chemically controlled: The first of many neurotransmitter substances (acetylcholine) had been found. A long and tortuous journey then led to the conjecture that too much or too little of various neurotransmitters was implicated in many neurological and psychiatric conditions (cf. Parkinson's disease, schizophrenia, and bipolar disorder).

The further integration of psychology (and psychologists) into medical teams concerned with acquired cognitive and affective disorders can be illustrated from the career of Kurt Goldstein (1878–1965). Shortly after the outbreak of World War I, Goldstein was appointed medical director of the Frankfurt Hospital and Research Institute for the study of brain-injured soldiers. The institute rapidly developed into a major clinical centre for the diagnosis, treatment, and rehabilitation of military casualties suffering from neurological and psychiatric impairments. Goldstein insisted on treating 'the whole person' and, to that end, involved psychologists in all the work of the Institute: Adhémar Gelb, with whom Goldstein investigated reasoning after brain damage, and Egon Weigl, whose main interest was in the aphasias, were two of the more notable of Goldstein's psychologist collaborators. By one of those fierce ironies of European history, when Goldstein (1942) wrote *Aftereffects of brain injuries in war, their evaluation and treatment*, the United States had entered World War II and Goldstein was working in New York, an exile since 1933 from the Third Reich. But in America too, Goldstein stressed the crucial contributions that psychologists made to the assessment of cognitive impairments: He worked with Martin Scheerer on devising tests of abstract and concrete behaviour, and with Marianne Simmel on acquired disorders of reading. The latter work was an important precursor of current interest in the nature of paralexic errors. Goldstein's concept of 'biological intelligence' as a function of the frontal lobes has similarly been echoed in more recent work on 'fluid' intelligence (Duncan *et al.* 1995).

2 Present

By the end of the 1950s, psychologists had a secure role in all aspects of the assessment and rehabilitation of patients with cognitive disorders. Alexander Romanovitch Luria in Moscow, Oliver Zangwill in Edinburgh and then Cambridge, and Hans-Lukas Teuber in New York and Boston stand out among those who pioneered modern testing methods and laid the foundations of modern neuropsychology. Furthermore, physicians such as Norman Geschwind in Boston, Henri Hécaen in Paris, and Ennio De Renzi in Milan, sometimes in collaboration with psychologists, were instrumental in vitalizing post-war behavioural neurology.

Building upon the achievements of these seminal figures, the chapters that follow present an extensive and detailed overview of current knowledge relevant to clinical neuropsychology and best practice therein. This section can accordingly be fairly brief. Nonetheless, it may be useful to highlight some of the innovations that took place between Scoville and Milner's 1957 paper on the memory impairments of the patient H.M. and the consolidation and widespread adoption of functional neuroimaging to study both the healthy and the damaged brain in 2001. We also note some continuities with previous work, e.g. the involvement of psychologists in the study of traumatic brain injury (TBI). But nowadays—in the Western world at least—such injuries result more frequently from the impact of large projectiles (motor vehicles) than from small ones (bullets and shrapnel).

Clinical neuropsychology is now a recognized profession with most practitioners working with patients in hospitals and rehabilitation centres, or in private practice. By contrast, experimental neuropsychologists, typically university-based, have often worked with healthy participants in the laboratory, devising and testing theories of normal relationships between the brain and mental life. The distinction, however, has become increasingly blurred as experimental psychologists began seeing patients for research purposes and clinical neuropsychologists began to take a more lively interest in the theoretical foundations of their practice. This erosion of professional boundaries accelerated when the widespread revival of cognitive psychology in the 1960s gave renewed impetus to all manner of questions that had previously seemed of dubious propriety. The death of behaviourism, the birth of transformational grammar, and the inspiration of information theory and computer science renewed interest in the 'mind' as programmed software that 'ran' on the computer hardware (or more accurately, wetware) of the brain. Experimental psychologists were encouraged to propose and test models of cognitive competence and performance that allowed as many 'mental computations' as the tasks required and the empirical data would support.

Cognitive neuropsychology also underwent a renaissance in the 1960s and 1970s, driven by many of the same factors that had revitalized experimental psychology. The revival of commissurotomy (in the hands of Joe Bogen) for the relief of otherwise intractable epilepsy also drove an intense interest in the cerebral lateralization of cognitive functions (Sperry et al. 1969). The overall aim of the discipline was seen as effecting the integration of clinical neuropsychology (the principled description of disorders consequent, for the most part, upon demonstrable brain pathology) and normal cognitive psychology (the construction and empirical validation of general models of complex mental functions). The distinctive character of *cognitive neuropsychology* lies in the explicit endeavour to interpret disorders of cognition in relation to formal information-processing models of normal (brain/mind) systems.

Seen in this light, the study of pathologies of cognition serves a threefold purpose.

- Neuropathological fractionations of cognition impose strong constraints upon theories of the normal system. The striking dissociations of impaired and preserved performance seen after brain damage indicate which overt behavioural abilities must *not* be analysed together as manifestations of a single underlying function.

- The interpretation of pathological performance by reference to normal theory allows the investigator to move beyond the mere description of overt symptomatology to accounts of the underlying processes that are impaired.

- In any complex system, identical *overt* failures and errors can arise from malfunction of different underlying components. Such ambiguities must be resolved by linking the patterns of impaired and preserved performance to specified (and justified) information-processing components.

The relevance of this framework to the practical concerns of clinical neuropsychologists is clear. The obtaining of standardized scores on standardized tests may be a necessary step in examining the patient, but is not a sufficient one. One needs to know why this particular patient shows this particular pattern of vitiated and intact skills. One needs to understand the underlying impairments, not just to describe the overt signs and symptoms of cognitive breakdown. Initially, observations made within this framework were systematized by 'box-and-arrow' diagrams that would have seemed entirely familiar to late nineteenth-century behavioural neurologists (compare, for example, Lichtheim 1885 and Marshall and Newcombe 1973). More recently, such models have been implemented in a computationally more rigorous form (Coltheart *et al.* 1993; Plaut and Shallice 1993).

Progress was first made in the description and interpretation of reading disorders (Marshall and Newcombe 1966) and verbal short-term memory (Warrington and Shallice 1969). But the approach characteristic of cognitive neuropsychology progressively colonized all the traditional domains of behavioural neurology: disorders of language (Caplan and Hildebrandt 1988); object- and face-recognition (Farah 1990; Young 1992); calculation (Butterworth 1999); spatial cognition (Robertson and Marshall 1993); praxis (Rothi *et al.* 1997); episodic memory (Schacter 1996); and planning and executive control (Rabbitt 1997). Eventually, it even became possible to admit to an interest in the neurobiology of consciousness, although the most striking results to date seem to concern what the mind/brain can achieve without conscious awareness (Weiskrantz 1997).

Early work that mapped the performance of individual patients on to (normal) models of the impaired domain quickly showed that the habitual symptom complexes of behavioural neurology (Broca's aphasia, dyslexia with dysgraphia, retrograde amnesia, associative agnosia, ideational apraxia, etc.) fractioned into a wide variety of clinically distinct (and theoretically meaningful) forms. Furthermore, in some domains, knowledge of lesion locus (the traditional correlate of behavioural syndromes) was judged to be irrelevant to the description of pathology-induced cognitive breakdown. The contribution of psychologists to the work of neurosurgical teams concerned with the relief of epilepsy by cortical ablation constitutes the most notable exception to this latter generalization

(Scoville and Milner 1957), although it was the horrendous memory impairment of *one* patient, H.M., that first showed the importance of this work. The success of 'radical' cognitive neuropsychology soon became apparent from the insights it gave into the structure of impaired mental functions, and the way in which it drove justified changes to models of *normal* cognition.

Current work has to a large extent preserved a keen distrust of syndromes (except as clinical shorthand), and single-case studies continue to play a supreme role in theoretical innovation and in the evidential support and disconfirmation of cognitive models. In this respect, contemporary studies greatly resemble those of the first golden age (Marshall and Newcombe 1984). Nevertheless, the importance of group studies is now recognized when, for example, effect sizes are small or when correlational analysis of patterns of impaired and preserved performance is demanded (Gurd 2000; Newcombe and Marshall 1988). In some instances, large samples become interesting in their own right. For example, in a major follow-up of World War II veterans, Newcombe (1969) showed that, although selective impairments were frequent after missile injury to the brain, 'no generalized intellectual deterioration was detected in these men as a group'. Interest in neuroanatomical and neurophysiological localization has also grown, driven in the first place by the widespread availability of computerized tomography (CT) and magnetic resonance imaging (MRI) and, more recently, by advances in functional brain imaging using such techniques as positron emission tomography (PET), functional MRI, and magnetoencephalography (MEG) (Frackowiak *et al.* 1997; Cabeza and Kingstone 2001).

With respect to rehabilitation, the 1970s and 80s saw the revival of efforts to produce rational therapies and (even more importantly) rational evaluations of efficacy. An important randomized UK trial of speech therapy for aphasia gave somewhat mixed results: David *et al.* (1982) found that patients seen by professional speech therapists and by untrained volunteers seemed to recover at much the same rate and that patients who started treatment late made as much progress as those who started earlier. Such results suggested that therapies might be more effective if explicitly tailored to the strengths and weaknesses of the individual patient as assessed by a detailed neuropsychological examination.

This single-case approach to therapy for cognitive impairments drew heavily upon arguments that had previously been advanced as to why the description and interpretation of neuropsychological symptoms should be based upon the performance of individual patients and case-series. The polytypic syndromes characteristic of behavioural neurology may not be an appropriate knowledge-base on which to plan therapy. What is required in the first place are longitudinal single-subject experimental designs that can evaluate the efficacy of treatment in the individual. Potentially effective treatments can then be tested on larger samples in a case-by-case fashion. A number of such protocols are now available, including reversal and withdrawal designs, multiple baseline designs, and crossover treatment designs (cf. Willmes and Deloche 1997). Preliminary results from the new theoretically motivated therapies can be found in Riddoch and Humphreys (1994) and Berndt and Mitchum (1995).

It is not yet clear whether long-term, generalized gains actually accrue from such behavioural retraining of cognitive deficit or attempted substitution of alternative strategies that bypass the deficit (Shallice 2000). Knowing what is wrong does not automatically lead to knowing what should be done to ameliorate the problem.

3 Future

Predicting the future and extrapolating current trends are enterprises that have somewhat different risks attached. It is the latter that we will essay here. What can confidently be predicted, however, is that clinical neuropsychologists will not be short of work in the foreseeable future (cf. Denes and Pizzamiglio 1999).

Populations (in the developed world at least) are growing ever more elderly and hence suffering more and more from neurodegenerative diseases that have a potentially disastrous impact on cognitive functions and quality of life. When better cognition-enhancing drugs (and transplants) become available, it will be necessary to measure their true efficacy, to distinguish any pharmacological amelioration of performance from placebo effects, and to check for unforeseen side-effects. In younger populations, autoimmune deficiency syndrome (AIDS)-related cognitive impairments are analogous to those associated with neurosyphilis in the nineteenth century, with drug-resistant strains of human immunodeficiency virus (HIV) becoming more and more common. As with the diseases of ageing, significant work will be required to assess the efficacy of new drugs upon cognitive decline in AIDS. The impact of the Human Genome Project will no doubt increase substantially as more knowledge becomes available about neurological and psychiatric conditions whose onset is multiply determined by genetic and epigenetic susceptibility, developmental conditions, and environmental stressors.

The paradigms characteristic of cognitive neuropsychology will undoubtedly make further inroads into our understanding of psychiatric and other 'functional' disorders (Frith 1992). In this context, we note with alarm the high proportion of seemingly 'neurological' conditions for which no organic disorder can be found that would explain the patient's hemiparesis, somatosensory loss, visual field constriction, etc. (Halligan *et al.* 2001). We are already seeing a significant revival of interest in the neurobiology of the emotions (LeDoux 1992) and greater concern with how mood and affect interact with problem-solving and decision-making (Damasio 1999). The study of grossly disturbed reasoning and delusion formation should also yield major advances in the relatively near future. It is perhaps in the domain of psychiatric and affective disorders that functional neuroimaging techniques and analysis procedures will have one of their most important clinical applications. Advances in the calculation of functional or effective connectivity between brain regions will help imaging techniques to address more directly the functional architecture of cognition, praxis, and affect and their disorders. Nonetheless, we must stress that there is no substitute for the controlled observation of the patient's behavioural strengths and weaknesses. Brain imaging is not an alternative to neuropsychological practice and, in some instances, the neuropsychological examination may even be a better guide to the anatomical localization of deficit.

We can also look forward to further insights into the social brain in its natural habitat (Brothers 1997; Cacioppo *et al.* 2002). Too often in the past, clinicians have regarded the individual patient and his or her test scores as the primary 'object' of neuropsychological practice. Without in any way wishing to deny the importance of the individual, we emphasize that the 'subject' of our discipline is the person in his or her social and environmental setting. At the moment, it could be embarrassing to inquire too deeply into the ecological validity of many of our neuropsychological measures and rehabilitation programmes. In too many instances we only pay lip service to the distinctions between impairment (abnormality of function), disability (the effects of impairment on ability), and handicap (the effects of disability in interaction with the patient's physical and social environment). A future in which we paid more attention to how our patients (or are we now only allowed to say 'clients'?) functioned in the kitchen, the department store, the office, the bingo club, and the dinner party would be 'a consummation devoutly to be wished' (but cf. Foundas *et al.* 1995).

Acknowledgements

We are grateful to Graham Beaumont for allowing us to use suggestions from his unpublished manuscript on the history of clinical neuropsychology.

Selective references

Berndt, R.S. and Mitchum, C.C. (eds.) (1995). *Cognitive neuropsychological approaches to treatment of language disorders.* Lawrence Erlbaum Associates, Hove, East Sussex.

Brothers, L. (1997). *Friday's footprint: how society shapes the human mind.* Oxford University Press, New York.

Butterworth, B. (1999). *The mathematical brain.* Macmillan, London.

Cabeza, R. and Kingstone, A. (eds.) (2001). *Handbook of functional neuroimaging of cognition.* MIT Press, Cambridge, Massachusetts.

Cacioppo, J.T., Berntson, G.G., and Adolphs, R. (eds.) (2002). *Foundations in social neuroscience.* MIT Press, Cambridge, Massachusetts.

Caplan, D. and Hildebrandt, N. (1988). *Disorders of syntactic comprehension.* MIT Press, Cambridge, Massachusetts.

Coltheart, M., Curtis, B., Atkins, P., and Haller, M. (1993). Models of reading aloud: dual-route and parallel-distributed-processing approaches. *Psychol. Rev.* **100**, 589–608.

Damasio, A.R. (1999). *The feeling of what happens: body and emotion in the making of consciousness.* Harcourt Brace, New York.

David, R., Enderby, P., and Bainton, D. (1982). Treatment of acquired aphasia: speech therapists and volunteers compared. *J. Neurol., Neurosurg., Psychiatry* **45**, 957–61.

Denes, G. and Pizzamiglio, L. (eds.) (1999). *Handbook of clinical and experimental neuropsychology.* Psychology Press, Hove, East Sussex.

Duncan, J., Burgess, P.W., and Emslie, H. (1995). Fluid intelligence after frontal lobe lesions. *Neuropsychologia* **33**, 261–8.

Farah, M. (1990). *Visual agnosia.* MIT Press, Cambridge, Massachusetts.

Foundas, A.L., Macauley, B.L., Ramer, A.M., Maher, L.M., Heilman, K.M., and Rothi, L.J.G. (1995). Ecological implications of limb apraxia: evidence from mealtime behavior. *J. Int. Neuropsychol. Soc.* **1**, 62–6.

Frackowiak, R.S.J., Friston, K.J., Frith, C.D., Dolan, R.J., and Mazziotta, J.C. (1997). *Human brain function*. Academic Press, San Diego.

Frith, C.D. (1992). *The cognitive neuropsychology of schizophrenia*. Lawrence Erlbaum Associates, Hove, East Sussex.

Goldstein, K. (1942). *After effects of brain injuries in war*. Heinemann, London.

Gurd, J.M. (2000). Verbal fluency deficits in Parkinson's disease: individual differences in underlying cognitive mechanisms. *J. Neurolinguistics* **13**, 47–55.

Halligan, P.W., Bass, C., and Marshall, J.C. (eds.) (2001). *Contemporary approaches to the study of hysteria: clinical and theoretical perspectives*. Oxford University Press, Oxford.

Howard, D. and Hatfield, F.M. (1987). *Aphasia therapy: historical and contemporary issues*. Lawrence Erlbaum Associates, Hove, East Sussex.

LeDoux, J.E. (1992). *The emotional brain*. Simon and Schuster, New York.

Lichtheim, L. (1885). On aphasia. *Brain* **7**, 433–84.

Lillie, M.C. (1998). Cranial surgery dated back to Mesolithic. *Nature* **391**, 354.

Marshall, J.C. and Newcombe, F. (1973). Patterns of paralexia: a psycholinguistic approach. *Journal of Psycholinguistic Research* **2**, 175–199.

Marshall, J.C. and Newcombe, F. (1966). Syntactic and semantic errors in paralexia. *Neuropsychologia* **4**, 169–76.

Marshall, J.C. and Newcombe, F. (1984). Putative problems and pure progress in neuropsychological single case studies. *J. Clin. Neuropsychol.* **6**, 65–70.

Newcombe, F. (1969). *Missile wounds of the brain: a study of psychological deficits*. Oxford University Press, Oxford.

Newcombe, F. and Marshall, J.C. (1988). Idealization meets psychometrics: the case for the right groups and the right individuals. *Cogn. Neuropsychol.* **5**, 549–64.

Plaut, D.C. and Shallice, T. (1993). Deep dyslexia: a case study of connectionist neuropsychology. *Cogn. Neuropsychol.* **10**, 377–500.

Poppelreuter, W. (1917/1990). *Disturbances of lower and higher visual capacities caused by occipital damage*. Clarendon Press, Oxford.

Rabbitt, P. (ed.) (1997). *Methodology of frontal and executive function*. Psychology Press, Hove, East Sussex.

Riddoch, M.J. and Humphreys, G.W. (eds.) (1994). *Cognitive neuropsychology and cognitive rehabilitation*. Lawrence Erlbaum Associates, Hove, East Sussex.

Robertson, I.H. and Marshall, J.C. (eds.) (1993). *Unilateral neglect: clinical and experimental studies*. Lawrence Erlbaum Associates, Hove, East Sussex.

Rothi, L.J.G., Ochipa, C., and Heilman, K.M. (1997). *A cognitive neuropsychological model of limb praxia and apraxia*. Psychology Press, Hove, East Sussex.

Schacter, D.L. (1996). *Searching for memory: the brain, the mind, and the past*. Basic Books, New York.

Scoville, W.B. and Milner, B. (1957). Loss of recent memory after bilateral hippocampal lesions. *J. Neurol. Neurosurg., Psychiatry* **20**, 11–21.

Shallice, T. (2000). Cognitive neuropsychology and rehabilitation: is pessimism justified? *Neuropsychol. Rehabil.* **10**, 209–17.

Sperry, R.W., Gazzaniga, M.S., and Bogen, J.E. (1969). Interhemispheric relationships: the neocortical commissures; syndromes of hemisphere disconnection. In *Handbook of clinical neurology*, Vol. 4 (eds. P.J. Vinken and G.W. Bruyn), pp. 273–90. Elsevier, Amsterdam.

Warrington, E.K. and Shallice, T. (1969). The selective impairment of auditory verbal short-term memory. *Brain* **92**, 885–96.

Weisenberg, T. and McBride, K.E. (1935). *Aphasia: a clinical and psychological study*. The Commonwealth Fund, New York.

Weiskrantz, L. (1997). *Consciousness lost and found: a neuropsychological exploration.* Oxford University Press, Oxford.

Willmes, K. and Deloche, G. (eds.) (1997). *Methodological issues in neuropsychological assessment and rehabilitation.* Psychology Press, Hove, East Sussex.

Young, A.W. (1992). Face recognition impairments. *Phil. Trans. R. Soc. Lond. B* **335**, 47–54.

Part 2

Methodological issues

Chapter 2

Basic concepts and principles of neuropsychological assessment

Jonathan J. Evans

1 Assessment objectives

Neuropsychological assessment is concerned with identifying the cognitive, emotional, and behavioural consequences of brain dysfunction. This type of assessment is used to address a number of different questions.

1.1 Is there evidence of organic brain dysfunction?

Despite considerable technological advances, it is not always possible to diagnose brain dysfunction purely on the basis of evidence from brain imaging, neurophysiological assessment, or other physical tests. In some cases, cognitive impairment is the only indicator of a pathological process. The most common situation of this sort involves identifying whether someone who complains of a memory problem is suffering from an organic brain disease such as dementia of the Alzheimer's type or a mood disorder such as depression. A question that occurs frequently in medico-legal cases is whether someone who has experienced a mild head injury or whiplash has suffered a brain injury sufficient to affect cognitive processing.

1.2 What is the nature and extent of cognitive impairment?

In some cases, the existence of brain dysfunction is not in dispute, but the nature and extent of any cognitive impairment needs to be clarified through more detailed neuropsychological assessment. Neuropsychological assessment is used to identify both cognitive impairment and areas of relative cognitive strength. Some neurological disorders present with specific patterns of neuropsychological impairment and therefore neuropsychological assessment may also contribute to differential diagnosis. One of the duties of the Neuropsychologist is to enable the patient to understand, or make sense of, his or her cognitive strengths and deficits.

1.3 What are the practical consequences of cognitive impairment?

A comprehensive neuropsychological assessment should address the practical or functional consequences of cognitive impairment for the individual in terms of limitations on the ability to participate in activities of daily living, work, education, leisure, and social relationships. In some circumstances the main question for the assessment is simply whether or not a person is suffering with some form of brain dysfunction, but it is always useful to consider what practical impact particular cognitive, emotional, or behavioural problems might have on the individual's life. For this purpose the use of questionnaires such as symptom checklists or rating scales relating to the performance of everyday tasks are often useful. When possible, it is helpful to observe the patient in practical situations. Although this inevitably produces only qualitative information, if used in combination with standardized test data it is likely to produce more accurate predictions about the practical consequences of brain injury. Neuropsychological assessment is used in forming an opinion regarding a person's capacity to manage his or her affairs, particularly financial affairs, or consent to treatment.

1.4 How are an individual's mood and behaviour affected by brain dysfunction?

Although the central focus of neuropsychological assessment is cognition, the neuropsychologist should also examine the impact of brain dysfunction on mood, personality, and behaviour. There are two major reasons why an assessment of mood is essential.

+ The presence of a mood disorder, caused directly or indirectly by brain injury, is an important area of psychological assessment in its own right.

+ A mood disorder may have a significant impact on performance on cognitive tests and therefore must be taken into account when interpreting test results.

1.5 Does cognitive performance change over time?

A further use for neuropsychological assessment is in measuring change over time. This might involve charting the process of decline in cognitive functioning associated with progressive disorders such as Alzheimer's disease, monitoring recovery from head injury or stroke, or measuring fluctuations in cognitive performance in conditions such as epilepsy. One problem with the use of neuropsychological tests for monitoring change is that many tests are vulnerable to practice effects. A practice effect occurs when the patient who is tested for a second, third, or fourth time on the same test improves simply because of increased familiarity with the test materials and test demands, rather than as a result of any real change in the underlying cognitive skill. This is particularly the case if tests are repeated within a matter of a few weeks, but practice effects may last a lot longer. One solution is to use parallel versions of tests on each occasion, though the number of neuropsychological tests with multiple parallel tests remains very small.

1.6 What are the implications of the pattern of cognitive strengths and weaknesses for the rehabilitation process?

Information about cognitive strengths and weaknesses is used in planning rehabilitation interventions. The presence of severe impairments in some areas of cognition will have implications for the types of intervention that are possible (e.g. external aid or self-initiated mental strategy) or the way in which patients learn new information or skills.

Information about areas of retained cognitive strength can help to plan how to compensate for deficits. The most straightforward example of this occurs when an individual has intact visual memory and impaired verbal memory, or vice versa. Rehabilitation efforts may then involve helping the individual to develop compensatory strategies using the intact system. Performance on cognitive tests, however, is not the best way of measuring the impact of rehabilitation, at least not in the post-acute stages. Rehabilitation at this stage is primarily concerned with helping individuals to cope with or compensate for cognitive deficits and improve practical performance in everyday life. In other words, the aim is usually to reduce the activity limitations imposed by the impairment, rather than reducing the impairment. Using a measure of impairment is therefore unlikely to reflect functional gains made in rehabilitation.

1.7 How might cognitive function be affected by neurosurgery?

One specialist role for neuropsychological assessment is in examining the potential impact on cognitive functioning of surgery carried out, (e.g. for the relief of epilepsy). The Wada assessment involves temporarily shutting down each cerebral hemisphere by an injection of sodium amobarbital. The effect on cognitive processes, particularly language and memory, can then be assessed and the information used to inform clinical decision-making about the appropriateness of a surgical intervention.

1.8 How is cognitive function affected by medication?

Many medicines affect cognitive performance. Neuropsychological assessment may be used to monitor the effect of starting a particular medication. Medications, such as those used in the management of epilepsy, Parkinson's disease or psychosis may affect cognition negatively, or sometimes positively, and neuropsychological assessment may therefore contribute to clinical decision making in relation to prescribing or managing cognitive side effects.

2 Approaches to assessment—behavioural neurology and neuropsychology

In the behavioural neurology approach, observable signs or symptoms are used as indices of brain pathology. However, whilst some patterns of behaviour are clearly absent in the person with no neurological condition and only occur in the context of brain lesions, many forms of cognitive impairment do not fit this dichotomy. For most cognitive skills, there is a continuum of performance in the non-neurological population. Nevertheless, the skilled observer can determine a large amount of information from relatively short interactions with the patient. By spending time talking with or observing the patient, it is possible to identify deficits in a number of cognitive domains. Short bedside tests can also be useful in highlighting the presence of some disorders. However, qualitative observation is usually not sufficient to judge the severity of impairment and may not detect certain forms of more subtle cognitive dysfunction at all.

2.1 The standardized test

The main tool of the neuropsychological assessment is the standardized, or psychometric test. Psychometric tests are tasks that have been designed to assess specified cognitive functions and are administered in a standardized fashion defined in a test manual. Such tests have been given to a normative sample group in order that the performance of the patient can be compared with that of a representative reference or 'normal control group', (i.e. individuals who have not suffered any form of neurological condition). The typical scores of the normal control group are used to produce 'norms'. The statistical properties and issues of validation of such tests are considered in Chapter 3. Suffice it to say here that a test is considered to have 'good norms' if the reference group is representative of the general population in terms of all factors likely to influence test performance (e.g. age, level of education, gender). Sometimes, if a particular factor is likely to have a large influence on test performance, separate sets of norms are provided for each category of that factor (e.g. different age bands). With norms available, the performance of the patient can be compared with the average performance of individuals of a similar age, taking into account how much variability there is in 'normal' performance. Test scores are expressed in terms of a 'standard score' or a percentile. A standard score is a measure of the distance of the patient's score from the average of the reference group, taking into account the amount of variability in the scores of the reference group. A percentile is the percentage of the reference group who score the same as, or less than, the patient.

Standardized tests are the most effective tools for quantifying impairments. However, whenever possible, it is also useful to use information from observation of the patient carrying out practical or functional tasks. Some areas of cognitive function are relatively poorly assessed by standardized tests. For example, many of the formal, structured, and time-limited standardized tests may be insensitive to problems of initiation, problem-solving, and sustained attention associated with executive functioning. Although more sensitive, ecologically valid standardized tests are emerging, the qualitative information gained from a task such as planning and preparing an unfamiliar meal can help formulate the patient's impairments. Furthermore, given that one task of the neuropsychologist is to identify the practical or functional consequences of brain injury, supporting evidence from functional situations makes this process a lot easier, and more valid.

3 Assessment prerequisites

Before proceeding with a neuropsychological assessment involving the administration of standardized tests, a number of prerequisites must be checked.

3.1 Concentration

The patient must be able to concentrate for at least the time needed to administer any one test. Most full neuropsychological assessments take several hours to complete, although testing is usually carried out over several shorter sessions. However long the assessment session, it is always necessary for the examiner to be attentive to how well the patient is able to concentrate on task instructions and on carrying out the test. An injury-related impairment in attention might make the patient distractible and unable to sustain attention to the task in hand. Pain, particularly headaches, will impair concentration. Preoccupation with worrying thoughts associated with anxiety or depression can be distracting. Fatigue is also a common problem after brain injury and cognitively demanding tests may cause the patient to fatigue rapidly. Poor sleep may mean that the patient is fatigued even before an assessment has begun. Therefore, when testing is likely to proceed over a long time period, it is necessary to ensure that adequate breaks are taken.

3.2 Comprehension

The patient must also be able to comprehend the task instructions for any test given. This does not mean that some tests cannot be given to a person with verbal comprehension difficulties since, of course, the administration of language tests is one means of identifying the presence of receptive dysphasia. Nevertheless, if a test is given to a patient who cannot understand what he or she is required to do, then the results of that test will be invalid. These issues highlight the fact that there are no pure tests of any one cognitive function. For example, verbal memory tests are dependent upon adequate language skills so that, if a memory test involves remembering a short story and the patient does not understand the content of the story, the test results will reflect the patient's language deficits rather than testing memory functioning. Similarly, visual memory tests are dependent upon adequate perceptual skills so there is little point testing a person's memory for a complex design by asking the patient to draw the design from memory if the person cannot adequately copy the design.

3.3 Motivation and effort

A further issue is the motivation of the patient to engage in the assessment process. Brain injury can cause motivational problems directly when the centres in the brain responsible for drive and initiation of activity are damaged. In more extreme forms of this disorder the patient may experience an inability to initiate action unless prompted at every stage. In less extreme forms, the patient may simply not apply him or herself to the task in the same way that it is reasonable to assume that most normative subjects would have done. Once again, therefore, this would result in test results reflecting lack of effort more than the cognitive skill under scrutiny.

Alternatively, motivation problems may be a result of a mood disorder. The patient who is depressed may not feel able to make an effort during testing and the results of the patient's performance may overestimate the level of impairment. Whilst this issue can affect performance on almost any cognitive test, certain tests are more vulnerable to the effects of motivational problems. For example, tests of memory such as story recall may be more sensitive to motivation problems than tests that use recognition of information as the means of assessing whether information is remembered.

3.3.1 Motivation by hopes of secondary gain

Sometimes a patient is motivated by secondary gain to perform more poorly than determined by the level of impairment that actually exists. This is most likely to occur in the context of medicolegal assessments when the level of a patient's compensation award is dependent upon the severity of the impairment or forensic settings when judgement of a person's mental capacity is involved. In such situations the person may be compliant with the assessment process, but may attempt to 'fake bad'. This might be in the context of the patient actually having no cognitive deficit at all or, more probably, in the context where the patient is attempting to exaggerate the severity of a genuine impairment. While examples of frank malingering are quite rare, it is necessary to consider the possibility that insufficient effort has been applied in any assessment, particularly in any medicolegal assessment (cf. Halligan, Bass & Oakley 2003).

This issue can be addressed in several ways. First, the examiner needs to be attentive to the situation where the severity of the complaints of the patient appears to be inconsistent with the severity of the injury. However, it is not possible to rely on this type of comparison alone since the relationship between injury severity indicators, such as length of coma or posttraumatic amnesia, and cognitive or functional impairments is not straightforward. For this reason, it is important to use tests that have been specifically designed to identify the patient who is not applying a normal level of effort. Most tests of this sort rely on the assumption that such patients will have a limited knowledge of the typical consequences of brain injury on cognitive functioning or have a poor knowledge of test procedures. As a result of this test naivety the patient may produce a performance that is significantly worse than that of most genuinely impaired patients. In some cases, performance on tests is inconsistent with level of functioning in daily life (i.e. patient is severely impaired on tests, but everyday functioning is not affected). For further discussion of the assessment of feigned or non-credible performance, (cf. Boone 2007).

4 Contra-indicators to assessment validity

Even when the assessment prerequisites have been checked, several other factors can significantly affect a patient's performance on neuropsychological tests. Groth-Marnat (2000, p. 95) lists 18 factors that could render the results of neuropsychological tests invalid.

- Physical problems may affect performance. In addition to pain, which will affect concentration, sensory or motor disturbances are likely to affect performance speed.
- Intoxication with alcohol or recreational drugs may impair cognition, as will some prescription medications (cf. Powell, 2004).
- Current or pre-existing psychiatric disorder or learning disability will affect results.
- Congenital or pre-existing neurological conditions including prior brain injury, insult, or epilepsy are also relevant factors.
- People for whom the language in which they are tested is not their first language may be disadvantaged.
- Some tests are considered to be culturally biased, which will compromise the results of someone whose cultural background is different.
- A patient may appear motivated to comply with testing, but assessment reveals suboptimal effort which may invalidate results from tests administered.

◆ The performance of patients may vary from one testing session to another for a variety of reasons and therefore the neuropsychologist must be cautious in interpreting the results from just one session.

It is critical therefore that the neuropsychologist assesses for the presence of any of these factors and considers carefully their potential impact on each individual assessment.

5 The assessment process

5.1 Review of information provided by the referrer

The assessment process begins with a review of the information provided by the referrer. Sometimes a great deal of information is available, including a detailed clinical history, brain imaging data, and results of neurological evaluation. At other times, the only information may be that the patient is complaining of a particular problem (e.g. difficulty in remembering names or appointments), or that the patient has experienced a particular incident (e.g. a mild head injury).

5.2 Interviewing the patient and his/her relative or carer

Upon arrival the patient should be helped to feel at ease. Neuropsychological assessment is often a lengthy process, which can be upsetting for people who may be faced with difficulties of which they are only partially aware. Thus, the need to maintain their cooperation is vital. An initial interview is used to establish the patient's perspective on the problems, the history, and the impact of the problems on daily living. In addition to the patient, it is usually necessary to interview a relative or carer who knows the patient well. Whilst it is important to obtain the patient's view of the problems, difficulties with insight or memory may mean that this personal account may be inaccurate or limited in scope. Many clinicians will use a semi-structured interview format for this clinical interview. Symptom checklists are also useful in prompting patients and relatives to report problems that may otherwise be forgotten or unstated. It is helpful to interview the patient's relative without the patient being present, so that the relative has the opportunity to express concerns that would otherwise not be discussed through embarrassment or protecting the feelings of the patient.

5.3 Administration of standardized tests

5.3.1 The use of cognitive screening tests

There are many different tests designed to provide a brief screening assessment of cognitive function. Cullen *et al.* (2007) reviewed 39 such tools, noting that they are typically used for one of three main purposes; (1) brief assessment in the doctor's office; (2) large scale community screening; (3) domain specific screening to guide further assessment. The Mini-Mental State Examination (MMSE; Folstein *et al.*, 1975) is the most ubiquitous in clinical practice, though tools which assess a broader range of cognitive domains than the MMSE, such as the Addenbrookes Cognitive Examination – Revised (ACE-R; Mioshi *et al.* 2006), are now being used more widely. For whatever purpose they are used, interpretation of results from cognitive screening tests should be cautious. Some patients present with a clear history of neuropsychological difficulties and are impaired on the screening test, while others perform well on the screening test and have few or no everyday problems. In these situations interpretation is straightforward, though even when there is clear evidence of dysfunction, more detailed assessment may be useful to clarify areas of specific deficit and retained abilities. Some patients will present with everyday difficulties, but perform well on a screening test, whilst others may be impaired on a screening test, but present with everyday neuropsychological problems. In these two situations, further evidence must be collected via more detailed neuropsychological and, where possible, neuropsychological assessment.

There is no universally agreed set of tests used for neuropsychological assessment. Some clinical neuropsychologists routinely use a screening test at the start of the assessment process as a means of formulating initial hypotheses about areas of cognitive strength and impairment (before proceeding to a more detailed examination). Other neuropsychologists prefer to routinely administer a fixed battery of tests to systematically address all cognitive domains in reasonable detail - in this situation, the screening test would be of little or no use. These two approaches to assessment have been characterized as the 'hypothesis-testing' approach and the 'big battery' approach (see Miller 1992; Lezak *et al.* 2004; Groth-Marnat 2000).

5.3.2 The 'big battery' versus the individualized hypothesis-testing approach

The big battery approach uses, as the name implies, a battery of tasks that is designed to assess most types of cognitive skill on the premise that, if a deficit is present, the battery will detect it. The main disadvantage of this approach is that it can be too time-consuming and may not assess some types of cognitive skill in sufficient detail to fully formulate the impairment.

By contrast, the individualized, hypothesis-testing approach is based on the particular question posed in the assessment. Information available prior to and during the assessment about the patient's strengths and weaknesses is used to select tests to assess in detail particular areas of deficit. For example, the main question in some assessments is whether or not brain damage is present. In this case the clinician will try to select those tests that are most sensitive to any form of brain injury. However, these tests are often not the best ones for making predictions concerning the 'real-life' impact of cognitive impairment. If predicting everyday problems and guiding rehabilitation are the main issues, then other tests may be selected. The main disadvantage of the hypothesis-testing approach is that the clinician is vulnerable to failing to assess a particular cognitive skill because a deficit is not readily apparent.

In practice, most clinicians probably use a combination of these approaches, by selecting a broad set of tasks designed to screen most areas of cognitive skill (or using a specifically designed screening test), and incorporating other tests as needed on the basis of test performance, the complaints of the patient or others, or the particular assessment question.

5.3.3 The importance of good normative data

A further issue for test selection is the importance of using well standardized tests that therefore have good normative data. Although the importance of accompanying information concerning performance in everyday life has been emphasized, the standardized test provides objective evidence of the nature and extent of cognitive impairment. Certain groups are not well represented in most normative samples for cognitive tests (e.g. people with low pre-morbid intellectual ability or very old people). In such cases the neuropsychologist must be cautious in test interpretation.

6 Cerebral organization and laterality

The brain is not cognitively symmetrical. While some cognitive processes are represented in both cerebral hemispheres, others are more localized to one or other hemisphere or to particular areas within a hemisphere. This is consistent with the currently prevailing view that many cognitive functions are modular in nature and that different cognitive modules rely on different brain regions.

The asymmetry of cerebral organization is most strikingly illustrated with language skills, which for most people are localized to the left hemisphere. It is also illustrated by the phenomenon of handedness, whereby one hand is 'dominant' in terms of being used for tasks requiring higher levels of fine motor skill. Handedness is typically assessed through questions about which hand or foot is used for various tasks or by asking the patient to perform or mime tasks such as writing or throwing and kicking a ball.

The majority of right-handed people (95%) have language skills in the left hemisphere, but the picture is more complex for left-handers, with most (around 80%) also having language on the left, some on the right, and some with language represented bilaterally. The identification of the speech dominant hemisphere is most critical when surgical procedures are planned, but for these purposes laboratory assessments such as the Wada technique are used.

With the advent of more sophisticated imaging techniques, the usefulness of assessing handedness, in combination with cognitive test performance, for the purposes of lesion location has diminished. Although there are reported group differences in cognitive strengths between left- and right-handers, such differences are at best modest and are unlikely to be helpful when accounting for patterns of performance on an individualized basis. The assessment of cerebral dominance can, however, help with the interpretation of patterns of neuropsychological test results. The assessment of handedness becomes most relevant when an unexpected pattern of performance on cognitive tests is shown (e.g. when a patient with a right hemisphere lesion demonstrates significant language disorder).

7 Specific cognitive skills examined during the neuropsychological assessment

The following sections describe in brief the cognitive skills that are the subject of neuropsychological assessment. More detailed accounts of the assessment process in each cognitive domain are provided in the following chapters. Some of these areas are not assessed in detail unless there are indications of possible problems, though the clinician should be attentive to difficulties that require more detailed examination. The section begins with a discussion of the importance of assessing pre-morbid functioning.

7.1 Premorbid functioning

In the neurologically normal population there is a wide range of ability in almost all forms of cognitive skill. Brain injury *can* lead to performance on a cognitive test that is worse than that of almost any person who has not suffered a brain injury. However, it is also possible for a person who pre-morbidly functioned at a high level of ability to suffer an impairment, while his or her test score remains within a normal range. While the score is not abnormal in relation to the general population, it is abnormal for that individual. When evaluating a patient's scores on any cognitive test, it is therefore necessary to consider what the patient's expected score would have been *before* the brain injury.

Most people will not have had any form of cognitive assessment pre-morbidly and therefore pre-injury performance has to be estimated. The three most common ways of doing this are to use:

◆ general demographic information (age, years of education, social class);

◆ the individual's best performance on any of the cognitive tests presented;

◆ a test that is usually resistant to the general effects of brain injury.

The most commonly used tests for estimating pre-morbid ability are those that examine performance reading words with atypical grapheme to phoneme relationships. Such tests include the Wechsler Test of Adult Reading (WTAR; Wechsler 2001) and the National Adult Reading Test, 2nd edition (Nelson and Willison 1994). These tests have been shown to correlate highly with performance on measures of general intelligence such as the Wechsler Adult Intelligence Scale (Wechsler 1999) in a normative sample and so can be used to estimate pre-morbid intellectual level, except where there is evidence of a pre- or post-morbid dyslexia. An alternative test of this sort is the Spot the Word subtest, from the Speed and Capacity of Language Processing Test (Baddeley *et al.* 1992). Spot the Word is a lexical decision task in which pairs of words are presented, only one of which is real, with the task being to identify the real word.

7.2 Current intellectual functioning

Most clinicians will administer a test, or battery of tests, designed to capture an individual's general level of intellectual functioning. The Wechsler Adult Intelligence Scale (WAIS; now in its third edition) is the most widely used tool for this purpose. The main aims of using such a battery are to provide a means of identifying whether an individual is likely to have suffered deterioration in cognitive performance in relation to estimates of pre-morbid functioning and to highlight particular areas of deficit that may need further investigation.

It is worth noting that neither the WAIS nor its subsequent incarnations were designed as neuropsychological assessment tools and poor performance on any one subtest cannot be used to diagnose a deficit in a particular cognitive domain. A formulation of a patient's impairments must be developed by careful analysis of the pattern of performance over a range of tests. While the WAIS can be used to determine an intelligence quotient (IQ) score (which is compared with estimates of pre-morbid IQ in the identification of brain dysfunction), in the neuropsychological context one must be cautious in expressing performance on a range of tests in terms of an IQ score. This is because a cognitive deficit in just one domain may lead to an extremely poor performance on a small number of subtests, while performance on other tests remains entirely normal. The averaging process used to calculate the IQ score could therefore mask a severe impairment in just one domain. Crawford (2004) makes a cogent argument that the primary level of analysis of WAIS III performance should be at the level of the Indexes (Verbal Comprehension, Perceptual Organisation, Working Memory, Processing Speed) as these are empirically derived and have superior reliability.

7.3 Memory

A range of different types of memory function must be assessed. (cf. Chapters 9 and 10.)

7.4 Attention and concentration

The terms attention and concentration are used interchangeably to refer to the ability to focus upon a particular stimulus and to maintain that stimulus in mind, sometimes over an extended period of time. (cf. Chapters 5 and 6.)

7.5 Speech, language, and communication skills

Although speech, language, and communication skills are often the domain of the speech therapist/pathologist, in the clinical setting it is necessary for the neuropsychologist to have a good knowledge of the nature of aphasic (language) disorders and dysarthia (impaired articulation), since these problems will impact on performance on other tests and be relevant to considerations of the functional impact of cognitive impairments. (cf. Chapters 13,14, 15 and 16.)

7.6 Visuospatial perception and constructional skills

Brain injury may cause visual field disorders, problems with visual acuity, spatial contrast sensitivity, visual (light and dark) adaptation, colour perception, figure–ground separation, or movement perception. Some of these problems can be addressed in opthalmological or neurological examinations and, if such problems are suspected to be present, then appropriate referral should be made. Other visual perception deficits such as agnosia, prosopagnosia, and unilateral neglect are examined within the neuropsychological assessment. (cf. Chapters 7 and 11.)

7.7 Executive functioning

Executive functioning refers to the ability to plan and problem-solve, self-monitor, and regulate behaviour (see Chapters 19 and 20).

7.8 **Mood, personality, and behaviour**

Direct consequences of brain injury may arise when the regions of the brain responsible for emotional processing or emotional control have been damaged. Indirect consequences arise from the stress of adjusting to losses of cognitive or physical functioning, role, or relationships.

Emotional lability is a common consequence of brain injury. Irritability and anger control are major problems for many patients. Although diagnostically controversial, some people with brain injury suffer from posttraumatic stress syndrome. While they do not usually remember the accident or injury, a small number of individuals suffer flashbacks to isolated memory fragments (islands of memory) of the event or perhaps waking in hospital, which for some is itself traumatic.

Attributions made by relatives concerning changes in personality are often related to changes in levels of inhibitory control and initiative. Those people who are disinhibited, more impulsive, and emotionally labile, or those who are unable to initiate activity in the same way, are those who are most commonly described as having changed in personality.

8 **Conclusion**

There are no pure tests of any single cognitive skill. The formulation of a patient's pattern of cognitive strengths and weaknesses is a complex task involving the assimilation of information from a wide range of different sources including the detailed history of the client's presenting problems and pre-morbid functioning, results from standardized tests and functional observation, and an assessment of the mood and motivation of the patient. Many problems experienced after brain injury or illness are very obvious from a short conversation with the patient. Some problems may be revealed by brief cognitive screening tools, but others are much more subtle, albeit no less disabling, and require more detailed assessment.

Selective references

Baddeley, A.D. Emslie, H. and Nimmo-Smith, I. (1992). *The Speed and Capacity of Language Processing Test*. Pearson, Oxford.

Boone, K.B. (2007). *Assessment of Feigned Cognitive Impairment*. Guilford Press, New York.

Crawford, J. (2004). Psychometric foundations of neuropsychological assessment. In *Clinical neuropsychology: a practical guide to assessment and management for clinicians* (eds. L.H. Goldstein and J.E. McNeil), pp. 99–119. Wiley, Chichester, West Sussex.

Cullen, B., O'Neill, B., Evans, J.J., Coen, R.F. and Lawlor, B.A. (2007). A review of screening tests for cognitive impairment. *Journal of Neurology, Neurosurgery and Psychiatry*, **78**, 790–799.

Folstein, M.F., Folstein, S.E. and McHugh, P.R. (1975). "Mini-Mental State". A practical method for grading the cognitive state of patients for the clinician. *Journal of Psychiatric Research*, **12**, 189–198.

Groth-Marnat, G. (2000). *Neuropsychological assessment in clinical practice*. John Wiley and Sons Inc, New York.

Halligan, P.W., Bass, C. and Oakley, D. (2003). *Malingering and Illness Deception*. Oxford University Press, Oxford.

Lezak, M.D., Howieson, D.B and Loring, D.W. (2004). *Neuropsychological Assessment*, 4th edn. Oxford University Press, Oxford.

Miller, E. (1992). Some basic principles of neuropsychological assessment. In *A handbook of neuropsychological assessment* (ed. J.R. Crawford, D.M. Parker, and W.W. McKinlay), pp. 10–11. Lawrence Erlbaum Associates, Hove, East Sussex.

Mioshi, E., Dawson, K., Mitchell, J., Arnold, R. and Hodges, J. (2006). The Addenbrookes Cognitive Examination Revised (ACE-R): a brief cognitive test battery for dementia screening. *International Journal of Geriatric Psychiatry,* **21**, 1078–1089.

Nelson, H. and Willison, J. (1994). *National Adult Reading Test*, 2nd edn. NFER, Windsor.

Powell, J. (2004). The effect of medication and other substances on cognitive functioning. In *Clinical neuropsychology: a practical guide to assessment and management for clinicians* (eds. L.H. Goldstein and J.E. McNeil), pp. 99–119. Wiley, Chichester, West Sussex.

Wechsler, D. (1999). *Wechsler Adult Intelligence Scale*-Third *Edition*. Harcourt, San Antonio, TX

Wechsler, D (2001). *Wechsler Test of Adult Reading*. Harcourt, San Antonio, TX.

Chapter 3

The methodological and statistical foundations of neuropsychological assessment

Klaus Willmes

1 Basic psychometric considerations

Neuropsychological tests are not different from psychological tests in general, as far as psychometric aspects are concerned. *Psychometrics* is a specific domain of measurement in psychology concerned with the assignment of numerals to one (or several) property/ies of objects or events according to fixed rules. Measurement proper (or a scaling process) occurs when a quantitative value is assigned to the sample of behaviour collected with a test from which test users draw inferences about the amount or extent of the theoretical construct (trait) that is taken to be characteristic of a person.

- Unlike physical attributes, psychological attributes of a person cannot be measured directly.
- Psychological attributes are constructs or hypothetical concepts the existence of which can never be confirmed in an absolute way nor is there universal acceptance how to measure any construct.
- The degree or extent to which some psychological construct is characteristic of a person can only be inferred from limited samples of that person's behaviour.
- Before any measurement of a construct can be made, one has to establish an operational definition (i.e. a rule of correspondence between the theoretical construct and observable behaviours that may be considered indicators of the construct).
- Any measurement obtained is always subject to error.
- The units of measurement on the measurement scales are not well-defined *per se*.
- The measurements on one construct must also have demonstrated relationships to other constructs within a theoretical system.

In psychology, a *test* is a standard procedure for obtaining a sample of behaviour from some specific domain. One can furthermore make a distinction between:

- (aptitude, achievement, proficiency) tests, with which one can obtain a behavioural sample of a person's *optimal* performance,
- questionnaires or inventories collecting a person's *typical* performance,

- sampling typical performance with a standard schedule and list of behaviours in a naturalistic setting (e.g. observation checklists).

2 The classical test theory model

Test theory is concerned with methods for estimating the extent to which the specifics of assessment of psychological functions influence the measurements in a given situation and with methods for minimising these problems.

2.1 Basic properties

Most neuropsychological tests - as the majority of psychological tests in general - are constructed along the rational of the *classical test theory model* or *classical true score model* (Gulliksen 1987, Lord and Novick 1968) with a subject's observed score assumed to be additively composed of a true performance level and a random error.

Basic properties and principles of the classical test theory model

- The *observed score* random variable X_{ij} (denoting the hypothetical distribution of potential scores) for subject i in test j is composed additively of the subject's true score T_{ij} for test j and the error random variable E_{ij}:

$$X_{ij} = T_{ij} + E_{ij}.$$

- The *true score* can be interpreted as the average of observed scores obtained over an infinite number of repeated test administrations (i.e. the expected value) with the same test.

- The test score of a different examinee represents another random variable with a potentially different true score.

- The expected value of the error variable E_{ij} is zero.

- In a population of examinees the expected error is zero, as well as the correlation between true score and error score.

2.2 Reliability

In order to obtain information about how closely related observed score and true scores are for some examinee in a given test (dropping the index j for the moment) one has to make use of the *reliability coefficient* ρ. The higher the reliability, the better the observed score represents the true score. The reliability coefficient is defined as the ratio of true score variance $\sigma^2(T)$ to observed score variance $\sigma^2(X)$ in the population of examinees:

$$\rho = \sigma^2(T)/\sigma^2(X) \; ; \; 0 \le \rho \le 1.$$

The reliability coefficient ρ is the square of the *reliability index* ρ_{XT} which denotes the correlation between true and observed scores. The above expression does not have practical value because true scores are not directly observable. Different approaches to actually assessing reliability are parallel test-, split half-, and retest reliability, as well as measures of consistency.

Different approaches to determining reliability

Parallel test reliability

This is the correlation between parallel tests. In classical true score theory two tests *A* and *A'* are defined as *parallel* when

— each examinee has the same true score on both forms of the test

— the error variances for the two forms are identical.

(Due to these properties, parallel tests also have identical observed score means and variances. The more general assumption of *essential τ-equivalence*, i.e. the true scores may only differ by a fixed constant across all subjects, is also sufficient.)

— With the additional assumption of uncorrelated error variables for the two separate tests the reliability coefficient is identical to the correlation between both observed variables *X, X'*:

$$\rho_{XX'} = \text{corr}(X, X') = \rho_{XT}^2.$$

Retest-reliability:

This is a measure of the correlation between two administrations of the same test; may only be interpreted as a reliability coefficient, if the assumptions of parallel tests are satisfied. In particular, the identity (except for an inter-individually constant term in essentially τ-equivalent measures) of true scores across the two measurement occasions for each person may be problematic; it calls for the absolute stability of inter-individual differences (with respect to the theoretical (true score) variable of interest.

Split-half reliability:

This measure of the correlation of the item totals of a test split into two halves may only be interpreted as a reliability coefficient, if the assumptions of parallel (more general: essentially τ-equivalent) tests are satisfied for both test halves. Since there are only half of the items in each part, reliability will be underestimated. The reliability ρ^* of the full-length test is:

$$\rho^* = 2\rho/(1+\rho); \text{ e.g. } \rho = 0.80, \text{ then } \rho^* = 1.60/1.80 = 0.89.$$

There are many ways to split a test (e.g. odd vs. even items; first vs. second half, etc.).

Different approaches to determining reliability (*continued*)

The last formula represents a special case of the general *Spearman-Brown (prophecy) formula* for modifying the number of items in a test by a factor K ($K = 2$ in the split-half case); the reliability coefficient ρ^* for the modified length test is:

$$\rho^* = K\rho/(1+(K-1)\rho).$$

Standardized item alpha reliability coefficient

This measures the average correlation ave(ρ) between all $K(K-1)/2$ pairs of *parallel* items scaled to a test of length K:

$$\rho^* = K\,\text{ave}(\rho)/(1+(K-1)\,\text{ave}(\rho)).$$

Cronbach alpha coefficient of consistency

This is a lower bound to standardized item alpha ρ^* for non-parallel items:

$$\alpha = (K/(K-1))(1-\Sigma\sigma_l^2/\sigma_X^2).$$

where σ_l^2 is the variance of the l-th item and σ_X^2 the variance of the total score. In case of parallel (more generally: essentially τ-equivalent) items, the right-hand side in the last formula is identical to $\rho_{XX'}$ with X denoting the total score (or arithmetic mean) of the K items.

In the case of dichotomous items, Cronbach alpha equals Kuder-Richardson Formula-20 (KR-20). For more details, see Crocker and Algina (1986) and Suen (1990).

Reliability of difference score

Let $D = X - Y$; assuming uncorrelated errors among X and Y,

$$\rho_{DD'} = \left(\rho_{XX'}\sigma_X^2 + \rho_{YY'}\sigma^2 - 2\rho_{XY}\sigma_X\sigma_Y\right)/\left(\sigma_X^2 + \sigma_Y^2 - 2\rho_{XY}\,\sigma_X\sigma_Y\right).$$

In case of parallel measures, $\rho_{DD'} = 0$.

Example (with identical variances): $\rho_{XX'} = 0.90$, $\rho_{YY'} = 0.95$ and $\rho_{XY} = 0.70$ gives $\rho_{DD'} = 0.75$ only; but a low correlation $\rho_{XY} = 0.30$ would yield a higher $\rho_{DD'} = 0.89$.

The *reliability of a difference score* may be of particular interest when diagnostic decisions have to be based on the difference $D = X - Y$ between two measures. Often, the reliability of the difference score is less than the one of both original measures. Rather, reliable difference scores will result when one chooses measures that are both highly reliable, but are not highly correlated. In case of correlated error variables or a correlation between X and $X - Y$, the reliability of the difference score may be higher than for either of the two measures.

The techniques for assessing reliability described so far cannot capture all relevant aspects of reliability estimation. Most restrictive is the assumption of just one non-differentiated error component (resp. one undifferentiated source of unreliability) in the classical true score model.

Generalizability theory, as a generalisation of reliability theory, allows for the introduction of several sources of unreliability (cf. Crocker and Algina 1986, Chapter 8).

2.3 Standard error of measurement and standard error of estimate

One important diagnostic question is how measurement errors have an influence on the interpretation of an individual person's scores. The exact size of error in a given score cannot be determined, but classical test theory allows for computing the expected variation of an individual subject's observed score around the true score, the *standard error of measurement*, i.e. the square root σ_E of the error variance. If one additionally assumes that the error variable E follows a normal distribution, a person's true score lies within the confidence limits of $X - \sigma_E$ and $X + \sigma_E$ with a probability of about 68%. The standard error of measurement will not be identical for all examinees and σ_E expresses the average of all examinees' individual standard errors; thus the standard error of measurement provides an interval for the average examinee. Furthermore, the confidence interval has the same width irrespective of the value of X, i.e. the uncertainty about the exact value of the true score is assumed to be the same for poor, medium and good performance.

Another relevant error, the *standard error of estimate*, is defined as the discrepancy between an examinee's observed score on one test and the predicted score on a parallel form of that test.

Standard error of measurement and standard error of estimate

- The *standard error of measurement* is related to observed score variance and reliability coefficient:

$$\sigma_E = \sigma_X \sqrt{(1 - \rho_{XX'})}.$$

Often, the 95%-confidence interval for the true score around the observed score X is reported for a test and it is computed as:

$$X \pm 1.96\sigma_E.$$

Example: with $\sigma_X = 10$ and $\rho_{XX'} = 0.91$, the standard error is $\sigma_E = 10\sqrt{(1 - 0.91)} = 3$.

- The *standard error of estimate* is:

$$\sigma_{XX'} = \sigma_X \sqrt{(1 - \rho_{XX'}^2)}.$$

The standard error of measurement is less than the standard error of estimate except for the case of perfect or zero reliability; in the example $\sigma_{XX'} = 4.15$.

2.4 **Normative data, standardization**

An examinee's raw score usually cannot lead to useful interpretations or inferences. For example, with 40 items in a visual discrimination test (composed of 50 items) answered correctly, a statement about visual discrimination ability depends on the difficulty of the test and/or the performance of other similar examinees.

♦ The use of *norms*, i.e. an external reference, helps to enhance interpretability of scores.

♦ A *normative score* provides information about an examinee's performance in comparison to the (total) score distribution of some reference group or norm sample representing a well-defined population. It is required to describe the normative sample with respect to demographic characteristics (gender, age, educational background). In neuropsychology, characteristics of the pathological condition will be of interest as well: etiology, size and site of brain lesion, time post onset, (clinical) syndrome assignment, etc. One also has to decide on the normative sample size, since it determines how adequately the normative sample represents the reference population.

♦ The *percentile rank* (PR) is one common type of normative score, denoting the percentage of examinees in the norm sample scoring below or identical to a given raw score. Although the PR is easy to interpret, one has to consider that the PR scale is a non-linear transformation of the raw score scale with the same gain in raw scores possibly indicating a varying gain in PR scores at different locations on the raw score scale.

♦ A *normalized z-scale* is often constructed in the case of a non-normal raw score distribution by identifying a certain PR with the corresponding quantile of the standard normal distribution. In case of more marked deviations from a normal raw score distribution this procedure will introduce substantial distortion often at the lower and/or upper end of the raw score scale.

♦ *Linear z-scores* are derived from raw scores in the case of their distribution being normal and they are further transformed into *standard norms* with means and standard deviations that lend themselves to an easy interpretation.

In the case of dependence of test performance on age or education (school grade), separate norms for different age or education sub-populations or grade and age equivalents are determined. Another approach is to determine the (linear) regression of age on the raw score for the whole standardization sample and compute a correction score.

Norms

♦ The *percentile rank* of a raw score x is defined as:

$$PR(x) = 100\%(\text{cum}f_x + f_x/2)/N,$$

where cum f_x is the cumulative frequency for all scores less than the score of interest, f_x is the frequency of the score of interest, and N is the normative sample size. Usually, the PR is rounded to the nearest integer number.

Norms (*continued*)

- *Normalized z-scale* (mean zero, standard deviation one): a certain *PR* is identified with the corresponding quantile of the standard normal distribution, i.e. with that *z*-score below which *PR* percent of a normally distributed trait are to be found.

- *Linear z-score and standard norms*: linear transformation of raw score *x* in normative sample:

$$z = (\text{raw score } x - \text{mean raw score})/\text{standard deviation of raw scores.}$$

For better interpretability, linear transformation $L + Kz$ into a standard norm with mean L and standard deviation K:

$T = 50 + 10z$ (T-score) $\qquad W = 10 + 3z$ (Wechsler scaled score)

$Z = 100 + 10z$ (Standard score) $\quad C = 5 + 2z$ (Centile score)

$IQ = 100 + 15z$ (Deviation IQ)

2.5 Validity

- *Validity* is the potential of the true score to reflect what a test intends to assess; in most cases this is an unobservable trait or psychological construct. Validity has always been regarded as the most fundamental and important property of psychometric instruments. The validity of a test is the extent to which it measures what it purports to measure. Generally, the chosen measure and its related true score only quantify some relevant aspect of a construct; it can never be fully captured by one or a few measures. A measure cannot simply be classified as being valid or invalid in an absolute fashion, rather validity is a relative property always to be considered with respect to some intended purpose. Validity is an overall evaluative judgement, founded on empirical evidence and theoretical rationales, of the adequacy and appropriateness of inferences and actions based on test scores (Messick in Wainer and Braun 1988, p. 33).

- *Validation* describes the process by which a test developer collects evidence to support the types of inferences that may be drawn from test scores.

Changes in emphasis and orientation towards validity have taken place in the history of psychometrics with an emphasis on the concept of construct validity in more recent times. Key validity issues are the interpretability, relevance, and utility test of scores.

Three main aspects of validity are generally discerned:

- *Construct validity* refers to a mutual verification of a measurement instrument and the theory of the construct it is intended to measure by way of testable hypotheses. There are several approaches to *construct validation*. Most of them are related to analyzing the pattern and size of correlations implied by consequences from the theoretical conceptions or the differentiation between groups in terms of theoretically implied expected differences (see Crocker and Algina 1986, pp. 232–4).

- *Criterion-related* (or criterion) *validity* refers to relating one measure of a construct to another measure of the same construct or some 'gold standard', if available. The criterion can take several forms:
  - — *Concurrent* validity is looked for in the case of another measure of accepted validity;
  - — *Predictive* validity captures the relation of a measure with some aspect of the expected future, a major aspect of screening and prognostic measures.
- *Content validity* – often employed with achievement tests - refers to how well one can draw inferences from an examinee's test score to a larger item domain similar to those belonging to the actual test instrument. Content validation is often based on expert ratings about how well the generation of items from some performance domain has been specified and how well the actual items reflect that domain. Several indices have been proposed to quantitatively summarize expert decisions about item adequacy (cf. Crocker and Algina 1986, pp. 221–2).

Validity coefficient

Validity coefficient: the correlation between the true score T_X of a test variable X and the true score T_Y of a second variable Y (e.g. a criterion variable):

$$\rho(T_X, T_Y) = \rho(X,Y)/\sqrt{\rho_{XX'}}\sqrt{\rho_{YY'}}.$$

This equation is also called the *correction for attenuation*. It also follows that

$$\rho(X,Y) \le \sqrt{\rho_{XX'}}\sqrt{\rho_{YY'}},$$

indicating that only reliable measures can present with a high validity coefficient.

3 Criterion-referenced measurement

In cognitive neuropsychological single-case studies with specifically tailored assessment procedures for some cognitive functions, another type of testing approach, criterion-referenced testing, is employed at least implicitly. A *criterion-referenced test* ascertains a person's status with respect to a well-defined behavioural domain (Berk 1980). The principle concern is to obtain rigorous and precise domain specifications to maximize the validity and interpretability of a person's domain score (e.g. test of simple arithmetic: visually presented addition tasks '$a + b = ?$' requiring a written number as the answer; explicitly state the range of numbers to be employed, whether carrying is required, etc.). In tests constructed according to the classical test theory model, less rigorous specifications are the rule and item selection is dominated by empirical aspects, e.g. item difficulty and item discriminability (i.e. its correlation with the total score).

3.1 Basic concepts

- *Content validity* is taken to be the major criterion for item generation and item selection. A test is called *content valid* if it (completely) contains or represents a universe (domain) of items.

- A *domain* is defined either by exhaustive enumeration of its elements or, more often, by stating its properties via generation rules that an item from that particular domain has to fulfil.

- A *representative* item sample from that domain constitutes an actual test.

- A domain is usually *stratified* (structured) according to one or more aspects in a hierarchical or completely crossed fashion with representative item samples drawn from each stratum (subdomain) or combination of strata.

As a test author one has to decide which of these parameters one wants to vary systematically and which parameters one is willing to ignore or control for by allocating items with these properties at random to the strata or strata combinations. Representativeness can often be obtained by drawing a random sample of prespecified size from the subset.

- *Content valid parallel tests* can be generated by drawing distinct representative samples from the domain of interest.

- For a specified domain, the *degree of competence* (achievement, proficiency, ability) for a subject i can be defined as the probability p_i of correctly answering items from that domain. Empirically, the level of competence is estimated from a representative sample of items from that domain. The properties of the ability estimate are dependent on the particular test model used (e.g. the binomial model; see below).

- Persons can also be characterised according to their *mastery/non-mastery* with respect to a domain. Mastery can operationally be defined as holding if the competence level p_i is no less than some (lower-bound) *criterion probability* p_c, often fixed at some high value of $p_c = 0.90$ resp. 0.95 or even 0.99.

Mastery and criterion-referenced testing thus relate a person's test performance to an *absolute* level of competence, not to a *relative* distribution of scores across some reference population, as in the classical true score model.

3.2 The binomial test model

- The *binomial distribution* gives the probability for the number x of critical events in n independent replications ($0 \leq x \leq n$) of the same chance experiment with a constant probability p for the critical event to happen (e.g. critical event 'head up' in each of n tosses of a regular coin).

- The *binomial model* is invoked implicitly when the competence level is estimated from dichotomously scored items using the relative frequency of items solved correctly as its estimate. But even for very homogeneous domains it is unrealistic to assume identical item difficulties.

- The '*sampling model*' version of the binomial model is more adequate. With a new random sample of items drawn from a domain to assess a new subject, the total score correct follows a binomial distribution across subjects even for items with varying difficulty. With PC-based item generation facilities there is no principled limitation to proceeding this way. The assumption of (local) stochastical independence among items (independent replications of the same chance experiment) cannot be tested in a single subject. Nevertheless, care can be taken not to choose a sequence of items that provokes practice, fatigue, or learning/transfer effects.

◆ The most simple *mastery decision* is based on the exact $(1-\alpha)$–confidence interval around the observed relative frequency of items scored correct: if the upper confidence limit $> p_c$, then the individual competence level p_i is compatible with mastery. More complicated decision rules also taking into account the error of falsely declaring non-mastery have been proposed as well.

(Example: $n = 80$ items, $x = 72$ correct for person i; competence level estimate $= 72/80$ $= 0.9$; exact 95%-confidence interval $(0.8124, 0.9558)$, computed using StatXact (Mehta and Patel 1999) or using software available for free via the internet; decision of mastery, since $p_c = .95$ is covered by the confidence interval.)

3.3 Operational definition of performance dissociation

◆ The concept of mastery can be employed to empirically demonstrate the intactness of some processing components and/or routes in a cognitive neuropsychological model.

◆ The criterion referenced measurement approach, utilizing the binomial model in combination with exact statistical tests for dichotomous scores (Fisher's exact test for 2×2 tables, exact version of the McNemar test), can be employed to give an operational definition and a procedure for detecting (double) dissociation of performance in individual patients, also distinguishing *classical, strong, and trend dissociations* as proposed by Shallice (1988, Chapter 10):

◆ *Classical* dissociation: performance in some task A well below the normal range and much inferior to task B within the normal range (possibly close to the pre-morbid level).

— For tasks with almost no variability in normal subjects, adopt a very high level of mastery ($p_c = 0.99$) for competence level p_B in task B; for tasks with more variability in competence among healthy controls, p_c to be equated with some low quantile in the score distribution of normal subjects (Table 3.1).

— Much lower competence level p_A for task A, e.g. compatible with chance level for multiple-choice items, definitely significantly lower than task B (e.g. using Fisher's exact test).

— Moreover, a large effect size (difference h between arcsin-transformed p_B and p_A) to be actually observed to warrant adequate statistical power (e.g. $1-\beta = 0.95$; Cohen 1988).

◆ *Strong* dissociation: performance in some task A well below the normal range and much inferior to task B also below the normal range.

— Standards for effect size the same as for a classical dissociation.

Table 3.1 Operational definition of different levels of dissociation using two tasks A (impaired performance) and B (better preserved performance) with dichotomous items (employing the exact Fisher test)

	Dissociation		
	Classical	**Strong (robust)**	**Trend**
Requirement	For the better preserved competence p_B in task B ($p_B = p_C$)		
1. Normal performance at ceiling	$p_C = 0.99$	$p_C = 0.80$ (definitely below normal performance)	p_C definitely below normal performance
2. Normal performance with variability	p_C related to e.g. 25%-quantile of normal performance, if known, or fixed arbitrarily	p_C below normal performance, if known, or fixed arbitrarily	p_C definitely below normal performance
Requirement	For the poorer competence $p_A < p_B$ in task A; determination of number of items such that effect size h can be attained with test power $1 - \beta$ for type-I error $\alpha = 0.05$ one-tailed		
Planned effect size*	large: $h = 0.8$	large: $h = 0.8$	medium: $h = 0.5$
Planned test power	$1 - \beta = 0.95$	$1 - \beta = 0.95$	$1 - \beta = 0.80 - 0.95$
Empirical effect size	large	large	medium

* $h = 2\arcsin\sqrt{p_B} - 2\arcsin\sqrt{p_A}$; standards for high and medium proposed by Cohen (1988)

- *Trend* dissociation: degree of competence for both tasks well below mastery levels.
  - Number of items large enough for good statistical power in comparison of competence levels
  - Effect size less than for the other types of dissociations (e.g. medium).
- *Double dissociation*: two complementary dissociations in two different patients; for exclusion of resource artefacts falsely indicating a double dissociation, reject 4 null hypotheses such that: (i) within pt. 1: competence task $B >$ task A, (ii) within pt 2: task $A >$ task B as well as (iii) for task A: pt. 2 > pt. 1, (iv) for task B: pt. 1 > pt 2. A worked-out example can be found in Deloche and Willmes (2000).

3.4 Reliability

Reliability of a criterion-referenced test comprises two aspects: reliability of domain score estimation and reliability (consistency) of mastery classification, which is of more interest when a test is primarily used for mastery classification(s) (cf. Crocker and Algina 1986, pp. 197–212).

4 Probabilistic test models

4.1 Basic considerations

There are three attitudes towards the construction of measurement instruments (Rost 1988):

- The test score of a measurement instrument is chosen to be the sum total of the item scores and granted interval scale properties per fiat taken to be justified empirically if it provides a powerful predictor for some relevant criterion measure ('*validity pragmatism*').

◆ The use of total scores is justified via deriving standardised or normative scores for some reference population ('*norm pragmatism*').

◆ Every assignment of numbers to persons requires a formal model stating testable assumptions and properties for that assignment ('*model priority*').

Almost all tests and scales in neuropsychological assessment are lacking a firm measurement basis (cf. Wade 1992, Chapter 2); e.g. for the Barthel-Index (cf. Wade 1992) the differential weighting of items and use of different numbers of scale points per item has not been justified psychometrically, nor has it been shown that the total score expresses a position on a *uni-dimensional* (latent psychological) continuum. On the other hand, e.g. the Glasgow Coma Scale has been shown to lack uni-dimensionality (Koziol and Hacke, 1990). Since the ground-breaking publication of the probabilistic test theory model (latent trait model) for dichotomous item scores by Rasch (1960, 1980) and its several extensions to polytomous items (general term: *item response theory* (IRT); cf. Wright and Masters 1982; Rost and Langeheine 1997) there is no principled excuse for skipping the stage of analysing the measurement properties, in particular the uni-dimensionality, of a new test or scale. Otherwise, assigning a total score over items to some patient may provide invalid information about the level of ability/competence/typical behaviour. Willmes (1997) has shown the *partial credit model*, a very general model for polytomously scored items (Masters 1982), to hold within each of the different item groups making up the Subtest Written Language of the Aachen Aphasia Test (AAT) with a ($m =$) 4-point graded item scoring.

4.2 The dichotomous Rasch model

In item response theory a mathematical model equation specifies how examinees at different ability levels respond to an item. The *item characteristic curve* (ICC) reveals how the probability P(+) of responding correctly to an item depends on the latent uni-dimensional trait θ that is assumed to underlie performance in the dichotomous items constituting a test.

◆ For the Rasch model one has the following (logistic) ICC (see Figure 3.1):

$$P(+,\theta) = \exp(\theta - \sigma_i)/(1 + \exp(\theta - \sigma_i))$$

The *ability* β_n of a person n and the *difficulty* σ_i of an item i are measured on the same unidimensional (interval) scale θ. The item difficulty is the point on the latent dimension where $P(+,\theta) = 0.5$.

◆ In a *uni-dimensional* test, statistical dependence among items can be accounted for by a single latent trait: For a specified θ, characterising a homogeneous subpopulation of examinees with that extent or amount of the latent trait, items are statistically independent (*local stochastical independence* property).

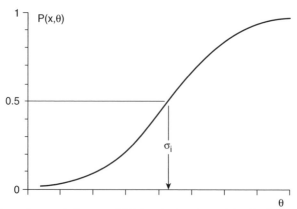

Fig. 3.1 Logistic item characteristic curve (ICC) for the Rasch model with dichotomous item scores; item difficulty σ_i is the point on the latent dimension for θ with $P(+,\theta) = 0.5$.

- If the above model holds, estimation of β_n only requires the *number* of items scored correctly irrespective of the actual pattern of items solved correctly. Likewise, estimation of item difficulty σ_i requires only the number of examinees with a correct solution for item i.

- In the case of model adequacy, item difficulty can be estimated in a *specifically objective* way, i.e. the item difficulty estimate (resp. person ability estimate) is independent of the distribution of person ability estimates (resp. distribution of item difficulty estimates) in the sample.

(For details on estimation procedures and a discussion of the concept of specific objectivity, cf. Wright and Masters (1982).)

A practical restriction to the use of the Rasch model is the rather substantial number of subjects (usually $n > 100$) to be examined for sufficiently precise parameter estimation and testing of model adequacy. For a demonstration of the unidimensionality and application of the Rasch model to the Token Test see Willmes (1981). An informative homepage with references to IRT publications and software is http://www.winsteps.com/.

5 **Individual case classification**

Classification procedures allocate a single subject to a certain pre-specified group. The most common questions in clinical neuropsychological diagnostic examinations:

- How is a patient doing in relation to a normative sample of healthy subjects (assignment of *deficit* yes/no); possibly after adjustment for age and/or educational level?

- To which group does a patient belong among a set of explicitly stated populations?

Soundness of classification is important in clinical work when providing a nosological label or a statement about the normality/deficit status. Preferably, the assignment to a population is qualified with a probability statement. It is often also reasonable to include a 'non-classifiable' alternative.

5.1 **Normality judgement**

Normality can be approached from the perspective of:

* *mastery*, with the level of performance judged in relation to some task inherent standard,

* *statistical normality*, with performance judged in relation to a (large) group of similar subjects:

  — Separate norms for different combinations of demographic variables are rare, a viable way is to work with one fixed norm but adjust an original raw score x_i of patient i by means of a (multiple linear regression) model equation specifying the influence of demographic variables:

  $$\text{adjusted } x_i = x_i + b_1(\text{age} - \text{mean age}) + b_2(yrs \text{ school}_i - \text{mean yrs school}).$$

  — The adjusted score is then related to the norm data from the healthy reference population.

  There are several ways to reach a decision about (statistical) normality:

* Tolerance limits, i.e. limits within which a given percentage (e.g. 95%) of the population is expected to be observed, together with control of the inferential risk involved because only a limited standardisation sample from the population is considered:

  — *Outer tolerance limit*: If the subject's score falls outside the limits, a decision with a controlled risk about non-normality can be made. In neuropsychology, often a uni-directional tolerance limit is required; non-normality is only related to the region of poor performance.

  — *Inner tolerance limit*: If the subject's score falls inside the limits, the decision is 'normal'.

* For scores in the gap between both limits no control of the inferential risk is possible.

  — *Parametric* tolerance limits require the true distribution of original scores to be known or to be estimable from a big sample. After correction for the influence of demographic variables, scale properties of adjusted scores degenerate for scales with fixed upper and lower scores.

  — *Nonparametric* (one-sided) tolerance limits specify that above the value of the r-th ranked observation in the standardisation sample there is at least a pre-specified proportion of the population with an error risk specified apriori (cf. Capitani and Laiacona 2000); e.g. the 10th ranked score for a sample of $n = 321$ equals the one-sided outer tolerance limit for the lowest 5% of the population with a risk of 5% that a larger proportion of normal subjects performs below the limit. This way of specifying tolerance limits also works with the ranks of adjusted scores.

  There are also ways to set bi- or multivariate (non-)parametric tolerance limits.

* Operationally declaring a *PR* or standard norm score to constitute the (one-sided) cut-off between normality and non-normality; e.g. *PR* = 1, 5 or 10 or norm scores 2, 2.5, or 3 standard deviations below the mean norm score. In cognitive neuropsychology,

frequently a cut-off has even been determined deliberately from a small normative sample simply taking the mean minus 2, 2.5 or 3 standard deviations as a cut-off.

- Inferential statistical decision about significantly worse performance in comparison to a (small) healthy control sample (approach advocated by Crawford and coworkers, see below).

5.2 Classification based on discriminant analysis

Discriminant analysis (DA) methods use an allocation rule, determined with previous samples from explicitly specified populations that optimises the classification of examinees to either one of a set of populations, preferably with a probability statement. It is desirable to also have a 'non-classifiable' statement when the allocation probability for any of the populations considered falls below some operationally set cut-off value. The allocation rule may be based on *parametric* (linear or quadratic) discriminant functions assuming the data to be (multivariate) normal in the different populations or on *nonparametric* techniques, which estimate the true distributions from the sample data and use a general Bayes theorem for the computation of the allocation probabilities (cf. Willmes 1985).

5.3 Deficit measurement

The notion of *deficit* presupposes some ideal, normal or premorbid level of performance against which the actual functioning of a patient may be compared.

- Both *normative standards* and *individual comparison standards* are used.
- *Direct methods* of individual comparison standards presuppose premorbid test scores, school grades or other data to be available; but they are often non-existent or very difficult to obtain.
- *Indirect methods* aim at estimating the original ability level based on historical and observational data; this provides only shaky evidence in most cases.
- Consequently, different approaches to estimating the missing information from the test scores actually obtained have been used: e.g. premorbid intellectual ability level estimated from a vocabulary score or reading performance, but they all have substantial problems as discussed in Lezak (1995, pp. 102–5).
- Inferential statistical decision about significantly deviant performance in comparison to a (small) healthy control sample without explixit reference to premorbid level (approach advocated by Crawford and coworkers, see below).

6 Psychometric single-case analysis

A comprehensive inferential statistical approach was suggested by Huber (1973) for:

- comparison of performances within an individual subject's profile of standardised test scores;
- comparison of two individual performance profiles, e.g. before and after some intervention (see Willmes 1985, for an application; a free PC-program CASE123 for psychometric single-case analysis is available from willmes@neuropsych.rwth-aachen.de).

6.1 **Basic concepts**

6.1.1 Roots

Zubin's postulates (1950) for the statistical treatment of intraindividual observations are as follows.

- ◆ Each individual, in particular if not from the healthy population, has to be treated as an independent 'universe', not to be classified prematurely into one patient group.
- ◆ Each subject is characterised by a given level and degree of variability *of performance.*
- ◆ Internal or external causes (spontaneous recovery, disease progression or therapeutic intervention) may affect either level or scatter of performance or both.

6.1.2 Principle idea

Treat diagnostic hypotheses about a person's identity of *true* scores (true performance levels) in two (sub) tests like other statistical hypotheses e.g. about the identity of parameters of distributions (e.g. t-test: identity of means from two normal distributions).

6.1.3 Connection to classical test theory model

The observed score X_{ij} of subject i in test j is considered a one-element random sample from the distribution of potentially observable scores; it is assumed to be additively composed of the person's true score T_{ij} (individual true performance level) and error E_{ij} (about that true level). An individual diagnostic examination cannot provide information concerning variability, and repetitive testing is not feasible as well.

6.1.4 Fundamental homogeneity assumption

Identity of the test specific error variance σ_{ij}^2 is assumed to hold across all subjects of the reference population for which normative data and reliability information have been obtained; in this case, the test specific error variance is identical to the square of the standard error of measurement, i.e. $\sigma_{ij}^2 = \sigma(X_j)(1-\rho_{jj})$, for the particular test j with $\sigma^2(X_j)$ the raw score variance in the reference population and ρ_{jj} a reliability coefficient (internal consistency, split-half or parallel test reliability) for test j. Both are regularly available in a test manual. Normative data must be available for the general normal (healthy) population and/or for some (well defined) patient population(s).

6.1.5 Concept of τ-standardisation

For a comparison of performance across subtests, only standard scores can be employed, since different subtests will usually show differences in difficulty. Diagnostic hypotheses are concerned with the identity of true scores, e.g. $T_{ij} = T_{ih}$. But identity of true raw scores only implies identity of true standardised scores if the reliability of both tests is identical (see Huber 1973). In the case of differences between subtest reliabilities, an additional transformation, the so called τ-*standardisation*, has to be carried out on the standardised score Y_{ij}^x (x denoting observed score standardisation), which provides the best estimate Y_{ij}^τ of true standardised performance:

$$Y_{ij}^\tau = Y_{ij}^x / \sqrt{\rho_{ij}} + L(1-1/\sqrt{\rho_{ij}}).$$

The higher a test's reliability the smaller is the difference between both types of standardised scores. In the case of identical reliabilities, ordinary x-standardised scores, as described above, will suffice and the same (average) reliability estimate ρ from the subtests involved is considered.

6.1.6 Choice of error probabilities

When deciding on diagnostic null hypotheses about true standardised scores by means of inferential statistical procedures, type-I and type-II errors occur just as with any statistical test. In the case of diagnostic hypotheses, commitment of type-II errors, i.e. overlooking some difference in true performance levels, may have more detrimental consequences for a patient than committing type-I errors, i.e. falsely declaring an observed difference in standardised scores to be indicative of a true difference in performance. Therefore, a more liberal default type-I error level of $\alpha = 10\%$ is recommended as default.

6.1.7 Practical requirements

Good reliability estimates for all (sub)tests in the profile (> 0.85 approximately) and normative data from a large standardisation sample ($n > 400$–500).

There are two aspects when testing for differences in performance:

- *Reliability aspect*: Is a performance difference unlikely due to errors of measurement alone?

- *Aspect of diagnostic validity*: In the case of a reliable difference, what is the probability of observing a still larger difference in the reference population?

If that probability is $< 20\%$, this difference in performance is taken to be *diagnostically valid*, i.e. potentially indicative of some relevant piece of diagnostic information (e.g. *dissociation*, see below).

6.2 Individual profile analysis

When analysing a performance profile of m subtests, level, scatter, and shape can be discerned:

- *Profile level*: weighted mean h_i^τ of τ-standardised subtest scores with higher reliability implying more weight.

- *Profile scatter*: overall differences among m subtest performances are assessed via the sum of reliability-weighted squared differences between subtest scores and profile level. In the case of significant profile scatter (value $> 90\%$-quantile of X_{m-1}^2-distribution), the profile is declared *real*, i.e. representing true performance level differences.

- *Profile shape*: to be analysed in more detail for a real profile under the reliability aspect.

  — Without a specific (neuro-) psychological hypothesis concerning relations of subtest performances, all $M = m(m-1)/2$ *pairwise comparisons* of subtests (j, h) are carried out with individual type-I error adjustment such that overall, the type-I error $<10\%$ (Holm 1979).

— A *linear contrast* of two non-overlapping groups of subtests, I with m_1 (≥ 1) and II with m_2 (≥ 1) ($m_1 + m_2 \leq m$) may be diagnostically more interesting (e.g. comparing verbal and non-verbal subtests in an intelligence test battery or expressive and receptive subtests in some aphasia test). Technically, the profile level h_{iI}^τ resp. h_{iII}^τ for subgroups I and II is computed and the linear contrast $\psi_i^\tau = h_{iI}^\tau - h_{iII}^\tau$ determined.

— Profile shape may additionally be analysed under the diagnostic validity aspect.

6.3 Intra-individual profile comparison

Psychometric single-case analysis also offers a way of comparing two profiles of the same subject or patient examined twice in the course of some neurological condition, possibly before and after some phase of therapy or training, or perhaps in a follow-up examination some time after an intervention, in order to find out whether performance has improved, stabilised or deteriorated again. Three steps of analysis may be discerned:

6.3.1 Global profile comparison

— *Profile identity*: identity of two profiles for the same test-battery – both in level and shape – are assessed via the sum of reliability weighted squared subtest differences between examinations 1 and 2. In the case of significant deviation from identity (value > 90%-quantile of χ^2_m-distribution), one proceeds to profile comparisons of level and shape.

— *Identity of profile levels*: the difference of both profile levels is tested for deviation from zero. Depending on the diagnostic hypothesis, this test is one-sided (improvement after therapy or due to expected spontaneous recovery resp. deterioration after some progressive disorder) or two-sided (e.g. stability at follow-up).

— *Identity of profile shapes*: for a pure comparison of profile shapes, the sum of level-difference adjusted squared subtest differences between examinations 1 and 2 is assessed. In the case of a significant shape difference (value > 90%-quantile of χ^2_{m-1}-distribution), additional comparisons serve to study these differences in profile scatter in more detail.

6.3.2 Specific comparisons for profile shape differences

— Without a specific (neuro-)psychological hypothesis, a change of the relation in performance between a pair (j, h) of subtests from examination 1 to examination 2 is carried out for all $M = m(m-1)/2$ pairs of subtests, applying Holm's adjustment for multiple testing.

— If a specific change in the performance pattern can be expected as a consequence of some intervention or disease progress, the same linear contrast ψ_i^τ may be compared between both examinations 1 and 2, i.e. $\delta_i^\tau = \psi_{i1}^\tau - \psi_{i2}^\tau$ is tested for a deviation from zero.

6.3.3 Comparison of all profile components

A more conventional comparison between two profiles - in the case of no identity - that does not involve relations between profile components simply asks whether true subtest performance has changed between two examinations. Again, these comparisons may be one- or two-sided, and adjustment for multiple testing, applying Holm's procedure, is required.

6.4 Specific applications in neuropsychology

- *Performance dissociation*: In order to back-up a selective sparing/impairment of some cognitive function one can examine whether true performance in that specific subtest *s* is reliably *and* diagnostically validly above/below all or a subset of all other subtests. One computes all $m-1$ (or a smaller subset) pairwise differences $Y_{ij}^{\tau} - Y_{is}^{\tau}$, which all must be reliable (one-tailed) using Holm's procedure and have diagnostic validity probabilities $< 20\%/(m-1)$.

- *Specific therapy effects*: test for a predicted change of some specific (set of) linear contrast(s) after an intervention period by carrying out one (or several) specific profile comparisons: e.g. this approach has been chosen to substantiate the assumed presence of primary progressive aphasia (Poeck and Luzzatti 1988): Besides language impairments revealed in an aphasia test it was shown that a linear contrast comparing language bound subtests of an intelligence test battery with non-language bound ones was reliable and diagnostically valid at initial clinical testing. But in the course of disease progression the strong discrepancy between both subtest groups became significantly smaller at an overall lower performance level.

- *Definition of responders*: The profile comparison methods may be used to generate operational criteria for identifying responders to some specific intervention, a more promising approach than only looking for significant group differences.

7 Comparison of a single case to a small control or normative sample

There is a comprehensive inferential statistical approach available, suggested by Crawford and co-workers (see http://www.abdn.ac.uk/~psy086/dept/SingleCaseMethodology.htm, also providing access to free software) for the intermediate case of comparison between an individual patient's performance and a small or modestly sized control sample, mostly consisting of healthy subjects more or less well matched for relevant demographic and other properties (sex, age, education, etc.). One encounters two basic problems when relating a patient's performance to that of a matched control sample:

- detection of a performance deficit for a single patient

- detection of a significant difference in performance for a single patient possibly for the demonstration of a dissociation of function.

7.1 Performance deficit

The performance score x^* of an individual patient on some performance measure X is related to the arithmetic mean $\bar{x}$ and the standard deviation s_X in the control sample via a "modified" t-test with $df = n-1$ proposed by Crawford and Howell (1998) for the single case context:

$$t = \frac{x^* - \bar{x}}{s_x\sqrt{\dfrac{n+1}{n}}}$$

◆ This test allows one to examine the research hypothesis at a prespecified type-I error level α that a patient does not belong to the population of control subjects via probing the null hypothesis that the patient's performance score is indeed an observation from the control population (mirroring the reliability aspect of the psychometric single-case approach).

◆ There is also a method using the exact p-value of the modified t-test (Crawford and Garthwaite 2002) for computing confidence limits on the probability of obtaining a still more deviant score than the patient's performance x^* in the control population (mirroring the diagnostic validity aspect).

(Example: Let the score of the patient be $x^* = 50$ in an 80-item task with arithmetic mean 70 and standard deviation 10 in a control group consisting of $n = 20$ matched subjects. Program SINGLIMS.EXE provides $t(19) = -1.952$ with a one-tailed $p = 0.033$ indicating a significantly decreased performance, with the 95%-confidence interval for the estimated percentage = 3.29% of the control population falling below the patient's score comprising 0.29%–11.07%. Since the upper limit of the confidence interval is small, i.e. below 20%, this performance difference may be considered a performance deficit.)

7.2 Difference in performance

Different tasks in single-case studies often comprise different numbers of items and/or show differences in difficulty, most probably resulting in different arithmetic means and standard deviations for two tasks A and B, to be meaningfully compared with reference to some processing model.

◆ For a reasonable comparison of both tasks it is mandatory to use standardized scores only.

◆ The test statistic t_D with $df = n - 1$ as proposed by Crawford, Howell and Garthwaite (1998) is composed of the individual patient's performance difference in terms of standardized scores z_X and z_Y for both observed score variables X und Y - using the means and standard deviations for X and Y in the control sample of size n - divided by the standard error of that difference, which contains the correlation r_{XY} among both measures in the control sample:

$$t_D = (z_X - z_Y)/\sqrt{((2 - 2r_{XY})(n+1)/n)}.$$

◆ Only if the standard deviations and the correlation of both measures were treated as parameters – not reasonable for small control samples - the test statistic t_D would have a t-distribution. Garthwaite and Crawford (2004) have proposed a revised standardised difference test (program RSDT.EXE) with a more complicated looking test statistic that does not contain parameters and may well be approximated by a t-distribution with $df = n - 1$.

(Example: Let the scores of the patient be $x^* = 20$ resp. $y^* = 50$ in a 60-item task A resp. 70-item task B with arithmetic mean 50 (resp. 55) and standard deviation 10 (resp. 5) in a control group of $n = 20$ matched subjects with correlation $r_{XY} = 0.70$ among both tasks in the control sample. The individual standardized scores are $z_X = -3$ resp. $z_Y = -1$. Program RSDT.EXE provides $t(19) = 2.394$ with a two-tailed $p = 0.027$ indicating a significant performance difference, with an estimated percentage $= 1.357\%$ in the control population for a more extreme difference between the poorer performance on task A as compared to task B.)

- The test for individual differences between tasks A and B can be combined with the test for a performance deficit in task A with respect to task B to allow for an operational definition of a classical performance dissociation. Let the performance on task A be assumed to be the impaired one. For a classical dissociation one has to show that the following set of criteria is fulfilled:
  — a significant difference in performance between tasks A and B
  — a deficit for task A and no deficit for task B.

(Example: Using the data from the example before, program DISSOCS.EXE provides the same results as before for the comparison aspect as well as the following for the deficit aspect: for task A $t(19) = -2.928$ with a one-sided $p = 0.004$ (95%-confidence interval from 0.003% to 2.559%) there is a performance deficit but not for task B with $t(19) = -0.976$ and one-sided $p = 0.19$.)

A complementary definition of a classical dissociation for another patient can be given by just exchanging the labels task A and B, thus also providing an operational definition for a classical double dissociation if the criteria for both complementary single dissociations are fulfilled. It has been demonstrated via simulations that the operational criteria have a very small probability of falsely identifying a subject from the control sample as showing a classical dissociation and that the criteria are quite robust in cases of skewed score distributions in the control sample. Likewise, there is only a small probability of misclassifying a patient with equivalent deficits in both tasks as presenting with a classical dissociation. The power to detect a classical dissociation is quite low in most cognitive neuropsychological single-case research since the single patient is compared to a rather small control sample which usually also shows considerable interindividual differences in performance (except for easy tasks which lead to ceiling effects). Power gets higher for pairs of tasks with sizeable correlations in the control population and with increasing sample size.

Selective references

Berk, R. A. (ed.) (1980). *Criterion*-referenced *measurement*. The Johns Hopkins University Press, Baltimore, MD.

Capitani, E. and Laiacona, M. (2000). Classification and modelling in neuropsychology: from groups to single cases. In *Handbook of neuropsychology*, 2nd Edition, Vol. 1 (eds. F. Boller, J. Grafman, and G. Rizzolatti), pp. 53–76. Elsevier, Lisse.

Cohen J. (1988). *Statistical power analysis for the behavioral sciences* (2nd ed.). Lawrence Erlbaum Associates, Hillsdale, NJ.

Crawford, J. R. and Garthwaite, P. H. (2002). Investigation of the single case in neuropsychology: Confidence limits on the abnormality of test scores and test score differences. *Neuropsychologia*, **40**, 1196–1208.

Crawford, J. R. and Howell, D. C. (1998). Comparing an individual's test score against norms derived from small samples. *The Clinical Neuropsychologist*, **12**, 482–486.

Crawford, J. R., Howell, D. C. and Garthwaite, P. H. (1998). Payne and Jones revisited: Estimating the abnormality of test score differences using a modified paired samples t-test. *Journal of Clinical and Experimental Neuropsychology*, **20**, 898–905.

Crocker, L. and Algina, J. (1986). *Introduction to classical and modern test theory*. Harcourt Brace Jovanovich College Publishers, Fort Worth, TX.

Deloche, G. and Willmes K. (2000). Cognitive neuropsychological models of adult calculation and number processing: the role of the surface format of numbers. *Eur. Child Adolesc. Psychiatry*, **9**, Suppl 2 II, 27–40.

Garthwaite, P.H. and Crawford, J.R. (2004). The distribution of the difference between two *t*-variates. *Biometrika*, **91**, 987–994.

Gulliksen, H. (1987). *Theory of mental tests*. Lawrence Erlbaum Associates, Hillsdale, NJ.

Holm, S. (1979). A simple sequentially rejective multiple test procedure. *Scandinavian Journal of Statistics*, **6**, 65–70.

Huber, H. P. (1973). *Psychometrische Einzelfalldiagnostik*. Beltz, Weinheim.

Lezak, M. D. (1995). *Neuropsychological assessment* (3rd ed.). Oxford University Press, New York.

Lord, F. M. and Novick, M. R. (1968). *Statistical theories of mental tests scores*. Addison-Wesley, Reading, MA.

Masters, G. N. (1982). A Rasch model for partial credit scoring. *Psychometrika*, **47**, 149–174.

Mehta, C. and Patel, N. (1999). *StatXact4 for Windows – User manual*. CYTEL Software Corporation, Cambridge, MA.

Poeck, K. and Luzzatti, C. (1988). Slowly progressive aphasia in three patients. The problem of accompanying neurological deficit. *Brain*, **111**, 151–168.

Rost, J. (1988). *Quantitative und qualitative probabilistische Testtheorie*. Huber, Bern.

Rost, J. and Langeheine, R. (eds.) (1997). *Applications of latent trait and latent class models in the social sciences*. Waxmann, Muenster.

Shallice, T. (1988). *From neuropsychology to mental structure*. Cambridge University Press, Cambridge.

Suen, H. K. (1990). *Principles of test theories*. Lawrence Erlbaum Associates, Hillsdale, NJ.

Wade, D. T. (1992). *Measurement in neurological rehabilitation*. Oxford University Press, Oxford.

Wainer, H. and Braun, H. I. (eds.) (1988). Test validity. Lawrence Erlbaum Associates, Hillsdale, NJ.

Willmes, K. (1981). A new look at the Token Test using probabilistic test models. *Neuropsychologia*, **19**, 631–645.

Willmes, K. (1985). An approach to analyzing a single subject's scores obtained in a standardized test with application to the Aachen Aphasia Test (AAT). *Journal of Clinical and Experimental Neuropsychology*, **7**, 331–352.

Willmes, K. (1997). Application of polytomous Rasch models to the Subtest Written Language of the Aachen Aphasia Test (AAT). In *Applications of latent trait and latent class models in the social sciences* (eds. J. Rost, and R. Langeheine), pp. 127–137. Waxmann, Muenster.

Wright, B. D. and Masters, G. N. (1982). *Rating scale analysis*. Mesa Press, Chicago, IL.

Zubin, J. (1950). Symposium on statistics for the clinician. *Journal of Clinical Psychology*, **6**, 1–6.

Chapter 4

Principles of cognitive rehabilitation

Nicole D. Anderson, Gordon Winocur, and
Heather Palmer

1 Overview

Cognitive rehabilitation can be defined as an intervention in which patients and their
families work with health professionals to restore or compensate for cognitive deficits,
thereby improving the patients' everyday functioning. Three features of this working
definition are important.

- Cognitive rehabilitation is a team effort. The patient's awareness of his/her deficit
  and his/her motivation to improve, the family's involvement and support, and the
  therapists' expertise are all crucial elements for a successful outcome.

- An important theoretical distinction in cognitive rehabilitation is whether the aim
  is to restore function to its original level, or to compensate for lost functioning. This
  distinction will be discussed in greater detail later in this section.

- The ultimate goal of cognitive rehabilitation is to facilitate meaningful and measurable
  improvements in patients' everyday functioning, be it functional, academic, vocational, social, or recreational. Later in this chapter we discuss the need to build these
  aspects of everyday functioning into rehabilitation practice.

Dixon and Bäckman (1999) argue that the need for rehabilitation ('compensation' in
their terms) arises when there is a mismatch between a person's actual performance levels
on the one hand, and environmental demands on the other. Various causes of such
a mismatch exist. Some of these are developmental (e.g., autism, learning disabilities,
schizophrenia), some are acquired (e.g., traumatic brain injury, stroke, neurodegenerative diseases such as Alzheimer's), and some occur as part of the normal aging process.
This review focuses on cognitive rehabilitation for adults. See Ylvisaker *et al.* (2005) for
a recent review of cognitive rehabilitation for children.

The International Classification of Functioning, Disability, and Health (World Health
Organization, 2001) describes three levels of functioning: body functions structures,
activities, and participation. In the context of cognitive neuropsychology:

- Impairment refers to damaged brain structures (e.g., frontal lobe damage) or
  neuropsychological functions (e.g., executive dysfunction);

- Activity limitations refer to changes in an individual's ability to carry out day-to-day
  behaviours (e.g., preparing a meal);

- Participation restrictions refer to changes in an individual's involvement in various life arenas (e.g., work or social engagements).

An individual's impairments and the presence of personality or psychological factors (e.g., depression) can result in activity limitations and/or participation restrictions. In addition, the environment or social setting can contribute to participation restrictions (e.g., barriers to vocational training).

Cognitive programs that emphasize retraining of abilities aim to improve functioning of a damaged structure or underlying process, while those that focus on compensatory mechanisms aim to minimize activity limitations. Cognitive rehabilitation may also focus on participation restrictions insofar as their root is psychological or the effect of an environment that does not facilitate effective functioning (e.g. a cluttered workspace). Generally, however, participation is best addressed in practical ways in multidisciplinary settings that include social workers and/or occupational therapists.

The distinction between treating impairments or activity limitations is important on two counts. Treatments of the underlying neuropsychological impairments are often artificial and therefore must demonstrate transfer to 'real life' situations to be justifiable. Treatments of activity limitations, on the other hand effectively bypass this step because they focus on the functional consequences of impairments in a reality-based context. The second important difference between impairment- and activity-oriented treatments pertains to assumptions about the underlying brain mechanisms involved in recovery.

Cognitive retraining approaches assume that treatment helps to speed spontaneous neural recovery or promote neural plasticity and/or regeneration. That is, a restorative process is assumed. By contrast, compensatory approaches assume that treatment helps to induce neural substitution or functional reorganization, whereby undamaged brain regions assume the function of damaged regions. Later in this chapter we will discuss the use of neuroimaging tools to help explicate the neural mechanisms of functional improvement.

Wilson (2002) argues that while cognitive rehabilitation has grown from disparate models of cognitive and neural functioning, what is truly needed is a comprehensive model that encompasses neural, cognitive, behavioural, emotional and psychosocial components in order to best identify problems, target treatments, explain mechanisms of recovery, and evaluate outcome. Holistic and multidimensional approaches to cognitive rehabilitation discussed later in this chapter are best geared to meet this goal.

2 Issues in cognitive rehabilitation

2.1 Factors affecting rehabilitation outcome

A number of factors affect rehabilitative outcome including neurological symptoms, neuropsychological status, psychosocial status, background history and supports (see Box 4.1).

2.1.1 Neurological symptoms

The location, size, and type of lesion are critical determinants of cognitive consequences and the likelihood of recovery. The natural history of TBI recovery depends on whether the head injury is diffuse or focal, with recovery from diffuse injury following a more stereotypic course (coma, post-traumatic amnesia [PTA], post-acute recovery), and recovery from focal injury being more dependent on the lesion location and size (Katz and Mills 1999). Coma severity (typically measured by the Glasgow Coma Scale), coma duration, and

---

Box 4.1 Factors affecting rehabilitative outcome

Neurological Symptoms

- Location, Type, and Extent of Lesion
- Secondary Effects (e.g., edema, increased intracranial pressure, hematoma)
- Coma Severity and Duration
- Post-Traumatic Amnesia Duration

Neuropsychological Functioning

- Attention
- Memory
- Language Functioning
- Visual-Spatial Skills
- Motor Skills
- Problem-Solving/Mental Flexibility
- Information Processing Speed

Psychosocial Factors

- Awareness of Deficit
- Motivation
- Coping Style
- Anxiety and Depression

Background History and Supports

- Age
- Personality
- Premorbid Level of Functioning
- Social Supports
- Financial Supports

PTA duration have been identified as significant predictors of functional outcome from diffuse TBI (c.f. Sherer *et al.* 2007, for a detailed analysis of these indicators). Secondary effects of trauma such as edema, increased intracranial pressure, and hematomas can add variability to recovery prognosis (c.f. Katz and Mills 1999, for a more complete discussion of primary and secondary effects). Moreover, progressive atrophy in both gray and white matter can occur up to a year post-injury, perhaps contributing to neuropsychological and functional difficulties (Bramlett and Dietrich 2007; Sidaros *et al.* 2009).

2.1.2 Neuropsychological status

A comprehensive neuropsychological evaluation (see box 4.1 above) is recommended, to determine which skills have been compromised and need to be rehabilitated versus those skills which survived and can be recruited to compensate for lost functioning. Deficits in executive functioning and sustained attention pose particular challenges for the patient's ability to engage in effortful, extended cognitive rehabilitation, and to reintegrate into social and vocational activities. Nevertheless, it must be noted that most standard neuropsychological tests assess cognitive impairments rather than disabilities. Hence, they are modest predictors of functional outcome, although some measures (e.g., general cognitive screens and executive control measures) appear to correlate with more complex functional activities (e.g., medical decision making) (Royall *et al.* 2007). The last couple of decades saw attempts to create more ecologically valid neuropsychological tests. These include the Rivermead Behavioural Memory Test (Wilson *et al.* 1985), the Test of Everyday Attention (Robertson *et al.* 1994), and the Behavioural Assessment of the Dysexecutive Syndrome (Wilson *et al.* 1996). In addition, Wilson (1995) stresses the importance of direct assessment of everyday problems via interviews, questionnaires, observation, and the patient and family's recording of the difficulties encountered.

2.1.3 Psychosocial factors

It is widely known that psychosocial status and lifestyle affect cognitive function in vulnerable populations and hence these factors need to be addressed in treatment programs (e.g., Winocur, Moscovitch, and Freedman, 1987; Mateer, Sira and O'Connell 2005). Prigatano (2005) has conducted considerable research into the relationship between patients' awareness of their functional disabilities and their ability to benefit from rehabilitation. Poor awareness can lead to passive or resistant behaviour in therapeutic settings. Different approaches have been taken to help improve awareness and/or motivation. These include

- patient and family education about common sequelae of brain injury (Anderson 1996);
- records of patients' behaviour (through logs or videotape) to provide the patient with a more objective view of their behaviour (Mateer 1999);
- psychotherapy to help patients cope with their disabilities (Ben-Yishay and Diller 1993; Mateer and Sira 2006).

Psychological problems, including anxiety, depression, social withdrawal, loneliness and changes in personality are commonly associated with brain injury (Morton and

Wehman 1995; Prigatano *et al.* 1998). Poor psychosocial adjustment (e.g., Dawson *et al.* 1999; Fields *et al.* 1998) and avoidant coping (Krpan *et al.* 2007) are related to poorer cognitive functioning in areas such as attention, memory and information processing speed. In addition locus of control, self-efficacy and optimism appear to influence rehabilitative outcome (Dawson and Winocur, 2008). These and related findings have led to widespread agreement that problems with awareness, motivation, emotion, and personality need to be addressed as part of any comprehensive cognitive rehabilitation program (e.g., Mateer *et al.* 2005; Prigatano 2005; Williams *et al.* 1999; Wilson 1995).

2.1.4 Background history and supports

Although the patients' background characteristics and social supports play an important role in rehabilitative outcome, they are rarely, with the exception of patients' age (younger individuals have a more positive recovery after brain injury), integrated into rehabilitation therapies or outcome evaluations in an objective way. Studies demonstrating the importance of premorbid patient characteristics have found that patients with poor outcome following mild TBI were likely to have had past neurological and psychiatric problems as well as other life stressors (Ponsford *et al.* 2000; Wagner *et al.* 2002). Similarly, a number of studies have documented reductions in patients' social support networks following TBI (Morton and Wehman 1995); reductions which may negatively affect recovery outcome (Lezak 1995). To address these needs, Ruff and Camenzuli (1991) recommend a multi-axial classification system to help identify factors that may influence rehabilitative outcome. This classification system includes premorbid and current emotional, psychological, psychosocial, and vocational status; factors that should be considered prior to establishing outcome goals and expectations.

2.2 Issues in rehabilitation design and outcome assessment

How rehabilitation is designed and outcomes assessed, are complicated issues and the reader is referred to several excellent reviews on the subject (e.g., Cicerone 2008; Sohlberg and Raskin 1996). Here, we limit our discussion to three primary issues.

2.2.1 Individual versus group approaches

Group sessions have the benefit of being more economical, as well as affording greater development of interpersonal adaptation and acceptance of impairments (Caetano and Christensen 1997; Wilson 1995). However, controlled trials examining the efficacy of group versus individual therapy are lacking (Wilson and Moffat 1992). Given that patients vary widely in their neurological, cognitive, and emotional status, a strong case can be made for tailoring programs to meet individual needs (Sohlberg and Raskin 1996; Wilson 1995), although individual programs suffer the disadvantages of being costly and inefficient, and depriving patients of valuable group support. Moreover, the evidence regarding outcome is mixed. One recommended solution is to offer a combination of individual and group rehabilitation (e.g., Cicerone *et al.* 2000; Prigatano 1997; Wilson 1997).

The efficacy of individual or group therapy approaches can be assessed with either single-subject or group designs. Single-subject designs need not be limited to a sample size of one, as the design can be applied repeatedly to multiple patients to establish generalization across subjects. Some investigators prefer single-subject designs, given the sizeable variability among patients in neurological, psychosocial, and cognitive terms (e.g., Sohlberg and Mateer 1989a), however group designs typically entail more uniform therapy practices across individuals. Once again, a combined individual/group approach that examines both group and individual effects may be advisable.

2.2.2 Control groups

The inclusion of appropriate control groups is essential in order to demonstrate the efficacy of rehabilitation. Only the treatment should differ between the control and treatment groups, and patients who desire treatment should be randomly assigned to treatment or control groups in order to avoid selection biases related to factors such as motivation, education, and age. Park and Ingles's (2001) meta-analysis of attention retraining studies revealed that, on average, pre- to post-treatment gains were significant only in studies that did not include a control group, thus indicating that the bulk of the gains reflected practice effects. Moreover, control groups tend to fare better in randomized controlled trials than in observational studies (Sacks, Chalmers, and Smith 1982), thereby inflating treatment effects in the latter group. While this difference has been interpreted in terms of participant selection effects, in the case of a waitlist control design, there may also be negative consequences to having an anticipated treatment delayed (c.f. Winocur *et al.* 2007a). One way to minimize this undesired effect is to provide the control group either with standard care or some alternate activity equal in therapist and interpersonal interaction to the treatment, so that the general effects of being in a therapeutic milieu are equated.

2.2.3 Generalization

The need to show generalization to other similar tasks and to everyday functioning is perhaps the most important issue in cognitive rehabilitation research. With few exceptions (c.f., Hall and Cope 1995), most studies have not even attempted to show generalization to everyday functional or psychosocial aspects of life, despite the fact that this is the ultimate goal of cognitive rehabilitation. Instead, most studies have examined whether training generalizes to similar but untrained cognitive tasks, and have found transfer only when the training and target tasks require very similar underlying processes (Cicerone *et al.* 2000; Park and Ingles, 2001).

There are several approaches to the issue of generalization (Stokes and Baer 1977). Historically, investigators have been content to assume somewhat optimistically, that their treatments will generalize in a meaningful way. Far preferable (to this 'train and hope' approach) is to build generalization into training from the outset; that is a 'train to generalize' approach. Sohlberg and Raskin (1996) recommend that therapists use everyday stimuli in training and conduct training in a variety of settings in order to facilitate generalization. Ruff and Camenzuli (1991) and High *et al.* (1995) recommend seeking generalization, not only to similar activities in everyday life, but also to psychosocial improvements.

3 Approaches to cognitive rehabilitation

There are three traditional approaches to cognitive rehabilitation:

- cognitive retraining;
- compensatory approaches;
- holistic approaches.

Recently, we have witnessed the emergence of a multidimensional approach which in a sense borrows from each of these, and attempts to organize their essential features into integrated, formalized programs. In addition, it is necessary to consider the pharmacological approach, for its inherent value, and because of the potential benefits from combining drug and behavioural therapies. Regardless of orientation, the goal of each approach is to rehabilitate cognitive functioning over and above that which might occur naturally with the passage of time, or through generalized practice. Each approach is reviewed in turn.

3.1 Cognitive retraining

Retraining programs usually involve repeated practice of specific cognitive exercises designed to strengthen basic skills (e.g., attention, encoding) that are essential for more complex cognitive function. This approach is continuing to develop and one promising adaptation is a scaffolding approach whereby training begins with basic processes and progresses to more complex skills. The approach is clearly reflected in Sohlberg and Mateer's (1989a) 'process oriented' model in which component processes presumed to mediate particular cognitive skills are trained in a hierarchical order, such that progressively more complex processes are trained as learning occurs. Within each level of training, skills are repetitively practiced under the assumption that repeated practice in a structured setting is a necessary component for strengthening and re-automatizing cognitive skills (Mateer 1999).

A specific example of the process-oriented model is Sohlberg and Mateer's Attention Process Training, which includes training in various aspects of attention including sustained, selective, alternating, and divided attention (1989a; 2001; Park *et al.* 1999; and c.f., Gray and Robertson 1989, and Sturm *et al.* 1997, for similar approaches). The efficacy of attention training has been demonstrated in a number of studies showing improvements on independent, untrained tasks that were presumed to tap the same functions (c.f. Mateer 1999, for a review). Subsequent developments of this model (Sohlberg *et al.* 1993) added methods to enhance patients' monitoring of their attention performance in order to improve self-control over other cognitive weaknesses.

While direct retraining has historically been ineffective when targeted at memory functioning (Sohlberg and Mateer 2001), one memory retraining paradigm developed for older adults holds considerable promise. Based on evidence that aging disrupts conscious effortful memory for prior events in their spatial-temporal context (recollection) but leaves intact automatic memory for prior events devoid of contextual information (familiarity), Jennings and Jacoby (2003) devised a recollection training paradigm. Participants studied a list of words, and then performed a yes-no recognition test on a new list, consisting of the studied as well as new, unstudied words. Each of the new words was presented twice during the recognition test. Participants were instructed to respond "yes" only to studied words. Repeated new words elicited a feeling of familiarity; a familiarity which needed to be offset by recollection of the words' original context (i.e., as a new, unstudied word) (Jennings and Jacoby 1997). Training began with just a couple of words intervening before the new word was repeated (the "lag"). This progressed over 28 sessions (15 min per session), held over seven days of training, until the lag was gradually increased (as participants met criterion performance). By the end of training, the older participants were responding correctly at an average lag of 28 words, suggesting vast improvement in the ability to recollect information. Moreover, Jennings and her colleagues (Jennings *et al.* 2005) later showed that the recollection training benefits did transfer to other tasks requiring recollection (e.g. as n-back and self-ordered pointing). As indicated by positive results from an initial study of 10 individuals with acquired brain injury (Lillie and Mateer 2006), this type of memory training technique seems to benefit any individual with recollection impairments (although clearly, further evidence is required).

3.2 Compensatory approaches

Compensatory approaches are based on the principle that individuals can offset reduced cognitive abilities by utilizing different ways of performing a task. Internal strategies can help individuals to make the necessary effort required to solve a problem. Such techniques place considerable demands on the individual's ability to use them appropriately. However, as West (1995) points out, one added benefit of such effort is the increased attention to task. With external strategies, the goal is to identify environmental objects which can assume some of the demands normally placed on cognitive processing. The following are some examples of compensatory techniques thought to be of value in cognitive rehabilitation.

3.2.1 Internal strategies

To varying degrees, normal adults depend on well-established internal strategies to support learning and memory. Cognitively impaired patients are less able to do this, but are able to benefit from direct training. Numerous strategies involving verbal and visual aids, organization of information and executive skills training are available. Their usefulness depends partly on the type of information to be remembered.

One example of an internal strategy that makes use of visual aids comes from the work of Yesavage and his colleagues (1983, 1990). They successfully trained older adults to use a face-name strategy in which one identifies a salient facial feature (e.g., a ruddy nose), creates a concrete image transformation of a person's name (e.g., a rose for 'Rosie'), and then forms an interactive visual image of the facial feature and the name transformation (e.g., a rose in place of her nose). While this kind of approach has been used successfully for individuals with mild memory problems (c.f., Troyer *et al.* 2006), it has generally been less successful for patients with moderate to severe memory impairments (e.g., Gade 1994; but c.f., Kaschel *et al.* 2002). The familiar method-of-loci, in which a visual image is associated with each of a series of locations or items on a list, is another example of the use of interactive imagery, due to its difficulty however, it is seldom practical for use with brain injured individuals (Richardson 1995).

Improved memory performance has also been reported following spaced retrieval training. Sohlberg and Mateer have successfully applied spaced retrieval techniques to train prospective memory – the ability to remember to do things in the future (1989a; Sohlberg *et al.* 1992a, 1992b). In this technique, individuals are trained to recall information at progressively longer intervals. The principle is that this experience facilitates the spontaneous use of efficient retrieval strategies.

Internal strategies that make use of verbal mediators such as forming semantically meaningful associates or easily connected rhymes of material to be remembered, are considered useful in learning people's names, or short words lists and sequences (e.g., 'Thirty days hath September…'). For longer lists or more complex material, creating a story can be a useful aid. The idea here is to devise personalized associations to each of the items that can be represented in meaningful and integrated ways, and easily accessed at retrieval. Other learning techniques encourage the organization of new information (i.e., into units of a manageable size or by taxonomic categories). Identifying as many contextual features as possible can also be useful for purposes of registering or encoding new information, and providing effective retrieval cues during recall.

There has been considerable debate concerning the value of training brain-damaged people to use internal strategies, and the extent to which, in the absence of other forms of training, they generalize from the training environment (Prigatano *et al.* 1998; Wilson and Kapur 2008). Wilson (1995) emphasizes that relatives, therapists, and teachers can use these strategies to help facilitate memory-impaired individuals' learning. At the same time, there is evidence that severely brain-damaged patients with limited potential for recovery, can benefit (to some degree) from intensive internal-strategy training (Thoene and Glisky 1995).

Techniques designed to rehabilitate executive skills have been used effectively with patients who have relatively small brain lesions and moderate cognitive impairment. One technique is to help patients regulate their behavior through self-instruction, wherein one talks his/her way through an activity in order to maintain appropriate attention (Cicerone and Wood 1987; Cicerone and Giacino 1992; Ownsworth and McFarland 1999; Meichenbaum 1977). This technique helps individuals to gain control over thought processes needed to plan and regulate behaviours appropriately.

Robertson's (1996) 'Goal Management Training' program was also designed to reduce executive impairments related to frontal lobe damage. This is a manual-based protocol for helping patients organize their behaviour and execute tasks in a goal-directed manner.

Patients are taught that successful task completion requires the implementation of several related strategies:

- evaluating the current situation and generating appropriate goals;
- selecting goals;
- parsing overall goals into sub-goals;
- learning and retaining the goals and sub-goals;
- evaluating outcome against the goals.

Goal Management Training is an intensive program that places considerable demands on patients' residual skills. Nevertheless, there is some evidence that it can be effective. Levine *et al.* (2000) demonstrated the utility of this method in a real-life setting. They described a single-case study of a woman recovering from meningo-encephalitis. Despite normal performance on standard neuropsychological tests of memory and executive functioning, she performed poorly on the more naturalistic tests of everyday attention and memory (described earlier in this section). One of her chief complaints was difficulty managing meal preparations. After Goal Management Training, there was a significant reduction in her number of cooking errors. For example, she was more likely to assemble the necessary ingredients, and better able to follow the sequence of a recipe, keep to the task, and get back on track when sidetracked. The primary advantage of this strategy is its applicability to everyday activities that require self-regulated, organized behaviour (c.f., Von Cramon *et al.* 1991).

3.2.2 External strategies

External strategies make use of objects in the environment to compensate for cognitive deficits. A simple approach is to design environments with built-in cues that reduce disorientation and help navigation. For example, lines painted on floors or ceilings can help guide in-patients to the cafeteria. Labels on cabinets, maps in buildings, and doors painted different colours are other examples of orientation cues. Effective treatments for executive dysfunction have included:

- using checklists to facilitate appropriate task sequencing in vocational settings;
- providing concurrent verbal feedback to reinforce and shape behaviour (Burke *et al.* 1991);
- cueing to improve self-initiation (Sohlberg *et al.* 1988);
- introducing response cost methods to decrease disinhibited behavior (Alderman *et al.* 1995).

In the memory domain, external aids include common reminders such as lists, calendars, and alarm clocks, and a 'memory place' in which important objects such as glasses, keys, and wallets are kept (West 1995).

Harris (1978) argued that external aids should meet three criteria.

- They should be active, rather than passive. Passive cues like calendars require one to initiate a checking behaviour, and initiating action is problematic for brain-injured individuals. Active cues, such as those that employ alarms, draw attention to the cue.

- They should be timely. That is, the cue should draw attention at the appropriate time when an action must be performed.
- They should be specific. A string around a finger may remind someone that they need to do something, but it does not specify which activity should be performed.

A very practical external memory aid is a memory book. Memory books often contain sections for personal information (e.g., name, address, phone number), a calendar, daily schedule, and 'things to do' list. Additional sections are added as needed (e.g., medication lists). Sohlberg and Mateer (1989b) described a rehabilitation approach to memory book training that involves three stages:

- Acquisition. In this phase, patients are taught the name, purpose, and proper use of each section of the memory book.
- Application. In this phase, patients practice the use of each section by following the therapist's role-playing instructions.
- Adaptation. In this phase, the use of the book is transferred to naturalistic settings.

Sohlberg and Mateer present a case study illustrating the success of this method (c.f. Burke *et al.* 1994).

Newer technology has provided increasingly portable and powerful memory aids. Wilson *et al.* (2001) describe the efficacy of an easy-to-use pager system that cues memory-impaired individuals when particular actions must be performed. Devices such as a Palm Pilot® or BlackBerry® offer even more flexibility, and their efficacy in memory rehabilitation has received some attention (Dry *et al.* 2006; Gentry 2008; Kim *et al.* 1999). Technology can have drawbacks, however. Many of these devices are expensive, and the risk of losing them must be considered. In addition, as electronic aids become more flexible, there are greater opportunities for confusion and interference during learning. Investigators and therapists are advised to restrict training to the essential functions afforded by the devises and to use training methods that prevent errors during learning. Examples of such methods are described in the next section.

3.2.3 Domain-specific techniques

Domain-specific approaches capitalize on preserved cognitive domains, or systems, to train functions that are normally mediated by other, impaired systems. For example, amnesics are severely impaired on tests of explicit memory (e.g., free recall), but perform normally on tests of implicit memory in which no reference is made to a previous event but where past experience nevertheless influences current behaviour (e.g., Schacter and Graf 1986). Specifically, amnesics would not be able to recall many words from a previously presented list. However, if provided with the first few letters of each word and asked to complete these 'word stems' with the first word that came to mind, amnesics would be as likely as healthy individuals to provide words that had been presented earlier. That is, their implicit memory for the previous event is intact, despite the fact that their explicit memory for past events is severely impaired.

Two approaches are based on these principles.

◆ In the method of vanishing cues (Glisky *et al.* 1994), memory-impaired people are provided with enough cues to allow successful performance, and as learning occurs, cues are gradually withdrawn. This method has been successfully employed to teach amnesics new computer skills (Glisky *et al.* 1986a, 1986b, 1994), but a meta-analysis found that when averaged across studies, the benefits of vanishing cues are small and non-significant (Kessels and de Haan 2003).

◆ A similar approach is the errorless learning procedure. Baddeley and Wilson (1994) observed that once a memory-impaired patient makes an error, he or she is more likely to repeat that error. They reasoned that the preserved implicit memory system is poorly equipped to resolve the interference. A number of investigators have demonstrated that errorless learning is more effective than standard conditions in which errors are allowed (c.f. Clare and Jones 2008).

3.3 **Holistic approaches**

In contrast to retraining and compensatory approaches, holistic approaches are more broadly concerned with the overall human condition. As such, they address cognitive, social, emotional, and functional issues that result from brain impairment. Holistic programs aim for practical benefits by emphasizing self-awareness with the aim of creating more insight into the changes that have taken place following brain injury. These include:

◆ self-regulatory skills in coping with social and cognitive demands;

◆ feelings of well-being that relate to confidence and self-esteem;

◆ communication skills considered essential to successful social interactions.

The holistic approaches are predicated on several key assumptions:

◆ Cognitive therapies must not be isolated from other therapies (physical, psychological) that are essential to functional rehabilitation;

◆ Cognitive interventions must proceed in sequential fashion from lower levels to more complex functions;

◆ The disorganized and sometimes chaotic nature of thought processes in brain-damaged people necessitate an orderly and structured therapeutic program;

◆ because the problems of brain-injured people are highly personalized, treatment must be as individualized as possible (c.f., Ben-Yishay 1996).

Holistic programs involve both group and individual therapy, often extend for years, and are demanding in terms of resources and commitment on the part of the patient. Individuals participate in intensive remedial intervention that includes simple drills and retraining exercises, as well as learning compensatory techniques. An important objective is that patients gain an appreciation of their strengths and weaknesses, and the practical limitations imposed by their brain damage. The expectation is that they will then be better equipped to restructure their lives in realistic ways.

Two prominent holistic programs are those developed by Ben-Yishay (1978), a pioneer in the field, and Prigatano (1986). Ben-Yishay's approach is characterized by the creation of a 'therapeutic community' in which the patients, members of the therapeutic team, family and significant others, work together to promote the rehabilitative process. Prigatano follows a similar approach but attaches great importance to the psychosocial consequences of neuropsychological disturbances. Prigatano's program focuses on residual function and is guided by the philosophy that optimal use of these functions can be achieved if the patient has psychologically adjusted to the injury-induced changes and is coping effectively. While there is continuing need to evaluate the holistic approach, evidence from several studies points to significant benefits to TBI patients in terms of neuropsychological test performance, vocational status, and emotional functioning (Cicerone *et al.* 2008; Prigatano *et al.* 1998; Salazar *et al.* 2000).

3.4 Multidimensional approaches

The recognition that cognitive impairment is a multi-faceted problem, as reflected in the holistic approach, is also apparent in the emergence of multidimensional rehabilitation programs that take into account combinations of biological, social, and psychological factors that impact on cognitive expression in individuals with brain dysfunction. In addition to their broad approaches, these programs share a number of important features. For example, they are evidence-based in that they attempt to integrate accepted clinical practice with empirically-derived theory of cognitive processes and cognitive impairment. Each has been evaluated by a rigorous randomized control trial that includes short- and long-term outcome assessment under carefully controlled conditions. In contrast to traditional individualized programs, which can extend for years and are resource-intensive, these programs are delivered in small-groups over relatively brief time periods.

Interestingly, the major multidimensional cognitive rehabilitation programs were developed initially for normal older adults and tested successfully in this population. However, the considerable overlap in the cognitive profiles of cognitively impaired populations suggests that in principle, brain-damaged individuals with mild to moderate cognitive loss could also benefit from such programs. Two different treatment approaches are as follows.

3.4.1 Specific-process training strategy

The specific-process approach is guided by the rationale that improvement in designated functional domains is best achieved by cognitive retraining that selectively targets those domains. Programs that follow this approach have been influenced heavily by studies that demonstrated relationships between improvements in specific cognitive abilities and improvements in performance in various everyday activities (Jobe *et al.* 2001). The first such approach to be reported in detail is the SIMA project (Oswald *et al.* 1996), in which 390 older adults living in the community were assigned to one of three following training conditions:

◆ memory: general competence, which focused on coping with everyday problems;

◆ psychomotor: to improve visuo-motor coordination and response time;

◆ memory + psychomotor: general competence + psychomotor.

After a nine-month training program, there was evidence that participants benefited in the specific areas in which they were trained, although there was little generalization to other areas. Memory training appeared to have the strongest effect and, when it was combined with psychomotor training, resulted in some protection against cognitive decline.

In 1998, the Advanced Cognitive Training for Independent and Vital Elderly (ACTIVE) program was launched as a multi-centre trial in which 2802 independent-living older adults received a six-week training program directed at memory skills, reasoning abilities, or speed of information-processing (Jobe *et al.* 2001; Ball *et al.* 2002). Outcome measures included basic cognitive functions in the training domains, everyday tasks (e.g., financial management, driving skills), health-related activities (e.g., quality of life, mobility, health services utilization), and instrumental activities of daily living.

The trial was conducted over a three year period with outcomes assessed immediately (< 10 days), 12 months, and 24 months after training. Relative to baseline, each intervention resulted in improved performance in its targeted domain. As in the SIMA study, there was no evidence of generalization to non-trained cognitive abilities *or* to performance of everyday tasks. Participants in the speed of processing and reasoning groups, but not the memory groups, exhibited improvement on quality of life measures that were still manifest five years post-training (Wolinsky *et al.* 2006). Finally, a sub-group of 193 memory-impaired individuals representing all three training conditions was identified and compared to the remaining unimpaired participants. The memory-impaired participants showed typical gains after receiving reasoning or speed of processing training but, interestingly, not following memory training. This unexpected pattern which may have reflected the heterogeneity of the impaired population, underscores the need for caution in applying training programs designed for a particular population to other populations.

3.4.2 Comprehensive training strategy

A team of scientists and clinicians at the Rotman Research Institute in Toronto took a different approach to developing a multidimensional cognitive rehabilitation program (Stuss *et al.* 2007; Winocur *et al.* 2007 a, b; Craik *et al.* 2007; Levine *et al.* 2007). Their program is guided by a general model of strategic processing which assumes that cognitive tasks, whether they involve straight-forward aspects of learning and memory or complex problem solving, require strategic thought directed at achieving a particular goal. Cognitively-impaired individuals are limited in their ability to apply strategies spontaneously and, unlike normal young adults, fail to adjust to the fact that conscious effort is now required. An essential premise is that, with direction and insights gained from the program, participants' use of effective strategies would increase and their overall cognitive performance would improve.

The protocol divides into three, four-week modules:

- memory skills training; in which various, mainly internal, memory strategies of the kinds described in section 3.2.1 are taught and applied to everyday life situations

◆ practical task training; an adaptation of Levine *et al.*'s (2000) Goal Management Training program, which focuses on strategies for performing everyday cognitive tasks;

◆ psychosocial training in which the aim is to enhance psychological well-being and confidence in participants' ability to follow a strategic approach in problem solving.

The trial was conducted on 49 community-dwelling, normal older adults, following a multiple baseline, cross-over design that allowed for between- and within-group comparisons to evaluate training effects. Memory, practical task planning, and psychosocial status were evaluated before training, immediately and six months after the completion of training. Notwithstanding the small sample size, significant gains were achieved in all three domains. Notably, there were improvements in performing simulated real-life tasks which reflected generalization of improved cognitive skills to everyday situations. Training-related benefits were maintained over the long-term. On some measures, there was progressive improvement over the six-month follow-up period, suggesting that participants were continuing to practice and benefit from techniques acquired during rehabilitation training.

The results of the Rotman trial add to those of the ACTIVE and SIMA trials and reinforce the value of the multi-dimensional approach. At the same time, they raise important questions. Future research will determine whether focusing on specific processes or following a more comprehensive strategy will be more efficacious, or whether circumstances (e.g., type of patient, availability of resources) will dictate treatment selection. Also to be resolved is the suitability of the respective protocols for different clinical populations. The ACTIVE trial indicated that caution must be exercised in attempting such applications. The Rotman protocol has been revised for individuals with diagnosed cognitive impairment and trials involving brain-damaged populations are underway. Related to this, the programs were designed for individuals with age-related cognitive decline or relatively mild impairment. It remains to be seen whether the programs can be adapted to patients with more severe cognitive impairment and co-existing mental health problems.

Finally, an important question relates to how well such programs work in combination with pharmacological therapies. As indicated below, the use of cognitive-enhancing drugs (eg., anti-cholinesterase, methylphenidate) to treat cognitive impairment is increasing, and there is some evidence of added benefits in patients with Mild Cognitive Impairment when such treatment is combined with cognitive training. Systematic study, including appropriate control groups, is needed to determine whether there are benefits to combining drug therapy with multidimensional cognitive rehabilitation over and above those to be gained from each form of treatment on its own.

3.5 Pharmacological Approach

Drug therapy in the treatment of cognitive impairment derives, of course from the medical model. The origins of this approach are in the cholinergic hypothesis (Bartus 1982), which relates memory loss (i.e. of the type seen in old age, Mild Cognitive Impairment, and the early stages of Alzheimer's disease), to a depletion of acetylcholine levels in basal forebrain and hippocampal brain regions. As a result, several drugs, notably donepezil (Aricept), rivastigmine (Excelon), galantamine (Reminyl), were developed to increase cholinergic function by increasing the supply of a key enzyme – choline acetyltransferase. The drugs, which are widely used, are well tolerated. Several studies, including some randomized control trials, have shown that they can help stabilize and improve cognitive function in individuals experiencing mild to moderate memory loss (Farlow *et al.* 2000; Mohs *et al.* 2001; Gauthier *et al.* 2002; Raskind *et al.* 2004). Some studies suggest that cholinergic drugs may be effective in treating memory impairment following TBI (Cardenas *et al.* 1994; Walker *et al.* 2004).

In terms of relative effectiveness, the Cochrane Dementia and Cognitive Impairment Group recently published separate meta-analyses of double-blind randomized control trials of donepezil (Birks and Harvey, 2006), galantamine (Loy and Schneider 2007), and rivastigmine (Birks *et al.* 2000). Each was associated with significant cognitive improvement relative to placebo treatment, and there seemed to be little difference in over-all efficacy (see also Hogan *et al.* 2004). The few studies that attempted to compare directly the effects of the different cholinergic drugs (e.g., Hogan *et al.* 2004; Wilcock *et al.* 2003; Wilkinson *et al.* 2002), have not yielded definitive conclusions.

Not all studies have reported positive effects of cholinergic treatment. In a recent review, Lanctôt *et al.* (2003) identified several factors that may affect outcome. These include APOε4 status, post-treatment autonomic responses, disease status, neuropsychiatric profile, and several biological markers, including CSF metabolites, and the metabolic status of the amyloid precursor protein. This suggests that only a subset of memory-impaired individuals can benefit from cholinergic treatment, which underscores the need to characterize those individuals.

Other cognitive-enhancing drugs whose effects are mediated by different pharmacological pathways are becoming available. Memantine, an NMDA receptor antagonist, has been approved recently in the USA and Canada. There is evidence that memantine may be effective in relatively advanced stages of Alzheimer's disease (Reisberg 2003), and a study by Tariot (2004) suggests that its effectiveness may increase when combined with donepezil. Finally, methylphenidate, a CNS stimulant that acts on dopaminergic and serotinergic systems is being used increasingly to treat cognitive impairment in various clinical populations, including ADHD (Szobot *et al.* 2003), TBI (Kaelin *et al.* 1996), brain tumour (Meyers *et al.* 1998), and stroke (Goldstein 2003).

The overall consensus is that cholinergic drugs and other approved drugs do offer cognitive benefits to at least some individuals with Alzheimer's disease and possibly other cognitively impaired people as well. The gains are often modest and there are conflicting findings but the results to date can be viewed as promising. Further investigation of the cognitive enhancing properties of pharmacological agents is clearly warranted.

4 New directions in rehabilitation

4.1 Range of service

Cognitive rehabilitation as a field has primarily developed with the needs of individuals with acquired brain injuries in mind. Increasingly however, patients with cognitive impairments due to much broader array of etiologies are also requesting rehabilitation (see box 4.2 below).

Box 4.2 Etiologies of focus in adult cognitive rehabilitation

- Traumatic Brain Injury
- Stroke and White Matter Disease
- Aphasia and other language disorders
- Healthy Aging
- Healthy Working Adults
- Dementia and Mild Cognitive Impairment
- Multiple Sclerosis
- Epilepsy
- Attention Deficit Hyperactivity Disorder
- Schizophrenia and Schizotypy
- Mood Disorders
- Pain
- Addiction
- Cancer and cancer treatment

One area of particular focus is the cognitive effects associated with cancer and cancer treatment. Cognitive disruption following cancer diagnosis and treatment is becoming universally accepted by patients, health care professionals and researchers. In one study, as many as 75% of breast cancer patients experienced cognitive changes as a result of cancer and cancer treatment (Weineke and Dienst, 1995). This research is limited by methodological challenges and the lack of standardization of neuropsychological tests (Vardy *et al.* 2007). The following neurocognitive changes are most common:

- verbal and visual memory;
- attention/concentration;
- language;
- motor skills;
- mental slowing;
- difficulties multi-tasking;
- ability to organize.

This cluster has lead some to suggest that frontal-subcortical networks are particularly vulnerable to cancer treatment effects (Wefel *et al.* 2004).

The mechanisms for cognitive change following cancer diagnosis and treatment are largely unknown. One obvious culprit is the direct effects of radiation or chemotherapy.

Cranial irradiation can cause cognitive deficits, even dementia (Taphoorn and Klein, 2004), and patients receiving high dose chemotherapy are at greater risk for cognitive disruption following treatment than patients receiving low dose chemotherapy (Schagen *et al.* 2006; Stewart *et al.* 2008; Van Dam *et al.* 1998). However, not only do many cancer patients experience cognitive loss in the absence of any radiation or chemotherapy treatment, research has found *pre-treatment* neuropsychological impairments in Stage 1–3 breast cancer patients relative to Stage 0 patients and healthy controls (Ahles *et al.* 2007). This would suggest that either the cancer itself, or psychosocial effects such as anxiety, depression and post traumatic stress disorder (Hermelink *et al.* 2007), and a host of other factors (e.g., impact of surgery and anesthesia; comorbid illnesses) may play a role. Fortunately, long term post-treatment cognitive changes seem to persist in only a subset (17%–34%) of cancer survivors treated with chemotherapy (Ahles and Saykin, 2007).

Considerable effort has been placed on rehabilitation for these changes, with rehabilitation in pediatric and adolescent cancer patients leading the way (c.f. Butler and Mulhern, 2005). As an example from the adult population, Ferguson *et al.* (2007) administered Memory and Attention Adaptation Training (MAAT) to 29 women (averaging 8 years post-chemotherapy for stage 1 and 2 breast cancer). MAAT consisted of a workbook and four individual monthly visits. The 30–50 minute individual monthly visits involved a review of the patients current knowledge of cancer-associated memory problems, identification of 'at risk' situations where memory failures arise, and learning and practicing both internal and external compensatory strategies specific to the kinds of mistakes they were prone to make. Application of the strategies in their home environments via homework assignments provided additional opportunities to rehearse and consolidate the information learned. Telephone contacts between the monthly visits served as reminders and additional support for applying the strategies. Participants were assessed on:

- quality of life;
- depression;
- anxiety;
- self reported cognitive complaints;
- measures of attention/concentration;
- spatial memory;
- verbal memory;
- language;
- executive function.

Assessment occurred at four points during the study; baseline, immediately following the program, 2 months and 6 months following the program. Significant improvement over baseline was observed at each assessment on measures of verbal memory and processing speed complimented by a significant reduction in self-reported daily cognitive complaints. This group now has a large scale study currently underway with expectations of promising results.

Although the research into cognitive changes associated with cancer is in its infancy, great strides have been made in a short time. Given the improvement in mortality rates associated with cancer (specifically breast cancer), the need for efficacious cognitive rehabilitation programs is becoming increasingly vital.

4.2 Use of neuroimaging tools

A large number of studies have used neuroimaging tools to explore the neural correlates of cognitive difficulties associated with TBI, stroke, aging, and dementia, but only more recently have these tools been applied to studying the neural correlates of performance gains associated with rehabilitation. In the previous edition of this book, we reviewed Robertson and Murre's (1999) framework integrating rehabilitation and neural recovery. In short, they argued that recovery depends on a number of factors including the extent to which an underlying neural network is disrupted, the extent to which the neural network is distributed versus localized, and the type of stimulation affecting recovery (bottom-up versus top-down). Research on practice-related plasticity in healthy individuals provides some support for the notion that neural change (or recovery) depends on these factors (c.f. Kelly *et al.* 2006). Practice of simpler cognitive tasks (e.g., sensorimotor tasks) generally *increases* task-related activation, usually involving more extensive areas of activation (e.g., broader activation of primary motor cortex) after practice of a finger-to-thumb opposition sequence (Karni *et al.* 1995). By contrast, practice of complex cognitive tasks (e.g., working memory) generally *decreases* task-related activation, most notably in prefrontal and parietal regions, suggesting a decreased reliance on top-down control processes (Erickson *et al.* 2007).

The same principles may not apply in the case of training effects on brain activations in brain injured individuals. Sturm *et al.* (2004) explored brain activation during an attention task before and after alertness training in individuals who had suffered a right-hemisphere stroke. Training was associated with increased activation in right frontal and parietal regions activated at baseline by a healthy control group. Meinzer *et al.* (2008) found similar perilesional increases in activation following language training after stroke. Kim *et al.* (2009) reported reduced activation of middle and inferior prefrontal cortex and increased activation of the anterior cingulate after attention training following TBI. All three studies suggest that training effects were mediated more by restoration ("normalized" activation patterns) than by compensation (recruitment of additional brain areas). However, the pattern of results is likely to depend on a complex interplay among factors such as etiology, particular aspects of training (e.g., duration and frequency), and time-since-injury. Compensation may be more likely in the case of slowly developing etiologies such as aging (c.f. Cabeza 2002). In patients with acute injuries, compensation may precede restoration, as Saur *et al.* (2006) found for language recovery following stroke. Although the use of neuroimaging tools is too new to draw conclusions about the neural mechanisms of recovery and rehabilitation, we expect significant progress in this regard in the coming years.

4.3 **Incorporation of adjuvant interventions**

The results from recent studies have identified two factors that have fairly profound effects on cognitive and neural functioning that have yet to be incorporated into cognitive rehabilitation: physical fitness and diet. Studies in non-human animals have identified that physical exercise promotes neural angiogenesis, neurogenesis, and up-regulation of neuroprotective molecules (e.g., brain-derived neurotrophic factor) (c.f. Kramer *et al.*, 2008). When sedentary older adults are engaged in aerobic training (particularly if combined with strength and flexibility training), cognitive improvements are noted especially in executive abilities (Colcombe and Kramer 2003). Aerobic training during an attentional control task yields increased activation in prefrontal and parietal regions (Colcombe *et al.* 2004), as well as in grey matter volumetric increases in prefrontal and superior temporal regions (c.f. Kramer *et al.*, 2008). In terms of diet, both proper intake of particular micronutrients (e.g., vitamins, antioxidants, folate) and *low* intake of particular macronutrients (saturated fats and cholesterol) are associated with better cognitive functioning; this due possibly to the role of these nutrients in neurovascular health (Greenwood 2003). These benefits of physical exercise and diet intervention may enhance the efficacy of cognitive rehabilitation programs. Preliminary support for this idea comes from a study by Small *et al.* (2006), which combined exercise, diet, stress reduction, and mnemonics interventions in a group of middle aged adults, and found improvements in verbal fluency and activation of prefrontal regions. Future studies will help to identify the particular combinations that best facilitate recovery or improvement of functioning and the combinations best tailored to different client groups.

5 Conclusion

Despite the relatively new development of cognitive rehabilitation as a clinical discipline, the studies reviewed above provide grounds for optimism. The refinement of standard approaches offer more reasons to be optimistic but perhaps the most encouraging development is the growing willingness to combine the best of the various approaches. The result is the emergence of holistic and multidimensional approaches which have been associated with positive outcomes. Equally encouraging is the broad consensus that cognitive rehabilitation programs must be evidence-based and derive from solid empirical and theoretical bases (Cicerone *et al.* 2005).

Acknowledgements

Work on this chapter was supported by grants from the Alzheimer Society of Canada awarded to N. D. Anderson and from the Canadian Institutes of Health Research awarded to G. Winocur. We thank Brian Mainland for his editorial assistance.

Selective references

Ahles, T. A. and Saykin, A.J. (2007). Candidate mechanisms for chemotherapy-induced cognitive changes. *Nature Reviews Cancer*, 7, 192–201.

Ahles, T. A., Saykin, A.J., McDonald, B.C., Furstenberg, C.T., Cole, B.F., Hanscom, B.S., Mulrooney, T.J., Schwartz, G.N., and Kaufman, P.A. (2008). Cognitive function in breast cancer patients prior to adjuvant treatment. *Breast Cancer Research and Treatment*, **110**, 143–52.

Alderman, N., Fry, R. K., and Youngson, H. A. (1995). Improvement of self-monitoring skills, reduction of behaviour disturbance and the dysexecutive syndrome: Comparison of response cost and a new programme of self-monitoring training. *Neuropsychological Rehabilitation*, **5**, 193–221.

Anderson, S. W. (1996). Cognitive rehabilitation in closed head injury. In *Head injury and postconcussive syndrome* (eds. M. Rizzo and D. Tranel), pp. 457–68. Churchill Livingstone, New York.

Baddeley, A. and Wilson, B. A. (1994). When implicit learning fails: Amnesia and the problem of error elimination. *Neuropsychologia*, **32**, 53–68.

Ball, K., Berch, D. B., Helmers, K. F., Jobe, J. B., Leveck, M. D., Marsiske, M., Morris, J. N., Rebok, G. W., Smith, D. M., Tennstedt, S. L., Unverzagt, F. W., Willis, S. L., (2002) the Advanced Cognitive Training for Independent and Vital Elderly Study Group. Effects of cognitive training interventions with older adults: A randomized controlled trial. *Journal of the American Medical Association*, **288**, 2271–81.

Bartus, R., Dean, R., Beer, B., and Lippa, A. (1982). The cholinergic hypothesis of geriatric memory dysfunction. *Science*, **217**, 408–17.

Ben-Yishay, Y. (1978). Working approaches to remediation of cognitive deficits in brain damaged persons. *Rehabilitation Monograph No. 59*. New York University Medical Centre, New York.

Ben-Yishay, Y. (1996). Reactions on the evolution of the therapeutic milieu concept. *Neuropsychological Rehabilitation*, **6**, 327–43.

Ben-Yishay, Y. and Diller, L. (1993). Cognitive remediation of traumatic brain injury: Update and issues. *Archives of Physical Medicine and Rehabilitation*, **74**, 204–13.

Birks, J., Grimley Evans, J., Iakovidou, V., and Tsolaki, M. (2000). Rivastigmine for Alzheimer's disease. *Cochrane Database of Systematic Reviews*, Issue 4, Article CD001191.

Birks, J. S. and Harvey, R. (2006). Donepezil for dementia due to Alzheimer's disease. *Cochrane Database of Systematic Reviews*, Issue 1, Article CD001190.

Bramlett, H. M., and Dietrich, W. D. (2007). Progressive damage after brain and spinal cord injury: Pathomechanisms and treatment strategies. *Progress in Brain Research*, **161**, 125–41.

Burke, J. M., Danick, J. A., Bemis, B., and Durgin, C. J. (1994). A process approach to memory book training for neurological patients. *Brain Injury*, **8**, 71–81.

Burke, W. H., Zencius, A. H., Wesolowski, M. D., and Doubleday, F. (1991). Improving executive function disorders in brain-injured clients. *Brain Injury*, **5**, 241–52.

Butler, R. and Mulhern, R. (2005). Neurocognitive interventions for children and adolescents surviving cancer. *Journal of Pediatric Psychology*, **30**, 65–78.

Cabeza R. (2002). Hemispheric asymmetry reduction in older adults: The HAROLD model. *Psychology and Aging*, **17**, 85–100.

Cabeza, R., and Nyberg, L. (2000). Imaging cognition II: An experimental review of 275 PET and fMRI studies. *Journal of Cognitive Neuroscience*, **12**, 1–47.

Caetano, C. and Christensen, A.-L. (1997). The design of neuropsychological rehabilitation: The role of neuropsychological assessment. In *Neuropsychological rehabilitation: Fundamentals, innovations, and directions* (ed. J. León-Carrion), pp. 63–72. GR/St. Lucie Press, Delray Beach, FL.

Cardenas, D. D., McLean, A., Farrell-Roberts, L., and Baker, L. (1994). Oral physostigmine and impaired memory in adults with brain injury. *Brain Injury*, **8**, 579–87.

Cicerone, K. D. (2008). Principles in evaluating cognitive rehabilitation research. In *Cognitive neurorehabilitation: Evidence and application* (2nd ed.) (eds. D. T. Stuss, G. Winocur, and I. H. Robertson), pp. 106–18. Cambridge: London, England.

Cicerone, K. D., Dahlberg, C., Kalmar, K., Langenbahn, D. M., Malec, J. F., Bergquist, T. F., Felicetti, T., Giacino, J. C., Harley, J. P., Harrington, D. E., Herzog, J., Kneipp, S., Laatsch, L., and Morse, P. A.

(2000). Evidence-based cognitive rehabilitation: Recommendations for clinical practice. *Archives of Physical Medicine and Rehabilitation*, **81**, 1596–615.

Cicerone, K.D., Dahlberg, C., Malec, J.F., Langenbahn, D.M., Felicetti, T., Kneipp, S., Ellmo. W., Kalmar, K., Giacino, J.T., Harley, J.P., Laatsch, L., Morse, P.A., and Catanese, J. (2005). Evidence-based cognitive rehabilitation: Updated review of the literature from 1998 through 2002. *Archives of Physical Medicine and Rehabilitation*, **86**, 1681–92.

Cicerone, K. D. and Giacino, J. C. (1992). Remediation of executive function deficits after traumatic brain injury. *Neurorehabilitation*, **2**, 12–22.

Cicerone, K. D., Mott, T., Azulay, J., Sharlow-Galella, M. A., Ellmo, W. J., Paradise, S., and Friel, J. C. (2008). A randomized controlled trial of holistic neuropsychological rehabilitation after traumatic brain injury. *Archives of Physical Medicine and Rehabilitation*, **89**, 2239–49.

Cicerone, K. and Wood, J. (1987). Planning disorder after closed head injury: A case study. *Archives of Physical Medicine and Rehabilitation*, **68**, 111–5.

Clare, L. and Jones, R. S. (2008). Errorless learning in the rehabilitation of memory impairment: A critical review. *Neuropsychological Review*, **18**, 1–23.

Colcombe S. and Kramer, A. F. (2003). Fitness effects on the cognitive function of older adults: A meta-analytic study. *Psychological Science*, **14**, 125–30.

Colcombe, S. J., Kramer, A. F., Erickson, K. I., Scalf, P., McAuley, E., Cohen, N. J., Webb, A., Jerome, G. J., Marquez, D. X., and Elavsky, S. (2004). Cardiovascular fitness, cortical plasticity, and aging. *Proceedings of the National Academy of Sciences USA*, **101**, 3316–21.

Craik, F. I., Winocur, G., Palmer, H., Binns, M. A., Edwards, M., Bridges, K., Glazer, P., Chavannes, R., and Stuss, D. T. (2007). Cognitive rehabilitation in the elderly: Effects on memory. *Journal of the International Neuropsychological Society*, **13**, 132–42.

Dawson, D., Winocur, G., and Moscovitch, M. (1999). The psychosocial environment and cognitive rehabilitation in the elderly. In *Cognitive neurorehabilitation* (eds. D. T. Stuss, G. Winocur, and I. H. Robertson), pp. 94–108. Cambridge, New York.

Dawson, D. R. and Winocur, G. (2008). Psychosocial considerations in cognitive rehabilitation. In *Cognitive neurorehabilitation: Evidence and application* (2nd ed.) (eds. D. T. Stuss, G. Winocur, and I. H. Robertson), pp. 232–49. London, England.

Dixon, R. A. and Bäckman, L. (1999). Principles of compensation in cognitive neurorehabilitation. In *Cognitive neurorehabilitation* (eds. D. T. Stuss, G. Winocur, and I. H. Robertson), pp. 59–72. Cambridge, New York.

Dry, A., Colantonio, A., Cameron, J. I., and Mihailidis, A. (2006). Technology in the lives of women who live with memory impairment as a result of a traumatic brain injury. *Assistive Technology*, **18**, 170–80.

Erickson, K. I., Colcombe, S. J., Wadhwa, R., Bherer, L., Peterson, M. S., Scalf, P. E., Kim, J. S., Alvarado, M., and Kramer, A. F. (2007). Training-induced functional activation changes in dual-task processing: An fMRI study. *Cerebral Cortex*, **17**, 192–204.

Farlow, M., Anand, R., Messina, J. Jr., Hartman, R., and Veach, J. (2000). A 52-week study of the efficacy of rivastigmine in patients with mild to moderately severe Alzheimer's disease. *European Neurology*, **44**, 236–41.

Ferguson, R. J., Ahles, T., Saykin, A.J., McDonald, B.C., Furstenberg, C.T., Cole, B.F., and Mott, L.A. (2007). Cognitive-behavioral management of chemotherapy related cognitive change. *Psycho-Oncology*, **16**, 772–7.

Fields, J. A., Norman, S., Straits-Tröster, K. A., and Tröster, A. I. (1998). The impact of depression on memory in neurodegenerative disease. In *Memory in neurodegenerative disease: Biological, cognitive, and clinical perspectives* (ed. A. I. Tröster), pp. 314–37. Cambridge, New York.

Gade, A. (1994). Imagery as a mnemonic aid in amnesia patients: Effects of amnesia subtype and severity. In *Cognitive neuropsychology and cognitive rehabilitation* (eds. M. J. Riddoch and G. W. Humphreys), pp. 571–89. Erlbaum, Hillsdale, NJ.

Gauthier, S. (2002). Advances in the pharmacotherapy of Alzheimer's disease. *Canadian Medical Association Journal*, **166**, 616–23.

Gentry, T. (2008). PDAs as cognitive aids for people with multiple sclerosis. *American Journal of Occupational Therapy*, **62**, 18–27.

Glisky, E. L., Schacter, D. L., and Butters, M. A. (1994). Domain-specific learning and remediation of memory disorders. In *Cognitive neuropsychology and cognitive rehabilitation* (eds. M. J. Riddoch and G. W. Humphreys), pp. 527–48, Erlbaum, Hillsdale, NJ.

Glisky, E. L., Schacter, D. L., and Tulving, E. (1986a). Computer learning by memory-impaired patients: Acquisition and retention of complex knowledge. *Neuropsychologica*, **24**, 313–28.

Glisky, E. L., Schacter, D. L., and Tulving, E. (1986b). Learning and retention of computer-related vocabulary in amnesic patients: Method of vanishing cues. *Journal of Clinical and Experimental Neuropsychology*, **8**, 313–28.

Goldstein, L. B. (2003). Amphetamines and related drugs in motor recovery after stroke. *Brain Injury*, **17**, 685–94.

Gray, J. and Robertson, I. (1989). Remediation of attentional difficulties following brain injury: Three experimental single case studies. *Brain Injury*, **3**, 163–70.

Greenwood, C. E. (2003). Dietary carbohydrate, glucose regulation, and cognitive performance in elderly persons. *Nutrition Reviews*, **61**, S68-S74.

Hall, K. M. and Cope, D. N. (1995). The benefit of rehabilitation in traumatic brain injury: A literature review. *Journal of Head Trauma Rehabilitation*, **10**, 1–13.

Harris, J. E. (1978). External memory aids. In *Practical aspects of memory* (eds. M. M. Gruneberg, P. E. Morris, and R. N. Sykes), pp. 172–9, Academic Press, London.

Hermelink, K., Untch, M., Lux, M.P., Kreienberg, R., Beck, T., Bauerfeind, I., and Münzel, K. (2007). Cognitive function during neoadjuvant chemotherapy for breast cancer: Results of a prospective, multicenter, longitudinal study. *Cancer*, **109**, 1905–13.

High, W. M., Boake, C., and Lehmkuhl, L. D. (1995). Critical analysis of studies evaluating the effectiveness of rehabilitation after traumatic brain injury. *Journal of Head Trauma Rehabilitation*, **10**, 14–26.

Hogan, D. B., Goldlist, B., Naglie, G., and Patterson, C. (2004). Comparison studies of cholinesterase inhibitors for Alzheimer's disease. *Lancet Neurology*, **3**, 622–6.

Jennings, J. M. and Jacoby, L. L. (1997). An opposition procedure for detecting age-related deficits in recollection: Telling effects of repetition. *Psychology and Aging*, **12**, 352–61.

Jennings, J. M. and Jacoby, L. L. (2003). Improving memory in older adults: Training recollection. *Neuropsychological Rehabilitation*, **13**, 417–40.

Jennings, J. M., Webster, L. M., Kleykamp, B. A., and Dagenbach, D. (2005). Recollection training and transfer effects in older adults: Successful use of a repetition-lag procedure. *Aging, Neuropsychology, and Cognition*, **12**, 278–98.

Jobe, J. B., Smith, D. M., Ball, K., Tennstedt, S. L., Marsiske, M., Willis, S. L., Rebok, G. W., Morris, J. N., Helmers, K. F., Leveck, M. D., and Kleinman, K. (2001). ACTIVE: A cognitive intervention trial to promote independence in older adults. *Controlled Clinical Trials*, **22**, 453–79.

Kaelin, D. L., Cifu, D. X., and Matthies, B. (1996). Methylphenidate effect on attention deficit in the acutely brain-injured adult. *Archives of Physical Medicine and Rehabilitation*, **77**, 6–9.

Karni, A., Meyer, G., Jezzard, P., and Adams, M. M. (1995). Functional MRI evidence for adult motor cortex plasticity during motor skill learning. *Nature*, **377**, 155–8.

Kaschel, R., Della Sala, S., Cantagallo, A., Fahlböck, A., Laaksonen, R., and Kazen, M. (2002). Imagery mnemonics for the rehabilitation of memory: A randomised group controlled trial. *Neuropsychological Rehabilitation*, **12**, 127–53.

Katz, D. I. and Mills, V. M. (1999). Traumatic brain injury: Natural history and efficacy of cognitive rehabilitation. In *Cognitive neurorehabilitation* (eds. D. T. Stuss, G. Winocur, and I. H. Robertson), pp. 279–301. Cambridge, New York.

Kelly, C., Foxe, J. J., and Garavan, H. (2006). Patterns of normal human brain plasticity after practice and their implications for neurorehabilitation. *Archives of physical medicine and rehabilitation*, **87**, S20–9.

Kessels, R. P. C. and de Haan, E. H. F. (2003). Implicit learning in memory rehabilitation: A meta-analysis on errorless learning and vanishing cues methods. *Journal of Clinical and Experimental Neuropsychology*, **25**, 805–14.

Kim, H. J., Burke, D., Dowds, M. M., and George, J. (1999). Utility of a microcomputer as an external memory aid for a memory-impaired head injury patient during in-patient rehabilitation. *Brain Injury*, **13**, 147–50.

Kim, Y.-H., Yoo, W.-K., Ko, M.-H., Park, C.-h., Kim, S. T., and Na, D. L. (2009). Plasticity of the attentional network after brain injury and cognitive rehabilitation. *Neurorehabilitation and Neural Repair*, **23**, 468–77.

Kramer, A. F., Erickson, K. I., and McAuley, E. (2008). Effects of physical activity on cognition and brain. In *Cognitive neurorehabilitation: Evidence and application* (2nd ed.) (eds. D. T. Stuss, G. Winocur, and I. H. Robertson), pp. 417–34. London, England.

Krpan, K. M., Levine, B., Stuss, D. T., and Dawson, D. R. (2007). Executive function and coping at one-year post traumatic brain injury. *Journal of Clinical and Experimental Neuropsychology*, **29**, 36–46.

Lanctôt, K. L., Herrmann, N., Yau, K. K., Khan, L. R., Liu, B. A., LouLou, M. M., and Einarson, T. R. (2003). Efficacy and safety of cholinesterase inhibitors in Alzheimer's disease: A meta-analysis. *Canadian Medical Association Journal*, **169**, 557–64.

Levine, B., Robertson, I., Clare, L., Carter, G., Hong, J., Wilson, B. A., Duncan, J., and Stuss, D. T. (2000). Rehabilitation of executive functioning: An experimental-clinical validation of Goal Management Training. *Journal of the International Neuropsychological Society*, **6**, 299–312.

Levine, B., Stuss, D. T., Winocur, G., Binns, M. A., Fahy, L., Mandic, M., Bridges, K., and Robertson, I. H. (2007). Cognitive rehabilitation in the elderly: Effects on strategic behavior in relation to goal management. *Journal of the International Neuropsychological Society*, **13**, 143–52.

Lezak, M. D. (1995). *Neuropsychological assessment* (3rd ed.). Oxford: New York.

Lillie, R. and Mateer, C. A. (2006). Constraint-based therapies as a proposed model for cognitive rehabilitation. *The Journal of Head Trauma Rehabilitation*, **21**, 119–30.

Loy, C. and Schneider, L. (2007). Galantamine for Alzheimer's disease and mild cognitive impairment. Cochrane Database of Systematic Reviews, **1**.

Mateer, C. A. (1999). The rehabilitation of executive disorders. In *Cognitive neurorehabilitation* (eds. D. T. Stuss, G. Winocur, and I. H. Robertson), pp. 314–32. Cambridge, New York.

Mateer, C. A., and Sira, C. S. (2006). Cognitive and emotional consequences of TBI: Intervention strategies for vocational rehabilitation. *NeuroRehabilitation*, **21**, 315–26.

Mateer, C. A., Sira, C. S., and O'Connell, M. E. (2005). Putting Humpty Dumpty together again: The importance of integrating cognitive and emotional interventions. *Journal of Head Trauma Rehabilitation*, **20**, 62–75.

Meichenbaum, D. (1977). *Cognitive behavior modification: An integrative approach*. Plenum, New York.

Meinzer, M., Flaisch, T., Breitenstein, C., Wienbruch, C., Elbert, T., and Rockstroh, B. (2008). Functional re-recruitment of dysfunctional brain areas predicts language recovery in chronic aphasia. *Neuroimage*, **39**, 2038–46.

Meyers, C. A., Weitzner, M. A., Valentine, A. D., and Levin, V. A. (1998). Methylphenidate therapy improves cognition, mood, and function in brain tumor patients. *Journal of Clinical Oncology*, **16**, 2522–7.

Mohs, R. C., Doody, R. S., Morris, J. C., Ieni, J. R., Rogers, S. L., Perdomo, C. A., and Pratt, R. D. (2001). A 1-year, placebo-controlled preservation of function survival study of donepezil in AD patients. *Neurology*, **57**, 481–8.

Morton, M. V. and Wehman, P. (1995). Psychosocial and emotional sequelae of individuals with trau-matic brain injury: A literature review and recommendations. *Brain Injury*, **9**, 81–92.

Oswald, W. D., Rupprecht, R., Gunzelmann, T., and Tritt, K. (1996). The SIMA-project: Effects of 1 year cognitive and psychomotor training on cognitive abilities of the elderly. *Behavioural Brain Research*, **78**, 67–72.

Ownsworth, T. L. and McFarland, K. (1999). Memory remediation in long-term acquired brain injury: Two approaches in diary training. *Brain Injury*, **13**, 605–26.

Park, N. W. and Ingles, J. L. (2001). Effectiveness of attention rehabilitation after an acquired brain injury: A meta-analysis. *Neuropsychology*, **15**, 199–210.

Park, N. W., Proulx, G., and Towers, W. (1999). Evaluation of the Attention Process Training pro-gramme. *Neuropsychological Rehabilitation*, **9**, 135–54.

Ponsford, J., Willmott, C., Rothwell, A., Cameron, P., Kelly, A.-M., Nelms, R., Curran, C., and Ng, K. (2000). Factors influencing outcome following mild traumatic brain injury in adults. *Journal of the International Neurological Society*, **6**, 568–79.

Prigatano, G. P. (1986). Personality and psychosocial consequences of brain injury. In *Neuropsychological rehabilitation after brain injury* (eds. G. P. Prigatano, D. J. Fordyce, H. K. Zeiner, J. R. Roueche, M. Pepping, and B. C. Woods), pp. 29–50, Johns Hopkins University Press: Baltimore, MD.

Prigatano, G. P. (1997). Learning from our successes and failures: Reflections and comments on "Cognitive Rehabilitation: How it is and how it might be". *Journal of the International Neuropsychological Society*, **3**, 497–9.

Prigatano, G. P. (2005). Disturbances of self-awareness and rehabilitation of patients with traumatic brain injury: A 20-year perspective. *Journal of Head Trauma Rehabilitation*, **20**, 19–29.

Prigatano, G. P., Glisky, E. L., and Klonoff, P. S. (1998). *Cognitive rehabilitation for neuropsychiatric dis-orders* (eds. P. W. Corrigan and S. C. Yudofsky), pp. 223–42, American Psychiatric Press, Washington, DC.

Raskind, M. A., Peskind, E. R., Truyen, L., Kershaw, P., and Damaraju, C. V. (2004). The cognitive benefits of galantamine are sustained for at least 36 months: A long-term extension trial. *Archives of Neurology*, **61**, 252–6.

Reisberg, B., Doody, R., Stöffler, A., Schmitt, F., Ferris, S., and Möbius, H. J. (2003). Memantine in moderate-to-severe Alzheimer's disease. *New England Journal of Medicine*, **348**, 1333–41.

Richardson, J. T. E. (1995). The efficacy of imagery mnemonics in memory remediation. *Neuropsychologia*, **33**, 1345–57.

Robertson, I. H. (1996). *Goal management training: A clinical manual*. PsyConsult: Cambridge, England.

Robertson, I. H. and Murre, J. M. J. (1999). Rehabilitation of brain damage: Brain plasticity and princi-ples of guided recovery. *Psychological Bulletin*, **125**, 544–75.

Robertson, I. H., Ward, A., Ridgeway, V., and Nimmo-Smith, I. (1994). *The Test of Everyday Attention*. Thames Valley Test Corporation, Flempton, UK.

Royall, D. R., Lauterbach, E. C., Kaufer, D., Malloy, P., Coburn, K. L., and Black, K. J. (2007). The cog-nitive correlates of functional status: A review from the Committee on Research of the American Neuropsychiatric Association. *Journal of Neuropsychiatry & Clinical Neurosciences*, **19**, 245–69.

Ruff, R. M. and Camenzuli, L. F. (1991). Research challenges for behavioral rehabilitation: Searching for solutions. In *Cognitive rehabilitation for persons with traumatic brain injury: A functional approach* (eds. J. S. Kreutzer and P. H. Wehman), pp. 23–34. Brooks, Baltimore.

Sacks, H., Chalmers, T. C., and Smith, H. Jr. (1982). Randomized versus historical controls for clinical trials. *American Journal of Medicine*, **72**, 233–40.

Salazar, A. M., Warden, D. L., Schwab, K., Spector, J., Braverman, S., Walter, J., Cole, R., Rosner, M. M., Martin, E. M., Ecklund, J., and Ellenbogen, R. G. (2000). Cognitive rehabilitation for traumatic brain injury: A randomized trial. *The Journal of the American Medical Association*, **283**, 3075–81.

Saur, D., Lange, R., Baumgaertner, A., Schraknepper, V., Willmes, K., Rijntjes, M., and Weiller, C. (2006). Dynamics of language reorganization after stroke. *Brain*, **29**, 1371–84.

Schacter, D. L. and Graf, P. (1986). Preserved learning in amnesic patients: Perspectives from research on direct priming. *Journal of Clinical and Experimental Neuropsychology*, **8**, 727–43.

Schagen, S. B., Muller, M.J., Boogerd, W., Mellenbergh, G.J., and van Dam, F.S.A.M. (2006). Change in cognitive function after chemotherapy: A prospective longitudinal study in breast cancer patients. *Journal of the National Cancer Institute*, **98**, 1742–5.

Sherer, M., Struchen, M. A., Yablon, S. A., Wang, Y., and Nick, T. G. (2008). Comparison of indices of TBI severity: Glasgow Coma Scale, length of coma, and post-traumatic amnesia. *Journal of Neurology, Neurosurgery, and Psychiatry*, **79**, 678–85.

Sidaros, A., Skimminge, A., Liptrot, M. G., Sidaros, K., Engberg, A. W., Herning, M., Paulson, O. B., Jernigan, T. L., and Rostrup, E. (2009). Long-term global and regional brain volume changes following severe traumatic brain injury: A longitudinal study with clinical correlates. *Neuroimage*, **44**, 1–8.

Small, G. W., Silverman, D. H. S., Siddarth, P., Ercoli, L. M., Miller, K. J., Lavertsky, H., Wright, B. C., Bookheimer, S. Y., Barrio, J. R., and Phelps, M. E. (2006). Effects of a 14-day healthy longevity lifestyle program on cognition and brain function. *Americal Journal of Geriatric Psychiatry*, **14**, 538–45.

Sohlberg, M. M., Johnson, L., Paule, L., Raskin, S. A., and Mateer, C. A. (1993). *Attention process training II: A program to address attention deficits for persons with mild cognitive dysfunction*. Association for Neuropsychological Research and Development, Puyallup, WA.

Sohlberg, M. M. and Mateer, C. A. (1989a). *Introduction to cognitive rehabilitation: Theory and practice*. Guilford, New York.

Sohlberg, M. M. and Mateer, C. A. (1989b). Training use of compensatory memory books: A three stage behavioral approach. *Journal of Clinical and Experimental Neuropsychology*, **11**, 871–87.

Sohlberg, M. M. and Mateer, C. A. (2001). *Cognitive rehabilitation: An integrative neuropsychological approach*. New York: Guilford.

Sohlberg, M. M. and Raskin, S. A. (1996). Principles of generalization applied to attention and memory interventions. *Journal of Head Trauma Rehabilitation*, **11**, 65–78.

Sohlberg, M. M., Sprunk, H., and Metzelaar, K. (1988). Efficacy of an external cuing system in an individual with severe frontal lobe damage. *Cognitive Rehabilitation*, **6**, 36–40.

Sohlberg, M. M., White, O., Evans, E., and Mateer, C. A. (1992a). Background and initial case studies into the effects of prospective memory training. *Brain Injury*, **5**, 129–38.

Sohlberg, M. M., White, O., Evans, E., and Mateer, C. A. (1992b). An investigation of the effects of prospective memory training. *Brain Injury*, **5**, 139–54.

Stewart, A., Collins, B., Mackenzie, J., Tomiak, E., Verma, S., and Bielajew, C. (2008). The cognitive effects of adjuvant chemotherapy in early stage breast cancer: A prospective study. *Psycho-Oncology*, **17**, 122–30.

Stokes, T. F. and Baer, D. M. (1977). An implicit technology of generalization. *Journal of Applied Behavior Analysis*, **10**, 349–67.

Sturm, W., Willmes, K., Orgass, B., and Hartje, W. (1997). Do specific attention deficits need specific training? *Neuropsychological Rehabilitation*, **7**, 81–103.

Sturm W., Longoni, F., Weis, S., Specht, K., Herzog, H., Vohn, R., Thimm, M., and Willmes, K. (2004) Functional reorganisation in patients with right hemisphere stroke after training of alertness: A longitudinal PET and fMRI study in eight cases. *Neurology*, **42**, 651–7.

Stuss, D. T., Robertson, I. H., Craik, F. I. M., Levine, B., Alexander, M. P., Black, S., Dawson, D., Binns, M. A., Palmer, H.; Downey-Lamb, M., and Winocur, G. (2007). Cognitive rehabilitation in the elderly: A randomized trial to evaluate a new protocol. *Journal of the International Neuropsychological Society*, **13**, 120–31.

Szobot, C. M., Ketzer, C., Cunha, R. D., Parente, M. A., Langleben, D. D., Acton, P. D., Kapczinski, F., and Rohde, L. A P. (2003). The acute effect of methylphenidate on cerebral blood flow in boys with attention-deficit/hyperactivity disorder. *European Journal of Nuclear Medicine and Molecular Imaging*, **30**, 423–26.

Taphoorn, M. J., and Klein, M. (2004). Cognitive deficits in adult patients with brain tumours. *Lancet Neurology*, **3**, 159–68.

Tariot, P. N. (2004). Memantine for patients with Alzheimer's disease: Reply. *Journal of the American Medical Association*, **291**, 1695.

Thoene, A. I. T. and Glisky, E. L. (1995). Learning of name-face associations in memory impaired patients: A comparison of different training procedures. *Journal of the International Neuropsychological Society*, **1**, 29–38.

Troyer, A. K., Häfliger, A., Cadieux, M. J., and Craik, F. I. M. (2006). Name and face learning in older adults: Effects of level of processing, self-generation, and intention to learn. *Journals of Gerontology: Series B: Psychological Sciences and Social Sciences*, **61B**, P67-P74.

Van Dam, F.S., Schagen, S.B., Muller, M.J., Boogerd, W., Wall, E., Fortuyn, M. and Rodenhuis, S. (1998). Impairment of cognitive function in women receiving adjuvant treatment for high-risk breast cancer: High-dose versus standard-dose chemotherapy. *Journal of the National Cancer Institute*, **90**, 210–8.

Vardy, J., Wefel, J.S., Ahles, T.A., Tannock, I.F. and S. B. Schagen, S.B. (2007). Cancer and cancer-therapy related cognitive dysfunction: An international perspective from the Venice cognitive workshop. *Annals of Oncology*, **19**, 623–9.

von Cramon, D. Y., Matthes-von Cramon, G., and Mai, N. (1991). Problem-solving deficits in brain-injured patients: A therapeutic approach. *Neuropsychological Rehabilitation*, **1**, 45–64.

Wagner, A. K., Hammond, F. M., Sasser, H. C., and Wiercisiewski, D. (2002). Return to productive activity after traumatic brain injury: Relationship with measures of disability, handicap, and community integration. *Archives of Physical Medicine and Rehabilitation*, **83**, 107–14.

Walker, W., Seel, R. T., Gibellato, M., Lew, H., Cornis-Pop, M., Jena, T., and Silver, T. (2004). The effects of Donepezil on traumatic brain injury acute rehabilitation outcomes. *Brain Injury*, **18**, 739–50.

Wefel, J. S., Kayl, A. E., and Meyers, C. A. (2004). Neuropsychological dysfunction associated with cancer and cancer therapies: A conceptual review of an emerging target. *British Journal of Cancer*, **90**, 1691–6.

Weineke, M.H. and Dienst, E.R. (1995). Neuropsychological assessment of cognitive functioning following chemotherapy for breast cancer. *Psycho-Oncology*, **4**, 61–6.

West, R. L. (1995). Compensatory strategies for age-associated memory impairment. In Handbook of memory disorders (eds. A. D. Baddeley, B. A. Wilson, and F. N. Watts), pp. 481–500. Wiley, Chicester, UK.

Wilcock, G., Howe, I., Coles, H., Lilienfeld, S., Truyen, L., Zhu, Y., Bullock, R., and Kershaw, P. (2003). A long-term comparison of galantamine and donepezil in the treatment of Alzheimer's disease. *Drugs and Aging*, **20**, 777–89.

Wilkinson, D. G., Passmore, A. P., Bullock, R., Hopker, S. W., Smith, R., Potocnik, F. C., Maud, C. M., Engelbrecht, I., Hock, C., Ieni, J. R., and Bahra, R. S. (2002). A multinational, randomized, 12-week, comparative study of donepezil and rivastigmine in patients with mild to moderate Alzheimer's disease. *International Journal of Clinical Practice*, **56**, 441–6.

Williams, W. H., Evans, J. J., and Wilson, B. A. (1999). Outcome measures for survivors of acquired brain injury in day and outpatient neurorehabilitation programmes. *Neuropsychological Rehabilitation*, **9**, 421–36.

Wilson, B. A. (1995). Management and remediation of memory problems in brain-injured adults. In *Handbook of memory disorders* (eds. A. D. Baddeley, B. A. Wilson, and F. N. Watts), pp. 451–79. Wiley, Chicester, UK.

Wilson, B. A. (1997). Cognitive rehabilitation: How it is and how it might be. *Journal of the International Neuropsychological Society*, **3**, 487–496.

Wilson, B.A. (2002). Toward a comprehensive model of cognitive rehabilitation. *Neuropsychology Rehabilitation*, **12**, 91–110.

Wilson, B. A., Alderman, N., Burgess, P., Emslie, H., and Evans, J. J. (1996). *The Behavioral Assessment of the Dysexecutive Syndrome*. Thames Valley Test Corporation, Flempton, UK.

Wilson, B. A., Cockburn, J., and Baddeley, A. D. (1985). *The Rivermead Behavioural Memory Test*. Thames Valley Test Corporation, Bury St. Edmunds, UK.

Wilson, B. A., Emslie, H. C., Quirk, K., and Evans, J. J. (2001). Reducing everyday memory and planning problems by means of a paging system: A randomised control crossover study. *Journal of Neurology, Neurosurgery & Psychiatry*, **70**, 477–82.

Wilson, B. A., and Kapur, N. (2008). Memory rehabilitation for people with brain injury. *Cognitive neurorehabilitation: Evidence and application* (2nd ed.) (eds. D. T. Stuss, G. Winocur, and I. H. Robertson), pp. 522–40. Cambridge: London, England.

Wilson, B. A. and Moffat, N. (1992). The development of group memory therapy. In *Clinical management of memory problems* (2nd ed.) (eds. B. A. Wilson and N. Moffat), pp. 243–73. Chapman and Hall, London, UK.

Winocur, G., Moscovitch, M., and Freedman, J. (1987). An investigation of cognitive function in relation to psychosocial variables in institutionalized old people. *Canadian Journal of Psychology*, **41**, 257–269.

Winocur, G., Craik, F. I., Levine, B. Robertson, I. H., Binns, M. A., Alexander, M., Black, S., Dawson, D., Palmer, H., McHugh, T., and Stuss, D. T. (2007a). Cognitive rehabilitation in the elderly: Overview and future directions. *Journal of the International Neuropsychological Society*, **13**, 166–171.

Winocur, G., Palmer, H., Dawson, D., Binns, M. A., Bridges, K., and Stuss, D. T. (2007b). Cognitive rehabilitation in the elderly: An evaluation of psychosocial factors. *Journal of the International Neuropsychological Society*, **13**, 153–65.

Wolinsky, F. D., Unverzagt, F. W., Smith, D. M., Jones, R., Stoddard, A., and Tennstedt, S. L. (2006). The ACTIVE cognitive training trial and health-related quality of life: Protection that lasts for 5 years. *Journals of Gerontology: Series A: Biological Sciences and Medical Sciences*, **61A**, 1324–29.

World Health Organization (2001). *International classification of functioning, disability and health*. Author, Geneva.

Yesavage, J. A., Rose, T. L., and Bower, G. H. (1983). Interactive imagery and affective judgments improve face-name learning in the elderly. *Journal of Gerontology*, **38**, 197–203.

Yesavage, J. A., Sheikh, J. I., Friedman, L., and Tanke, E. (1990). Learning mnemonics: Roles of aging and subtle cognitive impairment. *Psychology and Aging*, **5**, 133–7.

Ylvisaker, M., Adelson, P. D., Brago, L. W., Burnett, S. M., Glang, A., Feeney, T., Moore, W., Rumney, P., and Todis, B. (2005). Rehabilitation and ongoing support after pediatric TBI: Twenty years of progress. *Journal of Head Trauma Rehabilitation*, **20**, 95–109.

Part 3

Neuropsychological impairments

Chapter 5

Assessment of attention

Joke Spikman and Ed van Zomeren

1 Introduction

Attention is a broad concept that has been defined in various ways. In everyday daily language it is often used to mean concentration, which refers to selective looking or listening; effortful processes. Thus, attention has two broad dimensions: *selectivity* and *intensity*. These dimensions are readily visible in the spotlight metaphor: attention can be directed like a spotlight to illuminate a certain object, while the intensity of the light may vary. Attention can be seen as a quality of information-processing; perception, processing, storage, retrieval and use of information are optimal when the system is directed properly and when the required level of intensity is present. Thus, attention can be defined as the state of a processing system that is optimally tuned in terms of selectivity and intensity. The concept of attention is closely related to speed of information processing. As the capacity of the information processing system is too limited to process all available information, selection of relevant information is essential.

It is important to note that despite this definition, attention is not a unitary concept. Our definition already distinguishes two dimensions. When attentional behaviour is described, several additional task-related terms appear (for example, when investigators speak of divided attention or sustained attention). In fact, different taxonomies of attention have been proposed, some of them psychological (Mirsky *et al.* 1991; van Zomeren and Brouwer 1994), and others based on neuroanatomy (Mesulam 1985; Posner and Petersen 1990). The existence of these different approaches inspires two caveats.

- General statements about 'the attention' of a patient should be avoided. The situation (or the task) to a large extent determine which aspects of attention will be essential and whether deficits will become apparent. A patient's attention may be adequate for a social chat, but inadequate for driving a car through dense traffic in rush hour. Thus, statements about the attention of a patient should always be qualified in terms of the specific task and situation.

- The assessment of attention should never be limited to performance on a single task. For example, recording of simple reaction time can tell us something about the basic speed of processing in a particular patient, but tells us little or nothing about his or her ability to react flexibly on a dual task, or to sustain attention over half an hour.

In practice, the clinician will be interested in certain aspects of attention, depending on the type of brain damage involved and the practical questions to be addressed. In the assessment of epileptic patients transient cognitive impairments may be critical, whereas in stroke patients hemi-neglect will be most relevant. In head-injured patients the clinician might want to study speed of information-processing. Practical questions may include fitness to drive (in which divided attention is important), in educational situations (in which sustained attention to a task in a noisy environment is essential). Hence, the selection of attention tests should be made relevant to the patient's neurological diagnosis, and daily life (including occupational risks).

2 Ways of assessing attention

As a mental construct, attention can only be measured indirectly, since, in Section 1, attention can be defined as a quality in the subject's perception, processing, storing, retrieval and use of information. This implies that attention has to be measured through other behaviours (e.g., by studying the efficiency of visual search or the speed of visuo-motor responses). In this sense one could say, 'There are no tests of attention.' The ideal paradigm for studying the attentional component of a particular activity consists of a task with two conditions (and a variation that taps a certain aspect of attention). For example, focused attention can be tested by presenting the same task twice i.e. with and without distraction by irrelevant stimuli. The best known paradigm in this regard is the *Stroop Colour Word Test*, where speed of colour naming is measured twice; the second time under distraction by word meaning. Hence the efficiency of a certain aspect of attention is expressed as a difference between two time scores. Unfortunately, difference scores raise a number of metric and reliability problems, among them decreased reliability. Solutions to such problems differ in their clinical usefulness, but the use of ratio scores seems more fruitful than covariance analyses (Spikman *et al.* 1996; Zoccolotti and Caracciolo 2002).

A second problem is that most available clinical tests tap more than one aspect of attention. A time score obtained in a visual search task may reflect both the speed of processing of visual information, and higher-order aspects of attention such as strategy and flexibility.

A third problem concerns the fact that there is a gap between attention tests and everyday life situations that tap the same attentional aspects. Ideally, assessment of attention should have ecological validity, that is, predictive value for the patient's daily life functioning. This does not necessarily imply that attention tests should look like daily life tasks. Rather, they should require the same cognitive abilities as daily life situations do.

2.1 Observation and rating

The oldest approach to the assessment of attention as a psychological construct is *clinical observation*. Observation has obvious advantages: it does not require any equipment, and it hardly requires extra time, since it is integrated into the natural contact between clinician and patient. During bedside conversation or an apparent social chat on the way to the neuropsychology department, the psychologist may observe whether the patient is alert and attending to the environment and the investigator, or whether there are signs of hemi-neglect or drifting attention (Stuss and Benson 1986). During formal assessment one may note whether patients are distracted by noises from outside, and whether they are attending adequately to tasks that in themselves, are not considered attention tests.

Observation can be standardized by the use of *rating scales*. The Neurobehavioral Rating Scale, devised by Levin *et al.* (1987), contains a few items aimed at attention. The scale has satisfactory inter-judge reliability and validity. A questionnaire that can be filled out by patients and their relatives is the Cognitive Failures Questionnaire (Broadbent *et al.* 1982). A Rating Scale of Attentional Behaviour (RSAB) was developed by Ponsford and Kinsella (1991). This instrument uses 5-point scales to record the frequency of attentional problems in patients. Its validity and usefulness were demonstrated in a rehabilitation institute where professionals (speech therapists and ergotherapists) rated aspects attention in head-injured patients. The RSAB has a high inter-rater reliability (0.91).

2.2 Categorization of attention tests

Any review of attention tests is confronted with an organizational challenge. Although division into focused attention, divided attention, and sustained attention may appear useful, it is actually an unsatisfactory approach. As mentioned above, several taxonomies of attention have been proposed and the choice of a particular one for the organization of assessment methods is always arbitrary. Also, there is evidence from statistical studies that shows that concepts that seem quite useful for the description of behaviour (such as divided attention or sustained attention), are not necessarily supported by the evidence from factor analyses of large series of subjects tested on attention tests. Spikman *et al.* (2001) studied the construct validity of well known attentional concepts, listing several statistical studies that showed little agreement on useful factors. It appeared that each investigation produced new factors and hence new constructs. Still, two main factors were noted to appear, albeit under various names, in most of the statistical studies:

- speed or processing capacity;
- control or working memory.

Thus, a distinction on an empirical statistical basis is available. In our own experience, this is quite helpful for the analysis of attention problems in head-injured subjects (Spikman *et al.* 2001). However, it also seems useful for the practical categorization of attention tests. The two concepts of speed and control are not completely independent: control processes occur at a certain speed and these processes may slow down in cases of brain damage. Moreover, changes in processing speed may affect control: when speed of processing increases or decreases, this will bring changes in the amount and nature of control required.

The relative weights of speed and control can vary from task to task. This is partly due to *task characteristics* or task demands. Some tasks are experienced as easy and proceeding almost 'on their own' once they have been started. For example, finger tapping performance is an easy, repetitive motor task requiring very little control—the only control required is to monitor one's tapping speed. On the other hand, writing a letter of application requires intensive control, although speed is rarely essential. Generally speaking, control requirements are maximal in unstructured tasks that cannot be tackled using routine responses. Control invariably implies working memory activity, in which rules for the performance of the task need to be kept activated. A second task characteristic is the time pressure involved.

Another source of variation is *subject characteristics*, in particular, learning effects. In general, the amount of control required decreases as a function of task learning. In fact, many well-trained tasks require so little control that we consider them to be automatized and not requiring much effort. Learning to drive is a good example of a task consisting of many subtasks which require control and a great deal of effort (in the first lessons), but which becomes highly automatized in the experienced driver. A second important characteristic is speed/accuracy trade-off.

Thus, the distinction between speed and control is related to the distinction between time pressure and structure. This allows us to look at attention tests on three levels: the operational level, the tactical level and the strategic level.

2.2.1 Operational level

At this level speed is the main factor, while control is minimal. Time pressure is high as patients are either instructed to work as quickly as possible, or are presented with stimuli at a high rate. On the other hand, the task presented to the subject is highly structured, signals and responses are simple and unambiguous, and through instruction the subject knows exactly what to do. Attention can be tested at a basic level, here with time being the essential dependent variable. At this level, the subject can do little other than 'pay attention and try to be quick'. Performance on these basic tasks may be called stimulus-driven (see Table 5.1). Because the task stimuli direct subjects on what to do the working memory load is minimized.

2.2.2 Tactical level

At this level, both time pressure and structure are intermediate. Tasks are more complicated and being fast is no longer sufficient for optimal performance. A certain amount of control is required, because the stimuli are often ambiguous, but the operation to be performed on them is specified in the instructions. For example, subjects are instructed to ignore distracting stimuli, or to divide their attention while reacting to two kinds of symbols. At this level, subjects have to find a personal speed/accuracy trade-off (i.e. a balance between working speed and error rate). Performance on this level can be considered

Table 5.1 Characteristics of the three levels of attention tests

Level	Time pressure	Structure of task
Operational	High	Highly structured, stimulus-driven
Tactical	Intermediate	Partially structured, memory-driven
Strategic	Low	Unstructured, strategy-driven

memory-driven, since instructions and rules for performance must be kept activated in working memory.

2.2.3 Strategic level

At this level, time pressure is minimal but subjects have to find their own approach for an optimal performance of the task. Hence, instructions do not dictate completely what should be done and, in this sense, these tests of attention offer less structure than tests that are aimed at the operational and tactical levels. Basically, the subject has to apply his or her own strategy (i.e. performance is strategy-driven).

3 The operational level: speed of information-processing

At this level time scores are essential although errors do not assume any importance. An example would be the recording of simple reaction times in response to either visual or auditory stimuli. Neurological patients may be slow on this task, but the signals are clear and the responses are so simple that errors are extremely rare and thus not useful as assessment. What one tries to assess at this level is the basic speed of information-processing.

3.1 Assessing mental slowness

Reaction time recordings (as they feature in many computerized test batteries), are an excellent method of assessing basic mental speed. However, it is important that the task permits total reaction time to be split into decision and movement components, in order to disentangle the confounding effects of peripheral slowness on central slowness. The test forms S1-S5 of the *Reaction Test* in the Vienna Test System allow for this possibility (Schufried, 2006). Reliabilities (Cronbach's Alpha) for these tests vary between .83, and .98 for the reaction times, and between .84 and .95 for the motor times. Apart from reaction times, the clinician may use the basic conditions of well known clinical tools such as *Trailmaking A*, and word reading and colour naming of the *Stroop Colour Word Test*. Test–retest reliability is satisfactory for both tests, ranging from 0.70 to 0.90 for *Trailmaking A*, and from 0.83 to 0.91 for reading and colour naming in the Stroop test (Spreen and Strauss 1991). Also, the subtest *Digit Symbol* from the Wechsler Adult Intelligence Scale (WAIS)-R can be used for the assessment of mental speed.

As noted in Section 1, no attention test ever taps one aspect of attention only. This will be clear from the tests mentioned above: many of them require some visuo-motor skill. A second important point is that the assessment of speed of processing requires finely graded norms. In particular, age is an important factor. Generally speaking, processing speed decreases with increasing age. For some tasks, gender is also important. For example, men react slightly faster than women to simple signals. Thus, the clinician should take age and sex into account when testing attention in the basic sense of speed of processing.

Theoretically, the question of *domain-specific slowness* can be raised. In the clinical literature, mental slowness is usually discussed as a global phenomenon that manifests itself in all task domains and all sensory modalities. In practice, this simplification seems justified. In case of diffuse injury to the brain or of (more or less) diffuse degenerative processes such as Alzheimer's disease, the slowness indeed manifests itself in all aspects of behaviour. Even in the case of focal damage such as that caused by stroke or neoplasm, a general mental slowness is often noted and confirmed on subsequent testing. However, it is conceivable that a focal lesion may disrupt or slow down specific processes only, (e.g. the manipulation of verbal information in the case of left hemisphere damage in right-handed subjects).

4 The tactical level: focused and divided attention

In tests at this level, subjects are still expected to work as quickly as possible, but more control is required in order to prevent errors. A good example would be *Trailmaking B*. While in *Trailmaking A* the instruction is rather straightforward—to connect numbered circles by a pencil line—in *Trailmaking B* a certain load is placed on working memory in which two sequences have to be kept active, i.e. the alphabet and the numbers from 1 to 13. As the correct response depends on keeping track in both sequences and using them alternately, there is ample opportunity for making errors. As far as visuo-motor behaviour is required, *Trailmaking B* is roughly comparable to *Trailmaking A*. Hence, the fact that healthy subjects need more than twice the time required for A when doing B reflects the far greater amount of control involved in the latter condition of the test.

On the tactical level, the distinction between tests of *focused* and *divided* attention is useful.

♦ The concept of focused attention can be applied whenever the subject has to respond selectively, i.e. when irrelevant stimuli are present;

♦ The concept of divided attention refers to task situations in which there are more subtasks that have to be performed simultaneously or that require more than one type of response.

In the 1990s, two batteries of attention tests were presented that assess attention mainly at the tactical level. Both of them can be seen as attempts to approach assessment with a firm theoretical basis and well-defined concepts and both of them originated in Europe. Zimmerman and Fimm (1993) devised the *Test for Attentional Performance* (TAP), a computerized battery with unusual psychometric qualities. While each subtest was based on the relevant theoretical literature, the authors have made an effort to make the tasks feasible in a clinical setting, in terms of ease of administration, standardization of instructions, and solid normative data. Among its subtests are tests of Divided Attention, a Go/No go task and Visual Scanning. The psychometric characteristics of the TAP are discussed extensively by Zimmermann and Fimm (2002).

A second useful battery of attention tests was presented in 1994 by Robertson *et al.* The *Test of Everyday Attention* (TEA) is marked by its attempt to demonstrate ecological validity. Like the TAP, the TEA attempts to assess attention from a sound theoretical background, but its outward appearance is quite different. While the TAP is computerized, the TEA requires minimal instrumentation as its visual tasks are paper-and-pencil while the acoustic tasks require a tape recorder for presentation. Ecological validity is created by choosing tasks that closely resemble daily life situations. The validity of the TEA has been studied in cerebrovascular accident (CVA) and head-injured patients and can be judged as satisfactory. The reliability of all subtests is good, with the exception of Telephone Search while Counting.

4.1 Assessing focused attention

When irrelevant stimuli can act as distractors, subjects have to focus on the relevant ones. Visual search tasks are attention tests that require some selectivity, as all stimuli are irrelevant except the ones designated as targets. In *Trailmaking A*, all numbered circles are to be regarded as 'noise' except the number that the subject is searching for. An important distinction should be made between structured and unstructured fields of search. Visual search tasks with a structured field are easier, i.e. require less control, than tests with an unstructured field. For example, some letter cancellation tasks present letters in horizontal lines, and the *d-2 test* (Brickenkamp 1981) also presents its stimuli in convenient lines. In contrast, some visual search tasks present quasirandom fields, thus forcing the subjects to scan the field according to their own insight. *Trailmaking* is a good example, but tests for the detection of hemi-neglect also make use of unstructured fields (e.g., the *Bells test*, Gauthier *et al.* 1989). The *Test of Everyday Attention* (Robertson *et al.* 1994) contains two visual search tasks assessing focused attention with ecological validity and satisfactory reliability—Map Search and Telephone Search. In the first of these subtests, the subject is required to search for gas stations or restaurants on a real map; in the second the subject has to find certain items in a telephone directory.

Many visual search tasks allow the clinician to consider the speed/accuracy trade-off in patients, by studying number of errors in relation to speed. For example, in our own laboratory we found that severely head-injured patients were working slowly but accurately on *the Bourdon dot configuration test* (van Zomeren and Brouwer 1994).

In most visual search tasks, all distractors are present simultaneously. A classic test of focused attention, the *Continuous Performance Test*, presents distractors successively in time, while the subject is on the look-out for the target letter A. This test also has a condition requiring slightly more control by working memory—in the XA condition, the letter A is a target only when it is preceded by an X.

The S3 and S4 test forms in the *Reaction Test* of the Vienna Test System (Schuhfried, 2006) can also be considered to be tasks measuring focused attention because the subject must only react to a specific stimulus combination and inhibit responses to irrelevant stimulus configurations.

Distractors differ greatly in their distracting power. In the case of visual search, it is usually quite easy to search for a target while processing all other stimuli very superficially only. A good example of a strong distractor is found in the classic *Stroop* paradigm, where stimuli have two features: a colour and a word meaning that conflicts with the colour. As reading is highly automatized, the instruction to focus on the colours of the words creates a strong response interference that is measured in a slowing of performance, compared to that in simple colour naming. For this interference subtask of the Stroop, reliability coefficients of 0.89 and 0.91 have been reported (Spreen and Strauss 1991).

4.2 Assessing divided attention

The classic paradigm to test divided attention is a dual task, in which a subject is instructed to perform two or more tasks simultaneously. In some tests this involves mainly switching between two or more response tracks or modalities, thus requiring flexibility, in others this involves the combination of several activities under time pressure in order to produce the correct response. The complexity of such tasks may vary greatly, depending on the amount of control required in each subtask. Park *et al.* (1999) demonstrated that divided attention is impaired in head-injured subjects when the tasks require controlled processing, but not when the tasks can be carried out relatively automatically. Unfortunately, the dual-task paradigm has hardly been used in clinical assessment. The *Test of Everyday Attention* (TEA, Robertson *et al.* 1994) contains the subtest Telephone Search while Counting, in which subjects have to find items in a telephone directory while at the same time counting the number of tones in a tape-recorded series. Unfortunately, reliability of the dual-task decrement effect was not high; satisfactory in two groups of non-brain-damaged subjects (0.59 and 0.61) but somewhat lower in a group of patients with cerebrovascular accidents (0.40).

A typical example of a task requiring switching between two response modes is the *Trailmaking B*, in which the subject has to keep track both of the numbers as well as the letters while alternating between them. Correction for the confounding effect of visuo-motor slowness is allowed by using the B:A ratio; several authors (Mitrushina, 2005) found a ratio score greater than 3 reflecting deficient performance on part B indicating a problem with alternating switches.

The *Determination Test* (DT) of the Vienna Test System (Schuhfried, 2006) requires the division of attention between different stimulus modalities, namely visual and acoustic, as well as between different response possibilities, namely pressing a hand button or a foot pedal. It was found that the test discriminated between groups of neurological and psychiatric patients and a group of healthy controls.

A well known instrument is the *Paced Auditory Serial Addition Task* (PASAT; Gronwall and Sampson 1974). This presents series of 61 digits to the subject, with the instruction to add the last digit to the preceding one, giving the answer aloud. This task can be seen as a divided attention task, as subjects are dividing their processing capacity over several activities: listening, adding, answering, and keeping track in their working memory. However, the smaller the inter-stimulus interval (ISI), the more these subtasks will overlap in time and consequently, the more the ability to divide attention is required. Several studies have demonstrated the validity of PASAT (i.e. sensitivity to the effects of head injury, and factor analytic evidence of loading on an attention/concentration factor). Gronwall and Sampson claimed that performance on PASAT was not related to arithmetic ability (or general intelligence), but this claim has been challenged. As Zoccolotti and Caracciolo (2002) put it: 'The overall picture seems to reveal a mild to moderate link between general intellectual abilities and performance on the PASAT. Clinicians should consider this finding and further research might allow for a possible adjustment of normative data based on the general intelligence g factor.'

5 The strategic level: supervisory control

Testing attention on the strategic level meets with a paradox: strategy can be deployed only in an unstructured situation, but a test requires standardization and hence structure. As a result of this paradox, it is hard to find paradigms that truly assess the higher aspects of attention, i.e. supervisory attentional control. Still, there are a few instruments that can be recommended.

5.1 Assessing supervisory control

The oldest of these is the *Wisconsin Card Sorting Test* (Lezak 1995). In this task, the subject has to change his or her response set on the basis of feedback by the experimenter. That is, while sorting cards according to a principle originally chosen by the subject (e.g. colour of symbols on the cards), from a certain point in the process the experimenter no longer confirms the sortings, now indicating that the subject is sorting cards on the wrong pile. Thus, the subject has to find a new principle (e.g. number of symbols on the cards). This shifting can be seen as requiring higher order flexibility, which links it to attention on the strategic level. There exists an extensive literature on the validity of the WCST and its revised versions. While originally it was believed that the WCST was especially sensitive to frontal brain damage, this view has been criticized with good arguments.

Shallice (1988) devised the *Tower of London test*. This test, derived from an oriental puzzle game, is closely connected to the theoretical model of the Supervisory Attentional System as proposed by the same author. Three coloured beads (red, blue, and yellow) have to be arranged on three sticks of increasing length, in order to reach a certain pattern in a prescribed number of moves. There are restrictions in the handling of the beads, e.g. one may handle only one of them at a given time, and they may not be put down on the table. The solving of each puzzle item requires some thinking ahead and practically always a certain bead has to be placed temporarily on a stick that is not its final destination. Thus, subjects have to plan their moves and to suppress impulsive 'solutions', and in this regard it might tap supervisory attentional control. Unfortunately, normative data are lacking and both validity and reliability are unknown.

Thirdly, located within a battery called the *Behavioural Assessment of the Dysexecutive Syndrome* (BADS; Wilson *et al.* 1996), there is an interesting task called the *Six Elements Test*. In this task, subjects are given 10 minutes to perform six tasks. They are expected to use this limited time wisely and to respect certain shifting rules. For example, the six tasks fall in three categories but the subject is not allowed to shift from task A to B within the same category. The Six Elements Test is largely unstructured, as it does not tell the subject how to divide the available time over the different tasks. Hence, it offers good opportunity to observe the subject's strategy. In particular, the test has a strong ecological appeal as it enables us to judge whether the subject is paying attention to passing time—there is a little clock on the desk counting down the minutes and seconds.

Finally, the BADS also contains the *Zoo Test*, in which subjects have to visit a number of sites in a certain order, while respecting certain rules. Finding the correct route requires planning and overview in a fairly complex situation, and thus the task taps aspects of supervisory control.

5.2 Testing the strategic level in daily life

Still, these four tests are far removed from essential attentional strategies in daily life. What one would like to test is the subject's ability to attend to highly relevant but unpredictable cues in an unstructured situation. For example, attention for nonverbal cues in the social domain is essential for the maintaining of smooth relationships, both in private life and in professional situations. However, it is hardly possible to devise standardized situations that deserve the name of 'test' and that will yield objective and quantified information on these higher aspects of attention. Spikman *et al.* (2000) attempted to assess executive functioning in head-injured patients in a chronic stage (2–5 years after injury) by observing them when they were trying to find their way through the University Hospital in Groningen. It was recorded how these subjects used available information (signs) and searched for additional information by addressing passers-by and hospital staff. Spikman *et al.* found that their head-injured subjects, were less efficient in the search for and use of information, and needed more cues to carry on with the task. Within this group, patients with frontal lesions (detected by neuroimaging) had poorer performance. With respect to the *Executive Route Finding Task* (Boyd and Sautter 1993) which assesses 'attention for sources of additional information', it may be viewed as a test of attention on the strategic level.

Recently, Spikman and colleagues developed a new, ecologically valid test, called the *Executive Secretariat Task* (EST), measuring higher order control in a daily life situation. In this three-hour task, a job assessment procedure is simulated. The subject is left alone in a room with a box in which a series of simple secretarial assignments, which have to be organized and executed, some with a deadline. No cues are provided about how to carry out the assignments, but necessary materials and information are all available, and at fixed times, the 'manager', sitting in the room next door, can be asked questions. During the assessment, the subject is interrupted with an urgent new assignment. It was found that this test was sensitive to executive dysfunctioning in TBI as well as stroke patients (Spikman *et al.* 2007).

6 Sustained attention and sustained control

The term 'sustained attention' refers to assessment on a longer timescale than usual, covering intervals from 10 to 30 minutes. A distinction should be made between high event-rate tasks and low event-rate tasks. In the former subjects are kept quite busy, in the latter they are exposed to a boring situation and their main task is to maintain an adequate level of alertness in order to detect rare and subtle stimuli. The former type of task is called a *continuous performance test*; the latter type a *vigilance test*.

Unfortunately, in clinical practice it is often concluded that 'sustained attention is poor' when a patient is performing below standard, for whatever reason, on a lengthy test. In most cases, this will be unjustified. Even when patients are reacting slowly on a continuous reaction time (RT) task or missing many signals in a vigilance task, it may well be that they are sustaining their 'poor' attention quite well. Conclusions about sustained attention should be based on time-on-task effects (TOTs). These are changes in performance over time, and sustained attention may be considered insufficient when a patient shows an abnormal TOT, i.e. abnormally increasing response times or an abnormal increase of missed signals or errors. To detect such deterioration, the duration of the test should be divided in blocks (e.g. of 5 minutes each).

The demands of a sustained attention test depend on whether the task is self-paced or experimenter-paced. In other words, who determines the time pressure? If one uses a prolonged visual search task such as the *Bourdon dot configuration test* (lasting 12 to 15 minutes) subjects choose their own speed of working. Many well known tests, however, are experimenter-paced (e.g. the *Continuous Performance Test*). The essential difference, of course, is that time pressure cannot be influenced by the subjects in experimenter-paced tasks.

Another important feature of sustained attention tests is the amount of control required. In our experience, brain-damaged subjects can usually deal with prolonged tasks if these are self-paced and require little control (see Fig. 5.1). On the other hand, head-injured patients very frequently complain of increased mental fatigue, indicating that they cannot concentrate long on daily-life tasks that require some mental effort. This suggests that

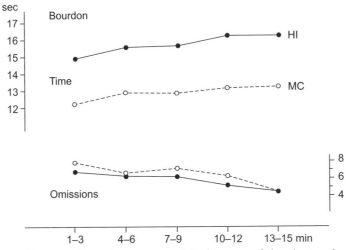

Fig. 5.1 A case of low speed but adequate control. Performance of chronic stage head-injured patients (HI), and matched controls (MC) on a visual search task (Bourdon) lasting 15 minutes. In this self-paced task, subjects have to search for groups of four dots, in lines that contain 25 groups of three, four, and five dots. Patients need about 3 seconds more per line than control subjects, but at this working speed their accuracy is normal; their response curves are strikingly similar and no special time-on-task effects are visible in the head-injured group.

prolonged control is the key feature in the question of sustained attention in subjects with brain lesions.

6.1 Tests assessing sustained attention

The classical test for the assessment of sustained attention is the *Continuous Performance Test* (Rosvold *et al.* 1956) in which subjects have to react to the target letter A in a long random series of letters. The TAP battery (Zimmermann and Fimm 1993, 2002) contains a useful *Vigilance Test* in an auditory and a visual format, with adequate norms. The Test of Everyday Attention (Robertson *et al.* 1994) contains subtests that can be conceived as tests for sustained attention. The first of these is *Lottery*, in which subjects have to listen for their 'winning number' that ends in '55'. They are presented with a 10-minute tape recorded list of numbers such as BC 143 and LD 967, and their task is to write down the two letters preceding all 10 target numbers. The other subtest is *Elevator Counting*, which has an unusually short timescale, and which operationalises the concept in a highly specific way via counting strings of audio taped tones. The tasks have an interesting link with neuroanatomy (i.e. the right frontal lobe). Both subtests have a satisfactory validity and reliability.

The TAP contains sustained-attention related paradigms such as Alertness and Vigilance. In the subtest Alertness, the difference between reaction times with and without warning signal is calculated. The subtest Vigilance presents a classic vigilance task (i.e. a quite boring situation in which the subject is required to watch a monotonously moving line for 15 or 30 minutes, and to push a button whenever an irregularity in this movement occurs).

Robertson and Manly (1997) devised a paradigm that is not yet available as a formal test, but might turn out to be quite useful—the *Sustained Attention for Response Test* or SART. This offers a high-event-rate situation, in which subjects have to react continuously to a random series of digits (0 to 9) appearing on a screen. Only the digit 3 is a non-target, i.e. a response to any 3 should be suppressed. As the digits come at a high rate, approximately one per second, the responding quickly gets automatised, with the result that subjects are lured into reacting to the non-target 3 ('Oops!'). Robertson and Manly demonstrated that their paradigm has some validity in the study of head-injured subjects: these patients do not sustain their control as well as healthy subjects.

7 Hemi-inattention

Hemi-neglect or hemi-inattention differs from other impairments of attention by its basic nature: it is a disturbance in a preconscious aspect, i.e. our normally symmetrical orientation with respect to the outside world. This biological prerequisite is realized by a cortico–limbic–reticular loop and thus it can be disturbed by lesions at different anatomical levels (Mesulam 1985). Hemi-inattention, or neglect of one-half of the outer world, can manifest itself in all sensory domains and also in the motor domain. Clinically most important, however, is visual-spatial hemi-inattention. This is seen most frequently after lesions in the right hemisphere, in which case patients fail to attend to the left side of space and/or their body and this failure cannot be explained by primary sensory or motor deficits.

7.1 Assessing hemi-inattention

The first method of assessment is *observation*. A patient may bump into furniture on the left side or against the left doorpost. During testing, it can happen that the patient overlooks the first words or coloured stimuli in the Stroop Colour Words Test.

7.1.1 Line bisecting and drawing

For formal testing of neglect a large array of tests is available (Lezak 1995). A classic method of assessment of neglect is *line bisecting*, in which subjects have to mark the centre point of a horizontal line by placing an X on it (Marshall and Halligan 1990). Patients with left-sided neglect tend to deviate to the right pole of the lines, as they are not aware of the left half of these lines. Another paper-and-pencil approach of neglect is *drawing*: patients will often leave their drawings of a clock, star, or flower incomplete on the left side (Halligan and Marshall 1997). For obvious reasons, objects that are more or less symmetrical are most suitable for the judgment of hemi-inattention.

7.1.2 Visual search tasks

Next, neglect can be assessed with *visual search tasks* with either structured or unstructured fields. Structured fields consist of lines of stimuli as in some Letter Cancellation Tests, while unstructured fields present quasi-random arrays of stimuli such as the Star Cancellation Test or the Bells Test. In the latter, target stimuli are in fact grouped into seven columns and a ratio for neglect can be calculated based on numbers of omissions in 3 columns on the left versus 3 on the right side (Vanier *et al.* 1990).

7.1.3 Reading tests

Visual neglect can also be assessed with reading tests, in which words on the far left are neglected by the subject. A special case is the *Indented Paragraph Reading Test* (Caplan 1987) in which the first word of each line is indented from 0 to 25 spaces. This lay-out precludes the possibility that the neglecting subject could form a compensatory 'spatial set', as each refixation from the end of one line to the beginning of the next requires a separate act of controlled scanning.

7.1.4 Tests measuring lateral bias and extinction

The *Grey Scales task* (Mattingley *et al.* 1994) was designed to assess the early automatic orienting of attention towards the ipsilesional side of space. The Grey scale is a semi-continuous horizontal scale of different grey shades varying between black and white. The subject is presented with sheets of paper with two vertically aligned rectangular grey scales of equal length, whereby the pairs are the mirror reverse of each other. The subject is asked to judge which of the two appears overall darker; the upper or the lower scale. Test performance can be qualified in terms of a rightward or leftward bias. Tant *et al.* (2002) found that this test was specifically sensitive in detecting hemi-neglect.

The *Test of Attentional Performance* (Zimmermann and Fimm 2001) contains a subtest in which 3-digits numbers are presented that are distributed randomly over the screen of a personal computer. Among these, there are target numbers that seem to flicker, as their value is changing at a high rate. Subjects have to react to these apparently moving targets. As neglect patients attend predominantly to the non-target stimuli in the ipsilesional visual field, they miss the critical stimuli on the left half of the screen due to extinction.

7.1.5 The Behavioural Inattention Test

For those who want to study neglect extensively, Wilson *et al.* (1987) developed an attractive battery called the *Behavioural Inattention Test*. This test is composed partly of traditional hemi-neglect tests such as letter cancellation and line bisection, but it also contains tasks with a clear ecological validity, such as telephone dialing, coin sorting, and map navigation. For the set of conventional subtests, reliability is satisfactory ($r = 0.75$) while for the behavioural set it is excellent (test–retest $r = 0.97$).

8 Cognitive rehabilitation of attention

A more detailed review of the cognitive rehabilitation of attention is provided in Chapter 6. However, a few remarks can be made. First, the clinical neuropsychologist can advise his patients on how to cope with their attentional limitations (i.e. coach them in the 'management of slowness', Spikman 2001). This boils down to supplying general *guidelines* that will be useful in various daily life tasks and situations. In Section 2.2 it was argued that the attentional demands of a given task situation are determined by two task characteristics: time pressure and structure. Thus, several guidelines can be formulated to reduce time pressure and improve the structure of tasks.

- Avoid or reduce time pressure.
- Create structure.
- Keep subtasks separate when possible.
- Avoid interruptions.
- Determine priorities in advance.

Strategies

This approach has been formalized and validated by Fasotti *et al.* (2000) who devised a training called *Time Pressure Management* (TPM). This compensatory strategy training TPM teaches patients how to deal with their slowness. It consists of a general self-instruction ('Let me give myself enough time to do the task') followed by four specific steps in the form of questions the patient has to ask himself. These steps are as follows.

1. Anticipate time pressure by analysing stages in the task where two or more things have to be done at the same time.

2. Make a plan for things that can be done before the actual task begins.

3. Make an emergency plan to deal as quickly and effectively as possible with overwhelming time pressure.

4. Make regular use of the anticipatory plan and the emergency plan.

Fasotti *et al.* demonstrated that head-injured patients could learn this strategy and apply it to a new task, which consisted of reproducing the relevant information of a videotaped short story.

As described in Section 2.2, performance on a task is also determined by subject characteristics, in particular learning and *experience*. The history of attention training has shown that 'attention in general' cannot be trained by stimulation or repetition. Time and again, it was found that training effects do not, or do not sufficiently, generalize to attention-demanding tasks in daily life. In contrast, task-specific training can be effective: it is possible to teach subjects to attend to relevant aspects within a given daily life task, even when this effect does not generalize. Hence, for the cognitive rehabilitation of attention, two options seem to exist: strategy training or task-specific training (cf. Fasotti and Spikman 2002).

Selective references

Brickenkamp, R. (1981). *Test d-2, Aufmerksamkeits-Belastungstest*. Hogrefe Verlag, Göttingen.

Broadbent, D.E., Cooper, P.F., FitzGerald, P., and Parkes, K.R. (1982). The Cognitive Failures Questionnaire (CFQ) and its correlates. *Br. J. Clin. Psychol.* **21**, 1–16.

Caplan, B. (1987). Assessment of unilateral neglect: a new reading test. *J. Clin. Exp. Neuropsychol.* **9**, 359–64.

Fasotti, L., Kovacs, F., Eling, P.A.T.M., and Brouwer, W.H. (2000). Time pressure management as a compensatory strategy training after closed head injury. *Neuropsychol. Rehabil.* **10**, 47–65.

Fasotti, L. and Spikman, J.M. (2002). Cognitive rehabilitation of central executive disorders. In *Neuropsychological rehabilitation: a cognitive approach* (ed. W.H. Brouwer, A.H. van Zomeren, I.J. Berg, J.M. Bouma, and E.H.F. de Haan), pp. 107–23. Boom, Amsterdam.

Gauthier, L., Dehaut, F., and Joannette, Y. (1989). The Bells Test: a quantitative and qualitative test for visual neglect. *Int. J. Clin. Psychol.* **11**, 49–54.

Gronwall, D. and Sampson, H. (1974). *The psychological effects of concussion*. Auckland University Press, Auckland.

Halligan, P.W. and Marshall, J.C. (1997). The art of visual neglect. *Lancet* **350**, 139–40.

Levin, H.S., High, W.M., and Goethe, K.E. (1987). The neurobehavioral rating scale: assessment of the behavioral sequelae of head injury by the clinician. *J. Neurol., Neurosurg., Psychiatry* **50**, 183–93.

Lezak, M.D. (1995). *Neuropsychological assessment*. Oxford University Press, New York.

Marshall, J.C. and Halligan, P.W. (1990). Live bisection in a case of visual neglect: Psychophysical studies with implications for theory. *Cognitive Neuropsychology* **7**, 107–30.

Mattingley, J.B., Bradshaw, J.L., Bradshaw, J.A., and Nettleton, N.C. (1994). Residual rightward attentional bias after apparent recovery from right hemisphere damage: implications for a multicomponent model of neglect. *J. Neurol., Neurosurg., Psychiatry* **57**, 597–604.

Mesulam, M.M. (1985). *Principles of behavioral neurology*. Davis, Philadelphia.

Mirsky, A.F., Anthony, B.J., Duncan, C.C., Ahearn, M.B., and Kellam, S.G. (1991). Analysis of the elements of attention: a neuropsychological approach. *Neuropsychol. Rev.* **2**, 109–45.

Mitrushina, M., Boone, K.B., Razani, J., and D'Elia, L.F. (2005). *Handbook of normative data for neuropsychological assessment*. Oxford University Press, Oxford.

Park, N.W., Moscovitch, M., and Robertson, I.H. (1999). Divided attention impairments after traumatic brain injury. *Neuropsychologia* **37**, 1119–33.

Ponsford, J. and Kinsella, G. (1991). The use of a rating scale of attentional behaviour. *Neuropsychol. Rehabil.* **1**, 241–57.

Posner, M.I. and Petersen, S.E. (1990). The attention system of the human brain. *Ann. Rev. Neurosci.* **13**, 182–96.

Robertson, I.H. and Manly, T. (1997). *Oops! The Sustained Attention for Response Test, SART.* *Neuropsychologia*, **35**, 747–58.

Robertson, I.H., Ward, T., Ridgeway, V., and Nimmo-Smith, I. (1994). *The Test of Everyday Attention.* Thames Valley Test Company, Bury St. Edmunds.

Rosvold, H.E., Mirsky, A.F., Sarason, I., Bransome, E.D., and Beck, L.H. (1956). A continuous performance test of brain damage. *J. Consult. Psychol.* **20**, 343–50.

Schuhfried, G. (2006). *The Vienna Test System. Reaction Test and Determination Test.* Available at: http://www.schuhfried.at

Shallice, T. (1988). *From neuropsychology to mental structure.* Cambridge University Press, Cambridge.

Spikman, J.M. (2001). *Attention, mental speed and executive control after closed head injury: deficits, recovery and outcome.* Doctoral thesis, University of Groningen.

Spikman, J.M., van Zomeren, A.H., and Deelman, B.G. (1996). Deficits of attention after closed head injury: slowness only? *J. Clin. Exp. Neuropsychol.* **18**, 755–767.

Spikman, J.M., Deelman, B.G., and van Zomeren, A.H. (2000). Executive functioning, attention and frontal lesions in patients with chronic CHI. *J. Clin. Exp. Neuropsychol.* **22**, 325–38.

Spikman, J.M., Kiers, H.A.L., Deelman, B.G. and Van Zomeren, A.H. (2001). Construct validity of concepts of attention in healthy controls and closed head injured patients. *Brain and Cognition* **47**, 446–60.

Spikman, J.M., Hol-Steegstra, A.,Rietberg, H., Vos, S., Boelen, D., and Lamberts, K.F. (2007). The executive secretariat task (EST); a real-life, ecologically valid measurement of executive functioning. *Brain Impairment*, **8**, 223.

Spreen, O. and Strauss, E. (1991). *A compendium of neuropsychological tests.* Oxford University Press, New York.

Stuss, D.T. and Benson, D.F. (1986). *The frontal lobes.* Raven Press, New York.

Tant, M.L., Kuks, J.B., Kooijman, A.C., Cornelissen, F.W., and Brouwer, W.H. (2002). Grey scales uncover similar attentional effects in homonymous hemianopia and visual hemi-neglect. *Neuropsychologi*, **40**, 1474–1481.

Vanier, M., Gauthier, L., and Lambert, J. (1990). Evaluation of left visuospatial neglect: norms and discrimination power of two tests. *Neuropsychology* **4**, 87–96.

Wilson, B.A., Cockburn, J., and Halligan, P. (1987). *Behavioural Inattention Test.* Thames Valley Test Company, Titchfield.

Wilson, B.A., Alderman, N., Burgess, P.W., Emslie, H., and Evans, J.J. (1996). *BADS—Behavioural Assessment of the Dysexecutive Syndrome.* Thames Valley Test Company, Bury St. Edmunds.

van Zomeren, A.H. (1981). *Reaction time and attention after closed head injury.* Doctoral dissertation, University of Groningen.

van Zomeren, A.H. and Brouwer, W.H. (1994). *Clinical neuropsychology of attention.* Oxford University Press, New York.

Zimmermann, P. and Fimm, B. (1993). *Testbatterie zür Erfassung von Aufmerksamkeitsstörungen,* Version 1.02. Psytest, Freiburg.

Zimmermann, P. and Fimm, B. (2002). A test battery for attentional performance. In *Applied neuropsychology of attention* (ed. M. Leclercq and P. Zimmermann), pp. 110–51. Psychology Press, London.

Zoccolotti P. and Caracciolo B. (2002). Psychometric characteristics of attention tests in neuropsychological practice. In *Applied neuropsychology of attention* (ed. M. Leclercq and P. Zimmermann), pp. 152–85. *Psychology Press*, London.

Chapter 6

The rehabilitation of attention

Tom Manly, Jessica Fish, and Ian H. Robertson

1 Overview

In recent years there have been considerable developments in how we understand attention. Of most relevance to the clinical field is the view that attention is not a single entity
but rather a fractionated set of brain processes that are vulnerable to selective damage.
With a clearer idea of what we are looking at, the role of attention in influencing clinical
outcome is becoming increasingly apparent - both as a function in its own right and as
essential adjunct to the useful expression of other abilities.

As we will discuss, attention and other 'central' functions cannot be observed directly.
The scientific inferential techniques of neuropsychology and clinical neuropsychology
are essential in determining how these processes operate (and break down) and in developing specific assessments. The contribution of a particular impairment to difficulties
faced by patients in daily life is not always clear. In the rehabilitation of attention, as with
any deficit, a broader psychological perspective that takes into account co-existing impairment, pre-morbid factors and the psychosocial context of a patient is vital. Pharmacological
interventions for attentional disorders, at least for adults with neurological damage, are at
a relatively early stage (cf. Warden *et al.*, 2006). Although very useful developments may
take place in this respect, the role of the neuropsychologist in careful assessment and
targeted rehabilitation is likely to remain crucial in fostering positive outcomes.

Here we examine various attempts to enhance the natural recovery of attentional processes, or to better manage the consequences of impairment, following brain injury
acquired in adulthood. The results we review give grounds for cautious optimism.
However, rehabilitation is about working with patients to achieve functional goals in
everyday life. If the promising findings showing changes on neuropsychological tests are
to usefully filter through to clinical care, the extent to which these translate into meaningful functional improvements must be evaluated.

2 Contemporary views of attention

Improvements in quantification often trigger theoretical advances. In the case of
attention, such quantification is inherently difficult. We cannot measure what happens
when people attend in the abstract, so we must give them an activity to perform (read a
passage, press a button, name colours and so forth). Variations in all the other abilities
necessary for this task may well be just as influential as our 'hidden' attention system in

determining performance. One way around this problem, and one that has probably underpinned much of the resurgence in scientific interest in attention over the past few decades, is to infer 'its' presence from the systematic variation in performance under different attentional conditions. A simple and highly influential example of this approach can be found in visual cueing paradigms. Here participants are asked to keep their gaze fixated at the centre of a screen and to press a button as soon as they see a target appear. Whilst for the most part they will have no idea where this will be (and therefore should ideally monitor the whole screen), on a few trials they receive a helpful cue as to the most probable location. Such cues, when accurate, result in significant reductions in reaction times and, when inaccurate, in significant increases. As all other aspects of the task remain constant, these differences can be attributed to the participants prioritising signals from one location - in other words - the movement of spatial attention (Posner, 1980). A similar approach focusing on decrement and enhancement underpins many other areas such as the effect of distraction, the effect of time, and the consequences of attempting to perform two tasks simultaneously.

Such methods have led to much clearer accounts of the capacities and limitations of normal human attention and, when combined with the study of brain damaged patients, neuroimaging and neurophysiological techniques, to the neural basis of these abilities. Reviewing the area in 1990, Posner and Petersen proposed three key principles of attentional function;

> "First... the attention system of the brain is anatomically separate from the data processing systems that perform operations on specific inputs even when attention is oriented elsewhere. In this sense, the attention system is like other sensory and motor systems. It interacts with other parts of the brain but maintains its own identity. Second, attention is carried out by a network of anatomical areas. It is neither the property of a single centre, nor a general function of the brain operating as a whole... Third, the areas involved in attention carry out different functions and these specific computations can be specified in cognitive terms." (p.26)

They proposed that these different functions included; as discussed, the capacity to prioritise signals from one spatial location (*spatial attention*); to prioritise some forms of information and to suppress others on the basis of a functional goal or a stored representation of a target (*selective or focused attention*); and to self-maintain an alert, ready to respond state (*arousal/sustained attention*). This and similar taxonomies (e.g. Van Zomeren *et al.*, 1984; Mirsky *et al.*, 1991; Cohen & Kaplan, 1993) are of course provisional and vulnerable to further fractionation. The most important clinical implication is that deficits can arise that are exclusively or predominantly attentional in nature and that quite distinct forms of impairment profile (with quite different functional implications) can arise depending on the location and extent of damage. This should influence how we perform assessment and how we go about rehabilitation.

3 A note on terminology

There is a great deal of conceptual overlap between the fields of attention, executive function and aspects of working memory - and whether one or other is used is often more to do with terminological or theoretical preference than any imagined hard division. For example, the executive functions of the brain can be seen as resulting from a 'Supervisory Attentional System' (Norman & Shallice, 1980) or attention viewed as the product of a Central Executive (Baddeley, 1993). Certainly for rehabilitation it is often of greater use to specify more clearly what a patient actually has difficulty with (e.g. finds it difficult to follow conversations in noisy environments, fails to follow or adjust plans) than to subsume such problems beneath any of these higher order theoretical categories.

4 Attention and outcome

As attention in one form or another pervades almost all aspects of our cognitive life, we would expect far-reaching consequences of serious impairment. As the assessment of attention becomes more widespread, evidence supporting this contention is increasingly apparent. For example improvements in attention, as indexed by simple reaction time, are one of the earliest predictors of emergence from posttraumatic amnesia following traumatic brain injury, consistent with a general role in 'bootstrapping' the rest of the cognitive system (Wilson *et al.*, 1999). Further down the line, persistent problems in attention are associated with poor social and occupational outcome (Brooks & McKinlay, 1987; McPherson *et al.*, 1997; Woischneck *et al.*, 1997).

In learning to cope with the consequences of brain damage, patients need to be aware of when they are experiencing difficulties, to focus on rehabilitation techniques and, often, to learn new strategies to get around problems. In each stage impairments in attention are likely to undermine progress. In addition to these functional properties there is now evidence that the neural correlates of 'paying attention' may play a more direct role in the recovery and organisation of damaged circuits. Attention has been observed to modulate or 'gate' activity in primary sensory areas of the brain (Desimone & Duncan, 1995). This has been reported in vision (Moran & Desimone, 1985), audition (Woldorff *et al.*, 1993), and in somatosensory perception (Drevets *et al.*, 1995). The role of such inputs in influencing synaptic connectivity is suggested by both animal (Recanzone *et al.*, 1993) and now human studies. Pascual-Leone and colleagues, for example, found that areas of the motor cortex associated with a particular action were enlarged following purely mental practice of this skill (Pascual-Leone *et al.*, 1995).

Such factors may account for why the ability to attend and maintain a focus of attention may form a good predictor of recovery in other capacities. To take one example, Robertson and colleagues found that sustained attention function assessed at two months post-stroke formed a significant predictor of motor function and ability to perform activities of everyday living two years later (Robertson *et al.*, 1997b; cf. Ben-Yishay *et al.*, 1968).

One very important reason for us to target attention deficits, therefore, is that in addition to any direct effects, their presence may undermine recovery in of other capacities and prevent the useful expression of abilities that may be relatively intact.

5 **A note on rehabilitation**

Clinical neuropsychology largely developed from (or in a parallel with) the academic discipline of cognitive neuropsychology. However, the two fields should have very different priorities. In order to constrain models, cognitive psychology requires more and more focused assessments capable of isolating one or other specific capacity. For clinical neuropsychology an important aim is to predict difficulties in everyday life, for which such specific assessments may, at times, be rather ill-suited (cf. Wilson, 1999; Burgess *et al.*, 1998). The same difficulty can pervade what is viewed as rehabilitation. For many cognitive psychologists, rehabilitation is most interesting if it helps to constrain a model of the function in question, e.g. that a particular rehabilitative gambit might improve working memory as indexed by digit span performance. In contrast, patients - and therefore clinicians - should be most interested in what improves outcome at the level of functional goals. Having a long digit span might be nice for all sorts of reasons but it doesn't (in itself) get you to the shops.

In this chapter we therefore adopt a broad definition of rehabilitation that encompasses interventions at a number of levels; the restitution or enhancement of basic function, training in compensatory strategies and the use of environmental aids. While our focus is on research that allows conclusions about specific interventions, it almost goes without saying that for individual patients a combination of approaches directed at achieving *his or her* particular goals is desirable.

6 **Unilateral neglect**

Unilateral neglect (or hemi-spatial neglect) is one of the most striking and extensively studied forms of attentional impairment. Perhaps not coincidentally, it is also the area where rehabilitation is most advanced. Unilateral neglect refers to a difficulty in detecting, acting on or even thinking about information from one side of space. Patients may fail to notice food on the left side of their plate, fail to dress or wash the left side of their body, have difficulty in imagining the left side of familiar objects and, in some cases, even deny ownership of their own left limbs. Although classically associated with lesions to the right posterior parietal cortex (Heilman & Watson, 1977; Vallar & Perani, 1986), neglect has been observed following damage to a variety of brain structures including the right prefrontal cortex and subcortical areas (Damasio *et al.*, 1980; Mesulam, 1981; Samuelsson, *et al.*, 1997; Karnath *et al.*, 2001).

6.1 **The natural recovery of neglect**

An attentional neglect of contralesional space is less prevalent and markedly less persistent following damage to the left, compared with the right hemisphere (Bowen McKenna & Tallis 1999). Estimates regarding number of people with right hemisphere stroke who show neglect in the acute stage vary considerably depending on the sensitivity of the tests applied and when the measurement is taken. In one study 84% of patients were missing information on the left 3 days after their stroke (Stone *et al.*, 1993), while other estimates are closer to 50% (Bowen, *et al.*, 1999; Farne *et al.*, 2004; Buxbaum *et al.*, 2004).

An example of unilateral neglect

Joan suffered a right hemisphere stroke in July of 1999 that left her with quite extensive damage to the right parietal and temporal cortices. After an initial period in which she was very confused, staff at the hospital noted her tendency to keep her trunk, head and eyes oriented to the right. Often she would fail to notice people approaching her from the left (unless they were able to attract her attention by raising their voices) and would be unable to locate objects such as her teacup if it was to the left of her bed-table. Although her language and memory appeared relatively unaffected by the stroke she had great difficulty in making any sense of what she read. Sometimes she appeared very confused, for example, claiming after she had been moved to a different bed, that she was no longer in the same hospital. Although she was capable of making some movements with her left arm, hand or leg she largely ignored them. When asked by the psychologist to imitate an action with her left hand, she simply performed it with her right. Joan required help with washing and dressing and in navigating her wheelchair around the ward.

Four months after her stroke, Joan's persistent problems with left space were having serious implications for her rehabilitation sessions. The physiotherapists found it very difficult to get her to focus on left-sided movements and the occupational therapists found that many activities that she would have been able to perform without thinking, such as making a sandwich, were now an almost insurmountable ordeal. Unless there was to be a considerable change in these symptoms, the chances of Joan being able to return to an independent lifestyle were slim.

This variability also pervades estimates of persistence. While some patients certainly undergo quite rapid spontaneous recovery, a review of relevant studies reported that, on average, 42% of right hemisphere patients will continue to show neglect at 3–6 months post-stroke (Bowen *et al.*, 1999).

An important question in thinking about rehabilitation is whether the spontaneous improvements in neglect take place primarily because of recovery of the underlying systems (e.g. through a reduction in diaschitic effects) or through the operation of compensatory mechanisms. Goodale, Milner, Jakobson, and Carey (1990) studied a group of nine right hemisphere patients twenty-one weeks after they had experienced a stroke. None of the patients now showed clinically significant signs of neglect and were able to reach for visual targets with the same accuracy as a control group. However, when the reach trajectories were analysed, significant deviations into right space were observed - deviations that were only corrected just before the hand reached the target. In addition, when patients were asked to estimate and reach towards the mid-point between two targets, significant rightward deviations were again apparent. Taken together with the results of Mattingley *et al.* (1994), this suggests that underlying distortions in the representation of space may persist in some or many cases but be masked in most day-to-day activity.

There is some evidence to suggest that these compensatory processes make demands on limited capacity resources. Robertson and Frasca (1992), for example, worked with patients who had apparently recovered from many aspects of neglect. When performing a simple reaction time task to left- and right-sided stimuli, no clear spatial bias was apparent. When however, they were asked to simultaneously perform another attentionally demanding task, reaction times to left sided targets were disproportionately compromised. Bartolomeo (2000) recently found that dual task interference with a spatial task was relatively greater for 'recovered' neglect patients than for patients still showing clinical evidence of the disorder (who, by inference, were not yet using a compensatory strategy). In a later section we will return to limitations in *non-spatial* attentional capacity as a marker of persistent neglect.

Spontaneous reductions in neglect therefore occur for the majority of patients without the need for specific intervention - and compensation for a persistent spatial bias appears to be one mechanism underpinning these changes. Many patients who do not show spontaneous improvement are, however, able to become temporarily more aware of left sided information if cued to do so (e.g. Riddoch & Humphreys, 1983; Mattingley *et al.*, 1993). The investigation of whether chronic patients can be trained to make compensatory ocular scans has therefore been central to rehabilitation in this area.

6.1.1 Scanning training

Early attempts at encouraging leftward ocular scans, such as asking patients to find the left side of a line of text before trying to read it, tended to show significant improvements on the trained materials, but little generalisation to other activities (Lawson, 1962; Seron *et al.*, 1989; Wagenaar *et al.*, 1992; Robertson, 1990). At times the specificity could be striking, in one case not even transferring between two different editions of the same book (Lawson, 1962). Although such failure to generalise does not preclude a useful rehabilitation effect, needing to train in each and every important context that a patient encounters would have clear resource implications.

It is possible that one barrier to generalised improvements in these studies lay not in the methods used per se, but in the diversity and duration of training. Pizzamiglio *et al.*, (1992) provided scanning training to thirteen patients between three and thirty-four months post-stroke. The training, which took place over 40 sessions, included a wide variety of scanning tasks with cues (such as warning tones, flashing lights to the left of the display) being systematically faded as performance improved. Significant improvements were observed on the trained tasks and, most importantly, on untrained measures and life-like structured activities. Subsequent evaluation using a full randomised-controlled design verified the efficacy of these techniques (Antonucci *et al.*, 1995).

6.1.2 Forcing attention to the left: Non-volitional leftward scanning methods

Neglect is known to operate within different spatial frameworks. Patients may, for example, neglect the left side of objects within an array despite the represented (right) side of those objects being to the left of the array as a whole (object-centred neglect; Driver and Halligan, 1991), or show dissociation between the degree of spatial bias between near (within arms reach) and far space (Halligan and Marshall, 1991). There is also strong evidence of a distortion within egocentric co-ordinates and, in particular, a displacement of subjective body-midline to the right (Karnath, 1994).

We discussed how the spontaneous compensatory strategies adopted by apparently recovered neglect patients appear to use limited capacity resources - which for some patients are a rather scarce commodity. A number of interventions are known, however, to induce distortions in the perception of (egocentric) space with healthy individuals regardless of their intentions. These include optokinetic stimulation, caloric vestibular stimulation, neck muscle vibration and prism lens adaptation. In each case, the basis of the effect is to use idiosyncrasies of the sensory system to induce an illusion that you are in a different location or are moving in a different direction to what is actually the case. By these means, the compensatory responses of the brain in the opposite direction have the potential for rehabilitation or training gains. In optokinetic stimulation, for example, patients are asked to perform a task against a moving background (e.g. dots on a computer monitor moving in a coherent direction) which gives the illusion that one is moving in the other direction, like the illusion that one's own train is moving when a nearby train, filling the view from the window, is moving in the opposite direction (Pizzamiglio et al., 1990). The patients' responses take into account this 'movement' and can therefore be biased in the opposite direction. Similarly, caloric vestibular stimulation (CVS) and neck muscle vibration induce the illusion of that you are rotating in a certain direction by imposing a temperature gradient between the left and right vestibular system (in practice irrigating the contralesional ear with cold water and/or the ipsilesional ear with warm water (Cappa et al., 1987; Rubens, 1983) or by vibration of the posterior neck muscle on the contralesional side (Karnath et al., 1993) respectively.

Such interventions have been theoretically useful in calibrating the spatial biases of neglect, but the generally short-lived effects and requirement for less-than-portable apparatus have led to pessimism about their role in rehabilitation. Early optimism that optokinetic stimulation may enhance scanning training, for example, was not supported by clinical trial data. (Pizzamiglio et al., 2004). However, it is possible that they may serve an important role as part of a more general training programme, particularly where patients have difficulty in exerting even temporary corrective control over neglect (Antonucci et al., 1995). Beis et al. (1999), for example, used patches to occlude the right-visual field as a means of forcing increased awareness of left space. Three months after training the technique was associated with significantly improved eye-movements and performance of everyday activities (compared with patching of the entire left eye and a no treatment control).

While the full implications of these techniques for rehabilitation, and in particular the improvement of functional activity, have yet to be explored, we turn to another intervention based on a displacement illusion that has been the subject of intense activity over recent years: adaptation to rightward deviating prism lenses.

6.1.3 Prism adaptation (PA) training

Prism lenses worn as spectacles induce an optical deviation, making an object that is straight ahead appear to be, say, to the right. When first wearing such glasses, if asked to reach for the straight-ahead object, individuals will tend to miss (the misdirection reflecting the rightward distortion). The error is clearly visible and is generally corrected within a few attempts. After multiple reaching trials, the brain's automatic adaptation to this distortion is apparent when the glasses are removed and errors occur for a short time in the opposite direction. Rossetti *et al.* (1998) investigated the effect of asking patients with left neglect to make repeated reaches to left and right arms-length targets over 5 minutes, while wearing rightward deviating prism glasses. Once the glasses were removed, the patients showed significantly reduced rightward bias on spatial tasks. What was surprising was that these benefits persisted for at least 2 hours. In the largest clinical study to have examined PA training, benefits persisted for at least 6 weeks after cessation of training (Frassinetti *et al.*, 2002). Prism training, it appeared, could be used to re-calibrate neglect patients' sense of space. Benefits for some, but not all patients, have subsequently been reported on a variety of spatial measures and in various modalities (e.g. Farne *et al.*, 2002; Jacquin-Courtois *et al.*, 2008; McIntosh *et al.*, 2002; Rode *et al.*, 2001; Rode *et al.*, 1998). A recent review claimed, while conceding that further controlled studies were required, that PA was the treatment of choice for neglect (Luaute *et al.*, 2009). It is easy to see why, if effective, it is an attractive therapy. The equipment required is relatively cheap and is only required for training rather than as a prosthesis, meaning that in principle at least, one set of goggles could be used by many patients. Similarly, the training can be performed by anyone who can follow the basic instructions.

In terms of the mechanisms of PA training, it has been suggested that the beneficial effects stem from adaptive re-calibration of one's spatial representation caused by the disruptive experience of the PA procedure. Relatively few functional imaging studies have so far addressed this question, although Clower *et al.* (1996) found, in neurologically healthy volunteers, that posterior parietal cortex (PPC) is specifically involved in this re-calibration process. In a more recent PET study, Lauate *et al.* (2006b) scanned 5 neglect patients performing a line bisection judgement task, both before and after completing one session of PA training. They looked specifically for brain areas where rCBF changes pre- and post-training covaried with the observed behavioural change exerted by PA. Increases were observed in three clusters – the left globus pallidus and left thalamus; the dentate nucleus of the right cerebellum and lobule V of the right cerebellar hemisphere; and BA 19 in the left occipital lobe, and BA37 in left fusiform gyrus. Decreased rCBF was seen in two clusters, the first in the left medial temporal lobe and the second in the right posterior parietal lobe (precuneus, BA37). The authors proposed that PA prompted short-term sensorimotor plasticity through recruitment of intact brain regions involved in normal visuospatial attention (cerebellum, dentate nucleus, thalamus, globus pallidus, parts of the ventral stream). Based on observations of patients with PPC and cerebellar lesions, Pisella *et al.* (2006) suggested that the cerebellum is principally involved in the realignment component of PA (and leads to persistent and generalised benefits), whereas posterior parietal cortex is involved in a more strategic component of PA. Their proposed mechanism of PA benefits in neglect patients is that error-signals produced by the PA procedure are processed in left occipital cortex, eliciting spatial realignment processes in the right cerebellum, which subsequently modulate projections to frontal, temporal and posterior parietal cortices in the undamaged hemisphere.

As the popularity of PA based therapy has grown, however, a number of studies have now failed to identify any beneficial effects (e.g. Morris *et al.*, 2004; Rousseaux, Bernati, Saj & Kozlowski, 2006). A recent placebo-controlled RCT of PA for neglect (Nys *et al.*, 2008) demonstrated that neglect patients in the acute phase (2–23 days post-stroke) receiving PA training for four consecutive days improved on 2/4 measures of spatial performance (line bisection and letter cancellation, but not line cancellation or scene copying) compared with patients undergoing an identical training procedure with placebo glasses. However, there was no detectable difference between prism and placebo-training groups on either conventional or ecological tests at one-month follow-up. Such appropriate controls for the general effects of therapy are important and suggest that when and for whom PA benefits occur remains an important research area. As we will discuss further, an interesting question given the association between persistent neglect and a range of non-spatial capacity limitations is whether an intervention that operates exclusively on the spatial aspects of the disorder will provide the hoped for general improvements in outcome.

6.1.4 Limb-activation

Influential views of spatial attention suggest that it is intimately linked with the preparation for action (e.g. Rizzolatti & Camarda, 1987; Allport, 1992). It is certainly the case that changes in the motor context (e.g. the difference between reaching to point and reaching to pick up) can exert a significant influence on the degree of spatial bias shown by neglect patients (Robertson *et al.*,1995a). Halligan and Marshall (1989) reported that when a patient used his left hand to perform a spatial task he showed significantly less neglect of left space than when he used his right. Robertson and colleagues systematically examined these effects. In particular they controlled for the inevitable out of sight whilst performing a spatial task that required only a verbal (naming) response (Robertson & North, 1992; Robertson & North, 1993; Robertson & North, 1994; Robertson *et al.*, 1994).

The results of this series of studies are summarised in Figure 6.1 overleaf. They show that the most significant reductions in left-sided omissions are associated with the left hand moving within left space (defined relative to the patient's midline). Movement of the right hand within left space, or of the left hand within right space produced much less dramatic effects, and simultaneous movements of both hands abolished any benefits of left limb movement.

The important question is whether this striking experimental effect can be extended into improving everyday function. Two recent studies suggest that this is the case. Robertson and colleagues developed a portable 'neglect alert device' to prompt patients to continue to make left hand movements (a buzzer sounded if the button was not pressed regularly). Significant improvements in a number of everyday spatial activities (including combing the hair and navigating around a hospital route) coincided with the onset of training (Robertson *et al.*, 1998a). Wilson *et al.* (2000) worked with a 62 year old man whose very severe left neglect (including of his own body) was seriously affecting his ability to take care of himself. To create an ecological measure his morning washing

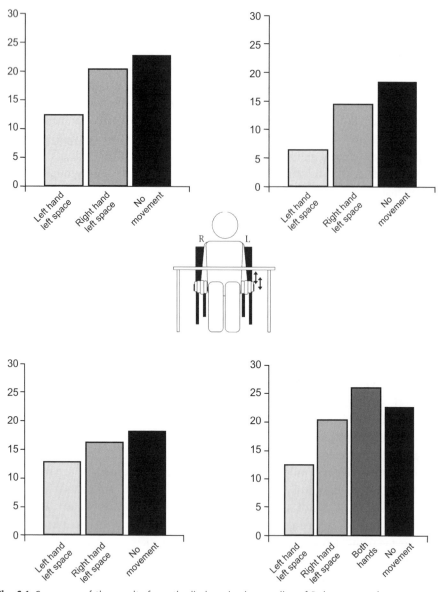

Fig. 6.1 Summary of the results from the limb activation studies of Robertson and colleagues.Unseen movement of the left hand to the left side of the body is associated with a reliable reduction in spatial attention bias. Movement of the left hand on the right, or of the right hand on the left produces less striking effects (units are the number of target omissions made by the patients).

routine was divided into distinct steps (washing both arms, washing both legs and so on). The measure of his independence was the number of prompts he required to complete each stage (prompts were given if activity stopped for 20 seconds). As shown in Figure 6.2, after a 10 day baseline the introduction of limb activation training was associated with a significant increase in his independence. Importantly, as was the case for some patients in Robertson *et al.*'s study, these gains were well maintained even when formal training had stopped. It seems possible, therefore, that in some cases the initial encouragement to use the left hand enhances awareness of left space, which in turn leads to greater spontaneous use of the left hand. By this means, a positive feedback loop could be established that maintains and enhances the effect.

6.1.5 Sustained attention training

From reading textbooks in neuropsychology, one might imagine that the only difficulty experienced by patients with unilateral neglect is their curious lack of awareness of left space. This is rarely the case. Clinically, one very noticeable feature of such patients is the immense difficulty they can have remaining engaged in *any* task, regardless of its spatial content. This impression is supported by research showing that patients with neglect have particularly poor sustained attention, even when compared to other patients with right hemisphere lesions (Robertson *et al.*, 1997a; Samuelsson *et al.*, 1988).

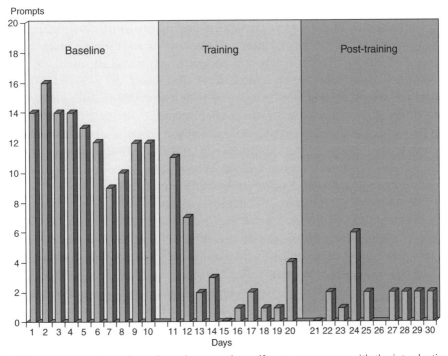

Fig. 6.2 Improvement in independence in a morning self-care programme with the introduction of limb activation training.

As with leftward cueing and use of the left hand, experimental evidence that the associated deficits of neglect and poorly maintained alertness were *functionally* connected may inform a different approach to rehabilitation. Such evidence emerged from a study in which patients were occasionally alerted by a loud tone as they performed a spatial task. Although the tone had no predictive value for whether a target would appear on the left or right, when presented it completely abolished (and is some cases even reversed) the neglect (Robertson *et al.*, 1998b).

Robertson *et al.* (1995b) examined whether longer term training in self-maintaining an alert, 'ready to respond' state could reduce neglect. In the training patients were asked to perform various non-spatial and rather tedious activities. Every so often (with the patient's prior consent) the therapist would bang the table top - both to cause an involuntary alerting effect and to cue the patients to say to themselves "WAKE UP!" or "ATTEND". In line with a procedure first described by Meichenbaum & Goodman (1971; cf. Meichenbaum & Cameron, 1973) the external cueing was progressively faded. In a multiple baseline x patient design (a method of controlling for spontaneous improvements), one week of daily training produced significant reductions in neglect on non-trained measures (Robertson *et al.*, 1995b). A similar type of self-alerting training, using biofeedback, has recently been found to improve sustained attention in adults with Attention Deficit Hyperactivity Disorder (O'Connell *et al.*, 2008) suggesting that wider application of such techniques is warranted.

Following a related rationale, Thimm *et al.* (2006) studied the behavioural effects of a 3-week computerised alertness-training program in a group of 7 neglect patients, along with fMRI correlates of such effects. Though benefits consistent with a beneficial effect of training were found on behavioural measures of spatial bias, and these were accompanied by increased fMRI activation in networks associated with spatial attention, the behavioural benefits disappeared once training had ceased (although the increased fMRI activations remained). Further work in this area is clearly needed to determine whether maintenance of such short-term benefits can be promoted.

At least four very different approaches have therefore produced significant rehabilitative results with unilateral neglect. Unilateral neglect is a highly fractionated set of symptoms that can arise from damage to a variety of brain areas. More research is needed in clarifying the applicability of these methods to different manifestations of spatial bias - and indeed whether the effects may be additive in some cases. A recent Cochrane review (Bowen & Lincoln, 2007) concluded that there was some evidence that interventions for neglect could improve performance on tests of spatial ability (i.e. at the impairment level), but that there was no available evidence of an effect on measures of disability (i.e. that the benefits translated to improvements in functionality). The authors pointed out that these rather negative findings were the result of paucity of randomized control trial (RCT) evidence and an over-emphasis on changes in test scores rather than functional disability. While there are positive indications from studies employing non-RCT methods, in order for definitive statements to be made regarding efficacy, studies that are adequately randomized, with blind assessment, and include measures of functional handicap need to be conducted.

7 Non-spatial attention

An example of non-spatial attention

Brian was a well-educated man in his mid 40's. In 1995 he suffered a serious head injury in a road accident that left him in coma for 3 days. In many ways his recovery was remarkable. Over two years his performance on tests of reasoning and memory returned to above average levels. Unfortunately, it was only when Brian returned to work that his remaining deficits became apparent. His job required a great deal of flexibility. In order to achieve goals and meet deadlines he would need to keep track of a changing situation, re-prioritise, and switch between one activity and another. It was precisely this level of organisation that Brian now found so difficult. He was now highly distractible and would leave jobs unfinished or fail to notice crucial details that he had omitted. At home he found it difficult to complete simple jobs without needing constant reminders and was described by his wife as often drifting into a world of his own. Despite retaining many of his premorbid abilities, Brian was now very frustrated by his inability to harness these effectively in order to achieve goals.

7.1 A behavioural, goal based approach

Our discussion of unilateral neglect has focused on interventions designed to improve underlying ability, as this can represent a more general solution to the functional problems experienced by the patient. When the underlying problems are less clearly understood, as is the currently the case for many forms of non-spatial attention, it can be more appropriate to tackle a specific activity. Wilson and Robertson (1992), for example, adopted a behavioural approach in working with a man whose severe head injury had left him with problems in 'keeping his mind' on what he was reading. Initially the man was asked to monitor how many times his attention slipped when he was reading. In training he was initially encouraged to read for only very brief periods. If these were completed without slip the duration of the subsequent session was increased by ten percent. Following 160 sessions over 40 days, the goal of reliably reading for 5 minutes without a slip was attained. Most importantly, the number of slips reported when reading material relevant to his job had also significantly reduced, even though this had not been directly trained.

This systematic, shaping approach does not tell us a great deal about the underlying nature of the difficulties experienced by the patient. There was also little evidence that the training produced any improvements in other activities in this case (although this can be very hard to measure). It does show, however, that appropriate reinforcement and learning can modulate the consequences of poor attention and offers a technique that could be easily applied to many situations.

7.2 Improving attention through general training

We have seen how, in the case of scanning training for spatial neglect, the duration of rehabilitation may be crucial (Pizzamilio et al., 1992). The revolution in computer technology and price over the last three decades has made long periods of systematic and reflexive training increasingly possible. For researchers, the use of computers to 'deliver' therapy also means that exposure to treatment can be highly standardised - improving the interpretation of particular factors that can promote performance change.

In a study by Gray *et al.* (1992), thirty-one patients with reported attention difficulties were randomly allocated to one of two conditions. One consisted of approximately 15 hours of computerised training including; a) a reaction time task with feedback on speed; b) a task requiring the identification two identical digit strings from a briefly presented array of 4; c) a digit-symbol translation task; and d) a colour-word Stroop task. The other was 15 hours of recreational computing. Immediately following the 3–9 week training, the experimental group showed significant improvements on two *non-trained* tasks relative to the controls (the WAIS-R Picture Completion subtest, requiring visual search and reasoning, and the Paced Auditory Serial Addition Task (PASAT), widely considered as primarily a measure of processing speed (Gronwall & Sampson, 1974). At six months follow-up, the benefits on these measures had been maintained and, in addition, further untrained measures were showing training benefit (backward digit span, mental arithmetic, and WAIS-R Block Design).

As the groups were well matched on task performance prior to training, the results suggested both that the training had produced generalised improvements and that a 'sleeper effect' led to continued improvement beyond the training period. While little evidence exists on this, it is possible to speculate that such effects emerge both through consolidation of the learning and from the increased exposure to attentionally demanding situations consequent upon initial improvements.

The results are persuasive in suggesting a specific effect that, thanks to the well matched control group, cannot be interpreted in terms of generalised recovery. The generalisation to *functional activities* of everyday life was not, however, examined in this study.

7.3 Training specific attention functions

We have discussed how attention has been viewed as a fractionated set of processes. In a strong form of this argument, training one form of attention may have minimal consequences for another. Sturm *et al.* (1997) examined this by randomly allocating 38 stroke patients to different training programmes. The programmes, now published as part of the "AIXTENT" training package, were made up of separate modules targeting a particular form of attention. They used this idea to evaluate a programme in which all participants received training but in which the modules were completed in different orders.If attentional functions were relatively encapsulated, they argued, observed improvements should broadly follow the order of training.

Each of the exercises was in the form of a computer game that became more challenging as performance improved. Alertness, for example, was trained using a motorbike simulation while selective attention required the patients to 'shoot' one but not another form of target. Improvements were evaluated on an untrained computerised measure (Zimmermann *et al.*, 1993). After approximately 56 hours of training the hypothesis was substantially supported. The detection rate for targets in the untrained test battery vigilance task was significantly improved only after vigilance training and not following training in selective or divided attention. Similarly, reaction times in the selective attention test were improved following selective, but not sustained attention training. As might be expected, some crossover effects were also observed. Performance on the divided attention task, for example, was significantly enhanced following training in selective, as well as divided, forms of attention. Note that this training procedure was the same as that used in the previously discussed study examining alertness training for neglect (Thimm *et al.*, 2006). Comparable results were obtained in a further study of effects of the AIXTENT training in people with multiple sclerosis (Plohmann *et al.*, 1998). Further studies, with appropriate controls, are clearly warranted.

Sohlberg *et al.* (2000) conducted a randomised control crossover trial to evaluate the efficacy of another form of attention training, referred to as Attention Process Training (APT). Participants received 24 hours of APT over 10 weeks, with the sessions involving completion of non-computerised tasks taxing different aspects of attention (e.g. detecting target sounds within distractor noise, listening to a sentence and alphabetising the component words). The control condition involved a total of 10 hours of brain injury education and supportive listening, over 10 weeks. Across the whole group, benefits specific to APT were seen in two tests of "executive attention" (the Paced Serial Addition Task PASAT (Gronwall & Sampson, 1974), and the Sternberg (1966) memory for locations test). In a subset of participants with poor vigilance performance, APT-specific improvements were also seen on the Stroop (1935) and Trail Making Tasks (Reitan & Wolfson, 1985). There were also benefits of APT on self-reported attention and memory functioning.

A recent development has been the working memory (WM) training studies of Klingberg and colleagues. Olesen *et al.* (2004) reported that subjects who engaged in around 40 minutes of repeated practise on three working memory tasks over 5 weeks showed faster and more accurate responses on WM tasks in comparison with untrained participants. Crucially, there was some evidence of generalised benefits to *untrained* tasks including the Stroop task and the Raven's Matrices fluid intelligence measure. These changes were accompanied by increased fMRI activation during WM performance in the right middle frontal gyrus, right inferior parietal cortex and bilateral intraparietal sulcus. Based on this work, a training program, RoboMemo© (Cognitive Medical Systems AB, Stockholm), has been developed, and its effects have been evaluated in two recent randomised controlled trials. The program involves various WM tasks, some visuo-spatial WM (effectively computerised versions of the corsi-block task), and three verbal tasks (remembering phonemes, letters or digits). In all tasks, the difficulty level is titrated to match individual WM span. The first study, an RCT with blind assessment and a stringent placebo-control, involved 56 children with ADHD (Klingberg *et al.*, 2005). Participants were randomly assigned to either experimental or control arms of the trial, with children in the former group being subjected to either 40 minutes of RoboMemo training for 25 days, and those in the latter group, an equivalent period of training on the same software, but without automatic titration of task difficulty (e.g. just repeating 2–3 item span tasks). Benefits specific to the experimental training were seen in a variety of untrained tests of WM, as well as on the Stroop task and Raven's matrices, and were maintained at 3-month follow-up. Parent-ratings of ADHD symptoms also improved with training, and were also maintained at follow-up.

Westerberg *et al.* (2007) reported similar findings in a small (n=18) RCT involving adults in the chronic (>1 year) phase post-stroke. Here, the experimental training was the same as that described in Klingberg *et al.* (2005), but training effects were determined by comparison with a no-training (passive) control group – an obvious limitation of the study. Performance on two untrained tests of WM, the PASAT and the Ruff (1992) 2 and 7 test (assessing sustained and selective attention) all improved disproportionately in the training group. Futhermore, self-reported lapses in attention and memory as indexed by the Cognitive Failures Questionnaire also decreased with training.

Taken together, there is certainly promising evidence that repeated (and ideally progressive) training in attentional and WM tasks, if carried out over a sufficient period of time, can produce generalised changes in function as assessed on untrained tasks and, crucially, in people's reports of everyday difficulties.

7.4 Environmental support for attention

Within specialist clinical settings it is possible to organise the environment in a way that minimises demands on patients' deficient attentional and executive skills (e.g. reducing distraction, having a very set schedule, keeping a written record of an agreed plan, systematic reinforcement of goal-directed behaviour). Such techniques can be useful in helping very severely impaired patients to control inappropriate behaviour and to focus on other important rehabilitation goals (cf. Alderman & Ward, 1991; Alderman & Burgess, 1994; Alderman, 1996) - but are clearly inappropriate for many patients with less severe problems. Recently we have been examining whether it is possible to introduce 'portable' environmental support for attention that is compatible with (and hopefully enhances) independence. This type of approach is neatly demonstrated in a case study by Evans *et al.* (1998). They describe a patient who had suffered bilateral damage to the frontal lobes following a subarachnoid haemorrhage. Although on many standard IQ and memory tests her function was relatively well preserved, in everyday life she had great difficulty in achieving goals and was highly dependent on the support of others. In particular (as has been described in a number of frontal patients) she appeared to get overly caught up in whatever activity she was currently performing to the severe detriment her other essential activities. The patient was given an electronic pager that had originally been designed for memory-impaired patients, which remotely sent messages to cue an important activity (The 'Neuropage' system; Hersch & Treadgold, 1994; Wilson *et al.*, 1997, 2001). In this case, its introduction significantly improved her capacity to begin goal directed activity, often without her needing to see the content of the message. It appeared that this environmental intrusion was acting to refocus her attention on her goals - and once this had occurred, her other intact capacities allowed her to achieve them.

To investigate these effects at a group level we (Manly *et al.*, 2002) developed a modification of the 'Six Elements Test' (Shallice & Burgess, 1991) in which patients were asked to perform a number of tasks associated with running a hotel (calculating bills, ordering conference labels alphabetically, proof-reading a tourism leaflet and so on). As with the Six Elements, the key feature was that the total time available for the test (15 minutes) was far less than the time required to fully complete each component task. In order to comply with the goal of trying *some* of *each* activity in the test, patients would therefore need to plan at the outset to switch tasks with a certain regularity and to keep this goal actively in mind throughout the test. As with the patient reported by Evans *et al.* the key error made by the traumatically brain injured patients we worked with was to become so engrossed in one activity that this goal was neglected.

The patients were administered two versions of the task in random order one week apart. During one session we told the patients that they would periodically hear a rather salient bleeping noise - and that this was a reminder to them to think about what they were doing in the task. In this group, not only did the presence of the tone significantly improve their performance, it had now become indistinguishable from that of healthy control participants. This result was useful in ruling out a number of other causes of poor performance in the test such as failure to understand the task or remember what the plan was. Most importantly it suggests that, even if attention could not be directly improved, its functional consequences on complex activities can be minimised. We recently demonstrated a similar beneficial effect on the everyday prospective memory performance of a group of patients with acquired executive impairments by sending randomly timed text messages to participants' mobile phones (Fish *et al.*, 2007). As mobile phone and palmtop technology is increasingly available, and more frequently used by patients with brain injury, such interventions may become all the more important.

8 Summary

The scientific study of functions that are *specifically* attentional are at an early stage, but have begun to inform improved assessment and rehabilitation for neurological patients. Perhaps the most important development lies in seeing attention not as a single entity but as a set of processes that are vulnerable to separate damage and which can have very different consequences. As assessment has improved, the negative impact that poor attention has on recovery and outcome is increasingly clear - evidence that makes interventions designed to enhance natural recovery in these systems a particularly pressing clinical goal.

We have reviewed different approaches to working with attentional deficits; attempting to improve underlying function, targeting particular behavioural/functional goals, and using external aids to maximise residual function. Work with unilateral neglect is by far the most advanced. Four separate interventions, training patients to make compensatory left-ward scans, encouraging use of the left hand and arm, prism adaptation therapy, and teaching self-alerting techniques have all produced generalised improvements - other techniques exploiting new experimental effects may well follow. Although often more loosely defined, work with non-spatial attentional functions has also produced positive results. It has been demonstrated that systematic practice and reinforcement can shape attentive behaviour - perhaps to a much greater degree than has proved possible in the rehabilitation of memory (Wilson, 1999). Carefully evaluated computer training packages have produced clear improvements in attentional function, and there are now hints that these changes indeed translate to improvements in everyday function.

A key feature in a number of the studies we have considered seems to lie in the duration of training. Whether the processes necessary to enhance basic function are learning new strategies, using different neural pathways to achieve the same ends, or plastic re-organisation within damaged areas, effects should not be expected within a few sessions.

For researchers, clinicians, and most particularly, patients, careful evaluation of interventions is essential. Showing changes in well controlled experimental designs and using targeted neuropsychological measures is essential in understanding the specific relationship between what we do and any improvements, but this is not, in itself, rehabilitation. Many of our operational definitions of attention have been imported from cognitive psychology and the relationships between these entities and everyday difficulties can sometimes be obscure. While it defies belief to argue that we have cognitive capacities that are only tapped by neuropsychological tasks and untouched in daily life, a great deal more work is needed in examining the impact of particular deficits and the functional consequences of any improvements that we might help bring about.

Selective references

Alderman, N. (1996). Central Executive Deficit and Response to Operant Conditioning Methods. *Neuropsychological Rehabilitation*, **6**(3), 161–186.

Alderman, N., and Burgess, P. W. (1994). A comparison of treatment methods for behaviour disorder following Herpes Simplex Encephalitis. *Neuropsychological Rehabilitation*, **4**(1), 31–46.

Alderman, N., and Ward, A. (1991). Behavioural treatment of the dysexecutive syndrome: reduction in repetitive speech using response cost and cognitive overlearning. *Neuropsychological Rehabilitation*, **4**(4), 65–80.

Allport, A. (1992). Attention and control: Have we been asking the wrong questions? A Critical review of twenty-five years. pp. 183–218 in D. E. Meyer and S. Komblum (Eds.), *Attention and Performance (Vol. XIV)*. Cambridge, Mass: MIT Press.

Antonucci, G., Guariglia, C., Judica, A., Magnotti, L., Paolucci, S., Pizzamiglio, L., and Zoccolotti, P. (1995). Effectiveness of neglect rehabilitation in a randomized group study. *Journal of Clinical and Experimental Neuropsychology*, **17**, 383–389.

Baddeley, A. D. (1993). Working memory or working attention. In A. D. Baddeley and L. Weiskrantz (Eds.), *Attention: Selection, Awareness and Control: A Tribute to Donald Broadbent* (pp. 152–170). Oxford: Oxford University Press.

Bartolomeo, P. (2000). Inhibitory processes and spatial bias after right hemisphere damage. *Neuropsychological Rehabilitation*, **10**(5), 511–526.

Beis, J. M., Andre, J. M., Baumgarten, A., and Challier, B. (1999). Eye patching in unilateral spatial neglect: Efficacy of two methods. *Archives of Physical Medicine and Rehabilitation*, **80**, 71–76.

Ben-Yishay, Y., Diller, L., Gerstman, L., and Haas, A. (1968). The relationship between impersistence, intellectual function and outcome of rehabilitation in patients with left hemiplegia. *Neurology*, **18**, 852–861.

Bowen, A. and Lincoln, N.B. (2007). Rehabilitation for spatial neglect improves test Performance but not disability. *Stroke*, **38**, 2869–2870.

Bowen, A., McKenna, K., Tallis, R.C. (1999). Reasons for variability in the reported rate of occurrence of unilateral spatial neglect after stroke. *Stroke*, **30**, 1196–1202.

Brooks, D. N., and McKinlay, W. (1987). Return to work within the first seven years of severe head injury. *Brain Injury*, **1**, 5–15.

Burgess, P. W., Alderman, N., Evans, J., Emslie, H., and Wilson, B. A. (1998). The ecological validity of tests of executive function. *Journal of the International Neuropsychological Society*, **4**, 547–558.

Buxbaum, L. J., Ferraro, M. K., Veramonti, T., Farne, A., Whyte, J., Ladavas, E., Frassinetti, F., Coslett, H.B. (2004). Hemispatial neglect: Subtypes, neuroanatomy and disability. *Neurology*, **62**, 749–756.

Cappa, S. F., Sterzi, R., Vallar, G., and Bisiach, E. (1987). Remission of hemineglect and anosognosia during vestibular stimulation. *Neuropsychologia*, **25**, 775–782.

Clower, D. M., Hoffman, J. M., Votaw, J. R., Faber, T. L., Woods, R. P. and Alexander, G. E. (1996). Role of posterior parietal cortex in the recalibration of visually guided reaching. *Nature*, **383**, 618–621.

Cohen, R. A., and Kaplan, R. F. (1993). Attention as a multicomponent process - neuropsychological validation. *Journal of Clinical and Experimental Neuropsychology*, **15**(3), 379.

Damasio, A. R., Damasio, H., and Chui, H. C. (1980). Neglect following damage to frontal lobe or basal ganglia. *Neuropsychologia*, **18**, 123–132.

Desimone, R., and Duncan, J. (1995). Neural mechanisms of selective visual attention. *Annual Review of Neuroscience*, **18**, 193–221.

Drevets, W. C., Burton, H., Videen, T. O., Snyder, A. Z., Simpson, J. R., and Raichle, M. E. (1995). Blood flow changes in human somatosensory cortex during anticipated stimulation. *Nature*, **373**, 249–252.

Driver, J., and Halligan, P. W. (1991). Can visual neglect operate in object-centred co-ordinates? An affirmative single-case study. *Cognitive Neuropsychology*, **8**, 475–496.

Evans, J. J., Emslie, H., and Wilson, B. A. (1998). External cueing systems in the rehabilitation of executive impairments of action. *Journal of the International Neuropsychological Society*, **4**, 399–408.

Farne, A., Buxbaum, L. J., Ferraro, M., Frassinetti, F., Whyte, J., Veramonti, T., Angeli, V., Coslett, H. B., and Ladavas, E. (2004). Patterns of spontaneous recovery of neglect and associated disorders in acute right brain-damaged patients. *Journal of Neurology, Neurosurgery and Psychiatry*, **75**, 1401–1410.

Farne, A., Rossetti, Y., Toniolo, S., Ladavas, E. (2002). Ameliorating neglect with prism adaptation: visuo-manual and visuo-verbal measures. *Neuropsychologia*, **40**, 718–729.

Fish, J., Evans, J.J., Nimmo, M., Martin, E., Kersel, D., Bateman, A., Wilson, B.A., & Manly, T. (2007) Rehabilitation of executive dysfunction following brain injury: "Content-free" cueing improves everyday prospective memory performance. *Neuropsychologia*, **45**, 1318–30.

Frassinetti, F., Angeli, V., Meneghello, F., Avanzi, S., and Ladavas, E. (2002). Long-lasting amelioration of visuospatial neglect by prism adaptation. *Brain*, **125**, 608–623.

Goodale, M. A., Milner, A. D., Jakobson, L. S., and Carey, D. P. (1990). Kinematic analysis of limb movements in neuropsychological research: subtle deficits and recovery of function. *Canadian Journal of Psychology*, **44**, 180–195.

Gray, J. M., Robertson, I. H., Pentland, B., and Anderson, S. I. (1992). Microcomputer based cognitive rehabilitation for brain damage: a randomised group controlled trial. *Neuropsychological Rehabilitation*, **2**, 97–116.

Gronwall, D. M. A., and Sampson, H. (1974). *The Psychological Effects of Concussion*. Auckland: Auckland University Press.

Halligan, P. W., and Marshall, J. C. (1989). Laterality of motor response in visuo-spatial neglect: a case study. *Neuropsychologia*, **27**, 1301–1307.

Halligan, P. W., and Marshall, J. C. (1991). Left neglect for near but not far space in man. *Nature*, **350**, 498–500.

Heilman, K. M., and Watson, R. T. (1977). The neglect syndrome - a unilateral deficit of the orienting response. pp. 285-302 in S. Harnad, R. W. Doty, L. Goldstein, J. Jaynes, and G. Krauthamer (Eds.), *Lateralisation in the Nervous System.* New York: Academic Press.

Hersh, N. A., and Treadgold, L. G. (1994). NeuroPage: the rehabilitation of memory dysfunction by prosthetic memory and cueing. *Neurorehabilitation,* 4, 187–197.

Jacquin-Courtois, S., Rode, G., Pisella, L., Boisson, D., and Rossetti, Y. (2008). Wheel-chair driving improvement following visuo-manual prism adaptation. *Cortex,* 44, 90–96.

Karnath, H. O. (1994). Subjective body orientation in neglect and the interactive contribution of neck muscle proprioception and vestibular stimulation. *Brain,* 117, 1001–1012.

Karnath, H. O., Christ, K., and Hartje, W. (1993). Decrease of contralateral neglect by neck muscle vibration and spatial orientation of trunk midline. *Brain,* 116, 383–396.

Karnath, H. O., Ferber, S., and Himmelbach, M. (2001). Spatial awareness is a function of the temporal not the posterior parietal lobe. *Nature,* 411, 950–953.

Klingberg, T., Fernell, E., Olesen, P. J., Johnson, M., Gustafsson, P., Dahlstrom, K., Gillberg, C. G., Forssberg, H., Westerberg, H. (2005). Computerized training of working memory in children with ADHD–a randomized, controlled trial. *Journal of the American Academy of Child and Adolescent Psychiatry,* 44, 177–186.

Lawson, I. R. (1962). Visual-spatial neglect in lesions of the right cerebral hemisphere: A study in recovery. *Neurology,* 12, 23–33.

Luauté, J., Halligan, P., Rode, G., Jacquin-Courtois, S., Boisson, D. (2006a). Prism adaptation first among equals in alleviating left neglect: a review. *Restorative Neurology and Neuroscience,* 24, 409–418.

Luaute, J., Michel, C., Rode, G., Pisella, L., Jacquin-Courtois, S., Costes, N., Cotton, N., le Bars, D., Boisson, D., Halligan, P., and Rossetti, Y. (2006b). Functional anatomy of the therapeutic effects of prism adaptation on left neglect. *Neurology,* 66, 1859–1867.

Manly, T., Hawkins, K., Evans, J. J., Woldt, K., and Robertson, I. H. (2002). Rehabilitation of Executive Function: Facilitation of effective goal management on complex tasks using periodic auditory alerts. *Neuropsychologia,* 40, 271–181.

Mattingley, J. B., Bradshaw, J. L., Bradshaw, J. A., and Nettleton, N. C. (1994). Residual right attentional bias after apparent recovery from right hemisphere damage: implications for a multicomponent model of neglect. *Journal of Neurology, Neurosurgery and Psychiatry,* 57, 597–604.

Mattingley, J. B., Pierson, J. M., Bradshaw, J. L., Phillips, J. G., and Bradshaw, J. A. (1993). To see or not to see: The effects of visible and invisible cues on line bisection judgements unilateral neglect. *Neuropsychologia,* 31, 1201–1215.

McIntosh, R. D., Rossetti, Y., Milner, A. D. (2002). Prism adaptation improves chronic visual and haptic neglect: A single case study. *Cortex,* 38, 309–320.

McPherson, K., Berry, A., and Pentland, B. (1997). Relationships between cognitive impairments and functional performance after brain injury, as measured by the functional assessment measure (FIM+FAM). *Neuropsychological Rehabilitation,* 7(3), 241–257.

Meichenbaum, D., and Cameron, R. (1973). Training schizophrenics to talk to themselves: a means of developing attentional control. *Behaviour Therapy,* 4, 515–534.

Meichenbaum, D., and Goodman, J. (1971). Training impulsive children to talk to themselves: a means of developing self-control. *Journal of Abnormal Psychology,* 77, 115–126.

Mesulam, M. M. (1981). A cortical network for directed attention and unilateral neglect. *Annals of Neurology,* 10, 309–325.

Mirsky, A. F., Anthony, B. J., Duncan, C. C., Ahearn, M. B., and Kellam, S. G. (1991). Analysis of the elements of attention: A neuropsychological approach. *Neuropsychology Review,* 2, 109–145.

Moran, J., and Desimone, R. (1985). Selective attention gates visual processing in the extrastriate cortex. *Science*, **229**(782–784), 782–784.

Morris, A. P., Kritikos, A., Berberovic, N., Pisella, L., Chambers, C. D., and Mattingley, J. B. (2004). Prism adaptation and spatial attention: A study of visual search in normals and patients with unilateral neglect. *Cortex*, **40**, 703–721.

Norman, D. A., and Shallice, T. (1980). *Attention to Action: Willed and automatic control of behaviour*. Centre for Human Information Processing (Technical Report No. 99).

Nys, G.M., de Haan, E. H., Kunneman, A., de Kort, P.L., and Dijkerman, H.C. (2008). Acute neglect rehabilitation using repetitive prism adaptation: A randomised placebo-controlled trial. *Restorative Neurology and Neuroscience*, **26**, 1–12.

O'Connell, R. G., Bellgrove, M. A., Dockree, P. M., Lau, A., Fitzgerald, M., and Robertson, I. H. (2008). Self-Alert Training: Volitional modulation of autonomic arousal improves sustained attention. *Neuropsychologia*, **46**, 1379–1390.

Olesen, P. J., Westerberg, H., and Klingberg, T. (2004). Increased prefrontal and parietal activity after training of working memory. *Nature Neuroscience*, **7**, 75–79.

Pascual-Leone, A., Dang, N., Cohen, L. G., Brasilneto, J. P., Cammarota, A., and Hallett, M. (1995). Modulation of muscle responses evoked by transcranial magnetic stimulation during the acquisition of new fine motor skills. *Journal of Neurophysiology*, **74**, 1307–1345.

Pisella, L., Rode, G., Farne, A., Tilikete, C., Rossetti, Y. (2006). Prism adaptation in the rehabilitation of patients with visuo-spatial cognitive disorders. *Current Opinion in Neurology*, **19**, 534–542.

Pizzamiglio, L., Antonucci, G., Judica, A., Montenero, P., Razzano, C., and Zoccolotti, P. (1992). Cognitive rehabilitation of the hemineglect disorder in chronic-patients with unilateral right brain-damage. *Journal of Clinical and Experimental Neuropsychology*, **14**(6), 901–923.

Pizzamiglio, L., Fasotti, L., Jehkonen, M., Antonucci, G., Magnotti, L., Boelen, D., and Asa, S. (2004). The use of optokinetic stimulation in rehabilitation of the hemineglect disorder. *Cortex*, **40**, 441–450.

Pizzamiglio, L., Frasca, R., Guariglia, C., Incoccia, C., and Antonucci, G. (1990). Effect of optokinetic stimulation in patients with visual neglect. *Cortex*, **26**, 535–540.

Plohmann, A. M., Kappos, L., Ammann, W., Thordai, A., Wittwer, A., Huber, S., Bellaiche, Y., and Lechner-Scott, J. (1998). Computer assisted retraining of attentional impairments in patients with multiple sclerosis. *Journal of Neurology, Neurosurgery and Psychiatry*, **64**, 455–462.

Posner, M. I. (1980). Orientating of attention. *Quarterly Journal of Experimental Psychology*, **32**, 3–25.

Posner, M. I., and Petersen, S. E. (1990). The attention system of the human brain. *Annual Review of Neuroscience*, **13**, 25–42.

Recanzone, G. H., Schreiner, C. E., and Merzenich, M. M. (1993). Plasticity in the frequency representation of primary auditory cortex. *Journal of Neuroscience*, **13**, 87–103.

Reitan, R. M., and Wolfson, D. (1985). *The Halstead-Reitan Neuropsychological Test Battery: Theory and Clinical Interpretation*. Tucson, AZ: Neuropsychology Press.

Riddoch, M. J., and Humphreys, G. W. (1983). The effect of cueing on unilateral neglect. *Neuropsychologia*, **21**, 589–599.

Rizzolatti, G., and Camarda, R. (1987). Neural circuits for spatial attention and unilateral neglect. In M. Jeannerod (Ed.), *Neurophysiological and Neuropsychological Aspects of Neglect*. Amsterdam: North Holland Press.

Robertson, I. (1990). Does computerized cognitive rehabilitation work? A review. *Aphasiology*, **4**(4), 381–405.

Robertson, I. H., and Frasca, R. (1992). Attentional load and visual neglect. *International Journal of Neuroscience*, **62**, 45–56.

Robertson, I. H., Hogg, K., and McMillan, T. M. (1998a). Rehabiliation of Unilateral Neglect: Improving Function by Contralesional Limb Activation. *Neuropsychological Rehabiliation*, **8**(1), 19–29.

Robertson, I. H., Manly, T., Beschin, N., Haeske-Dewick, H., Hömberg, V., Jehkonen, M., Pizzamiglio, L., Shiel, A., Weber, E., and Zimmerman, P. (1997a). Auditory Sustained Attention is a Marker of Unilateral Spatial Neglect. *Neuropsychologia*, **35**, 1527–1532.

Robertson, I. H., Mattingley, J. M., Rorden, C., and Driver, J. (1998b). Phasic alerting of neglect patients overcomes their spatial deficit in visual awareness. *Nature*, **395**, 169–172.

Robertson, I. H., Nico, D., and Hood, B. (1995a). The intention to act improves unilateral neglect: two demonstrations. *Neuroreport*, **7**, 246–248.

Robertson, I. H., and North, N. (1992). Spatio-motor cueing in unilateral neglect: the role of hemispace, hand and motor activation. *Neuropsychologia*, **30**, 553–563.

Robertson, I. H., and North, N. (1993). Active and passive activation of left limbs: influence on visual and sensory neglect. *Neuropsychologia*, **31**, 293–300.

Robertson, I. H., and North, N. (1994). One hand is better than two: motor extinction of left hand advantage in unilateral neglect. *Neuropsychologia*, **32**, 1–11.

Robertson, I. H., Ridgeway, V., Greenfield, E., and Parr, A. (1997b). Motor recovery after stroke depends on intact sustained attention: A 2-year follow-up study. *Neuropsychology*, **11**(2), 290–295.

Robertson, I. H., Tegnér, R., Goodrich, S. J., and Wilson, C. (1994). Walking trajectory and hand movements in unilateral left neglect: A vestibular hypothesis. *Neuropsychologia*, **32**(12), 1495–1502.

Robertson, I. H., Tegnér, R., Tham, K., Lo, A., and Nimmo-Smith, I. (1995b). Sustained attention training for unilateral neglect: Theoretical and rehabilitation implications. *Journal of Clinical and Experimental Neuropsychology*, **17**, 416–430.

Rode, G., Rossetti, Y., Boisson, D. (2001). Prism adaptation improves representational neglect. *Neuropsychologia*, **39**, 1250–1254.

Rode, G., Rossetti, Y., Li, L., and Boisson, D. (1998). Improvement of mental imagery after prism exposure in neglect: A case study. *Behavioural Neurology*, **11**, 251–258.

Rossetti, Y., Rode, G., Pisella, L., Farne, A., Li, L., Boisson, D., and Perenin, M. T. (1998). Prism adaptation to a rightward optical deviation rehabilitates left hemispatial neglect. *Nature*, **395**, 166–169.

Rousseaux, M., Bernati, T., Saj, A., Kozlowski, O. (2006). Ineffectiveness of prism adaptation on spatial neglect signs. *Stroke*, **37**, 542–3.

Rubens, A. B. (1985). Caloric stimulation and unilateral visual neglect. *Neurology*, **35**, 1019–1024.

Ruff RM, Niemann H, Allen CC, Farrow CE, Wylie T (1992). The Ruff 2 and 7 selective attention test: A neuropsychological application. *Perceptual and Motor Skills*; **75**:1311–1319.

Samuelsson, H., Hjelmquist, E., Jensen, C., Ekholm, S., and Blomstrand, C. (1988). Nonlateralized attentional deficits: An important component behind persisting visuospatial neglect? *Journal of Clinical and Experimental Psychology*, **20**(1), 73–88.

Samuelsson, H., Jensen, C., Ekholm, S., Naver, H., and Blomstrand, C. (1997). Anatomical and neurological correlates of acute and chronic visuospatial neglect following right hemisphere stroke. *Cortex*, **33**, 271–85.

Seron, X., Deloche, G., and Coyette, F. (1989). A retrospective analysis of a single case neglect therapy: A point of theory. In X. Seron and G. Deloche (Eds.), *Cognitive Approaches to Neuropsychological Rehabilitation* (pp. 236–289). Hillsdale NJ: Laurence Earlbaum Associates.

Shallice, T., and Burgess, P. (1991). Deficits in strategy application following frontal lobe damage in man. *Brain*, **114**, 727–741.

Sohlberg, M. M., McLaughlin, K. A., Pavese, A., Heidrich, A., and Posner, M.I. (2000). Evaluation of Attention Process Training and Brain Injury Education in Persons with Acquired Brain Injury. *Journal of Clinical and Experimental Neuropsychology*, **22**, 656–676.

Sternberg, S. (1966). High-speed scanning in human memory. *Science, 153*, 652–654.

Stone, S. P., Halligan, P. W., and Greenwood, R. J. (1993). The incidence of neglect phenomena and related disorders in patients with an acute right or left hemisphere stroke. *Age and Ageing, 22*, 46–52.

Stroop, J.R. (1935). Studies of interference in serial verbal reactions. *Journal of Experimental Psychology, 18*, 643–662.

Sturm, W., Willmes, K., Orgass, B., and Hartje, W. (1997). Do specific attention deficits need specific training? *Neuropsychological Rehabilitation, 7*(2), 81–103.

Thimm, M., Fink, G. R., Kust, J., Karbe, H. and Sturm, W. (2006). Impact of alertness training on spatial neglect: A behavioural and fMRI study. *Neuropsychologia, 44*, 1230–1246.

Vallar, G., and Perani, D. (1986). The anatomy of unilateral neglect after right-hemisphere stroke lesions: A clinical/CT scan correlation study in man. *Neuropsychologia, 24*, 609–622.

Van Zomeren, A. H., Brouwer, W. H., and Deelman, B. G. (1984). Attentional deficits: The riddles of selectivity, speed and alertness. In D. N. Brooks (Ed.), *Closed Head Injury. Psychological Social and Family Consequences*. Oxford: Oxford University Press.

Wagenaar, R. C., Wieringen, P. C. W. V., Netelenboss, J. B., Meijer, O. G., and Kuik, D. J. (1992). The transfer of scanning training effects in visual attention after stroke: five single case studies. *Disability and Rehabilitation, 14*, 51–60.

Warden, D. L., Gordon, B., McAllister, T. W., Silver, J. M., Barth, J. T., Bruns, J., *et al.* (2006). Guidelines for the pharmacologic treatment of neurobehavioral sequelae of traumatic brain injury. *Journal of Neurotrauma, 23*, 1468–1501.

Westerberg, H., Jacobaeus, H., Hirvikoski, T., Clevberger, P., Ostensson, M.-L., Bartfai, A., and Klingberg, T. (2007). Computerised working memory training after stroke – a pilot study. *Brain Injury, 21*, 21–29.

Wilson, B. A. (1999). *Case studies in neuropsychological rehabilitation*. Oxford: Oxford University Press.

Wilson, B. A., Evans, J. J., Emslie, H., Balleny, H., Watson, P. C., and Baddeley, A. D. (1999). Measuring recovery from post traumatic amnesia. *Brain Injury, 13*(7), 505–520.

Wilson, B. A., Emslie, H. C., Quirk, K., and Evans, J.J. (2001). Reducing everyday memory and planning problems by means of a paging system: a randomised control crossover study. *Journal of Neurology, Neurosurgery and Psychiatry, 70*, 477–482.

Wilson, B. A., Evans, J. J., Emslie, H., and Malinek, V. (1997). Evaluation of NeuroPage: a new memory aid. *Journal of Neurology, Neurosurgery, and Psychiatry* (Vol. 63, pp. 113–115).

Wilson, C., and Robertson, I. H. (1992). A home-based intervention for attentional slips during reading following head injury: a single case study. *Neuropsychological Rehabilitation, 2*, 193–205.

Wilson, F. C., Manly, T., Coyle, D., and Robertson, I. H. (2000). The effect of contralesional limb activation training and sustained attention training for self-care programmes in unilateral spatial neglect. *Restorative Neurology and Neuroscience, 16*(1), 1–4.

Woischneck, D., Firsching, R., Ruckert, N., Hussein, S., Heissler, H., Aumuller, E., and Dietz, H. (1997). Clinical predictors of the psychosocial long term outcome after brain injury. *Neurological Research, 19*(3), 305–310.

Woldorff, M. G., Gallen, C. C., Hampson, S. A., Hillyard, S. R., C Pantev, Sobel, D., and Bloom, F. E. (1993). Modulation of early sensory processing in human auditory cortex during auditory selective attention. *Proceedings of the National Academy of Science, USA, 90*, 8722–8726.

Zimmermann, P., North, P., and Fimm, B. (1993). Diagnosis of attentional deficits: Theoretical considerations and presentation of a test battery. In F. Stachowiak (Ed.), *Developments in the assessment and rehabilitation of brain damaged patients*. Tubingen: G Narr-Verlagg.

Chapter 7

Assessment of perceptual disorders

L.D. Kartsounis

1 Sensation and perception

For many centuries philosophers have been asking questions about the validity of human experiences in that things are not always what they seem. More strikingly, perhaps, we have experiences in the absence of actual physical stimulation, e.g. hypnagogic hallucinations are not uncommon within the normal population (Collerton *et al.* 2005). In addressing these matters, a distinction should be made between sensation and perception. The senses capture information from the environment in various forms of physical energy (*stimulus*). They accomplish this via specially dedicated receptors of a single cell or a group of cells. The receptors convert this energy into appropriate neural signals (*sensory transduction*). Subsequent elaborations and interpretations of the neural signals in different parts of the brain (broadly referred to as *perceptual processes*) enable one to become aware of external stimulation. It is often forgotten that we do not solely derive our experience of the outside world from our senses.

1.1 Principles of assessment of perceptual disorders

The neural events taking place between sensory stimulation and interpretation are normally experienced as 'automatic'. This 'automaticity' may be lost with brain damage/disease (injury, stroke, tumour, anoxia, degenerative disorder). The affected patient is then unable to analyse environmental stimuli meaningfully. Neurologists, neuropsychologists, and other professionals are asked to identify the deficit(s) responsible for the breakdown—a task often akin to a detective's work.

For the assessment of perceptual impairments the examiner needs to be acquainted with the chain of events between sensory stimulation and awareness of stimuli. It requires sound understanding of both the nature of stimuli as sounds, sights or smells and the abilities of humans to discriminate disparate types of neural signals. Different techniques have been developed for the assessment of perceptual skills as they relate to physical stimuli (*psychophysics*). Some testing procedures have been refined into standardized formal tests. However, from time to time, procedures may need to be invented 'on the spot'. Clearly, these procedures are not in keeping with mental test theory and lack normative data. The implicit assumption in these cases is that there is discontinuity between normal and abnormal performance that can readily and universally be understood.

When perceptual skills are assessed, a range of constitutional, cultural, and other factors ought to be taken into account, including the following.

- Individuals may vary in their ability to distinguish different stimulus signals due to primary sensory deficits. Some people have defects in the eyes that prevent them from experiencing the full range of colours. Others have defects in their ears or tongues and are unable to experience aspects of sounds (e.g. pitch) and taste (e.g. bitter).

- With advancing age, senses become less sensitive and perceptual experiences become 'bland'.

- The state of the perceiver may influence the perception of a stimulus. The experience of the warmth of water in a basin does not depend on the temperature in the water alone but on the perceiver's own state at the time. If his or her hand had previously been in hot water, the water of the basin would feel cold and vice versa (John Locke).

- Cognitive processes (memories, expectations, etc) and emotional states (anxiety, mood disorders, etc) may influence perceptions.

- A patient may be unable to comply with the demands of tests due to deficits in skills different to those being examined, (e.g. severe language problems), would hinder a patient responding appropriately to tests of tactile sensitivity.

In clinical practice the assessments of perceptual skills are undertaken by different professionals. Neurological examinations include the assessment of sensory organs (eye, ear, nose), perception of pain, touch, etc. in different parts of the body. From a neuropsychological point of view the best known types of perceptual deficits are:

- auditory;
- tactile;
- visual.

A common term, 'agnosia', may be applied to all of them, implying inability to know or interpret sensory experiences.

2 Auditory recognition deficits

This is a group of disorders consisting of impairments in the ability to recognize verbal and nonverbal sounds. They may arise as a result of damage or dysfunction in different parts of the auditory system through which sounds are being processed. The auditory system includes the *outer ear,* the *middle ear* and the *inner ear* where neural impulses are generated (sensory transduction) and are transmitted to the brain via the *auditory nerve.* The auditory nerve branches into several pathways projecting to the brain stem and to other parts of the brain and then they reconvene at the auditory cortex. Each pathway processes different aspects of auditory information. Auditory perceptual deficits may be due to *conduction* loss or *neural* damage. The former relates to a disorder in the outer ear or in the middle ear due to wax, infection or otosclerosis, (i.e. immobilization of the small bones in the middle ear). Conduction loss may partially be remedied by hearing aids, mainly amplifying the sounds of speech. At central processing the range of sound frequencies over which cells respond become narrow. A *cortically deaf* patient may present with a range of auditory perceptual deficits, including abnormal pure tone, sound localization, and temporal auditory analysis.

The term '*auditory sound agnosia*' refers to a loss of the ability to recognize common sounds (e.g. bell ringing, dog barking, and train, that is not due to cortical deafness). When asked to identify these sounds the patient makes mistakes, e.g. a telephone ring may be interpreted as a sound of a railroad crossing. Auditory agnosia is often associated with bilateral lesions in the region of the superior temporal lobe (Griffiths, 2002). More generally, auditory agnosia occurs in the context of bilateral temporo-parietal pathology or bilateral subcortical pathology (Taniwaki *et al.* 2000).

2.1 Word deafness (verbal auditory agnosia)

There are more neurons dedicated to analyzing frequencies involved in speech (200–8000 hz) than other types of sounds. The term '*pure word deafness*' refers to the impairment in analysing/understanding spoken words in the context of preserved recognition of non-verbal sounds and relative preservation of spontaneous speech, reading, and writing. Unlike patients with primary comprehension problems (transcortical sensory aphasia), those with pure word deafness deficits are impaired on word repetition tasks. Word deafness is associated with bilateral pathology of the primary auditory cortex or of the underlying deep white matter (Tanaka *et al.* 1991). The critical lesions are thought to disconnect Wernicke's areas from auditory input. This is in keeping with observations indicating that the patients are neither deaf nor aphasic.

Despite the adjective 'pure', clinical experience suggests that word deafness may be associated with impairment in temporal resolution of auditory stimuli or abnormal click-fusion thresholds, although the predominant deficit involves spoken word stimuli. It is critical that the clinician establishes the integrity of primary auditory perceptual skills before a diagnosis of word deafness is made. As a first step, ask the patient to discriminate softly spoken words or finger snaps. For proper delineation of a patient's auditory sensory/perceptual skills, however, an audiological assessment is required. This includes measures of pure tone audiometry and speech detection thresholds. Provided significant auditory sensory deficits and aphasia are excluded, the assessment for word deafness may proceed by asking the patient to discriminate whether spoken pairs of words and non-words are the same or different (house/*house* versus house/*mouse*, pef/*bef*) (e.g. Kay *et al.* 1992). These tests require special care.

- Prevent lip reading.
- Make sure the patient is able to 'hold' in mind and compare two items.
- Stimulus pairs may differ according to the examiner's voice and accent (use a native speaker with clear articulation).
- It may be difficult to convey to the patient the requirements of the test and you will need to use pictorial material to demonstrate the nature of the task.

2.2 Auditory amusia

This refers to a loss of the ability to recognize familiar music (well-known melodies or a particular voice). Both hemispheres contribute to music appreciation and the anatomical correlates of amusia are multiple, underpinning the multifactorial nature of music (Stewart *et al.* 2006). Given also the wide range of individual differences in innate ability and musical education/exposure, the assessment of auditory amusia is very difficult. Melody perception, however, may be assessed by various subtests of the Seashore Test of Musical Talent.

3 Tactile recognition deficits

The tactile system is the largest sensory system in the body. A multitude of different kinds of receptors give rise to sensations of touch, texture, mechanical consistency, heat / cold and pain. The skin in the human hand, in particular, contains thousands of "mechanoreceptors" (receptors sensitive to mechanical pressure) that, together with a complex set of muscles, explore the surface of an object. The perceptual processes that underpin tactile object recognition are not well understood and may be differentially affected by different classes of object properties (Bohlhalter *et al.* 2002). Generally, impairments in tactile object recognition skills should be diagnosed in the absence of significant somatosensory impairment, neglect, aphasia, or dementia.

The somatosensory cortex receives touch information from the thalamus and this is further processed and elaborated in other parts of the cortex. Each hemisphere receives information from the contralateral side of the body. Related to the sense of touch is the information about the positions of our limbs, known as **proprioception (kinaesthesis).** The receptors of proprioception are in the muscles, tendons and joints. Tactile information is closely associated with proprioception and they both contribute to the representation of an object.

Tactile agnosia as a selective disorder has been the subject of dispute in the past, not least due to lack of precise quantitative measures. In clinical practice a useful guide to the assessment of disorders of touch is by Caselli (1997). According to this scheme, somaesthetic functions may be divided into basic, intermediate, and complex types

- *Basic* somaesthetic impairments include light touch, position sense, vibration, two-point discrimination, pain perception, and temperature (usually assessed by neurologists).
- *Intermediate* somaesthetic impairments include texture discrimination and simple form discrimination that is part of *astereognosis* (usually assessed by neurologists, sometimes by neuropsychologists).
- *Complex* somaesthetic impairments are disorders of pure forms of tactile agnosia, with preserved basic and intermediate functions. Tactile agnosia is usually associated with damage to parietal operculum.

As implied above, somaesthetic deficits are unilateral and the examiner may use a patient's good hand as control. Tactile agnosia may initially be assessed by light touch, position sense, etc. Patients are asked to discriminate texture and basic form by touch (e.g. between different kinds of edges, flat and curved surfaces). If they pass these tests (reflecting basic and intermediate skills), ask them to name objects by touch. Each object (e.g. a cassette tape) is placed randomly in either hand. Tests of tactual memory may be added, e.g. 'Which is smoother an almond or a walnut', to ensure that the deficit is specific to the tactile modality (cf. Reed *et al.* 1996). If patients are aphasic they will have difficulty in naming objects placed in either hand. When they have a specific difficulty in naming objects palpated with only one hand, tactile agnosia may be inferred.

4 Visual object recognition deficits

About 40 percent or more of the human brain is thought to be involved in vision (Werner *et al.* 2007). In keeping with this, visual object recognition deficits are more common (than those in other sensory modalities) to clinical neuropsychological practice. They are also much better understood and hence, in this review, they are presented in greater detail.

The optic nerve is formed by the axons of the retinal ganglion cells. At the optic chiasm, fibers from the inner half of each retina cross over and enter the contralateral hemisphere. Each eye, therefore, projects visual information to each hemisphere. Each visual pathway travels backwards to the Lateral Geniculate Body (LGB) that may be considered as a subdivision of the thalamus. The LGB transmits information to the visual cortex and this final part of the optic pathway is known as **"optic radiation"** (or **"geniculo-calcarine tract"**). The optic radiation is commonly compromised by vascular disorders or brain tumours, giving rise to a variety of visual object recognition deficits. It is noted that lesions that interrupt the visual pathways may also cause different visual field defects, depending on the lesion site, of which the clinical neuropsychologist needs to be aware during patient assessment.

4.1 Historical background

The first descriptions of visual object recognition disorders can be traced to the nineteenth century. In 1890 Lissauer made a distinction between deficits in the ability to consciously perceive stimuli, versus inability to ascribe meaning to what is perceived. He referred to them as *aperceptive* and *associative* 'mindblindness', respectively. Similarly, in 1891 Freud made a distinction between deficits of sensation and disorders of '*gnosis*' (knowledge)—hence the term '*agnosia*' (without knowledge). This terminology has largely survived but there is no general agreement as to what the term 'perceptual' (as in aperceptive mindblindness) denotes. For some cognitive neuropsychologists it encapsulates a wide range of deficits ranging from early visual processing to high-level object recognition impairments (e.g. Farah 1990, Humphreys, and Riddoch 1987). For others (including the present author) the term refers to more circumscribed deficits that arise after satisfactory early visual processing is accomplished and before meaning is ascribed to stimuli (see McCarthy and Warrington 1990). This is not just a theoretical point—the distinction between early visual (cortical) deficits and aperceptive deficits corresponds to different anatomical correlates and is therefore of diagnostic significance (Table 7.1). There is a wider ongoing debate regarding the classification of impairments in visual cognition. Unlike cognitive psychologists, visual physiologists and anatomists appear reluctant to accept notions of high-level visual 'agnosic' deficits. Instead, they consider them to signify impairments in integrating sensory information or accessing long-term memory. Moreover, it has recently been suggested that the thin retina tissue in the eye is capable of parsing visual information into a dozen discrete components. That is, it is thought that a significant amount of preprocessing occurs inside the eye, which subsequently sends a series of partial representations ("movies") to the brain for interpretation (Werblin and Roska, 2007). For the diagnosis of patients, however, we can continue to rely on the clinically validated neuropsychological model of object recognition deficits, as outlined in this chapter and represented in Table 7.1.

4.2 Caveats

The assessment of deficits in object recognition needs to be flexible and adaptable to the individual patient. A patient's performance may be impaired as a result of deficits in other cognitive domains.

◆ A test involving drawing for example, may primarily be failed due to motor deficits (sensory/motor weaknesses, dyspraxia), or planning (executive) problems.

◆ Visual object recognition tests may be failed due to sensory deficits, visuospatial neglect, severely restricted visual fields, or impairments in eye movements. The latter include disorders involving subcortical/brainstem structures and frontal eye fields (e.g. Luria 1976).

◆ Tests dependent on verbal responses may not be appropriate for dysphasic patients.

Table 7.1 Object recognition deficits

Early visual processing	Visual agnosias	
	Aperceptive	**Associative**
Acuity	Inability to access structure/spatial properties of visual stimuli	Inability to access meaning of visual stimuli
Eye fixation (visual disorientation)		
Movement (akinetopsia)		
Shape discrimination		
Figure/ground discrimination		
Colour (achromatopsia)		
Texture		
Anatomical correlates		
Posterior brain (occipital lobes)	Right post-Rolandic hemisphere	Inferior left post-Rolandic
No hemispheric asymmetry		hemisphere

When multiple deficits are present, one needs to validate observations with additional testing (this requires considerable expertise, and at times, inventiveness by the examiner).

It should always be remembered that visual object recognition impairments may be due to a variety of deficits, although the outcome is the same. They range from *early visual (cortical) processing disorders* to high-level deficits relating to the structure and identity of objects (*visual agnosias*).

4.3 Early visual processing disorders

Early visual processing skills are organized in a modular form. They involve specialized areas of the posterior part of the brain that code different properties, including colour, size, basic shape, and movement. Given their segregation, these skills may be selectively impaired with brain damage/disease in the occipital lobes (*partial cortical blindness*). There is no asymmetry between the two hemispheres at this level of visual processing. Early visual processing deficits are generally assessed with tests measuring physical differences between two or more stimuli.

4.3.1 Acuity

Occipital lobe damage may affect visual acuity similarly to disorders of the eye or optic nerve. There may be effects on the ability to detect the presence or absence of light, different changes in contrast sensitivity, and a target varying in size. A significant impairment in one of these aspects of acuity results in deficits in object recognition by sight. Acuity can be assessed by Snellen charts and other similar ophthalmological instruments.

When assessing visual acuity the ability of the patient to cope with the demands of commonly used acuity charts needs to be considered. Patients with lesions in the posterior areas of the brain may perform poorly for reasons other than poor acuity. They may find it difficult to fixate on or scan visual targets due to *visual disorientation* (below), *visuospatial neglect, or simultanagnosia* (inability to perceive more than one stimulus at a time). The acuity of these patients may be assessed with a test comprising simple shapes (square, circle, triangle) decreasing in size. Each target stimulus is presented individually and the clinician obtains good visual acuity measures (James *et al.* 2001).

4.3.2 Visual disorientation

This term refers to a difficulty in visually localising the position or distance of objects in space. As a result, the patient may bump into things and does not show the normal blink response when the hand of the examiner is moved rapidly towards his/her face. Related to this deficit is *optic ataxia,* a visuo-motor disorder, in which the patient has a specific difficulty in reaching (by hand) visual targets under visual guidance (Perenin and Vighetto, 1988). Both these types of early visual processing deficits are associated with lesions in the occipito-parietal boundaries (McCarthy and Warrington, 1990, Karnath and Perenin, 2005). In clinical work, the term "Balint's syndrome" in association with posterior cortical lesions is also encountered. This term lacks specificity in that it is thought to give rise to the aforementioned and additional deficits, including problems of inattention/neglect and a difficulty in processing objects that are seen sequentially at the same location (Malcolm and Barton, 2007).

To assess visual disorientation, ask the patient to count or point to random arrays of dots (e.g. Counting Dots test, Visual Object and Space Perception (VOSP) battery; Warrington and James 1991), or to pick up small items (e.g. paper clips) from a desk. You may also ask the patient to reach with the index finger towards a visual target in different parts of space, or to judge which of two differently coloured tokens or small objects placed on a desk is nearer/further from him/her. Patients with visual disorientation are impaired in all these tasks. Those with optic ataxia are only impaired on tasks involving reaching targets by hand under visual guidance.

4.3.3 Movement

The ability to locate points in space (Section 4.3.1) dissociates from the ability to detect movement of stimuli in space. A selective impairment in the perception of movement (*akinetopsia*) is very rare and associated with lateral occipitotemporal lesions. The perception of motion is thought to be *retinotopically* organized (confined to one visual field contralateral to the lesion).

Zihl *et al.* (1991) described a female patient who was able to locate targets in space but was unable to detect their movements. Visual scenes appeared to her as a series of static snapshots. She was unable to perceive traffic or to use motion as a cue when attempting to pour liquid.

For the assessment of akinetopsia, record what a patient reports when observing moving objects in space, e.g. vehicles. The patient may report a car in positions A and B but not between these two points. Milder forms of this disorder need to be studied with special equipment in ophthalmological departments.

4.3.4 Size

Some patients may be able to recognize small but not 'large' visual stimuli, e.g. letters of the alphabet (Kartsounis and Warrington 1991). This disorder may be independent of any sensory problems, including restrictions in visual fields.

Assessment of size perception:

◆ Ask the patient to judge whether lines of the same or different lengths are the same or not. Present pairs of lines in random order, one pair at a time. To control for possible visual field defects or inattention, the lines may be printed horizontally, vertically, and in other directions.

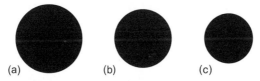

Fig. 7.1 Circles for a size discrimination test.

Fig. 7.2 Efron shapes matched for total surface.

- Ask the patient to judge whether pairs of simple geometric shapes (e.g. circles) are of the same size or not (Fig. 7.1). Randomly present the same and different pairs of shapes.

4.3.5 Shape/form

Patients may become impaired in form perception due to bilateral occipital lesions. These patients may have good visual acuity and be able to perceive colours, match surface textures, and locate obstacles in space.

Efron (1968) described a patient who was unable to recognize objects and his impairment was attributed to this fundamental deficit. Efron devised a shape discrimination test comprising stimuli of squares and oblongs matched for total surface area and contrast (simplified form of the test in Fig. 7.2). Each test stimulus is presented individually and the patient is asked to indicate whether it is a square or an oblong.

Research has indicated that certain visual skills may support action but not conscious discrimination of stimuli. A patient described by Milner and colleagues performed at chance level in discriminating a square from an oblong pattern of equal area, up to a ratio of 1:2. Despite her lack of awareness of shapes, she was able to reach and pick up solid rectangular blocks of different widths without difficulty. Her grip was perfectly precalibrated (aperture between her index finger and thumb) during midreach for a skilled grasp. These observations are consistent with the notion that there are two visual systems, one serving action (dorsal stream) and the other serving visual discrimination and cognition (ventral stream) (Milner 1997). (For implications of these notions on conscious experience, see Goodale and Milner, 2004.)

4.3.6 Figure—ground discrimination

Early visual processing skill involves figure—ground discrimination. This enables the viewer to analyse the defining outlines of a stimulus and its background separately. Impairments of this skill are associated with occipital lesions and may dissociate from form perception deficits (Kartsounis and Warrington, 1991; Davidoff and Warrington 1993). A test for the assessment of figure—ground discrimination deficits is included in the VOSP (Warrington and James 1991) (Fig. 7.3(a)).

Several other tasks can be used for the assessment of this disorder. Ask the patient to identify line drawings of simple geometric shapes, e.g. a square, circle or triangle, each

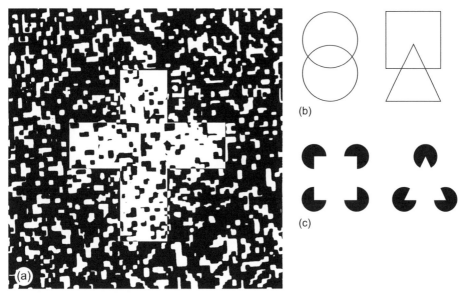

Fig. 7.3 Examples of figure ground discrimination tests. (a) Adapted from VOSP. (b) Overlapping geometric shapes. (c) Kanizsa type figures.

printed separately on a card. If the patient performs this task satisfactorily, then proceed with overlapping drawings comprising geometric shapes. Patients with figure—ground discrimination impairment may fail to report whole shapes or report parts of them (Fig. 7.3(b)). They may similarly be impaired in perceiving subjective contours (Fig. 7.3(c)).

4.3.7 Colour

Achromatopsia refers to impairment in colour perception. A patient may be unable to see colour at all or perceive colours as lacking in intensity. Impairments in colour perception are associated with occipitotemporal lesions. They may be confined to one visual field contralateral to a lesion (retinotopic).

Assessment of colour perception:

◆ Exclude congenital abnormalities.

◆ Ask the patient to name, match colour patches, or arrange them in a series according to brightness or saturation.

— The *Holmgren Wool Test* consists of pieces of wool that the patient is asked to sort according to their hues.

— The *Farnsworth–Munsell 100-Hue and Dichotomous Test for Color Vision* (Farnsworth 1943) is a more demanding task requiring the patient to arrange in the appropriate sequence coloured small counters (matched for saturation and brightness) according to hue.

— The *Ishihara plates* can also be used for testing colour vision but they may not be sensitive to milder cases of achromatopsia.

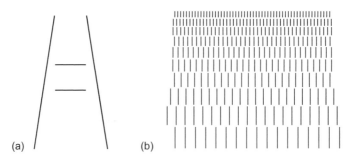

Fig. 7.4 (a) Perspective influences perceived size. (b) Texture gradient.

Unlike patients with retinal coloured blindness, achromatopsic patients are impaired in all sectors of the spectrum, although discrimination of shades of grey may be preserved.

◆ For some patients who are unable to cope with tasks involving a large number of items (above), a new test has been devised. It comprises arrays of a few colour patches of the same hue varying in brightness, including one colour patch of 'medium' brightness but of different hue. The patient is asked to indicate which patch is the odd one out (James *et al.* 2001).

Patients with left posterior lesions may have normal colour vision but are impaired in naming/comprehending colour names. Others may present with a loss of colour knowledge (*colour agnosia*). These patients find it difficult to accurately colour with crayons black and white drawings of objects, fruit, animals (e.g. a frog may be painted blue). These tests require special care—a deficit in object recognition (Section 4.4) may confound results.

4.3.8 Texture

Psychology textbooks refer to different examples of illusory phenomena whereby perspective (impression of depth) influences perceived size (Fig. 7.4(a)). However, surfaces that recede in depth (Fig. 7.4(b)) and have a visible texture, e.g. the grain in wood, may have additional effects. Texture gradients may provide precise information about the distances of surfaces and the sizes of stimuli on these surfaces. Abrupt changes in texture gradient may signal the presence of edges and corners, and strongly influence the perception of stimuli (Gibson 1950). It is likely that texture perception is selectively preserved or impaired in the same way as other early visual processing skills.

Assessment of texture perception:

◆ Ask the patient to describe stimuli with different texture gradients. Impairment is identified when the patient is unable to perceive the effects of texture (analogous deficit to the inability to perceive illusory phenomena).

4.4 **Higher visual recognition disorders**

These deficits refer to visual agnosias for *objects* or *faces* (*prosopagnosia*). The diagnosis of these disorders presupposes well preserved primary sensory and early visual processing systems (Section 4.3). Higher visual recognition problems are due to a failure in attainment of a coherent structured percept (*structural perception*) or in assignment of meaning to an object or face (*semantic processing*).

4.4.1 Structural perception of objects

In life, objects are encountered in unlimited variations. Normally, we are able to recognize them both in prototypical, and in a range of unconventional views and lighting conditions. This ability relates to *object constancy*, which may become impaired with right post-Rolandic lesions.

Patients with this disorder (*aperceptive agnosia*) are unable to process the necessary information for the attainment of coherent spatial properties of objects. It is thought that there is stored representation of objects (*object-centred representation*) with information about volume and structure of familiar objects. When this information cannot be accessed, the patient cannot identify degraded (or rotated) versions of familiar objects. In non-optimal conditions this results in misidentification of objects.

For the assessment of deficits in structural perception ('*visual perceptual deficits*' proper) a variety of test materials can be used, examples of which can be seen in Fig. 7.5. Many perceptual tasks are dependent on the ability of the patient to communicate verbally. The Object Decision test (one of the tests in VOSP) does not require verbal responses and can be used for the assessment of aphasic patients (the patient is simply required to point to target stimuli). Other tests may also be used without requiring the patient to respond

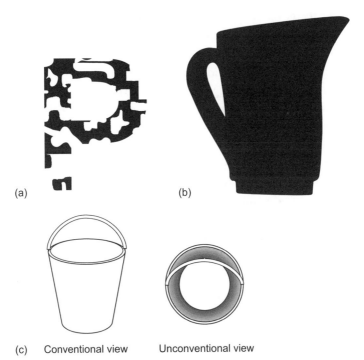

(a) (b)

(c) Conventional view Unconventional view

Fig. 7.5 Examples of perceptual tests. (a) Incomplete letter. (b) Silhouette of object. (c) Conventional view; unconventional view of object.

verbally—ask the patient to match incomplete stimuli, with their complete versions, e.g. incomplete letters, with alternative 'solid' letters.

4.4.2 Semantic processing of objects

Patients with a disorder in semantic processing (*associative visual agnosia*) perform satisfactorily on early visual processing and perceptual tests (Sections 4.3 and 4.4.1). They are able to copy objects and pictures of stimuli but fail to say what they are. Their problem is not a naming deficit. This reflects their inability to provide accurate information about the uses of objects, colour, and size and where they can be found. These patients cannot indicate whether two visually distinct examples of the 'same' object, e.g. two types of glass, have identical function. However, they may be able to identify objects by touch. Associative visual agnosia does not necessarily affect all types of visual stimuli, e.g. face recognition may be spared. Studies in the past suggested that semantic processing deficits are associated with bilateral posterior brain lesions. More recently, single-case studies of agnosic patients with unilateral left posterior (inferotemporal) lesions have superseded the earlier reports (e.g. McCarthy and Warrington 1986). That unilateral left posterior lesions are sufficient to give rise to associative visual agnosia is also indicated from group studies—patients with right posterior hemisphere lesions are impaired on perceptual tasks; patients with left posterior lesions are impaired on matching tasks.

Assessment of associative visual agnosia:

- Present patients with pictures or models of animals, tools, or other objects and ask them to name them, ask them about their properties and where they can be found. A naming test that includes different categories of stimuli can be used for this purpose (McKenna 1997).

Beware. Patients may be unable to identify objects by name due to *optic aphasia.* Both visual and verbal semantic knowledge may be preserved but a disconnection between these two cognitive domains prevents the patient from naming an object. Patients with optic aphasia are able to demonstrate the use of objects by other (nonverbal) means.

- Present patients with pictures of a wide range of objects (e.g. kitchen items, tools, sport equipment, animals, means of transport) and ask them to sort them according to use or the category to which they belong.

- Real and unreal objects (comprising configurations of features of objects that may or may not be encountered in the real world) can also be used (Riddoch and Humphreys 1993; Fig. 7.6). Ask patients to say whether these items exist in the real world or not.

- Ask patients to choose which one of two pictures relates to a target picture (Fig. 7.7). A test using this technique is the *Pyramids and Palms Trees Test* (Howard and Patterson 1992). The distractors in this task are chosen to be similar to the items matched so that the patient finds it difficult to choose simply on the basis of visual similarity.

4.4.3 Structural perception of faces

Impairments in recognition of familiar faces are collectively referred to as *prosopagnosia.* These are thought to be distinct deficits in visual recognition. The core deficit lies in a

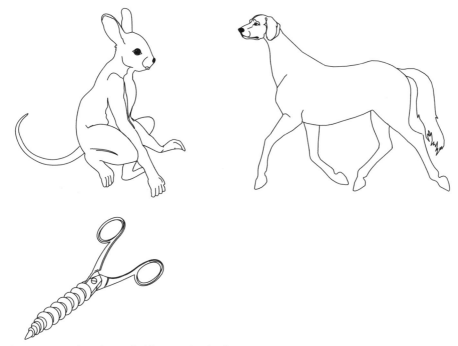

Fig. 7.6 Examples of unreal objects and animals.

selective, faulty perceptual analysis of faces (other types of visual stimuli may be perceived normally). This disorder is associated with lesions in the posterior regions of the right hemisphere.

Assessment of deficits in the structural perception of faces:

◆ Patients may be assessed on tasks involving photographs of three or more faces differing in sex or age ('who is the oldest?'), with faces photographed from different viewpoints or with same/different expressions ('is it the same or a different person?'). Patients affected by structural deficits find it difficult to tackle these tasks or are very slow in their responses, tending to use a feature-by-feature analysis.

◆ More formally, structural disorders in face recognition can be assessed with the *Benton Facial Recognition Test* (Benton *et al.* 1978). Patients are required to find a target face amongst six alternative faces shown in different viewpoints and different lighting conditions.

4.4.4 Semantic processing of faces

Patients with this type of prosopagnosia are capable of passing structural perceptual tests (Section 4.4.3) but are unable to recognize familiar faces. They may be able to recognize them by other features, including their voices, hairstyles, and clothing. Semantic deficits in face recognition can be assessed using photographs of family members, friends, and well known public figures.

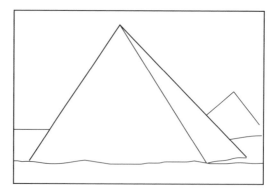

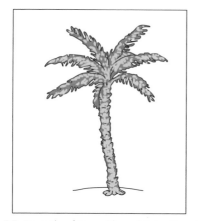 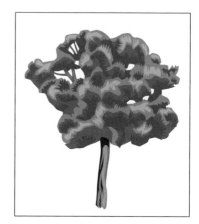

Fig. 7.7 Example of Pyramids and Palm Trees Test.

A test for assessing face recognition ability has been devised by Young and colleagues (Ellis *et al.* 1989). It consists of two sets of public figures, one comprising 20 very well known people (e.g. Margaret Thatcher, John Wayne) and another comprising 20 'low-familiarity' faces (e.g. Marlene Dietrich and Max Bygraves). A further set of 20 comprises unfamiliar faces. The test requires that each face is first rated for familiarity on a 7-point scale ('totally unfamiliar'–'highly familiar'). The subject is then asked to provide the known person's profession and name. This is a sensitive test, yielding quantitative measures at different levels of familiarity, leading to complete recognition of a face. It is limited by the fact that 'familiar' faces need to be updated. Another potential critical variable that may confound results is the individual patient's media exposure (or lack thereof) (e.g. Kapur *et al.* 1999).

Prosopagnosic patients may show covert recognition skills for faces. Although unable to identify faces verbally, they may show differential electrodermal responses to familiar and unfamiliar faces involving correct and incorrect face–name pairings. They may also show different reaction times and memory performance towards familiar versus unfamiliar faces. However, these techniques are not readily accessible to the clinical neuropsychologist (and are usually used as research tools).

4.4.5 False recognition of faces

A complementary deficit to prosopagnosia may be observed in patients with right frontal lesions, that is, 'recognition' for unfamiliar faces. This type of deficit is considered to be due to an impairment in strategic memory retrieval and monitoring, typical of patients with frontal lesions.

4.4.6 Recognition of emotional expressions

The ability to recognize emotional expressions may dissociate from the ability to identify faces. Patients with right hemisphere damage are more likely to be impaired than those with left hemisphere damage. They may become impaired in recognizing the emotion of fear (following amygdalectomy) and disgust (presymptomatic patients with Huntington's disease). For the assessment of these disorders clinicians may use a test by Young *et al.* (2002) or devise their own stimuli depicting unambiguous emotions. For a greater variety of emotional expressions see e.g. Ekman *et al.* (1972).

5 Conclusion

The implicit assumption in the above review is that visual object recognition skills have a hierarchical and parallel organization (Table 7.1). In ordinary clinical practice however, object recognition disorders are 'random'. The question arises as to where a clinician should start when assessing a patient with object and/or face recognition problems.

The first consideration is to obtain information on potential sensory problems, visuospatial neglect, aphasia, etc. that may at least partly account for perceptual/agnosic deficits. As a general rule, clinicians should be alert to the complaints and errors patients make during other tasks involving picture interpretation. They may 'misname' (misperceive) common objects or give 'don't know' answers when asked to name them. Questions about the properties/uses of these stimuli may elicit further information about the underlying impairments—e.g. whether these reflect language or visual recognition deficits. Patients' answers may also suggest the level of the visual recognition deficit.

- If they refer to very limited, basic features of an object when shown a picture (e.g. 'there is a line here and another one there…'), it may be assumed that the disorder reflects an early visual processing deficit. Formal tests of early visual processing should then be the starting point (e.g. point localization to exclude visual disorientation, form perception, figure/ground discrimination).

- If patients are able to indicate the basic structural form of a stimulus but fail to identify it correctly, their deficits are more likely to be of a higher order. In these cases the assessment should start with tests of apperceptive agnosia (object decision, incomplete letters tasks, and other degraded stimuli).

- When perceptual skills are found to be well preserved, proceed with tests of associative agnosia (questions about properties of objects, matching tasks, etc.) (Table 7.2).

Clearly, when a patient is known to be grossly impaired in analysing a wide range of real stimuli, including objects, faces, etc., testing should begin with early visual processing tasks.

Table 7.2 Tests of object recognition deficits

Early visual processing	Visual agnosias	
	Aperceptive	Associative
◆ *Acuity* Snellen charts, Queen Square*	Incomplete Letters, Object Decision, Silhouettes (VOSP)	Questions *re* names, colour, size location, functions of objects (pictures/models)
◆ *Visual disorientation* Point Localization, Dot Counting *Size*: see Fig. 7.1	Stimuli shown from unconventional views (BORB)	Sorting of stimuli (pictures/ models) according to category
◆ *Shape*: see Fig. 7.2	*Copying tasks*	Matching objects that are visually dissimilar but have the same function
◆ *Figure/ground* VOSP		The Pyramids and Palm Trees Test
◆ *Colour* Holmgren Wool Test, Farnsworth–Munsell 100-Hue Test, Queen Square*, Ishihara		
◆ *Texture*: see Fig. 7.4(b)		

*Queen Square Cortical Vision Screening Test.

If the patient fails these tests, there is no need for tests of visual agnosias either of the aperceptive or associative type—any agnosia diagnosed in this context would be 'pseudo-agnosia' (Warrington 1985).

The assessment methods outlined above are adequate for the identification of the main types of impairments in object recognition. Occasionally, and for a more precise definition of a deficit, the clinician may need to devise a series of new tests. In doing so, both the precise nature of a deficit may be delineated and refinement in our knowledge of object recognition may be attained. This knowledge can then be harnessed for the development of more sensitive and accurate methods of assessment.

Selective references

Benton, A. L., Hamsler, K., Varney, N. R., and Spreen, O. (1978). *Contributions to neurological assessment*. Oxford University Press, New York.

Bohlhalter, S., Fretz, C. and Weder, B. (2002) Hierarchical versus parallel processing in tactile object recognition. *Brain*, **125**, 2537–48.

Caselli, R. J. (1997). Tactile agnosia and disorders of tactile perception. In *Behavioural neurology and neuropsychology* (ed. T.E. Feinberg and M.J. Farah), pp. 277–88. McGraw-Hill, New York.

Collerton, D., Perry, E. and McKeith, I. (2005). A novel Perception and Attention Deficit model for recurrent complex visual hallucinations. *Behavioral and Brain Sciences*, **28** (6), 737–57.

Davidoff, J. and Warrington, E. K. (1993). A dissociation of shape discrimination and figure–ground perception in a patient with normal acuity. *Neuropsychologia* **31**, 83–93.

Ellis, A. W., Young, A. W., and Critchley, E.M.R. (1989). Loss of memory for people following temporal lobe damage. *Brain* **112**, 1469–83.

Farah, M.J. (1990). *Visual agnosia*. MIT Press, Cambridge, MA.

Farnsworth, D. (1943). Farnsworth–Munswell 100-Hue and Dichotomous Test for Color Vision. *J. Opt. Soc. Am.* **33**, 568–78.

Gibson, J. J. (1950). *The perception of the visual world*. Houghton-Mifflin, Boston.

Goodale, M. A. and Milner, A. D. 2004. *Sight unseen: An exploration of conscious and unconscious vision*. Oxford University Press, Oxford.

Griffiths T. G. (2002). Central Auditory Pathologies. *British Medical Bulletin*, **63** (1), 107–120.

Howard, D. and Patterson, K. (1992). *The Pyramids and Palm Trees Test*. Thames Valley Test Company, Bury St Edmunds.

Humphreys, G. W. and Riddoch, M. J. (1987). *To see or not to see: a case study of visual agnosia*. Lawrence Erlbaum, London.

James, M., Plant, G. T., and Warrington, E. K. (2001). *The Queen Square Cortical Vision Screening Test*. Thames Valley Test Company, Bury St Edmunds.

Kapur, N., Thompson, P., Kartsounis, L.D., and Abbott, P. (1999). Retrogade amnesia: clinical and methodological caveats. *Neuropsychologia* **37**, 27–30.

Karnath, H. D. and Perenin, M. T. (2005). Cortical control of visually guided reaching: Evidence from patients with optic ataxia. *Cerebral Cortex* **15**(10), 1561–69.

Kartsounis, L. D. and Warrington, E. K. (1991). Failure of object recognition due to a breakdown of figure–ground discrimination in a patient with normal acuity. *Neuropsychologia* **29**, 969–80.

Kay, J., Lesser, R. and Coltheart, M. (1992). *Psycholinguistic assessments of language processing in aphasia*. Lawrence Erlbaum Associates, Hove, East Sussex.

Luria, A.R. (1976). *The working brain, an introduction to neuropsychology*. Penguin Books, Middlesex.

McCarthy, R. A. and Warrington, E. K. (1986). Visual associative agnosia: a clinico-anatomical study of a single case. *J. Neurol. Neurosurg. Psychiatry* **49**, 1233–40.

McCarthy, R. A. and Warrington, E. K. (1990). *Cognitive neuropsychology, a clinical introduction*. Academic Press, London.

McKenna, P. (1997). *The Category-Specific Names Test*. Psychology Press, Hove, East Sussex.

Malcolm, G. L. and Barton, J. J. S. (2007). "Sequence agnosia" in Balint's syndrome: Deficits in visuo-temporal processing after bilateral parietal damage. *Journal of Cognitive Neuroscience* **19**, 102–8.

Milner, A. D. (1997). Vision without knowledge. *Phil. Trans. R. Soc. Lond. B, Biol. Sci.* **352**, 1249–56.

Perenin, M. T. and Vighetto, A. (1988). Optic ataxia. *Brain* **111**(3), 643–74.

Reed, C. L., Caselli, R. J., and Farah, M. J. (1996). Tactile agnosia: underlying impairment and implications for normal tactile object recognition. *Brain* **119**, 875–88.

Riddoch, M. J. and Humphreys, G. W. (1993). *Birmingham Object Recognition Battery (BORB)*. Lawrence Erlbaum Associates, Hove, East Sussex.

Stewart, L., von Kriegstein, K., Warren D.J. and Griffths, T.D. (2006) Music and the brain. *Brain* **129**, 2533–53.

Tanaka, Y., Kamo, T., Yoshida, M. and Yamadori, A. (1991). So-called cortical deafness. *Brain* **114**, 2385–2401.

Taniwaki, T., Tawaga, K., Sato, F. and Iino, K. (2000). Auditory agnosia restricted to environmental sounds following cortical deafness and generalized auditory agnosia. *Clinical Neurology and Neurosurgery* **102**, 156–62.

Warrington, E. K. (1985). Agnosia: the impairment of object recognition. In *Handbook of clinical neurology*, Vol 45 (ed. P.J. Vinken, G.W. Bruyn, and H.L. Klawans), pp. 333–49. Elsevier Science Publishers, Amsterdam.

Warrington, E. K. and James, M. (1991). *Visual Object and Space Perception Battery (VOSP)*. Thames Valley Test Company, Bury St Edmunds.

Werblin, F, and Roska, B. (2007). The movies in our eyes. *Scientific American*, **296**, 55–61.

Werner J. S, Pinna, B. and Spillmann L. (2007). Illusory color and the brain. *Scientific American*, **296**, 70–75.

Young, A., Perrett, D., Calder, A., Sprengelmeyer, R. and Ekman, P. (**2002**) *Facial Expression of Emotion: Stimuli and Tests*. Thames Valley Test Company, Bury St Edmunds.

Zihl, J., Von Cramon, D., and Schmid, C.H. (1991). Disturbance of movement vision after bilateral posterior brain damage. *Brain* **114**, 2235–52.

Chapter 8

Recovery and treatment of sensory perceptual disorders

C. Groh-Bordin and G. Kerkhoff

1 Basic principles of perceptual (re)-learning

In an early survey of studies about learning in the three main modalities, Gibson (1953) showed that nearly any sensory or motor ability can be improved considerably by training in healthy subjects. More recently, the neural changes within the sensory cortices have been described as the neural substrate of such perceptual learning processes (cf. Gilbert *et al.* 2001; Fahle 2005). This cortical plasticity can be assumed to be a prerequisite for sensory-perceptual relearning after brain damage. However, the capacity for full recovery through training is often limited by several factors, (e. g. aetiology, age, and size of lesion), as well as the affected modality and the preserved sensory ability. In any case, perceptual rehabilitation accounts for some basic principles which are briefly illustrated below.

Principles of treatment in sensory perceptual neurorehabilitation

- **Restitution**. Direct, repetitive training of the impaired function is expected to promote improvements that are important in themselves, but also relevant for other related abilities (e.g. training of basic somatosensory abilities not only improves these abilities, but also has positive effects on motor performance since somatosensory perception is important for motor control; see Section 3.2). The efficacy of restitutive treatments is more limited in "lower" cortical areas (e.g. primary sensory cortex) than in "higher cortical areas" (parietal lobe; Buonomano and Merzenich 1998).

- **Compensation**. Utilization of a spared function to compensate for a deficit; e.g. in patients with homonymous scotomata the treatment of visual scanning and reading effectively reduces everyday problems associated with the field cut (bumping into obstacles or persons, slow reading) but has little effect on the field defect itself. Compensation techniques are widely used in sensory perceptual rehabilitation because restitution of elementary sensory deficits is often strictly limited due to the relatively fixed brain topography of primary sensory cortical representations (primary visual, auditory, or somatosensory cortices).

> **Principles of treatment in sensory perceptual neurorehabilitation** *(continued)*
>
> ◆ **Substitution**. Use of technical/prosthetic devices to compensate for a deficit (e.g. use of special light-absorbing glasses in patients with blinding, to reduce the amount of light). Also, environmental changes designed to adapt the patient's environment optimally to those deficits that cannot be cured by restitution or compensation treatments (e.g. modifying the house of a patient to improve his spatial orientation and reduce falls).
>
> ◆ **Combination of Principles**. In sensory perceptual neurorehabilitation it is often necessary and fruitful to combine any of the principles listed above to maximize the outcome for the patient.

In the following sections of this chapter, information on recovery from and treatment techniques for sensory perceptual disorders in the visual, somatosensory, and auditory modalities will be provided.

2 Visual disorders

Visual-perceptual disorders occur after brain damage in about 30% of patients with cerebrovascular disorders and some 50% of patients with traumatic brain injury (TBI). Consequently, routine screening of the various types of visual deficits is necessary for rehabilitation planning. Non-neglecting patients can easily be assessed using the following questionnaire (and respond correctly in 95% of the cases) (see Table 8.1).

2.1 Visual acuity

Primary and secondary causes of impaired static visual acuity have to be distinguished before initiating treatment.

◆ *Primary causes:* Bilateral postchiasmatic lesions (Frisén 1980) may cause between partial and total loss of visual acuity in both eyes which cannot be corrected by glasses. This is often associated with bilateral visual field defects (Kerkhoff 1999).

◆ *Secondary causes:* Disturbed visual exploration, fixation difficulties due to Balint's syndrome, impaired contrast sensitivity, eccentric fixation due to cerebral hypoxia, or nystagmus. Impairments in acuity for moving targets (dynamic acuity) are caused by deficient smooth pursuit eye movements (Haarmeier and Thier 1999).

2.1.1 Recovery

Recovery is frequent in patients with secondary, but rare in those with primary causes of disturbed visual acuity. As impaired acuity affects all subsequent visual activities as well as neuropsychological testing, treatment of the secondary causes should be started immediately.

2.1.2 Treatment

The following short interventions can be given (cf. Kerkhoff 2000)

◆ *Bilateral postchiasmatic lesion:* Use magnification software (for PCs), or screen reading machines for permanent enlargement of printed text, pictures, and letters.

Table 8.1 Schema for the anamnesis of visual disorders after acquired brain lesions. Insert the questions in the table into the following phrase: "Have you experienced … since your brain lesion?" (Based on Kerkhoff *et al.* 1990)

Question	Purpose of Question, Underlying Disorder
1. … any changes in vision …?	- Awareness of deficits? Information about case history
2. … diplopia …? transiently/permanently?	- Type of gaze palsy? If transient: fusional disorder?
3. … reading problems …? … syllables/words missing, change of line, reduced reading span …?	- Hemianopic alexia? Differential diagnosis of neglect dyslexia, aphasic alexia, or pure alexia
4. … problems in estimating depth on a staircase …? … reaching with your unimpaired hand for a cup, hand, door handle …?	- Depth perception? Optic ataxia?
5. … bumping into obstacles …? … failure to notice persons …? at which side?	- Visual exploration deficits in homonymous visual field disorders?
6. … blinding after exposure to bright light …?	- Foveal photopic adaptation?
7. … dark vision …? … that you need more light for reading … ?	- Foveal scotopic adaptation?
8. … blurred vision …? transiently/permanently?	- Contrast sensitivity? Acuity? Fusion?
9. … that colours look darker, paler, less saturated …?	- Colour hue discrimination? Impaired contrast sensitivity?
10. … that faces look darker, paler, unfamiliar …?	- Face discrimination/recognition disorders?
11. … problems in recognizing objects …?	- Object discrimination/recognition disorders?
12. … problems in finding your way in familiar/ unfamiliar environments …?	- Topographic orientation deficits?
13. … visual hallucinations (stars, dots, lines, fog, faces, objects …) or illusions (distorted objects, faces …) …?	- Simple or complex visual hallucinations, illusions? Awareness about illusory character?

- *Visual exploration deficit*: Improve visual search by providing the patient with a systematic (horizontal or vertical) saccadic search strategy. Acuity will improve when visual search is more systematic, quicker and when omissions are reduced (see Section 2.5.2).

- *Nystagmus*: Calm nystagmus with orthoptic (prisms) or pharmacological means (Straube and Kennard 1996).

- *Spasmodic fixation* (Balint's syndrome): Test acuity with single letter charts; acuity for single letters should be normal. Furthermore, improving simultaneous perception by repetitive treatment enlarges the useful field of view (Perez *et al.* 1996) and improves activities of daily living.

- *Dynamic visual acuity*: Treat smooth pursuit eye movements in the horizontal domain (left, right) for different velocities. The recognition of moving objects is important for vocational tasks (Gur and Ron 1992) and mobility in the environment. It improves in parallel with the increase of smooth pursuit gain.

2.2 Spatial contrast sensitivity (CS), foveal photopic and scotopic adaptation, visual discomfort

Spatial CS denotes the ability to discriminate between striped patterns (gratings) of differing luminance (contrast) and stripe width (spatial frequency). It is often impaired in posterior brain lesions (80%, Bulens *et al.* 1989).

- Foveal photopic adaptation means the continuous adapting to a brighter illumination;
- scotopic adaptation means the adaptation to a darker illumination than the present one.

Both processes are dissociable and impaired in some 20% of patients with posterior cerebral artery infarctions or cerebral hypoxia (Zihl and Kerkhoff 1990).

2.2.1 Recovery

- *Contrast Sensitivity*: Rapid recovery in the majority of patients; permanent deficits in about 20%.
- *Adaptation*: No recovery (even after years) present in the patients tested so far (Zihl and Kerkhoff 1990).

2.2.2 Treatment

- *Impaired CS*: CS can be trained effectively in normal subjects but this has never been tried in brain damaged patients. In those 20% with permanent deficits the use of additional, indirect lighting is helpful because it improves contrast.
- *Isolated loss of photopic adaptation or combined disorder*:
  — Avoid direct lighting, use dimmer to adjust light individually;
  — Avoid flickering neon lights;
  — Use sun glasses outside buildings;
  — Avoid continuously adapting sun glasses (Varilux) because they are too expensive and too slow in readapting inside a building.
  — Car driving at night ("blinding") is not advisable.
- *Isolated loss of scotopic adaptation*: Increase indirect lighting by additional light bulbs, use dimmer to adjust lighting individually.

2.3 Stereopsis and convergent fusion

Local and global stereopsis are reduced in patients with occipital, parietal or temporal brain lesions and impair manual activities in near space (reaching and grasping, technical work, depth perception), which is relevant for vocational rehabilitation. Convergent fusion is a prerequisite of stereopsis and refers to the fusion of the left and right eye's image to one combined (fused) picture of the world. Fusion is impaired in some 20% of patients with posterior vascular lesions and about 1/3 of TBI patients (Kerkhoff 2000). Patients with impaired fusion have severe reading problems after some 10 minutes. They rapidly develop diplopia and are impaired in all near-work activities.

2.3.1 Recovery

The percentage of patients showing recovery is unknown in stereopsis. In TBI patients with fusional disorders 3/4 have persistent disorders for years after their injury (Hart 1969).

2.3.2 Treatment

Fusion and stereopsis can be trained together using simple orthoptic or binocular devices (Kerkhoff and Stögerer 1994) within the following treatment plan:

- *Anamnesis*: Asthenopic disorders (eye pressure, fatigue in reading or PC-work), blurred vision, problems in near-work activities?
- *Therapy*: Improvement of fusion and stereopsis by repetitive display of dichoptic images with increasing disparity angle; 8-20 sessions advisable.
- *Outcome*: Favourable in 80% of patients; improvements in reading duration, stereopsis and fusional range; relief from asthenopia; better functioning in vocational life.
- *Exclusion criteria*: Premorbid deficits in binocular integration; permanent diplopia with angle >15°.

2.4 Visual discomfort

Looking at homogeneous, regular patterns like lines, written text, flagstones or stripes of a certain spatial frequency (3-4 cycles per degree visual angle, Wilkins 1986) elicit unpleasant sensations (termed "visual discomfort"), blurred vision and headaches in some healthy subjects, but much more so in patients with cerebral visual disorders. Visual discomfort in brain lesioned patients may reduce sustained visual activities considerably and lead to asthenopic symptoms.

2.4.1 Recovery

Unknown.

2.4.2 Treatment

In reading, visual discomfort can be eliminated by using a simple mask that covers all lines except the one that is currently read.

2.5 Homonymous visual field disorders (VFDs)

VFDs are present in 20–30% of all neurological patients in neurorehabilitation centers. Visual field sparing is 5° or less in 70% of them (Zihl and von Cramon 1986). VFD patients may present with three types of associated deficits: visual exploration deficits, reading disorders and visuospatial deficits.

- *Visual exploration deficit*: Time-consuming, inefficient visual search due to loss of overview and unsystematic search strategies; numerous, small-amplitude staircase-saccades in blind hemifield; omissions of targets in blind field

  (Zihl 1995a, Pambakian *et al.* 2000, 2004).

- *Hemianopic reading disorder:* Slow reading with few errors in VFDs with field sparing < 5°, also present in paracentral scotomas and quadrantanopia; reading of short, single words is normal (no aphasia or alexia; Zihl 1995b, Leff *et al.* 2000).

- *Visuospatial deficits:* Subjective midline (in line bisection) is shifted towards the blind field (horizontally in left/right VFDs, vertically in altitudinal VFDs) in 90% of patients (Kerkhoff 1993, Barton and Black 1998); this shift is also evident in daily life (walking through doorways, sitting in front of a table).

2.5.1 Recovery

Field recovery is present in the first 2–3 months post-lesion in up to 40% of the patients with a stable aetiology (Zhang *et al.* 2006). After 6 months postlesion, spontaneous recovery is extremely unlikely (Zihl and von Cramon 1986, Zhang *et al.* 2006).

2.5.2 Treatment

Since field recovery is very limited, restorative field training is appropriate only in a very small group of patients (detailed below). For the majority of VFD patients (95%) compensatory visual field treatment of the associated disorders in reading and visual scanning is advocated (see Table 8.2).

Recently, Bologninie *et al.* (2006) have suggested cross-modal (visual-auditory) training for the improvement of reading and scanning in hemianopia. Here, visual and auditory targets are presented time-locked in different locations of the visual field, and the patient has to saccade to them. This is an effective additional training.

Ineffective or disadvantageous therapies:

- Prisms are in most cases useless for the treatment of VFDs because patients become confused. However, in selected cases small prisms fitted to a spectacle have been found useful.

- Compensatory head shifts towards the scotoma (either spontaneously adopted by the patient or instructed by staff) are of *no use* in the rehabiltation of VFDs, because they lead to visual exploration deficits in the ipsilesional visual field, stays of the neck muscles, and delay treatment progress in visual scanning training (Kerkhoff *et al* 1992).

- Training of 'blindsight' in VFDs is probably not a useful therapy (Zihl and Kennard 1996) because it does not lead to improved functioning in daily life.

In the last decade, restorative visual field training has been revived after publication of advantageous results following new training procedures (Kasten *et al.* 1998). However, numerous replication studies have not found significant visual field enlargements (Nelles *et al.* 2001, Pambakian *et al.* 2004, Reinhard *et al.* 2005). Table 8.3 summarizes the main findings of the discussion. The results clearly suggest that compensatory visual field training is advisable for 95% of patients with visual field defects, whereas restorative field training is only promising when lesions are incomplete and a high degree of visual capacities (light, motion, form, or colour perception) are preserved in specific regions of the scotoma (Kerkhoff 2000).

Table 8.2 Summary of compensatory (hemianopic reading and visual exploration training) and restorative (visual field training) approaches in patients with postchiasmatic scotoma

---

Compensatory visual field training: hemianopic reading training

---

1. **Anamnesis:** change of line, types of errors (omissions, substitutions, problems with long words or numbers), maximum reading duration, asthenopic disorders

2. **Type of Treatment:** improvement of oculomotor reading strategies to substitute the lost parafoveal visual field; tachistoscopic reading of single words, moving window technique, floating words, search for words in a text, scanning reading technique, training of numbers with embedded zeros; variation of physical and linguistic parameters: word length and frequency, position on screen (left, centre, right), number of words, presentation time, complexity of text, variation of instructions

3. **Transfer:** reading of newspapers, books, own manuscripts; text editing on a PC, increase of maximal reading duration

4. **Outcome and follow-up:** increase in reading speed; 500% reduction in reading errors; partial field recovery (mean 5 °) in 1/3 of patients

---

Compensatory visual field training: visual exploration training

---

1. **Anamnesis:** limited overview, bumping into persons and obstacles, defective orientation in visual space, e.g. crowded situations, traffic

2. **Type of Treatment:** increase amplitude and velocity of saccadic eye movements towards scotoma: variation of size, reduction of saccadic reaction time; discourage head movements or compensatory head shifts; teach systematic, spatially organized (horizontal or vertical) visual search strategy on wide-field displays; start search in blind field; use visual displays requiring serial and parallel search; possibly combination with other stimulation devices (optokinetic stimulation); alternative account: audiovisual (crossmodal) training (see text for details)

3. **Transfer:** treat orientation in clinic, own urban district, new environments, management of *visual* ADLs: find objects on table or in room, find therapist's room, find objects in supermarket, cross street, use public traffic, find way home

4. **Outcome and follow-up:** reduction of omissions and search time; partial field recovery (mean: 5–7 °) in 34% of patients

---

Restorative visual field training

---

1. **Anamnesis:** residual visual capacities (often movement of a stimulus) in regions of scotoma; search for amblyopic transition zones (with partially preserved function) which are most likely candidates for field recovery; however, such transition zones are present only in some 10–20% of patients.

2. **Type of Treatment:** improvement of saccadic localization at field border or in amblyopic transition zone; recognition of colour, form, orientation, or luminance of the target

3. **Transfer:** improvement in reading und subjective awareness of visual problems

4. **Outcome and follow-up:** mean field increase: 5–10°; stability at follow-up; 70% of patients have a field recovery < 5°

2.6 Visual hallucinations

Simple, formed, visual hallucinations (light dots, bars, lines, stars, fog, coloured sensations, etc.; Lance 1976) are frequently reported by patients (only when questioned systematically!) with posterior vascular lesions, and occur most frequently following occipital lesions. More complex visual hallucinations and illusions are rare and most often associated with temporal lobe lesions (Kölmel 1984, 1985).

Table 8.3 A comparison of compensatory versus restorative visual field training

	Compensatory visual field training (reading, saccadic scanning training)	Restorative visual field training
Objective visual field enlargement after treatment?	+, 0–5° in a subgroup of patients, no field improvement in the majority of patients	+, 2–5° in computer-based campimetry, no field enlargement (0.0°) in fundus-controlled visual field tests
Objective improvements in reading and visual scanning?	+++, 20–50% improvement in reading (speed and errors)	+, 8% improvement in reading (speed)
Subjective improvements in visual activities of daily living?	+++, great improvements in 90% of patients treated	+, small improvements
Number of required treatment sessions?	++, 25–50 hours (for reading and scanning training)	+++, 100–150 hours
Vocational improvements after therapy?	+++, return to job in >90 % of treated hemianopic patients	?
Costs?	++ (max 1000 Euro for software)	+++, 5000 Euro for software

Legend: + (small), ++ (medium), +++ (high), ? (not known)

2.6.1 Recovery

Recovery is rapid and complete in 95% of patients, so that at 6 weeks postlesion the occurrence is quite rare (Kölmel 1984, 1985).

2.6.2 Treatment

As hallucinations and illusions are irritating but mostly transient phenomena, therefore information to and reassurance of the patient are important.

- *Inform your patient*: Visual hallucinations are quite normal but *transient* phenomenon after a vascular brain lesion.

- *Calm your patient*: Most patients experiencing simple hallucinations know that they perceive erroneous visual stimuli not present in the outer visual world. Tell the patient that he/she is not going mad. If necessary, demonstrate to the patient that hallucinations can be provoked in any person by pressing the eye-ball (pressure phosphenes) or when suddenly rising from a supine position (blood-pressure-related).

- *Complex vs. simple hallucinations*: Complex visual scenes have a higher reality character than simple hallucinations, and are therefore more frightening for the patient. These patients are very reluctant to talk about their experience because they fear being misdiagnosed as a psychiatric case. Note, that psychiatric patients more frequently experience *auditory* versus *visual* hallucinations, while the opposite holds true for patients with organic visual hallucinations following posterior brain lesions. Furthermore, brain damaged patients very rarely report "hearing voices".

- *Persistent visual hallucinations*: Check whether there is an epileptic focus (EEG), the possibility of a new infarction developing, or a psychiatric disease.

2.7 Colour perception

Colour and form perception can be impaired within a scotoma after postchiasmatic VFD, or within central vision after postchiasmatic lesions of various aetiologies (Meadows 1974; Zeki 1990). The deficit in central vision may range from a subtle deficit in hue discrimination (often with unilateral occipitotemporal lesions) to a nearly total achromatopsia after bilateral lesions.

2.7.1 Recovery

Recovery of colour and form vision within a scotoma are often observed in patients with partial field recovery (Zihl and von Cramon 1985). As a rule, the progression of visual recovery (if there is one!) in VFDs is as follows:

Light detection → light localization → brightness discrimination → form discrimination → colour perception.

Hence, colour vision is the last to recover. In those patients with colour vision deficits in central vision, no recovery has been reported over six years in one study (Pearlman *et al.* 1979).

2.7.2 Treatment

- *Defective colour vision in visual field regions*: In patients with residual colour perception in a scotoma and incomplete lesions, improvement of colour discrimination can be trained by displaying coloured targets at the field border and having the patient saccade to them and discriminate the colour (as described in Table 8.2, visual field training).
- *Defective colour perception in central vision:* Forced discrimination of differently coloured forms is partially effective in cerebral anoxia, however with limited transfer to non-trained colours (Merrill and Kewman 1986). Often, the patients can learn to base their colour judgments on other cues such as the brightness or saturation despite permanently impaired hue discrimination.

2.8 Visual form recognition

Recognition deficits for simple visual forms (rectangle, square, triangle, etc.) without a semantic dimension (such as real objects) is only observed in patients with extensive bilateral or diffuse-disseminated, posterior brain lesions. When present, the patients are unable to discriminate simple geometric forms equated for total luminance (Milner *et al.* 1991). The rareness of the disorder is due to the fact that it occurs most often after extensive anoxic brain damage.

2.8.1 Recovery

Recovery is often incomplete or even absent, possibly due to the bilateral or diffuse-disseminated lesions in cerebral anoxia or carbon monoxide poisoning. The case reported by Sparr *et al.* (1991) showed the disorder to be stable for more than 40 years. Recovery may be more likely in patients with cerebrovascular aetiologies and/or unilateral lesions.

2.8.2 Treatment

Visual form recognition can be improved by repetitive discrimination training for simple geometric forms equated for total luminance. Verbal or computerized feedback is essential, as are progressive increase in the similarity of the stimuli to be discriminated. As a result, visual form discrimination of simple geometric forms but also of line drawings and partially of photographs displaying real objects is improved, along with increased visual acuity and contrast sensitivity. Treatment can be accomplished either with self-constructed paper-made stimuli, or with computerized devices which give detailed quantitative feedback and allow variations of colours, sizes and forms (c. f. Kerkhoff and Marquardt 1998).

2.9 Visual object and face perception

The inability to recognize visual objects (visual agnosia) and faces (prosopagnosia) are rare conditions, occurring probably in less than 1% of all neurological patients (Zihl and Kennard 1996). Both types of agnosia occur most frequently after bilateral occipitotemporal lesions (Farah 1990). In object agnosia, a more perceptual (apperceptive agnosia) and a more conceptual (associative agnosia) subform are usually distinguished. The former indicates a deficit in perceptual object discrimination; the latter implies a loss of semantic knowledge related to visually presented objects (Farah 1990).

2.9.1 Recovery

Detailed case reports about recovery are rare. Partial recovery in the recognition of real life objects has been occasionally noted, while recognition of photographs of objects or faces rarely improves. Recovery is particularly unlikely in anoxic brain damage, probably due to the widespread diffuse lesions and the additional cognitive impairment impeding the acquisition of compensatory strategies (Sparr *et al.* 1991). Partial recovery is more likely in traumatic or vascular lesions and in those few cases with unilateral right sided lesions showing face agnosia (Farah 1990).

2.9.2 Treatment

Controlled treatment studies are rare. Zihl and Kennard (1996) noted improvement of object and face discrimination on photographs and in real life in three patients following an intensive (120 hours) treatment procedure focusing on the specific search for key features of objects or faces. Furthermore, the use of context information (knowledge about objects and faces and the relevant social situation) is advisable and helpful for these patients.

2.10 Visual motion perception

Relative impairments of visual motion perception may occur after focal lesions of the motion centre in the occipito-parieto-temporal cortex, but permanent deficits are probably rare, and even in these patients only relative (frequency of relative deficits: 13%, Schenk and Zihl 1997). However, many brain damaged patients subjectively report problems in estimating the velocity and position-changes of moving vehicles in traffic (as a pedestrian, or in a car). This may result either from impaired motion perception (linearly or in depth), disturbed visuospatial perception, or a combination of both.

2.10.1 Recovery

Little is known about recovery. In those rare patients with bilateral lesions, no recovery has been reported (Zihl *et al.* 1991), while those with unilateral lesions may show recovery. Even the motion-blind patient reported by Zihl *et al.* (1991) readapted to moving stimuli in daily life by certain compensatory techniques, despite her permanent motion deficit under laboratory conditions.

2.10.2 Treatment

Due to the rarity of severe impairments in visual motion processing and the probable multiplicity of cortical and subcortical areas involved in visual motion perception, treatment approaches have not been developed. However, the treatment of an associated ability, that is, smooth pursuit eye movements when tracking a moving target, is useful for improving visual scanning on PC-screens and visual orientation in daily life (Gur and Ron 1992). Treatment can be accomplished by use of a large PCscreen, where the subject follows a moving target in different directions with a stabilized head. Target velocity should be adapted so that pursuit eye movements can be performed with relatively few catch-up saccades. In addition, a training of situations in daily life where motion is important (crossing a street, using a moving staircase), can improve orientation and reduce the likelihood of accidents due to reduced motion perception. Secondary cues may help to code visual motion of vehicles (i.e. by position or size changes), despite a stable impairment in motion processing under laboratory conditions.

3 Somatosensory disorders

Somatosensory deficits are present in the majority of hemiplegic patients and hence in about 30–40% of all stroke patients with unilateral lesions. Hermsdörfer *et al.* (1994) found in a large sample of 272 brain damaged patients, 29.8% had somatosensory disorders, and 37.9% subjectively reported somatosensory hallucinations, metamorphognosia, hypersensitivity, or pain. Of those patients impaired on somatosensory testing, the frequencies of differential deficits were:

- Impaired passive movement discrimination of fingers (82.7%), wrist (70.4%), elbow (51.8%), shoulder (48.2%)
- Impaired localisation of finger parts (55.5%)
- Impaired two-point discrimination of the index finger (53.1%)
- Impaired astereognosis (37.1%)
- Impaired detection of light finger touches (32.1%)

3.1 Recovery

Few systematic patient studies of recovery exist. Primate studies indicate substantial recovery of somatosensory dysfunctions spontaneously and after controlled treatment (Jenkins *et al.* 1990).

3.2 **Treatment**

The few controlled treatment studies for patients with tactile deficits indicate that these can be trained efficiently (Goldman 1966; Zane and Goldman 1966; Yekutiel and Guttman 1993; Carey and Matyas 2005). The following types of treatment are useful and have been evaluated quantitatively:

- *Retraining of different somatosensory functions*: Most somatosensory abilities can be trained (location of touch, sense of elbow position, two-point-discrimination, stereognosis) using the following therapeutic principles (Yekutiel and Guttman 1993):

  a) Improve awareness of sensory dysfunction by allocating attention to it;

  b) Start treatment with sensory tasks the patient *can do* in order to improve motivation and reduce frustration;

  c) Use or develop tasks that are interesting and relevant for the patient, which involve selective attention because this improves sensory functioning;

  d) Also use vision and the good hand during training to teach tactics and useful strategies of perception;

  e) Frequent rests are necessary.

One key feature of this approach is the implementation of systematic sensory training in relevant functional tasks. Examples of such tasks are: identification of line orientations; discrimination of shape, size, weight, or temperature of objects placed in patient's contralesional hand; identification of forms drawn with a pencil on the patient's hand/arm from a visually presented multiple-choice display (detailed in Yekutiel and Guttman 1993).

- *Tactile extinction training*: The objective is to improve the patient's attention to double simultaneous stimulation (DSS) of the hand's surface. For this purpose, either light touches of different fingers or positions on the hand or any other body region can be used. Patients are required to direct their attention to the touch on the impaired hand, which should be hidden from direct vision. The improvements obtained with this simple procedure are impressive, reducing tactile extinction of contralesional stimuli considerably (Goldman 1966; Zane and Goldman 1966). A critical therapeutic element is the focussing of attention towards the contralesional tactile stimulus and the relearning of the'twoness' of the DSS task.

- *Improvement of tactile functions by peripheral magnetic stimulation (RPMS)*: With this novel method the dorsal palm of the contralesional hand is stimulated magnetically (non-painfully). After a single (20 minute) stimulation session we found a 27% reduction in tactile extinction for different surfaces delivered to both hands, while a matched control group did not show any improvement (Heldmann *et al.* 2000). Probably, multiple stimulation sessions lead to stable and greater improvements. Subjectively, the patients report that they feel more in their contralesional arm; this could be especially helpful in patients with tactile neglect and unawareness of their contralesional hand/arm.

- *Optokinetic stimulation (OKS)*: OKS moving to the contralesional hemispace in patients with tactile neglect (Vallar *et al.* 1997) improves the subjective awareness of different angular arm positions (contra- and ipsilesional arm) and reduces tactile extinction (Nico 1999) transiently. Repetitive OKS over several sessions should improve tactile and kinaesthetic functions permanently.

- *Treatment combinations*: Although speculative, the combination of several treatments might be most effective and could improve the patient's self-awareness for the contralesional body side. Furthermore, the use of visual imagery might be helpful for patients with astereognosis since this process is helpful in tactile object recognition and mediated by the intact visual cortices (Deibert *et al.* 1999).

4 **Auditory disorders**

Significant alterations to a variety of auditory-perceptual functions have been reported following lesions below as well as beyond the medial geniculate bodies (auditory radiation). For the most part, the deficits can be categorized into *audio-spatial disorders* and *auditory feature discrimination* deficits, suggestive of modular processing in audition (Rauschecker 1998).

4.1 **Audiospatial disorders**

Among these, the following deficits have been reported, and will be summarized here together with the few findings about recovery and treatment.

4.1.1 Deviation of the subjective straight ahead or midline position

Patients with spatial neglect, often following right parietal lesions, show a significant shift of their subjective auditory midline in the horizontal plane in front and back space. This shift may be to the ipsilesional side in front and back space (Vallar *et al.* 1995), or ipsilesionally in front space and contralesionally in back space (Kerkhoff *et al.* 2006). Patients without neglect, but with homonymous hemianopia show the opposite, contralesional deviation (i. e. towards the scotoma; Kerkhoff *et al.* 1999).

- *Recovery*: During recovery from multimodal neglect the ipsilesional auditory midline shift often regresses. Likewise, during improvement of compensatory visual exploration functions in patients with homonymous visual field disorders (see 2.5.2), a reduction of the contralesional auditory midline shift is also observed.

- *Treatment*: Optokinetic stimulation (OKS) towards the neglected hemispace normalizes the auditory midline shift transiently and permanently after repetitive treatment (Kerkhoff *et al.* 2001).

4.1.2 General spatial uncertainty of auditory localization

Patients with visual neglect after right parietal lesions (Pavani *et al.* 2001) often have a general deficit in auditory localization (but not necessarily in detection) in their contralesional hemispace (horizontally and vertically). Patients undergoing cerebral hemispherectomy initially also show large localization errors in their contra-operated hemispace.

- *Recovery*: Zatorre *et al.* (1995) reported substantial recovery of auditory localisation in the contralesional hemispace in patients with unilateral hemispherectomy. Obviously, long-term experience can lead to a substantial reorganisation of the brain processes responsible for spatial hearing. Clinical experience in neglect patients indicates that localization accuracy improves as general attentional capacities improve (see Chapters 5, 6, 23).
- *Treatment*: No systematic studies are available. As in visuospatial neglect, sustained attention training may reduce the general uncertainty of neglect patients in auditory localization.

4.1.3 Auditory extinction of contralesional stimuli

This occurs after lesions of the auditory pathways in the temporal lobes (De Renzi *et al.* 1984) of either hemisphere, or in small lacunar lesions (Arboix *et al.* 1996).

- *Recovery*: Rapid recovery is found after frontal lobe lesions while persisting auditory extinction occurs following lesions of the auditory pathways (De Renzi *et al.* 1984).
- *Treatment*: No systematic studies are available.

4.1.4 Auditory motion processing

The right parietal cortex is involved in horizontal auditory motion perception (Griffiths *et al.*1998), and consequently right parietal cortex lesions impair auditory motion discrimination (Griffiths *et al.* 1996).

- *Recovery*: Unknown.
- *Treatment*: Unknown.

4.2 Deficits in auditory feature discrimination

The following deficits have been reported and will be summarized together with the few findings on recovery and treatment.

4.2.1 Cortical deafness

Cortical deafness is an extremely rare condition resulting either from brain-stem lesions, subcortical lesions disrupting the auditory pathways, or from bilateral temporal lobe lesions destroying the primary auditory cortex bilaterally (cf. Polster and Rose 1998). It comprises, as in cerebral blindness, the total or near-total inability to hear any sounds despite preserved afferent pathways to the primary auditory cortices.

Recovery: Some degree of recovery has been noted (Mendez and Geehan 1988). Usually, cortical deafness evolves into auditory agnosia, followed by selective auditory agnosia for certain tasks, pure word deafness, and/or amusia, and finally a residual disorder of temporal processing.

- *Treatment*: No treatments have been published due to the rareness of permanent deficits.

4.2.2 Auditory agnosia

Auditory agnosia is the inability to recognise auditorily presented sounds independent of any deficit of processing spoken language. This may include the inability to recognise environmental (i.e. different vehicles) and human sounds (coughing, baby cries), although perception and perceptual discrimination of these sounds is unimpaired, and peripheral hearing is normal as well. Generally, the disorder is thought to be analogous to the two types of visual object agnosia found after bilateral occipitotemporal lesions (apperceptive and associative agnosia, see 2.9). As in vision, a differentiation into a more perceptual deficit, probably most often found after right-hemispheric (temporal lobe) lesions, and a more associative-semantic deficit, most often seen in left-hemispheric lesions is made (Polster and Rose 1998).

- *Recovery*: Engelien *et al.* (1995) observed recovery in a case of auditory agnosia which was paralleled by activations (assessed with PET) in a large bilateral frontal, middle temporal, and inferior parietal network. Further, they noted activation of peri-infarct cortices which may enable recovery from auditory agnosia. In a case with "deaf-hearing" after bilateral auditory cortex lesions, directing selective attention to sound recognition improved auditory functions considerably and was paralleled by bilateral PET-activations in the lateral prefrontal, middle temporal, and cerebellar cortices (Engelien *et al.* 2000). In summary, selective attention may play a key role in adapting to auditory disorders. Surviving perilesional cortex, as well as more wide-spread cortical networks in both hemispheres may be critical for behavioural recovery.

- *Treatment*: Fechtelpeter *et al.* (1990) described a treatment for environmental sound recognition in a patient with auditory agnosia due to bilateral temporal lesions. The four-week treatment included the following elements and may be paradigmatic for similar cases:

  — *Sound imitation*: The patient had to imitate or actually perform a typical sound of an object (e.g. telephone) and was then later confronted with the tape-recorded sound of this object and asked to decide whether they were the same;

  — *Semantic association*: The patient had to associate a sound to a specific object out of a sample of ten visually presented objects;

  — *Auditory analysis*: The therapist taught the patient acoustic features of specific sounds (a starting car first makes a deep sound, and then interrupted sounds according to the different gears).

All treatment techniques effectively reduced the auditory deficits with a significant transfer to daily life in this case. These or similar, individually adapted techniques may be used to treat patients with auditory agnosia or more subtle perceptual deficits.

4.2.3 Pure word deafness

This is defined as the inability to process spoken words despite normal hearing thresholds and normal processing of auditory, non-language stimuli.

- *Recovery:* As mentioned above, pure word deafness often evolves into a more subtle auditory-perceptual disorder (Mendez and Geehan, 1988).
- *Treatment*: Unknown.

4.2.4 Nonverbal auditory perception and recognition disorders

Among these the following types of deficits have been described:

- *Phonagnosia*: Impaired recognition of familiar voices due to right hemispheric lesions (reviewed in Polster and Rose 1998).
- *Voice discrimination disorders*: Impaired perceptual discrimination of different voices (unfamiliar) after right temporal lesions (cf. Polster and Rose 1998).
- *Impaired perception of emotional prosody*: This occurs preferentially in right-hemispheric lesions and denotes the inability to understand affectively intoned speech (Ross 1981).
- *Impaired perception of pitch direction*: This occurs after right temporal lesions (Johnsrude *et al.* 2000).
- *Altered music perception*: This is mostly impaired after right or bilateral temporal lesions (cf. Polster and Rose 1998).
- *Nonrecognition of environmental sounds*: This occurs in right temporal lesions (cf. Polster and Rose 1998).
- *Temporal processing disorders*: These have been described in unilateral lesions of either hemisphere, but the left hemisphere is most critical for short acoustic transients.
- *Hypersensitivity to sounds*: This occurs in TBI patients (Waddell 1984) and is often coupled with hypersensitivity to light (blinding, see 2.2.2). The problem is important in work rehabilitation (avoid noisy workplaces!).
- *Recovery and treatment*: No systematic studies are available.

5 Conclusion

There is now growing evidence for the efficacy of cognitive rehabilitation in general (Cicerone *et al.* 2005), and visuoperceptual training in particular (Jutai *et al.* 2003), for patients with brain damage. Systematic treatments of somatosensory dysfunctions are just developing, despite their frequency and relevance to the patient. Nevertheless, the above mentioned techniques provide promising approaches towards significant improvements to the patients' disturbances (for further review, see Nowak and Hermsdörfer 2008). The consequences of auditory-perceptual deficits in daily life are increasingly well understood. Often it is assumed that most of these deficits can be compensated for easily, since either preserved auditory abilities may be used for compensation, or multiple cues are available in daily life. However, this view may be wrong, as many patients do not spontaneously report, and therefore fail to be aware of, their auditory deficits. Hence, the consequences for nonverbal communication are likely to be underestimated (as for example in neglect patients who seldom complain about their auditory deficits).

Selective references

Arboix, A., Junqué, C., Vendrell, P., and Marti-Vilalta, J. L. (1996). Auditory ear extinction in lacunar syndromes. *Acta Neurologica Scandinavica*, **81**, 507–511.

Barton, J. J. S., and Black, S. (1998). Line bisection in hemianopia. *Journal of Neurology Neurosurgery and Psychiatry*, **64**, 660–662.

Bellmann, A., Meuli, R., and Clarke, S. (2001). Two types of auditory neglect. *Brain*, **124**, 676–687.

Bisiach, E., Cornacchia, R., Sterzi, R., and Vallar, G. (1984). Disorders of perceived auditory lateralization after lesions of the right hemisphere. *Brain*, **107**, 37–54.

Bolognini, N., Rasi, F., Coccia, M., and Ladavas, E. (2005). Visual search improvement in hemianopic patients after audio-visual stimulation. *Brain*, **128**, 2830–2842.

Bouwmeester, L., Heutink, J., and Lucas, C. (2007), The effect of visual training for patients with visual field defects due to brain damage: a systematic review. *Journal of Neurology, Neurosurgery, and Psychiatry*, **78**, 555–564.

Bulens, C, Meerwaldt, J. D., Van der Wildt, G. J., and Keemink, C. J. (1989). Spatial contrast sensitivity in unilateral cerebral ischaemic lesions involving the posterior visual pathway. *Brain*, **112**, 507–520.

Carey, L. M., and Matyas, T. A. (2005). Training of somatosensory discrimination after stroke: Facilitation of stimulus generalization. *American Journal of Physical Medicine and Rehabilitation*, **84**, 428–442.

Cicerone, K. D., Dahlberg, C., Malec, J. F., Langenbahn, D. M., Felicetti, T., Kneipp, S., *et al.* (2005). Evidence-based cognitive rehabilitation: Updated review of the literature from 1998 through 2002. *Archives of Physical Medicine and Rehabilitation*, **86**, 1681–1692.

De Renzi, E, Gentilini,M., and Pattacini, F. (1984). Auditory extinction following hemisphere damage. *Neuropsychologia*, **22**, 733–744.

Deibert, E., Kraut, M., Kremen, S., and Hart, J. (1999). Neural pathways in tactile object recognition. *Neurology*, **52**, 1413–1417.

Engelien, A., Huber, W., Silbersweig, D. *et al.* (2000). The neural correlates of 'deaf-hearing' in man. Conscious sensory awareness enabled by attentional modulation. *Brain*, **123**, 532–545.

Engelien, A., Silbersweig, D., Stern, E. *et al.* (1995). The functional anatomy of recovery from auditory agnosia. A PET study of sound categorization in a neurological patient and normal controls. *Brain*, **118**, 1395–1409.

Fahle, M. (2005). Perceptual learning: Specificity versus generalization. *Current Opinion in Neurobiology*, **15**, 154–160.

Farah, M. (1990). Visual agnosia. Cambridge, Massachusetts, MIT Press.

Fechtelpeter, A., Göddenhenrich, S., Huber, W., and Springer, L. (1990). Ansätze zur Therapie von auditiver Agnosie. *Folia Phoniatrica*, **42**, 83–97.

Frisén, L. (1980). The neurology of visual acuity. *Brain*, **103**, 639–670.

Gilbert, C. D., Sigman, M., and Crist, R. E. (2001). The neural basis of perceptual learning. *Neuron*, **31**, 681–697.

Goldman, H. (1966). Improvement of double simultaneous stimulation perception in hemiplegic patients. Archives of Physical Medicine & Rehabilitation, **63**, 681–687.

Griffiths, T. D., Rees, A., Witton, C. *et al.* (1996). Evidence for a sound movement area in the human cerebral cortex. *Nature*, **383**, 425–427.

Griffiths, T. D., Rees, G., Rees, A. *et al.* (1998). Right parietal cortex is involved in the perception of sound movement in humans. *Nature Neuroscience*, **1**, 74–79.

Gur, S., and Ron, S. (1992). Training in oculomotor tracking, occupational health aspects. *Israel Journal of Medical Science*, **28**, 622–628.

Haarmeier, T., Thier, P. (1999). Impaired analysis of moving objects due to deficient smooth pursuit eye movements. *Brain*, **122**, 1495–1505.

Hart, C. T. (1969). Disturbances of fusion following head injuries. *Proceedings of the Royal Society of Medicine*, **62**, 704–706.

Heldmann, B., Kerkhoff, G., Struppler, A., and Jahn, Th. (2000). Repetitive peripheral magnetic stimulation alleviates tactile extinction. *NeuroReport*, **11**, 3193–3198.

Hermsdörfer, J., Mai, N., Rudroff, G., and Münßinger, M. (1994). Untersuchung zerebraler Handfunktionsstörungen. Borgmann Verlag, Dortmund.

Jenkins, W. M., Merzenich, M. M., Ochs, M. T. *et al.* (1990). Functional reorganization of primary somatosensory cortex in adult owl monkeys after behaviorally controlled tactile stimulation. *Journal of Neurophysiology*, **63**, 82–104.

Johnsrude, I. S., Penhune, V. B., and Zatorre, R. J. (2000). Functional specificity in the right human auditory cortex for perceiving pitch direction. *Brain*, **123**, 155–163.

Jutai, J. W., Bhogal, S. K., Foley, N. C., Bayley, M., Teasell, R. W., and Speechley, M. R. (2003). Treatment of visual perceptual disorders post stroke. *Topics in Stroke Rehabilitation*, **10**, 77–106.

Kasten, E., Wüst, St., Behrens-Baumann, W., and Sabel, B. A. (1998). Computer-based training for the treatment of partial blindness. *Nature Medicine*, **4**, 1083–1087.

Kerkhoff, G., (1993). Displacement of the egocentric visual midline in altitudinal postchiasmatic scotomata. *Neuropsychologia*, **31**, 261–265.

Kerkhoff, G., and Marquardt, C. (1998). Standardised analysis of visuospatial perception after brain damage. *Neuropsychological Rehabilitation*, **8**, 171–189.

Kerkhoff, G. (1999). Restorative and compensatory therapy approaches in cerebral blindness - a review. *Restorative Neurology and Neuroscience*, **15**, 255–271.

Kerkhoff, G. (2000). Neurovisual rehabilitation, recent developments and future directions. *Journal of Neurology, Neurosurgery, and Psychiatry*, **68**, 691–706.

Kerkhoff, G., Artinger F., and Ziegler, W. (1999). Contrasting spatial hearing deficits in hemianopia and spatial neglect. *NeuroReport*, **10**, 3555–3560.

Kerkhoff, G., Münssinger, U., Haaf, E. *et al.* (1992). Rehabilitation of homonymous scotomata in patients with postgeniculate damage of the visual system, saccadic compensation training. *Restorative Neurology and Neuroscience*, **4**, 245–254.

Kerkhoff, G., Schaub, J., and Zihl, J. (1990). The anamnesis of cerebral visual disorders after brain damage (German). *Nervenarzt*, **61**, 711–718.

Kerkhoff, G., and Stögerer, E. (1994). Recovery of fusional convergence after systematic practice. *Brain Injury*, **8**, 15–22.

Kerkhoff, G. (2003). Modulation and dehabilitation of spatial neglect by sensory stimulation. *Progress in Brain Research*, **142**, 257–271.

Kerkhoff, G., *et al.* (2006). Rotation or translation. *Neuropsychologia*, [vol? page numbers?]

Kölmel, H. W. (1984). Coloured patterns in hemianopic fields. *Brain*, **107**, 155–167.

Kölmel, H. W. (1985). Complex visual hallucinations in the hemianopic field. *Journal of Neurology, Neurosurgery, and Psychiatry*, **48**, 29–38.

Lance, J. W. (1976). Simple formed hallucinations confined to the area of a specific visual field defect. *Brain*, **99**, 719–734.

Leff, A. P., Scott, S. K., Crewes, H., Hodgson, T. L., Cowey, A., Howard, D. *et al.* (2000). Impaired reading in patients with right hemianopia. *Annals of Neurology*, **47**, 171–178.

Meadows, J. C. (1974). Disturbed perception of colours associated with localized cerebral lesions. *Brain*, **97**, 615–632.

Mendez, M. F., and Geehan, G. R. (1988). Cortical auditory disorders, clinical and psychoacoustic features. *Journal of Neurology, Neurosurgery, and Psychiatry*, **51**, 1–9.

Merrill, M. K., and Kewman, D. G. (1986). Training of color and form identification in cortical blindness, a case study. *Archives of Physical Medicine & Rehabilitation*, **67**, 479–483.

Milner, A. D., Perrett, D. I., Johnston, R. S. *et al.* (1991). Perception and action in visual form agnosia. *Brain*, **114**, 405–428.

Nelles, G., Esser, J., Eckstein, A., Tiede, A., Gerhard, H., and Diener, H. C. (2001). Compensatory visual field training for patients with hemianopia after stroke. *Neuroscience Letters*, **306**, 189–192.

Nico, D. (1999). Effectiveness sensory stimulation in tactile extinction. *Experimental Brain Research*, **127**, 175–182.

Nowak, D. A., and Hermsdörfer, T. (2008). Stroke. In D. A. Nowak and T. Hermsdörfer (Eds.), Sensorimotor Control of Grasping: Physiology and Pathophysiology. Cambridge: Cambridge University Press.

Pambakian, A. L., Mannan, S., Hodgson, T L., and Kennard, C. (2004). Saccadic visual search training: a treatment for patients with homonymous hemianopia. *J. Neurol. Neurosurg. Psychiatry*, **75**, 1443–1448.

Pambakian, A. L.M., Wooding, D. S., Patel, N., Morland, A B., Kennard, C., and Mannan, S. K. (2000). Scanning the visual world: a study of patients with homonymous hemianopia. *J. Neurol. Neurosurg. Psychiatry*, **69**, 751–759.

Pavani, F., Ladavas, E., and Driver, J. (2002). Selective deficit of auditory localisation in patients with visuospatial neglect. *Neuropsychologia*, **40**, 291–301.

Pearlman, A. L., Birch, J., Meadows, J. C. (1979). Cerebral color blindness, an acquired defect in hue discrimination. *Annals of Neurology*, **5**, 253–261.

Perez, F. M., Tunkel, R. S., Lachmann, E. A., and Nagler, W. (1996). Balints-Syndrome arising from bilateral posterior cortical atrophy or infarction - rehabilitation strategies and their limitation. *Disability and Rehabilitation*, **18**, 300–304.

Polster, M. R., and Rose, S. B. (1998). Disorders of auditory processing, evidence for modularity in audition. *Cortex*, **34**, 47–65.

Rauschecker, J. P. (1998). Parallel processing in the auditory cortex of primates. *Audiology and NeuroOtology*; **3**, 86–103.

Reinhard, J., Schreiber, A., Schiefer, U., Kasten, E., Sabel, B. A., Kenkel, S. *et al.* (2005). Does visual restitution training change absolute homonymous visual field defects? A fundus controlled study. *British Journal of Ophthalmology*, **89**, 30–35.

Ross, E. D. (1981) The aprosodias. Functional-anatomic organization of the affective components of language in the right hemisphere. *Archives of Neurology*, **38**, 561–569.

Schenk, Th., Zihl, J. (1997) Visual motion perception after brain damage, I. Deficits in global motion perception. *Neuropsychologia*, **35**, 1289–1297.

Sparr, S. A., Jay, M., Drislane, F. W., Venna, N. (1991) A historic case of visual agnosia revisited after 40 years. *Brain*, **114**, 789–800.

Spitzyna, G. A., Wise, R. J.S., McDonald, S. A., Plant, G. T., Kidd., D., Crewes, H., and Leff, A. (2007). Optokinetic therapy improves text reading in patients with hemianopic alexia. A controlled trial. *Neurology*, **68**, 1922–1930.

Straube, A., and Kennard, C. (1996). Ocular Motor Disorders. In, Brandt, T., Caplan, L. R., Dichgans, J., Diener, H. C., Kennard, C., editors. Neurological Disorders. Course and Treatment. San Diego, Academic Press, 101–11.

Vallar, G., Guariglia, C., Nico, D., and Bisiach, E. (1995). Spatial hemineglect in backspace. *Brain*, **118**, 467–472.

Vallar, G., Guariglia, C., and Rusconi, M. L. (1997). Modulation of the neglect syndrome by sensory stimulation. In, Thier P, Karnath H-O, editors. Parietal Lobe Contributions to Orientation in 3D Space. Berlin, Springer, 555–78.

Waddell, P. A., Gronwall, D. M.A. (1984). Sensitivity to light and sound following minor head injury. *Acta Neurologica Scandinavia*, **69**, 270–276.

Wilkins, A. (1986). What is visual discomfort? *Trends in Neurosciences*, **9**, 343–346.

Yekutiel, M., and Guttman, E. (1993). A controlled trial of the retraining of the sensory function of the hand in stroke patients. *Journal of Neurology, Neurosurgery, and Psychiatry*, **56**, 241–244.

Zane, M. D., and Goldman, H. (1966). Can response to double simultaneous stimulation be improved in hermiplegic patients? *Journal of Nervous and Mental Disease*, **142**, 445–452.

Zatorre, R. J., Ptito, A., Villemure, J-G. (1995) Preserved auditory spatial localization following cerebral hemispherectomy. *Brain*, **118**, 879–889.

Zeki, S. (1990). A century of cerebral achromatopsia. *Brain*, **113**, 1721–1777.

Zhang, X., Kedar, S., Lynn, J. J., Newman, N. J., and Viousse, V. (2006). Natural history of homonymous hemianopia. *Neurology*, **66**, 901–905.

Ziegler, W., Kerkhoff, G., ten Cate, D., Artinger, F., and Zierdt, A. (2001). Spatial processing of spoken words in aphasia and in neglect. *Cortex*, **37**, 754–756.

Zihl, J. (1995a). Visual scanning behavior in patients with homonymous hemianopia. *Neuropsychologia*, **33**, 287–303.

Zihl, J. (1995b). Eye movement patterns in hemianopic dyslexia. *Brain*, **118**, 891–912.

Zihl, J., von Cramon, D., Mai, N., and Schmid, C. (1991). Disturbance of movement vision after bilateral posterior brain damage. Further evidence and follow up observations. *Brain*, **114**, 2235–2251.

Zihl, J., Kennard, C. (1996). Disorders of higher visual functions. In, Brandt T, Caplan LR, Dichgans J, Diener HC, Kennard C, editors. Neurological Disorders. Course and Treatment. San Diego, Academic Press, 201–12.

Zihl, J., and Kerkhoff, G. (1990). Foveal photopic and scotopic adaptation in patients with brain damage. *Clinical Vision Sciences*, **2**, 185–195.

Zihl, J., and von Cramon, D. (1985).Visual field recovery from scotoma in patients with postgeniculate damage. *Brain*, **108**, 335–365.

Zihl, J., and von Cramon, D. (1986). Recovery of visual field in patients with postgeniculate damage. In, Poeck K, Freund HJ, Gänshirt H, editors. Neurology. Heidelberg, Springer, 188–94.

Further reading

Bouwmeester, L., Heutink, J., and Lucas, C. (2007). The effect of visual training for patients with visual field defects due to brain damage: a systematic review. *Journal of Neurology, Neurosurgery, and Psychiatry*, **78**, 555–564.

Kerkhoff, G. (2000). Neurovisual rehabilitation: recent developments and future directions. *Journal of Neurology, Neurosurgery, and Psychiatry*, **68**, 691–706.

Nowak, D. A., and Hermsdörfer, T. (2008). Stroke. In D. A. Nowak & T. Hermsdörfer (Eds.), *Sensorimotor Control of Grasping: Physiology and Pathophysiology*. Cambridge: Cambridge University Press.

Chapter 9

Neuropsychological assessment of memory disorders

Veronica Bradley and Narinder Kapur

1 Introduction

Memory difficulties are often the first and the most prominent sign of insidious or acute cerebral dysfunction, and may also represent the most common, or most notable, disability that remains after initial recovery from brain pathology. This is because of the wide range of brain regions that are usually involved in performing a memory task, even one that appears quite simple in its demands; at least one component of memory processing - encoding, storage or utilisation (retrieval, recognition, etc.) is likely to be affected. It follows that most neuropsychological assessments will include tests of memory, and the clinician will select tests that will enable him/her to answer questions that differ according to the context of the referral. When the main purpose of the assessment is diagnostic, consideration of the pattern of performance on memory tests and the severity of the memory deficit relative to deficits in other areas of cognitive functioning will enable an opinion to be given about the most likely cause of the impairment. For example, memory loss is the hallmark of the majority of presentations of Alzheimer's disease. In the early and middle stages of the illness the memory impairment will be marked in relation to other cognitive deficits, while in the cortico-subcortical dementias (which may accompany, for example, Parkinson's disease, Huntington's disease, and progressive supranuclear palsy) memory impairment may be more subtle and accompanied by characteristic executive deficits and slowing of response. Other questions that should be addressed in the diagnostic assessment are the following:

- To what extent can the patient continue with his/her normal activities?
- What coping strategies can be recommended on the basis of the strengths and weaknesses identified in the assessment?

The information obtained from the assessment may inform the decision to treat. For example, in normal pressure hydrocephalus, the extent to which cognitive impairment affects quality of life will be taken into account when the neurosurgeon discusses with the patient the benefits and risks of insertion of a shunt. Additionally, the presence of a co-occurring disorder will affect the risk-benefit ratio. A certain amount of information on prognosis can be given on the basis of a single assessment, but repeated assessment will provide additional information. Repeat assessment is essential when the requirement is to monitor the recovery or decline of memory function which occurs naturally or following medical/surgical intervention.

When the assessment is carried out for the purposes of rehabilitation the assessment results will help to identify areas of weakness that may be targeted in the rehabilitation programme, as well as preserved abilities that may help the patient to compensate for deficits. More generally, information about the patient's capacity to learn will always be helpful in determining the most fruitful approach to rehabilitation. For example, if there is relative preservation of learning, repeated instruction or repeated presentation of material may pay off. If there is little capacity to benefit from repeated presentation of material then external cues may need to be provided.

The effects of memory disorders on everyday life vary with the severity and nature of the disorder, from mild deficits that can be effectively managed with the help of memory aids (such as a diary or a notebook) to severe difficulties that render independent living impossible. It should, however, be borne in mind that even mild impairments can be quite disruptive for people whose jobs or personal circumstances require highly efficient memory processing. Kapur and Moakes (1995) describe the devastating effects of post-encephalitic amnesia on a young woman's everyday life. She regained some degree of quality of life, but a return to her job as a teacher was not possible. Household chores could be completed, but only by following a strict routine. Even the preparation of a shopping list was a problem because, as the authors point out, knowing that a particular item is needed requires memory. Different types of memory impairment can give rise to more circumscribed (and more easily managed) difficulties, such as inability to do mental arithmetic resulting from working memory deficit (Campbell and Conway 1995).

2 Memory: theoretical background and terminology

There is now a considerable body of research indicating that human memory is a multi-component system. Theories about different components of the system abound. For clinical purposes, a model developed from studies of dysfunctional memory resulting from neurological illness or insult is appropriate. Such a model also underpins a good deal of experimental work, including investigations of neurologically unimpaired subjects. Some components of the memory system, such as perceptual representation memory, which briefly records a visual or auditory image of a stimulus (termed iconic and echoic memory, respectively), have been investigated quite extensively in experimental studies, but are not readily testable in the clinical setting and will not be discussed here. In recent years, experimental studies using techniques such a positron emission tomography (PET) scanning and functional magnetic resonance imaging (fMRI) have enhanced our understanding of brain activity during both clinical and experimental tests. These developments have not yet fundamentally changed approaches to the assessment of memory disorders in the clinic, though they may do so in the future (Bigler 2001).

2.1 Terminology (Fig. 9.1)

2.1.1 Short- and long-term memory

A pervasive distinction in clinical and experimental studies of human memory is that between short- and long-term memory, though aspects of this distinction have been

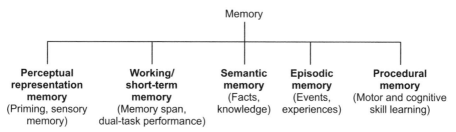

Fig. 9.1 Memory systems & associated components.

called into question (Ranganath and Blumenfeld, 2005). *Short-term memory* has typi-cally been used to refer to a system that stores a limited amount of information for a short period of time. Neuropsychologists should be aware that the medical profession, and indeed the general public, may have a rather different understanding of the term 'short-term memory'. They use it to refer to everyday episodic memory settings, covering events over a few hours, days or weeks, often using it as synonymous with the term 'recent memory'. They contrast this with memory for events that have occurred many years before, which in clinical settings is termed *long-term memory* or 'remote memory'. Most clinical and cognitive psychologists use the term 'short-term memory' or, more commonly, *working memory*, to refer to a set of processes for holding and manipu-lating in temporary store, over a period of seconds, information that has just been acquired.

2.1.2 Implicit versus explicit memory

Two further broad distinctions, based on testing methodology, have been made in mem-ory research. One distinguishes *implicit* from *explicit* memory. The terms do not describe memory systems as such, and are generally used to refer to varying states of awareness of the individual with respect to stored memories.

- *Implicit memory* is memory that is expressed through behavioural or physiological changes, where the individual has absent or limited conscious awareness of the informa-tion that has been stored. It usually includes tasks such as priming, conditioning, and skill learning. An important set of observations that gave rise to the concept of implicit memory indicates that amnesic patients who present with profound explicit memory impairment may be able to implicitly retain new information, or learn new skills. An example is the ability to learn to perform a pursuit rotor task where a moving target is tracked by a probe. *Implicit memory* has been extensively investigated experimentally. It is not routinely assessed in the clinical setting, partly because of the absence of standardised tests, but spared or impaired functioning may be detectable in the pattern of performance on certain tests, such as enhanced naming of pictures on repeat testing. Standardised tests of implicit memory have been considered but are not currently avail-able (see Section 5.3).

- The term *explicit memory* usually refers to memory that is consciously accessed, and covers most standard memory tasks.

2.1.3 Semantic and episodic memory

A further broad-ranging distinction is between *semantic* and *episodic* memory.

- The term *semantic memory* refers to an organized body of knowledge about words and concepts, and culturally and educationally acquired facts. It includes general knowledge, and covers a wide range of materials and modalities – familiar faces, language, and knowledge of the world.

- The term *episodic memory* generally refers to the encoding, storage, and utilization of memory for personally experienced events that can be related to specific spatial and temporal contexts.

2.1.4 Recent and remote memory

As indicated earlier, clinicians, particularly those working in medical settings, often distinguish between *recent* and *remote* memory.

- *Recent memories* are those stored within the last few hours, days or weeks, or even months.

- *Remote memories* date from childhood and early adulthood.

There is no clear cut-off point between the two, but the distinction is an important one in clinical neuropsychology, in that many patients with early-stage dementia will describe problems with recent memory in the context of preserved remote memory.

2.1.5 Anterograde and retrograde memory loss

Particularly relevant in clinical settings is the distinction between *anterograde* and *retrograde* memory loss.

- *Anterograde amnesia* is characterized by difficulty in acquiring new material and remembering events from the point at which neurological illness or traumatic injury to the brain occurred. Memory for events prior to the illness or injury may be unaffected, even when the anterograde amnesia is severe.

- The term *retrograde amnesia* is used when memory for events preceding the onset of brain damage is affected. The retrograde amnesia may cover a relatively short period (e.g. a few minutes or hours preceding a head injury) or can extend over decades. Conditions in which extensive retrograde memory loss can occur include Korsakoff syndrome, herpes simplex encephalitis, and late-stage dementia of the Alzheimer type.

2.1.6 Prospective memory

Prospective memory requires interaction between episodic memory and executive functions to enable an individual to remember to do something at a particular time in the future, or in relation to the occurrence of a particular event or activity in the future.

2.1.7 Material specificity

Another important concept is that of *material specificity*. Memory for nonverbal and verbal material may be differentially affected by neurological illness or injury. In general, verbal information is dealt with by the left cerebral hemisphere, and nonverbal information by the right, although it has been generally accepted that encoding and retrieval processes are not lateralised in this way. This position regarding encoding and retrieval processes has, however, been challenged, with a suggestion that encoding/retrieval differences may be as hemisphere-specific as other memory processes (Kennepohl *et al.* 2007).

2.1.8 Recall and recognition

Different techniques for the assessment of memory are available and some patients may be shown to be more or less impaired according to the type of test used. There is an important distinction to be made between *recall* and *recognition.*

- *Recall* is uncued retrieval and involves an active search process.

- In tests based on a *recognition* paradigm there is thought to be a familiarity and a recall component, since the individual selects from a number of stimuli that include the target (forced-choice) or states whether or not the stimulus presented is familiar (free-choice). Although tests developed for clinical use do not generally measure the extent to which explicit recollective processes are operating, relevant information can be obtained experimentally through the use of *remember-know* paradigms and through confidence judgements.

Recognition is almost always easier than recall, for the neurologically unimpaired as well as the neurologically impaired, and test norms reflect this. In some cases, e.g. certain cortico-subcortical or frontal presentations, recognition memory may be spared relative to recall, with discrepancies evident on standardized tests. Such differences in performance can be important diagnostic indicators.

Learning can occur after a single presentation, but the term is usually used in clinical neuropsychology to refer to tests in which there is repeated presentation and recall of material.

Recall or recognition is typically tested after a period of roughly 30 minutes (occasionally less) when a delayed trial is included. There are situations in which it would be helpful to assess *long-term anterograde forgetting*. In particular, some patients with a variety of temporal lobe epilepsy – transient epileptic amnesia (Butler *et al.* 2007) - sometimes report 'fading' memory of an event, such as a holiday or social occasion, which a relative or friend has said that they initially remembered quite well. Unfortunately, we do not have well-established norms for retrieval trials over weeks or months. Existing test materials may be used in this way, but interpretation will need to be carried out in the context of experimental studies (e.g. Blake *et al.* 2000) or locally-derived norms.

3 Assessment of memory: the clinical interview

In some types of referral, especially those with a diagnostic component and where the patient may have limited insight and/or memory for his difficulties, the presence of a relative/close friend/carer will be valuable. Two main sets of information should be sought:

- the memory symptoms which the patient or informant offers spontaneously;

- an indication of the patient's memory functioning gained from general questioning about recent autobiographical and public events, or recent factual knowledge such as names of grandchildren, personalities in the news, etc.

Once an account of symptoms has been given, specific probes may be made for symptoms such as the following:

◆ forgetting a telephone message;

◆ a high frequency of repetitive behaviour (repetitive questioning or repeating information in conversation) that cannot be explained by anxiety;

◆ losing track of conversation;

◆ forgetting to keep appointments;

◆ forgetting what has been read, or events in TV films/ soap operas;

◆ inability to navigate in familiar places.

The patient may be asked questions relating to his/her medical history (when she/he last saw the doctor, medication prescribed, and, if an inpatient, when she/he was admitted and what investigations have been carried out). Word-finding difficulties that could come under the rubric of semantic memory should also be probed. In the case of public events, it may be worth sampling both memory for famous personalities and memory for discrete events. This can be done by asking about a famous personality who has recently died and indirectly probing whether the patient knows that the personality is dead and how she/he died. In the case of a news event, it may be useful to start with a cue word to see if the patient can provide a news event relating to that word, and then probe for more specific information. Very accurate or very inaccurate responses to questions such as these may give a rough guide as to the direction in which more detailed memory assessment should proceed, although in some cases the responses may be equivocal, e.g. if there is patchy knowledge of recent news events in a patient who has little interest in the news and limited exposure to the news media. To obtain maximal information, this part of the clinical interview and its interpretation should be tailored to the individual patient.

The context in which the memory impairment is occurring is always relevant, and particularly so when assessment is carried out for diagnostic purposes. Marked variability in cognitive symptoms (eg. present in work but not in domestic settings), may point to psychological factors being important. Note whether the patient presents as alert or lethargic and whether there is evidence of affective disorder or test anxiety. Is the patient willing to persevere with difficult tasks or does she/he respond with frequent 'Don't know' or 'Can't remember' responses? The following questions should elicit useful diagnostic information:

◆ How severe is the memory impairment? To what extent has it necessitated a change in the patient's daily routine and ability to take part in activities that were once performed with ease?

◆ Has it affected ability to work or to engage in pastimes?

◆ Was the onset of the memory impairment sudden or gradual?

◆ Is the memory impairment consistently present or does it occur only on certain occasions?

◆ Is the memory impairment constant or are there fluctuations in severity?

- Has it been remarked upon by other members of the family? (The clinician may wish to obtain details in a separate interview.)

- Has it progressed over time?

- Is the memory impairment occurring in isolation, or is the patient aware of impairment of other cognitive functions? (Note that many impairments such as dyspraxia or dyscalculia may be experienced by the patient as memory problems –'I can't remember how to write letters of the alphabet'; I can't remember how to add up.')

- Are there accompanying physical or mental symptoms (e.g. headache, movement disorder, hallucinations)?

- Does sleep disturbance result in tiredness and poor concentration the following day?

- What is the patient's alcohol consumption? Does she/he take prescribed drugs or use recreational drugs? Has she/he been exposed to toxic chemicals?

Following assessment, the issue of consistency, both in terms of performance on different tests and the extent to which test performance is compatible with reported disruption to daily life, should be considered.

4 **Questionnaires and rating scales**

With a thorough clinical interview there is seldom a need to use formal questionnaires or rating scales. However, there may be occasions on which these may prove useful. For example, when assessment is carried out in a forensic and/or medico-legal setting, a normed questionnaire or rating scale may be considered more objective than interview data alone.

- The *Neurobehavioral Functioning Inventory*, devised by Kreutzer *et al.* (1999), includes a number of items relating to memory and has the advantage of there being two versions of the form, one for the patient and one for the family to complete. Responses to the items that make up the various scales, which include a Memory /Attention Scale, are summed and can be converted into standardized scores. The standardization sample is composed of pairs of patients and informants, the patients having sustained traumatic brain injury.

- The *Cognitive Symptoms Checklists,* developed by O'Hara *et al.* (1993), include a Memory Checklist, with questions divided according to different potential areas of difficulty, such as 'safety', 'money management', and 'time'. The completed checklist forms the basis for an in-depth clinical interview and has been designed with the setting of rehabilitation goals in mind.

- The *Cognitive Behaviour Rating Scales* (Williams 1987) are designed for completion by a relative or carer, and include a Memory Disorder Scale. This scale may be helpful in evaluating the cognitive sequelae of dementia.

- *The AD8 Scale* (Galvin *et al.* 2006, 2007a, 2007b) comprises a series of eight questions, which ask about problems in judgment, lack of interest in hobbies, repetitive speech, difficulties learning how to use a gadget, forgetting the month or year, difficulty handling complex financial matters, failure to keep appointments and daily frequency of memory/thinking difficulties. Galvin *et al.* (2007b) have suggested that in some situations, e.g. when given to an informant and combined with delayed word-list recall, this scale may be sensitive to subtle changes in the early stages of Alzheimer's disease.

In some cases, memory assessment procedures may have to be improvised. For example, in monitoring the effects of memory aids on everyday memory functioning, the clinician may wish to have a carer keep a daily diary of specific everyday memory lapses recorded before and after the therapeutic intervention.

5 Memory tests

5.1 Test selection

Issues of validity and reliability apply to the selection of all neuropsychological tests and will not be discussed here. The issue of *ecological validity* is also widely applicable, but can be particularly relevant to memory assessment, as everyday situations in which memory comes into play can be very hard to simulate. The question of ecological validity is especially important when critical decisions, e.g. about the patient's capacity to return to work or to live independently, are under consideration. A good understanding of the demands that will be made on the patient in a given setting and an awareness of the way in which the clinic differs from real-life settings are important. For example, during assessment the patient will be in a one-to-one situation that is deliberately kept as free from distraction as possible. This should give rise to optimal performance on formal tests but may be very different from a real-life situation in which there is extraneous noise and other competing demands on attention. Memory may need to be assessed sequentially to monitor recovery or rate of progression in degenerative illness. In this case, the existence of *parallel forms* of tests is invaluable. Finally, the severity of memory impairment may vary from mild forgetfulness to profound amnesia. Care must be taken to avoid *floor* and *ceiling effects*, which can occur if tests that are, respectively, too difficult or too easy for the patient are used.

Reference is made to specific tests in the sections that follow. The intention is not to supply an exhaustive list of tests suitable for assessing different aspects of memory, but to give examples. Where possible, examples are selected from tests or test batteries that are widely used and are likely to be readily available. In many cases, alternatives exist (for example the Memory Module of the Neuropsychological Assessment Battery, the Kaplan Baycrest Neurocognitive Assessment and the Hopkins Verbal Learning Test – Revised) that will do the job just as well. For details of such tests the reader is referred to test suppliers' websites (in particular the Professional Assessment Resources site –www.parinc.com and the Harcourt Assessment sites –www.harcourtassessment.com and www.harcourt-uk.com) as well as to books which review available tests such as Lezak *et al.* (2004) and Strauss *et al.* (2006).

5.2 Working memory/short-term memory

This is usually measured by span tasks. The *Wechsler Adult Intelligence Scale-III* (WAIS-III; Wechsler 1998a) and the *Wechsler Memory Scale-III* (WMS-III; Wechsler 1998b) contain verbal digit span tasks. The WAIS-III also contains a letter-number sequencing which is slightly more demanding than the 'digits backward' section of the digit span task. With regard to visuospatial span, the WMS-III contains a visual span task similar to the *Corsi Block-Tapping Test*, described by Milner (1971). Fourth UK versions of both tests are due for publication early in 2010.

Since the early 1970s, *dual task* paradigms have been used widely in experimental settings. Only a few tasks requiring dual tasking are available clinically. These are discussed in Chapter 5, of this volume.

5.3 Implicit memory

As noted earlier, this aspect of memory has traditionally been tested in the context of experimental studies rather than in clinical settings. Barbara Wilson and colleagues have taken steps towards the development of a formal test of implicit memory containing fractionated pictures and a stem completion task; the test (which was to have been standardised alongside the RBMT-III) is not currently under active development but may be published at a future date.

5.4 Semantic memory

- General knowledge is readily assessable using the 'Information'subtest of the WAIS-III. It is advisable to have details of the patient's educational history when interpreting test results as this test is education-related.

- Knowledge of word meanings can be assessed using the 'Vocabulary' and 'Similarities' subtests of the WAIS-III.

- Verbal semantic breakdown can show up on tests of confrontation object naming, such as the *Graded Naming Test* (McKenna and Warrington 1983, now available from Cambridge Cognition, address provided in Section 5.7; see Warrington 1997 for up-dated norms and Bird and Cipolotti 2007 for confirmation of its reliability and sensitivity in clinical populations) or the *Boston Naming Test* (Kaplan *et al.* 2001). These picture naming tests are sensitive to anomia (difficulty in naming), which can have a number of underlying causes. One cause is disturbance of comprehension – if a patient no longer has a store of semantic information about a visually presented object, she/he will be unlikely to be able to name it.

All of the above require a spoken response, which, in some cases, may render them inappropriate for use with aphasic patients.

- The *Pyramids and Palm Trees Test* (Howard and Patterson 1992), while not designed to assess semantic memory *per se*, is a useful test of a patient's ability to access detailed semantic representations from words and pictures. It is a matching test that does not require a spoken response. The authors provide normative data from control groups, and a cut-off score. Although the test has been used extensively with clinical populations, norms from these populations are not included in the manual, since it is the pattern of performance, rather than the subject's absolute score, that is felt to be important in understanding semantic impairment.

Throughout the last decade, there has been particular interest in the syndrome termed *semantic dementia*, a condition in which progressive impairment of semantic memory occurs in the absence of more widespread impairment of cognitive function; for example there is usually *relative* sparing of everyday episodic memory. Investigation of the deficits shown by patients with this disorder has enhanced our understanding of the semantic system (Hodges *et al.* 1992; Garrard and Hodges 2000). The tests described so far are (*inter alia*) routinely used in the neuropsychological diagnosis of semantic dementia, whether for clinical or research purposes. Two additional tests are described below:

- The *Speed and Capacity of Language Processing* (SCOLP) *Test* (Baddeley *et al.* 1992) is designed to provide a holistic measure of the efficiency of language comprehension. It includes the 'Speed of Comprehension Test', which is based on Collins and Quillian's (1969) 'Silly Sentences'. Simple statements about the world must be judged to be true or false.

- The *Autobiographical Memory Interview* (AMI) (Kopelman *et al.* 1990), as its title suggests, takes the form of a structured interview. It encompasses two components. The first is what the authors call 'personal semantic'. It assesses the patients' recall of facts about their earlier life. These facts, such as the pre-school address and the names of primary and secondary schools attended, are likely to have been acquired without conscious recollection of their acquisition – hence the inclusion of this part of the instrument in this section. The second component, relating to memory for personally experienced events, is discussed in Section 5.4.1.

5.5 Episodic memory

By far the greatest number of memory tests routinely used in the practice of clinical neuropsychology are tests of episodic memory. The majority are tests of recent memory. They require the patient to memorize information and retrieve it immediately after presentation or within half an hour or so. It is more difficult formally to test remote memory in the clinical setting but an instrument has been devised and will be discussed before looking at the range of tests of recent memory that are available. The examples of tests of recent episodic memory reflect the number and range available. Tests mentioned in Sections 5.5.2 and 5.5.3 are summarized in Table 9.1.

5.5.1 Remote episodic memory

The second component of the AMI (see Section 5.3) assesses the patients' recall of specific events in childhood and early adulthood, as well as memory for more recent personal events. A potential problem for a test of this type is the absence of any way of checking the accuracy of the patient's recall. Even if a relative or carer is present, she/he may not recall or be aware of certain incidents and events that have occurred in the patient's life. As part of their validation procedure the authors checked the accuracy of recall with relatives of patients in their validation sample. Although they concluded that the tendency was for patients' responses to be accurate on about 90% of occasions, the normative

Table 9.1 Tests of episodic memory

Test*	Measure						Age Range (years)	No. of parallel forms	Ceiling Effects possible	Suitable for use in severe deficit	Response required		Ecological validity a feature
	Recognition	Recall	Learning	Delayed recall		Prospective memory					Spoken	Complex motor	
				Short	Long†								
AMIPB Design Learning			+	+	+		18–75	2				+	
AMIPB Figure Recall		+			+		18–75	2				+	
AMIPB List Learning			+	+			18–75	2			+		
AMIPB Story Recall		+			+		18–75	2			+		
BMIPB Design Learning			+	+			16–89	4				+	
BMIPB Figure Recall		+			+		16–89	4				+	
BMIPB List Learning			+	+			16–89	4			+		
BMIPB Story Recall		+			+		16–89	4			+		
California Verbal Learning Test	+		+	+	+		16–89	2			+		

(continued)

Table 9.1 (continued) Tests of episodic memory

Test*	Measure						Age Range (years)	No. of parallel forms	Ceiling Effects possible	Suitable for use in severe deficit	Response required		Ecological validity a feature
	Recognition	Recall	Learning	Delayed recall		Prospective memory					Spoken	Complex motor	
				Short	Long†								
Camden Face Recognition	+						18–85		+	+			
Camden Paired Associate Learning			+				18–85		+	+	+		
Camden Pictorial Recognition	+						18–85		+	+			
Camden Topographical Recognition	+						18–85		+	+			
Camden Word Recognition	+						18–85		+	+			
Doors and People Verbal Recall		+	+	+			5–97 z			+	+		
Doors and People Verbal Recognition	+						5–97 z			+			
Doors and People Visual Recall		+	+	+			5–97 z			+		+	

Test		Age range	N					
Doors and People Visual Recognition	+	5–97 z						+
Rey Auditory Verbal Learning Test	+	13–97‡,§	3§	+		+	+	+
Rey–Osterreith Complex Figure	+×	6–89‡,§	2§	+	+⁋	+	+	+
RBMT Appointment	+	16–96 y	4	+	+⁋	+	+	
RBMT-E Appointment	+	16–76 y	2		+⁋	+	+	
RBMT-III Appointment	+	16–96 y	2	+	+⁋	+	+	
RBMT Belonging	+	16–96 y	4	+	+⁋	+	+	
RBMT-E Belonging	+	16–76 y	2		+⁋	+	+	
RBMT-III Belonging	+	16–96 y	2	+	+⁋	+	+	
RBMT Faces	+	16–96 y	4	+		+	+	
RBMT-E Faces	+	16–76 y	2	+		+	+	
RBMT-III Faces		16–96 y	2			+	+	
RBMT Message	+	16–96 y	4	+		+	+	
RBMT-E Message	+	16–76 y	2	+		+	+	
RBMT-III Message		16–96 y	2			+	+	

(continued)

Table 9.1 (continued) Tests of episodic memory

Test*	Measure						Age Range (years)	No. of par-allel forms	Ceiling Effects possible	Suitable for use in severe deficit	Response required		Ecological validity a feature
	Recognition	Recall	Learning	Delayed recall		Prospective memory					Spoken	Complex motor	
				Short	Long†								
RBMT Name		+					16–96 y	4	+	+	+		+
RBMT-E Name		+					16–76 y	2			+		+
RBMT-III Names							16–96 y	2		+	+		+
RBMT Pictures	+						16–96 y	4	+	+			+
RBMT-E Pictures	+						16–76 y	2		+			+
RBMT-III Pictures							16–96 y	2		+			+
RBMT Route		+		+			16–96 y	4	+	+			+
RBMT-E Route		+		+			16–76 y	2					+
RBMT-III Route							16–96 y	2		+			+
RBMT Story		+		+			16–96 y	4	+	+	+		+
RBMT-E Story		+		+			16–76 y	2			+		+
RBMT-III Story							16–96 y	2		+	+		+
Warrington RMT Faces	+						18–70						
Warrington RMT Words	+						18–70		+				
WMS-III** Face Recognition	+				+								

Test					Age range	
WMS-III** Family Pictures		+		+	16–89	+
WMS-III** List Learning	+	+	+	+	16–89	+
WMS-III** Logical Memory	+	+	+||	+	16–89	+
WMS-III** Paired Associate Learning	+	+		+	16–89	+
WMS-III** Visual Reproduction	+	+		+	16–89	+

* AMIPB, Adult Memory and Information Processing Battery; BMIPB, BIRT Memory and Information Processing Battery; RBMT, Rivermead Behavioural Memory Test (-E, extended version; -III, current revision); WMS, Wechsler Memory Scale.

† In most cases this is a 30-minute delay; the BMIPB delay is 40-minutes

‡ When normative studies are combined; individual studies have narrower ranges.

§ Readily available. Additional parallel forms and normative studies are in existence.

¶ Only a minimal spoken response required; could be used with aphasic patients.

|| One passage is presented twice and a learning slope calculation can be made.

× In the Meyers and Meyers (1995) version only.

ʸ Excluding modified children's versions.

ᶻ The new manual gives adult and child norms.

** The WMS-IV UK is due for publication early in 2010

sample was relatively small and, in clinical settings, a degree of caution should be exercised in interpreting patients' responses. Responses that are not obviously confabulatory (confabulatory responses may be bizarre and illogical or may not be consistent with other information which the patient has given) are scored as correct and, in theory, therefore, the instrument can be used with patients who are not accompanied by a relative or carer. However, the question of reliability of answers needs to be kept in mind, as well as the possibility that some autobiographical memories may be intact but are not tapped by the particular episodic memory items in the test.

5.5.2 Batteries and sets of tests assessing recent episodic memory

It is almost always necessary to administer a range of memory tests in order to obtain meaningful information about the status of a patient's memory functioning. When the purpose of assessment is to obtain a diagnostic profile, different tests are included to establish whether impairment is generalized or whether there are discrete areas of impairment, occurring in the context of preserved function in other areas.

A number of batteries that sample a range of abilities using different techniques are available. When there is a need to compare performance on different tests (e.g. those using nonverbal and verbal stimuli, it is worth selecting tests from the same set or battery where possible, since they will have been normed on the same population).

The Wechsler Memory Scales The Wechsler Memory Scales (WMS) are probably the best-known and most widely used batteries. They have expanded in scope since the original scale was published in 1945. Revisions in 1987 and 1998 brought the tests up to date. The fourth UK version is due for publication early in 2010. The WMS-III (Wechsler 1998b) is described here. It contains six primary subtests, used in calculating 'Index Scores' that are directly comparable with WAIS-III IQs.

+ Two of these, a verbal digit span task and a visual span task, are tests of working memory and have been discussed in Section 5.2.

+ The *Logical Memory* test comprises two short stories that are read to the patient. Free recall is required immediately after presentation and after a half-hour delay. It is also possible to examine recognition memory for the story.

+ The other primary test of verbal memory is a paired associate learning task, in which the patient is required to learn novel word associations over a number of trials and to respond with the second word of a pair when presented with the first.

+ On the nonverbal side, a series of 24 photographs of faces is presented. Memory for these faces is tested through recognition immediately and after a thirty minute delay – the patient is asked to pick out the target photographs from a set that includes distractors.

+ In the *Family Pictures* subtest, a family photograph and a series of scenes are presented. The patient is asked to recall who is in each scene, what they are doing, and where in the picture they are. This new addition to the battery was designed as a nonverbal analogue to the Logical Memory test, but it is not clear that it is entirely a test of nonverbal memory as a certain amount of verbal encoding could improve performance.

All of these tests require immediate and delayed recall. Although a half-hour delay is not particularly significant in terms of models of memory – both immediate and delayed trials test recent episodic memory – the inclusion of delayed recall trials is clinically significant. Performance in conditions such as Alzheimer's disease, in which material is lost over a delay, contrasts with performance in (e.g. the subcortical dementias or in anxiety states), in which there may be problems at the encoding stage, while material that is successfully encoded may be retained reasonably well over a delay.

Optional subtests in the WMS-III include

♦ a verbal learning task, in which the patient is asked to recall the contents of a 12-word list presented on four consecutive trials plus delayed recall and recognition trials;

♦ a nonverbal memory task, in which the patient is required to draw from memory a series of five designs, with delayed recall and recognition memory also assessed.

The battery is psychometrically quite complex, and a number of composite scores can be calculated in addition to the Index Scores. Administration of the entire battery to neurologically impaired patients is usually too demanding, but one advantage that this latest revision has over earlier versions is that norms for individual tests are available, so that the clinician can select appropriate tests from the battery when time constraints or lack of stamina on the patient's part preclude administration of the entire battery.

One disadvantage that the current revision does have is the absence of a parallel form, which was available for the first WMS. This means that interpretation of the results of repeated presentation within six months (or longer in some cases in which memory is reasonably well-preserved) is complicated by the possibility of practice effects.

The Rivermead Behavioural Memory Test (RBMT) The RBMT (Wilson *et al.* 1985) was devised specifically to meet the objection that many memory tests used in the clinical setting are adapted from laboratory-based tests and lack ecological validity. The test has been revised twice and an extended form produced (RBMT-E; Wilson *et al.* 1999). The most recent version (RBMT-III; Wilson *et al.* 2008) supersedes previous versions. It uses more up-to-date material, is designed to assess a wider range of abilities and provides revised normative data.

In addition to story recall, recall of names, and picture and face recognition tests, the RBMT-III also contains a number of subtests that are rather different from those contained in most other batteries, and that are felt to be closer to the everyday situations in which a patient might experience memory difficulties. One example is a subtest in which the patient is required to remember and follow a short route within the testing room. A number of tests of prospective memory are included (these are discussed in Section 5.6) and a test of the ability to learn a new skill has been added.

The original RBMT had four parallel versions to allow for repeated assessments; the RBMT-E and RBMT-III have two. The RBMT (its first revision), and the RBMT-E yield two scores; a screening score based on a pass/fail grading of each item, and a more detailed profile score. The scoring system for the RBMT-III is still under development. There is a children's version (RBMT-C; Wilson *et al.* 1991) which provides norms for children aged 5 years to 10 years 11 months.

The BIRT Memory and Information Processing Battery (BMIPB). The BMIPB (Coughlan *et al.* 2007; available from Dr M. Oddy, Kerwin Court, Five Oaks Rd, Slindon, Horsham, West Sussex RH13 0TP) has been developed under the auspices of the Brain Injury Rehabilitation Trust. It is modelled on the AMIPB (Adult Memory and Information Processing Battery: Coughlan and Hollows, 1985) but includes new features and is based on more extensive and up-to-date normative data. The battery uses entirely new material but the memory tests (story recall, word-list learning, figure recall and design learning) are similar to those in the AMIPB. There are some changes to the way in which tests are administered (for example, the interval between delayed and immediate recall of the story and figure has been extended from thirty to forty minutes) and there are useful additions in the form of recognition trials for the learning tasks.

The design learning test is felt to be a particularly good measure of nonverbal memory since it is very difficult to encode any part of the design verbally. Both learning tests, as previously, include a delayed recall trial following interference before administration of the newly-developed recognition trials. Norms are provided for each individual test. There is no overall memory quotient or composite score but this is in no way a disadvantage in clinical neuropsychological settings, where the focus is on relative strengths and weaknesses. The BMIPB has the advantage of four parallel forms and the test authors have given considerable thought to the issue of practice effects; the manual contains an extremely useful section on the subject and an accompanying CD enables the user to obtain, as a supplement to the percentile tables in the manual, continuous regression-based norms for each individual tested.

The Doors and People Battery. The Doors and People Battery (Baddeley *et al.* 1994) was designed principally to provide an improved measure of nonverbal episodic memory that would be acceptable to a wide range of subjects. It includes verbal recall and recognition tasks as well as nonverbal recall and recognition tests. Tests are relatively short and the battery is easy to administer. Norms are available for individual tests and an overall score. Scaled scores are also provided for nonverbal - verbal discrepancies and recall – recognition discrepancies.

There is now a children's version (Doors and People for Children; Baddeley *et al.* 2006). Changes to the adult test are minimal and the authors state that the adult test in its current form can be used with the child norms. The new manual provides both adult and child norms.

The Recognition Memory Test (RMT). This battery (Warrington 1984) contains only two subtests. The verbal test uses visually presented words and the nonverbal test uses faces. Both are forced-choice recognition memory tests. A discrepancy score can be calculated to assist the evaluation of differences between scores on the tests. Each test contains 50 items and, although they are easy to administer and usually quite pleasant from the patient's point of view, they are less suitable than some of the shorter tests for patients who have severe impairments of memory or problems with maintaining attention. However, there is the possibility of ceiling effects when the verbal test is used with very mildly impaired patients. As stimuli are visually presented, with a recognition testing format, it is an appropriate measure of memory for patients with certain types of language impairment. One disadvantage is the test's rather large intra-subject variability which makes it unsuitable for monitoring gradual change in degenerative or recovering conditions (Bird and Cipolotti 2007); another is the fact that the faces stimuli in the nonverbal test are somewhat dated.

The Camden Memory Tests. This set (Warrington 1996) contains five tests – two verbal and three nonverbal – that are intended to be presented individually and not as a battery. They are all presented visually. Four are forced-choice recognition tests and do not require a spoken response. The fifth is a paired-associate learning test that requires a single-word spoken response. These tests are shorter than the subtests of the Recognition Memory Test and include word and face recognition memory tests with similar formats. The least demanding is the 'Pictorial Recognition Memory Test' in which stimuli are photographs of London scenes. Selection of the target is made from unrelated distractors. This test is subject to ceiling effects when used with patients with mild or even moderate problems, but it is extremely useful for patients who have severe memory impairments or limited stamina in the early days following neurological insult. In relation to the latter group, all of the tests are easy to administer at the bedside. It may also be helpful in detecting memory loss due to reduced effort or motivational factors.

5.5.3 Individual tests assessing recent episodic memory

The Rey Auditory Verbal Learning Test (RAVLT). The RAVLT (Rey 1964) requires recall of an auditorily presented 15-word list over five learning trials. Delayed recall tests, following an interference trial, and a recognition test are provided. A number of parallel forms have been developed since the initial publication of the test. A selection of these can be found in Lezak (2004). Normative data are provided by Strauss *et al.* (2006). Schmidt (2003) has collected norms, validity studies and different administration and scoring procedures in a handbook.

The Rey-Osterreith Complex Figure. This test of visual recall was devised by Rey in 1941 and standardized by Osterreith in 1944 (papers translated by Corwin and Bylsma 1993). Taylor (1979) contributed a parallel form and scoring criteria. Until 1995 the test was not available from a commercial source. Information detailed enough to permit the clinician to design his/her own stimuli and score sheets are provided by Lezak (2004) and Strauss *et al.* (2006). A version is now commercially available (Meyers and Meyers 1995). Knight and Kaplan (2004) discuss clinical and research applications of the test (however this book is currently unavailable from the publishers).

The California Verbal Learning Test (CVLT). The CVLT (Delis *et al.* 2001) is another word-list learning task, which differs from the RAVLT and AMIPB list learning tasks in that stimuli are semantically related. In each list, items have been selected from a limited number of semantic categories and there are cued recall trials that ask for items within a given category. In the first edition of the test (Delis *et al.* 1987), items that could make up shopping lists were used, with the aim of increasing the test's ecological validity. This aspect of the test has been abandoned in the 2001 edition, in order to improve ease of understanding. Short- and long-delay recall is required and there is a long-delay recognition trial.

Norms are provided for a range of measures, such as vulnerability to interference and learning strategy. Computer-assisted scoring is an option. A children's version is available (Delis *et al.* 1994). The first edition of the test did not have a parallel form, but one was developed and published by Delis *et al.* (1991). The second edition has one parallel form, and this edition also includes a short form that roughly halves administration time.

5.6 Prospective memory

A number of items tapping prospective memory are included in the RBMT and RBMT-III (Wilson *et al.* 1985; Wilson *et al.* 2008, see Section 5.5.2). In the RBMT-III the patient must remember to:

- pick up and deliver a message.
- ask two questions relating to the near future when an alarm sounds.
- request the return of two belongings with information about their locations at a predetermined point.

The time-span over which the patient is required to remember varies for different items. It ranges from a few seconds for the immediate trial of memory for a route that includes remembering to pick up and deliver a message after a 25-minute time delay for remembering to ask questions when a timer rings; the request for the return of belongings must be made at the end of the session.

A welcome addition to prospective memory testing is the CAMPROMPT (Wilson *et al.* 2005). It includes six prospective memory tasks, three cued by time and three by events, to be carried out within a 25-minute period. The authors have devised tasks that are analogous to everyday tasks and patients are permitted to use their own strategies (such as making written notes) as memory aids. (An interesting finding in the standardisation studies is the importance of written notes; the test scores of patients who made full notes did not differ significantly from those of controls who made full notes, while patients who made no or partial notes differed significantly from controls.) A parallel form is provided. A note of caution in relation to this test is that dissociations between perceived/reported prospective memory dysfunction and objectively-measured prospective memory impairment have been described in experimental studies (e.g. Woods *et al.* 2007) although studies in which this dissociation has been reported have not used the CAMPROMPT. The CAMPROMPT manual reports correlations with some RBMT scores and other cognitive measures (but the issue of correlation with perceived prospective memory status or with recorded everyday prospective memory lapses is not addressed).

5.7 Computerized assessment

Computerized batteries that include tests of memory are available, but these tests have not been included as examples because, in spite of considerable interest in their development and use over the past 3 decades, none have yet come into general use in clinical settings. As mentioned previously, computer-assisted scoring is available for the CVLT, but this simply facilitates response recording and data analysis, and does not change the nature of the test in any way.

It is probable that administration of memory tests will be computer-assisted rather than fully computerized for the foreseeable future. An extremely sophisticated system would be required to capture qualitative data, give encouragement and reassurance, and deal with unexpected hitches in order to replace the clinician. Nevertheless, this may well be a growth area in the coming decade.

At present, the most readily available battery is probably the CANTAB Battery (available from Cambridge Cognition, Tunbridge Court, Tunbridge Lane, Bottisham, Cambridge CB25 9TU; cf. Robbins and Sahakian 1994), which has been developed and researched over many years. It has been designed primarily with applications for therapeutic trials in mind, but has been reported to be useful in some diagnostic settings – some clinical norms are now available. It includes tests of visuospatial and working memory. Like most computerized tests, it can be an expensive option.

5.8 Symptom validity in memory assessment

There are a number of ways in which the neuropsychologist may detect consciously or unconsciously poor motivation or lack of effort. Certain tests can be helpful in checking the validity of a memory complaint. A common indicator of a motivational problem is inconsistency between the patient's day-to-day functioning and performance on memory tests. The latter may show profound impairment, yet the patient is able to answer questions about certain recent events, or to cope independently at home.

Tests, such as Rey's *Memorization of 15 Items* (Rey 1964; cf. Lezak 2004), which are presented as demanding but are, in fact, quite easy for the patient who is not severely impaired, are likely to be failed by patients who are motivated to fail rather than to succeed. The forward digit span may be unexpectedly short and performance on forced-choice recognition tests, such as the RMT or Camden tests described above, can be revealing in that such a patient may score well below chance (cf. Halligan *et al.* 2003). Tests specifically designed to detect lack of effort are available. One of the most frequently used is the Test of Memory Malingering (Tombaugh 1996).

It is important to be aware that the assessment of motivation is complex, and no one test score in isolation can provide an answer to the question of whether or not the patient is adequately motivated. Test scores should be interpreted in the context of other information such as clinical history, symptom profile, radiological findings and so on.

5.9 **Normative data for older adults**

A helpful development over the last few years is the extension upwards of norms when new tests are developed or existing tests revised. WMS III norms are now provided for adults up to 89 years. Camden norms go up to 85 years, and the Doors and People standardization sample includes individuals up to 97 years. Testing the older adult is, in this respect, much easier than it was a decade ago when norms were often not available for the over-75s. Mayo's Older Americans Norms (Ivnik *et al.* 1992) have now been largely superseded by revisions of the WAIS and WMS. However, norms up to age 97 for the Rey AVLT may still be of value. Lezak (2004), Spreen and Strauss (1998), and Strauss *et al.* (2006) give additional test norms that are updated with each revision of their books. If appropriate age norms for a test are not provided in the test manual or in one of these volumes, it is worth checking journals for normative studies. The *Clinical Neuropsychologist* and the *Journal of Clinical and Experimental Neuropsychology* (both published by Swets and Zeitlinger) are good sources for such material.

Selective References

Baddeley, A., Emslie, H., and Nimmo-Smith, I. (1992). *The Speed and Capacity of Language Processing Test.* Thames Valley Test Company, Bury St Edmunds.

Baddeley, A., Emslie, H., and Nimmo-Smith, I. (1994). *Doors and People.* Thames Valley Test Company, Bury St Edmunds.

Baddeley, A., Emslie, H., and Nimmo-Smith, I. (2006). *Doors and People for Children.* Thames Valley Test Company, Bury St Edmunds.

Baddeley, A.D., Wilson, B.A., and Kopelman, M.D. (eds.) (2002). *Handbook of memory disorders,* 2nd edn. Wiley, Chichester.

Berrios, G.E., and Hodges, J.R. (eds.) (2000). *Memory disorders in psychiatric practice.* Cambridge University Press, Cambridge.

Bigler, E.D. (2001). The lesion(s) in traumatic brain injury: implications for clinical neuropsychology. *Arch. Clin. Neuropsychol.,* **16**, 95–131.

Bird, C.M., and Cipolotti, L. (2007). The utility of the recognition memory test and the graded naming test for monitoring neurological patients. *Brit J. Clin. Psychol.,* **46**, 223–234.

Blake, R.V., Wroe, S.J., Breen, E.K., and McCarthy, R.A. (2000). Accelerated forgetting in patients with epilepsy: evidence for an impairment in memory consolidation. *Brain,* **123**, 472–483.

Butler, C.R., Graham K.S., Hodges J.R., Kapur N., Wardlaw J.M., Zeman A.Z. (2007). The syndrome of transient epileptic amnesia. *Annals of Neurology,* **61**, 587–598.

Campbell,R., and Conway, M. (eds.) (1995). *Broken memories; case studies in memory.* Blackwell Publications, Oxford.

Collins, A.M., and Quillian, M.R. (1969). Retrieval time from semantic memory. *J. Verbal Learning Verbal Behav.,* **8**, 240–247.

Corwin, J., and Bylsma, F.W. (1993). Translations of excerpts from Andre Rey's Psychological examination of traumatic encephalopathy and P.A. Osterreith's The Complex Figure Copy Test. *Clin. Neuropsychologist,* **7**, 3–15.

Coughlan, A.K., and Hollows, S.E. (1985). *The Adult Memory and Information Processing Battery.* A.K. Coughlan, Psychology Department, St James's University Hospital, Leeds.

Coughlan, A.K., Oddy, M., and Crawford, J.R. (2007). *BIRT Memory and Information Processing Battery.* Brain Injury Rehabilitation Trust, Burgess Hill, Sussex.

Delis, D.C., Kramer, J.H., Kaplan, E., and Ober, B.A. (1987). *California Verbal Learning Test* (Version1). The Psychological Corporation, San Antonio, Texas.

Delis, D.C., Kramer, J.H., Kaplan, E., and Ober, B.A. (1994). *California Verbal Learning Test of Children*. The Psychological Corporation, San Antonio, Texas.

Delis, D.C., Kramer, J.H., Kaplan, E., and Ober, B.A. (2001). *California Verbal Learning Test*, 2nd UK edn. The Psychological Corporation, San Antonio, Texas.

Delis, D.C., McKee, R., Massman, P.J., *et al.* (1991). Alternate form of the California Verbal Learning Test: development and reliability. *Clin. Neuropsychologist*, **5**, 154–162.

Galvin, J.E., Roe, C. M., Powlishta, K. K., *et al.* (2005). The AD8: A brief informant interview to detect dementia. *Neurology*, **65**, 559–564.

Galvin, J.E., Roe, C.M., Xiong C., Morris, J.C. (2006). Validity and reliability of the AD8 informant interview in dementia. *Neurology*, **67**, 1942–1948.

Galvin, J.E., Roe, C.M., Morris, J.C. (2007a). Evaluation of cognitive impairment in older adults: combining brief informant and performance measures. *Archives of Neurology*, **64**, 718–724.

Galvin, J.E., Roe, C.M., Coats, M.A., Morris, J.C. (2007b). Patient's rating of cognitive ability: using the AD8, a brief informant interview, as a self-rating tool to detect dementia. *Archives of Neurology*, **64**, 735–730.

Garrard, P., and Hodges, J.R. (2000). Semantic dementia: clinical, radiological and pathological perspectives. *J. Neurol.*, **247**, 409–422.

Halligan, P.W., Bass, C., and Oakley, D. (2003). *Malingering and illness deception*. Oxford University Press, Oxford.

Hartley, T., Bird C.M., Chan, D., Cipolotti, L., Husain, M., Vargha-Khadem, F., Burgess, N. (2007). The hippocampus is required for short-term topographical memory in humans. *Hippocampus*, **17**, 34–48.

Hodges, J.R., Patterson, K., Oxbury, S., and Funnell, E. (1992). Semantic dementia. *Brain*, **115**, 1783–1806.

Howard, D., and Patterson, K. (1992). *The Pyramids and Palm Trees Test*. Thames Valley Test Company, Bury St Edmunds.

Ivnik, R.J., Malec, J.F., Smith, G.E., *et al.* (1992). Mayo's older Americans normative studies: updated AVLT norms for ages 56 to 97. *Clin. Neuropsychologist*, **6** (suppl.), 83–104.

Kaplan, E., Goodglass, H., Weintraub, S., and Segal, O. (2001). *Boston Naming Test*, 2nd edition. Pro-ed, Austin, Texas.

Kapur, N., and Moakes, D. (1995). Living with amnesia. In *Broken memories: case studies in memory* (ed. R. Campbell **and** M. Conway). Blackwell Publications, Oxford, 1–7.

Kennepohl, S., Sziklas, V., Garver, K.E., Wagner, D.D., and Jones-Gotman, M. (2007). Memory and the medial temporal lobe: Hemispheric specialization reconsidered. *NeuroImage*, **36**, 969–978.

Knight, J.A., and Kaplan, E. (eds.) (2004). *The handbook of Rey*-Osterreith *Complex Figure usage: clinical and research applications*. Psychological Assessment Resources, Lutz, Florida.

Kopelman, M., Wilson, B., and Baddeley, A. (1990). *The Autobiographical Memory Interview*. Thames Valley Test Company, Bury St Edmunds.

Kreutzer, J.S., Seel, R.T., and Marwitz, J.H. (1999). *Neurobehavioral Functioning Inventory*. The Psychological Corporation, San Antonio, Texas.

Lezak, M.D., Howieson, D.B., Loring, D.W., et al. (2004). *Neuropsychological assessment*, 4th edn. Oxford University Press, New York.

McKenna, P., and Warrington, E.K. (1983). *Graded Naming Test*. Cambridge Cognition, Cambridge, UK.

Meyers, J.E., and Meyers, K.R. (1995). *Rey Complex Figure Test and Recognition Trial*. Psychological Assessment Resources, Lutz, Florida.

Milner, B. (1971). Interhemispheric differences in the localisation of psychological processes in man. *Br. Med. Bull.*, **27**, 272–277.

Nichols, E.A., Y.-C. Kao, M. Verfaellie and J.D.E. Gabrieli (2006). Working memory and long-term memory for faces: evidence from fMRI and global amnesia for involvement of the medial temporal lobes. *Hippocampus*, **16**, 604–616.

O'Hara, C., Harrell, M., Bellingrath, E., and Lisicia, K. (1993). *Cognitive Symptom Checklists.* Psychological Assessment Resources, Lutz, Florida.

Ranganath, C., and Blumenfeld, R. (2005). Doubts about double dissociations between short- and long-term memory. *Trends in Cognitive Sciences*, **9**, 374–380.

Rey, A. (1964). *L'examen clinique en psychologie.* Presses Universitaires de France, Paris.

Robbins, T.W., and Sahakian, B.J. (1994). Computer methods of assessment of cognitive function. In *Principles and practice of geriatric psychiatry* (ed. J.R.M. Copeland, M.T. Abou-Saleh, and D.G. Blazer). Wiley, Chichester, 205–209.

Schacter, D.L., Wagner, A.D., and Buckner, R.L. (2000). Memory systems of 1999. In *Oxford handbook of memory* (ed. E Tulving and F. Craik). Oxford University Press, New York, 627–643.

Schmidt, M. (2003). *Rey Auditory Verbal Learning Test (RAVLT): A handbook.* Western Psychological Services, Los Angeles. Distributed by Psychological Assessment Resources, Lutz, Florida.

Spreen, O. and Strauss, E. (1998). *A compendium of neuropsychological tests*, 2nd edn. Oxford University Press, New York.

Strauss, E., Sherman, E.M., and Spreen, O. (2006). *A compendium of neuropsychological tests*, 3rd edn. Oxford University Press, New York.

Talmi, D., Grady, C.L., Goshen-Gottstein, Y., Moscovitch, M. (2005). Neuroimaging the serial position curve. A test of single-store versus dual-store models. *Psychological Science*, **16**, 716–723.

Taylor, L.B. (1979). Psychological assessment of neurosurgical patients. In *Functional Neurosurgery* (ed. T. Rassmussen and R. Marino). Raven Press, New York, 165–180.

Tombaugh, T.N. (1996). *Test of Memory Malingering.* MHS, Toronto, Ontario.

Tulving, E. and Craik, F. (eds.) (2000). *Oxford handbook of memory.* Oxford University Press, New York.

Warrington, E.K. (1984). *Recognition Memory Test.* NFER-Nelson, Windsor, Berkshire. Distributed by Psychological Assessment Resources, Lutz, Florida.

Warrington, E.K. (1996). *The Camden Memory Tests.* Psychology Press, Hove, East Sussex.

Warrington, E.K. (1997). The Graded Naming Test: a restandardisation. *Neuropsychol. Rehabilitation*, **7**, 143–146.

Wechsler, D. (1998a*). Wechsler Adult Intelligence Scale*-III. The Psychological Corporation, San Antonio, Texas.

Wechsler, D. (in press) *Wechsler Adult Intelligence Scale-IV.* Pearson Assessment, London.

Wechsler, D. (1998b). *Wechsler Memory Scale*-III. The Psychological Corporation, San Antonio, Texas.

Wechsler, D. (in press) *Wechsler Memory Scale-IV.* Pearson Assessment, London.

Williams, J.M. (1997). *Cognitive Behaviour Rating Scales.* Manual. Research edition. Psychological Assessment Resources Inc, Odessa, Florida.

Wilson, B.A., Cockburn, J., and Baddeley, A. (1985). *The Rivermead Behavioural Memory Test.* Thames Valley Test Company, Bury St Edmunds.

Wilson, B.A., Emslie, H., Foley, J., *et al.* (2005). *The Cambridge Prospective Memory Test.* Harcourt Assessment, London.

Wilson, B.A., Greenfield, E., Clare, L., *et al* (2008). *Rivermead Behavioural Memory Test*, 3rd edition. Pearson Assessment, London.

Wilson, B.A., Ivani-Chalian, R., and Aldrich, F. (1991). *Rivermead Behavioural Memory Test for Children Age 5-10 Years*. Thames Valley Test Company, Bury St Edmunds.

Wilson, B.A., Clare, L., Cockburn, J.M., Baddeley, A.D., Tate, R., and Watson, P. (1999). *Rivermead Behavioural memory Test – Extended Version*. Thames Valley Test Company, Bury St Edmunds.

Woods, S.P., Carey, C.L., Moran, L.M., *et al*. (2007). Frequency and predictors of self-reported prospective memory complaints in individuals infected with HIV. *Archives of Clinical Neuropsychology*, **22**, 187–195.

Chapter 10

The natural recovery and treatment of learning and memory disorders

Barbara A. Wilson

1 People with memory and learning disorders

This chapter focuses on people who have memory problems resulting from a neurological condition such as traumatic head injury, stroke, encephalitis, and hypoxic brain damage. It is not concerned with those who have developmental learning difficulties. Because learning is, to a large extent, dependent on memory, people with memory problems have difficulty learning new information. People with progressive neurological conditions such as Alzheimer's disease and multiple sclerosis also experience memory and learning difficulties and, although it is possible to reduce the everyday problems faced by these people (e.g., Clare and Woods 2001, Clare 2007), they will not be discussed here because they are not expected to recover or improve their functioning.

The typical person with memory and learning difficulties will have:

◆ a normal or nearly normal immediate memory when this is measured by forward digit span;

◆ difficulty learning and retaining most new information;

◆ a period of retrograde amnesia, i.e. a memory gap for a period preceding the insult.

Some will have normal functioning of other cognitive abilities and are said to have a pure amnesic syndrome. The majority will have additional cognitive deficits such as poor attention, word-finding difficulties, impaired problem-solving, and slowed information-processing.

2 What do we mean by recovery?

Recovery can be understood in several different ways. Finger and Almli (1988) see recovery as a complete regaining of the identical functions that were lost or impaired after brain injury. Few people with memory and learning disorders achieve recovery in this sense. Jennett and Bond (1975) regard recovery as resumption of normal life even though there may be minor neurological and psychological deficits. This is sometimes achievable for those with organic memory problems. Marshall (1985) defines recovery as the diminution of impairments in behavioural or physiological functions over time. Probably most people who sustain memory and learning deficits following non-progressive brain injury will show some diminution of their impairments over the first few days, weeks, or months. Kolb (1995) suggests that recovery typically involves partial recovery of function together with substitution of function. Wilson (1998, p. 281) defined recovery operationally as 'complete or partial resolution of deficits incurred as a result of an insult to the brain'.

The most common cause of brain damage (and memory impairment) in people under the age of 25 years is traumatic head injury. People incurring such injury usually undergo some, and often considerable, recovery. This is likely to be fairly rapid in the early weeks and months post injury, followed by a slower recovery that can continue for many years. A similar pattern may be seen following other kinds of non-progressive injury such as hypoxia, encephalitis, and cerebrovascular accident. In these latter cases, however, the recovery process may last months rather than years.

3 Factors affecting recovery

A number of factors influence the extent of recovery, some of which we can do nothing about once the damage has occurred. These include the age of the person at the time of insult, the severity of damage, the location of damage, the status of undamaged areas of the brain, and the premorbid cognitive status of the brain. Other factors such as motivation, emotions, and the quality of rehabilitation available can be manipulated.

3.1 Age

Age, often thought to be an important factor, is less clear-cut than many believe. Despite evidence to the contrary, there is a widespread belief that children recover from an injury to the brain better than adults. (Johnson et al 2003). This is known as the 'Kennard principle' after Kennard (1940) who showed that young primates with lesions in the motor and premotor cortex exhibited sparing and partial recovery of motor function. Even Kennard, however, recognized that such sparing did not always occur and that some problems became worse over time. Several studies have shown that younger children fare worse than older children (Forsyth *et al.* 2001, Konczak *et al.* 2005, Anderson *et al.* 2000, 2006 and Hessen *et al.* 2007). These findings suggest that younger children, particularly those below the age of two years, fare worse in the long term than older children. Those studies suggesting the opposite (Montour-Proulx *et al.* 2004) or suggest no difference (Mosch *et al.* 2005) are looking at children with focal rather than diffuse lesions.

Age, then, is just one factor in the recovery process that has to be considered alongside other perhaps more important factors, e.g.:

+ whether the lesion is focal or diffuse (Levin 2003);
+ the severity of the insult; (Catroppa and Anderson 2007);
+ the time since acquisition of the function under consideration (e.g. someone who has just learned to read at the time of the insult is more likely to show reading deficits than someone who learned to read many years before).

3.2 **Cognitive reserve**

The concept of 'cognitive reserve' refers to the fact that people with more education and high intelligence may show less impairment than those with poor education and low intelligence. Stern (2007) suggests that individuals with high intelligence may process tasks in a more efficient way. Consequently, in cases of Alzheimer's disease, task impairment manifests itself later in the disease in people with such cognitive reserve. He also says that most clinicians are aware of the fact that any insult of the same severity can produce profound damage in one patient and minimal damage in another. This may explain differences in recovery following non-progressive brain injury for, as Symonds (1937, p. 1092) said in an often quoted remark, 'It is not only the kind of head injury that matters but the kind of head.'

Stern (2007) argues that there is no direct relationship between the degree of damage and the clinical manifestation of that damage. He believes that there are two separate models of cognitive reserve namely a passive model dependent on brain size or neuronal count and an active model whereby the brain uses its cognitive processing strategies or compensatory techniques to deal with the damage.

Bigler (2007) believes that the passive model of cognitive reserve helps to explain not only the initial recovery from TBI but also recovery across the lifespan. Furthermore, the model allows us to understand why there is an increased risk of dementia in survivors of TBI. Schutz (2007) gives support to the active model of cognitive reserve in the description of nine highly successful survivors of severe TBI. These were far more successful than their peers in cognitive, academic and social achievements because they implemented procedures to minimize the impact of their deficits.

3.3 **Gender**

As long ago as 1987, it was suggested that female animals may be protected against the effects of brain injury at certain stages of their cycle due to the effects of oestrogen and progesterone (Attella *et al.* 1987). This was confirmed by Roof and Hall 2000). Potentially important for rehabilitation (Stein 2007), progesterone has been given to survivors of TBI with some suggestion that this leads to a better outcome (Wright *et al.* 2007). In addition, studies have looked at the long term outcome for females and males following TBI. There are conflicting reports with Ratcliff *et al.* (2007) suggesting that females do better, with Farace and Alves (2000) and Ponsford et al (2008) finding that the outcome for women was worse. The latter study controlled for Glasgow Coma Scale score, age and cause of injury. They found that females had a lower rate of survival and a lower rate of good outcome at 6 months post injury. The authors thought this reflected the lower rate of initial survival. They found no evidence that women did better and some evidence that they did worse.

4 **Mechanisms of recovery**

Insults to the brain cause rapid cell death and a disruption of functional circuits in the affected regions (Wieloch and Nikolich 2006). The effects of brain injury can remain active for days or weeks after the primary insult (Bramlett and Dietrich 2007), with progressive atrophy of both gray and white matter structures continuing up to a year post-insult. This could explain some of the long-term consequences observed in patients with TBI. Recovery from TBI is variable and far from uniform (Millis et al 2001). In some individuals recovery can continue for years (ibid).

The process of recovery is not well understood and probably involves different biological processes (Taupin 2006). Properties of plasticity of the central nervous system (CNS), such as the reorganization of the pre-existing network and axonal sprouting have all been implicated in recovery (ibid). Changes seen in the first few minutes (e.g. after a mild head injury) presumably reflect the resolution of temporary dysfunction without accompanying structural damage. This is akin to what Robertson and Murre (1999) refer to when they say that plastic reorganization may occur because of a rapidly occurring alteration in synaptic activity taking place over seconds or minutes. Recovery after several days is more likely to be due to resolution of temporary structural abnormalities such as oedema or vascular disruption (Jennett 1990), or to the depression of metabolic enzyme activity (Whyte 1990).

Recovery after months or years is even less well understood. Stein and Hoffman (2003) suggest several ways in which this might be achieved including regeneration, diaschisis, and plasticity.

4.1 Regeneration

Following brain damage, neurons initially begin to regrow, but this regrowth ceases as fibrotic scarring occurs preventing reconnection of severed neuronal pathways. Consequently, functional recovery from such injuries is poor (Logan *et al.* 2007). Voss *et al.* (2006), however, suggested that axonal regrowth may take place many years after severe brain injury leading, in at least one patient, to functional speech after he had been in a minimally conscious state for 19 years. For regeneration to take place, it is necessary for new cells and axons to survive, and integrate into existing neural networks (Johansson 2007). One way this may be achieved is through cell implantation. Ma *et al.* 2007 found that when injected directly into the brain, the cerebrospinal fluid or bloodstream, bone marrow stromal cells can promote recovery from TBI. The authors warn that although this is a promising treatment, there are still problems to be resolved. Indeed, Parr *et al.* (2007) say that the transplantation of bone marrow cells is unlikely to be a major factor in recovery from TBI and that other factors such as neuroprotection and enriched environments are likely to play a greater role. Taupin (2006) claims that after TBI and stroke new neuronal cells are generated at the sites of injury where they replace some of the degenerated nerve cells. And this represents an attempt by the CNS to regenerate itself.

There is now plenty of evidence that some regeneration of brain cells occurs after brain damage and the view held for many years that cerebral plasticity is severely restricted in the adult human brain is no longer credible. Taupin (2006) says there is a striking amount of neurological recovery in the months and years following brain damage despite often permanent structural damage. What is less clear however, is the extent to which regeneration can lead to functional gains in coping with real-life problems.

4.2 **Diaschisis**

Diaschisis is a term coined by von Monakow (1914, translated by Pribram, 1969). It assumes that damage to a specific area of the brain can result in neural shock or disruption elsewhere in the brain. The secondary neural shock can be adjacent to the site of the primary insult or much further away (Miller 1984). In either case, the shock follows a particular neural route. Similar to this, although not identical, is Luria's (1963) theory of inhibition. In inhibition, however, the shock is more diffuse and affects the brain as a whole. Robertson and Murre (1999, p. 547) interpret diaschisis as 'a weakening of synaptic connections between the damaged and undamaged sites, contingent on the reduced level of activity in the lesioned area'. Because cells in the two areas are no longer firing together, synaptic connectivity between them is weakened and this results in the depression of functioning in the undamaged but partly disconnected remote site. Reggia (2004) used a computational model to explain diaschisis. He suggests that it can be accounted for by a single model of hemispheric interactions.

4.3 **Plasticity**

While regeneration refers to the regrowth or repair of damaged areas of the brain, plasticity implies anatomical reorganization based on the idea that undamaged areas of the brain can take on the functions subserved by a damaged area. "Cerebral plasticity is the dynamic potential of the brain to reorganize itself during ontogeny, learning, or following damage" (Duffau 2006, p. 885). Until recently, this idea was discredited as an explanation for recovery in adults, although views are now changing. Bütefisch (2004) says that the human adult brain retains the ability to reorganize itself throughout life. Cecatto and Chadi (2007) suggest that behavioral experience and neuronal stimulation play a part in modifying the functional organization of remaining cortical tissue and leading to clinical improvements.

Robertson (2002) suggests that recovery is rapid for deficits that are subserved by multiple circuits such as unilateral neglect and slowest for deficits that are subserved by a more limited number of circuits such as hemianopia because fewer alternative pathways are available to take over the functioning of the damaged pathways. This could be the reason why language functions appear to show better recovery over time than memory functions (Kolb 1995). Robertson and Murre (1999), in a thought-provoking paper, suggest that plastic reorganization may occur because of:

- a rapidly occurring alteration in synaptic activity taking place over seconds or minutes;
- structural changes taking place over days and weeks.

The authors focus in particular on people who are likely to show recovery provided they have assistance and rehabilitation.

According to Robertson and Murre:

- there are some individuals who show autonomous recovery;
- others show very little recovery, even over a period of years;
- still others show reasonably good recovery provided they receive rehabilitation.

They refer to this as a triage of spontaneous recovery, assisted recovery, and no recovery. Robertson and Murre argue that the spontaneous recovery group do not need rehabilitation as they will get better anyway. They suggest that the strategy of choice for people in the no-recovery group is to teach compensatory approaches. Consequently, they focus on the assisted recovery group to address issues concerning brain plasticity. They also believe that the severity of the lesion maps on to this triage, with:

- mild lesions resulting in spontaneous recovery;
- moderate lesions benefiting from assisted recovery;
- severe lesions necessitating the compensatory approach.

Although heuristically useful, this idea may be too simplistic. For example, people with mild lesions in the frontal lobes could be more disadvantaged in terms of recovery than people with severe lesions in the left anterior temporal lobe. The former group might have attention, planning, and organization problems precluding them from gaining the maximum benefit from the rehabilitation on offer, whereas the latter group, with language problems, could show considerable plasticity by transferring some of the language functions to the right hemisphere.

Nevertheless, Robertson and Murre (1999) make some interesting arguments and present a model of self-repair in neural networks based on a connectionist model of recovery of function. Plaut (1996) also uses a connectionist model to predict recovery. He argues that the degree of relearning and generalization varies considerably depending on the lesion location, and this in turn has implications for the nature and variability of recovery. A more recent connectionist model looking at recovery of reading following brain damage is provided by Welbourne and Lambon-Ralph (2005). They believe that plasticity as reflected by changes in the pattern of connectivity is as important in recovery as is the pre-morbid structure of the reading system.

5 **How much recovery takes place?**

Kapur and Graham (2002) provide a review of recovery of long term episodic memory functioning and consider both single case and group studies. They look at the shrinkage of retrograde amnesia in individual patients with traumatic injury (which can be seen as one of the characteristics of post traumatic amnesia) and also look at patients with transient global amnesia. These conditions are temporary so we would expect some, perhaps substantial recovery to take place depending on the length of the PTA (Wilson *et al.* 1999). Indeed, this is confirmed in the group studies reported by Kapur and Graham. They conclude however, that recovery of memory function "remains a relatively uncharted map in the geography of cognitive neuroscience" (p. 245). Therefore we only have very tentative answers when we ask questions about recovery.

Another recent review of recovery is that by Kertesz and Gold (2003). Although this review is particularly concerned with recovery from aphasia, the authors briefly consider recovery of memory and also consider recovery from different diagnoses likely to give rise to memory problems such as traumatic brain injury and encephalitis. Like Kapur and Graham (2002), they look at shrinkage of retrograde amnesia and at recovery from Post Traumatic Amnesia, pointing out that prognosis of long term memory impairment is correlated with the length of PTA. They have little to say on recovery of memory functioning in people no longer in PTA but with more stable memory deficits.

A few studies have looked at the natural history of 'recovery' of memory functioning over a period of years. Vargha-Khadem et al. (1997) for example, report on three children who sustained early bilateral hippocampal damage. These children were followed for several years and showed reasonable levels of language and general knowledge despite remaining severely amnesic. Thus they were able to learn information despite their impoverished memories. Broman et al. (1997) also describe a child who became amnesic following a cardiac arrest when he was 8 years old. He sustained bilateral hippocampal lesions and was followed for 19 years. At that time he was still severely amnesic showing no recovery. The most famous amnesic patient in the world is probably H.M., reported initially by Scoville and Milner (1957), who appears to have shown no recovery since his original operation to relieve epilepsy. Wilson et al. (2008) also describe a man with a dense amnesia following herpes simplex encephalitis at the age of 45 years. The follow-up covered a 20-year period with no change in his memory functioning.

It is possible that memory shows less natural recovery over time than other functions such as language (Kolb 1995; Wilson 1998) and this is true for children and adults. Hughes et al. 2002 followed a child said to have made a dramatic recovery following near drowning. The child was submerged for 66 minutes and one report published 6 years post insult said she had 'recovered completely'. Neuropsychological assessment, at 12 years post insult when the girl was 14 years old however, found a global memory impairment.

Another factor appearing to influence recovery is the condition that caused the memory problem. People with head injuries often do better than people with other diagnoses. Newcombe (1996) for example, reported on a cohort of World War II veterans who survived missile wounds to the brain. This group has been followed since 1963 and is thus one of the most important follow-up studies of people with brain injury. Newcombe found a striking preservation of ability in the group as a whole, despite the fact that some members had selective impairments as a result of lesions in specific locations. In people with closed head injury (i.e. not from penetrating wounds), some have found that age and coma duration predict recovery (Zwaagstra et al. 1996), despite contradictory findings on age mentioned earlier. Fleming et al. (1997), like others, found that psychosocial problems are more persistent than physical problems one-year post-brain injury. People with encephalitis who remain with memory difficulties several months post insult appear to show less recovery over time. McGrath et al. (1997) found that 70% of encephalitis survivors showed memory impairment. The single-case studies of Wilson et al. (1995) and Funnell and de Mornay Davies (1996) found little change over time. A study looking at long-term outcome of 18 patients with hypoxic brain damage (Wilson 1996) found that, several years post insult, 11 had memory problems, usually together with other cognitive problems, and four were too severely intellectually impaired to be assessed on adult neuropsychological tests. Although recovery from stroke has been studied (e.g. Robertson *et al.* 1997), most studies focus on recovery of motor functions or attention. Robertson *et al.* found that ability to sustain attention was associated with better functional recovery.

6 Can we improve on natural recovery?

Although until recently it was believed that brain cells do not regenerate, Conover and Notti (2008) state that stem cells of the adult human brain support regeneration in the hippocampus through neuronal replacement. We have already seen that there is controversy as to how much, if any, functional recovery may take place through the replacement of stem cells, but it is certainly one area for further research that could enhance recovery of memory (Zeitlow *et al.* 2008). Animal studies have shown that it is possible to regenerate cells in the dentate gyrus through the provision of specific learning tasks (Griesbach *et al.* 2004) or through enriched environments (Dhanushkodi and Shetty, 2008; Döbrössy and Dunnett 2004). Thus it might be possible to enhance natural recovery through enriched environments and focused rehabilitation strategies. Furthermore, such programmes might indeed lead to neurogenesis in the human brain (see McMillan *et al.* 1999 and Ogden 2000 for further discussion). We now have the technology, through imaging procedures, to see whether it is possible to improve memory functioning (rather than relying primarily on compensatory approaches) and to see whether any observed behavioural change results in structural changes to the brain (Levin 2006). Grady and Kapur (1999) suggest that imaging studies may enable us to measure specific changes occurring in the brain during recovery and therefore allow us to determine whether recovery is the result of:

- reorganization within an existing framework; or
- recruitment of new areas into the network; or
- plasticity in regions surrounding the damaged area.

A few studies using imagery techniques to look at recovery from brain injury have appeared. One of the first papers in this area reported changes in regional cerebral blood flow (rCBF) after cognitive rehabilitation for people who had sustained encephalopathy following exposure to toxins (Lindgren *et al.* 1997). Later the same year, positron emission tomography (PET) was used to identify the neural correlates of stimulation procedures employed in the rehabilitation of people with dysphasia (Carlomagno *et al.* 1997). Laatsch *et al.* (1997, 1999) used single-photon emission computerized tomography (SPECT) to evaluate rCBF during recovery from brain injury. The authors suggested that specific changes in rCBF appeared to be related to

- the location of the injury;
- strategies used in cognitive rehabilitation.

Continued improvements in the three patients in the 1997 study were documented in rCBF, functional abilities, and cognitive skills up to 45 months post insult. A further study by Laatsch *et al.* (2004) showed that improvements following Cognitive Rehabilitation could be detected by fMRI.

In 1998, Pizzamiglio *et al.* used functional imaging to monitor the effects of rehabilitation for unilateral neglect. The brain regions most active after recovery were almost identical to the areas active in control participants engaged in the same tasks. This would appear to support the view that some rehabilitation methods repair the lesioned network and do not simply work through compensation or behavioural change.

A recent paper by Baxter *et al.* (2007) described a patient with non-paraneoplastic limbic encephalitis who had severe anterograde amnesia with subsequent recovery. They used fMRI to show increased hippocampal activation before and after recovery. Does this happen after memory rehabilitation? We do not yet know the answer to this question, but there is a growing interest in determining:

- whether attempts to restore memory functioning and attempts to help people compensate result in structural changes to the brain;
- whether any changes seen are different depending on the approach employed.

In reality, of course, the two approaches are not mutually exclusive and a combination of the two may prove to be the most practically useful.

7 Is treatment effective in helping people with memory and learning difficulties?

Perhaps the people who have done the major investigations into the efficacy of cognitive rehabilitation are Cicerone and his colleagues (Cicerone *et al.* 2000 and 2005). They looked at several cognitive domains including attention difficulties, visuo-spatial deficits, apraxia, language and communication problems, memory deficits, executive functioning, problem solving and awareness. On the issue of retraining versus compensation they found that retraining was effective for some cognitive functions for example, language whereas compensations were necessary for others such as memory deficits. Their overall conclusion was "There is now a substantial body of evidence demonstrating that patients with TBI or stroke benefit from cognitive rehabilitation" (Cicerone *et al.* 2005 p. 1689). These authors also state that "Future research should move beyond the simple question of whether cognitive rehabilitation is effective, and examine the therapy factors and patient characteristics that optimize the clinical outcomes of cognitive rehabilitation" (p. 1681). Halligan and Wade (2005) provide a summary of much of the work on the effectiveness of rehabilitation for cognitive deficits.

There would appear to be four major approaches to cognitive rehabilitation:

- cognitive retraining through stimulation or exercises;
- strategies derived from cognitive-neuropsychological theoretical models;
- techniques combining methodologies and theories from a number of different fields (particularly behavioural psychology, neuropsychology, and cognitive psychology);

- holistic approaches that address social and emotional problems alongside the cognitive ones.

The nature of these approaches together with their strengths and weaknesses are addressed in further detail by Wilson (1997*a, b*).

7.1 Compensatory approaches

There is increasing evidence to suggest that rehabilitation can improve cognitive functioning (Cicerone *et al.* 2005). In the field of memory disorders a good review is provided by Sohlberg *et al.* (2007). The method of choice for reducing everyday problems (rather than improving memory functioning) is probably to teach compensatory approaches. Several publications show that people with memory impairments can function independently if they are able to use strategies to get round their difficulties. Wilson *et al.* (1997) describe J.C., a young man who became densely amnesic following a ruptured aneurysm on the left posterior cerebral artery. Over a 10-year period, J.C. developed a sophisticated system of memory aids enabling him to live alone, hold down a job, and be totally independent despite the fact that he remains severely amnesic. The paper describes the natural history of the development of J.C.'s compensatory system, which began by his writing on scraps of paper a few weeks after his stroke and over time developing his highly successful system.

Another encouraging study describes the rehabilitation of a young woman who became amnesic following status epilepticus (Kime *et al.* 1996). This woman was taught to use a personal organizer (datebook), refer to it regularly, and monitor a number of daily events. Over a period of several weeks, she was able to learn the different sections of a datebook and use this to manage her life. After leaving the rehabilitation centre, she worked in a voluntary capacity (still using her system) and eventually was taken on as a paid employee.

Even with those people who are unable to return to work, memory compensations can assist independent living. One instrument that has been helpful to a number of memory-impaired people is NeuroPage®, an alphanumeric pager attached to a belt that sends out daily reminders. In a pilot study (Wilson *et al.* 1997), 100% of 15 people with memory and/or planning problems showed a statistically significant improvement in achieving everyday target behaviours (e.g. taking medication, feeding the dog, collecting children from school) with the pager than they had achieved during a baseline period. Further work with the pager showed how effective this could be for individuals (Evans *et al.* 1998; Wilson *et al.* 1999). Findings have since been replicated with a larger study of 143 people (Wilson *et al.* 2001) and diagnostic subgroups have also been reported including TBI (Wilson *et al.* 2005), encephalitis (Emslie *et al.* 2007), stroke (Fish *et al.*, 2008) and children (Wilson *et al.*). An interesting new development for helping people with prospective memory difficulties is reported by Fish *et al.* 2007.

7.2 'Errorless' learning

In addition to compensations in the form of external memory aids, techniques for improving learning in memory-impaired people are a major part of rehabilitation. It has been demonstrated that people with amnesia learn better if they are prevented from making mistakes during the learning process (Baddeley and Wilson 1994). Most of us benefit from trial-and-error learning if we can remember our previous mistakes. People with amnesia, of course, cannot do this because once a mistake has been made, it may be strengthened or reinforced or be indistinguishable from the correct response. Consequently, it is better to prevent the incorrect response being made in the first place. Following the original Baddeley and Wilson (1994) paper, several studies have been carried out applying the 'errorless learning' principle to teaching real-life tasks (Wilson *et al.* 1994; Clare 2003; Campbell *et al.* 2007). In a meta-analysis of Errorless Learning Kessels and De Haan (2003) found a large effect size of EL. Akhtar *et al.* (2006) showed the method was also useful for people with mild cognitive impairment. Page *et al.* (2006) suggest that the benefits of errorless learning are dependent on the implicit memory system which is normal or nearly normal in most amnesic patients. Although a number of questions, both clinical and theoretical, remain to be answered about 'errorless learning', the principle would appear to be better than trial-and-error learning for teaching people with memory difficulties useful information to help them cope in everyday life.

7.3 A holistic approach

Finally, holistic programmes for helping people with memory problems would address emotional problems such as anxiety and depression together with any cognitive deficits. Such programmes feature both group and individual therapy embedded in a goal-planning approach to reduce emotional and cognitive problems. The goals would be negotiated between clients/patients, family members, and staff. Long-term goals are those that should be achieved by the time of discharge from the rehabilitation programme and short-term goals are the steps taken to reach the long-term goals. Thus, long-term aims might be to:

◆ 'develop a system for scheduling appointments';
◆ learn how to use a computer program for managing one's finances;
◆ learn the location of the nearest bank;
◆ reduce anxiety about meeting new people.

Short-term objectives for 'developing a system for scheduling appointments' might include:

◆ the occupational therapist accompanying the client to purchase an electronic organizer;
◆ the psychologist using an errorless learning procedure to teach the client how to enter an appointment;
◆ the client learning how to check a message when the alarm sounds;
◆ in the memory group the client will practise using the machine to schedule appointments and respond appropriately.

Each long-term aim would require a different set of short-term objectives.

Examples of this approach with individual clients can be found in Wilson *et al.* (2002). The important aspects of the approach are:

◆ addressing both emotional and cognitive difficulties;

- involving the client/patient and the family in the decision-making process;
- setting goals which are of practical everyday value as well as being realistic and achievable;
- monitoring and recording progress, as well as reasons for failure in achieving certain goals.

Cicerone *et al.* (2004) say: "Intensive, holistic, cognitive rehabilitation is an effective form of rehabilitation particularly for persons with TBI who have previously been unable to resume community functioning" (p. 943).

8 Summary and conclusions

People with memory problems typically show some resolution of deficits acquired as a result of an insult to the brain. Following traumatic brain injury the recovery process can continue for a number of years. In other conditions, such as encephalitis or hypoxic brain damage, the recovery process may not continue for such a long period. Age may have some bearing on the amount of recovery attainable, but other factors, such as whether the lesion is focal or diffuse, and the amount of time since the skill was originally learned will also play a part.

The mechanisms of recovery are not well understood but several processes may be involved including regeneration of brain cells, diaschisis, and plasticity or reorganization of brain functions. Memory functions certainly show some recovery in the early days and weeks following an insult to the brain and, once again, the amount of recovery may depend on the cause of the brain damage (e.g. traumatic brain injury or encephalitis). It is not clear to what extent brain areas involved in memory can regenerate and whether such regeneration can be influenced by enriched environments, rehabilitation programmes, or other specific training strategies. Imaging techniques may enable us to answer some of these questions.

Rehabilitation can certainly reduce some of the everyday problems faced by people with memory deficits. Helping them to compensate for their poor memory skills is, at present, one of the most fruitful methods. Technology, including a new paging system, has significantly enhanced the ability to carry out everyday tasks in a recent randomized control cross-over design with 143 brain-injured people. Errorless learning techniques (i.e. avoiding trial-and-error learning) have proved beneficial in helping people to learn more efficiently. Holistic programmes addressing both emotional and cognitive problems are recommended in the rehabilitation of people with memory and learning difficulties, particularly when embedded in a goal-planning approach.

Selective references

Akhtar, S., Moulin, C.J.A., and Bowie, P.C.W. (2006). Are people with mild cognitive impairment aware of the benefits of errorless learning? *Neuropsychological Rehabilitation*, **16**, 323–346.

Anderson, V.A., Catroppa, C., Morse, S., Haritou, F., and Rosenfeld, J. (2000). Recovery of intellectual ability following traumatic brain injury in childhood: Impact of injury severity and age at injury. *Pediatric Neurosurgery*, **32**, 282–290.

Anderson, V.A., Dudgeon, P., Haritou, F., Catroppa, C., Morse, S.A., Rosenfeld, J.V. (2006). Understanding predictors of functional recovery and outcome 30 months following early childhood head injury. *Neuropsychology*. **20**, 42–57.

Attella, MJ, Nattinville, A., and Stein, D.G. (1987). Hormonal state affects recovery from frontal cortex lesions in adult female rats. Behav. Neural Biol. **48**, 352–367.

Baddeley, A.D., and Wilson, B.A. (1994). When implicit learning fails: amnesia and the problem of error elimination. *Neuropsychologia*, **32**, 53–68.

Baxter, L, Spencer, B, Kerrigan, J.F. (2007). Clinical application of functional MRI for memory using emotional enhancement: Deficit and recovery with limbic encephalitis. *Epilepsy and Behaviour*, **11**, 454–459.

Bigler, E.D. (2007). Traumatic brain injury and cognitive reserve. In Y. Stern (ed) *Cognitive Reserve: Theory and Applications*. Taylor and Francis, New York. [Bramlett & Dietrich 2007 – to be completed]

Broman, M., Rose, A.L., Hotson, G., and Casey, C.M. (1997). Severe anterograde amnesia with onset in childhood as a result of anoxic encephalopathy. *Brain*, **120**, 417–433.

Bütefisch, C.M. (2004). Plasticity in the Human Cerebral Cortex: Lessons from the Normal Brain and from Stroke. *Neuroscientist*, **10**, 163–173.

Campbell L., Wilson F.C., McCann, J., Kernahan, G., Rogers, R.G. (2007). Single case experimental design study of Carer facilitated Errorless Learning in a patient with severe memory impairment following TBI. *NeuroRehabilitation*, **22**, 325–333.

Carlomagno, S., VanEeckhout, P., Blasi, V., Belin, P., Samson, Y., and Deloche, G. (1997). The impact of functional neuroimaging methods on the development of a theory for cognitive remediation. *Neuropsychol. Rehabil.*, **7**, 311–326.

Catroppa, C., and Anderson, V.A. (2007). Recovery in memory function, and its relationship to academic success, at 24 months following pediatric TBI. *Child Neuropsychology*, **13**, 240–261.

Cecatto, R.B., Chadi, G. (2007). The importance of neuronal stimulation in central nervous system plasticity and neurorehabilitation strategies. *Functional Neurology*, **22**, 137–143.

Cicerone, K.D., Dahlberg, C., Kalmar, K., Langenbahn, D.M., Malec, J.F., Bergquist, T.F., Felicetti, T. (2000), Morse, P.A. [Date] Evidence-based cognitive rehabilitation: Recommendations for clinical practice. *Archives of Physical Medicine and Rehabilitation*, **81**(12), 1596–1615.

Cicerone, K.D., Mott, T., Azulay, J., Friel, J.C. (2004). Community integration and satisfaction with functioning after intensive cognitive rehabilitation for traumatic brain injury. *Archives of Physical Medicine and Rehabilitation*, **85**, 943–950.

Cicerone, K.D., Dahlberg, C., Malec, J.F., Langenbahn, D.M., Felicetti, T., Kneipp, S., Ellmo, W., Catanese, J. (2005). Evidence-based cognitive rehabilitation: Updated review of the literature from 1998 through 2002. *Archives of Physical Medicine and Rehabilitation*, **86**, 1681–1692.

Clare, L. (2007). Neuropsychological rehabilitation and people with dementia. Hove: Psychology Press.

Clare, L., and Woods, B. (eds.) (2001). Neuropsychological rehabilitation: special issue on cognitive rehabilitation in dementia. Psychology Press, Hove.

Clare, L. (2003). Cognitive rehabilitation in early-stage dementia. *Research and Practice in Alzheimer's Disease*, **7**, 97–102.

Conover, J.C, and Notti, R.Q. (2008). The neural stem cell niche. *Cell and Tissue Research*, **331**, 263–269.

Dhanushkodi, A., Shetty, A.K. (2008). Is exposure to enriched environment beneficial for functional post-lesional recovery in temporal lobe epilepsy? *Neuroscience and Biobehavioural Reviews* (in press).

Döbrössy, M.D., and Dunnett, S.B. (2004). Environmental enrichment affects striatal graft morphology and functional recovery. *European Journal of Neuroscience*, **19**, 159–168.

Duffau, H. (2006). Brain plasticity: From pathophysiological mechanisms to therapeutic applications of encephalitic patients. *Neuropsychological Rehabilitation*, **17**, 567–581.

Evans, J.J., Emslie, H., and Wilson, B.A. (1998). External cueing systems in the rehabilitation of executive impairments of action. *J. Int. Neuropsychol. Soc.* **4**, 399–408.

Farace, E., and Alves, W.M. (2000). Do women fare worse? A metaanalysis of gender differences in outcome after traumatic brain injury. *Neurosurgical focus [electronic resource]*, **8**(1), pp. e6.

Finger, S., and Almli, C.R. (1988). Margaret Kennard and her 'Principle' in historical perspective. In *Brain injury and recovery: theoretical and controversial issues* (ed. S. Finger, T.E. LeVere, R. Almli, and D.G. Stein), pp. 117–32. Plenum Press, New York.

Fish, J., Evans, J.J., Nimmo, M., Martin, E., Kersel, D., Bateman, A., Wilson, B.A, Manly, T. (2007). Rehabilitation of executive dysfunction following brain injury: "Content-free" cueing improves everyday prospective memory performance. *Neuropsychologia*, **45**, 1318–1330.

Fish, J., Manly, T., Emslie, H., Evans, J.J., and Wilson, B.A. (2008). Compensatory strategies for acquired disorders of memory and planning: Differential effects of a paging system for patients with brain injury of traumatic versus cerebrovascular aetiology. *Journal of Neurology, neurosurgery and psychiatry*, **79**, 930–935.

Fleming, J.M., Strong, J., Ashton, R., and Hassell, M. (1997). A one-year longitudinal study of severe traumatic brain injury in Australia using the Sickness Impact Profile. *J. Head Trauma Rehabil.*, **12**, 27–40.

Forsyth, R.J, Wong, C.P., Kelly, T.P., Borrill, H., Stilgoe, D., Kendall S., Eyre, J.A. (2001). Cognitive and adaptive outcomes and age at insult effects after non-traumatic coma. *Archives of Disease in Childhood*, **84**, 200–204.

Funnell, E., and De Mornay Davies, P. (1996). JBR: a reassessment of concept familiarity and a category-specific disorder for living things. *Neurocase*, **2**, 461–474.

Grady, C.L., and Kapur, S. (1999). The use of imaging in neurorehabilitative research. In *Cognitive neurorehabilitation: a comprehensive approach* (ed. D.T. Stuss, G. Winocur, and I. Robertson), pp. 47–58. Cambridge University Press, New York.

Griesbach, G.S. Hovda, D.A., Molteni, R., Wu, A., Gomez-Pinilla, F. (2004). Voluntary exercise following traumatic brain injury: brain-derived neurotrophic factor upregulation and recovery of function. *Neuroscience*, **125**, 129–139.

Halligan, P.W., Wade, D.T., (eds.) (2005). *Effectiveness of rehabilitation for cognitive deficits*. Oxford: Oxford University Press.

Hessen, E., Nestvold, K., Anderson, V.A. (2007). Neuropsychological function 23 years after mild traumatic brain injury: A comparison of outcome after paediatric and adult head injuries. *Brain Injury*, **21**, 963–979.

Hughes, S.K., Nilsson, D.E., Boyer, R.S., Bolte, R.G., Hoffman, R.O., Lewine J.D., Bigler, E.D. (2002). Neurodevelopmental outcome for extended cold water drowning: a longitudinal case study. *JINS*, **8**, 588–596.

Jennett, B. (1990). Scale and scope of the problems. In *Rehabilitation of the adult and child with traumatic brain injury* (ed. M. Rosenthal, E.R. Griffith, M.R. Bond, and J.D. Miller), pp. 3–7. F.A. Davis and Co, Philadelphia.

Jennett, B., and Bond, M. (1975). Assessment of outcome after severe brain damage. *Lancet*, **1**, 480–484.

Johansson, B.B. (2007). Regeneration and plasticity in the brain and spinal cord. *Journal of Cerebral Blood Flow and Metabolism*, **27**, 1417–1430.

Johnson, D.A., Rose, F.D., Brooks, B.M., Eyers, S. (2003). Age and recovery from brain injury: Legal opinions, clinical beliefs and experimental evidence. *Pediatric Rehabilitation*, **6**(2), pp. 103–109.

Kapur, N., Graham, K. (2002). Recovery of memory functioning In Baddeley A.D., Kopelman M., Wilson B.A. (Eds) *The Handbook of Memory Disorders: second edition*. Chichester: John Wiley & Sons.

Kennard, M.A. (1940). Relation of age to motor impairment in man and subhuman primates. *Archives of Neurology and Psychiatry*, **44**, 377–397.

Kertesz, A.G., and Gold, B.T. (2003). *Recovery of cognition*. [Journal?]

Kessels, R.P.C., and De Haanm E.H.F. (2003). Implicit Learning in Memory Rehabilitation: A Meta-Analysis on Errorless Learning and Vanishing Cues Methods. *Journal of Clinical and Experimental Neuropsychology*, **25**, 805–814.

Kime, S. K., Lamb, D.G., and Wilson, B.A. (1996). Use of a comprehensive program of external cuing to enhance procedural memory in a patient with dense amnesia. *Brain Injury*, **10**, 17–25.

Kolb, B. (1995). *Brain plasticity and behaviour*. Lawrence Erlbaum, Hillsdale, New Jersey.

Konczak, J., Schoch, B., Dimitrova, A., Gizewski, E., and Timmann, D. (2005). Functional recovery of children and adolescents after cerebellar tumour resection. *Brain*, **128**, 1428–1441.

Laatsch, L., Jobe, T., Sychra, J., Lin, Q., and Blend, M. (1997). Impact of cognitive rehabilitation therapy on neuropsychological impairments as measured by brain perfusion SPECT: a longitudinal study. *Brain Injury*, **11**, 851–863.

Laatsch, L., Pavel, D., Jobe, T., Lin, Q., and Quintana, J.-C. (1999). Incorporation of SPECT imaging in a longitudinal cognitive rehabilitation therapy programme. *Brain Injury*, **13**, 555–570.

Laatsch, L.K., Thulborn, K.R., Krisky, C.M., Shobat, D.M., Sweeney, J.A. (2004). Investigating the neurobiological basis of cognitive rehabilitation therapy with fMRI. *Brain Injury*, **18**, 957–974.

Levin, H.S. (2003). Neuroplasticity following non-penetrating traumatic brain injury. *Brain Injury*, **17**, 667–674.

Lindgren, M., Osterberg, K., Orbaek, P., and Rosen, I. (1997). Solvent-induced toxic encephalopathy: electrophysiological data in relation to neuropsychological finding. *J. Clin. Exp. Neuropsychol.*, **19**, 772–83.

Logan, A., Oliver, J.J., Berry, M. (2007). Growth factors in CNS repair and regeneration. *Progress in Growth Factor Research*, 379–391, 393–405.

Luria, A.R. (1963). *Recovery of function after brain injury*. Macmillan, New York.

Ma, J., Zhang, C-G., Li, Y. (2007). Bone marrow stromal cells transplantation for traumatic brain injury. *Journal of Clinical Rehabilitative Tissue Engineering Research*, **11**, 2932–2935.

Marshall, J.F. (1985). Neural plasticity and recovery of function after brain injury. *Int. Rev. Neurobiol.*, **26**, 201–247.

McGrath, N., Anderson, N.E., Croxson, M.C., and Powell, K.F. (1997). Herpes simplex encephalitis treated with acyclovir: diagnosis and long-term outcome. *J. Neurol. Neurosurg. Psychiatry*, **63**, 321–326.

McMillan, T.M., Robertson, I.H., and Wilson, B.A. (1999). Neurogenesis after brain injury. *Neuropsychol. Rehabil.*, **9**, 129–33.

Miller, E. (1984). *Recovery and management of neuropsychological function*. Wiley, Chichester.

Millis, S.R., Rosenthal, M., Novack, T.A., Sherer, M., Nick, T.G, Kreutzer. J.S., High jr.,W.M., Ricker J.H. (2001). Long-term neuropsychological outcome after traumatic brain injury. *Journal of Head Trauma Rehabilitation*, **16**, 343–355.

Montour-Proulx, I., Braun, C.M.J., Daigneault, S., Rouleau, I., Kuehn, S., Oeégin, J. (2004) Predictors of intellectual function after a unilateral cortical lesion: Study of 635 patients from infancy to adulthood. *J. Child. Neurology*, **19**, 935–943.

Mosch, S.C., Max, J.E., Tranel, D. (2005). A Matched Lesion Analysis of Childhood Versus Adult-Onset Brain Injury Due to Unilateral Stroke: Another Perspective on Neural Plasticity and Recovery of Social Functioning. *Cognitive & Behavioral Neurology*, **18**, 5– [page].

Newcombe, F. (1996). Very late outcome after focal wartime brain wounds. *J. Clin. Exp. Neuropsychol.* **18**, 1–23.

Ogden, J.A. (2000). Neurorehabilitation in the Third Millenium: new roles for our environment, behaviors, and mind in brain damage and recovery. *Brain Cogn.*, **42**, 110–112.

Page, M., Wilson, B.A., Shiel, A., Carter, G., and Norris, D. (2006). What is the locus of the errorless-learning advantage? *Neuropsychologia*, **44**, 90–100.

Parr, A.M., Tator, C.H., Keating, A. (2007). Bone marrow-derived mesenchymal stromal cells for the repair of central nervous system injury. *Bone Marrow Transplantation*, **40**, 609–619.

Pizzamiglio, L., Perani, D., Cappa, S.F., Vallar, G., Paolucci, S., Grassi, F., Paulesu, E., and Fazio, F. (1998). Recovery of neglect after right hemispheric damage: H2(15)O positron emission tomographic activation study. *Arch. Neurol.* **55**, 561–568.

Plaut, D. (1996). Relearning after damage in connectionist networks: towards a theory of rehabilitation. *Brain Language*, **52**, 25–82.

Ponsford, J.L., Myles, P.S., Cooper, D.J., McDermott, F.T., Murray, L.J., Laidlaw, J., Cooper, G. (2008). Gender differences in outcome in patients with hypotension and severe traumatic brain injury. *Injury*, **39**, 67–76.

Ratcliff, J.J., Greenspan, A.I., Goldstein, F.C., Stringer, A.Y., Bushnik, T., Hammond, F.M., Novack, T.A., Wright, D.W. (2007). Gender and traumatic brain injury: Do the sexes fare differently? *Brain Injury*, **21**, 1023–1030.

Reggia, J.A. (2004). Neurocomputational models of the remote effects of focal brain damage. *Medical Engineering and Physics*, **26**(9 SPEC.ISS.), 711–722.

Robertson, I.H. (1999). Theory-driven neuropsychological rehabilitation: the role of attention and competition in recovery of function after brain damage. In *Attention and performance XVII: Cognitive regulation of performance: interaction of theory and application* (ed. D. Gopher **and** A. Koriat), pp. 677–696. MIT Press, Cambridge, Massachusetts.

Robertson, I.H. (2002). Cognitive neuroscience and brain rehabilitation: A promise kept. *Journal of Neurology Neurosurgery and Psychiatry*, **73**, 357.

Robertson, I.H., and Murre, J.M.J. (1999). Rehabilitation after brain damage: brain plasticity and principles of guided recovery. *Psychol. Bull.* **125**, 544–575.

Robertson, I.H., Ridgeway, V., Greenfield, E., and Parr, A. (1997). Motor recovery after stroke depends on intact sustained attention: a two-year follow-up study. *Neuropsychology*, **11**, 290–295.

Roof, R.L., and Hall, E.D. (2000). Gender differences in acute CNS trauma and stroke: Neuroprotective effects of estrogen and progesterone. *Journal of Neurotrauma*, **17**, 367–388.

Schutz, L.E. (2007). Models of exceptional adaptation in recovery after traumatic brain injury: A case series. *Journal of Head Trauma Rehabilitation*, **22**, 48–55.

Scoville, W.B., and Milner, B. (1957). Loss of recent memory after bilateral hippocampal lesions. *J. Neurol., Neurosurg. Psychiatry*, **20**, 11–21.

Sohlberg, M.M., Fickas, S., Hung P.F, and Fortier, A. (2007). A comparison of four prompt modes for route finding for community travellers with severe cognitive impairments. *Brain Injury*, **21**, 531–538.

Stein, D.G. (2007). Brain damage, sex hormones and recovery: A new role for progesterone and estrogen? *Trends in Neurosciences*, **24**, 386–391.

Stern, Y. (2007). Cognitive Reserve:Theory and Applications. Taylor & Francis, New York.

Symonds, G.P. (1937). Mental disorder following head injury. *Proc. R. Soc. Med.* **30,** 1081–1094.

Taupin, P. (2006). Adult neurogenesis and neuroplasticity. *Restorative Neurology and Neuroscience,* **24,** 9–15.

Vargha-Khadem, F., Gadian, D. G., Watkins, K.E., Connelly, A., Van Paesschen, W., and Mishkin, M. (1997). Differential effects of early hippocampal pathology on episodic and semantic memory. *Science,* **277,** 376–380.

von Monakow, C. (1914). *Die Lokalisation im Grosshirn und der Abbau der Funktion durch kortikale Herde.* J. F. Bergmann, Wiesbaden.

Voss, H.U., Ul g, A.M., Dyke, J.P., Watts, R., Kobylarz, E.J., McCandliss, B.D., Heier, L.A., Schiff, N.D. (2006). Possible axonal regrowth in late recovery from the minimally conscious state. *Journal of Clinical Investigation,* **116,** 2005–2011.

Welbourne, S.R., Lambon-Ralph, M.A. (2005). Using computational, parallel distributed processing networks to model rehabilitation in patients with acquired dyslexia: An initial investigation. *Aphasiology,* **19,** 789–806.

Wieloch, T., and Nikolich, K. (2006). Mechanisms of neural plasticity following brain injury. *Current Opinion in Neurobiology,* **16,** 258–264.

Whyte, J. (1990). Mechanisms of recovery of function following CNS damage. In *Rehabilitation of the adult and child with TBI,* 2nd edn (ed. M. Rosenthal, E.R. Griffith, M.R. Bond, and J.D. Miller), pp. 79–87. F.A. Davis and Co, Philadelphia.

Wilson, B.A. (1996). Cognitive functioning of adult survivors of cerebral hypoxia. *Brain Injury.* **10,** 863–874.

Wilson, B.A. (1997). Cognitive rehabilitation: how it is and how it might be. *J. Int. Neuropsychol. Soc.,* **3,** 487–496.

Wilson, B.A. (1998). Recovery of cognitive functions following non-progressive brain injury. *Curr. Opin. Neurobiol.,* **8,** 281–287.

Wilson, B.A., Emslie, H.C., Quirk, K., and Evans, J.J. (2001). Reducing everyday memory and planning problems by means of a paging systtem: a randomised control cross over study. *Journal of Neurology, Neurosurgery and Psychiatry,* **70,** 477–482.

Wilson, B.A., Baddeley, A.D., Evans, J.J., and Shiel, A. (1994). Errorless learning in the rehabilitation of memory impaired people. *Neuropsychol. Rehabil.,* **4,** 307–326.

Wilson, B.A., Evans, J.J., and Keohane, C. (2002). Cognitive rehabilitation: a goal planning approach. *Journal of Head Trauma Rehabilitation,* **17,** 542–555.

Wilson, B.A., Evans, J.J., Emslie, H., and Malinek, V. (1997). Evaluation of NeuroPage: a new memory aid. *J. Neurol., Neurosurg., Psychiatry,* **63,** 113–115.

Wilson, B.A., Emslie, H., Quirk, K., and Evans, J. (1999). George: learning to live independently with NeuroPage®. *Rehabil. Psychol.,* **44,** 284–296.

Wilson, B.A., Evans, J.J., and Keohane, C. (2002). Cognitive Rehabilitation: A Goal-Planning Approach. *Journal of Head Trauma Rehabilitation,* **17,** 542–555.

Wilson, B.A., Emslie, H., Quirk, K., Evans, J., and Watson, P. (2005). A randomised control trial to evaluate a paging system for people with traumatic brain injury. *Brain Injury,* **19,** 891–894.

Wilson, B.A., Kopelman, M., and Kapur, N. (2008). Prominent and persistent loss of self-awareness in amnesia: delusion, impaired consciousness or coping strategy? (Neuropsychological Rehabilitation), **18,** 527–540.

Wright, D.W., Kellermann, A.L., Hertzberg, V.S., Clark, P.L., Frankel, M., Goldstein, F.C., Salomone, J.P., and Stein, D.G. (2007). ProTECT: A Randomized Clinical Trial of Progesterone for Acute Traumatic Brain Injury. *Annals of Emergency Medicine*, **49**, 391–402.e2.

Zietlow, R., Lane, E.L., Dunnett, S.B., and Rosser, A.E. (2008). Human stem cells for CNS repair. *Cell and Tissue Research*, **331**, 301–322.

Zwaagstra, R., Schmidt, I., and Vanier, M. (1996). Recovery of speed of information processing in closed-head-injury patients. *J. Clin. Exp. Neuropsychol.*, **18**, 383–393.

Chapter 11

Assessment and treatment of disorders of visuospatial, imaginal, and constructional processes

Lilianne Manning

1 Introduction

The usual screening neuropsychological batteries have practically ignored the assessment of visuospatial, imaginal, and constructional deficits. The general tendencies underlying current approaches consist of:

- an early *assessment* of these functions;
- the introduction of everyday life parameters, particularly, in *rehabilitation*.

The first tendency can be achieved by adding simple measures in order to increase the sensitivity of routine tests and guide the clinician to detect, from the very beginning of the assessment, one or more nonverbal disorders of the type covered in this chapter. An example is the enhancement of the sensitivity of the Mini Mental Status Examination by adding a clock drawing.

The second current tendency, studying the relationships between a given disorder and some measures of activity in daily living, implies the construction of highly targeted programmes based on both the patient's description (whenever possible) of his/her most disabling symptom(s) and a comprehensive assessment of deficits *and* preserved cognitive functions. It is worthwhile noting that everyday function can improve with the appropriate treatment without there being any improvement in cognitive test scores. The current 'ecological' concern also consists of using assessment and rehabilitation based on virtual environment technology when working with the real environment is impossible or unsuitable (e.g. for elderly patients) and when the aim of the programme cannot be achieved by using traditional neuropsychological methods. It basically consists of dynamic three-dimensional stimulus environments, in which a wide range of nonverbal deficits can be recorded, particularly concerning visual, topographical, and constructional processes.

2 Defects in visuospatial processes

Visuospatial processing ability can be defined as the capacity to localize objects in relation
to each other in space and to know the location of single objects with respect to oneself.
The major clinically different forms of visuospatial disorders are:

- visual disorientation;
- defective complex visuospatial processing;
- unilateral visual neglect;
- Balint's syndrome.

Balint's syndrome is triggered predominantly by attentional defects as is visual neglect—
however, the latter can also be of an intentional and representational nature. Balint's
syndrome and visual neglect are both dealt with elsewhere in this volume (see Chapter 8).
Several other less frequently observed visuospatial deficits, such as impaired performance
on mazes, have not been included in this section. The two forms of visuospatial disorders
covered here are visual disorientation and defective complex visual processing.

2.1 Visual disorientation

2.1.1 Clinical presentation

Patients are unable to localize single objects, and act as if they were blind.

- They have marked difficulty in directing voluntary eye movements towards an object.
  Patients asked to look at the examiner's face look at many different points and are
  unable to 'stop' voluntarily at the face in front of them. *⊃ Problem for Ax during CAT, WAB.*
- They also have problems in reaching for or pointing to an object. They will almost
  invariably position the hand at the wrong distance in one or more of the three spatial
  dimensions. This deficit, observed despite the object actually being seen, is called *optic
  ataxia*. Note that patients with optic ataxia have no difficulty in localizing their own
  body parts. If the patient succeeds (often with help) in picking up food with a fork, he/
  she will bring it with no hesitation whatever to his/her mouth.
- Attentional processes are also impaired (see Chapters 5 and 6).

2.1.2 Brain damage localization

The brain damage is usually observed in the dorsal, occipitoparietal projections, i.e. the
'where' pathway. Lesions are generally bilateral, though there are some reports of visual
location deficit in the hemi-field contralateral to the lesion. Visual disorientation, after
either bilateral or unilateral lesions, is rare and its most severe form is found in patients
with Balint's syndrome.

2.1.3 Diagnosis

The diagnosis of visual disorientation, i.e. impaired single-object localization, applies
to the patient who, besides normal visual acuity, is able to localize external sounds (e.g.
correctly pointing to the source of a voice while blindfolded) and tactile stimulation on

his/her own body. This is necessary to rule out motor deficits and demonstrate accurate body sensations and normal use of body parts.

2.1.4 Assessment – Strategies

A neuropsychological examination should only be conducted in patients who have successfully completed an ophthalmological examination.

- Ask the patient to look at an object and to point at an object or a dot on a sheet of paper to test *simple localization.*
- Assess *depth discrimination* by asking him/her to estimate distance of objects in the natural environment and by showing the patient two objects either on the same horizontal plane or on different planes, one of the objects being clearly closer to him/her. Can the patient say whether or not they are at the same distance? Carry out the same task moving the patient's finger from one object to the other. This tactile test should be normal.
- To test *size discrimination* place different sized real objects at the same distance from the patient. Can he/she say which is larger? The number of trials and the comparative size of the objects presented will depend on the initial results.
- *Optic ataxia* needs two conditions of testing:
  - First, ask the patient to reach out and grasp an object that he/she is looking at.
  - Second, repeat the manoeuvre but with a screen (a file or similar) placed between the patient's head and his/her arm to prevent him/her from seeing the hand movement.

  Optic ataxic patients succeed in the second condition only.
- Test the patient's *spatial scan* and single-point localization using a dot-counting task. Norms exist for different groups of brain-damaged patients and normal controls (Warrington and James 1991).

2.1.5 Recovery and rehabilitation

Spontaneous recovery has been observed after unilateral right hemisphere damage. 'Improvement' of visuospatial difficulties has been observed after non-specific training programmes on visual material reflecting a general increase in the level of attention and awareness. Rehabilitation programmes in patients presenting impaired visual fixation, difficulty in scanning dot arrays, and inability to reach objects on visual guidance have been carried out. New rehabilitation programmes can be developed to improve on existing programmes provided that the rationale behind the intervention, the articulation of stages, and the time required to obtain results are all compatible with the case at hand. See, for example, Zihl (2000, pp. 107–32). His rationale was to improve localization of objects by fixating and reaching. He designed a progressively complex training scheme, the last stage being reading treatment demanding a very high level of visual control of eye movement. The whole programme took nearly 100 sessions. The results are encouraging. The patient improved her vision in everyday life, and improved fixation and localization helped her to achieve better identification of objects.

Case report

Patient H.B., a 63-year-old woman, obtained a Verbal IQ of 100 (Wechsler Adult Intelligence Scale (WAIS-R). She was able to name objects from a description but unable to carry out the Performance IQ. This combination of preliminary results both oriented the interview and indicated a test of visual process. She showed poor visual acuity but relatively well preserved ability to perceive shapes. Colour and face perception were preserved. Preliminary *visual orientation* was tested by asking her to point to a finger and to 1 cm diameter coloured dots presented one by one in different positions on a sheet of white paper. Her performance was markedly impaired. It was observed that she retained the ability to localize points on her body and the source of the examiner's voice with eyes closed. These few results suggested that both diffuse neurodegenerative processes and shape disorders could be ruled out and pointed to a *differential diagnosis* of visual disorientation. It was decided to carry out several of the tests described above (see Section 2.1.4).

2.2 Complex visuospatial processing

Disorders in complex visuospatial processing are subdivided into two types:

+ topographical disorientation;
+ spatial analysis deficits.

2.2.1 Topographical disorientation

Clinical presentation This deficit considerably hinders patients' everyday life. Characteristically, they have difficulty in finding their way from one location to another, despite intact basic visual processes. Moreover, they may present preserved topo-graphical visual recognition and memory—they are able to recognize places while getting lost on familiar and/or simple routes or have difficulty in finding objects at home. The opposite pattern of performance, i.e. loss of topographical recognition and preserved spatial knowledge, results in an inability to recognize buildings and places while managing accurate accounts of journeys.

Brain localization Predominantly right parietal damage.

Diagnosis Diagnosis is based on interviews with the patient and a relative or carer about the extent and characteristics of topographical disorientation.

+ Does the patient get lost in *familiar* surroundings?
+ Is he/she unable to learn *new* simple routes?
+ Was his/her way-finding good before the illness?

Take into account the fact that this disorder can be either a feature of dementia or a selective impairment with other functions well preserved (see 'Recovery and rehabilitation' in this section).

Assessment Ask patient questions such as:

+ How did you get here?

+ Can you tell me how to get from X to Y? (X and Y being two places familiar to the patient).

+ How do you go from this room to your ward?

+ Can you describe your home/flat/room?

Maps or plans are often used for the patient to locate well known places in his/her country or city. It can also be useful to present a large square on a sheet of paper, to represent the patient's bedroom, and ask him/her to locate furniture, doors, and windows.

Recovery and rehabilitation

+ Patients having difficulty in locating items in their familiar places benefit from written lists, e.g. of contents of cupboards.

+ Patients getting lost on familiar routes can be helped by photographs of prominent environmental cues to be used as landmarks.

+ Written instructions are also useful for some patients.

+ To increase meaningful associations concerning well delimited locations of daily journeys between several places, teach the patient simple mnemonics combining names of streets and their location.

+ A further real-life orientated treatment consists of walking with the patient in familiar surroundings, briefly or for a few minutes (depending on the patient's degree of deficit), then asking him/her to go back to the starting point. The length of time and the number of changes of direction are gradually increased. Finally, the patient can be asked to draw the route.

Rehabilitation programmes are more frequently constructed (and reported) when topo-graphical disorientation is isolated rather than embedded in a diffuse clinical picture. However, it is important to bear in mind that the isolated presentation can be the result of combined effects of several impairments such as space perception and nonverbal memory. Treatment can focus on one of these. When deciding on the type of treatment it is helpful to have the patient's description of the most disabling symptom in his or her everyday life.

2.2.2 Spatial analysis deficits

+ *Clinical presentation.* These deficits are often only revealed through testing. Patients suffering from spatial analysis deficits have difficulty in position discrimination and/or line orientation discrimination. Detection of discrimination impairments requires fairly elaborate tasks (see 'Assessment' in this section).

+ *Brain localization.* Predominantly right parietal damage.

+ *Diagnosis* of spatial analysis deficits is based on quantitative results in a series of specially constructed tests.

Assessment The following tests assessing the patient's capacity to perceive the relative position of objects in two-dimensional space have been standardized (Warrington and James 1991).

- *Position Discrimination* consists of sets of two adjacent horizontal squares, one with a dot printed in the centre and one with a dot slightly off-centre. Ask the patient to point to the dot that is in the centre (cut-off, 17/20). Carry out the next task even if the patient's performance is normal.

- *Number Location* consists of sets of two non-adjacent squares placed one above the other. The bottom square contains one single dot corresponding to one of the randomly placed nine numbers of the top square. Ask the patient to say or point to the number that matches the position of the dot (cut-off, 7/10).

- *Cube Analysis*. The patient has to interpret three-dimensional space in two-dimensional representations (see Fig. 11.1). Ask the patient to count the number of solid bricks (cut-off, 6/10).

- Discrimination of *line orientation* is tested with a graded difficulty task consisting of two figures, one above the other, showing a 'sun ray' of lines of different orientation: the top figure shows two 'rays', the bottom figure shows 11 'rays' covering 180°. Ask the patient to match the two lines of the top figure to those that have the same slant in the 'sun ray' bottom figure. The task is fairly sensitive and provides norms for groups of brain-damaged patients and normal controls (Benton *et al.* 1983, pp. 56–62). (See Table 11.1 for a synopsis.)

Recovery and rehabilitation Measurement of specific visuospatial abilities at time of admission may help the rehabilitation prognosis.

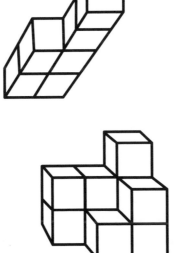

Fig. 11.1 Example of stimuli from a spatial analysis test, the Cube Analysis task (Warrington and James 1991). (Reproduced with permission of the publisher Pearson Assessment. (2009) Copyright © 1991. All rights reserved. No part of this publication may be reproduced or transmitted in any form or by any means electronic or mechanical, including photocopy, recording or any information or retrieval system, without permission in writing from the publisher.)

Table 11.1 Visuospatial processes: synopsis of deficits and tests

Visuospatial disorientation	Complex visual processing	
	Topographical deficits	Spatial analysis deficits
Simple item localization	'How did you get here?'	Position Discrimination
Depth discrimination	'Go from X to Y'	Number Location
Size discrimination	'Show me … on this map'	Cube Analysis
Reaching out tests	'Draw your flat/room'	Line Orientation Test

- Treatment could be attempted using the tactile versions of the cube analysis subtest or the line orientation test, with patients presenting deficits on spatial analysis in the visual modality only.

- A treatment using the tactile and the visual modalities consists of fitting different shapes into the correct holes in a board, as quickly as possible.

- Computer-generated virtual environments that can be explored in real time could be used to treat acquired visuospatial deficits.

- Finally, patients with some musical abilities could benefit from a rehabilitation programme combining increasing levels of difficulty, figures of cubes (of the type presented in Fig. 11.1), and musical isomers. It has been suggested that the latter facilitate visuospatial relations since the same holistic processes appear to be at work both in the perception of musical contour and in mental manipulations of two-dimensional figures.

Case report

Patient C.S., a 73-year-old woman, obtained a verbal IQ of 99 and a performance IQ of 87 (WAIS-R). Naming on description was very good. Verbal recognition memory was adequate (it was orally presented). She was unable to recognize unusual views of common objects but recognized 20/20 when the canonical view was presented. This result led to her being asked to perform several visuoperceptual tasks (not commented on here) and visuospatial tasks. Concerning the latter, she failed the Position Discrimination test (8/20), and the Cube Analysis task (2/10). These preliminary results suggested that there was a deterioration affecting, in particular, perceptual and visuospatial skills, with verbal abilities remaining relatively intact. A further assessment session was decided with a view to obtaining a complete cognitive profile.

3 Deficits in imaginal processes

There are two forms of imaginal deficits: deficits in visual imagery and in spatial imagery. Visual or spatial imagery can be selectively impaired.

3.1 Visual imagery

Visual imagery is defined as the conscious reproduction of previously experienced events and objects, their shape, colour, size, and any other visual attributes that we know.

- *Clinical presentation.* Patients may not realize that the brain lesion has induced a loss of imaginal visual attributes. On the contrary, they may be surprised not to be able to perform some tests. Loss of visual imagery may be observed together with visual agnosia or in the context of preserved visual recognition. Patients frequently also have right homonymous hemianopsia. Right hemiplegia and/or language disturbances (particularly shortly after a stroke) can also be present.

- *Brain damage localization.* Left posterior lesions.

- *Diagnosis.* Loss of visual imagery can be diagnosed only if the capacity to copy models and describe their visual characteristics is preserved (see Manning 2000).

3.1.1 Assessment

- Ask the patient to draw from memory and then to copy from canonical models, objects such as a cube, a flower, etc. This very simple and informative task can be carried out even at bedside.

- Ask the patient questions rich in visual attributes (e.g. 'what's the name of the bird with a hooked beak, large, flat face, round head, large eyes, and soft plumage?') and questions concerning functions only (e.g. 'the bird that stays awake all night long, flies, and hoots?'). Results are fairly straightforward: patients with no aphasic symptoms and impaired visual imagery fail selectively the 'visual' questions.

- Present the patient with coloured line drawings of canonical views of animals. Ask the patient to indicate whether the tail of the animal is long or short relative to its body in each of the following three conditions:

  — the perceptual control condition, in which the patient has to respond while looking at the depicted animal; if failed, the test should be discontinued;

  — the test situation proper, in which the tail of the animal is masked;

  — the auditory condition, where only the name of the animal is given.

This test allows comparisons to be drawn between the patient's ability to conjure up mental images from incomplete visual items and from auditory input. Patients with genuine loss of visual imagery will fail the test on the last two conditions.

- To test visual imagery of *colours*, administer the following tests:

  — Control condition. Present the patient with 10 different coloured patches. Ask him/her to point to the same coloured patch as indicated by the examiner on a set of identical coloured patches distributed differently. If the patient fails this task, discontinue the colour examination.

  — Present the patient with 10 or more uncoloured canonical line drawings and a good set of crayons. Ask him/her to fill in the line drawings with the appropriate colour.

— Auditory condition. Ask the patient the colour of different fruits (cherry, banana, tangerine), animals (tiger, elephant, parrot), and personal objects (his/her toothbrush, front door, car).

3.1.2 Recovery and rehabilitation

A treatment using nonvisual information consists of a series of familiar (e.g. spoon, key, watch) and less familiar objects (e.g. stapler, funnel, pair of goggles) to be *tactilely* explored by the patient. Objects' surfaces, or part of them, are covered with fabrics of different textures, which are associated with colours. Instruct the patient to describe the shape, imagine the colour (from the texture), imagine the object on a table, in a bag, near the window, etc.

The issue of imaginal rehabilitation is crucial for patients with artistic activity. Copying sufficiently elaborated models may allow the patient to re-acquire at least some of his/her technical and artistic skills. Models to be copied, which should be very well known to the patient, could be presented with progressively fewer parts as training of visual imagery progresses.

3.2 Spatial imagery

Spatial imagery is the ability to conjure up images of the location and structure of objects in three dimensions. The capacity to manipulate images is crucial to mental spatial transformations.

- *Clinical presentation.* It is not unusual for patients with spatial imagery deficits to say that they have more difficulty in 'working things out' than they used to before the brain accident.
- *Brain damage localization.* Left posterior lesions.
- *Diagnosis.* Deficits in spatial imagery are diagnosed if the patient fails tests of mental transformations, regardless of his/her ability or inability to conjure up visual images.

3.2.1 Assessment

- Present the patient with a sheet of paper containing capital letters in random order, half of them upside-down. Ask the patient to indicate which letters are the right way up. This is probably the easiest task and it is useful to start with it in order to reduce anxiety in patients who feel ill at ease when asked to perform spatial tasks.
- Ask the patient to imagine a capital letter and to count the corners. This task is sensitive enough to indicate if extended testing on spatial imagery is necessary.
- Give orally a series of letters, with (Q, G, etc.) or without (L, E, etc.) curves. Ask the patient to imagine them in the upper-case form and to indicate whether or not they have curves.
- Present a series of drawings of a man holding a black disc sometimes in his right and sometimes in his left hand. The figure should be shown upright or upside-down and from the front or from behind. Ask the patient to indicate in which hand the 'manikin' is holding the black disc. This rotation task is particularly useful in cases of association

of visual and spatial imagery, since the task elicits mental transformation but not generation of mental images.

3.2.2 Recovery and rehabilitation

A tactile training device utilizing a board with rotated, made fast letters can be used to treat spatial imagery.

4 Deficits in constructional processes

Constructional processes involve the ability to produce properly organized 'constructions' such as drawings and building tasks, i.e. to assemble patterns of simple arrangements made up of blocks, tokens, or sticks. They involve the ability of normal visual and motor systems to execute visuomotor tasks.

Clinicians use the term 'constructional apraxia' for convenience rather than as a term with a precise meaning. Different factors may provoke constructional difficulties. However, the symptoms are sufficiently distinctive to be defined independently of other classical apraxias and visuoperceptive deficits (see Andrewes 2001, pp. 35–81).

4.1 Clinical presentation

The patient is unable to grasp the way in which the component elements relate to the final model to be (re)-produced, and then to fit the components together in the correct spatial organization.

4.2 Brain localization

Either right or left parietal lesions. Incidence is higher after a right injury (right: left ratio of 3 : 1) and the deficit is more severe in right and bilaterally injured patients. Independently of the side, the predominantly posterior localization of lesions is confirmed by significant correlations between the damaged neural substrate of Brodmann's area 18 and constructional ability.

◆ *Left lesions* result in oversimplification of the model within the context of a relatively preserved spatial relation. The *cause* is failure in the organization of actions necessary for constructing tasks.

◆ *Right lesion* patients produce overelaborate, often irrelevant fragments showing spatial disorganization. The *cause* is failure in the organization of space.

4.3 Diagnosis

The patient's inability to perform drawing and construction tasks occurs in the context of the following preserved functions:

◆ visual form perception;

◆ spatial localization;

◆ ideomotor praxis.

Although 'pure' constructional apraxic patients are rarely encountered in everyday practice, at least a *relative* preservation of the above functions must be demonstrated before this can be diagnosed.

Note that relatively complex tasks make demands on sustained attention and therefore could be performed defectively without any clinical significance for constructional processes (e.g. the Complex Rey Figure Test). Should this be the case, base diagnosis on easier tasks (e.g. copy of a cube). Likewise, aphasic patients should have demonstrated their understanding of the verbal instructions before a constructional disability is diagnosed.

4.4 **Assessment**

+ Ask the patient to carry out a spontaneous drawing. Note that it can be difficult to score drawings produced on verbal command (right lesion patients may produce marked lateral neglect drawings; left lesion patients may be unable to perform—see Section 4.2.).

+ If this is the case, ask him/her to draw a bicycle (see Lezak 1995, pp. 74–81) and to comment on as many details as possible about the way in which the different parts relate to each other. (For example, a right parietal patient produced an elaborate defective bicycle with the pedals close to the saddle. Asked how she made it work, she told me, 'you have to bend your knees up'. Her verbal response was tailored to the defective relation of a component part to the whole, which she was unable to correct.)

+ Ask the patient to copy a line drawing, an abstract design such as the Rey Complex Figure. Scoring procedures for this and some other copying tasks (e.g. the copying section of the Benton Visual Retention Test; Benton 1962) are reliable and norms exist for different groups of brain-damaged patients and normal individuals (but see Section 4.2). Time of completion can be important for the qualitative analysis.

+ To assess greater demands on the spatial component of perception than those made by the drawing tests, present block construction tests. They test three-dimensional construction processes, which call upon a particular set of functions since they elicit deficits not shown on two-dimensional tests. The Benton Constructional Test, which has detailed norms, is frequently used together with two simple tasks from the Stanford–Binet battery, the Tower and the Bridge. The latter two tasks are useful for severely impaired patients.

+ The Block Design test (WAIS subtest or similar) is one of the most frequently used clinical tools. The patient is normally instructed to reproduce the models within a time limit since this is an IQ subtest for which norms are reliable and can be found in many different countries. However, when the task is used to assess constructional processes, no time limit should be imposed.

+ Constructing stick patterns and copying from stick patterns are both rapid and less demanding tasks, but norms are not readily available. Qualitatively, despite their simplicity, they have proved sensitive to constructional impairment.

The common and characteristic factor among these constructional tasks is that they all need to be carried out in extrapersonal space. On this basis, it is useful to bear in mind that right- and left-damaged patients fail constructional tests for different reasons: an inability to correctly organize the parts of an object and an inability to analyse those parts, respectively.

Note that visuoconstructional processes need to be assessed by at least two different tests, mainly due to only moderate intertest correlation coefficients and differing test sensitivity. Analysis of this latter point showed that clinicians relying on the WAIS Block Design alone could easily underestimate a high percentage of constructional apraxia patients whose impaired performance is apparent on the more sensitive Rey Complex Figure Test. A final point concerns constructional processes in neurodegenerative diseases. In demented patients of the Alzheimer type, impairments in constructional tests requiring access to semantic and lexical knowledge (e.g. drawing or constructing something meaningful) are present in the early phase of the disease, while impairments in constructional tests that do not require that access (e.g. copying the Rey Complex Figure) become evident in later phases. Digressions from this general pattern of deficits may prompt the clinician to envisage the administration of extended constructional batteries aiming at clarifying an early involvement of the posterior associative cortex in the onset of Alzheimer dementia in a given patient. In patients suffering from Parkinson's disease, performance on constructional tasks, particularly copying a cube, is associated with mobility in daily life and social cognition.

4.5 Recovery and rehabilitation

Spontaneous recovery has been observed in two-thirds of patients. The size of the lesion is not related to the rate of recovery from constructional disability. There is a difference in average recovery depending on the side of brain injury. Patients in the left-hemisphere group show better recovery a few months postonset than the right-hemisphere group. Rehabilitation programme reports are virtually non-existent in the literature. Compared to language or memory deficits, the inability to reproduce a line drawing or build a tower seems insignificant. 'Pure' cases are extremely rare and, whenever an intervention is reported, it is in the context of either motor or visuoperceptive impairments. Patients may never complain of being unable to reproduce patterns since this ability mostly involves non-ecological tasks.

Some empirical suggestions to be taken into account in a tailor-made rehabilitation programme follow.

◆ Analyse the patient's constructional errors concerning the whole, the parts, and the 'boundedness'. Observe the effects of time constraints. Some tasks (e.g. Block Design) are usually timed. It may be useful to obtain a score for standard time limit completion and a separate score for performance with no time constraints. However marginally patients may benefit from the extra time allowed them in terms of improved performance, comparisons of productions with and without a time limit might be helpful in determining whether different types of difficulty appear in each situation.

Table 11.2 'What to test and when': suggestions for everyday clinics for patients whose medical files and referral requests do not specify the symptoms (see text for more information)

Patient's characteristics	Suggested disorder to be tested
Defective pointing to and copying tasks; preserved shape recognition	Visual disorientation
Defective way and objects finding; preserved memory	Topographical disorientation
Defective or weak score on any subtest of the VOSP in routine examination	Visuospatial analysis disorder
Defective drawings from memory; preserved copies from models	Loss of visual imagery
Explicit complaint or loss of visual imagery	Loss of spatial imagery
Defective score on the Block Design task on routine assessment	Constructional apraxia

◆ Concerning daily life treatment, it is useful to bear in mind that

— there is a correlation between the WAIS-R Block Design subtest (see above) and meal preparation skills;

— some patients suffering from constructional apraxia may have difficulty in dressing (not the full-blown dressing apraxia picture), because a portion of the inability to dress is perceptual, not motor in origin. Constructional praxis treatment may produce some gains in the ability to dress.

Finally, computer-aided training programmes are available. The 'Visuoconstructive Abilities KONS' (Visuoconstructive Abilities Kons 1997) is intended for patients with mild or moderate constructional apraxia whose memory is preserved. The programme consists of 18 levels of difficulty. The authors state that the adaptive nature of the programme allows a great deal of variation in training. This has the advantage of ensuring maximum adjustment per patient, whose improvement is recorded. However, the programme makes no provision for quantitative data for groups of patients.

Table 11.3 Examples of treatments reported to have had positive effects on the patient's everyday life (see text for more information)

Disorder	Treatment	Everyday life
Visual disorientation	Fixating and reaching objects	Improved 'vision' in familiar surroundings
Topographical disorientation	Written lists and instructions	Find objects at home
	Mnemonics to create associations	Find familiar routes
	Back to the starting point task	Find familiar routes
Loss of visual imagery in artists	Copy and complete well-known pictures	Helps artistic production
Constructional apraxia	Training in constructional tasks	Meal preparation
		Ability to dress

5 Conclusion

- The deficits referred to in this chapter reflect a disturbance of the *processing* of sensory information, the sense organs usually remaining intact.
- Deciding 'What to test and when' considers both impaired and preserved functions, as shown in Table 11.2.
- To ensure that the patient receives appropriate treatment these syndromes must be diagnosed as early as possible. Table 11.3 lists the treatments that have been shown to have beneficial effects on everyday life.

Selective references

Andrewes, D. (2001). *Neuropsychology from theory to practice*. Psychology Press Ltd, Hove, East Sussex.

Benton, A. (1962). The visual retention test as a constructional praxis test. *Confina Neurologica* **22**, 141–55.

Benton, A., Hamsher, K., Varney, N., and Spreen, O. (1983). *Contributions to neuropsychological assessment*. Oxford University Press, New York.

Lezak, M. (1995). *Neuropsychological assessment*, 3rd edn. Oxford University Press, New York.

Manning, L. (2000). Loss of visual imagery and defective recognition of parts of wholes in optic aphasia. *Neurocase* **6**, 111–28.

Visuoconstructive Abilities KONS. (1997). *REHA COM*. Schuhfried, Moedling.

Warrington, E. and James, M. (1991). *The Visual Object and Space Perception Battery*. Thames Valley Test Company, Bury St Edmunds.

Zihl, J. (2000). *Rehabilitation of visual disorders after brain injury*. Psychology Press, Hove, East Sussex.

Chapter 12

Assessing disorders of awareness and representation of body parts

Carlo Semenza

1 Introduction

Disorders of awareness and representation of body parts traditionally encompass a number of very heterogeneous pathological conditions, whose link with one another share a common intuition that something about the representation of body has been damaged. This chapter acknowledges this tradition in the absence of a better way to cover the whole topic in a clinical handbook. Some provisos, however, must precede the description of single pathological entities.

For some time, the common factor grouping together these different behavioural pathologies was their effect on the so-called 'body schema'. This largely underspecified concept has enjoyed an immense, undeserved, and potentially damaging popularity. First, the concept has always been very vague. Second, a large variety of symptoms have been attributed to a 'disturbance of body schema' and then used to prove the validity of the concept. The circularity of this line of reasoning was first pointed out by Poeck and Orgass (1971), but it took several years for neuropsychologists to become aware of this problem and avoid the concept. Serious theorizing about disorders of bodily awareness and representation must thus be regarded, with the exception of a few studies, to be the result of a relatively recent enterprise that has taken place, over the past 3 decades. This whole matter is dealt with, in detail, in several recent reviews (e.g. Denes 1989; Semenza 2001).

Quite apart from poor theorizing, the field has also suffered from inappropriate procedures and a failure to demonstrate body specificity for the effects emerging from clinical investigations. These all have seriously hampered traditional assessment and the theoretical conclusions derived from such methods. A good example is the request to draw one's own body as a method to test a subject's knowledge and sensory experience of their 'body schema'. Typically, such a procedure, suggested by authorities such as Schilder (1935), ignored the fact that drawing abilities were spared in all cases.

2 Overview: the variety of pathologies (representation and awareness)

One reason for the neglect of theory in the field is that the most significant pathological conditions (Table 12.1) are, in general, rare and often difficult to spot, especially since most patients do not spontaneously complain about them.

Table 12.1 Disorders of body representation and awareness

Autotopagnosia
Somatosensory hallucinations and illusions
Hemisomatagnosia (personal neglect) and related disorders
Allochiria
Somatoparaphrenia
Extinction of contralesional stimuli to bilateral stimulation
Distal extinction on unilateral double stimulation
Altered muscular proprioception
Proprioceptive deafferentation
Deafferentation after parietal lesions
Alien hand syndrome (including Anarchic Hand)
Phantom limb and related disorders
Body-specific cognitive biases in eating disorders

- The clearest example of body-specific representation disorder is *autotopoagnosia*, a rare condition where the patient cannot locate body parts on verbal command. The neuropsychological instruments used to detect such a disorder are paradigmatic and were developed from principled criteria. Consequently, they will be mentioned first.

- Hemisomatoagnosia or personal neglect and related disorders such as allochiria and extinction of contralesional stimuli to bilateral tactile stimulation are traditionally ascribed to malfunctioning of body awareness. Distal extinction on uni-lateral double stimulation is another interesting condition with a different clinical meaning. This group of quite commonly observed disturbances have been extensively investigated and clinicians can therefore profit from a large repertory of clinical tools.

- The alien hand syndrome, though sometimes overlapping conceptually with hemiso-matoagnosia, is an uncommon cluster of symptoms wherein involuntary limb movements are coupled with a sense of estrangement from or of personification of the limb.

- Somatosensory hallucinations and illusions mainly consist of the experience of a larger, a smaller, or even a duplicated body. Some patients also report being 'unable to recognize their body boundaries' or their posture. There is no established assessment for these disorders, most reports being anecdotal. They will, therefore, not be discussed here, except for the more common ones, i.e. those associated with personal neglect that concern the contralesional side of the body.

- The consequences of altered muscular proprioception, proprioceptive deafferentation, and deafferentation after parietal lesion will also be described here, although well reported cases are extremely rare.

- Consciousness of missing body parts, i.e. phantom limb and related phenomena, constitutes a less traditional domain for neuropsychological investigation, since no direct damage to the brain is involved (despite considerable reorganization of the cortical representation of missing body parts). A detailed assessment of these conditions, rather frequent in amputees, depends on careful observational and experimental studies.

◆ Finally, *body-specific cognitive biases in eating disorders* will be considered. The reason for including this is not that these problems are treated as 'body schema' or 'body image' disorders. However, it has been recently shown that such biases (basically consisting of misjudgements of size and weight) can be body-specific. These observations were derived from, among other things, neuropsychological data.

Theoretically motivated rehabilitation of all the above disorders has rarely been attempted, except in the case of personal neglect, and often only in severe cases, where the condition dramatically interfered with everyday life.

3 Autotopagnosia

Autotopagnosia is the inability to locate body parts in response to command. The nature of this disturbance is not well understood in terms of the mental representations and cognitive processes involved.

The main preoccupation for researchers has been to make sure that the observed phenomenon is related to experience of the body. This deficit has to be the primary deficit, i.e. it should not result from other cognitive disorders. In its assessment, as in any case of agnosia, other sources of error should be ruled out. It is therefore important to make sure that aphasia, attentional deficits (e.g. neglect), visual or tactile agnosia, apraxia, or reaching disturbances, as well as more peripheral motor and sensory disorders, cannot explain the observed inability. Other more subtle and less well known deficits must equally be ruled out, such as the inability to isolate parts from a whole—a rare disorder that, in the past, was thought to be the basis of what seemed, in all other respects, to be true cases of autotopagnosia (De Renzi and Scotti 1970)

The term 'autotopagnosia' itself is not without problems. As Gerstman (1942) observed, and as the prefix 'auto' implies, 'autotopagnosia should, in principle, refer to a difficulty in indicating one's own body parts and not the body parts of other persons, of mannequins or drawings of a body'. Gerstman proposed the term 'somatotopagnosia' to include difficulties with the body parts of others. Indeed, no reported case has been shown where the difficulty only concerns one's own body parts and not also those of other people. Thus, in a strict sense, pure autotopagnosia has never been described. The arguably more correct term 'somatotopagnosia', however, was never fully adopted, and 'autotopagnosia' remains the currently used name for the disorder.

A detailed theoretical treatment of autotopagnosia and the operational tasks used to reveal such a disturbance has never been attempted. Available empirical evidence, however, suggests that specific transcoding mechanisms support the localization of body parts. Various input (verbal, visual, tactile) and output (motor, verbal) modalities are involved, with or without the mediation of a body-specific representation in semantic memory. Both spatial and functional components have been identified as constituents of this representation (see later in this section), although it is still unclear as to what proportion these contribute and which tasks tap which component.

Assessment of the few known cases of autotopagnosia (Table 12.2) has been performed using four specific tasks (Semenza and Goodglass 1985; Semenza 2001; Semenza and Delazer, 2003) and several control tasks.

3.1 **Pointing tasks**

The request to point to body parts is the task that originally uncovered autotopagnosia as a clinical entity, when the subject showed an inability to carry it out. This task should be assessed in at least two conditions: a *verbal* and a *nonverbal* one. Failure in the verbal condition only may be attributed to aphasia (though not necessarily in an uninteresting way: if found to be specific for the names of body parts, for instance, a comprehension disorder would be a relatively rare category-specific aphasia).

Several transcoding subtests, varying in stimulus and response, are also required in order to:

- ascertain whether the symptom concerns parts of one's own and also those of other's bodies (though so far the two deficits have never been found to dissociate);

- be reasonably sure that the problem is not one of isolating one part within the whole (see later for further testing).

Table 12.2 Transcoding tasks used in the assessment of autotopagnosia

Stimulus	Example	Response
Pointing tasks		
Verbal command	'Show me the ear'	Pointing to self Pointing to other person Pointing to drawing (full size) Pointing to drawing (single parts)
Nonverbal command	Examiner touches self Examiner touches the patient (who must keep the eyes closed) Examiner shows a picture of isolated parts	Pointing to self Pointing to other person Pointing to drawing (full size) Pointing to drawing (cut-out single parts)
Verification tasks	'Am I touching the ear?'	Yes/no (verbal or nonverbal indication)
Construction tasks	From pieces of puppets, etc.	
Description tasks		
Structural description	'Is the nose above or below the mouth?' 'Is the wrist next to the forearm?'	
Functional description	'What is the nose for?' 'Is the nose for smelling?'	

Of particular importance are tests in which the patient is touched while keeping his/her eyes closed and then requested to point to the stimulated part on someone else's body. The observed difficulty in this task allowed Semenza and Goodglass (1985) to conclude that authentic, body-specific, autotopagnosic errors could be detected after left-hemisphere brain damage.

Classification of the patient's errors is important and is indeed necessary to understand the nature of the mental representation whose disturbance is thought to result in the problem. Semenza and Goodglass (1985) divided autotopagnosic errors into three types of categories.

- *Contiguity (spatial) errors*, same limb as stimulus or face–head response for a face–head stimulus; this group includes errors that reflect misreaching.

- *Conceptual errors.* Different types of errors are included under this label: joint for joint, eye–ear–nose substitutions and *contiguity errors* where alternative response choices are presented as cut-out parts in a multiple choice display. This last type of error is not classified as spatial because it cannot possibly result from a spatially vague indication. It is indeed likely to derive from a disorder in the conceptual representation or in its output.

- *Random* errors include all the remaining.

A prevalence of conceptual or contiguity errors may indicate the type of autotopagnosia. It has been recently recognized that, in some of the reported cases (e.g. I.S. in Semenza 1988), a conceptual component is crucial to the defect, while in other cases (e.g. patients V.M. and D.A. in Denes *et al.* 2000) the spatial component appears to be overwhelming.

A sufficient number of body parts must appear in pointing tests (Semenza and Goodglass used 18), including parts of the head, of the limbs, and of the trunk. For special purposes, the investigator may want to include less prominent parts like wrists, nails, etc. No dissociation concerning these parts has, however, been described.

3.2 Verification tasks

Published cases of autotopagnosia have reported patients who perform this task flawlessly. Thus autotopagnosia does not affect recognition for body parts but rather affects transcoding tasks that include pointing to body parts as an output.

3.3 Construction tasks

These tasks require the subject to build up a two- or three-dimensional body (or just a head; Ogden 1985) from separate pieces. Typically, autotopagnosics cannot perform these tasks and tend to miss correct positions. Ogden's patient, for instance, put the ears where the eyes should go and vice versa or put the mouth at the top of the head.

Patients are invariably unhappy with their performance and appear puzzled on completion. They cannot, however, tell what exactly is wrong with their construction. While this behaviour underlines the importance of the spatial component, it also suggests that a functional component must be disturbed as well. Since simple recognition of single body parts (as shown in verification tasks) is unaffected, it appears that knowledge of their exact function, which would allow the patient, for instance, to spot a hand/foot confusion, is less than intact.

3.4 Description tasks

These tests are meant to tap knowledge of body parts as stored in the semantic system. Such tests require at least two different kinds of description: that of structural attributes and that of functional attributes. Either questions requiring a categorical response (yes/no) or more open questions involving different degrees of difficulty have been used. Questions implying structural descriptions include:

- Is the wrist next to the forearm?
- Is the mouth above or below the nose?
- Where is the elbow?

Examples of questions implying functional descriptions include:

- Is the mouth for eating?
- What is the mouth for?

Unfortunately, no published study of autotopagnosia has pursued a thorough investigation using these or similar tasks. Patients seem to be more disturbed on structural items than on functional ones. An isolated deficit for 'description' tasks has never been reported.

3.5 Control tasks

Body specificity should be the only defining feature of autotopagnosia. It is thus necessary to collect evidence of the patient's ability to locate parts of other complex objects. If the patient fails also in this task, he/she cannot be considered a 'genuine' autotopoagnosic. If the deficit cannot be attributed to more general problems, such as reaching inabilities, visual agnosia, etc., it must be attributed to the 'inability to locate parts within a whole', cases of which were described by De Renzi and Scotti (1970) and by De Renzi and Faglioni (1963) and never reported since.

A good control task was used in Semenza's (1988) study. The patient was asked to locate on verbal command parts of a bike, a shoe, and a pair of glasses. In a nonverbal condition, the same parts on the object were first pointed to by the examiner—the patient had then to point to the equivalent part on a different object of the same kind, but with a different shape. For instance the examiner pointed to the heel of a heavy boot and the patient had to point to the heel of a high-heeled elegant lady's shoe. Patient I.S. was flawless in both the verbal and the nonverbal condition.

Control tasks should also be devised for construction and description tasks. In the case of 'construction' tasks, a dissociation is unlikely to be found because constructional apraxia is likely to be a concurrent deficit. The diagnosis of autotopagnosia thus rests mainly on pointing tasks. Selective deficits or a selective sparing within semantic memory of bodily knowledge (functional and/or structural) have never been properly investigated.

4 Personal neglect and related disorders (see Chapter 6)

Unilateral spatial neglect and a number of less frequent but often associated disorders are a relatively common consequence of right hemisphere lesions (and, in particular, stroke). In addition to extrapersonal space and peripersonal space, unilateral neglect may affect one-half of the patient's body. This condition is called *personal neglect* or *hemisomatagnosia*. According to Bisiach and Vallar (2000), this phenomenon is less frequent than extrasomatic neglect. Somatic and extrasomatic neglect are usually found in association, but double dissociations have been observed. While, however, severe extrasomatic neglect may be found in many patients where somatic neglect is absent, severe somatic neglect unaccompanied by neglect of extrasomatic space is very infrequent (Bisiach *et al.* 1986; Bisiach and Vallar 2000).

Selective personal neglect mostly occurs after right-sided lesions. However, neglect of the right personal space may also be a consequence, in the early phases of the disease (Peru and Pinna 1997), of a left-sided lesion. Indeed, it often occurs in the form of paroxysmal symptomatology, most frequently in the course of epilepsy or migrane (De Renzi 1982). For further details concerning localization, including symptoms raising after left-sided lesions, the reader is referred to Bisiach and Vallar's (2000) review.

In the absence of relevant primary motor deficits, unilateral neglect may affect motor functions of contralateral limbs. In this condition automatic movements may, however, be relatively preserved.

4.1 Related disorders

4.1.1 Allochiria

Allochiria is a disorder, often associated with unilateral visual neglect, wherein tactile stimuli delivered to the contralesional side of somatic (or extrasomatic) space are referred to the symmetrical location on the ipsilateral side. Less frequently, analogous phenomena may be observed in the auditory or in the visual modality (but see Halligan *et al.* 1995).

4.1.2 Anton–Babinski's syndrome

A frequently associated disorder is *anosognosia* for deficits contralateral to the lesion, known as *Anton–Babinski's syndrome*. While Anton (1899) first noted this condition, Babinski (1914) recognized it as resulting from a focal cortical lesion. This disorder may or may not be accompanied by a generalized anosognosia for illness. This condition has been observed to double dissociate from somatosensory and motor neglect (Bisiach *et al.* 1986; Stone *et al.* 1993).

Patients who are anosognosic for deficits contralateral to their lesion may show all degrees of severity, from minimization to obstinate denial of illness or of possession of the affected limb, even in the face of demonstrations by the examiners. Furthermore, delusions and confabulation concerning the affected side may appear (*somatoparaphre-nias*; Gerstman 1942), a typical instance of which is the attribution of a plegic limb to the examiner or to other people (Bottini *et al.* 2002). Other pathological attitudes include showing indifference (*anosodiaphoria*; Babinski 1914), an expression of dislike for the affected side (*misoplegia*), and *personification*, where affected limbs are spoken about in third person (he, she, etc.). These delusions may even include the belief that another person lies permanently on the affected side (Zingerle 1913; Nightingale 1982). This 'person' may elicit intense emotion and even erotic sensations. Concrete examples of delusions described in the literature are reported in Table 12.3.

4.1.3 Extinction of contralesional stimuli on bilateral stimulation (or double simultaneous stimulation)

This may be found in patients who can otherwise detect single contralesional stimuli (Oppenheim 1911; Bender *et al.* 1948; Head and Holmes 1911; Denny Brown *et al.* 1952). This phenomenon has been reported to occur in the tactile, auditory, visual, and olfactory modalities. While it equally affects all modalities, double dissociations have been reported (De Renzi *et al.* 1984; Vallar *et al.* 1994) among modalities and with personal and extrapersonal neglect.

Table 12.3 Examples of somatoparaphrenic delusions reported in the literature

- '[The left side of my body] belongs to a woman lying beside me' (Zingerle 1913)

- 'My old left hand began to shrink and a new hand has emerged, becoming fleshier and more voluminous' 'I have a nest of hands in my bed' (Ehrenwald 1930)

- '[This arm] is not mine: I found it in the bathroom, when I fell. It's not mine because it's too heavy; it should be yours. I can move and do everything; when I feel it too heavy, I put it on my stomach. It doesn't hurt me, it's kind.' (Rode *et al.* 1992)

- 'They took two fingers and joined them back together. The left hand, it's cut down the centre, but it still functions quite well. It's a nice hand.'

  'It's difficult ... to live with a foot that isn't yours .... I came to the conclusion that it was a cow's foot .... But .I adopted it.'

  My mother has a suitcase and there are at least three pairs of fingers in there, and they are all functional ... we brought them through the customs. The customs men were all shocked when they saw these fingers in a box. It wasn't conducive to good relations.'

  I could never tell why the doctors were so interested in amputating my arms, or my fingers ... or my legs.' 'I wake up with this arm lying in my bed with me ... but I remember the hairs and this nick here, and I realize it's my arm. It was a bit strange and disconnected. It had come loose from its bindings and was covered in blood. Not a nice thing. Sometimes it goes away ... It goes back to my mother's suitcase where it belongs ....'

The same patient four years later:

  'A few years ago it was somebody else's leg, not mine. To start with, I didn't think that my left arm and leg were my own. I thought that the left foot I kept in a box under my bed ... for safe keeping, for later ... and that solved the problem ... It's all very well to laugh at it now, but at the time it was pretty bloody terrifying, to say the least.' (Halligan *et al.* 1995)

Since Zingerle's (1913) early work, disorders related to spatial neglect, collectively labelled as *dyschiria*, have been viewed as a consequence of a disturbance of the conscious representation of one side of the body and (though with less emphasis, as Bisiach and Vallar 2000 have noted) of the extrapersonal environment. The appeal to the notion of the body schema as a cue to the understanding of the conditions (e.g. Brain 1941; Critchley 1953; Gerstman 1942) has been common in the past and, as Bisiach and Vallar (2000) have noted, may be considered the basis for Bisiach's own representational account (Bisiach and Luzzatti 1978; Bisiach 1995, 1999).

All these phenomena, however, have also been interpreted in terms of an attentional disorder. Whether attention is involved *per se* or as attention to an internal representation is still an open question (which, to a certain extent, reconciles attentional and representational interpretation of the phenomena). As Kinsbourne (1995) argued, if awareness of the body derived from selective attention to somatosensory input to various body parts, there would be no need for the *ad hoc* construct of a separate 'body schema'.

Whatever the interpretation, and despite the tradition of its inclusion in body schema disorders, personal neglect and related problems seem to say little about the content and the format of bodily representation—except to prove the independence of this representation from other representational contents and to be indicative of an analogous non-prepositional quality. This disturbance may be viewed as complementary to phantom limb sensation. Taken together the two disturbances may indeed be suggestive of a system, hardwired somewhere in the brain, imparting signals that 'this is my body, it is part of me'. One such system is considered by Melzack (1992) as a component of the 'neuromatrix' responsible for phantom sensations.

4.2 Clinical assessment

Patients with personal neglect may show the condition in various degrees of severity. Sometimes only a careful neuropsychological examination may detect the phenomenon. In other cases the presentation is more dramatic. The patient may be unable to dress properly, leaving one-half of the body unclothed, and showing signs of personal care only on one side, leaving the contralateral side very untidy. Proper assessment should contain at least a *checklist* of these behavioural anomalies related to body usage.

- When not so severe, the presence of personal neglect may be assessed by asking patients to touch contralesional body parts using the unaffected ipsilateral hand, or through tasks involving the patient's body, such as using a comb. Light touches or even pinprick stimulation of the afferent side may also be used. Patients may still deny pinprick stimulation while showing movements aimed at avoiding it.

- *Motor* neglect may be assessed (Bisiach and Vallar 2000) by requiring the patients *to extend their hands* or *to squeeze the examiner's fingers placed within the palms of their hands*. Motor neglect may vanish if the patient is invited to attend the neglected limb or is actively prevented from moving the non-neglected one.

- In order to systematically assess personal neglect, Cocchini *et al.* (2001) recently developed the *Fluff Test*. This test requires subjects to remove white cardboard circles

(2 cm in diameter) attached by velcro, at regular intervals, located to the front of their clothes. These stickers are distributed, on both the right and the left side, along the central body areas, the legs, and the arm that is not performing the task. The subject sits blindfolded whilst the circles are attached. Still blindfolded they are asked to remove all the stickers. The percentage of targets detached from each side is then calculated. Normative data are available.

Somewhat surprisingly, Cocchini *et al.* (2001) found no correlation and a double dissociation of the Fluff Test with the *Comb and Razor/Compact Test* (Beschin and Robertson 1997), a test requiring exploration of the face area. Their interpretation for this dissociation is still speculative. Further research is required to clarify this issue as well as the role of motor neglect in failing the test.

♦ *Self-evaluation tests* (Marcel and Tegner 1994; Berti *et al.* 1996) and *structured interviews* (e.g. Cutting 1978) that require the patient to carefully describe their problem may be useful in cases of anosognosia and somatoparaphrenia. Patients affected by these disorders may show dissociations in verbal reports on their abilities. They may consistently exhibit the belief that their affected limbs are perfectly functioning while showing, in contrast, a realistic self-evaluation. For example Berti *et al.*'s (1998) patient, C.C., assigned a score of 2/10 to her own ability to lift a glass with her left hand but, at the same time, claimed that she could perform the task perfectly.

As Halligan *et al.* (1995) pointed out, it is of the utmost importance to elicit full accounts of what such patients believe their condition to be. Such irrationalities may be important cues to the patients' mental contents. The evolution of symptoms over time may also be revealing. Halligan *et al.* (1995), reporting detailed abstracts of subsequent interviews with a somatoparaphrenic patient, showed how most symptoms could be interpreted as a delusional way of coping with new, unfamiliar sensations.

♦ *Extinction* is generally assessed by symmetrically presenting two identical stimuli at the same time. However (Critchley 1953), the phenomenon may appear even with different and asymmetrical stimulation (see, for instance, the 'face–hand test'; Fink and Bender 1952). Sometimes the contralesional stimulus is not entirely neglected, but just misperceived. Different types of material have been also used. Schwartz and co-workers (1979) used the Quality Extinction Test, which consisted of two sets of various common materials such as sandpaper, tin foil, velvet, etc. One set consisted of test items each of which was made entirely of the same material ('whole items') while the other consisted of items made up of two different materials side-by-side ('half and half items'). In the test, each item is brushed against the subject's fingers so that both hands are stimulated simultaneously. Stimulation with the 'half-and-half' is arranged so that a different material stimulates each hand at the same time. An 'extinction' trial is recorded if the subject names only one when in fact two have been presented. The total score is derived by subtracting the number of omissions made by the other hand and converting the difference into a percentage. Errors in naming are not scored.

4.3 **Rehabilitation (see Chapter 6)**

Patients with severe and persisting unilateral neglect are seriously handicapped in every-day life and rehabilitation should therefore be attempted as soon as possible. Neglect is not only handicapping, but it has been demonstrated (Denes *et al.* 1982) to interfere in general rehabilitation. A major obstacle to rehabilitation efforts is the frequent co-occurrence of anosognosia.

Rehabilitation of unilateral neglect has been attempted with different techniques and different success (see Zoccolotti 1999; and Robertson and Halligan 1999 for comprehensive reviews). They mostly consist of repeated lateralized stimulation to the affected side and, in general, employ a series of sensory suggestions orientating or anchoring the patient's attention to the side of the target stimuli.

Visual stimuli have been most frequently used but somatosensory-proprioceptile and vestibular stimulation has also been employed with some improvement. Vestibular stimulation, in particular (Rubens 1985; Cappa *et al.* 1987; Vallar *et al.* 1990; Bisiach *et al.* 1991; Rode *et al.* 1992), has been shown to temporarily reduce remission of unilateral neglect phenomena, including somatoparaphrenic delusions and even associated motor deficits.

Most current attempts are made on patients affected by both personal and extraper-sonal neglect, without clear efforts to distinguish the two conditions. Positive results are (with some notable exceptions, e.g. Halligan *et al.* 1992) generally reported. The effects of treatment have been shown to surpass those of spontaneous recovery, to be specific for neglect, to be stable over time after dismissal, and to extend to tasks not involved in treatment, at least when rehabilitation is protracted enough (Antonucci *et al.* 1995; see Chapter 6, this volume).

4.4 **Distal extinction to unilateral double tactile stimulation**

Patients may show extinction of the distal stimulus on unilateral tactile double stimulation (Denny Brown *et al.* 1952; Bender *et al.* 1948). This phenomenon is relatively little known, although it has been considered an early sign of diffuse brain damage (e.g. dementia). Cohn (1951), however, described it as a common finding in 3–5-year-old normal children. Typically, subjects are stimulated on the face and on the hand, the face stimulus being invariably the one resistant to the extinction. Other locations (e.g. shoulder and hand) may be chosen and a rostral dominance is invaed, the foot will be dominant (Bender *et al.* 1948).

5 **Alien hand syndrome (see Chapter 20)**

The alien hand syndrome is a loosely defined cluster of symptoms, characterized by involuntary movements of a limb in conjunction with an experience of estrangement from and personification of the limb itself (see Blakemore *et al.* (2002)). The limb is perceived as having a will of its own, though ownership is seldom denied. While the syndrome concerns upper limbs, it may affect the legs.

The underlying pathology involves lesions of two types.

* In the *anterior type*, the damage is either to the left frontal lobe and to the anterior corpus callosum or to the corpus callosum alone. In the first case the right, dominant limb is affected, while in the second case the symptomatology is found in the left limb.

* In the less frequent, *posterior type*, the damage consists of corticobasal degeneration or, in a few cases, of posterior vascular damage. The anatomical substrate is the parietal and posterofrontal cortex and the corresponding subcortical areas, bilaterally. Recently, however, Martì-Fabregas *et al.* (2000) have described a patient with a vascular lesion limited to the right parietal lobe. Generally, if not exclusively, posterior cases have been found to involve the nondominant limbs.

The clinical presentation includes several phenomena. The following is taken from Fisher (2000).

* Failure to identify an upper limb as one's own on palpating it behind the back or with the eyes closed. As Fisher (2000) observes, this was the original definition.

* Movement of a limb that the patient regards as foreign, unwilled, strange, uncooperative. The limb seems to act on its own, outside the patient's control. It may actively contradict the other limb (see Della Sala *et al.* (1991)).

* Stereotyped 'reflex' motor activity of the 'frontal' type: reaching out, groping and grasping with inability to release, utilization behaviour, tactile and visual oral reactions.

* Other: withdrawal of a limb; flinging movement of optico-sensory ataxia.

Alien hand symptoms following corticobasal lesions may be distinguished insofar as involuntary movements are typically non-purposeful and non-conflictual, and include such behaviours as arm levitation and finger-writhing (Bundick and Spinella 2000). The corticobasal, posterior variety, therefore, does not include 'frontal' symptoms.

Patients with alien hand are usually alert, cooperative, interested, and aware of the movements requested. Their reaction to their symptomatology varies from frustration and torment to amusement. Concrete examples of alien hand behaviour described in literature are provided in Table 12.4.

6 **Altered muscular proprioception**

The role of muscular proprioception and its contribution to bodily representation emerges from observations of patients suffering from proprioceptive deafferentation due to peripheral pathologies and deafferentation due to central lesions. These patients are extremely rare and no routine clinical assessment is available. However, existing detailed descriptions of the phenomenon suggest the framework for proper testing procedures (Cole and Paillard 1995; Paillard *et al.* 1983).

One type of patient has been observed with a very selective and complete loss of large sensory fibres, while motor and small sensory fibres are left intact. Muscular proprioception

Table 12.4 Examples of alien hand behaviour

- [On order to pick an object with the right hand] Picking the object, the right hand approaches it and pauses, the left hand comes over to approach the object, and then both hands pick the object (left hemisphere infarction; Liepmann 1900).

- Put on clothes with the right hand and pull them off with the left hand.

  Open a drawer or a door with the right hand and simultaneously push it shut with the left hand. Dry the clean dishes and then put them back in the pan to be washed again.

  When thirsty fill a glass with water and then pour it out (following callosotomy; Akelaitis 1945).

- Inability, on verbal command, to place the left hand behind the head or to use it to point to something.

  Reaching across with the right hand to grab the left hand and place it in proper position (following callosotomy; Gazzaniga et al. 1962).

- Failure to recognize as one's own one of the hands, usually the left, when the hands were out of sight (callosal tumour; Brion and Jedynak 1972).

- Hands fighting each other: holding an envelope, each hand independently and simultaneously tries to hold and to release it, tugging at it, sometimes for as long as 10 minutes (anterior cerebral artery infarction; Watson and Heilman 1983).

- The right hand pays for an item in a store, the left hand withdraws the money; while purchasing something else the left hand picks up an orange (ruptured anterior cerebral artery; Papagno and Marsile 1995).

- While the left hand takes food to the mouth with the fork, the right hand brings the knife towards the eye with the risk of injury (corticobasal degeneration; Lhermitte et al. 1925).

- The left hand has a tendency to levitation and the fingers wander 'like the tentacles of an anemone' (corticobasal degeneration; Gibb et al. 1989).

---

is lost but vestibular information as well as the senses of pain and temperature is retained.

These patients express the feeling of using their bodies as tools, relying heavily on visual feedback, concentration, and intellectual effort. Motor automatism is apparent to them. If their vision is precluded, their ability to preshape the grip posture to the size and shape of a target would be absent.

On clinical examination, these patients may be asked, when blindfolded, to point to a part of their skin where a thermal stimulus (which they perceive) had been delivered. They could not carry out such a task. In dramatic contrast, however, they would be able to verbally designate the point ('over my elbow') and later to show it precisely on the picture of a human body.

Patients with parietal lesions may suffer from deafferentation of a body area. For instance, in the case reported by Paillard et al. (1983), a parietal lesion provoked deafferentation of the forearm. The patient was unable, when blindfolded, to detect the presence of a tactile stimulus on the affected area, but was surprisingly able to indicate the place of stimulation with the other hand. Paillard et al. considered this phenomenon to be the equivalent of blindsight in the tactile modality.

7 Phantom limb and related phenomena

Most amputees experience the continued existence of the amputated limb or body part. Detailed descriptions of all aspects of this phenomenon, including the history of condition, may be found in Ramachandran and Hirstein (1998), Ramachandran and Rogers Ramachandran (2000), Semenza (2001) and Halligan (2002). This chapter is only concerned with clinical assessment and attempts at rehabilitation.

Phantoms involve not only limbs but also other body parts such as breasts, male genitalia, or facial parts like the jaw. Amputation is not essential for the occurrence of such phantoms. They have been reported in conditions such as brachial plexus avulsion, spinal cord damage, and even single spinal anaesthesia. Even patients with congenital absence of limbs experience phantoms.

Phantom sensations are spontaneous but may also be evoked with appropriate stimulation not only of the stump but also of distant body areas. For instance, the stimulation of the ipsilateral side of the face may evoke sensations in phantom hands (e.g. Halligan *et al.* (1993) and Halligan *et al.* 1999). Referred sensations are often topographically organized and may be modality-specific. Thus, for example, hot, cold, vibration, rubbing, metal, or massage are felt as hot, cold, vibration, rubbing, metal, or massage at precisely localized points of the phantom limb. Such sensations can occur even hours after amputation.

A thorough interview should be carried on to assess phantom limb phenomena, considering all the main factors characterizing phantoms. (see Fraser, Halligan, Robertson and Kirker 2001) Phantom sensations seem to vary considerably in their intensity and veridicality. The size and form of missing parts may change over time. The vividness of the phantom sensation is typically enhanced by imaginary tasks performed with the phantom limb. The phantom may change in form or disappear in consequence of particular movements, e.g. bringing the stump near to a wall. Absent limbs seem to coordinate with the rest of the body in movement.

Patients may be able to provide a correct evaluation of the size, length, and weight of the missing part; in other cases the missing part may be perceived as shortened or in a bizarre, anatomically impossible position. 'Islands' of phantom sensation may be all the patient feels, e.g. phantom hands may be felt as suspended in mid-air. A common distinctive phenomenon that occurs over time is 'telescoping'—a phantom may gradually retract in such a way that, in the end, peripheral parts seem to join to the stump.

Pain is the most typical feature of phantom sensation and occurs in approximately 70% of cases. When severe it is described as burning, cramping, or shooting. Complex sensations may also accompany phantoms—patients with lower cord injury may report the sensation of defecation; phantom penises experience ejaculation.

A less frequent and less known phenomenon is the felt presence of and hallucinatory belief in the real existence of supernumerary body parts. Such a condition may paradoxically coexist with denial of hemiplegia and feeling of nonbelonging of the contralesional limb (Halligan *et al.* 1993).

7.1 Rehabilitation attempts

Phantom limb phenomena appear dependent on neural reorganization after amputation or the equivalent (besides already indicated references, see, on this point, Karl *et al.* 2001).

On the basis of findings that phantom limb pain is closely associated with plastic changes in the primary somatosensory cortex and on animal data that show that behaviourally relevant training alters the cortical map, Flor *et al.* (2001), have recently devised a sensory discrimination training programme for patients with intractable phantom limb pain. The programme consists of 10 daily 90-minute sessions of feedback-guided sensory training, in which patients have to discriminate the frequency or the location of high-intensity nonpainful electric stimuli applied in a random fashion through electrodes attached to their stump. After this training, patients showed a significant improvement in discriminating both the location and the frequency of the stimuli as well as a significant reduction of pain.

Ramachandran and Rogers-Ramachandran (1996) required phantom limb patients to look at the reflection of their intact hand mirror-reflected on the felt location of their phantom hand. The patients were thus able, while moving the intact hand, to receive visual feedback that the phantom hand was obeying commands. A number of patients appeared to benefit from repeated use of such procedures, in that they were relieved of spasms and cramps, with elimination of associated pain.

8 Body-specific cognitive biases in eating disorders

Mental anorexia and bulimia have been considered to be disorders of body schema. Modern investigators, however, quite rightly believe (see a review by Hsu and Sobkiewic 1991) that this ida is unfounded. Nonetheless subjects affected by eating disorders have been shown to be unable to correctly judge the size of their bodies. This problem is nowadays attributed to a 'cognitive bias' that is thought to commonly accompany eating disorders (Thompson 1990).

Typically, patients with eating disorders have been found to misjudge hip-to-hip, armpit-to-armpit, and cheekbone-to-cheekbone distances or the size of the waist. Waist size and hip-to-hip distance seem the most likely to be grossly misjudged.

Despite the variety of detection techniques, surprisingly little has been done so far to ascertain with proper control conditions whether misjudgement of size is indeed body-specific as has been always assumed. A few investigations (e.g. Slade and Russell 1973; Franzen *et al.* 1988; Probst *et al.* 1998a,b) required estimation of the size of small tridimensional objects or of the length of short lines. While these control conditions seemed to indicate that, indeed, size misjudgements are body-specific, the choice of measures is far from being satisfactory, since in most investigations control distances are grossly different from body distances. No weight estimation has been properly controlled. No comparison has been made between misjudgements of one's own body and of other people's bodies, whether of females or males. No control has ever been made on the modality of response (e.g. whether verbal responses differ from nonverbal responses). Comparisons between different types of anorexia and bulimia have been rare (Probst *et al.* 1998*a,b*).

No routine clinical instruments are, therefore, available for evaluating cognitivebiases in eating disorders. Ideally, however, their proper assessment should take into consideration the above observations.

Selective references

Akelaitis, A.J. (1945). Studies on the corpus callosum IV. Diagonist dyspraxia in epileptics following partial and complete section of the corpus callosum. *Am. J. Psychiatry* **101**, 594–9.

Anton, G. (1899). Uber die Selbstwahrnehmung der Herderkrankungen des Gehirns durch den Kranken bei Rindenblindheit und Rindentaubheit. *Arch. Psychiatrie Nervenkrankh.* **32**, 86–127.

Antonucci, G., Guariglia, C., Judica, A., Magnotti, L., Paolucci, S., Pizzamiglio, L., and Zoccolotti, P. (1995). Effectiveness of neglect rehabilitation in a randomised group study. *J. Clin. Exp. Neuropsychol.* **17**, 386–9.

Babinski, J. (1914). Contribution a l'étude des troubles dans l'hémiplégie cérébrale. *Rev. Neurologique* **31**, 365–7.

Bender, M.L., Wortis, S.B., and Cramer, J. (1948). Organic mental syndrome with phenomena of extinction and allesthesia. *Arch. Neurol. Psychiatry* **59**(3), 273–91.

Berti, A., Ladavas, E., and Della Corte, M. (1996). Anosognosia for hemiplegia, neglect dyslexia and drawing neglect. Clinical findings and theoretical considerations. *J. Int. Neuropsychol. Soc.* **2**, 426–40.

Berti, A., Ladavas, E., Stracciari, A., Giannarelli, C., and Ossola, A. (1998). Anosognosia for motor impairment and dissociations with patients' evaluation of the disorder: theoretical considerations. *Cogn. Neuropsychiatry* **3**(1), 21–44.

Beschin, N. and Robertson, I.H. (1997). Personal versus extrapersonal neglect: a group study of their dissociation using a reliable clinical test. *Cortex* **33**, 379–84.

Bisiach, E. (1995). Unawareness of unilateral neurological impairment and disordered representation of one side of the body. *Higher Brain Function Res.* **15**, 113–40.

Bisiach, E. (1999). Unilateral neglect and related disorders. In *Handbook of clinical and experimental neuropsychology* (ed. G. Denes and L. Pizzamiglio), pp. 479–96. Psychology Press, Hove, East Sussex.

Bisiach, E. and Luzzatti, C. (1978). Unilateral neglect of representational space. *Cortex* **14**, 129–33.

Bisiach ,E. and Vallar, G. (2000). Unilateral neglect in humans. In *Handbook of neuropsychology* (ed. F. Boller, J. Grafman, and G. Rizzolatti), Vol. 1, pp. 459–502. Elsevier Publishers, Amsterdam.

Bisiach, E., Perani, D., Vallar, G., and Berti, A. (1986). Unilateral neglect: personal and extrapersonal. *Neuropsychologia* **24**, 759–67.

Bisiach, E., Rusconi, M.L., and Vallar, G. (1991). Remission of somatoparaphrenic delusion through vestibular stimulation. *Neuropsychologia* **29**, 1029–31.

Bottini, G., Bisiach, E., Sterzi, R. and Vallar, G. (2002). Feeling Touches in someone else's hand. *Neuroreport* **13**, 249–52.

Blakemore, S.J., Wolpert, D.M., and Frith, C.D. (2002). Abnormalities in the awareness of action. *Trends Cogn. Sci.* Jun 1; **6**(6), 237–42.

Brain, W.R. (1941). Visual disorientation with special reference to lesions of the right hemisphere. *Brain* **84**, 244–72.

Brion, S. and Jedynak, C.P. (1972). Troubles du transfert interhémispherique (callosal disconnection) a propos de 3 observations de tumeurs du corps calleux. Le signe de la main étrangère. *Rev. Neurologique* **4**, 273–90.

Bundick, T. and Spinella, M. (2000). Subjective experience, involuntary movement, and posterior alien hand syndrome. *J. Neurol., Neurosurg., Psychiatry* **68**, 83–5.

Cappa, S., Sterzi, R., Vallar, G., and Bisiach, E. (1987). Remission of hemineglect and anosognosia after vestibular stimulation. *Neuropsychologia* **25**, 775–82.

Cocchini, G., Beschin, N., and Jehkonen, M. (2001). The Fluff Test: a simple task to assess body representation neglect. *Neuropsychol. Rehabil.* **11**, 17–31.

Cohn, R. (1951). On certain aspects of the sensory organization of the human brain. *Neurology* **2**, 119–22.

Cole, J. and Paillard, J. (1995). Living without touch and peripheral information about body position and movement: studies with deafferented subjects. In *The body and the self* (ed. J.L. Bermudez, A.J. Marcel, and N. Eilan), pp. 245–66. MIT Press, Cambridge, Massachusetts.

Critchley, M. (1953). *The parietal lobes.* Edward Arnold, London.

Cutting, J. (1978). Study of anosognosia. *J. Neurol., Neurosurg., Psychiatry* **41**, 548–55.

Della Sala, S., Marchetti, C., and Spinnler, H. (1991). Right-sided anarchic (alien) hand: a longitudinal study. *Neuropsychologia*, 1113–27.

Denes, G. (1989). Disorders of body awareness and body knowledge. In *Handbook of neuropsychology* (ed. F. Boller and J. Grafman), Vol. 2, pp. 207–27. Elsevier Publishers, Amsterdam.

Denes, G., Semenza, C., Stoppa, E., and Lis, A. (1982). Unilateral spatial neglect and recovery from hemiplegia. A follow-up study. *Brain* **105**, 543–52.

Denes, G., Cappelletti, J.Y., Zilli, T., Dalla Porta, F., and Galliana, F. (2000). A category-specific deficit of spatial representation: the case of autotopagnosia. *Neuropsychologia* **38** (4), 345–50.

Denny Brown, D., Meyer, J.S., and Horenstein, S. (1952). The significance of perceptual rivalry resulting from parietal lesions. *Brain* **75**, 433–71.

De Renzi, E. (1982). *Disorders of space exploration and cognition.* Wiley and Sons, New York.

De Renzi, E. and Faglioni, P. (1963). Autotopoagnosia. *Arch. Psicol., Neurol. Psichiatria* **24**, 1–34.

De Renzi, E. and Scotti, G. (1970). Autotopagnosia: fiction or reality? Report of a case. *Arch. Neurol.* **23**, 221–7.

De Renzi, E., Gentilini, M., and Pattacini, F. (1984). Auditory extinction following hemisphere damage. *Neuropsychologia* **22**, 733–44.

Eherenwald, H. (1930). Verandertes Erleben des Korperbildes mit konsekutiver Wahnbildung bei linkseitiger Hemiplegie. *Monatschr. Psychiatrie Neurologie* **75**, 89–97.

Fink, M. and Bender, B. (1952). Perception of simultaneous tactile stimuli in normal children. *Neurology* **3**, 27–34.

Fisher, C.M. (2000). Alien hand syndrome: a review with the addition of six personal cases. *Can. J. Neurol. Sci.* **27**, 192–203.

Flor, H., Denke, C., Schaefer, M., and Grusser, S. (2001). Effect of sensory discrimination training on cortical reorganisation and phantom limb pain. *Lancet* **357**, 1763–4.

Franzen, V., Florin, I., Schneider, S., and Meier, M. (1988). Distorted body image in bulimic women. *J. Psychosom. Res.* **32**, 445–50.

Fraser, C.M., Halligan, P.W., Robertson, I.H. and Kirker, S.G. (2001). Characterizing Phantom limb phenomena in upper limb amputees. *Prosthet Orthot Int* **25**, 235–42.

Gazzaniga, M.S., Bogen, J.E., and Sperry, R.W. (1962). Some functional effects of sectioning the cerebral commissures in man. *Proc. Natl Acad. Sci., USA* **48**, 1765–9.

Gerstman, J. (1942). Problems of imperception of disease and of impaired body territories with organic lesions. Relation to body scheme and its disorders. *Arch. Neurol. Psychiatry* **48**, 890–913.

Gibb, W.R.G., Luthert, P.J., and Marsden, C.D. (1989). Corticobasal degeneration. *Brain* **112**, 1171–92.

Halligan, P.W., Donegan, C.A., and Marshall, J.C. (1992). When a cue is not a cue? On the intractability of visuospatial neglect. *Neuropsychol. Rehabilitation* **2**, 283–93.

Halligan, P.W., Marshall, J.C., and Wade, D.Y. (1993). Three arms: a case study of supernumerary phantom limb after right hemisphere stroke. *J Neurol Neurosurg Psychiatry* **56**(2), 159–66.

Halligan, P.W., Marshall, J.C., and Wade, D.T. (1995). Unilateral somatoparaphrenia after right hemisphere stroke. A case description. *Cortex* **31**, 173–82.

Halligan, P.W., Marshall, J.C., Wade, D.T., Davey, J., and Morrison, D. (1993). Thumb in cheek? Sensory reorganization and perceptual plasticity after limb amptation. *Neuroreport* **4**(3), 233–6.

Halligan, P.W., Zeman, A., and Berger, A. (1999). Phantoms in the brain. *Br. Med. J.* **319**, 587–8.

Halligan, P.W. (2002). Phantom limbs: the body is mind. *Cog. Neuropsychiatry* **7**, 251–68.

Head, H. and Holmes, G. (1911). Sensory disturbances from cerebral lesions. *Brain* **34**, 102–254.

Hsu, L.K.G. and Sobkiewicz, T.A. (1991). Body image disturbance: time to abandon the concept for eating disorders? *Int. J. Eating Disorders* **10**, 15–30.

Karl, A., Birbaumer, N., Lutzenberger, W., Cohen, L.G., and Flor, H. (2001). Reorganization of motor and somatosensory cortex in upper extremity amputees with phantom limb pain. *J. Neurosci.* **21**, 3609–18.

Kinsbourne, M. (1995). Models of consciousness: serial or parallel in the brain?. In *The cognitive neurosciences* (ed. M. Gazzaniga), pp. 1321–9. MIT Press, Cambridge, Massachusetts.

Lhermitte, J., Lévy, G., and Kyriako, N. (1925). Les perturbations de la représentation spatiale chez les apraxiques—a propos de deux cas cliniques d'apraxie. *Rev. Neurologique* **2**, 586–600.

Liepmann, H. (1900). Der Krankeit der Apraxie, motorischen Asymbolie. *Monatschr. Psychiatrie Neurologie* **11**, 15–44, 102–32, 182–97.

Marcel, A.J. and Tegner, R. (1994). Knowing one's plegia. Poster presented at the XII European Workshop on Cognitive Neuropsychology, Bressanone, Italy.

Martì-Fabregas, J., Kulisevsky, J., Barò, E., Mendoza, G., Valencia, C., and Martì-Villalta, J.L. (2000). Alien hand sign after a right parietal infarction. *Cerebrovasc. Dis.* **10**, 70–2.

Melzack, R. (1992). Phantom limbs. *Sci. Am.* **187**(4), 90–6.

Nightingale, S. (1982). Somatoparaphrenia: a case study. *Cortex* **18**, 463–7.

Ogden, J.A. (1985). Autotopagnosia. Occurrence in a patient without nominal aphasia and with an intact ability to point to parts of animals. *Brain* **108**, 1009–22.

Oppenheim, H. (1911). *Textbook of nervous diseases*. Foulis, Edinburgh.

Paillard, J., Michel, F., and Stelmach, G. (1983). Localization without content. A tactile analogue of blind-sight. *Arch. Neurol.* **40**, 548–51.

Papagno, C. and Marsile, C. (1995). Transient left-sided alien hand with callosal and unilateral fronto-mesial damage: a case study. *Neuropsychologia* **33**, 1703–9.

Peru, A. and Pinna, G. (1997). Right personal neglect following a left hemisphere stroke. A case report. *Cortex* **33**, 585–90.

Poeck, K. and Orgass, B. (1971). The concept of the body schema: a critical review and some experimental results. *Cortex* **7**, 254–77.

Probst, M., Vandereycken, W., Van Coppenolle, H., and Pieter, G. (1998a). Body size estimation in anorexia nervosa patients, the significance of overestimation. *J. Psychosom. Res.* **44**, 451–6.

Probst, M., Vandereycken, W., Vanderlinden, J., and Van Coppenolle, H. (1998b). The significance of body size estimation in eating disorders: its relation with clinical and psychological variables. *Int. J. Eating Disorders* **24**(2), 167–74.

Ramachandran, V.S. and Hirstein, W. (1998). The perception of phantom limbs. The D.O. Hebb Lecture. *Brain* **121**, 1603–30.

Ramachandran, V.S. and Rogers Ramachandran, D. (1996). Synesthesia on phantom limbs induced with mirrors. *Proc. R. Soc. London B* **273**, 377–86.

Ramachandran, V.S. and Rogers Ramachandran, D. (2000). Phantom limbs and neural plasticity. *Arch. Neurol.* **57**, 317–20.

Robertson, I.H. and Halligan, P.W. (1999). *Spatial neglect*. Psychology Press, Hove, East Sussex.

Rode, G., Charles, N., Perenin, M.T., Vighetto, A., Trillet, M., and Aimard, G. (1992). Partial remission of hemiplegia and somatoparaphrenia through vestibular stimulation in a case of unilateral neglect. *Cortex* **28**, 203–8.

Rubens, A.B. (1985). Caloric stimulation and unilateral neglect. *Neurology* **35**, 1019–24.

Schilder, P. (1935). *The image and the appearance of the human body*. International Universities Press, New York.

Schwartz, A.S., Marchok, P.L., Kreinick, C.J., and Flynn, R. (1979). The asymmetric lateralization of tactile extinction in patients with unilateral cerebral dysfunction. *Brain* **102**, 669–84.

Semenza, C. (1988). Impairment in localization of body parts following brain damage. *Cortex* **24**, 443–9.

Semenza, C. (2001). Disorders of body representation. In *Handbook of neuropsychology* (ed. R.S. Berndt), Vol. 3, pp. 285–303. Elsevier Publishers, Amsterdam.

Semenza, C. and Delazer, M. (2003). Pick's cases studies on bodily representation (1908, 1915, 1922). A retrospective assessment. In *Classic cases in neuropsychology*, Vol. 2 (ed. C. Code, C. Wallesch, Y. Joanette, and A.R. Lecours), pp. 233–40. Psychology Press, Hove, East Sussex.

Semenza, C. and Goodglass, H. (1985). Localization of body parts in brain injured subjects. *Neuropsychologia* **23**, 161–75.

Slade, P. and Russell, G.F.M. (1973). Awareness of body dimensions in anorexia nervosa: cross-sectional and longitudinal studies. *Psychol. Med.* **3**, 188–99.

Stone, S.P., Halligan, P.W., and Greenwood, R.J. (1993). The incidence of neglect phenomena and related disorders in patients with an acute right or left hemisphere stroke. *Age Ageing* **22**, 46–52.

Thompson, J.K. (1990). *Body image disturbances: assessment and treatment*. Pergamon Press, New York.

Vallar, G., Rusconi, M.L., Bignamini, G., Geminani, G., and Perani, D. (1994). Anatomical correlates of visual and tactile extinction in humans: a clinical CT study. *J. Neurol., Neurosurg., Psychiatry* **57**, 464–70.

Vallar, G., Sterzi, R., Bottini, G., Cappa, S., and Rusconi, M.L. (1990). Temporary remission of left hemianesthesia after vestibular stimulation. A sensory neglect phenomenon. *Cortex* **26**, 123–31.

Watson, R.T. and Heilman, K.M. (1983). Callosal apraxia. *Brain* **106**, 391–403.

Zingerle, H. (1913). Ueber Stoerungen der Wahrnehmung des eigenen Koerpers bei organischen Gehirnerkrankungen. *Monatsschr. Psychiatrie Neurol.* **34**, 13–36.

Zoccolotti, P. (1999). Visual, visuospatial, and attentional disorders. In *Handbook of clinical and experimental neuropsychology* (ed. G. Denes and L. Pizzamiglio), pp. 875–86. Psychology Press, Hove, East Sussex.

Chapter 13

The assessment of acquired spoken language disorders

Claus-W. Wallesch, Helga Johannsen-Horbach, and Gerhard Blanken

1 Introduction

The acquired language and speech disorders comprise aphasia, speech apraxia, dysarthria, and language impairments in dementia and confusional states. Only the first three conditions will be considered here.

1.1 Definitions

1.1.1 Aphasia

The aphasias are disorders of language processing resulting from acquired focal brain pathology. The underlying pathology affects the cerebral representations of linguistic rules and language-specific information. In most instances, aphasia is a supramodal deficit (i.e. both language production and perception, both spoken and written, are affected). However, due to the existence of cognitive pathways that only subserve written, but not spoken language, written language disorders will be treated separately (see Chapter 17). Also, disorders of written language processing may occur in the absence of aphasia (e.g. in pure alexia or neglect dyslexia). In its strict use, the term 'aphasia' is reserved for patients who suffer from circumscribed pathology, and in whom language dysfunction constitutes a focus of cognitive impairment. (Therefore, the frequent and characteristic language impairment with dementia of the Alzheimer type would only be termed aphasia in the broader sense.)

The aphasias affect the cerebral representation of a developed language system. They are therefore separated from disorders of language acquisition ('developmental dysphasia'). (The term 'childhood aphasia' is restricted to the effects of brain damage upon language functions that had been acquired previously.)

1.1.2 Speech apraxia

The existence and definition of speech apraxia have been intensely debated. Today a majority of researchers and clinicians accept its existence and Darley's definition: 'An articulatory disorder resulting from impairment, as a result of brain damage, of the capacity to program the positioning of speech musculature and the sequencing of muscle movements for the volitional production of phonemes. No significant weakness, slowness, or incoordination in reflex and automatic acts.' (Darley, 1969, cited Rosenbek, 1993). Speech apraxia very rarely occurs in isolation; usually it is combined with Broca's or global aphasia (see Chapter 15).

1.1.3 Dysarthria

The term 'dysarthria' is used to describe the effects of a sensorimotor disorder resulting from neurological pathology on respiratory, phonatory and articulatory functions involved in speech sound production. It has been argued that 'dysarthrophonia' or even 'dysarthrophonopneumia' may be terminologically more adequate, but these terms have not found entrance into clinical use. Dysarthria may co-occur with aphasia, especially acute nonfluent, Broca's, and global aphasia.

2 Aphasia

2.1 Epidemiology

Aphasia is a common symptom of cerebral disease with an incidence of about 1/1000 (not including transient aphasia as a symptom of TIA), and a prevalence of about 2/1000. Its most frequent cause is ischemic infarction in the territory of supply of the left middle cerebral artery (about 75%). Other causes are hemorrhage, tumor, trauma, infarctions in other territories, cerebral infections (herpes encephalitis), and circumscribed atrophic pathology.

2.2 Symptoms of aphasia

Clinically and in aphasia test batteries, the analysis and description of an aphasic patient's language performance is based on two types of observations:

- the analysis of his/her linguistic and communicative performance in conversation,
- the comparison of linguistic proficiency across modalities using tasks such as repetition, oral and written naming, writing to dictation, reading aloud, speech and script comprehension.

2.2.1 Spontaneous speech

In spontaneous speech, deficits and errors are analyzed on the levels of phonology, lexicon/semantics and syntax. Other important dimensions are the fluency of language production and the presence of repetitive speech. Usually, the accuracy and speed of articulation and prosodic features are also described. For a glossary of neurolinguistic terminology, see Table 13.1.

The phonological structure of an utterance includes the appropriateness of phoneme selection and combination in order to form the sound structure of words. Impairment of phoneme production as such is not an aphasic symptom but would indicate the presence of dysarthria or speech apraxia (whether the interface between linguistic and sensorimotor processes can be defined so rigidly, is being intensively debated).

Table 13.1 Glossary of aphasic symptoms

Speech Automatism	the automatic and compulsive production of the same phrase, word, neologism, syllable or sound, contrary to intention
Agrammatism	reduction of grammatical elem ents, such as inflections and function words (e.g. prepositions)
Echolalia	repetition of utterances of the communication partner, frequently with adequate changes denoting the speaker ('How are you?'– 'How am I?').
Jargon, phonemic or neologistic	phonemic paraphasia occurs to an extent that speech is incomprehensible
Jargon, semantic	semantic paraphasia occurs to an extent that speech is incomprehensible
Neologism, phonemic	a word is incomprehensible because of phonemic paraphasia
Paraphasia, phonemic	substitution, omission, addition, or perseveration of a phoneme or error of phoneme sequence
Paraphasia, verbal	substitution of a presumably intended word by another
Paraphasia, semantic	substitution of a presumably intended word by a meaning related one
Perseveration	the recurrent production of a previous response out of context
Stereotypy	the repetitive and stereotyped use of a communicatively acceptable word or phrase without propositional meaning (e.g. 'yes', 'my God', 'I don't know', 'such is life') in the position of a pause

The phonological structure of a word may be altered by omissions, substitutions, the addition of phonemes, errors of sequence and perseverations. Some aphasics strenuously attempt to correct their phonological output, be it comprehensible or not. Both the production of phonemic paraphasias and disorders of output monitoring and correction may result in the characteristic behaviours of 'conduite d'approche' and 'conduite d'écart', (i.e. approximations and digressions from the target: e.g. trutle – tertle – turtle – trullet (naming a turtle)). Words that are phonemically so distorted that they are incomprehensible, are termed 'phonemic neologisms'. The term 'phonemic or neologistic jargon' is used, when the patient's speech is incomprehensible because of phonemic paraphasia.

The analysis of lexical and semantic structure includes the processes of word access, word selection and the differentiation of word meanings. Impaired word-finding is a symptom of all types of aphasia, but also of more diffuse pathology such as dementia and impaired consciousness. It may also occur in normal speakers, especially under stress, distraction, fatigue and intoxication. Word finding difficulties may manifest themselves as pauses, in the use of circumlocutions, or in the discontinuation of the phrase. The term 'verbal paraphasia' describes the incorrect use of a word. Verbal paraphasias can be related to the target by meaning similarity, form similarity, or both. Also (seemingly) unrelated verbal paraphasias can occur. Usually meaning related errors ('semantic paraphasias') form the most frequent type of word substitution. Semantic paraphasias typically stem from the target's semantic category (e.g. 'bus' for 'lorry' – close semantic paraphasia), or can be otherwise semantically associated (by situation, function etc.). If productions are rendered incomprehensible by semantic paraphasia, the term 'semantic jargon' is used.

Traditionally, syntactic errors in aphasia are classified as 'agrammatic' and 'paragrammatic'. Because pathological stereotypies may be grammatically appropriate, the analysis of the use of syntax is based only on newly created propositional utterances. An error is classified as agrammatic when a necessary grammatical element, such as a bound inflectional morpheme, a function word, or an auxiliary verb in a complex verb phrase is missing. In severe cases of agrammatism, the patient almost exclusively uses nouns, verbs in the infinite form such as the present and past participles, adjectives and adverbs. Function words, such as prepositions, and inflections are greatly reduced or lacking. In paragrammatism, grammatical rules are applied. Patients inflect nouns and verbs and use function words, but their speech deviates from the grammatical norm. Sentence structures are typically long and complex. Sentence boundaries may become obscured ('when I came home is my favourite place').

Fluency and nonfluency (Kertesz, 1979) denote two prototypes of aphasic patients:

- the nonfluent aphasic struggles with every word and gives the impression of great effort required for speech production;

- the fluent aphasic exhibits little or no effort but usually produces many empty phrases or many paraphasic errors.

The fluency/nonfluency dimension is especially helpful for the description of acute aphasia.

There are various types of repetitive speech that may occur in aphasic language productions. The most common are speech automatism (recurring utterances), echolalia, perseveration and stereotypy (for definitions, see Table 13.1). From a clinical point of view, it is important to note that speech automatisms almost exclusively occur in aphasia, whereas echolalia, perseveration and stereotypy also occur with non-aphasic brain pathology and even in non brain-damaged persons (cf. Wallesch, 1990).

2.4 Performance in language modalities

Although it is a great simplification in view of neural networks, the Wernicke (1874) - Lichtheim (1885) model (Fig. 13.1) has had a great influence upon aphasiology. In this model, (spoken) language is processed by three interconnected components: a sensory center for auditory word forms, a center for speech-motor word forms, and a (semantic) concept center. Wernicke did not localize the concept center in a circumscribed brain region, but assumed its representation in the interconnection of various association areas. The assumed connection between the sensory and the motor speech centers provided the ability to repeat without semantic analysis, and also control and monitoring of speech output. The link between sensory and concept center, was necessary for comprehension, and that between concept and motor speech center for naming. With the exception of the concept center, a parallel (or subordinate construction) was hypothesized for written language processing. On the historical basis of the Wernicke-Lichtheim model,

Table 13.2 Error types in visual confrontation naming and their functional basis (based on Linebaugh, 1990)

Type	Functional basis
Delayed naming	slowed activation or selection of lexical target
Self-correction	recognition of error
Circumlocution	failure to retrieve lexical target, alternative production of semantic information
Near semantic paraphasia	retrieval of a lexical entry semantically related to the target
Unrelated word	failure to access appropriate target
Visually related word	error in visual object analysis
Perseveration	failure to inhibit a previous response
Gesture	compensation for failure to retrieve lexical target
No response	

the vast majority of aphasia assessment batteries include the tasks of repetition, naming, and comprehension, in most instances both at the word and the sentence level.

Table 13.2 summarizes error types in visual confrontation naming. For neurolinguistic analysis, naming has the advantage that the lexical target is known and errors can be more easily analyzed linguistically than in spontaneous speech. Naming contains fewer degrees of freedom than spontaneous speech. Therefore, some aphasics may find naming comparatively easy. On the other hand, in most naming situations, only one response is appropriate. Aphasics with prominent disturbances of word access (e.g. with anomic aphasia) may be particularly impaired in naming (e.g. 'I cannot tell its name, but we have similar chairs at home'). Some patients have a specific impairment of visual object naming as compared to naming with other presentation modalities. This condition is called 'optic aphasia' (Coslett and Saffran, 1989). Its functional basis is a disconnection of the language region from the visual association cortex as it may occur with posterior watershed infarctions. These patients can easily be identified by their ability to produce names in response to questions (e.g. 'what do you open a lock with?').

In repetition, semantic and lexical search processes are usually not critically involved. Some patients however, may have to rely on a semantic route in this task (Katz and

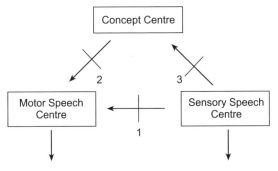

Fig. 13.1 The Wernicke-Lichtheim model.

Goodglass, 1990); they cannot repeat nonwords (phoneme sequences that do not constitute a meaningful word in the respective language). The assessment of repetition should include stimuli of varying length, and lexical as well as nonlexical items. A focal deficit of repetition may indicate a deficit of auditory-verbal short term memory; an impairment of the memory for sequence, or of the transformation of a phonological representation into a phonetic string. The latter explanation is similar to the anatomical assumption of a disconnection between receptive and expressive speech areas to account for repetition deficits (Geschwind, 1965).

Intactness or only mild impairment of spoken language comprehension is often wrongly assumed in aphasic patients, as the patient may make use of situational cues. In formal assessment, forced choice decision tasks are often easier for the patient than those that demand production, both with respect to linguistic and neuropsychological processing demands (Wallesch and Kertesz, 1993). To compensate for this effect, aphasia test batteries such as the Boston Diagnostic Aphasia Examination (Goodglass and Kaplan, 1972), the Western Aphasia Battery (Kertesz, 1979), or the Aachen Aphasia Test (Huber et al., 1983/1984) use norms derived from aphasic patients to assign scaled scores or values.

2.5 Syndromes of aphasia

The term 'syndrome' denotes the statistical co-occurrence of a cluster of symptoms. It is not imperative that all symptoms of a syndrome be present in a given patient. The statistical cluster is supposed to indicate an underlying cause of the various symptoms. Poeck (1983) pointed out that the underlying pathophysiological basis of the aphasia syndromes may rather be the vascular anatomy of the cerebral language representations rather than 'natural' linguistic structures.

Statistical cluster analysis reveals that most (about 70 to 80%) of aphasic patients are grouped together and that these clusters relate to the clinical syndromes of acute and chronic aphasia (Kertesz, 1979, Huber et al., 1983, Wallesch et al., 1992). Generally, patients with non-ischemic aphasia syndromes correspond much less both to the clusters and clinical syndromes of chronic aphasia than do patients with ischemic stroke.

To increase confusion even further, a number of different classification systems are used. These can be grouped into three types:

+ modality – oriented: Syndromes are distinguished on the basis of assumed dissociations across modalities, resulting in categories such as 'motor'/'sensory' or 'expressive'/'receptive'. Recent examples are the classification systems of Goodglass and Kaplan (1972), and Kertesz (1979).

+ Anatomically-oriented with syndromes such as 'anterior' vs. 'posterior' (Benson, 1967). Often, atypical aphasia syndromes are denoted by anatomical terms, e.g. 'subcortical' or 'thalamic' aphasia.

+ According to the linguistic deficit. A very simple classification into 'fluent' and 'non-fluent' aphasia (Benson, 1967) is based upon speed of production and phrase length. The classification system described in more detail below is based on cluster analyses of the results of aphasia tests, and therefore on the linguistic deficit.

Table 13.3 Differences between acute and chronic vascular aphasia

	acute	chronic
Time post onset	few weeks	many months
Pathophysiology	penumbra and diaschisis enlarges functional lesion	cerebral reorganisation reduces functional deficit
Neuropsychology	additional disorders of consciousness, attention and awareness	compensation, reorganisation
Psychology	distress	coping
Social role	illness	handicap

The syndromes of acute and chronic aphasia will be treated separately. Obviously, there is no dichotomous distinction. However, acute aphasia (i.e. aphasia syndromes seen in the acute hospital), differs in many ways from chronic aphasia, seen in rehabilitation and afterwards (Table 13.3). These differences explain the syndromatic instability of some types of acute aphasia.

2.5.1 Syndromes of acute aphasia

Patients suffering from acute aphasia present symptoms of acute focal pathology in combination with the effects of diffuse cerebral dysfunction (Table 13.3), such as reduced consciousness, attentional impairment and rapid fluctuations in performance. The deficits preclude detailed linguistic and neuropsychological assessment. Kertesz (1979) and Wallesch et al. (1992) analyzed groups of patients 3 to 6 weeks after onset of aphasia by means of cluster analysis. The results of both studies converge with respect to syndromes of acute aphasia by finding clusters of

1 mild aphasia with prominent word-finding difficulty,
2 mild aphasia with prominent comprehension deficit,
3 moderate aphasia with prominent repetition impairment ('acute condution aphasia'),
4 marked aphasia with preserved repetition ('acute transcortical motor aphasia'),
5 severe aphasia with preserved comprehension,
6 severe aphasia with deficits in all modalities.

Clusters 1) and 2) are usually fluent, 4) 5) and 6), nonfluent. Type 3) is fluent in stereotypies and mainly nonfluent in propositional utterances and repetition ('acute conduction aphasia'). A development towards chronic Wernicke's aphasia occurred in clusters 3) and 5), but not in 2) (Wallesch et al., 1992). A large number of patients from cluster 6) develop Broca's aphasia, and most patients from cluster 5) become anomic (Kertesz, 1984). The frequency of a change of symptomatology ('Syndromwandel') speaks against the use of the terminology of chronic aphasia syndromes in the acute stage.

Notwithstanding, Pedersen et al. (2004) applied the Western Aphasia Battery (Kertesz 1982) to 270 consecutive clinically aphasic patients within the first week after stroke and

Table 13.4 Change in type of aphasia from first week to one year follow-up in survivors (data from Pedersen *et al.* 2004)

At follow-up	Global	Broca's	Wernicke's	Transcort. Motor	Conduction	Anomic	No aphasia
Within first week:							
Global	22%	35%	7%			22%	15%
Broca's		18%		9%		36%	36%
Wernicke's			18%		36%	27%	18%
Transcort. Sensory						17%	83%
Conduction					14%	14%	71%
Anomic						38%	62%

also the battery's scoring system that forcibly assigns each patient to an aphasic syndrom. Table 13.4 shows that there were great changes in syndrome allocation between first week and one-year follow-up. Each aphasia syndrome encountered during the first week was compatible with full recovery. Except for those classified as global within the first week, a majority of each other syndrome recovered fully or changed into anomic aphasia within one year post stroke.

Among the acute aphasias, one may encounter syndromes that do not occur in the chronic stage. One of these is acute phonemic paraphasia with sometimes largely preserved comprehension, which is a rare but not unusual finding with subcortical infarctions involving the ventrolateral (Wallesch, 1997) or anteromedian (Carrera *et al.*, 2004) thalamus. Language disorders resulting from thalamic lesions are often confounded by perseveration and fluctuating impairments of attention and consciousness that are particularly frequent with lesions of the nonspecific thalamic nuclei. Acute semantic paraphasia with variable degrees of comprehension deficit have been described with lesions of the left head of caudate and anterior limb of the internal capsule (for a review, see Wallesch, 1997). The underlying pathophysiology has been related to the lesion of thalamocortical projections involved in gating the processing of multiple lexical choices.

In the first hours and day after stroke or trauma, many patients are mute. Neurological mutism can result from aphasia, but also from severe apraxia, paresis, akinesia or disorders of attention or motivation. An analysis of nonverbal communication and comprehension may guide the initial differential diagnosis.

2.5.2 Syndromes of chronic vascular aphasia

As has been pointed out, the classical aphasia syndromes describe best the symptomatology of stroke patients who have suffered a functional deficit due to a circumscribed lesion at one point in time and who have developed adaptive and maladaptive compensatory strategies consequently.

Global aphasia The term 'global' denotes that all language processes are severely affected. Propositional language is either almost absent, or reduced to single words or phrase fragments and is produced with great effort. Few stereotyped phrases may be preserved and used adequately in some situations. A subgroup of patients are able to produce highly overlearned sequences such as prayers, series such as the days of the week, or popular songs. With echolalia as an additional syndrome-nonspecific symptom, repetition may be quite good. Speech automatisms (recurring utterances) can frequently (though not necessarily) be observed in global aphasia and seem to supersede intended more adequate utterances which in some cases can be realized by superior writing performance (see Blanken *et al.*, 1990).

Global aphasia is the result of severe damage to the cerebral language representation in the area of supply of the left middle cerebral artery. Lesions of the deep periventricular white matter and/ or the basal ganglia seem to be of special importance. Global aphasia is a syndrome of older patients; subjects below the age of about 40 are likely to develop Broca's aphasia even with very large infarcts.

Broca's aphasia The syndrome of Broca's aphasia is different from the clinical status (global aphasia) and functional interpretation (similar to the modern concept of speech apraxia) of Broca's original patients. The principal feature of Broca's aphasia is a reduction of linguistic proficiency on the phonological (simplification of phonemic structure), lexical (word-finding difficulty) and syntactic (agrammatism) levels. Of these, the agrammatic deficits are quite specific for the syndrome and have been proposed to constitute an axial symptom. Severe agrammatism leads to the so-called 'telegraphic style' with a lack of function words and inflection forms ('skiing – bang – head – sick'). In mild cases, the patients' productions may be characterized only by a reduction in the use of subordinate clauses, multiple objects, or complex verb forms. In these cases, a premorbidly more elaborate use of language should be established. Case reports of patients with quite specific morphological or syntactic deficits however, contradict a unitary view of agrammatism (Nadeau, 1988).

Patients suffering from Broca's aphasia exhibit a deficit of lexical retrieval with time-consuming, laborious attempts at word finding. Phonological assembly and articulation are slowed down. A combination with speech apraxia is common. In a clinical situation, the comprehension deficit is mild. It has been shown that most patients have comprehension problems similar to their expressive symptomatology, namely a prominent impairment with the understanding of grammatical constructions (Grodzinsky *et al.*, 1999).

In the majority of cases, Broca's aphasia develops from a very severe deficit in all modalities, in most instances in a youngish (younger than 60 years) patient who suffers from a large infarct in the territory of the left middle cerebral artery. Their improvement indicates that reorganisation (activation of lexical representations outside the damaged language region) and compensatory strategies (e.g. telegraphic style) contribute to the syndromes phenomenology.

Wernicke's aphasia This syndrome is characterized by its prominent 'para-symptomatology', phonemic and semantic paraphasia, neologisms or jargon, and paragrammatism.

Speech production is usually fluent, with few attempts at error correction. With phonemic jargon, the syntactic structure cannot be analyzed, although the presence of such structure can often be inferred, as undistorted function words frequently stand out and segment the utterance (Buckingham & Kertesz, 1976) and inflectional morphemes may be used on neologisms. If the lexical content is sufficiently comprehensible, syntactic violations such as sentence blendings, choice of inadequate functors and inappropriate inflections can be detected. Generally, language comprehension is more impaired in Wernicke's than in Broca's aphasia, although jargon may occur with little comprehension deficit.

Fluent paraphasic aphasia is frequent in the first two weeks post onset (20% - Willmes and Poeck, 1984) but rare among chronic aphasics (3% in the same series). Most patients develop towards anomic or unspecific residual aphasia. This finding probably also indicates a process of reorganisation by reestablishing monitoring and output control. The most common cause of chronic Wernicke's aphasia is posterior cerebral infarction in patients who are either elderly or have diffuse or multifocal brain pathology in addition.

Anomic aphasia The core symptom of anomic aphasia is deficient lexical access and/or retrieval. Phonology and syntax are only mildly affected. The word-finding impairment results in pauses, circumlocutions, closely related semantic paraphasias, evasion of the target word by use of empty phrases or fillers without specific meaning ('thing'), circumscriptions by verbal or nonverbal means, or discontinuation of the ongoing phrase followed by variation of the statement. Most of these strategies are communicatively acceptable. The deficit becomes striking, when only one lexical response is acceptable, such as in naming.

Anomic aphasia usually results from a lesion in the posterior border regions of the core language area. In most cases, the temporoparietal junction or the inferior parietal lobe is affected. Anomic aphasia is relatively frequent with non-ischemic pathology, such as tumor or trauma.

Conduction aphasia Conduction aphasia was predicted by the Wernicke-Lichtheim model (Fig. 13.1) as a disconnection between the sensory and motor language centers. Wernicke predicted rather a deficit of output monitoring and control than a disorder of repetition (Köhler *et al.*, 1998). Within the diagnositic category of conduction aphasia, two different types of patients have been distinguished (Shallice and Warrington, 1977):

- those with a prominent repetition deficit due to an impairment of phonological short-term memory (Caramazza *et al.*, 1981)
- those with an impairment of phonological output programming for single words which together with relatively preserved monitoring results in frequent attempts at correction (conduites d'approche) which can be most prominent in repetition (Kohn, 1984).

Only the latter patients form 'pure' cases of conduction aphasia. However, many conduction aphasics show deficits at both levels of performance. Conduction aphasia is frequent in the acute and rare in the chronic stage. When encountered with acute aphasia, its prognosis is good. Its association with a lesion of the arcuate fascicle, the anatomical connection between Wernicke's and Broca's area, is disputed.

The transcortical aphasias The syndromes of transcortical motor, sensory and mixed transcortical aphasia are characterized by their preserved ability to repeat. They were predicted by the Wernicke-Lichtheim model as disorders in which the direct connection between sensory and motor speech areas was left intact.

Patients suffering from transcortical motor aphasia show greatly reduced language production, except for repetition, and rather preserved comprehension. This syndrome is usually encountered with lesions of the left frontal lobe outside Broca's area, especially in the vicinity of the supplementary motor area on the medial surface, and with lesions of the left basal ganglia. It has been related to a nonlinguistic mechanism involving initiative for speech. Repetition is least affected, because it involves the fewest degrees of freedom (Goldberg, 1985).

Both transcortical sensory and mixed transcortical aphasia are rare. Patients are characterized by disinhibited echolalia. Most patients decribed in the literature have been demented. In transcortical sensory aphasia, language output is fluent with mainly semantic paraphasia. In mixed transcortical aphasia, language production is reduced to echolalia. Naming and comprehension are severely impaired in both syndromes. Mixed transcortical aphasia has been interpreted as an 'isolation of the speech area' (Geschwind et al., 1968), as these patients exhibit signs of linguistic processing in the absence of semantic analysis.

2.6 Diagnostic instruments

The experienced clinician does not require a formal test to detect the presence of aphasia and diagnose the syndrome. Tests subserve mainly three functions:

- establishing the severity of aphasia,
- analyzing the neurospychological or neurolinguistic structure of the patient's deficits as a basis for treatment planning and evaluation by a test battery,
- analyzing the effect of aphasia upon a patient's communication performance.

An overview over aphasia tests and their psychometric properties and problems is given by Willmes (1993).

The Token Test (de Renzi and Vignolo, 1962) is a simple and valid instrument to assess the severity of aphasia. It was originally designed as a test of language comprehension that would not include redundant information. The test consists of circles and squares of two different sizes and five different colours (Fig. 13.2), which the subject is required to point at or perform operations with at the request of the investigator. Contrary to the authors' intuition, the test scores correlate as highly with performance in expressive as in receptive language tasks.

The most frequently used aphasia test is probably the Boston Diagnostic Aphasia Examination (Goodglass and Kaplan, 1972). This battery includes 27 subtests that assess spoken and written language and associated functions. It provides norms from a collective

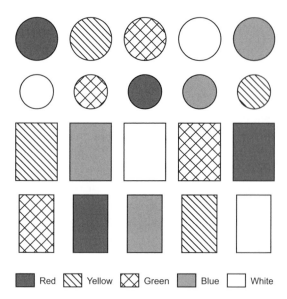

Fig. 13.2 The Token Test.　■ Red　◩ Yellow　⬚ Green　■ Blue　□ White

of aphasics as Z-scores and assigns the patient's aphasia syndrome on the basis of test results. The Aachen Aphasia Test (Huber *et al.*, 1984) assesses a more limited number of functions, but has psychometrical advantages, as it supports single-case statistics. Its English version has not been published. A brief, clinically oriented aphasia battery for nonspecialist use is the Frenchay Aphasia Screening Test (Enderby *et al.*, 1987).

A very detailed instrument for the assessment of aphasic symptoms is the PALPA (Psycholinguistic Assessment of Language Processing in Aphasia, Kay *et al.*, 1992). It provides an assessment of a wide variety of language processes intended for a mapping of single case deficits and dysfunctions on to a psycholinguistic model of normal language processing.

The Amsterdam-Nijmegen Everyday Language Test (ANELT, Blomert *et al.*, 1987) uses standardized everday situations in the form of role-plays to assess aphasics' communicative use of verbal and nonverbal means of communications.

3 **Speech apraxia**

Speech apraxia describes the pathology of brain-damaged persons whose speech is more affected by articulatory symptoms such as distortions, substitutions and dysprosody, than is explained by sensorimotor, language and cognitive deficits. The phenomenological boundaries of the apraxic dysfunction (e.g. towards dysarthria and conduction aphasia), remain unclear. The structure of the interface between linguistic and speech-motor processes is still unresolved. Speech apraxia has to be differentiated from oral (buccofacial) apraxia. Both conditions may co-occur but also occur separately.

Theoretically, speech apraxia denotes a deficit on the level of motor programming and execution that affects only speech-related movements. Sensomotorically, speech is organized differently from other motor acts, in that sensorimotor feedback plays only a neglegible role. On the phonetic level, speech apraxia is characterized by inconsistent errors variably related to the phonemic target, such as omission, substitution, distortion, addition and errors of sequence. The errors are influenced by articulatory complexity. There are also effects of propositionality: stereotyped productions, such as expletives, are less affected. Usually, the beginning of a word is more impaired than sounds within a word. This finding can be explained on the level of motor processing, because the transition probabilities from one phoneme to the next are smaller within words than at word onset.

A very characteristic symptom of speech apraxia is the occurrence of parapraxia. Parapraxia is defined as errors on the level of movement elements (e.g. omission of a necessary element, addition, permutation, substitution or perseveration). Without technical investigations, parapraxias can only be observed with the anterior articulators and inferred from the phonetic signal by an experienced examiner. Other typical symptoms are probed in order to check auditorily and somatosensorily whether type and place of articulation are correct.

3.1 Diagnostic instruments

There is no generally accepted clinical instrument for the assessment of speech apraxia (see Collins, 1989, and Rosenbek, 1993, for discussions). The same technical investigations may be used as with dysarthria (see below).

4 Dysarthria

The dysarthrias are disorders of the sensorimotor performance of speech acts which are characterized by disturbances in speech musculature control due to paresis, slowness, incoordination, altered tone or additional (dyskinetic) movements. They affect the respiration pattern required for speech, phonation, resonation, articulation and prosody. As with the sensorimotor speed and quality of other (e.g. hand) movements, a number of neurological impairments can cause dysfunction: lesions of the first (spastic paresis) and second (flaccid paresis and atrophy) motor neuron, ataxia, akinesia, dys- and hyperkinesia and sensory impairment. Accordingly, the dysarthrias are classified into a central and a peripheral paretic, a hypokinetic, an ataxic and a dyskinetic variety. Clinically, some frequent neurological diseases result in mixed forms, as more than one sensorimotor mechanism is affected, e.g. amyotrophic lateral sclerosis (ALS) combines first and second motoneuron degeneration and Multiple Sclerosis frequently includes both spastic and ataxic symptoms.

4.1 Types

Bilateral lesions of the first motoneuron of the corticobulbar tracts results in spastic (or central paretic) dysarthria; there is little spasticity in the involved muscles. It is characterized by impaired diadochokinetic motility of the articulatory musculature and a disinhibition of reflectory mass movements and synergisms (pathological laughter and crying, sucking etc.). Speech is laboured, monotonous and slow with imprecise consonants as the most prominent feature. It occurs in neurological diseases with prominent first motor neuron pathology, mainly diffuse or multifocal cerebrovascular disease ('pseudobulbar palsy').

The symptomatology of lesions of the second (peripheral) motor neuron (or the neuromuscular junction- myasthenia gravis, or diseases of the relevant musculature – e.g. muscular atrophy and dystrophy, polymyositis) depends on the affected nerves or muscles. With diffuse disease, such as in one form of ALS ('bulbar palsy'), bilateral affection of cranial nerves (e.g. Miller-Fisher syndrome) and mysathenia, speech is reduced in volume, monotonous, imprecise and hypernasal.

Hypokinetic dysarthria is phenomenologically similar to spastic dysarthria with imprecise articulation, slow speech, decreased prosody and often decreased loudness. Speech in Parkinson's Disease, the most frequent cause of hypokinetic dysarthria, is additionally characterized by variations in speech rate (tachyphasia) and rapid repetition of speech elements (palilalia).

Ataxic dysarthria is characterized by variable articulatory errors and imprecisions with frequent omissions, rapid changes in speech rate, pitch and loudness ('scanning speech') and inadequate respiratory patterns.

With dys- and hyperkinetic dysarthria, there is also a variable pattern of errors dictated by the involuntary movements. In view of the amount of dyskinesia, most patients articulate surprisingly well. A dissociation from respiration is typically, with phonation on inspiration, involuntary phonation and diminished control of pitch and loudness.

For a detailed description of the dysarthrias, Darley *et al.* (1975) is still a most valuable source.

4.2 Diagnostic instruments

Clinically, the most frequently used assessment instrument is the Frenchay Dysarthria Assessment (Enderby, 1983). It consists of a standardized investigation of speech and nonspeech motor acts of respiration, phonation, and speech and nonspeech movements of the articulators together with a rating of comprehensibility of the production of words, sentences and spontaneous speech. Normative data for groups of patients are provided and aid differential diagnosis.

In addition, speech related movements can be investigated by technical means, such as electroglottography, endoscopy, X-ray microbeam, and electromagnetic articulography, and phonetic signals by sound spectrography.

Selective references

Benson, DF (1967): Fluency in aphasia. *Cortex* **3**: 373–394.

Blanken, G, Wallesch, CW, Papagno, C (1990): Dissociations of language functions in patients with speech automatisms (recurring utterances). *Cortex* **26**: 41–63.

Blomert, L, Koster, C, van Mier, H, Kean, ML (1987): Verbal communication abilities of aphasic patients: The Everyday Language Test. *Aphasiology* **1**: 463–474.

Buckingham, HW, Kertesz, A (1976): Neologistic jargon aphasia. Amsterdam: Swets & Zeitlinger.

Caramazza, A, Basili, AG, Koller, JJ, Berndt, RS (1981): An investigation of repetition and language processing in a case of conduction aphasia. *Brain and Language* **40**: 235–271.

Carrera, E., Michel, P., and Bogousslavsky, J. (2004): Anteromedian, central, and posterolateral infarcts of the thalamus. Three variant types. *Stroke* **35**: 2826–2832.

Collins, MJ (1989): Differential diagnosis of aphasic syndromes and apraxia of speech. In: P. Square-Storer (ed.): *Acquired Apraxia of Speech in Aphasic Adults*. London: Taylor & Francis, pp. 87–114.

Coslett, HB, Saffran, EM (1989): Preserved object recognition and reading comprehension in optic aphasia. *Brain* **112**: 1091–1110.

Darley, FL, Aronson, AE, Brown, JR (1975): Motor speech disorders. Philadelphia: Saunders.

De Renzi, E, Vignolo, LA (1962): The token test: a sensitive test to detect receptive disturbances in aphasia. *Brain* **85**: 665–678.

Enderby, PM (1983): Frenchay Dysarthria Assessment. San Diego: College Hill.

Enderby, PM, Wood, VA, Wade, DT, Hewer, RL (1987): The Frenchay Aphasia Screening Test: a short, simple test for aphasia appropriate for nonspecialists. *International Journal of Rehabilitation Medicine* **8**: 166–170.

Geschwind, N (1965): Disconnection syndromes in animals and man. Part II. *Brain* **103**: 337–350.

Geschwind, N, Quadfasel, F, Segarra, J (1968): Isolation of the speech area. *Neuropsychologia* **6**: 327–340.

Goodglass, H, Kaplan, E (1972): The assessment of aphasia and related disorders. Philadelphia: Lea & Febiger.

Goldberg, E (1985): Supplementary motor area structure and function: Review and hypothesis. *Behavioral and Brain Research* **8**: 567–616.

Grodzinsky, Y, Pinango, MM, Zurif, E, Drai, D (1999): The critical role of group studies in neuropsychology: comprehension regularities in Broca's aphasia. *Brain and Language* **67**: 134–147.

Huber, W, Poeck, K, Weniger, D, Willmes, K (1983): Der Aachener Aphasie Test. Göttingen: Hogrefe.

Huber, W, Poeck, K, Willmes, K (1984): The Aachen Aphasia test. In: F.C. Rose (ed.): *Progress in Aphasiology*. New York: Raven, pp. 291–303.

Katz, RB, Goodglass, H (1990): Deep dysphasia: analysis of a rare form of repetition disorder. *Brain and Language* **39**: 153–185.

Kay, J, Lesser, R, Coltheart, M (1992): Psycholinguistic assessment of language processing in aphasia. Hove: Lawrence Earlbaum.

Kertesz, A (1979): Aphasia and associated disorders. New York: Grune & Stratton.

Kertesz, A (1982): Western Aphasia Battery. New York: The Psychological Cooperation.

Kertesz, A (1984): Recovery from aphasia. In: F.C. Rose (ed.): *Progress in Aphasiology*. New York: Raven, pp. 23–39.

Köhler, K, Bartels, C, Herrmann, M, Dittmann, J, Wallesch, CW (1998): Conduction aphasia - 11 classic cases. *Aphasiology* **12**: 865–884.

Kohn, S (1984): The nature of phonological disorders in conduction aphasia. *Brain and Language* **23**: 97–115.

Lichtheim, L (1885): Ueber Aphasie. Deutsches Archiv für klinische Medicin **36**: 204–268.

Linebaugh, CW (1990): Lexical retrieval problems: anomia. In: L.L. LaPointe (ed.): *Aphasia and Related Neurogenic Language Disorders*. New York: Thieme, pp. 96–112.

Nadeau, SE (1985): Impaired grammar with normal fluency and phonology. Implications for Broca's aphasia. *Brain* **111**: 1111–1137.

Pedersen, P.M., Vinter, K., and Olsen, T.S. (2004): Aphasia after stroke: type, severity and prognosis. Cerebrovascular Diseases **17**: 35–43.

Poeck, K (1983): What do we mean by 'aphasic syndromes'? A neurologist's view. *Brain and Language* **20**: 79–89.

Rosenbek, JC (1993): Speech apraxia. In: G. Blanken, J. Dittmann, H. Grimm, J.C. Marshall, C.W. Wallesch (eds.): *Linguistic Disorders and Pathologies*. Berlin, New York: De Gruyter, pp. 443–452.

Shallice, T, Warrington, EK (1977): Auditory verbal short-term memory impairment and conduction aphasia. *Brain and Language* **4**: 479–491.

Wallesch, CW (1990): Repetitive verbal behaviour: neurological and functional considerations. *Aphasiology* **4**: 133–154.

Wallesch, C.W. (1997): Symptomatology of subcortical aphasia. *Journal of Neurolinguistics* **10**: 267–275.

Wallesch, CW, Bak, T, Schulte-Mönting, J (1992): Acute aphasia – patterns and prognosis. *Aphasiology* **6**: 273–285.

Wallesch, CW, Kertesz, A (1993): Clinical symptoms and syndromes of aphasia. In: G. Blanken, J. Dittmann, H. Grimm, J.C. Marshall, C.W. Wallesch (eds.): *Linguistic Disorders and Pathologies*. Berlin, New York: De Gruyter, pp. 98–119.

Wernicke, C (1874): Der aphasische Symptomencomplex. Eine psychologische Studie auf anatomischer Basis. Breslau: Max Cohn & Weigert.

Willmes, K (1993): Diagnostic methods in aphasiology. In: G. Blanken, J. Dittmann, H. Grimm, J.C. Marshall, C.W. Wallesch (eds.): *Linguistic Disorders and Pathologies*. Berlin, New York: De Gruyter, pp. 137–152.

Willmes, K, Poeck, K (1984): Ergebnisse einer multizentrischen Untersuchung über die Spontanprognose von Aphasien vaskulärer Ätiologie. Nervenarzt **55**: 62–71.

Chapter 14

Motor speech disorders: an overview

Nick Miller

1 Motor speech disorders: what are they?

'Motor speech disorders' represents a general label applied to a set of distinct disruptions to speech output associated with neurological illness. There exists an array of subtypes of motor speech disorder, irrespective of whether one bases taxonomies on anatomy and physiology, neuropathology, acoustic-phonetic parameters, or models of speech output.

Motor speech disorders may arise from lesions of an isolated cranial nerve affecting a single articulator through to major systemic disorders implicating all movements of the vocal tract. The speech disorder can occur in isolation or present as one aspect of a complex cognitive-motor picture. Onset can be sudden (e.g. stroke; head-injury) or insidious (e.g. degenerative disorders, neoplams) over months or years. Speaking changes may emerge as late rare effects of some disorders, be an inevitable sequel of others, or constitute a sole or early harbinger of neoplastic, inflammatory, infectious, atrophic, metabolic or neurochemical changes (see below). In some cases one might expect recovery towards (not necessarily full) premorbid levels, in others decline is inexorable over longer or shorter time spans.

From the perspective of speech output processes or models, the label broadly encompasses two major subtypes of disorder: a) problems with higher cortical planning, supervision and execution of 'programmes' for speech movements; b) neuromuscular impairment of movements of the articulators (diaphragm, rib cage, larynx, soft palate, tongue, lips, jaw). Neuromuscular disorders arise from disturbances of neural transmission, problems with the electrochemistry of the nerve-muscle synapse and dysfunctions of muscles themselves. Cortical disturbances are claimed to underlie apraxia of speech and phonemic paraphasia, neuromuscular changes are associated with dysarthria. These terms are elaborated later. It will also become clear later that the distinction between cortical versus subcortical and peripheral impairments is an oversimplification. In particular, lesions associated with the cerebellum and basal ganglia may impact on programming and online monitoring of speech motor execution in addition to consequences for muscle tone, power and coordination (Spencer and Rogers, 2005, Ackermann *et al.*, 2007, Booth *et al.*, 2007).

Severity ranges from mild alterations perceptible only to the speaker or on sensitive instrumental analyses, through intelligible but non-normal sounding speech to total unintelligibility or muteness. One should add the rider that definitions of severity linked to objective assessments do not necessarily reflect perceived impact of changes by the speaker or their social circle. An apparently mild change judged on objective measures may produce severe psychosocial consequences for one speaker; an apparently severe impairment may be scarcely noticed by another.

An awareness of motor speech disorders is paramount not just for understanding them in their own right. They are important in neuropsychological assessment in that ignoring them may lead to an inaccurate picture because changes to speech mimic the presentation of certain cognitive, affective and neurobehavioural disorders (e.g. O'Keeffe *et al.*, 2007, Cannizzaro *et al.*, 2004, Duffy, 2006, Gorno-Tempini *et al.*, 2006, O'Sullivan *et al.*, 2008). On the other hand they may mask or distract from changes in these domains. Either way erroneous diagnoses will lead to mismanagement.

To provide a backdrop for discussion of assessment and differential diagnosis the following section offers a brief exposition of how normal speech production takes place.

2 Speech production

Essentially speech is produced by blowing air between the vocal cords and using the velum (soft palate), tongue and lips to shape the resultant sound into speech. More specifically, speech is produced through the muscles of the diaphragm, abdomen and ribcage modifying the rate and volume of inspiration and duration and pressure of expiratory airflow from the lungs. This air is used to drive the vocal cords, generating sound (phonation, voice) by causing the tensed, approximated vocal folds to vibrate (in the region of 130–140 times per second for adult males, 210–230 Hz for females). The sound directly from the larynx is akin to the sound produced from blowing two pieces of paper together or humming with tissue paper on a comb. This is transformed into what we hear as speech by amplification of the signal in the resonating chambers of the nasopharynx and oral cavity and modification of the signal by constricting (for continuant sounds such as f, v, s, l) or blocking (for plosive sounds such as p, b, t, g) the flow of air, or altering the shape and resonance of the oral cavity (for vowels).

The contrast between nasal and oral sounds (e.g. pairs such as m-w, m-b, n-d, n-l) is achieved by lowering or raising the velum to divert air predominantly through the nasal or the oral cavity. So-called voiced (e.g. b, d, g, v, z) and voiceless cognates (p, t, k, f, s) are contrasted in word initial positions (pea vs bee) in English according to millisecond differences in lag (voice onset time) between release of closures in the mouth and restart of vocal cord vibration. In word final position (lock vs log) perceived differences relate to duration of the preceding vowel. In some languages, standard British English for instance, an added perceptual clue for pairs such as b-p, t-d derives from the degree of aspiration that accompanies release, easily demonstrated by saying 'pea' and 'bee' onto the back of ones hand, where there should be a noticeable puff of air with 'pea' but not 'bee'.

Vowel contrasts rely on differing settings of the tongue tip and dorsum. For instance in standard British English the series 'heed, hid, head, had, hard, horde, hood, who'd' entails starting with the tongue tip raised, lowering it and switching to the dorsum gradually rising. Notice too the modifications to lip rounding-spreading that coordinate with the tongue changes and how 'abnormal' the vowels sound if one says 'heed' with rounded instead of spread lips and 'who'd' with spread instead of rounded.

Pitch (and changes in pitch, the intonation pattern of phrases) and voice quality are largely determined by the (changing) length, degree of tension and pattern of approximation of the vocal cords. Loudness (and contrasts in loudness for stressed versus unstressed syllables/words) derives from the balance between the respiratory driving force of the air (subglottal air pressure) and the level of resistance offered by the vocal cords (greater the pressure, tighter the cords, louder the voice). Voice quality (e.g. harsh, breathy, rich) is predominantly a function of the setting of the vocal cords and control of pharyngeal and oral resonance.

Respiration for speech is different to vegetative patterns. In the latter the ratio of inspiratory to expiratory phases is roughly 1:1. For speech this vegetative pattern must be overridden to effect a ratio of roughly 1:6–10 depending on the length, loudness and rate of the utterance. Inability to coordinate breathing with speech and with morpho-syntactic planning (Hixon and Hoit, 2005) can severely compromise intelligibility.

While the above schema has a neat simplicity to it, the process is actually highly complex. Speech motor control is the most complex activity humans (and probably any species) can achieve, in terms of the number of muscles and muscle groups needing to be coordinated; the rate and precision at which they have to be adjusted to sustain intelligible speech; the complex interaction at a minimum with phonological (sound system) processing to generate the right sound targets for required words, sentence level processing to produce correct breathing, stress and intonation patterns; and affective control to convey correct tone and feeling.

Table 14.1 summarises the chief changes one might hear when different parts of the vocal tract are impaired. As a rule of thumb impairments of respiration and phonation (larynx) compromise suprasegmental features of speech (loudness; pitch; stress patterns across words and phrases; intonation patterns; voice quality; affective expression), whilst tongue and lip disturbances perturb production of individual sounds (articulation). Given that there is a considerable amount of motor equivalence possibility in articulatory movements and redundancy in perception of speech sounds, a degree of compensation across the vocal tract on the part of the speaker, or ear of the listener may mask or neutralise disruptions to isolated speech subsystems. Where systemic conditions or extensive lesions affect multiple subsystems or where the underlying disruption is precisely to the ability to coordinate and compensate across subsystems, the ensuing speech disorder is liable to be correspondingly more pervasive and severe.

One must emphasize that communication is more than just speech and language. Facial expression and hand and arm gestures accompanying speech constitute an important component. Compromise to these can also have an effect on the intelligibility and acceptability of what is said (Munhall *et al.*, 2004, Garcia *et al.*, 2004).

3 **Motor speech disorders**

A broad distinction was made above between planning versus neuromuscular disorders of speech, with the former subsumed under the label apraxia of speech, the latter under dysarthria. The following sections look further at these distinctions and introduce some

Table 14.1 Broad associations between changes to articulator function and perceived voice and speech changes

Articulator	Possible changes affecting speech	Possible speech changes heard by listener
Lungs, chest wall, diaphragm: respiration	reduced breath capacity; problems controlling slow expiration; lack of coordination breathing-speech	frequent breaths, shorter phrases, reduced loudness or sudden bursts of loudness; speaking on residual air or on inspiration
Balance vocal cords-respiration	imbalance between normally well poised subglottal air pressure and laryngeal resistance	impaired control of loudness, stress patterns, intonation
Larynx: voice	uni- or bilateral cord weakness/paralysis; abrupt or persistent alterations to tone and stiffness in laryngeal muscles	control of pitch, loudness; altered voice quality towards whispery, weak or to strained, harsh, hoarse; inappropriate bursts of excessive loudness or whispers or inappropriate sudden pitch change
Velum (soft palate): resonance	velum unable to raise-lower (fast enough/sufficiently) to switch airstream from nasal to oral flow or vice versa	altered degree of nasality, more commonly to hypernasality
Tongue	hyper- or hypotonus; hyper- or hypokinesis; tremor; incoordination	perceived distortion, omission, addition, substitution of tongue sounds (t, d, n, l, r, s, z, sh, ch, j, k, g, vowels)
Lips	hyper- or hypotonus; hyper- or hypokinesis; tremor; incoordination	perceived distortion, omission, addition, substitution of lip sounds (p, b, f, v, m, w)
Mandible	hyper- or hypotonus; hyper- or hypokinesis; tremor; incoordination; hangs too far open	disordered movement unlikely to directly impact speech; may have significant knock-on effect on tongue and lip control, especially if they too are affected and unable to compensate for mandibular perturbation

of the subtypes within these categories that may pose particular differential diagnostic conundrums.

3.1 Apraxia of speech and phonemic paraphasia

The characteristic picture in apraxia of speech is of a person who knows what they want to say (no aphasia or general intellectual impairment; though usually apraxia of speech does co-occur with aphasia). They know the sounds they are trying to speak (no dissolution or inaccessibility of the sound system/phonology). They have full range, rate and power of movements of the articulators (no primary sensory-motor impairment). Yet, they are unable to combine these movements into an overall action plan and realisation of movements to produce the desired sounds for an utterance. In severe cases the person may be rendered mute. In less severe cases speech sounds are slow, laboured, hesitant, dysfluent, with visible groping movements of the tongue and lips and audible repeated attempts at starting a word as the person struggles to overcome the misdirected articulatory movements. In the mildest cases the problem may only be manifest when the person is fatigued, under time or emotional pressure, or on articulatorily more complex motor sequences.

Diagnosis represents a challenge, calling for referral to speech language pathology/therapy. Apraxia represents a disorder of learned, volitional action control (McNeil *et al.*, 2008). Consequently the apparent inability to produce target sounds and words and the relatively effortful, dysfluent speech in a consciously controlled, propositional context contrasts with the ability to utter the same targets more fluently and accurately in more reflexive, automatic, non-propositional contexts. The person cannot repeat after the examiner 'me' or 'tea' but shouts them clearly in response to 'Which of you's Jean?', 'Would you like coffee or tea?' The person can say 1-2-3-4-5 in the nursery rhyme, but fails to say 5-4-3-2-1; pronounce 'that's hard' clearly as an aside whilst struggling on a particular word, but then cannot repeat after the examiner 'that's hard' a minute later.

Perceptually, to the naked ear, the impression is that sounds are distorted (right target sound, but spoken in an atypical fashion, 'tea' is produced with heavy aspiration after the 't'), substituted ('table' sounds like 'kable'), omitted ('stamp' sounds like 'sam', 'magazine' like 'mazine'), added ('pay' sounds like 'pfay' or 'pshay'). The apparent substitutions may themselves sound distorted ('table' sounds like 'kyable'). Misorderings, anticipations or perseverations may occur (telephone is produced as 'feletone, felephone, teletone'). Parapraxic perseverations spread across utterances. In naming successive pictures of 'bus, car, horse', for instance, the person may pronounce them as 'bus, bar, brarse'. Stress and intonation patterns may also be disrupted – canOE is misstressed as CAnoe, magaZINE as maGAzine or with syllables separated off from each other – ma..ga..zine. Sound derailments are prominently inconsistent – e.g. the speaker is unable to say 'tea' on one occasion, can on another, one time it is mispronounced as 'key', another time as 'chee', another as 'stee'.

Contrary to earlier claims, these are not indications that the person has lost the concept of particular sounds, has misselected or misordered sounds. Rather the underlying cause is in the breakdown of planning and regulation of the movements to produce the auditory targets, in misphasing, misscaling the fine distinctions alluded to above (e.g. voice onset time, degree of aspiration, alternation of tongue tip and tongue dorsum gestures) that help distinguish between different sounds (Ziegler and von Cramon, 1986, Itoh *et al.*, 1982, Ziegler, 2001).

As well as contrasting with neuromuscular aetiologies, apraxia is traditionally seen as different to speech problems arising at the level of phonological impairment, variously labelled phonemic paraphasia, phonological output disorder or similar (Buckingham, 1998). There are indeed speakers who sound as if they make the same substitution, misordering, omission and addition derailments as apraxic speakers, with repeated run-ups at a word to try and reach the correct sounds, but who otherwise show normal rate of speech and intonation and in whom there is little or no perceptible distortion of sounds. This invites a distinction between a phonological, paraphasic, premotoric disruption to output planning versus a motoric apraxic breakdown.

Guidelines exist for how one might differentiate speakers clinically (McNeil *et al.*, 2008). However, none has found universal acceptance and application of principles to individual speakers in clinic remains more often than not decidedly problematic (McNeil *et al.*, 2008). Distinguishing the putative disruptions is fraught with controversy. This stems from competing theoretical positions on the relationship, interface (or not) between phonological, premotoric processes in speech planning and phonetic motoric processes, all further clouded by decades of terminological confusion (Lebrun, 1989). The result is opposing predictions from contrasting models of speech output (Levelt *et al.*, 1999, Ziegler, 2002a, Schwartz *et al.*, 2004, Kingston, 2007) and divergent approaches to assessment (Miller, 2002, McNeil *et al.*, 2008). Furthermore, with few exceptions (Guenther, 2006) models are highly underspecified concerning the nature of the premotor-motor interface and what constitutes (speech) motoric control. Current front runners for viable models that might inform the differentiation between planning type breakdowns come from views rooted in articulatory and gestural phonologies (Browman and Goldstein, 1992, Kingston, 2007).

The role of mirror neurons and new understandings of the relationship of input-output processes in phonology and the links between perception and action will doubtless advance understanding of what breakdowns underlie phonemic paraphasia and apraxia of speech and what their relationship is (Poeppel and Hickok, 2004, Arbib, 2006).

Table 14.2 offers some general rules of thumb hinting in the different directions. They do not represent a definitive diagnostic key. Detailed differential diagnosis would be the remit of speech language pathologists/therapists.

3.2 **Dysarthrias**

Dysarthria denotes a problem with articulation due to neuromuscular impairment (Duffy, 2005, McNeil, 2008, Yorkston, 2007). Neuromuscular disorders affect the tone, power and coordination of movements. The precise constellation of changes depends on site(s) of lesion. In turn the neuromuscular changes impact on the initiation, range, speed, strength, sustainability, steadiness and coordination of movements for speech. These changes are in turn associated with alterations to voice quality, pitch, loudness, stress patterns and intonation of words and phrases, resonance, articulation of speech sounds and the facial and gestural movements that accompany speech. They impact on the intelligibility and acceptability of speech and determine the willingness or ability of an individual to engage in communication.

Table 14.3 summarises the main areas of the central and peripheral nervous system more directly involved in speech motor control and the disruptions to speech associated with lesions in these areas following this medical model. In as far as speech motor control is dependent on or interacts with broader motor and cognitive processes – for example arousal, attention, memory, language – clearly more structures and pathways are involved than this, but these are considered the core components for speech. Given the rich bilateral crossed and uncrossed innervation of the speech musculature persisting and more severe disorders linked to upper motor neurone lesions are more likely to occur with bilateral insults, but lasting defects with unilateral lesions do happen (Duffy, 2005).

Dysarthric alterations to voice and speech are prominent aspects of several degenerative disorders – including Parkinson's disease, motor neuron disease/amyotrophic lateral

Table 14.2 Rules of thumb for differentiating between paraphasic and apraxic type speech

More to 'speech apraxic' picture	More to 'phonemic paraphasic' picture
Perceived errors are predominantly distortions, close substitutions or distorted substitutions that differ minimally from the target sound	Lot higher proportion of displacement errors and apparent distant substitutions
On diadochokinetic (DDK) tasks difficulties are apparent already on single syllable (/'ta'ta'ta/) repetitions (altered rhythm, drifting on and off target, effortfulness)	on DDK tasks perform normally on single syllable repetition, once the person has latched onto correct target, but fall down on alternating tasks (/'pa'ta'ka/)
On alternating tasks more likely to have perseveration errors (stuck on one target)	alternating tasks tend to be disrupted by sequence errors or distant substitutions
Perceptually involves all word classes	tends to be restricted to nouns, verbs, adjectives (content words)
If no aphasia, written language is fine. Aphasia usually present though, so not good differentiator	spelling errors generally accompany the speech problem
Performance to reading or repetition may be better than spontaneous speech, but this is not a reliable diagnostic feature for all speakers	reproduction conduction aphasic speakers are significantly worse on repeating words and sentences compared to spontaneous speech
Slow rate, even in on-target utterances	(near) normal rate in on-target utterances
Inability to increase rate whilst maintaining sound integrity	variable ability to increase rate and maintain sound accuracy, but rate within normal limits
Variable, but overall prolonged movement transitions	variable, but in normal limits movement transition durations
Variable, but abnormally long vowels in multisyllable utterances	variable but normal limits vowel duration in multisyllable utterances
Variable but increased movement durations for individual speech gestures in connected speech	variable, but within normal limits durations

sclerosis, Friedreich's ataxia, Huntington's disease, multiple system atrophy, and progressive supranuclear palsy (Hartelius *et al.*, 2006, Hillel *et al.*, 1999, O'Sullivan *et al.*, 2008, Sapir *et al.*, 2008, Tjaden, 2008, Yorkston, 2007). Changes to speech and voice may even be detectable in the prodromal phase or be the initial indication that something is awry (Stewart *et al.*, 1995, Harel *et al.*, 2004, Hillel *et al.*, 1999, Penner *et al.*, 2007, El Badawey *et al.*, 2008, Richter *et al.*, 2005). Dysarthria is common too in multiple sclerosis, several cerebellar disorders as well as some muscular dystrophies (de Swart *et al.*, 2004) (though these strictly speaking are not neurogenic speech disorders). In traumatic brain injury and stroke it may be one of many consequences of the incident or manifest as a sole sequel. Dysarthria can be found in association with viral (e.g. encephalitis), infectious (e.g. rheumatic fever, meningitis), metabolic (e.g. Wilson's disease) or iatrogenic conditions (recurrent laryngeal nerve damage during surgery; drug induced).

Table 14.3 Broad changes to speech associated with varying central and peripheral nervous system lesion sites

Neurological component	Speech motor control component affected	Associated disruption to speech
dominant temporal-parietal, insular, frontal cortex	planning, supervision/ execution of movements for speech	phonological disturbances, apraxia of speech (see text)
right temporal-parietal, frontal cortex	control of aspects of intonation	a-dysprosody (see text)
upper motor neuron, pyramidal pathways	transmission of impulses from primary motor cortex via cortical bulbar and cortical spinal tracts to lower motor neurons (LMN)	spastic dysarthria; hypertonus and spasticity of muscles; slowed, effortful voluntary movements, harsh 'strain-strangled' voice
basal ganglia	initiation, scaling, maintenance, alternation and smooth concatenation of movements	depending on which structures and functions affected: hypokinetic dysarthria: bradykinesia, rigidity, slowed, quiet, monotone, monoloud speech; hyperkinetic dysarthrias: chorea, dystonia, ballism, athetosis, tics, associated with erratic alterations to loudness, rate, articulation; tremor brings unstable tremulous voice or speech; palilalia
cerebellum	feedforward control and coordination and integration of movements; cognitive affective component	ataxic dysarthria: dysmetric (under- overshooting of movements), dysrhythmic, discoordinated, disintegrated flow of speech movements
lower motor neuron	transmission of nerve impulses from upper motor neuron to muscles	flaccid dysarthria: hypotonus of muscles: bilateral: weak, slowed, easily fatigued or absent movement unilateral: diplophonic voice, compensatory mechanisms may mean articulation not majorly affected
synaptic junction and muscular disorders	transmission of nerve impulses from LMN to muscles; muscle contraction	flaccid dysarthria: weak, slowed, easily fatigued or absent movement

The time course of speech changes in relation to other involvement may be diagnostically significant. Speech-voice examination may therefore offer a means of early detection and/or differentiation of underlying disorders.

4 Assessment of motor speech disorders

One's precise approach to assessment is shaped by the purpose of the exercise. It may be to establish if some kind of disorder is present; determine the type of disorder in terms of underlying neurological, neuromuscular, neuropsychological or neurolinguistic breakdown; differential diagnosis of which parts of the vocal tract are impaired and to what degree; identification of variables to target in intervention; or gauge the effects of a disorder on the individual's behaviour and quality of life. The following outlines some broad approaches to assessment that can accomplish these ends. It is taken as understood that a comprehensive examination sites speech within a broader investigation of affective, language and other relevant cognitive processes. In Britain and North America at least the person likely to undertake detailed speech investigations is the speech language pathologist/therapist.

Assessments can be divided according to ICF levels of measurement (Threats, 2008). This framework is followed here. More extensive expositions of assessment can be found elsewhere (Duffy, 2005, McNeil, 2008).

4.1 Impairment level assessment

This entails the assessment of the tone, power, rate and range of movements of the articulators for speech, as well as measures of steadiness (e.g. rhythmic or arhythmic tremor; athetosis) and consistency (patterns of (ir)regularity of changes in specific parameters over time, from second to second or different times of day).

There is some debate over whether the tasks best suited to accomplish impairment assessment are nonverbal tasks (e.g. stick tongue in and out; blow out cheeks), or whether speech and speech-like items are more valid (e.g. repeat word 'tea' 10 times as fast as possible; alternate between tea-key as fast as possible (Ziegler, 2003a, Ziegler, 2003b, McNeil, 2008). The objection to the former is that they may well disclose muscle weakness, altered range of movement and so forth, but these correlate only weakly with success or not on movements for speech. Hence the latter are generally preferred as delivering a more ecologically valid evaluation. Table 14.4 summarises some main techniques in appraisal of speech impairment.

Usual practice is to evaluate parameters in varying contexts, since performance can vary according to whether elicitation entails spontaneous speech, repetition or reading (Kempler and Van Lancker, 2002). Furthermore differences across these domains may be diagnostically relevant (McNeil 2008). Ideally, one assesses under varying cognitive loads. Performance may significantly deteriorate when competing tasks have to be carried out (Ho et al., 2002, Bunton and Keintz, 2008).

Helpful information may be obtained by observing the speaker/articulators at rest when not necessarily engaged in speaking. Can the speaker attain and sustain adequate posture for optimal breathing; are respiration and phonation impeded in other ways by e.g. hemiplegia, contractures, skeletal deformities, inappropriate seating/bed? Pain from whatever source may influence overall body posture as well as articulator positioning and movement. In- or expiratory stridor can point to particular pathologies and may indicate a referral for laryngoscopic or neurological investigation.

Tremor, writhing, and ballistic movements may interfere with any articulators. One records whether these are (ir)regular and (un)predictable; what triggers them; the degree of voluntary control the person has over them; whether they overflow from/to other articulators/body parts.

Table 14.4 Main approaches to assessment of speech impairment

Articulatory function	Main parameter(s)	Instrumental assessments	Non instrumental assessments
respiration	capacity, control of expiration	Ability to sustain breath out for 5" with straw at 5cm depth on water manometer (Hixon et al., 1982). Respiratory kinematics. Respiratory function.	Frequency of breaths on standard reading passage or counting to 30 at fixed rate. Length of sustained /a/ sound
voice and prosody	vocal cord closure patterns; loudness, pitch, voice quality	Acoustic analyses of pitch and amplitude perturbation; harmonics to noise ratio; range, mean and standard deviation of fundamental frequency and loudness	Perceptual ratings of voice quality (e.g Karnell et al., 2007), loudness and pitch variation suitability; ratings of ability to signal intonation patterns and stress contrasts
resonance	ability to produce nasal vs oral resonance and sounds	Nasality meter; acoustic measures of nasality	Ability to sustain differentiation of nasal-oral sounds on 10 repetitions of minimal pairs – e.g. no-doe, by-my, any-Eddie
tongue control	ability to reach and maintain articulatory contacts and precision	Strain gauges, force transducers; acoustic measure of articulation; duration, closure and consistency on diadochokinetic tasks; acoustic vowel space	Diadochokinetic (DDK, (Gadesmann and Miller, 2008; Ziegler, 2002b) measures of rate, range, sustainability and alternation of contacts for tongue tip and back – e.g. repetition of tea; key, tea-key; tea-see; see-she; pea-tea-key
lip control	as for tongue, mutatis mutandis	as for tongue	as for tongue, using words involving lip movements: pea, fee, be, V, we
Coordination across articulators	breathing with phonation; oral with laryngeal gestures; inter- and intra articulator timing (e.g. tongue tip-dorsum)	acoustic measures of voice onset time; timing of voice and respiration onset-offset; measures of coarticulation and syllabification	ability to make and sustain voiced-voiceless distinctions; articulatory rate (syllables per minute), pause duration and frequency on standard tasks give rough measures of overall fluency

Food left in the mouth and/or round the lips may indicate the speaker is unable to clear it because of a weak tongue, poor swallow, because they are not aware it is there from poor sensory awareness, or lack of attention or motivation.

4.2 Activity limitation

Measures here examine the consequences of impairment alterations for speech intelligibility and naturalness. Rating scales deliver rough and ready estimations of intelligibility but suffer from very poor intra- and inter-rater reliability (Schiavetti, 1992, Kreiman and Gerratt, 2000) and are wholly uninformative regarding targets for rehabilitation. Diagnostic intelligibility testing (Kent *et al.*, 1989) provides both a metric for overall severity and (the diagnostic part of the label) indications for therapy.

A speaker may have unimpaired or viable intelligibility, but alterations to how natural or disordered their voice, resonance, prosody and rate of speech are perceived, may act as limitations on activity. Presence of disruptive struggle to achieve intelligible speech may represent an additional feature curtailing communication either from the point of view of the speaker and how it impacts on them and their ability to adapt, or from the point of the listener and their ability to tolerate or adapt to the altered speech characteristics.

Whilst these factors can be assessed objectively (Table 14.4), their combined or separate effects on activity are typically rated on general scales of acceptability, disorderedness or naturalness, or more specific scales examining elements of prosody, voice quality, resonance (Karnell *et al.*, 2007).

4.3 Participation restriction and impact

Speech and voice changes, even mild, may alter a person's ability to enter into roles, places and activities they previously were able to, and/or alter listeners' reactions to the speaker with consequences for social participation (Miller *et al.*, 2006b, Yorkston *et al.*, 2007). Assessments of participation restriction gauge these factors. Well validated and reliable instruments specifically for speech are currently only under development (Eadie *et al.*, 2006, Walshe *et al.*, 2009). Some evaluations for voice impact exist (Karnell *et al.*, 2007). The semantic differential technique has been employed to effectively measure status and change in relation to communication (Miller *et al.*, 2008).

5 Other speech changes

Speech may be disrupted by a wide variety of neurological disturbances (Table 14.4). The following sections sketch a broad overview of some more common neurogenic speech changes, with a bias towards ones that may present some diagnostic conundrums, especially where the speech alterations occur in (relative) isolation from other signs and symptoms.

5.1 Dystonias

Dystonia is a neurogenic movement disorder characterized by repetitive, involuntary, sustained muscle contractions (Albanese, 2007). These can be limited to one area of the body or muscle (group), as in e.g. laryngeal or mandibular dystonias; involve two or more adjacent or non-contiguous areas of the body; or be generalized in nature. Movements may arise without apparent trigger, may be elicited as an overflow reaction to movements in unaffected body parts, or in action dystonias (below) only appear in response to highly specific eliciting conditions.

Although dystonias typically resolve over seconds or minutes, more severe fixed dystonias may lead to long term abnormal postures and contractures in the affected region.

Any focal dystonia involving muscles of speech (including breathing, larynx, jaw, soft palate, not just the more obvious facial and tongue sites) may compromise spoken output. Typically reactions involve a consistent movement pattern. Thus, an individual with mandibular dystonia, depending on which muscle (group) is affected, experiences the same opening, closing or lateral movement of the jaw, in the same direction, to the same degree.

Dystonic spasms are usually worsened by stress, emotional upset, or fatigue and improved with rest or sleep. A characteristic of dystonia is that patients may be able to temporarily suppress dystonic movements or feel they can release spasms by various compensatory tricks (sometimes termed gestes antagonistes) such as touching an affected or adjacent body part.

Task specific dystonias are triggered or severely exacerbated in response to specific voluntary movements. These highly specific or hidden triggers can lend a decidedly psychogenic air to the presentation, especially when they are combined with apparently 'bizarre' gestes antagonistes.

Amongst reported action dystonias several illustrate speech or facial movement related factors, including in response to wind instrument playing, auctioneering, praying, writing (Frucht et al., 2001, Rosset-Llobet et al., 2007, Das et al., 2007, Gaig et al., 2007, Scolding et al., 1995, Ilic et al., 2005). One cause of bruxism (teeth grinding) is dystonia (Singer and Papapetropoulos, 2006, Tan et al., 2004). Task specific dystonias may remain as such or may later emerge in other activities as the condition deteriorates (e.g. writers cramp spreads to eating behaviour or other activities involving arm control).

5.2 Spasmodic dysphonia

Probably the most prevalent action dystonia in relation to speech is spasmodic dysphonia (Baylor et al., 2007, Bender et al., 2004). The act of speaking induces dystonic spasms that either involuntarily draw the vocal cords together (adductor spasmodic dysphonia or adductor laryngeal dystonia) or apart (abductor variety). Whilst these varieties sometimes occur independently, most speakers evidence both ad- and abductor spasms.

Perturbations range from barely perceptible to severely debilitating. In mild cases in the adductor type the listener hears what sounds like a sudden hiccup or catch in the voice, or the 'huh' one might exclaim if suddenly experiencing a sharp pain. The more severe the state, the more symptoms resemble a strained voice quality, stuttering like blocks, right up to complete voice arrest as the speaker struggles to overcome hyperadduction. In the abductor variety in mild cases the listener may perceive voice breaks, sudden intrusive whispers or intermittent loss of volume and voicing, whilst at the severe end of the spectrum every endeavour to vocalise elicits an abductor spasm leading to complete voice loss.

In contrast to speech, vegetative functions such as laughing, throat clearing, yawning are frequently performed normally. As the problem is action induced, laryngoscopic examination of the larynx at rest demonstrates no abnormality. Requests to whisper, sing a note, say a high pitched /i/ may also not trigger a spasm. It is only during natural and sustained speech that the dystonic disruptions are likely to reveal themselves.

Such suggestions of normality may strengthen the impression of a psychogenic aetiology. This may be reinforced by the compensatory suppression or release gestures the individual has developed. Personal cases seen have performed a shaking movement of the head, pushed or pinched the thyroid cartilage, made a blowing movement with over rounded lips when their voice arrests, preceded utterances with a /hmm/ or a sniff, or 'covered' breaks with a cough. Others report patients who pressed their hand against the back of their head, or abdomen, or pulled their ear.

Onset is commonly in middle age. Symptoms gradually deteriorate over a few years. The person notices first what they might describe as catches of breath, little coughs or gasps. These progress to what are perceived as a more general hoarseness, or increasing whisperiness, eventually ending in the spasmodic disruptions described above. In association with nervous system damage onset may be sudden.

Apparent remission of symptoms followed by relapse is not uncommon. Speakers may report spasms are less or more severe at certain times of the day, week, or month, or in particular speaking situations, or with specific interlocutors. Symptoms may be ameliorated by tranquilizers or when under the influence of alcohol. While suggestive of a psychogenic origin, these features are all common findings in the dystonias and should not be used to confirm a psychiatric problem.

Whilst spasmodic dysphonia, contrary to earlier suppositions, is not of psychological aetiology speakers may nevertheless present with an overlay of psychological symptoms. Surveys unanimously point up the affective consequences of the disorder (Baylor *et al.*, 2005, Baylor *et al.*, 2007). Facing up to frightening progressive changes which you yourself seem unable to control, but which people, including medical staff, are only too willing to tell you is all in the mind; living with the stigma that attaches to such voice characteristics and associated 'bizarre' behaviours; loss of employment, loss of social standing; doubts about ones personal integrity and state of mind can for some all add together to foster depression, personality changes, breakdown of communication within the family, social circle and workplace.

Behavioural voice therapy has no effect on the underlying dystonia symptoms. Indeed, success from behavioural therapy is one indication of a likely psychogenic origin. The current treatment of choice is botulinum toxin injection of the affected muscles (Bender *et al.*, 2004). This can bring 4–6 months of symptomatic relief before a repeat injection is required.

5.3 Speech tics

Tics are recurrent, brief, intermittent, stereotypical movements which arise outside of or only under partial control of the individual – a blink of the eyes, shrug of the shoulders, twisting of the head, shouting of a sound or word. Tics that involve verbal or speech like behaviours, and/or nonverbal tics may interfere with speech production and communication generally.

Tics contrast with myoclonic conditions and seizures, and compulsive or ritualistic behaviours which may show themselves as compulsive spitting, touching, shouting, reciting over and again of words or sequences of words or sounds. They contrast with the repetitive stereotypies found in autism, some psychiatric disorders and in some post brain injury cases. Tics are not acquired habits or mannerisms, though it is important to be alert to the possibility that an apparent mannerism is a compensatory mask for an underlying tic or other movement disorder.

Simple tics involve one (uni- or bilateral) group of muscles (eye wink, pouting of the lips, sticking the tongue out), complex ones several groups, or indeed a whole behavioural sequence resembling a normal motor act (writing gesture, utterance of whole phrase, throwing, shaking the fist). Tic episodes can involve a sudden and rapid jerking movement (clonic tics) or a slower, held postural change (dystonic tics) or isometric contraction (tonic tics). Depending on the aetiology and severity they may be more or less constant, or intermittent – several times per day, per week, per month, or less frequent. The course may be transient (passes within a year) or stretches out chronically.

One of the commoner disorders linked to tics is Tourette syndrome (TS), a neurological disorder in which motor and phonic tics (Albin and Mink, 2006) are prominent. Phonic tics is a label coined to cover the fact that people with TS may manifest vocal (throat clearing, shouting, crowing, barking, squealing, gargling....) and speech (uttering specific speech sounds or words) behaviours, but tics may also include nonverbal sounds such as sniffing, lip smacking, clicks, blowing, sucking, raspberries. The repertoire of motor tics can encompass face twitching, nodding, shoulder shrugging, eye rolling and many more. Outbursts of foul language (coprolalia) (Van Lancker and Cummings, 1999) or obscene gestures (copropraxia), occur in around a third of patients. The mean age of onset is around 7 years (range ca. 3–12 years) though phonic tics commonly emerge somewhat later. For most people there is a lessening of tic severity or remission in late adolescence or adulthood.

Typically a sufferer shows multiple tics, either simultaneously, or over a short period of time, usually in bouts. The anatomical site (eyes, neck, face...) and type (e.g. vocal, speech) may alter over time, as can the frequency and complexity of the tics. Tics are involuntary in as far as at some stage the person is no longer able to resist their expression. However, around 4 out of 5 patients experience premonitory sensations. They have the feeling they need to blink, cough, shout, touch, or whatever, but are able for a period (minutes, an hour even) to suppress the compulsion. At the end of that time they have the urge they must perform the behaviour to release the tension. The precise timing of this release can have a degree of voluntary control.

One or more neuropsychiatric disturbances commonly coexist with the tics – including obsessive-compulsive thoughts or behaviour, attention deficit hyperactivity disorder, anxiety, depression, self injurious behaviour, and possibly personality disturbance. Whether they represent the expression of a common underlying factor with the tics or are comorbid for some other reason remains an ongoing debate. Language delay, reading disorder, and stuttering may also accompany the tics. Whether what is observed as stuttering is separate or coterminous with the tic behaviour is disputable (Ludlow and Loucks, 2003, Mulligan et al., 2003).

Speech tics in TS seldom impair intelligibility, in so far as they appear only in self-limiting bouts. However, in that they represent socially unacceptable behaviours and the height of symptoms peaks during the school years, the broader effects on communication may be considerable.

5.4 Palilalia

In palilalia a speaker appears to become stuck on a sound, word or phrase, repeating it over and over, typically a few times, but 15–20 repetitions in a row are not unknown. Generally repetitions are of final words, sounds or syllables. In attempting to say 'Pass me the salt' the person says 'pass me the salt the salt the salt the salt….'; 'I need the nurse' appears as 'I need the nurse-urse-urse-urse-urse. Characteristically iterations occur with a fixed, stereotypic intonation, with fading loudness and excursion of articulatory movements, and at least the perception that each successive repetition is faster than the previous (Borsel *et al.*, 2007, Benke and Butterworth, 2001). Speakers appear fully aware of the behaviour but are unable to inhibit it. The degree to which palilalia appears in a person's speech can vary according to task and linguistic unit, being more often heard in conversation, less so when repeating phrases after the examiner or on reading and automatic sequences.

Although the classical picture is the one just described, some writers have included under the label of palilalia all sorts of iterations of whole utterances, word initial sounds, and whole word repetitions (Benke and Butterworth, 2001) that more appropriately should be viewed as indicative of underlying language processing, apraxic, phonological or dystonic difficulties rather than the type of motor disruption causing the classical palilalic picture.

5.5 Tremor

Tremors of one kind or another occur as part of many neurological conditions, classically Parkinson's disease and essential tremor. Relatively isolated tremor like behaviours more liable to have a bearing on speech and voice are essential tremor and myoclonus of the palate, tongue or jaw (Silverdale *et al.*, 2008, Samuel *et al.*, 2004).

Essential tremor labels an isolated (i.e. not part of a more general condition), slowly progressive, chronic condition involving involuntary, rhythmic tremor of a body part. Commonly it commences in the hands or arms, but may go on (or rarely start) to involve the head, vocal cords and tongue. When the latter are involved, seldom before the seventh decade, disruption to speech and voice is possible. Hand tremor may impair writing or typing or render it entirely impossible.

Palatal myoclonus presents as a rhythmic contraction of either or both sides of the soft palate (Samuel *et al.*, 2004). Adjacent structures, and sometimes distantly the diaphragm and eyes, may also be involved, giving lingual or laryngeal myoclonus. At first the movement may be reported by the sufferer as a clicking in the ears (from contraction of the tensor veli palatini muscle which also opens the Eustachian tube). It may arise as an idiopathic, essential condition, typically in the 30–40 year age range, or symptomatically at any time after infarcts, trauma, tumour or infections, usually of the brainstem. Emergence of the myoclonus may be as long as one year post onset of the responsible illness. In essential palatal myoclonus the individual may be able to modify the tremor by intention or adopting compensatory neck positions, or mouth opening. It does not usually constitute a major cause of intelligibility loss.

5.6 Whisper and Mutism

Whispering and mutism do not constitute diagnostic entities. They are though a (occasionally sole) feature of numerous neurological aetiologies. Elective (sometimes termed selective) mutism, functional voice disorders and severe depression represent likely non-neurological aetiologies here contrasting with the neurological causes.

Mutism is present in the aptly named akinetic mutism, a condition linked to frontal lobe damage and characterized by a pronounced diminution of nearly all motor functions, including facial expression, gestures, and speech output. The person nevertheless remains apparently alert. Less extreme forms may be associated with a whispered voice. An isolated apraxia of the larynx has been claimed (Marshall *et al.*, 1988, Sieron *et al.*, 1995) where voluntary movements of the oral articulators remain intact but the person is unable to consciously initiate phonation. Non-conscious, spontaneous laryngeal sounds (e.g. cough, sigh, yawn) remain intact.

In what has been described as dynamic aphasia (Robinson *et al.*, 2006) attempts to elicit a spoken (or any) response from the individual may be met with muteness, or a severely delayed response that then appears in just a whisper, with the person apparently unable to sustain output beyond a few words before it fades again into silence. Whether dynamic aphasia represents a separate diagnostic entity or is merely a sign of frontal involvement remains unresolved. Progressive loss of voice ending in mutism is a profile reported in some cases of frontal and frontotemporal atrophy.

People with locked in syndrome (Smith and Delargy, 2005, Chisolm and Gillett, 2005) are unable to move any part of their body, including the vocal cords, except for eye movements and blinking. Hence they are mute. Being a disorder arising from brain stem pathology, cognition is usually intact. Individuals remain fully alert and may be able to acquire sophisticated alternative means of communication employing the intact eye and blinking movements.

A period of mutism is a common sequel early after stroke or head injury, especially frontal lesions. Over days or weeks this may resolve via a whispered voice (with or without aphasia) to dysarthric, apraxic or normal speech. Muteness arises as a transient and longer term sequel after some surgical interventions (e.g. commisurotomy, posterior fossa operations, especially in children). Transient muteness may be a manifestation of epileptiform seizures, either as one element of a complex pattern or as an isolated speech arrest.

Uni- and bilateral opercular lesions can cause muteness (Kuroda, 2007). The Francophone label – labio-facio-glosso-pharyngo-laryngo-paralysis (Foix Chavany Marie syndrome) – is more illustrative of the presenting motor picture of what some consider a cortical version of pseudobulbar palsy. There is paralysis of the lower face, masticatory, pharyngeal and laryngeal muscles, but, when it occurs in isolation, all other language (including writing) and neuropsychological functions remain intact. Characteristically there is no paralysis of upper or lower limbs and there is an automatic-voluntary dissociation. For instance the person is able to smile, swallow, lick their lips spontaneously, but not to command. Onset may be sudden (e.g. stroke) or progressive (e.g. frontal atrophy).

Whispered voice or total mutism may be present in the end stages of several degenerative neurological conditions, including motor neurone disease/amyotrophic lateral sclerosis, some cases of multiple sclerosis, multiple system atrophy, progressive supranuclear palsy and Parkinson's disease. In the latter three weak(ening) voice, problems with initiation or sustaining of phonation may be early signs of disease.

Bilateral vocal cord palsies render the speaker mute (Rubin and Sataloff, 2007). Unilateral cord palsies produce biplophonic phonation, but in an attempt to avoid the resultant unnatural sounding voice, speakers may compensate by speaking in only a whisper.

5.6.1 Prosody

Prosody refers to the general melody of speech derived from variation in the components of pitch, loudness, rate/duration. Linguistic prosody concerns the use of prosody to signal grammatical contrasts (e.g. 'That's MY coat' vs 'THAT'S my coat'; TOYshop vs toy SHOP; 'you're coming tomorrow!' vs 'you're coming tomorrow?'). Affective prosody concerns the emotional content of utterances expressed through manipulating pitch, loudness, duration (e.g. 'The sausage has fallen in the custard' spoken with an angry vs laughing vs sad tone; 'You're so kind' intended as a sincere vs ironic comment).

Linguistic a- or dysprosody may arise after left or right hemispheric lesions and can be disrupted by dysarthric and apraxic speech. Typically in phonemic paraphasia prosody is preserved. Affective aprosody is associated with right hemisphere lesions and some neurodegenerative conditions.

In expressive a- or dysprosody speakers are unable to signal the linguistic contrasts noted above and/or cannot convey emotional content. Speech may sound monotone, monoloud, monorate, or inappropriate stress and intonation patterns may appear. In receptive prosodic disturbances individuals fail to pick up or misunderstand prosodic cues to linguistic or affective meaning. Thus breakdowns in communication occur because the person fails to understand/produce the necessary linguistic marker to correctly convey/apprehend the meaning of an utterance or they misconstrue or listeners misinterpret the emotional intention – an ironic 'you're so kind' is taken as sincere; intended enthusiasm is heard as indifference.

An awareness of prosodic disturbances is important as a possible source of comprehension or expression problems and broader communication and interaction breakdown. It is also important as the flattened intonation and quiet, slow speech common in aprosodia, or instances of getting the 'wrong end of the stick' may be misinterpreted as signalling an underlying affective or neurobehavioural disorder when none is present. Alternatively changes may be falsely put down to disorders of attention, cognition or motivation (Blake et al., 2003).

6 Development of a foreign accent

People may be referred to clinic because they have acquired what appears to be a foreign accent. The vast majority of *published* cases are neurogenic, though psychogenic origins have recently been reported (Gurd *et al.*, 2001, Reeves *et al.*, 2007).

6.1 Re-emergence of a previous foreign accent

Speakers who migrated from one country to another, or even from a different part of the same country, may have lost the accent of their place of origin, yet after stroke or head injury they speak again with their former accent (Roth *et al.*, 1997, Seliger *et al.*, 1992). A possible neurolinguistic explanation given for this phenomenon is that it 'costs' someone (especially if they moved after the teenage years) in terms of processing resources, to alter a previous accent and maintain a new one. The new one may never become fully automatised. When processing resources are compromised from neurological damage, the ability to pay this cost is affected and the previously less costly pattern reemerges.

6.2 Acquired foreign accent syndrome

Here, after a neurological episode a person is perceived as speaking their native tongue with a foreign accent or different regional accent, despite the fact that they have never lived in that place, have no knowledge of the alleged base language and know no one who speaks with that accent. This is totally unrelated to issues of language change in bilingual or polyglot aphasia. FAS is as likely to be found in absolutely monolingual speakers as any others. The accent may be heard transiently for a few days or weeks or be permanent, unmodifiable by the speaker. Most reported cases have arisen from left hemisphere lesions, cortical and subcortical, but right hemisphere aetiologies are recorded (Dankovičová *et al.*, 2001, Miller *et al.*, 2006a). Aetiologies have included stroke, head injury, multiple sclerosis, vasculitis, and dystonia.

Sometimes listeners perceive a definite geographical accent. More usually listeners perceive only some generic 'Slav' or 'Southern' accent or disagree on where the accent comes from (Christoph *et al.*, 2004, Di Dio *et al.*, 2006). Typically speech does not contain all the features that might be linked to a given perceived accent and even features present may not necessarily appear constantly or consistently. Rather, impressions of being Italian, French or whatever can hinge on key features picked up by the listener (Gurd *et al.*, 1988). In as far as different listeners may focus on separate features, not every listener hears the same accent (one thinks it is French, the other Polish). In so far as features may be more or less prominent on different occasions, the same listener may judge an Italian accent one day, a German one the next. Hence the ease with which such behaviour is dismissed as psychiatric.

Detailed acoustic studies of people with FAS reveal a catalogue of changes associated with the altered accent. Changes can involve syllable structure (e.g. 'spy' sounds like 'suhpy'; 'big dog' like 'biguhdog', 'string' like 'trin'), prosodic alterations, or individual sounds (e.g. w sounds like v, r is rolled instead of burred). Many cases also have an accompanying mild agrammatism, word finding difficulty and slowed, hesitant speech, which lend an air of foreignness. No unifying factor explains all cases, except in most general terms that there are subtle perturbations to the speech output mechanism, at the level of planning or execution in either or both segmental (individual sounds) or suprasegmental (prosodic) features. The common denominator appears to be that the prominent changes to a speaker's speech are ones that listeners associate with an extant different accent or language. It is the disorder in the ear of the listener par excellence.

FAS is seldom linked with impaired intelligibility. This does not mean people with FAS do not experience problems with communicating. They may despair at the readiness of others to brand them as psychiatric cases, malingerers, posers; tire of the condescending 'foreigner talk' addressed to them; no longer tolerate the endless quips of family, friends and strangers at their expense; and most of all, mourn for their lost accent and what it meant for their identity and feeling of belonging (Miller, 2009).

7 Treatment

Medical and or surgical interventions can influence speech to a degree in some medical conditions (Duffy, 2005, McNeil, 2008), though in others may have no or a detrimental effect (Schulz, 2002, Sapir *et al.*, 2008). Speech language therapy can improve communication for most people with neurogenic motor speech disorders, including with degenerative conditions and with longstanding changes, even if improvement is seldom to a premorbid state.

Gains may be made through specific direct work on respiration, voice, resonance and articulation. Progress may come from introduction of techniques that influence speech overall (e.g. rate control techniques). On occasion, spoken communication has to be augmented by gestural, written or other instrumental means; or alternative non-verbal methods of communication sought.

While some treatment approaches for some conditions have well developed evidence bases for what works for whom when and how, definitive large scale studies or well controlled case series demonstrating efficacy for others have still to be carried out.

Selective references

Ackermann, H., Mathiak, K. and Riecker, A. (2007) The contribution of the cerebellum to speech production and speech perception. *The Cerebellum*, **6**, 202–213.

Albanese, A. (2007) Dystonia: clinical approach. *Parkinsonism and Related Disorders*, **13**, S356–S361.

Albin, R. and Mink, J. (2006) Recent advances in Tourette syndrome research. *Trends in Neurosciences*, **29**, 175–182.

Arbib, M. (2006) Aphasia, apraxia and the evolution of the language ready brain. *Aphasiology*, **20**, 1125–1155.

Baylor, C. Yorkston, K. and Eadie, T. (2005) The consequences of spasmodic dysphonia on communication-related quality of life. *Journal of Communication Disorders*, **38**, 395–419.

Baylor, C. Yorkston, K. Eadie, T. and Maronian, N. (2007) Psychosocial Consequences of botox Injections for Spasmodic Dysphonia. *Journal of Voice*, **21**, 231–247.

Bender, B. Cannito, M. Murry, T. and Woodson, G. (2004) Speech intelligibility in severe adductor spasmodic dysphonia. *J. Speech Language and Hearing Research*, **47**, 21–32.

Benke, T. and Butterworth, B. (2001) Palilalia and repetitive speech: Two case studies. *Brain and Language*, **78,** 62–81.

Blake, M., Duffy, J., Tompkins, C. and Myers, P. (2003) Right hemisphere syndrome is in the eye of the beholder. *Aphasiology*, **17,** 423–432.

Booth, J., Wood, L., Lu, D., Houk, J. and Bitan, T. (2007) The role of the basal ganglia and cerebellum in language processing. *Brain Research*, **1133,** 136–144.

Borsel, J., Bontinck, C., Coryn, M., Paemeleire, F. and Vandemaele, P. (2007) Acoustic features of palilalia. *Brain and Language*, **101,** 90–96.

Browman, C. P. and Goldstein, L. (1992) Articulatory Phonology - an Overview. *Phonetica*, **49,** 155–180.

Buckingham, H. (1998) Explanations for the concept of apraxia of speech. In M. Sarno (ed.) *Acquired aphasia*, 269–307.

Bunton, K. and Keintz, C. (2008) Use of dual task paradigm for assessing speech intelligibility in clients with Parkinson's disease. *J Medical Speech-Language Pathology*, **16,** 141–155.

Cannizzaro, M., Harel, B., Reilly, N., Chappell, P. and Snyder, P. (2004) Voice acoustical measurement of the severity of major depression. *Brain and Cognition*, **56,** 30–35.

Chisolm, N. and Gillett, G. (2005) The patient's journey: living with locked-in syndrome. *British Medical Journal*, **331,** 94–97.

Christoph, D., De Freitas, G., Dos Santos, D., Lima, M., Araujo, A. and Carota, A. (2004) Different perceived foreign accents in one patient after prerolandic hematoma. *European Neurology*, **52,** 198–201.

Dankovičová, J., Gurd, J., Marshall, J., Macmahon, M., Stuart-Smith, J., Coleman, J. and Slater, A. (2001) Aspects of non-native pronunciation in a case of altered accent following stroke (foreign accent syndrome). *Clinical Linguistics & Phonetics*, **15,** 195–218.

Das, C., Prabhakar, S. and Truong, D. (2007) Clinical profile of various sub-types of writer's cramp. *Parkinsonism and Related Disorders*, **13,** 421–424.

De Swart, B., Van Engelen, B., Van De Kerkhof, J. and Maassen, B. (2004) Myotonia and flaccid dysarthria in patients with adult onset myotonic dystrophy. *J Neurol Neurosurg Psychiatry*, **75,** 1480–1482.

Di Dio, C., Schulz, J. and Gurd, J. (2006) Foreign Accent Syndrome: In the ear of the beholder? *Aphasiology*, **20,** 951–962.

Duffy, J. (2005) *Motor speech disorders*, St Louis, Mosby.

Duffy, J. (2006) Apraxia of speech in degenerative neurologic disease. *Aphasiology*, **20,** 511–527.

Eadie, T., Yorkston, K., Klasner, E., Dudgeon, B., Deitz, J., Baylor, C., Miller, R. and Amtmann, D. (2006) Measuring communicative participation: A review of self-report instruments in speech-language pathology. *American Journal of Speech-Language Pathology*, **15,** 307–320.

EL Badawey, M., Punekar, S. and Zammit-Maempel, I. (2008) Prospective study to assess vocal cord palsy investigations. *Otolaryngology - Head and Neck Surgery*, **138,** 788–790.

Frucht, S., Fahn, S., Greene, P., O'brien, C., Gelb, M., Truong, D., Welsh, J., Factor, S. and Ford, B. (2001) The natural history of embouchure dystonia. *Movement Disorders*, **16,** 899–906.

Gadesmann, M. and Miller, N. (2008) Reliability of speech diadochokinetic test measurement. *International J Language Communication Disorders*, **43,** 41–54.

Gaig, C., Muñoz, E., Valls-Sole, J., Marti, M. and Tolosa, E. (2007) Eating-induced facial myoclonic dystonia probably due to a putaminal lesion. *Movement Disorders*, **22,** 877–880.

Garcia, J., Crowe, L., Redler, D. and Hustad, K. (2004) Effects of spontaneous gestures on comprehension and intelligibility of dysarthric speech. *J Medical Speech-Language Pathology*, **12,** 145–148.

Gorno-Tempini, M., Ogar, J., Brambati, S., Wang, P., Jeong, J., Rankin, K., Dronkers, N. and Miller, B. (2006) Anatomical correlates of early mutism in progressive nonfluent aphasia. *Neurology*, **67,** 1849–1851.

Guenther, F. H. (2006) Cortical interactions underlying the production of speech sounds. *Journal of Communication Disorders,* **39,** 350–365.

Gurd, J. Bessell, N. Bladon, R. and Bamford, J. (1988) A case of foreign accent syndrome, with follow-up clinical, neuropsychological and phonetic descriptions. *Neuropsychologia,* **26,** 237–251.

Gurd, J., Coleman, J., Costello, A. and Marshall, J. (2001) Organic or functional? A new case of foreign accent syndrome. *Cortex,* **37,** 715–8.

Harel, B., Cannizzaro, M., Cohen, H., Reilly, N. and Snyder, P. (2004) Acoustic characteristics of Parkinsonian speech: a potential biomarker of early disease progression and treatment. *Journal of Neurolinguistics,* **17,** 439–453.

Hartelius, L., Gustavsson, H., Astrand, M. and Holmberg, B. (2006) Perceptual analysis of speech in multiple system atrophy and progressive supranuclear palsy. *J Medical Speech*-Language *Pathology,* **14,** 241–247.

Hillel, A., Dray, T., Miller, R., Yorkston, K., Konikow, N., Strande, E. and Browne, J. (1999) Presentation of ALS to the otolaryngologist/head and neck surgeon: getting to the neurologist. *Neurology,* **53,** S22–S25.

Hixon, T., Hawley, J. and Wilson, K. (1982) An around the house device for the clinical determination of respiratory driving pressure: a note on making the simple even simpler. *J Speech Hearing Disorders,* **47,** 413–415.

Hixon, T. and Hoit, J. (2005) Evaluation and management of speech breathing disorders: principles and methods, Tuscon, Redington.

Ho, A., Iansek, R. and Bradshaw, J. (2002) Effect of a concurrent task on Parkinsonian speech. *J Clinical Experimental Neuropsychology,* **24,** 36–47.

Ilic, T. V., Potter, M., Holler, I., Deuschl, G. and Volkmann, J. (2005) Praying-induced oromandibular dystonia. *Movement Disorders,* **20,** 385–386.

Itoh, M., Sasanuma, S., Tatsumi, I. F., Murakami, S., Fukusao, Y. and Suzuki, T. (1982) Voice onset time characteristics in apraxia of speech. *Brain Language,* **17,** 193–210.

Karnell, M., Melton, S., Childes, J., Coleman, T., Dailey, S. and Hoffman, H. (2007) Reliability of clinician-based (GRBAS and CAPE-V) and patient-based (V-RQOL and IPVI) documentation of voice disorders. *Journal of Voice,* **21,** 576–590.

Kempler, D. and Van Lancker, D. (2002) Effect of speech task on intelligibility in dysarthria: a case study of Parkinson's disease. *Brain Language,* **80,** 449–64.

Kent, R., Weismer, G., Kent, J. and Rosenbek, J. (1989) Toward phonetic intelligibility testing in dysarthria. *J Speech Hearing Disorders,* **54,** 482–499.

Kingston, J. (2007) The phonetics-phonology interface. In Lacy, P. D. (Ed.) *Cambridge handbook of phonology.* Cambridge, CUP.

Kreiman, J. and Gerratt, B. (2000) Sources of listener disagreement in voice quality assessment. *J Acoustical Society America,* **108,** 1867–1876.

Kuroda, Y. (2007) Foix-Chavany-Marie syndrome: Case reports with literature review. *J Medical Speech*-Language *Pathology,* **15,** 137–147.

Lebrun, Y. (1989) Apraxia of speech: The history of a concept. In Square-Storer, P. (Ed.) *Acquired apraxia of speech in aphasic adults.* London, Taylor Francis.

Levelt, W., Roelofs, A. and Meyer, A. (1999) A theory of lexical access in speech production. *Behavioural Brain Sciences,* **22,** 1–75.

Ludlow, C. and Loucks, T. (2003) Stuttering: a dynamic motor control disorder. *J Fluency Disorders,* **28,** 273–295.

Marshall, R., Gandour, J. and Windsor, J. (1988) Selective impairment of phonation. *Brain Language,* **35,** 313–339.

McNeil, M. (Ed.) (2008) Clinical management of sensorimotor speech disorders, New York, Thieme.

Mcneil, M., Robin, D. and Schmidt, R. (2008) Apraxia of speech. In McNeil, M. (Ed.) *Clinical management of sensorimotor speech disorders*. New York, Thieme.

Miller, N. (2002) Neurological bases of apraxia of speech. *Seminars in Speech and Language*, **23**, 223–230.

Miller, N. (2009) Foreign Accent Syndrome – between two worlds, at home in neither. In Watt, D. **and** Llamas, C. (Eds.) *Language and identities*. Edinburgh, Edinburgh University Press.

Miller, N., Lowit, A. and O'Sullivan, H. (2006a) What makes acquired foreign accent syndrome foreign? *Journal Neurolinguistics*, **19**, 385–409.

Miller, N., Noble, E., Jones, D., Allcock, L. and Burn, D. (2008) How do I sound to me? Perceived changes in communication in Parkinson's disease. *Clinical Rehabilitation*, **22**, 14–22.

Miller, N., Noble, E., Jones, D. and Burn, D. (2006b) Life with communication changes in Parkinson's disease. *Age Ageing*, **35**, 235–239.

Mulligan, H., Anderson, T., Jones, R., Williams, M. and Donaldson, I. (2003) Tics and developmental stuttering. *Parkinsonism and Related Disorders*, **9**, 281–289.

Munhall, K., Jones, J., Callan, D., Kuratate, T. and Vatikiotis, E. (2004) Visual prosody and speech intelligibility - Head movement improves auditory speech perception. *Psychological Science*, **15**, 133–137.

O'Keeffe, F., Murray, B., Coen, R., Dockree, P., Bellgrove, M., Garavan, H., Lynch, T. and Robertson, I. (2007) Loss of insight in frontotemporal dementia, corticobasal degeneration and progressive supranuclear palsy. *Brain*, **130**, 753–764.

O'Sullivan, S. S., Massey, L. A., Williams, D. R., Silveira-Moriyama, L., Kempster, P. A., Holton, J. L., Revesz, T. and Lees, A. J. (2008) Clinical outcomes of progressive supranuclear palsy and multiple system atrophy. *Brain*, **131**, 1362–1372.

Penner, H., Miller, N. and Wolters, M. (2007) Motor speech disorders in three parkinsonian syndromes: a comparative study. *16th International Congress of Phonetic Sciences, Saarbrücken, August*, 1989–92.

Poeppel, D. and Hickok, G. (2004) Towards a new functional anatomy of language. *Cognition*, **92**, 1–12.

Reeves, R., Burke, R. and Parker, J. (2007) Characteristics of psychotic patients with foreign accent syndrome. *J Neuropsychiatry Clin Neurosci*, **19**, 70–76.

Richter, S., Schoch, B., Ozimek, A., Gorissen, B., Hein-Kropp, C., Kaiser, O., Hovel, M., Wieland, R., Gizewski, E., Ziegler, W. and Timmann, D. (2005) Incidence of dysarthria in children with cerebellar tumors: A prospective study. *Brain Language*, **92**, 153–167.

Robinson, G., Shallice, T. and Cipolotti, L. (2006) Dynamic aphasia in progressive supranuclear palsy: A deficit in generating a fluent sequence of novel thought. *Neuropsychologia*, **44**, 1344–1360.

Rosset-Llobet, J., Candia, V., Fabregas, S., Ray, W. and Pascual-Leone, A. (2007) Secondary motor disturbances in 101 patients with musician's dystonia. *J Neurol Neurosurg Psychiatry*, **78**, 949–953.

Roth, E., Fink, K., Cherney, L. and Hall, K. (1997) Reversion to a previously learned foreign accent after stroke. *Archives Physical Medicine Rehabilitation*, **78**, 550–2.

Rubin, A. and Sataloff, R. (2007) Vocal Fold Paresis and Paralysis. *Otolaryngologic Clinics of North America*, **40**, 1109–1131.

Samuel, M., Torun, N., Tuite, P., Sharpe, J. and Lang, A. E. (2004) Progressive ataxia and palatal tremor. *Brain*, **127**, 1252–1268.

Sapir, S., Ramig, L. and Fox, C. (2008) Speech and swallowing disorders in Parkinson disease. *Curr Opin Otolaryngol Head Neck Surg*, **16**, 205–10.

Schiavetti, N. (1992) Scaling procedures for the measurement of speech intelligibility. In Kent, R. (Ed.) *Intelligibility in Speech Disorders*. Amsterdam, Benjamins.

Schulz, G. M. (2002) The effects of speech therapy and pharmacological treatments on voice and speech in Parkinson's disease: A review. *Current Medicinal Chemistry*, **9**, 1359–1366.

Schwartz, M., Wilshire, C., Gagnon, D. and Polansky, M. (2004) Origins of nonword phonological errors in aphasic picture naming. *Cognitive Neuropsychology*, **21**, 159–186.

Scolding, N., Smith, S., Sturman, S., Brookes, G. and Lees, A. (1995) Auctioneers Jaw - a case of occupational oromandibular hemidystonia. *Movement Disorders*, **10**, 508–509.

Seliger, G., Abrams, G. and Horton, A. (1992) Irish brogue after stroke. *Stroke*, **23**, 1655–6.

Sieron, J., Westphal, K. and Johannsen, H. (1995) Apraxia of the Larynx. *Folia Phoniatrica*, **47**, 33–38.

Silverdale, M., Schneider, S., Bhatia, K. and Lang, A. (2008) The spectrum of orolingual tremor - proposed classification system. *Movement Disorders*, **23**, 159–167.

Singer, C. and Papapetropoulos, S. (2006) A comparison of jaw-closing and jaw-opening idiopathic oromandibular dystonia. *Parkinsonism and Related Disorders*, **12**, 115–118.

Smith, E. and Delargy, M. (2005) Locked in syndrome. *British Medical Journal*, **330**, 406–409.

Spencer, K. and Rogers, M. (2005) Speech motor programming in hypokinetic and ataxic dysarthria. *Brain Language*, **94**, 347–366.

Stewart, C., Winfield, L., Hunt, A., Bressman, S., Fahn, S., Blitzer, A. and Brin, M. (1995) Speech dysfunction in early Parkinson's disease. *Movement Disorders*, **10**, 562–5.

Tan, E., Chan, L. and Chang, H. (2004) Severe bruxism following basal ganglia infarcts. *J Neurological Sciences*, **217**, 229–232.

Threats, T. (2008) Use of the ICF for clinical practice in speech-language pathology. *International J Speech-Language Pathology*, **10**, 50–60.

Tjaden, K. (2008) Speech and swallowing in Parkinson's disease. *Topics in Geriatric Rehabilitation*, **24**, 115–126.

Van Lancker, D. and Cummings, J. L. (1999) Expletives: neurolinguistic and neurobehavioral perspectives on swearing. *Brain Research Reviews*, **31**, 83–104.

Walshe, M., Peach, R. and Miller, N. (2009) Dysarthria Impact Profile: Development of a Scale to Measure the Psychosocial Impact of Acquired Dysarthria. *International J Language Communication Disorders*. DOI: 10.1080/1368 2820802317536

Yorkston, K. (2007) The degenerative dysarthrias: A window into critical clinical and research issues. *Folia Phoniatrica*, **59**, 107–117.

Yorkston, K., Baylor, C., Klasner, E., Deitz, J., Dudgeon, B., Eadie, T., Miller, R. and Amtmann, D. (2007) Satisfaction with communicative participation as defined by adults with multiple sclerosis. *J Communication Disorders*, **40**, 433–451.

Ziegler, W. (2001) Apraxia of speech is not a lexical disorder. *Aphasiology*, **15**, 74–77.

Ziegler, W. (2002a) Psycholinguistic and motor theories of apraxia of speech. *Seminars in Speech and Language*, **23**, 231–244.

Ziegler, W. (2002b) Task-related factors in oral motor control: speech and oral diadochokinesis in dysarthria and apraxia of speech. *Brain Language*, **80**, 556–75.

Ziegler, W. (2003a) Speech motor control is task-specific: Evidence from dysarthria and apraxia of speech. *Aphasiology*, **17**, 3–36.

Ziegler, W. (2003b) To speak or not to speak: Distinctions between speech and nonspeech motor control - A reply to Ballard, Robin and Folkins. *Aphasiology*, **17**, 99–105.

Ziegler, W. and Von Cramon, D. (1986) Disturbed Coarticulation in Apraxia of Speech: Acoustic Evidence. *Brain Language*, **29**, 34–47.

Chapter 15

Treatment of spoken language disorders

Jane Marshall

1 Introduction

There are three broad types of speech disorder that can arise from brain damage: dysarthria; apraxia (or dyspraxia); aphasia (or dysphasia).

The first two affect the muscular control or coordination of speech. In contrast, aphasia is a language disorder. Here the speech impairment is part of a complex of symptoms, typically involving several aspects of communication (see Chapter 13).

The different speech disorders can coexist, e.g. a person may have both aphasia and dysarthria, or aphasia and apraxia. Also, the speech problem may be just one aspect of a more global neurological condition that carries further implications for communication. For example, dysarthrias often co-occur with generalized motor difficulties that make it difficult for the person to write or use technological aids.

Numerous treatments for neurological speech problems have been attempted, a selection of which are summarized below. Although diverse, these are underpinned by some common principles.

- Many therapies aim directly to recover lost skills or functions, e.g. through repeated and structured practice. If successful, these treatments may work by promoting a degree of neural reorganization.

- Alternatively or additionally, treatments may aim to compensate for the difficulties. Such compensations may be made by the person with the speech problem, by drawing upon retained skills, or they may be employed by those in the person's environment.

- The role of the environment in creating barriers for people with speech problems has been particularly emphasized in the therapy literature (e.g. Pound *et al.* 2000). As a result, many treatments focus as much on that environment as on the individual with the disorder.

2 Therapy for people with dysarthria

Dysarthria ranges from a mild loss of intelligibility, e.g. due to damage to a single cranial nerve, to complete anarthria, due to a severe loss of the neuromuscular control of speech. Prognosis is equally varied. Some individuals, e.g. those with vascular aetiology, may expect a good recovery, while others are coping with progressive and terminal conditions.

The social effects of dysarthria are wide-ranging, with implications for the person's working life, personal relationships, and family roles. There is no single 'dysarthria therapy'. Rather, clinicians employ a range of approaches, which vary across individuals, and within the treatment of the same individual over time.

2.1 Goals of therapy

Therapy aims to maximize the effectiveness, efficiency, and naturalness of communication (Duffy 1995). This entails a number of component aims.

- To restore or improve particular muscular functions, such as vocal cord closure. This is particularly relevant for those who can expect a degree of physiological recovery.
- To maintain neuromuscular function for as long as possible, e.g. in the case of some progressive disorders.
- To compensate for lost function, particularly when improvement of neuromuscular function is not achievable.
- To provide psychological support, e.g. to help the person deal with the profound life changes associated with dysarthria and, in some cases, plan for the progressive loss of speech. Support may consist of counselling, information and advice, and contact with relevant social and disability organizations.

2.2 Therapy regimes

Dysarthria calls for flexible therapy regimes. Some may be catered for in a single episode of intervention, while others require ongoing support, which changes in nature as the disease progresses. Therapy regimes should take account of the needs of family members, e.g. through relatives' support groups. Therapy settings should also be flexible. For example, therapy aiming to modify the person's environment is best conducted in that environment, some individuals may benefit from group therapy.

Individuals with complex neurological conditions typically receive input from a range of professionals. Coordination of multidisciplinary input is crucial.

2.3 The role of assessment in planning therapy

Assessment has many roles.

- *To probe the individual's view about their problem*, e.g. about what impairs intelligibility, what helps, what situations are most difficult, what strategies they are already using, and the role of others in either easing or exacerbating the problem. Ideally, therapy is client-driven, e.g. by targeting the aspects of speech that most concern them, or by building upon strategies that they have already started.
- *To identify a target for intervention*, e.g. by indicating which impairment to the speech mechanism most reduces intelligibility.
- *To identify an approach*, e.g. focal or mild impairments may benefit from a speech-orientated approach, while degenerative conditions usually call for compensatory techniques.
- *To identify factors that influence management decisions.* These include medical or personal factors such as fatigue that are likely to impact upon the individual's response to therapy.

- *To evaluate environmental factors.* Here client's insights can be supplemented with clinician observation, e.g. of the person's communication with significant others, and by structured questioning, e.g. about the layout of the home, social activities undertaken, and barriers confronted during those activities. This assessment is particularly crucial in planning communication-oriented approaches.

- *To provide a baseline against which to measure progress.* Baseline data may comprise quantitative or instrumental measures and/or intelligibility ratings. It should include measures of the dysarthric person's perspective, such as qualitative evaluations of their communication experiences.

2.4 Therapy approaches

2.4.1 Speech-orientated behavioural approaches (see examples in Table 15.1)

These involve exercises and drills aiming directly to improve neuromuscular function and hence speech. Tasks are hierarchically organized, progressing from readily attainable to more ambitious goals, and involve repeated and frequent practice. To achieve the latter, clinicians normally provide homework exercises. Ideally, the task is developed in

Table 15.1 Examples of speech-oriented approaches for dysarthria

Target parameter	Example exercises	Aim/rationale	Relevant dysarthria types
Respiration	Inspiritatory checking (Netsell 1992); the person is instructed to 'take a deep breath' and 'now let the air out slowly'	To improve breath support for speech and prevent air wastage, e.g. where there is reduced vocal cord adduction; uses the inspiratory muscles to maintain relatively constant subglottal air pressure	Flaccid Ataxic Hypokinetic
Phonation	Pushing, pulling, and lifting exercises (e.g. Aronson 1990); effortful movements, such as pushing against the arms of a chair, are coordinated with phonation	To maximize vocal cord adduction and possibly improve vocal cord strength; appropriate for people with uni or bilateral vocal cord weakness	Flaccid dysarthria only
Phonation	Lee Silverman Voice Therapy (e.g. Ramig et al, 2004)	To raise speech volume by improving self monitoring of vocal intensity and control over this parameter	Hypokinetic dysarthria associated with Parkinson's Disease
Articulation	Drill (Rosenbek and LaPointe 1985); an individual hierarchy of speech sounds is developed; targets are modelled by the clinician and cued, e.g. with illustrations of their production and hands on assistance in reaching articulatory placements; targets are practised and consolidated through drills	To improve accuracy and intelligibility in articulation; may promote compensatory strategies, e.g. by helping the person to attain acceptable articulatory substitutions for problem sounds	Flaccid Spastic Ataxic Hypokinetic Unilateral upper motor neuron

consultation with the dysarthric person, since self-directed therapy achieves better retention and generalization than purely clinician-led approaches (e.g. Wertz *et al.* 1984). Feedback is important, with specific feedback, outlining the type and locus of errors, being more useful than general comments about intelligibility (Till and Toye 1988). In some settings, feedback may include instrumental techniques (see Section 2.4.6).

A typical therapy cycle involves:

- discussion and explanation, including the rationale for the exercise and how it relates to the person's problem;
- practice with hierarchically structured tasks;
- feedback and self-evaluation;
- repeated practice, possibly at a more demanding level;
- practice of the target skill in communicative/conversational tasks.

2.4.2 Compensatory behavioural approaches (see examples in Table 15.2)

These aim to improve intelligibility without necessarily changing neuromuscular function. A good example is therapy that compensates for poor articulation by reducing speech rate.

2.4.3 Communication-oriented approach (see examples in Table 15.3)

This approach may be offered in isolation, or as a supplement to behavioural therapy. It aims to develop strategies, which can be adopted by both the dysarthic person and their listener, to facilitate communication, despite continuing problems with intelligibility. Strategies should be developed in the light of environmental assessment findings. The client, and significant others, should play a major role in developing the ideas and should be provided with opportunities to practise and modify the strategies in therapy sessions.

2.4.4 Prosthetic devices used in dysarthria therapy

A number of prostheses play a role in dysarthria therapy, ranging from 'low tech' materials, such as alphabet boards, to more sophisticated devices, such as artificial larynxes. Some prostheses are recommended when direct, behavioural therapy is unlikely to work. For example, hypernasality, due to velopharyngeal inadequacy, typically responds poorly to behavioural management (Duffy 1995; Theodorus and Thompson Ward 1998), but positively to palatal lifts (see Yorkston *et al.* 1988). These consist of a metal plate, fitting rather like a denture, with a posterior flap that aids elevation of the velum. Similarly, reduced volume, as occurs in hypokinetic dysarthria, may not be amenable to behavioural management, but might be assisted by a portable amplifier. Other devices can supplement behavioural approaches. A good example is a pacing board, which is a strip of wood marked with regular slots. This helps the client regulate speech rate by pointing to each slot as every word or syllable is produced.

2.4.5 Alternative and augmentative communication (AAC)

AAC includes some of the strategies and protheses that have already been discussed. Other tools include: symbol charts; photographic communication books; icons; word and alphabet charts; word-processing software; e-mail; speech synthesizers; portable, commercially available computer aids.

Table 15.2 Examples of compensatory behavioural approaches for dysarthria

Target parameter	Approach	Aim/rationale	Relevant dysarthria types
Respiration	Optimal breath group (Linebaugh 1983); Assessment establishes the number of syllables that can be produced comfortably on one breath; the client practises segmenting utterances according to this figure; drills may aim gradually to increase the optimal breath group	Improve coordination between speech and respiration	Flaccid Spastic Ataxic Hypokinetic
Rate	Pause modification (Yorkston *et al.*1988); pause boundaries are identified, e.g. in a written sentence or passage; the client practises saying the target passage with the identified pauses; pauses are sustained for a given time	Rate reduction improves intelligibility by allowing more time for articulation; modifying pauses reduces rate but preserves natural speech rythms; pauses are easier to modify than speech duration	Flaccid Spastic Ataxic Hypokinetic Unilateral upper motor neuron
	Alphabet board supplementation (Beukelman and Yorkston 1977; Crow and Enderby 1989); the person points to the 1st letter of each word as they say it, using an alphabet board; the technique is practised with utterances of increasing length and in conversational contexts	The alphabet board helps the person control speech rate; aided speech is more intelligible than unaided speech, both because rate is reduced and additional information supplied by the letter cue	All

Selection of AAC methods involves numerous factors such as client choice, attitudes to technology, cognitive and literacy skills, motor skills, and communicative need. The role of AAC for any individual may change over time. For example, people with progressive disorders may become increasingly dependent on AAC. In such cases, it is desirable to discuss and introduce possible methods before speech becomes unintelligible, so that the client is involved in the decision-making process.

2.4.6 Instrumental contributions to therapy

Dysarthric people have to regain control over a mechanism that, prior to the onset of their disabilities, was rapid and automatic. Such learning benefits from feedback, one source of which is instrumentation. A selection of instrumentation used in dysarthria therapy is summarized in Table 15.4.

Therapies incorporating instrumentation can bring about significant gains. For example, Thompson and Murdoch (1995) used kinematic instrumentation to provide a patient with feedback about respiration patterns, and so improved phonation times. Electromyographic (EMG) feedback has been used positively in the treatment of impaired velar fuction, and Visispeech in the treatment of parkinsonian dysarthria (Johnson and Pring 1990 and see

Table 15.3 Examples of communication-oriented strategies

Strategies adopted by the dysarthric speaker

- Convey how communication is to take place, e.g. by showing a card explaing the dysarthria and outlining the person's preferred communication method
- Establish the topic of conversation, e.g. by pointing to an icon or spelling the topic on an alphabet board; signal changes in topic
- Modify content and length of utterances, e.g. by limiting production to key words or by increasing redundancy
- Monitor listener's comprehension and check whether utterances have been understood

Strategies adopted by the listener

- Reduce environmental obstacles, such as background noise
- Adopt active listening, e.g. feed back what has been understood so far; be prepared to initiate repair when comprehension fails
- Encourage the dysarthric person to employ alternative approaches to communication, e.g. 'can you spell that word out for me?'

Strategies adopted by both the speaker and listener

- Maintain good eye contact
- Agree upon methods of feedback, e.g. some diads may adopt a gesture to signal when comprehension has failed;
- Agree upon repair strategies, e.g. some dysarthric speakers may ask listeners to guess targets, while others may prefer that they remain silent and wait for clarification. Some speakers may value explicit feedback about where intelligibility broke down

---

Theodoros and Thompson-Ward 1998 for review). Despite this, the application of instrumentation, at least in Britain, seems limited (Coventry *et al*. 1997).

2.4.7 Surgical and pharmacological approaches

In some settings treatments provided by speech and language therapists are supplemented by medical interventions, involving surgery or pharmacology.

Many surgical procedures are for disorders of phonation, and aim either to facilitate cord approximation, in the case of flaccid dysarthrias, or prevent hyperadduction, in the case of spastic dysarthrias (see summary in Table 15.5). Hypernasality, as a result of velopharyngeal incompetence, may be helped by phyaryngeal flap surgery, which, in effect, builds up the posterior pharyngeal wall and so facilitates closure with the velum (although the efficacy of this surgery is disputed; see Duffy 1995 for review).

Recent years have seen the increasing use of Deep Brain Stimulation as a treatment for Parkinson's Disease. This involves the surgical implantation of electrodes into the brain. These emit electrical pulses, in an attempt to inhibit abnormal brain signals. Although results have been encouraging for movement, effects on speech are variable and may even be negative (e.g.Farrell *et al* 2005; Gentil *et al* 2000; Tripoliti *et al* 2008).

Table 15.4 Examples of instrumentation used in dysarthria therapy

U Tube manometer	Measures air pressures generated by exhalation; used in therapy aiming to improve breath support for speech (e.g. Rosenbeck and LaPointe 1991)
Kinematic instrumentation	Records movement of the chest wall; can help dysarthric people improve respiratory function (Theodoros and Thompson-Ward 1998)
Visipitch, Visispeech, Speech viewer	Provide visual feedback about various vocal parameters, such as fundamental frequency, intensity, and duration; used in therapy for phonatory and prosodic disorders (e.g. Johnson and Pring 1990; Le Dorze *et al.* 1992)
Nasopharyngoscopes	Positioned in the nasal cavity to provide a view of the velopharyngeal sphincter from above during speech, and so offer feedback about the elevation of the velum; used in therapy for velopharyngeal disorders
Nasometer	Measures nasal and oral accoustic energy and so provides the patient with feedback about the degree of nasal resonance during speech; used in therapy for velopharyngeal disorders
EMG feedback	Provides feedback about muscle activity, e.g. of tongue, lip, and other facial muscles; used in therapy for articulation disorders

Many neurological conditions are managed with drug treatments that have associated benefits for speech, such as mestinon for myasthenia gravis. The specific pharmacological management of dysarthric speech requires further investigation, but might involve antispasticity medications and interventions to combat tremor and choreiform movements (see Rosenfield 1991). Clinicians need to be aware of the medication taken by patients and any associated side-effects for speech.

3 Therapy for apraxia of speech

There is a huge debate about the nature of speech apraxia (see Ballard *et al.* 2000). However, most agree that it is an impairment of volitional speech production in the face

Table 15.5 Examples of surgical procedures used in the treatment of dysarthria

Disorder	Treatment
Hyperadduction of vocal cords	Laryngeal nerve section (Dedo 1979). Paralyses one vocal cord and so prevents hyperadduction
	Injection of botulinum toxin into tyroarytenoid muscle (Aronson 1990) blocks release of acetylcholine from nerve endings, so denervating some of the thyroarytenoid muscle and preventing hyperadduction
Hypoadduction of vocal cords	Laryngoplasty (Koufman 1986). Implants cartilaginous material between the thyroid cartilage and inner thyroid perichondrium, so displacing the paralysed cord medially and facilitating cord approximation
	Teflon/collagen injection into submucosal tissue of paralysed vocal cord. Increases the bulk of cord and so facilitates approximation
Velopharyngeal incompetence	Pharyngeal flap surgery (Johns 1985)

of preserved linguistic and motor execution abilities. It differs from dysarthria in that there is no loss of strength or neuromuscular control. Rather the disorder is specific to the *planning* of speech movement.

Apraxia varies in severity. In mild cases, intelligibility may only be affected for long, phonologically complex words, or when rapid speech is attempted; while, severe apraxia can cause complete loss of speech.

Apraxia may occur in isolation, or with other communication problems, particularly aphasia. When other disorders are present the clinician has to decide which problem to treat. If the language problem is severe, this should be the focus of therapy. Conversely, apraxia should be treated if poor intelligibility is the main barrier to communication and if the person has sufficient language to benefit from improvements in speech.

Therapy for apraxia can aim to improve speech planning, and hence intelligibility, or to facilitate communication despite the speech problems. The former requires client-centred behavioural approaches. The latter takes more account of the communication environment and typically involves both the client and his or her key interactants. With many individuals, therapy tackles both aims, in sequence or parallel.

3.1 Therapies aiming to improve speech planning

Speech planning therapies typically involve repeated and structured practice of a hierarchy of speech sounds, normally progressing from single syllables/words, to phrases and more extended utterances. Therapy also seeks to extend skills from structured tasks to spontaneous production. A general hierarchy of difficulty is known to apply in apraxia (Darley *et al.* 1975). For example, within the consonants nasals are typically easiest, while affricates are more difficult, and clusters particularly so (although personal hierarchies may differ from the typical pattern). Therapy stimuli are designed in the light of this hierarchy. So, for example, drills may progress from /m/ + V words (May, more); to /m/ + V + /m/ words (maim, mime); to /m/ + V + C words (man, mine) and so on.

Some individuals with severe apraxia need help to phonate, before articulation drills can begin. Various techniques can be applied here, such as using a cough or sigh to elicit voice. Some may be able to use familiar songs or intoned speech, or automatic utterances such as counting or reciting the days of the week. One therapy for severe apraxia, the Voluntary Control of Involuntary Utterances, seeks to exploit islands of automatic speech, by bringing these under more conscious control.

A selection of programmes used in apraxia therapy is summarized in Table 15.6. Efficacy data for these programmes are variable. For example, Wambaugh and Doyle (1994) reviewed 28 treatment studies for apraxia of speech, and conclude that only eight achieved posttreatment retention of target skills, although since this review other studies have reported more positive outcomes (e.g. Freed *et al.* 1997; Wambaugh *et al.* 1998). One paper suggests that therapy should take more account of principles of motor learning, e.g. in the presentation of stimuli and feedback. When such principles are applied, better maintenance of effects may be achieved (Ballard *et al.* 2000). The most recent and comprehensive review of the Apraxia therapy literature also found variable outcomes (Wambaugh et al 2006 a & b) and substantial weaknesses that need to be addressed in future research (Wambaugh 2006).

Table 15.6 A selection of programmes used in treating apraxia of speech

Programme	Brief description	References
8 Step Continuum	A hierarchy of stimulus presentation ranging from imitation of the therapist to question/answer responses	Rosenbeck *et al.* 1973
Melodic Intonation Therapy (MIT)	Uses preserved singing skills to elicit speech, e.g. via 'intoned' utterances	Sparks *et al.* 1974
Prompts for Restructuring Oral Muscular Targets (PROMPT)	Uses physical prompts on the patient's face to facilitate articulation (e.g. tapping nose for nasal sounds)	Square *et al.* 1985; Freed *et al.* 1997
Minimal Pairs Treatment	Organized practice of minimal pair contrasts (e.g. 'sheet' versus, 'seat'; 'shame' versus, 'same', etc.)	Wambaugh *et al.* 1998
Intersystemic Facilitation/ Reorganization	Uses relatively intact systems to facilitate impaired systems; typically involves coupling speech with meaningful gestures, such as Amer-ind signs or finger tapping	See account in Wambaugh *et al.* (2006 b)

3.2 Communication-oriented approaches

These approaches aim to facilitate communication despite the impairment, and are rather similar to those used with dysarthric clients (see Table 15.3).

What are the clinical effects of apraxia therapy? As outlined above, some treatments may improve speech intelligibility, e.g. so that the person can clarify problem words or make better use of the phone. Compensatory approaches may enable apraxic people to participate more in conversation despite their problems, albeit in a new way. These approaches may also help the person recover from, or repair, communication breakdowns when they occur.

4 Remediation of spoken language impairments in aphasia

Aphasia causes diverse problems with spoken language. Some people cannot speak at all, or produce nothing but incomprehensible jargon. Those who can speak, may be frustrated by frequent word-finding blocks or problems in building sentences. Many aphasic people have reasonable comprehension, although not of abstract language or complex sentences; while others have virtually no understanding of speech. Aphasia also typically involves reading and writing problems (see Chapters 8 and 16).

Aphasia is typically a chronic condition, with initial severity being a strong predictor of outcome (Pedersen *et al.* 1995). A longitudinal study of 119 aphasic patients found that 43% still had significant aphasia at 18 months post onset; whereas only 24% had recovered (Laska *et al.* 2001). Clearly, therapy needs to respond to the long-term nature of the problem.

4.1 Setting goals in aphasia therapy

Goal-setting in aphasia therapy should start with the person (see Pound *et al.* 2000).

- ◆ What communication are they attempting, and what difficulties do they encounter?
- ◆ What would they like to be able to do?
- ◆ What do they see as their main skills?

Care-givers' views are also crucial, e.g. about what most impairs communication, and what strategies are being adopted by the aphasic person or by family and friends.

Through such questions, the therapist and aphasic person start to pinpoint likely goals for intervention. Assessment is conducted in the light of these goals, i.e. it aims to identify obstructions to realizing the goals and useful skills. This may well involve investigations of the person's language, but also evaluation of their environment and those in contact with the person. At the end of the process we should arrive at goals that are specific, realistic, measurable, and of benefit to the person's daily communication (see box below for an example of goal setting).

Goal setting in aphasia therapy: a case example (Maneta *et al.* 2001)

Phillip was 84 and had jargon aphasia following a stroke 5 years ago. Previous therapy aimed to improve his speech, but with little progress. Phillip lived with his wife, Florrie, but had few other social contacts.

In the initial discussion Florrie said that telling Phillip anything was a 'nightmare'. She had to repeat information several times, and even then could not be sure that he had got it. Misunderstandings were common and could lead to conflict, e.g. when Phillip felt that Florrie was keeping things from him. It was agreed that therapy should aim to reduce communication breakdowns at home.

Assessment aimed to identify the nature of Phillip's input problem, e.g. using tests of word discrimination and comprehension, and to explore reading, to see whether this could compensate for the difficulties. An interactive assessment also looked at how Phillip and Florrie were dealing with communication. Florrie was given a number of written questions to convey to Phillip, using any method of communication that she liked. The transaction was videoed and analysed.

Here are the main assessment findings.

- Phillip's auditory input was severely impaired. Although he could discriminate environmental sounds, he could not discriminate, recognize, or understand spoken words.

- Phillip's reading was much better than his auditory input. For example, he could match written words to pictures, but failed when the same words were spoken.

- The interactive assessment confirmed that communication often broke down. Florrie tried to help Phillip, e.g. by repeating words and phrases, but often this did not work. She rarely wrote information down, despite Phillip's good reading.

- The therapy goals were specified in the light of these findings.

- To improve Phillip's discrimination of speech sounds, at least in single words; If successful, this should enable him to recognize and comprehend spoken words more reliably, and so ease communication at home.

- To modify Florrie's communication with Phillip, e.g. so that she made more use of writing. This should reduce breakdowns and make exchanges between them more efficient and enjoyable.

4.2 Therapy for word comprehension problems

As suggested in the box, therapy may aim to alleviate the problems arising from a comprehension deficit. One approach aims directly to improve the person's input processing. The other aims to compensate for the problem, by changing the behaviours of those in the person's environment.

4.2.1 Direct therapy approaches

Therapy to improve word sound discrimination (Morris *et al.* 1996; Morris 1997)
Some comprehension problems arise from deficits in sound discrimination. This is signalled by difficulties with all auditory input tasks, including repetition, and particularly by an inability to discriminate minimal pairs, such as 'cat' and 'bat'. People with this problem benefit from visual cues, such as lip reading (Shindo *et al.* 1991).

The therapy developed by Morris *et al.* (1996) aimed to improve discrimination, using carefully structured minimal pair tasks and lip reading cues (see the box for examples of tasks). After therapy, both participants demonstrated gains, e.g. in repeating words, but not in comprehension. A similar approach was attempted by Maneta *et al.* (2001, and see the box below), but again with disappointing results. To date, studies suggest that improving sound discrimination is difficult and, even if progress is made, this may not benefit comprehension.

Examples of therapy tasks to improve word sound discrimination

Same/different judgements

- Two CV syllables are spoken by the therapist, e.g. /ka/ /ta/. The aphasic person indicates whether they are the same or different.

- Two VC syllables are spoken, e.g. /ak/ and /at/. The aphasic person indicates whether they are the same or different.

Matching spoken to written words

- The aphasic person is given a written word (e.g. 'car'). The therapist says a word that is either the same as the written word or minimally different (e.g. 'tar'). The aphasic person indicates whether the spoken word matches the written word.

- The aphasic person is given several rhyming written words (e.g. car, tar, par, etc.). The therapist says one word that then has to be matched with its written target.

Matching sounds to letters

- The aphasic person is given several written letters, e.g. T, K, B, etc. The therapist says a sound (e.g. /t/) that then has to be matched to one of the letters.

All the above tasks are presented first with lip-reading information (where the aphasic person is encouraged to watch the therapist's face), then with 'free voice' (where the aphasic person looks away).

Therapy to improve semantic processing Some comprehension problems appear to be due to a semantic disorder, as indicated by poor written and spoken comprehension, and comparable problems in production. In such cases, a semantic approach might be attempted, e.g. involving word to picture matching, picture and word categorization, and word association tasks. This approach was adopted by Grayson *et al.* (1997) with successful results. A subsequent stage of therapy successfully combined semantic and auditory therapy. For example, now the person had to match spoken words to pictures, but with rhyming foils (target: beer; distractors: deer and tear).

Another treatment study involved a client who could not access semantic information from spoken words, even though his comprehension of written words was good (Francis *et al.* 2001). Two forms of therapy were attempted. One only involved written words, e.g. a written word is presented with a written definition and then has to be copied. The other involved comparable tasks, but now with spoken words. Both treatments were effective, in that treated words were understood better after therapy than untreated words. However, the spoken word tasks produced more durable effects.

4.2.2 An indirect approach to comprehension therapy

Indirect therapies aim to advise friends and relatives about the aphasic person's difficulties, and help them communicate in ways that tap into their strengths (e.g. Lesser and Algar 1995). A good example can be found in Maneta *et al.* (2001; see the first box, this chapter). Phillip had much better reading than auditory comprehension. Despite this, his wife Florrie rarely wrote things down for him and, when she did, she tended to produce long sentences that were hard for Phillip to understand. Therapy demonstrated how to simplify information, using strategies like chunking information and writing only key words. In post therapy assessment there were fewer communication breakdowns between Phillip and Florrie and those that did occur were resolved more rapidly.

4.2.3 Summary and conclusions

Comprehension problems are difficult to treat, not least because the impairment may obscure the person's understanding of therapy. There is some evidence that input skills can be enhanced through treatment, but often such direct work needs to be combined with indirect interventions with friends and relatives. Maneta *et al.* (2001) show that simply advising friends and relatives to change their communication is often not enough. Family members need time, guidance, and practice to develop new skills.

4.3 Therapy for production problems

An almost ubiquitious production problem is anomia, or a word-finding deficit. Research has shown that word-finding can fail for different reasons (e.g. Howard and Orchard Lisle 1984, Kay and Ellis 1987), which suggests that therapy should be tailored to the particular processing needs of the individual. Another important finding is that anomia usually reflects problems of *access* rather than loss of vocabulary. We know this because people may achieve a word on one occasion, but not another. Also, aphasic people often benefit from cues (e.g. Howard *et al.* 1985), which may consist of the first sound of the word (phonological cues) or information about its meaning (semantic cues). This suggests that practice may recover more permanent access to words. Finally, we know that production is affected by numerous variables, such as word frequency, imageability, and age of acquisition (see Nickels 1997), which has implications for the selection of vocabulary in therapy.

4.3.1 Word finding therapy

A typical programme of word finding therapy entails repeated practice with a target group of words. These are carefully selected for their personal relevance, e.g. they may be associated with a particular interest or life goal. A second control group of words may be tested but not treated. The content of therapy reflects a person's skills and weaknesses. For example, semantic approaches might be used if there are felt to be semantic difficulties or if semantic cueing seems to prime access to words. The programme should be intensive, e.g. at least two sessions a week. After this, retention of the vocabulary is tested, typically with a picture naming assessment. This may be administered again, after a pause, to see whether gains have been maintained. Approaches to naming therapy are summarized below.

Semantic approaches Semantic tasks require the person to reflect upon the meaning of words, with the rationale that improved semantic processing may lead to better recovery of word forms (see examples in the box below). A number of studies demonstrate that repeated administration of such tasks can improve naming of the treated vocabulary, and with good maintenance of effects (e.g. Marshall *et al.* 1990; Nickels and Best 1996a,b). Best outcomes occur when semantic tasks are combined with exposure to target word forms (Le Dorze *et al.* 1994; Drew and Thompson 1999), i.e. the aphasic person should hear or see the target word, and think about its meaning.

Examples of semantic tasks to aid word finding

- *Word to picture matching* (e.g. Marshall *et al.* 1990). The person is given a picture, together with 5 written words comprising: the target, 2 words with similar meanings, and 2 words with similar forms. For example, the picture shows a television and the words are television, radio, computer, telescope, telephone. The person has to select the word that matches the picture and (optionally) read it aloud.

- *Semantic questions* (e.g. Barry and McHattie 1991). The person hears a question about each target word, which requires a yes/no answer. For example, 'is a microwave used for cooking food?'; 'does a microwave do the washing?'

- *Semantic associations* (Jones 1989). A target word is written in the centre of a piece of paper. Surrounding this are a number of other words that are either related or unrelated to the target. The person has to select the related words and explain their selection. For example, target word: car; words for selection: petrol, paraffin, garage, stable, wheels, rails, Ford, Microsoft.

Phonological therapy Phonological therapies work on the premise that exposure to the phonological properties of a word will prime access. Tasks typically involve repeated naming with phonological cues, i.e. ones that provide the first sound of the word or its rhyme (see box for an example). Phonological therapies can improve access to words and with good maintenance of effects (e.g. Raymer *et al*. 1993; Robson *et al*. 1998b).

A phonological therapy programme (Robson *et al*. 1998a)

Gillian had jargon aphasia with incomprehensible speech and severe word-finding problems. Speech was her priority for therapy, a decision endorsed by her husband.

The speech problem seemed due to impaired phonological access, in that comprehension was good and naming benefited from phonological cues. Gillian suggested that some phonological recovery might be taking place, which was rapidly fading, e.g. she said of one word-finding block: 'I had it there and then it went'. Gillian had good phonological skills on input, e.g. could discriminate minimal pairs like 'bat' and 'hat' and could repeat words.

Therapy aimed to build up her phonological knowledge about words. If successful, naming should improve.

- *Stimuli*. 50 words were chosen for personal relevance. They all began with one of 8 phonemes and had one or two syllables. Fifty untreated words acted as controls.
- *Materials*. Pictures of therapy items, a chart providing the written form of the 8 initial phonemes.

Task 1. Syllable structure

- The therapist said the target word and Gillian had to indicate whether it had 1 or 2 syllables, by pointing to the numbers on a sheet of paper
- Gillian was given a target picture. She had to think of its name and indicate how many syllables were contained in the name, by pointing to the numbers on the paper.

Task 2. Initial phoneme

- The therapist said a target word and Gillian had to point to its first phoneme on the chart.
- Gillian was given a target picture. She had to think of its name and point to its first phoneme on the chart.
- As in the previous step, but now Gillian was asked to say the name of the picture.

Outcome

Gillian's naming of both treated and control words improved and this was well maintained. Other language tasks that were unrelated to therapy were unchanged.

Relay therapy Therapy may use intact skills to access words 'in a new way'. A good example is given by Nickels (1992). T.C. had severe problems both in naming and reading aloud, although his writing was better. Therapy helped him to develop letter to sound matching skills, i.e. he learned to associate the letter 't' with the sound /t/, 'k' with /k/, and so on. One effect of this was to improve his reading. Another was to give him a new route to naming, in that he could imagine the written name of an object, think of its first letter, convert that into a sound, and so give himself a phonological cue. Sure enough, after therapy, T.C.'s spoken naming became almost as good as his written naming (for a similar approach, see White-Thomson 1999).

4.3.2 Therapies aiming to compensate for speech production problems

Some individuals may be unable to improve their word finding at all and, even when therapy is effective, often only treated words improve. Therefore, therapy should also develop strategies to compensate for the word-finding problem.

Strategies typically engage alternative forms of output. One candidate is writing, which has been used successfully even with severely aphasic people (e.g. Robson *et al.* 1998a, 2001; Beeson 1999). When writing is even more impaired than speech, nonverbal strategies, such as gesture and drawing, may be favoured (e.g. McIntosh and Dakin 1989; Sacchett *et al.* 1999; Rose, 2006).

A more comprehensive approach involves 'total communication' (Lawson and Fawcus 1999; Pound *et al.* 2000). Here the aphasic person is encouraged to communicate using any technique available to them, including speech, writing, drawing, communication books, facial expression, and gesture. Developing total communication is complex. Typically, the person is first made aware of the various communication options. They may need help with particular skills, e.g. to produce recognizable drawings or gestures. Constrained tasks, e.g. ones in which the person has to communicate a hidden word or picture using total communication, can further develop the skills. Finally, therapy often needs to encourage the generalization of skills to settings beyond the clinic, e.g. by involving relatives or through communication assignments.

4.3.3 Summary and conclusions

Therapy can help aphasic people recover access to words and with good maintenance of effects. Furthermore, aphasic people can take considerable control of this aspect of their therapy, since self-administered tasks can be very effective (Marshall *et al.* 1990; Nickels and Best 1996a,b). The aphasic person should also select the vocabulary for therapy.

Other findings are less encouraging. For example, naming therapy often only benefits treated words, with no carry-over to controls. This result is still useful, particularly if the words are carefully chosen. However, it indicates that therapy should include compensatory strategies such as total communication, which provide aphasic people with a resource for what is likely to be a chronic problem.

4.4 Connected speech and conversation

Aphasia may leave single-word processing relatively unscathed, but severely impair sentences. This makes it difficult for the person to deal with language about events and relationships, the typical subject of most conversations.

Sentence processing can fail for different reasons, e.g. some people have problems with the meaning relationships of sentences, while others have problems in building surface forms (see Marshall *et al.* 1999). Such variations have stimulated a range of sentence therapies, a selection of which are summarized in Table 15.7.

There is evidence that therapy can improve sentence production and comprehension. However, the extent of change is variable. Some studies only improved treated structures, while others also benefited untreated forms, and, while some treatments changed spontaneous production, this was not always the case (see Marshall, 2002 for a review of sentence therapy outcomes).

The above limitations suggest that sentence therapy alone may not necessarily improve the aphasic person's ability to converse. An alternative, or additional approach is to create conversational environments that are accessible to aphasic people despite their impairments. Typically, this involves training conversational partners, who may be volunteers or friends and relatives of the aphasic person (e.g. Kagan and Gailey 1993; Pound *et al.* 2000). Such trained interactants can make it possible for even severely aphasic people to participate in conversations, and so regain access to one of the primary social functions of language.

Another response to the problem of change is to provide aphasic people with a communication aid that enables them to capitalise on whatever language skills remain. One such aid is the 'Sentence Shaper' (Linebarger *et al* 2000). This computer device enables the person to record and other fragments of speech, so building up connected production. Practice with the aid has been shown to improve the grammatical cohension and complexity of speech, and to make it more informative (Linebarger *et al* 2007, McCall *et al* 2009).

4.5 Constraint Induced Aphasia Therapy

The above sections have outlined treatments for specific aphasic symptoms. A more generalist approach is Constraint Induced Aphasia Therapy (Pulvermuller et al 2001). Drawing on constraint therapies in other domains, this approach inhibits the use of compensary strategies, such as gesture, so requires the person to target speech. It involves practice of increasingly demanding speech acts within a highly intensive regime, i.e. at least 3 hours per day. Evaluations suggest that CIA may outperform other approaches, although it is difficult to know whether this is due to the constraint or intensity of practice.

4.6 Concluding comments

Aphasia therapy works. That is not to say that we can cure aphasia, but we can bring about numerous valuable changes, such as improved comprehension, word finding, and

Table 15.7 Examples of treatments for sentence processing disorders in aphasia

Approach	Rationale	Brief description of therapy content	References
Event Therapy	The aphasic person cannot determine the role structure of events, or who is doing what to whom	Making decisions about events shown on video, such as who instigated the action and who or what was changed by it	Marshall et al. (1993) Marshall (2009)
Mapping Therapy	The aphasic person has some syntactic skills, but cannot relate sentential word order to meaning	(i) Analysing written sentences, eg to find the verb, agent (instigator of action) and patient (person or object Changed by an action)	Jones (1986) Schwartz et al. (1994)
		(ii) Matching reversible sentences to pictures, such as 'the woman chases the man'	Mitchum et al. (1995) Rochon et al. (2005)
		(iii) Ordering sentence fragments to describe pictures	Byng (1988) Nickels et al. (1991)
		(iv) Interpreting and ordering 3 argument sentences, such as 'Bob lends £5 to John'	Marshall et al. (1997)
Verb Access Therapy	The sentence disorder is at least partly attributable to an impairment in verb retrieval	Naming verb pictures with cues; carrying out semantic tasks with verbs, such as odd one out tasks	Fink et al. (1992) Mitchum and Berndt (1994) Marshall et al. (1998) Marshall (1999) Conroy et al. (2006; 2009 a&b)
Syntax Training	The aphasic person has a morpho-syntactic impairment, or cannot generate the surface forms of sentences	Hierarchical and cued production of target sentence structures	Doyle et al. (1987) Helm Estabrooks et al. (1981) Helm Estabrooks and Ramsberger (1986)
Treatment of Underlying Forms	The aphasic person cannot process complex structures, like questions and passives, where sentence elements have been moved from their deep structure positions	Practising the production of complex forms, such as questions and clefts; forming complex sentences from simple ones	Thompson et al. (1993) Thompson and Shapiro (1995) Thompson et al. (1997) Ballard and Thompson (1999) Thompson 2008

sentence building. We can also change the behaviours of those in the aphasic person's environment, and so reduce the effects of the impairment. Of course, not all these aims can be achieved with all people. So one of the key skills of aphasia therapy is to identify an approach that is relevant for the person and has some chance of success. Above all, we need flexible therapy regimes that enable the aphasic person to tackle different goals at different stages of their recovery.

Selective references

Aronson, A. (1990). *Clinical voice disorders*. Thieme, New York.

Ballard, K. and Thompson, C. (1999). Treatment and generalisation of complex sentence production in agrammatism. *J. Speech, Language, Hearing Res.* **42**, 690–707.

Ballard, K., Granier, J., and Robin, A. (2000). Understanding the nature of apraxia of speech: theory, analysis, and treatment. *Aphasiology* **14**, 969–95.

Barry, C. and McHattie, J. (1991). Depth of semantic processing in picture naming facilitation in aphasic patients. Paper presented to the British Aphasiology Society Conference, Sheffield, September 1991.

Beeson, P. (1999). Treating acquired writing impairment: strengthening graphemic representations. *Aphasiology* **13**, 767–85.

Beukelman, D. and Yorkston, K. (1977). A communication system for the severely dysarthric speaker with an intact language system; *J. Speech Hearing Dis.* **42**, 265.

Byng, S. (1988). Sentence processing deficits: theory and therapy. *Cogn. Neuropsychol.* **5**, 629–76.

Conroy, P., Sage, K. and Lambon-Ralph, M. (2006). Towards theory driven therapies for aphasic verb impairments: A review of current theory and practice. *Aphasiology*, **20**(12), 1159–1185.

Conroy, P., Sage, K., and Lambon Ralph, M. (2009a). A comparison of word versus sentence cues as therapy for verb naming in aphasia. *Aphasiology*, **23**, 462–482.

Conroy, P., Sage, K., and Lambon Ralph, M. (2009b). Errorless and errorful therapy for verb and noun naming in aphasia. *Aphasiology*, **23**, 1311–1337.

Coventry, K., Clibbens, J., Cooper, M., and Rodd, B. (1997). Visual speech aids: a British survey of use and evaluation by speech and language therapists. *Eur. J. Dis. Commun.* **32**, 203–16.

Crow, E. and Enderby, P. (1989). The effects of an alphabet chart on the speaking rate and intelligibility of speakers with dysarthria. In *Recent advances in clinical dysarthria* (ed. K. Yorkston and D. Beukelman), pp. 99–107. Pro-Ed, Austin, Texas.

Darley, F., Aronson, A., and Brown, J. (1975). *Motor speech disorders*. Saunders, Philadelphia.

Dedo, H. (1979). Recurrent laryngeal nerve section for spastic dysphonia. *Annals of Otology, Rhinology and Laryngology* **85**, 451–9.

Doyle, P., Goldstein, H., and Bourgeois, M. (1987). Experimental analysis of syntax training in Broca's aphasia: a generalisation and social validation study. *J. Speech Hearing Dis.* **52**, 143–56.

Drew, R. and Thompson, C. (1999). Model-based semantic treatment for naming deficits in aphasia. *J. Speech, Language, Hearing Res.* **42**, 972–89.

Duffy, J. (1995). *Motor speech disorders: substrates, differential diagnosis and management*. Mosby, St Louis.

Farrell, A., Theodoros, D., Ward, E., Hall, B., and Silburn, P. (2005). Effects of neurosurgical management of Parkinson's disease on speech characteristics and oromotor function. *Journal of Speech, Language and Hearing Research*, **48**, 5–20.

Fink, R., Martin, N., Schwartz, M., Saffran, E., and Myers, J. (1992). Facilitation of verb retrieval skills in aphasia: a comparison of two approaches. *Clin. Aphasiol.* **21**, 263–75.

Francis, D., Riddoch, J., and Humphreys, G. (2001). Cognitive rehabilitation of word meaning deafness. *Aphasiology* **15**, 749–66.

Freed, D., Marshall, R., and Frazier, K. (1997). Long term effectiveness of PROMPT treatment in a severely aphasic speaker. *Aphasiology* **11**, 365–72.

Gentil, M., Pinto, S., Pollak, P., and Benabid, A. (2003). Effect of bilateral stimulation of the subthalamic nucleus on parkinsonian dysarthria. *Brain and Language*, **85**(2), 190–196.

Grayson, E., Hilton, R., and Franklin, S. (1997). Early intervention in a case of jargon aphasia: efficacy of language comprehension therapy. *Eur. J. Dis. Commun.* **32**, 257–76.

Helm-Estabrooks, N. and Ramsberger, G. (1986). Treatment of agrammatism in long-term Broca's aphasia. *Br. J. Dis. Commun.* **21**, 39–45.

Helm-Estabrooks, N., Fitzpatrick, P., and Barrisi, B. (1981). Response of an agrammatic patient to a syntax stimulation program for aphasia. *J. Speech Hearing Dis.* **47**, 385–9.

Howard, D. and Orchard Lisle, V. (1984). On the origin of semantic errors in naming: evidence from the case of a global dysphasic. *Cogn. Neuropsychol.* **1**, 163–90.

Howard, D., Patterson, K., Franklin, S., Orchard Lisle, V., and Morton, J. (1985). The facilitation of picture naming in aphasia. *Cogn. Neuropsychol.* **2**, 49–80.

Johns, D. (ed.) (1985). Surgical and prosthetic management of neurogenic velopharyngeal incompetency in dysarthria. In *Clinical management of neurogenic communication disorders*. Needham Heights MA, 153–78.

Johnson, J. and Pring, T. (1990). Speech therapy and Parkinson's disease: a review and further data. *Br. J. Dis. Commun.* **25**, 183–94.

Jones, E. (1986). Building the foundations for sentence production in a non-fluent aphasic. *Br. J. Dis. Commun.* **21**, 63–82.

Jones, E. (1989). A year in the life of EVJ and PC. Proceedings of the Summer Conference of the British Aphasiology Society Conference of the British Aphasiology Society, Cambridge.

Kagan, A. and Gailey, G. (1993). Functional is not enough: training conversational partners for aphasic adults. In *Aphasia treatment: world perspectives* (ed. A. Holland and M. Forbes). Singular, San Diego. 199–226.

Kay, J. and Ellis, A. (1987). A cognitive neuropsychological case study of anomia: implications for psychological models of word retrieval. *Brain* **110**, 613–29.

Koufman, J. (1986). Laryngoplasty for vocal cord medialization: an alternative to teflon. *Laryngoscope* **96**, 726–31.

Laska, A., Hellblom, A., Murray, V., Kahan, T., and Von Arbin, M. (2001). Aphasia in acute stroke and relation to outcome. *J. Intern. Med.* **249**, 413–22.

Lawson, R. and Fawcus, M. (1999). Increasing effective communication using a total communication approach. In *The aphasia therapy file* (ed. S. Byng, K. Swinburn, and C. Pound), pp. 61–74. Psychology Press, Hove, East Sussex.

Le Dorze, G., Dionne, L., and Ryall, S. *et al.* (1992). The effects of speech and language therapy for a case of dysarthria associated with Parkinson's Disease. *European Journal of Disorders of Communication*, **27**, 313–24.

Le Dorze, G., Boulay, N., Gaudreau, J., and Brassard, C. (1994). The contrasting effects of a semantic versus a formal-semantic technique for the facilitation of naming in a case of anomia. *Aphasiology* **8**, 127–41.

Lesser, R. and Algar, L. (1995). Towards combining the cognitive neuropsychological and the pragmatic in aphasia therapy. *Neuropsychol. Rehabil.* **5**, 67–92.

Linebarger, M., McCall, D., Virata, T. and Berndt, R. (2007). Widening the temporal window: Processing support in the treatment of aphasic language production. *Brain and Language*, **100**, 53–68.

Linebarger, M., Schwartz, M., Romania, J., Kohn S. and Stephens, S. (2000). Grammatical encoding in aphasia: Evidence from a processing prosthesis. *Brain and Language*, **75**, 416–427.

Linebaugh, C. (1983). Treatment of flaccid dysarthria. In *Current therapy of communication disorders: dysarthria and apraxia* (ed. W. Perkins), pp. 59–67. Thieme, New York.

Maneta, A., Marshall, J., and Lindsay, J. (2001). Direct and indirect therapy for word sound deafness. *Int. J. Language Commun. Dis.* **1**, 91–106.

Marshall, J. (1999). Doing something about a verb impairment: two therapy approaches. In *The aphasia therapy file* (ed. S. Byng, K. Swinburn, and C. Pound). Psychology Press, Hove, East Sussex.

Marshall, J. (2000). Framing ideas in aphasia: the need for thinking therapy. *The International Journal of Language and Communication Disorders*, **44**(1), 1–15.

Marshall, J. (2002). The assessment and treatment of sentence processing disorders: a review of the literature. In *Handbook of adult language disorders* (ed. A. Hillis), pp. 351–72. Psychology Press, New York.

Marshall, J., Pound, C., White-Thompson, M., and Pring, T. (1990). The use of picture/word matching tasks to assist word retrieval in aphasic patients. *Aphasiology* **4**, 167–84.

Marshall, J., Pring, T., and Chiat, S. (1993). Sentence processing therapy: working at the level of the event. *Aphasiology* **7**, 177–99.

Marshall, J., Chiat, S., and Pring, T. (1997). An impairment in processing verbs' thematic roles: a therapy study. *Aphasiology* **11**, 855–76.

Marshall, J., Pring, T., and Chiat, S. (1998). Verb retrieval and sentence production in aphasia. *Brain Language* **63**, 159–88.

Marshall, J., Black, M., and Byng, S. (1999). *Working with sentences: a handbook for aphasia therapists.* Winslow Press, Telford.

McCall, D., Virata, T., Linebarger, M. and Berndt, R. (2009). Integrating technology and targeted treatment to improve narrative production in aphasia: A case study. *Aphasiology*, **23**(4), 438–502.

McIntosh, J. and Dakin, G. (1989). *Restoration of communication through Amer-Ind.* Proceedings of the Summer Conference of the British Aphasiology Society, Cambridge.

Meinzer, M., Djundja, D., Barthel, G., Elbert, T. and Rockstroh, B. (2005). Long-Term Stability of Improved Language Functions in Chronic Aphasia after Constraint-Induced Aphasia Therapy. *Stroke*, **36**, 1462–1466.

Mitchum, C. and Berndt, R.S. (1994). Verb retrieval and sentence construction: effects of targeted intervention. In *Cognitive neuropsychology and cognitive rehabilitation* (ed. M. Riddoch and G. Humphreys), pp. 317–48. Lawrence Erlbaum Associates, Hove, East Sussex.

Mitchum C, Haendiges, A., and Berndt, R.S. (1995). Treatment of thematic mapping in sentence comprehension: implications for normal processing. *Cogn. Neuropsychol.* **12**, 503–547.

Morris, J. (1997). Remediating auditory processing deficits in adults with aphasia. In *Language disorders in children and adults* (ed. S. Chiat, J. Law, and J. Marshall), pp. 42–63. Whurr, London.

Morris, J., Franklin, S., Ellis, A., Turner, J., and Bailey, P. (1996). Remediating a speech perception deficit in an aphasic patient. *Aphasiology* **10**, 137–58.

Murdoch, B. (ed.) (1998). *Dysarthria: a physiological approach to assessment and treatment.* Stanley Thornes, Cheltenham.

Netsell, R. (1992). Inspiratory checking in therapy for individuals with speech breathing dysfunction. Presentation at American Speech-Language-Hearing Association Annual Convention.

Nickels, L. (1992). The autocue? Self-generated phonemic cues in the treatment of a disorder of reading and naming. *Cogn. Neuropsychol.* **9**, 155–82.

Nickels, L. (1997). *Spoken word production and its breakdown in aphasia.* Psychology Press, Hove, East Sussex.

Nickels, L. and Best, W. (1996a). Therapy for naming disorders (part 1).: principles, puzzles and progress. *Aphasiology* **10**, 21–47.

Nickels, L. and Best, W. (1996b). Therapy for naming disorders (part II).: specifics, surprises and suggestions. *Aphasiology* **10**, 109–36.

Nickels, L., Byng, S., and Black, M. (1991). Sentence processing deficits: a replication of therapy. *Br. J. Dis. Communication* **26**, 175–201.

Pedersen, P., Jorgensen, H., Nakayama, H., Raaschou, H., and Olsen, T. (1995). Aphasia in acute stroke—incidence, determinants and recovery. *Ann. Neurol.* **38**, 659–66.

Pound, C., Parr, S., Lindsay, J., and Woolf, C. (2000). *Beyond aphasia: therapies for living with communication disability.* Winslow Press, Telford.

Pulvermüller, F., Neininger, B., Elbert, T., Mohr, B., Rockstroh, B., Koebbel, P., and Taub, M. (2001). Constraint-Induced Therapy of Chronic Aphasia after Stroke. *Stroke*, **32**, 1621–1626.

Ramig, L., Fox, C, and Sapir, S. (2004). Parkinson's Disease: Speech and voice disorders and their treatment with the Lee Silverman Voice Treatment. *Seminars in Speech and Language*, **25**, 169–180.

Raymer, A., Thompson, C., Jacobs, B., and Le Grand, H. (1993). Phonological treatment of naming deficits in aphasia: model based generalisation. *Aphasiology* **7**, 27–53.

Rayner, H. and Marshall, J. (2003). Training Volunteers as Conversation Partners for People with Aphasia. *International Journal of Language and Communication Disorders*, **38**, 149–164.

Robson, J., Pring, T., Marshall, J., Morrison, S., and Chiat, S. (1998a). Written communication in undifferentiated jargon aphasia: a therapy study. *Int. J. Language Commun. Dis.* **33**, 305–28.

Robson, J., Marshall, J., Pring, T., and Chiat, S. (1998b). Phonological therapy in jargon aphasia: positive but paradoxical effects. *J. Int. Neuropsychol. Soc.* **4**, 675–86.

Robson, J., Marshall, J., Pring, T., and Chiat, S. (2001). Enhancing communication in jargon aphasia: a small group strudy of writing therapy. *Int. J. Language Commun. Dis.* **36**, 471–88.

Rochon, E., Laird, L., Bose, A. and Scofield, J. (2005). Mapping therapy for sentence production impairments in non fluent aphasia. *Neuropsychological Rehabilitation*, **15**(1), 1–36.

Rose, M. (2006). The utility of arm and hand gestures in the treatment of aphasia. *Advances in Speech Language Pathology*, **8**(2), 92–109.

Rosenbeck, J. and La Pointe, L. (1985). The dysarthrias: description, diagnosis, and treatment. In *Clinical management of neurogenic communication disorders* (ed. D. Johns), pp. 97–152. Allyn and Bacon: Needham Heights MA.

Rosenbeck, J., Lemme, M., Ahern, M., Harris, E., and Wertz, R. (1973). A treatment for apraxia of speech in adults. *J. Speech Hearing Dis.* **38**, 462–72.

Rosenfield, D. (1991). Pharmacologic approaches to speech motor disorders. In *Treating disordered speech motor control* (ed. D. Vogel and M. Cannito), pp. 27–77. Pro-Ed, Austin, Texas.

Sacchett, C., Byng, S., Marshall, J., and Pound, C. (1999). Drawing together: evaluation of a therapy programme for severe aphasia. *Int. J. Language Commun. Dis.* **34**, 265–89.

Schwartz, M., Saffran, E., Fink, R., Myers, J., and Martin, N. (1994). Mapping therapy: a treatment programme for agrammatism. *Aphasiology* **8**, 19–54.

Shindo, M., Kaga, K., and Tanaka, Y. (1991). Speech discrimination and lip reading in patients with word deafness or auditory agnosia. *Brain Language* **40**, 153–61.

Sparks, R., Helm, N., and Albert, M. (1974). Aphasia rehabilitation resulting from melodic intonation therapy. *Cortex* **10**, 303–16.

Square, P., Chumpelik, D., and Adams, S. (1985). Efficacy of the PROMPT system of therapy for the treatment of acquired apraxia of speech. In *Clinical Aphasiology Conference Proceedings* (ed. R.H. Brookshire), pp. 319–20.

Theodoros, D. and Thompson-Ward, E. (1998). Treatment of dysarthria. In *Dysarthria: a physiological approach to assessment and treatment* (ed. h. Murdoch). Stanley Thornes, Cheltenham.

Thompson, C. (2008). Treatment of syntactic and morphological deficits in agrammatic aphasia: Treatment of underlying forms. In R. Chapey (ed) *Language Intervention Strategies in Aphasia and Related Neurogenic Communication Disorders* (fifth edition). Baltimore: Lippincott, Williams and Wilkins.

Thompson, C. and Shapiro, L. (1995). Training sentence production in agrammatism: implications for normal and disordered language. *Brain Language* **50**, 201–24.

Thompson, C., Shapiro, L., and Roberts, M. (1993). Treatment of sentence production deficits in aphasia, a linguistic specific approach to wh-interrogative training and generalization. *Aphasiology* **7**, 111–33.

Thompson, C., Shapiro, L., Ballard, K., Jacobs, B., Schneider, S., and Tait, M. (1997). Training and generalized production of wh- and NP-movement structures in agrammatic aphasia. *J. Speech, Language, Hearing Res.* **40**, 228–44.

Thompson, E.C. and Murdoch, B. (1995). Treatment of speech breathing disorders in dysarthria: a biofeedback approach. Paper presented at the Australian Association of Speech and Hearing Conference, Brisbane, Queensland. [Quoted in Theodoros Thompson-Ward (1998).]

Till, J. and Toye, A. (1988). Acoustic phonetic effects of two types of verbal feedback in dysarthric speakers. *J. Speech Hearing Dis.* **53**, 449.

Tripoliti, E., Zrtnzo, L., Martinez-Torres I., Tisch, S., Frost, E., Borrell, E., Hariz, M. and Limousin, P. (2008). Effects of contact location and voltage amplitude on speech and movement in bilateral subtathalamic nucleus deep brain stimulation. *Movement Disorders*, **23**(16), 2377–2383.

Wambaugh, J. (2006). Treatment guidelines for apraxia of speech: Lessons for future research. *Journal of Medical Speech-Language Pathology*, **14**(4), 317–321.

Wambaugh, J. and Doyle, P. (1994). Treatment for acquired apraxia of speech: a review of efficacy reports. *Clin. Aphasiol.* **22**, 231–43.

Wambaugh, J., Kalinyak-Fliszar, M., West, J., and Doyle, P. (1998). Effects of treatment for sound errors in apraxia of speech and aphasia. *J. Speech Language Hearing Res.* **41**, 725–43.

Wambaugh, J., Duffy, J., McNeil, M., Robin, D. and Rogers, M. (2006a). Treatment guidelines for acquired apraxia of speech: A synthesis and evaluation of the evidence. *Journal of Medical Speech-Language Pathology*, **14**(2), 15–33.

Wambaugh, J., Duffy, J., McNeil, M., Robin, D. and Rogers, M. (2006b). Treatment guidelines for acquired apraxia of speech: Treatment descriptions and recommendations. *Journal of Medical Speech-Language Pathology*, **14**(2), 35–67.

Wertz, R., LaPointe, L., and Rosenbeck, J. (1984). *Apraxia of speech in adults: the disorders and its management.* Grune and Stratton, New York.

White-Thomson, M. (1999). Naming therapy for an aphasic person with fluent empty speech. In *The aphasia therapy file* (ed. S. Byng, K. Swinburn, and C. Pound). Psychology Press, Hove, East Sussex.

Yorkston, K., Beukelman, D., and Bell, K. (1988). *Clinical management of dysarthric speakers.* College Hill, San Diego

Chapter 16

Neuropsychological assessment and treatment of disorders of reading

J. Richard Hanley and Janice Kay

1 Introduction

Brain injury can disrupt the reading abilities of individuals whose performance was previously quite normal in a variety of different ways. In the sections that follow, some of the most common and the most theoretically important types of reading impairment are discussed. The review starts with descriptions of the peripheral dyslexias (pure alexia, letter-by-letter reading, neglect dyslexia) in which reading appears to be affected prior to the point at which the word is recognised as a familiar visual form. Descriptions then follow of central dyslexic impairments (deep dyslexia, phonological dyslexia, surface dyslexia, and reading in dementia) in which reading processes generally appear to be intact up to the point at which the meaning or pronunciation of a word must be generated.

A summary of these different types of acquired dyslexia together with some of their most important associated attributes can be found in Table 16.1. Although grouping patients into categories such as these provides an economical way of summarising a large body of literature, the extent to which they represent groupings that are scientifically useful is highly controversial. For example, the nature of the reading problems suffered by two individual patients who both fit the criteria for surface dyslexia may differ in fundamental ways (see section on *surface dyslexia*). Consequently, we would encourage clinicians to discover the precise point(s) at which an individual's reading ability has broken down rather than to worry unduly about precisely which type of acquired dyslexic label best fits them.

It must be acknowledged that at the present time there is considerable controversy as to which model is best to use when attempting to explain the reading impairments observed in acquired dyslexia. Coltheart (1985) advocated a three-route model that incorporated a *nonlexical* reading route and two separate *lexical* reading routes.

- The nonlexical route computes the pronunciation of a word on the basis of sub-lexical grapheme-phoneme correspondences (e.g. letter-sound associations). It is capable of reading accurately familiar and unfamiliar words whose pronunciation is consistent with those correspondences (often referred to as "regular" words).

- The lexical reading routes can recognise a previously learnt word by activating its representation in a store of familiar visual word forms ("orthographic lexicon").

— The *lexical-semantic* route involves accessing the word's meaning, and would be heavily involved in silent reading of text. If required, the pronunciation of the word can be accessed from its meaning.

— The *direct-lexical* route is based on direct connections between a word's visual form and its representation in a phonological lexicon. It would be heavily involved in reading aloud.

The lexical routes are equally capable of processing regular and irregular words so long as they have already been learnt, but are unable to deal with nonwords or unfamiliar words.

The status of the three-route model has been significantly strengthened by its successful implementation as a computational model capable of providing the pronunciation of written words (Coltheart *et al.* 1993, 2001) and simulating the effects of brain injury on word recognition. Nevertheless, the existence of the direct-lexical route is controversial; Hillis and Caramazza (1991) claim that the functions it provides can be performed by the interaction of the lexical-semantic and nonlexical routes.

A more radical alternative to the three-route model is provided by a connectionist computational model that is often referred to as the *triangle* model (Plaut *et al.* 1996;

Table 16.1 A summary of the impairments associated with different types of acquired dyslexia

Type of dyslexia	Impaired at reading	Characteristic responses to printed words	Ability relatively preserved	Common area(s) of brain injury
Pure alexia	All letters and words	No response or responds with unrelated words	Writing, recognition of orally spelled words	Left occipitotemporal, callosal Lesions
Letter-by-letter reading	Long words; individual letters	Very slow responses; speed affected by number of letters	Writing; recognition of orally spelled words	Left occipitotemporal, callosal Lesions
Neglect dyslexia	Words and/or text	Omissions or substitutions of letters on one side of word		Right parietal
Deep dyslexia	Nonwords; function words; words of low imageability	Semantic errors; visual errors; morphological errors	Reading of content words	Left frontotempo-roparietal
Phonological dyslexia	Nonwords	Visual errors	Reading of familiar words	Left anterior perisylvian
Surface dyslexia	Irregular words	Regularization errors; visual errors	Reading regular words; high frequency words, and nonwords	Left temporal lobe
Dementia	Irregular words; unusual nonwords	Regularization errors	Reading regular words	Left temporal lobe

Seidenberg and McClelland, 1989). Its advocates claim that it is not necessary to incorporate a separate nonlexical reading route. Plaut *et al.* argue that nonwords and regular words are generally read aloud via a direct orthography to phonology route (the triangle's first arm). Reading aloud of irregular words relies heavily on an orthography to semantics route (the triangle's second arm) and on the connections between semantics and phonology (the final arm of the triangle). Advocates of the triangle model (e.g. Patterson and Lambon Ralph, 1999) dispute the view that reading impairments reflect damage to mechanisms that are specific to reading. For example, Patterson and Lambon Ralph argue that:

- letter-by-letter reading reflects a primary visual impairment;
- surface dyslexia is caused by a semantic impairment;
- phonological dyslexia is the result of a phonological processing deficit.

The triangle model is clearly more parsimonious, but it is debatable whether its explanations of acquired dyslexia are equally plausible. For example, the triangle model has not provided a convincing account of why certain patients can read irregular words despite being ignorant of their meaning (see section on *reading impairment in dementia*).

Many of the conditions discussed in this chapter will affect profoundly how much pleasure can be derived from reading books or newspapers. This is particularly likely to be true of the peripheral dyslexias and of those central dyslexias that affect retrieval of a word's semantic representation. Where reading problems reflect a primary phonological impairment or word finding difficulty, however, individuals may continue to read books avidly (e.g. Hanley and McDonnell, 1997). Such cases demonstrate that comprehension of print can be entirely preserved even though the pronunciation of many familiar words can no longer be accessed when reading aloud.

In the sections that follow, we have included studies that attempt remediation of acquired reading problems. In determining whether to make use of any of these strategies, clinicians should bear in mind that they are likely to be time consuming and should be tailored precisely to the needs and abilities of the individual concerned. In addition, it must be borne in mind that statistically significant gains in terms of increased reading speed or accuracy do not necessarily reflect clinically significant improvements that will increase a patient's quality of life. It is also the case that the reading impairments experienced by some patients will improve spontaneously in the months that follow their illness or injury, although those of others appear to remain stable across all the years that they have been studied.

2 'Pure alexia' or 'alexia without agraphia'

2.1 Impairment

Detailed documented accounts of the impairments observed in pure alexia have been available since the end of the nineteenth century (Dejerine, 1892; Hinshelwood, 1895). Following a stroke, both of the patients described in these reports experienced sudden and complete loss of the ability to read any words despite intact speech production and

comprehension, normal object recognition and apparently unimpaired general intellectual functioning. Writing was entirely preserved in both patients (hence the term 'pure'
alexia), although neither of them was subsequently able to read back what they had
written. The reading problems did not appear to be the consequence of a basic visual
problem since acuity, colour vision and object naming were good when objects were presented in the preserved left visual field. Dejerine's patient could see letters clearly because
he could accurately copy and describe their visual form (e.g. he said that the letter Z
looked like "a serpent") but was completely unable to name them. Extremely poor naming of visually presented letters has consistently been observed in more recent reports of
pure alexic patients who are unable to read words aloud (Caplan and Hedley-White,
1974; Coslett and Saffran, 1989 1992; Miozzo and Caramazza, 1998; Mycroft *et al.* 2002).
However, all of these patients retained some ability to process letters:

- Caplan and Hedley-White's (1974) patient could correctly realign letter tiles that had
  been rotated away from their normal orientation.

- Coslett and Saffran's (1992) patient scored 10/10 at cross-case letter matching.

- Miozzo and Caramazza's (1998) patient was able to distinguish real letters from
  pseudo-letters and could identify canonical letter orientations.

- Mycroft *et al.'s* (2002) patient could perform cross-case matching of visually presented
  letters despite a complete inability to name them. This did not occur because the
  patient was suffering from an anomia for letter names because she was able to name
  letters perfectly when asked to recite the alphabet or spell words orally. This suggests
  that some pure alexic patients can access the abstract identity of visually presented
  letters despite being unable to name them.

2.2 Anatomical issues

The classical account of the anatomical correlates of pure alexia derives from Dejerine
(1892) and Geschwind (1965). A left hemisphere lesion produces a right-sided hemianopia which means that visual information from the right visual field cannot be processed
by the reading system in the left hemisphere. Dejerine argued that the location of the left
hemisphere lesion also made it impossible for visual information from the occipital lobe
in the right hemisphere to access the reading system. More recent accounts following
Geschwind (1965) argue that it is a lesion of the corpus callosum that prevents visual
information from the left visual field crossing from the right to the left hemisphere.

This view has been developed by Coslett and Saffran (1989, 1992). They demonstrated
that some patients are able to make lexical decisions (*is this a word or a nonword?*) and
retrieve some basic semantic information (e.g. *is this word the name of an animal?*) about
written words at above chance levels despite a complete inability to read words aloud.
Coslett and Saffran claim that there is a rudimentary right hemisphere reading system that
can perform lexical decisions and retrieve semantic information from visually presented
words despite being unable to name any words or letters. An intact right hemisphere reading system would also explain why some pure alexic patients who cannot name written

letters can access their abstract identity (see above). If words or letters are to be named, information about letter identity must be transferred across the corpus callosum to the left hemisphere (extremely difficult for pure alexics because of their callosal lesions).

Dejerine (1892) believed that the angular gyrus in the left hemisphere contained visual representations of words and letters. However, recent functional imaging suggests that the fusiform gyrus is more likely to be the locus of the visual word form area (Cohen *et al.* 2002), although there is controversy over its precise role in reading relative to other visual recognition tasks (Price and Devlin, 2003).

2.3 Remediation

Dejerine's patient died just over four years after his initial CVA never having recovered any ability to read words aloud. The only occasions when he correctly named a letter were when he traced over their visual form with his finger. The speed at which he could name letters this way was unfortunately too slow to allow words to be recognised during reading. This strategy has sometimes been reported in more recent accounts of pure alexia. For example:

- Case 3 (Benson *et al.* 1971) sometimes correctly identified a previously misnamed letter by tracing it with his finger.

- Maher *et al.* (1998) reported that a treatment for pure alexia based on finger spelling led to a 50% increase in reading speed with 100% accuracy.

An alternative remediation strategy is to attempt to teach pure alexic patients to name visually presented letters. If successful, this treatment should enable them to become letter-by-letter readers (see next section). Greenwald and Rothi (1998) report a successful therapy programme of this kind. They suggest that this remediation strategy is likely to be beneficial so long as the patient's ability to recognise orally spelled words is preserved. It is worth adding a cautionary note however. Hinshelwood (1900) subsequently reported that after approximately 6 months, his alexic patient started to attempt to relearn the alphabet. He practiced daily, and gradually came to read words "slowly and laboriously, spelling out the words letter by letter" (Hinshelwood 1900, page 13). Unfortunately, Hinshelwood (1917, page 5) finally reported that this man did not persevere with reading in this way because it "required such intense mental effort". Remediation strategies attempted by Mycroft *et al.* (2002) included an attempt to teach a patient a small set of high frequency words by sight, and an attempt to teach her to recognise groups of letters that co-occur frequently in English words. She was also taught to recite the alphabet in an attempt to find the name of the letter that she was looking at. Unfortunately, none of these strategies proved effective despite the patient's high motivation.

2.4 Assessment

Pure alexic patients will have great difficulty in reading aloud even simple lists of words (e.g. PALPA Test 29, Kay *et al.* 1992) or letters (e.g. PALPA Test 22). Writing of the same items to dictation should be preserved.

3 **Letter-by-letter reading**

3.1 **Impairment**

It is widely assumed that the nature of the deficit observed in letter-by-letter (LBL) reading is qualitatively similar to that found in pure alexia (see previous section), although there is little direct evidence to substantiate this claim. In LBL reading, words are often read aloud accurately but slowly and laboriously. Reading times increase in line with the number of letters in a word. For example, Patient DC (Hanley and Kay, 1996), who read relatively quickly for an LBL reader, took just over two seconds to read 3-lettter words aloud and approximately five seconds to read 9-letter words aloud. Patterson and Kay (1982) reported 3 patients who all took over 10 seconds on average to read a 3–4 letter word and over 30 seconds to read a 9–10 letter word. Nevertheless, the overwhelming majority of words were read correctly by these patients. The linear relationship between number of letters and reading times that is observed in LBL reading is not found in reading aloud by unimpaired individuals (Weekes, 1997). It suggests that, unlike normal readers, LBL readers are attempting to recognise a word by first naming its component letters. Consistent with this idea, some (though not all) LBL readers say the letter names aloud before the word is read.

There is widespread evidence that LBL reading is associated with severe letter recognition deficits. In a major review of LBL reading, Behrmann *et al.* (1998) found that 50/57 of the cases showed slow and error prone letter processing when letters were presented outside the context of words. The other seven were not tested on speeded tasks. As a consequence, they suggested that a letter processing deficit is of itself the cause of LBL reading. Nevertheless, there are at least two reasons why it appears unlikely that the key deficit is to the processing of single letters:

- ◆ LBL readers reported by Rosazza *et al.* (2007) and Warrington and Langdon (2002) were able to process single letters as accurately and quickly as controls.

- ◆ Lambon Ralph and Ellis (1997) and Crutch and Warrington (2007) reported individuals with *visual dyslexia* whose single letter processing was very poor and seemed to impair their ability to access visual word forms. Although these patients made a large number of errors in which the response was visually similar to the target word, neither of them showed any signs of LBL reading.

Following Patterson and Kay (1982), others have argued that the core impairment is a problem in recognising letters *in parallel* rather than a problem in recognizing single letters. There is a great deal of evidence which is consistent with this claim:

- ◆ Osswald *et al.'s* (2002) LBL reader found it more difficult to recognize words when letters were presented simultaneously than when they were presented sequentially.

- ◆ Kay and Hanley's (1991) LBL reader was slow at comparing the identities of visually presented letters when they were presented simultaneously but performed relatively quickly when the letters were presented sequentially.

- Despite being good at single letter processing, the LBL readers described by Behrmann and Shallice (1995), Rosazza *et al.* (2007) and Warrington and Langdon (2002) had difficulty in recognizing and naming sequences of letters.

Arguin *et al.* (2002) suggested that LBL readers tend to confuse the identity of letters in a word when attention must be directed to several letters simultaneously during parallel processing. Consistent with this claim, they showed that reading speed increased for LBL readers, but not for controls, when words were comprised of visually similar letters of high confusability. Conversely, the visual similarity of letters did not affect performance in LBL readers when letters in words were presented sequentially (Fiset *et al.* 2006). This finding suggests that the LBL strategy in which patients focus their attention on individual letters one at a time is employed to prevent confusion between simultaneously presented letters.

There are some similarities between LBL readers and patients with attentional dyslexia because, like LBL readers, attentional dyslexics are better at recognising letters that are presented singly than in arrays, and have been shown to read long words less accurately than short words (Price and Humphreys, 1993). However LBL readers do not typically make transpositional errors of the kind seen in attentional dyslexia (Shallice and Warrington, 1977) when reading simultaneously presented words (e.g. win fed > fin fed).

It has sometimes been claimed that the core impairment in LBL reading is a word-level deficit rather than a letter-level impairment, and that LBL reading reflects the compensatory use of the spelling system to read words aloud (Warrington and Shallice, 1980). Indeed Warrington and her colleagues have referred to LBL reading as "spelling dyslexia" (e.g. McCarthy and Warrington, 1990; Warrington and Langdon, 2002). The discovery of letter processing impairments (see above) and word superiority effects in some LBL readers (e.g. Bub *et al.* 1989; Reuter-Lorenz and Brunn, 1990) has cast doubt on this claim as a general account of LBL reading. Furthermore, spelling is severely impaired in some LBL readers, and it is sometimes impaired in a quite different way from reading (Hanley and Kay, 1992; Rapcsak, *et al.* 1990). It is conceivable, however, as Crutch and Warrington (2007) have argued, that there exists a small minority of LBL readers with good letter processing skills who adopt a serial letter processing strategy because of damage to visual word forms.

Some LBL readers appear to suffer from a clear word level deficit in addition to their parallel letter-processing deficit. Whereas some patients (termed "Type 1" LBL readers by Patterson and Kay, 1982) read words accurately given that they named the letters correctly, other patients (termed "Type 2" LBL readers by Patterson and Kay, 1982) made errors even when letters were named correctly. This suggests that Type 2 LBL readers have an additional impairment at the word form system level that is superimposed on top of their parallel letter processing problem. An additional lexical or post-lexical impairment can explain why LBL reading is sometimes associated with visual errors (Hanley and Kay, 1992), regularisation errors (Friedman and Hadley, 1992), semantic errors (Buxbaum and Coslett, 1996), and imageability effects (Behrmann *et al.* 1998).

There is considerable controversy over whether or not the parallel letter processing impairment in LBL reading is the consequence of a more basic visual processing impairment (see Patterson and Lambon Ralph, 1999; and Farah, 2000, for discussion). Crutch and Warrington (2007) suggested that visual crowding is an example of such a deficit. They reported an LBL reader who was much worse at letter naming when letters were flanked by additional letters or simple visual forms. Effects of flankers are observed in attentional dyslexia (Shallice and Warrington, 1977). However, unlike attentional dyslexics, Crutch and Warrington's LBL reader performed equally poorly when the flankers were drawn from categories such as numbers, consistent with the view that his letter processing deficit was caused by foveal crowding.

3.2 **Anatomical issues**

As is the case with pure alexic patients of the kind described in the previous section, LBL reading is frequently associated with lesions to the posterior part of the left hemisphere. Damage to the left occipito-temporal junction has been implicated as a probable cause of the difficulties experienced in recognising words as wholes (Leff *et al.* 2001). Additional left hemisphere injuries, it is assumed, will produce a right sided hemianopia. LBL reading is usually, though not invariably, also associated with lesions to the splenium of the corpus callosum (see Binder and Mohr, 1992 for further anatomical evidence concerning alexics who do and do not read words letter-by-letter).

Leff *et al.* (2001) have claimed that a right hemianopia that is caused by a lesion "affecting either primary visual cortex on the left, or its geniculostriate afferents" can of itself produce a reading impairment in patients with no left occipitotemporal damage, that can be confused with letter-by-letter reading. The impairment occurs because words can fall outside the patients' visual field and require one or more saccades before recognition is possible. In hemianopic alexia, they claim, reading times may show word length effects, but are quicker than for LBL readers (Leff *et al.* calculate a range of 51–162 msec. per letter) particularly with shorter words. They argue that it is important to diagnose hemianopic alexia accurately because there are remediation techniques available that can increase reading speed in these patients (Kerkhoff, 1992; Leff *et al.* 2000).

As in pure alexia, debate has centred on the precise role played by the left and right hemispheres in LBL readers. Shallice and Saffran (1986) showed that some LBL readers could make accurate lexical decisions and semantic classifications about visually presented words even when the words were presented so quickly that they could not be read by a LBL strategy. Similar abilities have been documented in some (but not all) LBL readers with whom these tasks have been attempted (Behrmann *et al.* 1998). Saffran and Coslett (1998) argue that LBL are using their right hemisphere reading system (see previous section) when they show these 'covert' effects. They claim that LBL reading involves the use of the damaged primary left hemisphere reading system, and that the left hemisphere inhibits the intact right hemisphere reading system. Behrmann *et al.* (1998), on the other hand, argue that residual activation within a damaged single reading system subserved by both left and right hemispheres could explain these effects so long as it is assumed that the system operates according to the principles of interactive-activation-and-competition models. McKeeff and Behrmann (2004) have shown that 'covert' effects are fairly fragile, consistent with the idea that they reflect the output of a damaged system. Lambon Ralph *et al.* (2004) provided evidence that preserved performance by Saffran and Coslett's (1998) LBL readers on 'covert' tasks may be due to the different nature of the response demands in tests of classification and overt word identification.

3.3 **Remediation**

A number of different remediation strategies have been attempted with LBL readers.

- Moyer (1979) and Moody (1988) employed multiple oral re-reading (MOR) in which the patient was encouraged to read the same passages of prose over and over again.
- Arguin and Bub (1994) employed a more theoretically driven technique by focusing on letter processing. They trained their patient to make cross-case matching decisions about pairs of letters in different sized letter fonts.
- Behrmann and McLeod (1995) attempted to treat their patient by encouraging her to identify the letters at the end of a word before saying it aloud.

These techniques generally led to increased reading speeds that were statistically significant. Unfortunately, none of them produced clinically effective increases in the time it took to read words aloud; reading speeds remained disappointingly slow.

- Sage *et al.* (2005) used an errorless learning technique in which an LBL reader was presented with a written word and listened to five presentations of the word's spoken form which he then repeated aloud. Strikingly, word level remediation led their patient to abandon the LBL strategy and start reading more quickly. However the new strategy also produced many more visual and semantic errors than had been observed prior to the treatment.

3.4 **Assessment**

Measure reading speed on a word list which manipulates letter length (e.g. PALPA Test 29, Kay *et al.* 1992).

4 **Neglect dyslexia**

4.1 **Impairment**

In neglect dyslexia, portions of the left side of text are sometimes omitted when passages are being read. When individual words are being read, initial letters may be

- omitted (e.g. *cage* > "age");
- substituted (e.g. *elate* > "plate");
- added (e.g. *pan* > "span").

Ellis *et al.*'s (1987) patient defined words consistent with her neglect error: (e.g. *rice* > "price . . . how much for a paper or something in a shop"). It is often assumed that neglect dyslexia is just one of a number of features associated with a more general neglect of contralesional space. However, neglect dyslexia has been observed in a number of cases without other features of neglect (e.g. Baxter and Warrington, 1983; Patterson and Wilson, 1990). In discussing these studies, Riddoch (1990) has pointed out that reading may be a particularly demanding task and that evidence of generalised neglect might have emerged with more stringent testing of other visual stimuli. Whether or not neglect dyslexia co-occurs with neglect of objects remains a controversial issue (Caramazza and Hills, 1990; Haywood and Coltheart, 2000).

There is clear evidence of fractionation of deficits within neglect dyslexia itself. Although word and text reading may both be affected in some patients, (e.g. Ellis *et al.* 1987), reading of single words can be impaired selectively (e.g. Costello and Warrington, 1991; Miceli and Capasso, 2001), and reading of text can be impaired selectively (Kartsounis and Warrington, 1989). Some patients make more neglect errors on nonwords than words (Arguin and Bub, 1997), but others show no lexicality effect (e.g. Ellis *et al.* 1987). When Ellis *et al.* (1987) rotated the page by 90 degrees, their patient no longer made any neglect errors. In contrast, patient NG (Caramazza and Hillis, 1990) continued to make errors affecting the initial letters in a word regardless of whether it was presented in vertical orientation, mirror image or inverted. Miceli and Capasso (2001) compared the performance of two neglect dyslexic patients using the same test materials and found that one of them (SVE) made approximately the same number of errors regardless of whether words were presented horizontally or vertically, whereas the other (MR) made much larger numbers with horizontal presentation, but no errors at all with vertical presentation.

Caramazza and Hillis (1990) suggested that any one of three distinct levels of representation (retina-centred, stimulus-centred, word-centred) involved in the early stages of word recognition might be affected in neglect dyslexia.

- The *retina-centred* level represents the visual shape and location of visual forms (letters) within the viewer's visual field. Patients with retina-centred impairments will make errors only to words that are presented in the left hemifield so long as central fixation is maintained.

- *Stimulus-centred* representation maintains orientation but codes the location of letters relative to each other irrespective of their absolute location in visual space. Patients with left-sided neglect associated with stimulus-centred impairments will make errors regardless of whether or not a word is presented to the left or right of fixation, but will not make errors on vertically presented words.

- The *word-centred* level represents the position and abstract identities of letters within a word irrespective of physical location (e.g. orientation). Patients such as SVE (Miceli and Capasso, 2001), who made neglect errors regardless of horizontal or vertical presentation, and whether or not the word was presented to the left or right of a fixation point, are considered by Caramazza and Hillis to have a word-centred neglect.

Haywood and Coltheart (2000) reviewed the performance of 14 previously reported neglect dyslexic patients who had been administered with suitable tests. They found that Caramazza and Hillis' theory provided a satisfactory account of all 14 of them.

4.2 **Anatomical issues**

Neglect dyslexia affecting the left side of text or words is generally associated with right occipito-parietal lesions. However, cases reported by Caramazza and Hillis (1990), Sieroff (1990), and Warrington (1991) all had left hemisphere lesions that correspondingly affected word endings and the right side of text.

4.3 **Assessment**

In neglect dyslexia, errors when reading words are visually related to the target word and consistently affect just one side of the word. In a patient with left-sided neglect, it is a good idea to use items that remain words when the first letter is omitted, and where the first letter can be substituted to make another word (e.g. cage, elate, peach, lever). Ellis *et al.* (1987) used a list of this kind.

5 **Deep dyslexia**

5.1 **Impairment**

Although the term "deep dyslexia" was first used by Marshall and Newcombe (1973), the first cases were reported as long ago as Low (1931) and Goldstein (1948) (see Marshall and Newcombe, 1980, for an historical review). Marshall and Newcombe (1966, 1973) investigated the types of word that their patients found most difficult to read, and examined systematically the nature of the errors that they made. They also attempted to explain their pattern of performance in terms of a model of reading derived from research in cognitive psychology. In so doing, Marshall and Newcombe provided a blueprint for subsequent cognitive neuropsychological investigations of acquired dyslexia.

Several decades of research into deep dyslexia have revealed a strikingly consistent pattern of reading impairment and associated language deficits (including agrammatism and phonological short-term memory problems). Deep dyslexics are almost completely unable to read nonwords and novel words aloud. They either respond with a visually similar real word or they make no response at all. The errors made by Marshall and Newcombe's patient (GR) included the following responses: *wux* > "don't know"; *nol* > "no idea"; *Zul* > "Zulu"; *wep* > "wet"; *dup* > "damp".

The probability that a familiar word can be read aloud correctly is closely related to its concreteness/imageability rating, with concrete words being much easier to read than abstract words. For example, LW (Newton and Barry, 1997) read correctly 19/30 highly concrete words (e.g. *house, snake*), but only 1/30 medium concrete words (e.g. *friend, joke*), 2/30 medium abstract words (e.g. *life, hint*), and 4/30 highly abstract words (e.g. *fate, hope*). Visual errors are most common on abstract words, with the incorrect response typically being of higher imageability than the target word (Shallice and Warrington, 1975). According to Paivio *et al.* (1968) imageability ratings are based on the capacity of a word to arouse *sensory experiences of objects, materials or persons,* whereas concreteness ratings are based on the extent to which a word *refers to objects, materials or persons experienced in the physical world.* According to Paivio *et al.* concreteness and imageability are highly intercorrelated (r = .83) and in deep dyslexia, they are almost certainly capturing the same dimension.

Several competing theoretical accounts have been proposed to explain the imageability effect in deep dyslexia:

- In Plaut and Shallice's (1993) influential computational model of deep dyslexic reading, it was assumed that abstract words contain fewer semantic features, and are therefore less resistant to semantic feature loss following brain injury than concrete words.

- Newton and Barry (1997) argued that abstract words tend to be more ambiguous than concrete words. They believe that ambiguity makes lexicalisation (the process whereby the phonological form of a word is accessed from its meaning) more difficult for abstract words.

- Crutch and Warrington (2005) suggest that abstract words tend to be represented in semantic memory in terms of their associations with related concepts (e.g. robbery-punishment). Concrete words, they argue, tend to be represented in terms of their similarity to other members of the same category (e.g cow-sheep). Consistent with this conceptualization, Crutch (2006) showed that in some deep dyslexics, semantic errors for abstract words tend to be associative errors (e.g. police > "evidence"), whereas semantic errors for concrete words tend to share more semantic features with the target word (e.g. bough > "branch"). Because they believe that concrete and abstract words are represented in qualitatively different representational systems, Crutch and Warrington's (2005) account can accommodate the double dissociation between deep dyslexia, and a patient who is better at reading abstract than concrete words (Warrington, 1981).

There is also a part of speech effect in deep dyslexia, whereby nouns are read better than adjectives, and adjectives are read better than verbs. However there is strong evidence that this effect only occurs when part of speech is confounded with imageability and/or frequency (Allport and Funnell, 1981; Barry and Richardson, 1988). Deep dyslexics also have particular problems with function words, often responding with a different function word (e.g. for > "and"; in > "the"; as > "he"). This problem occurs despite the fact that many function words are amongst the most common words in English. Deep dyslexic patients appear to have lost knowledge about the syntactic role of function words (e.g. Morton and Patterson, 1980).

The errors made by deep dyslexics when reading content words include:

- *semantic* errors, which are generally considered to be the hallmark of deep dyslexia. Examples include *uncle* read as "cousin" (Marshall and Newcombe, 1966), *hurt* read as "injure" (Shallice and Warrington, 1975) and *grass* read as "lawn" (Saffran and Marin, 1977). Semantic errors appear to occur with equal frequency in readers of shallow and deep orthographies (Beaton and Davies, 2007). Semantically related responses have been shown to be words that are earlier acquired than the targets (Gerhand and Barry, 2000). The majority of errors made by GR (Marshall and Newcombe, 1966) were semantic.

- *visual* errors in which a word is read as a word that shares letters with the target word. Examples include *crowd* read as "crown" (Marshall and Newcombe, 1966), *fixed* read as "mixed" (Shallice and Warrington, 1975), and *proof* read as "roof" (Saffran and Marin, 1977). Visual errors are the most common form of errors made by many deep dyslexic patients.

- Sometimes errors are *both* visual and semantic. Examples include *earl* read as "deaf" (Marshall and Newcombe, 1966), and *stream* read as "train" (Saffran and Marin, 1977).

- *derivational* errors (Marshall and Newcombe, 1966) in which the errors share a root morpheme with the target word (e.g. heat > "hot"). However, it must be borne in mind that morphological errors are also visually and semantically similar to the target word (for discussion of this issue, cf. Funnell, 2000).

In terms of the triangle model (Crisp and Lambon Ralph, 2006), deep dyslexia is associated with a severe general phonological processing deficit that affects reading, auditory repetition, and rhyme judgement. It follows that reading must rely on the orthographic to semantic route. In terms of the three-route model (Coltheart *et al.* 1993) deep dyslexics have suffered

- severe damage to the nonlexical reading route (hence abolished nonword reading).

- severe damage to the direct-lexical route whereby familiar words are connected with their pronunciation in a phonological lexicon because availability of this route would have allowed them to read aloud function words and words of low imageability.

It follows from both models therefore, that reading in deep dyslexia relies on semantic mediation. Newcombe and Marshall (1980) argued that semantic errors might be an automatic consequence of the output of the semantic route when it must operate in isolation. However, unimpaired individuals do not make semantic errors in picture naming (where the semantic route must also be operating without any phonological assistance) to anything like the same extent as a deep dyslexic patient such as GR (Marshall and Newcombe, 1966) made during reading.

This raises the important question of where precisely the impairment to the semantic reading route in deep dyslexia lies. Shallice and Warrington (1980) argued that at least three different types of deep dyslexia might exist.

- *input deep dyslexia* in which there is a difficulty in *accessing* intact semantic representations of low imageability words. Consistent with this account, Shallice and Coughlan (1980) described a deep dyslexic patient who was much better at auditory than written comprehension of low imageable words. Even though this patient performed poorly at visual lexical decision (Shallice and Coughlan, 1980), it seems unlikely that the primary cause of deep dyslexia could have a pre-semantic locus. As Shallice (1988) pointed out, if the impairment was to the word form system, it is difficult to see how imageability/concreteness could exert such an effect on deep dyslexic reading.

- *central deep dyslexia* in which there is said to be an impairment that affects the semantic representations themselves. Plaut and Shallice's (1993) computational model of deep dyslexic reading hypothesises that semantic features have been lost from semantic memory. There clearly are patients with central semantic deficits who make semantic errors on a variety of tasks (e.g. Hillis *et al.* 1990). However, although Crisp and Lambon Ralph (2006) did reveal evidence of written and auditory comprehension problems in three deep dyslexic patients, these impairments seemed to be too mild to be the sole cause of their semantic errors, and poor reading of abstract words. Moreover, Newton and Barry's (1997) review of the literature revealed that deep dyslexics often perform well at written comprehension so long as they are tested appropriately.

◆ *output deep dyslexia* in which there are problems in accessing the speech output system from intact semantic representations. Newton and Barry's review revealed widespread evidence of speech production problems in deep dyslexia. Consequently, they suggested that output problems are the primary cause of deep dyslexia.

In conclusion, the impairment to the semantic reading route in most cases of deep dyslexia is either to the semantic system itself or else to the connections between semantics and phonology. The relative importance of these two types of impairment remains controversial.

5.2 Anatomical issues

Extensive left hemisphere damage is frequently observed in brain scans of deep dyslexic patients. Lambon Ralph and Graham (2000) reviewed 48 articles examining deep dyslexia and found evidence of damage to the left fronto-temporo-parietal region in 44 of them. The lesions were generally large "encompassing at least the perisylvian area and often extending to include much of the left hemisphere". Their review also revealed that the majority of cases occurred as a consequence of cerebrovascular accident, although there were a small number of cases with head injury. There were no cases associated with dementia.

A crucial issue is whether the extensive left hemisphere damage means that reading depends on a secondary right hemisphere reading system. Coltheart (2000) pointed out that the right hemisphere hypothesis does not require that orthographic processing, semantic processing, and phonological processing are all carried out by the right hemisphere: "as long as any one of these three stages cannot be carried out by the left hemisphere, then some kind of right-hemisphere reading mechanism will be required if reading aloud is to be achieved." In fact, Coltheart claims that the results of brain imaging studies of deep dyslexic patients (Price *et al.* 1998; Weekes *et al.* 1997) are consistent with the view that orthographic processing and semantic processing are carried out initially in the right hemisphere. There is then, he argues, transmission of information from semantic areas in the right hemisphere to semantic areas in the left hemisphere followed by phonological processing in the left hemisphere leading to spoken word production.

5.3 Remediation

◆ De Partz (1986) attempted to improve the nonlexical reading skills of a French deep dyslexic patient. She taught him to blend phonemes to make words and nonwords, and re-taught him grapheme-phoneme correspondences by associating letters with the phonemes at the start of familiar words. Phonemes that are represented by more than one grapheme were taught by an ingenious series of mnemonics that made use of the patients preserved knowledge of whole word phonology. After nine months of intensive therapy, the patient's reading accuracy for nonwords had improved from zero to 90%. Reading of all types of familiar words also improved dramatically, although irregular words were often regularised (see section on *surface dyslexia*).

◆ Nickels (1992) used a similar technique with an English speaking patient. Unfortunately, he did not learn to blend phonemes together and so was unable to improve his ability to read nonwords and words of low imageability. The technique did, however, improve his ability to read words of high imageability, perhaps because knowledge of grapheme-phoneme associations enabled him to generate his own phonemic cues. These, in turn, may have enabled him to overcome word finding problems when trying to read high imageability words.

◆ Stadie and Rilling (2006) retrained a patient to blend phonemes who subsequently did show improved reading of trained words, untrained words and untrained nonwords. A separate lexically based treatment also improved reading of trained and untrained words.

◆ Hillis and Caramazza (1994) presented a series of theory-based studies that attempted to remediate lexical processing skills in patients who made semantic errors.

◆ The programmes used to improve phonological skills in phonological dyslexia (see next section) might also be effective with deep dyslexic patients.

5.4 Assessment

Investigate reading accuracy on words of low and high imageability (e.g. PALPA Test 31, Kay *et al.* 1992). Examine responses for evidence of semantic errors in particular. Examine reading accuracy on functors (e.g. PALPA Test 32) and nonwords (e.g. PALPA Test 36).

6 Phonological dyslexia

6.1 Impairment

The defining characteristic of phonological dyslexia is a selective impairment of the ability to read nonwords relative to real words. Relative preservation of the ability to read familiar words is probably the reason why phonological dyslexia was first reported relatively recently (Beauvois and Derouesne, 1979). Since then, cases of phonological dyslexia have been reported even in countries such as Spain which use a shallow alphabetic orthography (Cuetos *et al.* 1996), and Japan where a patient was described who could read familiar but not unfamiliar words that were written in the transparent syllabic script Kana (Sasanuma *et al.* 1996).

The level of the impairment in nonword reading ability can vary from one patient to another. For example, WB (Funnell, 1983) virtually never read a nonword correctly, whereas JD (Farah *et al.* 1996) read 25-30% of nonwords correctly. In general, however, nonword reading is somewhat better preserved in phonological dyslexia than it is in deep dyslexia, with some patients making errors that are phonologically similar to the target item. Detailed investigations of the nature of the nonword reading problem in 11 phonological dyslexics (Berndt *et al.* 1996) revealed that all of them experienced problems in:

+ graphemic parsing (how many phonemes does "auk" contain?).

+ grapheme-phoneme knowledge (providing the phonemes associated with single letters).

+ blending auditorily presented phonemes.

As phoneme blending does not involve reading, some have argued that phonological dyslexia is primarily the consequence of a phonological processing deficit that affects reading, rather than the consequence of an orthographic deficit per se (e.g. Friedman, 1995; Patterson and Marcel, 1992). Because nonwords have an unfamiliar phonological form relative to familiar words, these authors argue that nonwords will be particularly difficult for an impaired phonological system to generate from print. Consequently a purely phonological deficit will make reading of nonwords much more error prone than reading of familiar words. It is true that many individuals with phonological dyslexia do appear to suffer from a general phonological deficit that affects tasks that do not involve reading (for discussion, see Coltheart, 1996). However, recent studies by Caccappolo-van Vliet, Miozzo and Stern (2004), and Tree and Kay (2006) report exceptions to this pattern. Despite impaired nonword reading, Tree and Kay's patient performed well at phoneme segmentation and blending in the auditory modality, and appeared to have preserved phonological short-term memory skills. This patient's ability to read familiar words also appeared to be entirely preserved. Such a pattern of performance is clearly consistent with a selective orthographic impairment to a non-lexical reading route.

It is unusual for reading of familiar words to be entirely preserved in phonological dyslexia. Some patients show imageability effects (Farah *et al.* 1996), and patients such as AM (Patterson, 1982) are worse at reading function word than content words. The errors made by AM on content words were visual/morphological, and on function words were substitutions. Comprehension of familiar written words appeared to be entirely normal in AM (Patterson, 1982), who was able to make visual lexical decisions and make semantic classifications about written words as accurately as control subjects, despite poor nonword reading. WB (Funnell, 1983), on the other hand, was above chance but severely impaired on written comprehension tasks using words she could read aloud. In terms of three route models of reading (Coltheart *et al.* 1993), the obvious interpretation of these differences is that patients such as AM are reading via the lexical-semantic route whereas WB was reading via the direct-lexical route. However, advocates of two route models such as Hillis and Caramazza (1991), and Plaut *et al.* (1996) have attempted to argue that WB's reading of words might be explicable in terms of a partially functional semantic route and a partially functional phonological reading route.

Patients who recover from deep dyslexia sometimes turn into phonological dyslexics, consistent with the view that these two types of deep dyslexia are closely linked. For example, Klein *et al.*'s (1994) deep dyslexic patient remained bad at reading nonwords (though nonword reading *did* improve over time), but the semantic errors and imageability effect disappeared with reading of words returning close to normal levels. Several research groups have suggested that deep and phonological dyslexia may reflect opposite ends of a continuum of severity from deep dyslexia (relatively severe) to phonological dyslexia (relatively mild):

- ◆ Hanley and Kay (1997) suggested that the continuum may represent the severity of the impairment to the nonlexical route and that, as Hillis and Caramazza (1991) argue, even a partially functioning nonlexical route is able to inhibit semantic errors in phonological dyslexia.

- ◆ Friedman (1996) claimed that the continuum represents the severity of a semantic impairment.

- ◆ According to advocates of the triangle model (Crisp and Lambon Ralph, 2006), the severity of both the phonological deficit and the semantic deficit is critical. At one end of the continuum, isolated phonological impairments will produce nonword reading deficits (mild phonological dyslexia). Additional semantic deficits, or impaired semantic-phonological interactions, will lead to semantic errors and effects of imageability in reading (deep dyslexia).

6.2 Anatomical issues

In a review of 37 papers on phonological dyslexia, Lambon Ralph and Graham (2000) found consistent evidence of "damage focussed on the anterior perisylvian areas ranging from relatively circumscribed lesions typically of the left inferior, posterior frontal lobes to those patients with more extensive damage involving fronto-temporo-parietal areas". A small number of patients had posterior left hemisphere lesions affecting the occipito-temporo-parietal junction, and two had right hemisphere lesions. Apart from one case with head injury, one with Alzheimer's disease, one with Pick's disease, and one with hemispherectomy, all were associated with some form of cerebrovascular accident.

6.3 Remediation

Remediation is obviously a less pressing issue in a patient whose ability to read familiar words is relatively well preserved. Nevertheless, successful therapy programmes based on teaching of grapheme-phoneme correspondences (Kendall *et al.* 1998) and on teaching phonological awareness skills (Conway *et al.* 1998) have been reported. Gains were observed in both real word and nonword reading in these studies.

6.4 Assessment

Investigate reading accuracy on nonwords (e.g. PALPA Test 36, Kay *et al.* 1992). Compare reading aloud accuracy on matched words and nonwords (e.g. the items from PALPA 25).

7 Surface dyslexia

7.1 Impairment

Early accounts of surface dyslexic reading were provided by Marshall and Newcombe (1973) and have been the focus of intensive investigation ever since. Because English does not employ a transparent alphabetic writing system, written English contains many irregular words whose pronunciation cannot be reliably generated on the basis of grapheme-phoneme rules. The two cardinal features of surface dyslexia are greater problems in reading irregular words than regular words (a "regularity" effect) and regularised pronunciation of irregular words known as "regularisations" (e.g. *island* > "izland"; *trough* > "truff"; *come* > "comb"). For example, JC (Marshall and Newcombe, 1973) correctly read 67/130 (52%) regular words (e.g. *bite*), but only 41/130 (32%) irregular words (e.g. *come*). MK (Howard and Franklin, 1988) correctly read 90% of regular words (e.g. *shrug,*) and 67% of irregular words (e.g. *shove*). MP (Behrmann and Bub 1992) correctly read 100% regular words (e.g. *summer*), and 80% irregular words (e.g. *island*). Most of the errors made by MK and JC were regularisations, but JC also made some visual errors (e.g. *reign* > "region", *bargain* > "barge", *bike* > "bik"). It is therefore clear that the lexical reading route is impaired in surface dyslexia.

The nature of the impairment to the lexical route appears to differ from one patient to another (see Ellis *et al.* 2000, for detailed discussion). As Ellis *et al.* point out:

- some patients such as NW (Weekes and Coltheart, 1996) who was poor at distinguishing written words from nonwords, appeared to have difficulties in gaining access to the meaning of irregular written words.

- Others, such as MP (Behrmann and Bub, 1992), who had difficulties in understanding both spoken and written words, appeared to have a central semantic deficit.

- Finally, there appear to be surface dyslexic patients such as EST (Kay and Patterson, 1985), FM (Graham *et al.* 1994), and MK (Howard and Franklin, 1988) whose problems reflect a lexicalisation/word finding problem rather than a semantic deficit.

All surface dyslexics so far tested could read some irregular words correctly, however. In the case of MP (Behrmann and Bub, 1992), the ability to do so appeared to be related to word frequency. MP's ability to read regular words was unaffected by word frequency, but less common irregular words such as *anchor* and *echo* were read less accurately than more common irregular words such as *trouble* and *heart*.

It is sometimes claimed that nonword reading is normal in surface dyslexia, but this is true in only some of the published cases (e.g. Bub *et al.* 1985; Shallice *et al.* 1983; Weekes and Coltheart, 1996). MP, for example, read 42/44 nonwords correctly, but MK (Howard and Franklin, 1987) read only 25/30 nonwords correctly, and JC's nonword reading (Marshall and Newcombe, 1973) was poorer still. There is therefore no guarantee that surface dyslexia will be associated with an unimpaired nonlexical reading route. Nevertheless, the finding that nonword reading can be unimpaired in a patient such as MP despite poor reading of irregular words is of considerable theoretical significance. This is because it represents a double dissociation with phonological dyslexics such as WB

(Funnell, 1982) and provides evidence consistent with the view that the reading system contains functionally distinct lexical and nonlexical reading routes. MP has posed a severe challenge to computational models of reading that dispense with a separate non-lexical phonological reading route such as the triangle model (e.g. Plaut *et al.* 1996). It has not proved possible for the triangle model to reproduce the surface dyslexic symptoms observed in MP by lesioning a single phonological reading route. If a lesion to the phono-logical route is large enough to reduce performance on irregular words to the levels observed in MP, it will also severely damage reading of regular words and nonwords. Advocates of the triangle model therefore believe that irregular words are usually read aloud via the semantic pathway (see section on *reading impairments in dementia*).

Some surface dyslexics appear to comprehend words on the basis of the pronuncia-tion that they assemble. For example, JC (Newcombe and Marshall, 1973) read *begin* as "beggin" and defined it as "collecting money" and made comprehension errors on hom-ophones (Newcombe and Marshall, 1981). MK (Howard and Franklin, 1987), on the other hand, whose surface dyslexia appeared to reflect a post-semantic impairment read only 52% of a set of irregular words correctly but defined 88% of them accurately. For example, he defined *steak* as "good beef" but pronounced it as /stik/.

7.2 Anatomical issues

In a review paper, Vanier and Caplan (1985) found that surface dyslexia could occur following tumour, head trauma and stroke. Vanier and Caplan found that there was consistent evidence of damage to left temporal regions in published cases of surface dys-lexia. Damaged areas frequently included the insula and the putamen. It is also closely associated with left temporal pole atrophy in dementia (Gold *et al.* 2005) (see section on *reading impairments in dementia*).

7.3 Remediation

- A successful technique for treating the symptoms of surface dyslexia is to repeatedly present words that the patient cannot read together with a picture that provides infor-mation about what the word means (Byng and Coltheart, 1986; Coltheart and Byng, 1989). This technique might help strengthen representations within the orthographic lexicon and\or strengthen connections between the orthographic lexicon and the semantic system. Such a technique is less likely to achieve improvement in a patient whose reading difficulty is associated with speech production problems.

- Ellis *et al.* (2000) describe a technique in which the patient immediately hears a word's spoken form whenever the word is read incorrectly. The patient must then repeat the word whilst thinking about its meaning. Such a technique might prove successful in treating a number of different types of surface dyslexia.

7.4 Assessment

Compare reading accuracy on regular and irregular words (e.g. PALPA Test 35, Kay *et al.* 1992). Examine responses for evidence of regularisation errors.

8 Reading impairments in dementia

8.1 Impairment

The results from a number of studies reveal a very strong association between semantic dementia (progressive aphasia affecting semantic memory accompanying the temporal variant of fronto-temporal dementia) and surface dyslexia (see section on *surface dyslexia*). All 51 semantic dementia cases studied by Woollams *et al.* (2007) became surface dyslexic as their disease progressed. Graham *et al.* (1994) found that irregular words could be read aloud only if they could be matched with their appropriate picture; irregular words that could not be matched with pictures were not read accurately. These researchers claim that for most people oral reading of an irregular word requires access to the word's semantic representation, and that if the semantics for an item are missing or corrupted, it will not be read accurately. There is evidence that poor reading of irregular words in semantic dementia is associated with atrophy of the left temporal pole (Gold *et al.* 2005). As Gold *et al.* point out functional imaging studies have not shown this to be an area involved in reading aloud single words. They suggest therefore, that the left temporal pole provides a gateway to semantic representations which allow irregular words to be read aloud (Gold *et al.* 2005).

Nevertheless, there are a small number of patients with Alzheimer's disease (Lambon-Ralph *et al.* 1995; Schwartz *et al.* 1980) and semantic dementia (Cipolotti and Warrington, 1995; McKay *et al.* 2007) who are not surface dyslexic, despite semantic impairments. For example DC (Lambon Ralph *et al.* 1995) read correctly 40/42 of a list of irregular words but defined only 24/42 of them correctly, even though a fairly lax criterion was used for accepting definitions. Blazely *et al.* (2005) reported two patients with equivalent degrees of semantic memory loss, one of whom was, and one of whom was not, surface dyslexic. Woollams *et al.* (2007) believe that the semantic dementia patients who do not suffer from surface dyslexia reflect a small subset of the population who learned to read exception words without semantic mediation via direct orthographic to phonological connections. Unfortunately this claim is hard to test in the absence of any assessment of the way in which patients read exception words pre-morbidly.

Conversely, the existence of such patients has been taken (e.g. Blazely *et al.* 2005) to provide evidence that the reading system contains a direct-lexical reading route that does not require access to a word's meaning. Blazely *et al.* claim that the correlation between semantic dementia and surface dyslexia comes about because this route becomes incapacitated as the disease progresses. Only after the direct route is lost, they argue, will a patient's reading of exception words require semantic mediation. This account requires that the anatomical location of the direct lexical route is such that it will also be damaged around the time that semantic representations of words are disrupted by atrophy of inferior and anterior areas of the left temporal lobe. Opponents (Woollams *et al.* 2007) point out that no neuro-anatomical evidence currently exists to support this claim.

Two studies have reported effects of word length on the reading speed of patients with semantic dementia (Gold *et al.* 2005; Cumming *et al.* 2006). Cumming *et al.* reported that these effects are not as large as those observed in LBL reading (see earlier section), and that the dementia patients who showed length effects were less impaired on letter processing tasks and visuo-spatial tasks than LBL readers. As the semantic dementia patients were all surface dyslexic, it is likely that the length effect is a direct consequence of reading via the non-lexical route, rather than impaired parallel letter processing. Gold *et al.* did not observe abnormal word length effects in the reading of patients with Alzheimer's disease.

8.2 Assessment

The National Adult Reading Test (Nelson, 1982) was designed to provide a measure of pre-morbid IQ based on the assumption that irregular word reading is relatively immune to the effects of dementia. However, it is clear that performance on the NART is correlated with dementia severity (Patterson *et al.* 1994) and there are a number of reports of a decline on this test as the disease develops (e.g. Fromm *et al.* 1991; Paque and Warrington, 1995). Strain *et al.* (1998) suggest that decline on the NART can be observed as soon as the disease develops past the early stages, and Storandt *et al.* (1995) report a decline even in mild patients. Alzheimer patients have been shown to perform well at reading non-words unless they are orthographically unusual (Friedman *et al.* 1992), or phonologically unusual (Glosser *et al.* 1998).

Selective references

Allport, D.A. and Funnell, E. (1981). Components of the mental lexicon. *Philosophical Transactions of the Royal Society of London B*, **295**, 397–410.

Arguin, M. and Bub, D. (1994). Pure alexia: Attempted rehabilitation and its implications for interpretation of the deficit. *Brain and Language*, **47**, 233–268.

Arguin, M., Bub, D., and Bowers, J. (1998). Extent and limits of covert lexical activation in letter by letter reading. *Cognitive Neuropsychology*, **15**, 53–92.

Arguin, M., Fiset, S., and Bub, D. (2002). Sequential and parallel letter processing in letter-by-letter dyslexia. *Cognitive Neuropsychology*, **19**, 535–555.

Barry, C. and Richardson, J.T.E. (1988). Accounts of oral reading in deep dyslexia. In H. Whittaker (Ed) *Phonological Processes and Brain Mechanisms*. New York: Springer Verlag.

Baxter, D.M. and Warrington, E. (1983). Neglect dysgraphia. *Journal of Neurology, Neurosurgery and Psychiatry*, **46**, 1073–1078.

Beaton, A.A. and Davies, N.W. (2007). Semantic errors in deep dyslexia: does orthographic depth matter? *Cognitive Neuropsychology*, **24**, 312–323.

Beauvois, M-F. and Derouesne, J. (1979). Phonological alexia: Three dissociations. *Journal of Neurology, Neurosurgery and Psychiatry*, **42**, 1115–1124.

Behrmann, M. and Bub, D. (1992). Surface dyslexia and dysgraphia, Dual routes, single lexicon. *Cognitive Neuropsychology*, **9**, 209–251.

Behrmann, M. and McLeod, J. (1995). Rehabilitation for pure alexia. *Neuropsychological Rehabilitation*, **5**, 149–180.

Behrmann, M. and Shallice, T. (1995) Pure alexia. An orthographic not spatial disorder. *Cognitive Neuropsychology*, **12**, 409–454.

Behrmann, M., Plaut, D.C., and Nelson, J. (1998). A literature review and new data supporting an interactive view of letter by letter reading. *Cognitive Neuropsychology*, **15**, 7–51.

Benson, D.F., Brown, J., and Tomlinson, E.B. (1971). Varieties of alexia: Word and letter blindness. *Neurology*, **21**, 951–957.

Berndt, R.S., Haendiges, A.N., Mitchum, C.C., and Wayland, S.C. (1996). An investigation of nonlexical reading impairments. *Cognitive Neuropsychology*, **13**, 763–801.

Binder, J.R. and Mohr, J.P. (1992). The topography of callosal reading pathways. *Brain*, **97**, 1807–1826.

Blazely, A.M., Coltheart, M., and Casey, B.J. (2005). Semantic impairment with and without surface dyslexia: Implications for models of reading. *Cognitive Neuropsychology*, **22**, 695–717.

Bub, D., Black, S.E., and Howell, J. (1989). Word recognition and orthographic context effects in a letter-by-letter reader. *Brain and Language*, **36**, 357–376.

Buxbaum, L. and Coslett, H.B. (1996). Deep dyslexic phenomena in a letter-by-letter reader. *Brain and Language*, **54**, 136–167.

Byng, S. and Coltheart, M. (1986). Aphasia therapy research. In E. Helmquist and L.G. Nilsson (Eds) *Communication and Handicap*. Amsterdam: Elsevier.

Caccappolo-van Vliet, E., Miozzo, M., and Stern, Y. (2004). Phonological dyslexia without phonological impairment? *Cognitive Neuropsychology*, **21**, 820–839.

Caplan, L.R. and Hedley-White, T. (1974). Cueing and memory function in alexia without agraphia: A case report. *Brain*, **115**, 251–262.

Caramazza, A. and Hillis, A.E. (1990). Levels of representation, co-ordinate frames and unilateral neglect. *Cognitive Neuropsychology*, **7**, 369–389.

Chialant, D. and Caramazza, A. (1998). Perceptual and lexical factors in a case of letter-by-letter reading. *Cognitive Neuropsychology*, **15**, 203–238.

Cipolotti, L. and Warrington, E. (1995). Semantic memory and reading abilities: A case report. *Journal of the International Neuropsychological Society*, **1**, 104–110.

Coltheart M., Rastle K., Perry C., Langdon R., and Ziegler J. (2001). DRC: A dual route cascaded model of visual word recognition and reading aloud. *Psychological Review*, **108**, 204–256.

Coltheart, M. (1985). Cognitive neuropsychology and the study of reading. In M.I. Posner and O.S.M. Marin (Eds.) *Attention and Performance Volume 11*, Hillsdale NJ, Erlbaum.

Coltheart, M. (1996). Phonological dyslexia: Past and future issues. *Cognitive Neuropsychology*, **13**, 749–762.

Coltheart, M. (2000). Deep dyslexia is right-hemisphere reading. *Brain and Language*, **71**, 299–309.

Coltheart, M. and Byng, S. (1989). A treatment for surface dyslexia. In X. Seron and G. Deloche (Eds) *Cognitive Approaches to Neuropsychological Rehabilitation*. Hillsdale NJ: Erlbaum.

Coltheart, M., Curtis, B., Atkins, P., and Haller, M. (1993). Models of reading aloud: Dual-route *and* parallel-distributed processing approach. *Psychological Review*, **100**, 589–608.

Conway, T.W., Heilman, P., Rothi, L.J., Alexander, A.W., Adair, J., Crosson, B.A., and Heilman, K.M. (1998). Treatment of a case of phonological alexia with agraphia using the auditory discrimination in depth (ADD) programme. *Journal of the International Neuropsychological Society*, **4**, 608–620.

Coslett, H.B. and Saffran, E.M. (1989). Preserved object recognition and reading comprehension in optic aphasia. *Brain*, **112**, 1091–1110.

Coslett, H.B. and Saffran, E.M. (1992). Optic aphasia and the right hemisphere: A replication and extension. *Brain and Language*, **43**, 148–168.

Costello, A. and Warrington, E.K. (1987). Dissociation of visuo-spatial neglect and neglect dyslexia. *Journal of Neurology, Neurosurgery and Psychiatry*, **50**, 1110–1116.

Crisp, J. and Ralph, M.A. (2006). Unlocking the nature of the phonological-deep dyslexia continuum: The keys to reading aloud are in phonology and semantics. *Journal of Cognitive Neuroscience*, **18**, 348–362.

Crutch, S.J. (2006). Qualitatively different semantic representations for abstract and concrete words: Further evidence from the semantic reading errors of deep dyslexic patients. *Neurocase*, **12**, 91–97.

Crutch, S.J. and Warrington, E.K. (2005). Abstract and concrete concepts have structurally different representational frameworks. *Brain*, **128**, 615–627.

Crutch, S.J. and Warrington, E.K. (2007). Foveal crowding in posterior cortical atrophy. A specific early deficit affecting reading. *Cognitive Neuropsychology*, **24**, 843–866.

Crutch, S.J. and Warrington, E.K. (2007). Word form access dyslexia: Understanding the basis of visual reading errors. *Quarterly Journal of Experimental Psychology*, **60**, 57–78.

Cuetos, F., Valle-Arroyo, F., and Suarez, M.P. (1996). A case of phonological dyslexia in spanish. *Cognitive Neuropsychology*, **13**, 1–24.

Cumming, T.B., Patterson, K., Verfaellie, M., and Graham, K.S. (2006). One bird with two stones: Abnormal word length effects in pure alexia and semantic dementia. *Cognitive Neuropsychology*, **23**, 1130–1161.

De Partz, M.P. (1986). Re-education of a deep dyslexic patient: Rationale of the method and results. *Cognitive Neuropsychology*, **3**, 149–178.

Dejerine, J. (1892). Contribution _à l'étude anatomo-pathologique et clinique des différentes variétés de cécité verbale. *Mémoires de la Société Biologique*, **4**, 61–90.

Ellis, A.W., Flude, B., and Young, A.W. (1987). Neglect dyslexia and the early visual processing of letters in words and nonwords. *Cognitive Neuropsychology*, **4**, 439–464.

Ellis, A.W., Lambon Ralph, M.A., Morris, J., and Hunter, A. (2000). Surface dyslexia: Description, treatment and interpretation. In E. Funnell (Ed.) *Neuropsychology of Reading*, Hove UK: Psychology Press.

Farah, M.J. (2000). *The Cognitive Neuroscience of Vision*. Malden, MA: Blackwell.

Farah, M.J., Stowe, R.M., and Levinson, K.L. (1996). Phonological alexia: Loss of a reading specific component of the reading architecture? *Cognitive Neuropsychology*, **13**, 849–868.

Fiset D., Arguin M., and McCabe E. (2006). The breakdown of parallel letter processing in letter-by-letter dyslexia. *Cognitive Neuropsychology*, **23**, 240–260.

Friedman, R., Ferguson, S., Robinson, S., and Sunderland, T. (1992). Dissociation of mechanisms of reading in Alzheimers disease. *Brain and Language*, **43**, 400–413.

Friedman, R.B. (1996). Recovery from deep alexia to phonological alexia. *Brain and Language*, **52**, 114–128.

Friedman, R.B. and Hadley, J.A. (1992). Letter-by-letter surface alexia. *Cognitive Neuropsychology*, **9**, 185–208.

Friedman, R.B. (1995). Two types of phonological alexia. *Cortex*, **31**, 397–403.

Fromm, D., Holland, A.L., Nebes, R.D., and Oakley, M.A. (1991). A longitudinal study of word reading ability in Alzheimers disease: Evidence from the National Adult Reading Test. *Cortex*, **27**, 367–376.

Funnell, E. (1983). Phonological access in reading: New evidence from acquired dyslexia. *British Journal of Psychology*, **74**, 159–180.

Funnell, E. (2000). Deep dyslexia. In E. Funnell (Ed.) *Neuropsychology of Reading*, Hove UK: Psychology Press.

Gerhand, S. and Barry, C. (2000). When does a deep dyslexic make a semantic error? The roles of age-of-acquisition, concreteness, and frequency. *Brain and Language*, **74**, 26–47.

Geschwind, N. (1965). Disconnexion syndromes in animals and man. *Brain*, **88**, 237–294, 585–644.

Glosser, G., Friedman, R.K., Kohn, S.E., Sands, L., and Grugan, P. (1998). Cognitive mechanisms for processing nonwords: Evidence from Alzheimer's disease. *Brain and Language*, **63**, 32–49.

Gold, B.T., Bal.ota, D., Cortese, M.J., Sergent- Marshall, S.D., Snyder, A.Z., Salat, DH., Fischl, B., Dale, A.M., Morris, J.C., and Buckner R.L. (2005). Differing neuropsychological and neuroanatomical correlates of abnormal reading in early-stage semantic dementia and dementia of the Alzheimer type. *Neuropsychologia*, **43**, 833–846.

Graham, N., Hodges, J.R., and Patterson, K. (1994). The relationship between comprehension and oral reading in progressive fluent aphasia. *Neuropsychologia*, **32**, 299–316.

Greenwald, M.L. and Gonzalez-Rothi, L.J. (1998) Lexical access via letter naming in a profoundly alexic and anomic patient: A treatment study. *Journal of the International Neuropsychological Society*, **4**, 595–607.

Hanley, J.R. and Kay, J. (1996). Reading speed in pure alexia. *Neuropsychologia*, **34**, 1165–1174.

Hanley, J.R. and Kay, J. (1992). Does letter-by-letter reading involve the spelling system? *Neuropsychologia*, **30**, 237–256.

Hanley, J.R. and Kay, J. (1997). An effect of imageability on the production of phonological errors in auditory repetition. *Cognitive Neuropsychology*, **14**, 1065–1084.

Hanley, J.R. and McDonnell, V. (1997). Are reading and spelling phonologically mediated? Evidence from a patient with a speech production impairment. *Cognitive Neuropsychology*, **14**, 3–33.

Haywood, M. and Coltheart, M. (2000). Neglect dyslexia and the early stages of visual word recognition. *Neurocase*, **6**, 33–43.

Hillis, A. and Caramazza, A. (1991). Mechanisms for accessing lexical representations for output: Evidence from a category specific semantic deficit. *Brain and Language*, **40**, 106–144.

Hillis, A. and Caramazza, A. (1992). The reading process and its disorders. In D.I. Margolin (Ed.) *Cognitive Neuropsychology in Clinical Practice*. Cary: Oxford University Press.

Hillis, A. and Caramazza, A. (1994). Theories of lexical processing and rehabilitation of lexical deficits. In M. Riddoch and G. Humphreys (Eds) *Cognitive Neuropsychology and Cognitive Rehabilitation*. Hove UK, Erlbaum.

Hinshelwood, J. (1895). Word blindness and visual memory. *The Lancet*, **2**, 1564–1570.

Hinshelwood, J. (1900). *Letter, Word, and Mind-blindness*. London: Lewis and Co. Ltd.

Hinshelwood, J. (1917). *Congenital Word*-blindness. London: Lewis and Co. Ltd.

Howard, D. and Franklin, S. (1988). *Missing the Meaning*. Cambridge, Mass: MIT Press.

Kartsounis, L.D. and Warrington, E.K. (1989). Unilateral neglect overcome by cues implicit in stimulus displays. *Journal of Neurology, Neurosurgery and Psychiatry*, **52**, 1253–1259.

Kay, J. and Hanley, J.R. (1991). Simultaneous form perception and serial letter recognition in a case of letter-by-letter reading. *Cognitive Neuropsychology*, **8**, 249–273.

Kay, J. and Patterson, K. (1985). Routes to meaning in surface dyslexia In K. Patterson, J. Marshall and M. Coltheart (Eds) *Surface Dyslexia: Neuropsychological and Cognitive Studies of Phonological Reading*. Hove, UK: Erlbaum.

Kay, J., Lesser, R., and Coltheart, M. (1992). *Psycholinguistic Assessment of Language Processing in Aphasia*. London, Erlbaum.

Kendall, D.L., McNeil, M.R., and Small, S.L. (1998). Rule-based treatment for acquired phonological dyslexia. *Aphasiology*, **12**, 587–600.

Kerkhoff, G., Munsinger, U., Eberle-Strauss, G., and Stogerer, E. (1992). Rehabilitation of hemianopic alexia in patients with postgeniculate visual fields disorders. *Neuropsychological Rehabilitation*, **2**, 21–41.

Klein, D., Behrmann, M., and Doctor, E. (1994). The evolution of deep dyslexia. *Cognitive Neuropsychology*, **11**, 579–611.

Lambon Ralph, M.A. and Ellis, A.W. (1997). "Patterns of paralexia" revisited: Report of a case of visual dyslexia. *Cognitive Neuropsychology*, **14**, 953–974.

Lambon Ralph, M.A. and Graham, N.L. (2000). Acquired phonological and deep dyslexia. *Neurocase*, **6**, 141–143.

Lambon Ralph, M.A., Hesketh, A., and Sage, K.E. (2004). Implicit recognition in pure alexia: The Saffran effect - A tale of two systems or two procedures? *Cognitive Neuropsychology* **21**, 400–421.

Lambon-Ralph, M.A., Ellis, A.W., and Franklin, S. (1995). Semantic loss without surface dyslexia. *Neurocase*, **1**, 363–369.

Leff, A.P., Crewes, H., Plant, G.T., Scott, S.K., Kennard, C., and Wise, R.J.S. (2001). The functional anatomy of single-word reading in patients with hemianopic and pure alexia. *Brain*, **124**, 510–521.

Leff, A.P., Scott, S.K., Crewes, H., Hodgson, T., and Howard, D. (2000). Impaired reading in patients with right hemianopia. *Annals of Neurology*, **47**, 171–178.

Maher, L.M., Clayton, M.C., Barrett, A.M., Schober-Peterson, D., and Rothi, L.J.G. (1998). Rehabilitation of a case of pure alexia: Exploiting residual abilities. *Journal of the International Neuropsychological Society*, **4**, 636–647.

Marshall, J. and Newcombe, F. (1966). Syntactic and semantic errors in paralexia. *Neuropsychologia*, **2**, 169–176.

Marshall, J. and Newcombe, F. (1973). Patterns of paralexia: A psycholinguistic approach. *Journal of Psycholinguistic Research*, **4**, 175–199.

Marshall, J. and Newcombe, F. (1980). The conceptual status of deep dyslexia: An historical perspective. In M. Coltheart, K. Patterson and J. Marshall (Eds). *Deep Dyslexia*. London, Routledge.

McCarthy, R. A. and Warrington, E.K. (1990). *Cognitive neuropsychology. A Clinical Introduction*. London: Academic Press.

McKay, A., Castles, A., and Davis, C. (2007). The impact of progressive semantic loss on reading aloud. *Cognitive Neuropsychology*, **24**, 162–186.

McKeff, T.J. and Behrmann, M. (2004). Pure alexia and covert reading: Evidence from stroop tasks. *Cognitive Neuropsychology*, **21**, 443–458.

Miceli, G. and Capasso, R. (2001). Word-centred neglect dyslexia: Evidence from a new case. *Neurocase*, **7**, 221–237.

Miozzo, M. and Caramazza, A. (1998). Varieties of pure alexia: The case of failure to access graphemic representations. *Cognitive Neuropsychology*, **15**, 203–238.

Moody, S. (1988). The Moyer reading technique re-evaluated. *Cortex*, **24**, 473–476.

Morton, J. and Patterson, K. (1980). Little words-no. In M. Coltheart, K. Patterson and J. Marshall (Eds). *Deep Dyslexia*. London, Routledge.

Moyer, S.B. (1979). Rehabilitation of alexia: A case study. *Cortex*, **15**, 139–144.

Mycroft, R., Hanley, J.R., and Kay, J. (2002). Preserved access to abstract letter identities despite abolished letter naming in a case of pure alexia. *Journal of Neurolinguistics*, **15**, 99–108.

Nelson, H. (1983). *National adult reading test (NART)*. Windsor, UK: NFER.

Newcombe, F. and Marshall, J.C. (1980). Response monitoring and response blocking in deep dyslexia. In M. Coltheart, K. Patterson and J. Marshall (Eds). *Deep Dyslexia*. London, Routledge.

Newcombe, F. and Marshall, J.C. (1981). On psycholinguistic classification of the acquired dyslexias. *Bulletin of the Orton Society*, **31**: 29–46.

Newton, P. and Barry, C. (1997). Concreteness effects in word production but not word comprehension in deep dyslexia. *Cognitive Neuropsychology*, **14**, 481–509.

Nickels, L. (1992). The autocue? Self generated phonemic cues in the treatment of a disorder of reading and naming. *Cognitive Neuropsychology*, **9**, 155–182.

Osswald, K., Humphreys, G.W., and Olson, A. (2002). Words are more than the sum of their parts: Evidence for detrimental effects of word-level information in alexia. *Cognitive Neuropsychology*, **19**, 675–695.

Paque, L. and Warrington, E.K. (1995). A longitudinal study of reading ability in patients suffering from dementia. *Journal of the International Neuropsychological Society*, **1**, 517–524.

Patterson, K. (1979). What is right with deep dyslexic patients? *Brain and Language*, **8**, 111–129.

Patterson, K. (1982). The relation between reading and phonological coding: Furtherneuropsychological observations. In A.W. Ellis (Ed), *Normality and Pathology in Cognitive Function*. London: Academic Press.

Patterson, K. and Hodges, J.R. (1992). Deterioration of word meaning: Implications for meaning. *Neuropsychologia*, **30**, 1025–1040.

Patterson, K. and Kay, J. (1982). Letter-by-letter reading: Psychological descriptions of a neurological syndrome. *Quarterly Journal of Experimental Psychology*, **34A**, 411–441.

Patterson, K. and Lambon Ralph, M. (1999). Selective disorders of reading? *Current Opinion in Neurobiology*, **9**, 235–239.

Patterson, K. and Wilson, B. (1990). A rose is a rose or a nose: A deficit in initial letter identification. *Cognitive Neuropsychology*, **7**, 447–479.

Patterson, K.E. and Marcel, A. (1992). Phonological ALEXIA or PHONOLOGICAL alexia. In J. Alegria, D. Holender, J. Junca de Morais and M. Radeau (Eds.), *Analytic Approaches to Human Cognition*. Elsevier Science Publishers.

Plaut, D., McClelland, J., Seidenberg, M., and Patterson, K. (1996). Understanding normal and impaired word reading. *Psychological Review*, **103**, 56–115.

Plaut, D. and Shallice, T. (1993). Deep dyslexia, a case study of connectionist neuropsychology. *Cognitive Neuropsychology*, **10**, 377–500.

Price, C.J. and Devlin, J.T. (1993). The myth of the visual word form area. *Neuroimage* 19, 473–481.

Price, C.J. and Humphreys, G.W. (1993). Attentional dyslexia - the effect of co-occurring deficits. *Cognitive Neuropsychology*, **10**, 569–592.

Price, C.J., Howard, D., Patterson, K., Warburton, E.A., Friston, K., and Frackowiak, R.S.J. (1998). A functional neuroimaging of two deep dyslexic patients. *Journal of Cognitive Neuroscience*, **10**, 303–315.

Rapcsak, S.Z., Rubens, A.B., and Laguna, J.F. (1990). From letters to words: Procedures for word recognition in letter-by-letter reading. *Brain and Language*, **38**, 504–514.

Reuter-Lorenz, P.A. and Brunn, J.L. (1990). A prelexical basis for letter-by-letter reading. *Cognitive Neuropsychology*, **7**, 1–20.

Riddoch, M.J. (1990). Neglect and the peripheral dyslexias. *Cognitive Neuropsychology*, **7**, 369–389.

Rosazza, C., Appollonio, I., Isella, V., and Shallice, T. (2007). Qualitatively different forms of pure alexia. *Cognitive Neuropsychology*, **24**, 393–418.

Saffran, E.M. and Coslett, H.B. (1998). Implicit vs. letter-by-letter reading in pure alexia, a tale of two systems. *Cognitive Neuropsychology*, **15**, 141–165.

Saffran, E.M. and Marin, O.S.M. (1976). Reading without phonology: Evidence from aphasia. *Quarterly Journal of Experimental Psychology*, **29**, 515–525.

Sage, K.E., Hesketh, A., and Lambon Ralph, M.A. (2005). Using errorless learning to treat letter-by-letter reading: contrasting word versus letter based therapy. *Neuropsychological Rehabilitation*, **15**, 619–642.

Sasanuma, S. and Patterson, K. (1996). Phonological Alexia in Japanese: A Case Study. *Cognitive Neuropsychology*, **13**, 825–848.

Schwartz, M., Saffran, E.M., and Marin, O.S.M. (1980). Fractionating the reading process in dementia. In M. Coltheart, K. Patterson and J Marshall (Eds). *Deep Dyslexia*. London, Routledge.

Seidenberg, M.S. and McClelland, J. (1989). A distributed, developmental model of word recognition and naming. *Psychological Review*, **15**, 169–179.

Shallice, T. (1988). *From Neuropsychology to Mental Structure*. Cambridge, Cambridge University Press.

Shallice, T. and Coughlan, A.K. (1980). Word recognition in a phonemic dyslexic patient. *Quarterly Journal of Experimental Psychology*, **43**, 866–872.

Shallice, T. and Saffran, E. M. (1986). Lexical processing in the absence of explicit word identification: Evidence from a letter-by-letter reader. *Cognitive Neuropsychology*, **3**, 429–458.

Shallice, T. and Warrington, E.K. (1977). The possible role of selective attention in acquired dyslexia. *Neuropsychologia*, **15**, 31–41.

Shallice, T. and Warrington, E.K. (1980). Modality specific word comprehension deficits in deep dyslexia. *Journal of Neurology, Neurosurgery and Psychiatry*, **27**, 187–199.

Shallice, T. and Warrington, E.K. (1980). Single and multiple component central dyslexic syndromes. In M. Coltheart, K. Patterson and J Marshall (Eds). *Deep Dyslexia*. London, Routledge.

Sieroff, E. (1990). Focusing on/in visual-verbal stimuli in patients with parietal lesions. *Cognitive Neuropsychology*, **7**, 519–554.

Stadie, N. and Rilling, E. (2006). Evaluation of lexically and nonlexically based reading treatment in a deep dyslexic. *Cognitive Neuropsychology*, **23**, 643–672.

Storandt, M., Stone, K., and Labarge, E. (1995). Deficits in reading performance in very mild dementia of the Alzheimer type. *Neuropsychology*, **9**, 174–176.

Strain, E., Patterson, K., Graham, N., and Hodges, J.R. (1996). Word reading in Alzheimer's disease. *Neuropsychologia*, **36**, 155–171.

Tree J.J. and Kay J. (2006). Phonological dyslexia and phonological impairment: An exception to the rule? *Neuropsychologia*, **44**, 2861–2873.

Vanier, M. and Caplan, D. (1985). CT scan correlates of surface dyslexia. In K Patterson, J. Marshall and M. Coltheart (Eds) *Surface dyslexia: Neuropsychological and Cognitive Studies of Phonological Reading*. Hove, UK: Erlbaum.

Warrington, E. K. (1991). Right neglect dyslexia: A single case study. *Cognitive Neuropsychology*, **8**, 193–212.

Warrington, E.K. and Shallice, T. (1980). Word-form dyslexia. *Brain* **103**, 99–112.

Warrington, E.K. (1981). Concrete word dyslexia. *British Journal of Psychology*, **72**, 175–196.

Warrington, E.K. and Langdon, D.W. (2002). Does the spelling dyslexic read by recognizing orally spelled words? An investigation of a letter-by-letter reader. *Neurocase* **8**, 210–218.

Weekes, B. (1997). Differential effects of number of letters on word and nonword naming latency. *Quarterly Journal of Experimental Psychology*, **50A**, 439–456.

Weekes, B. and Coltheart, M. (1996). Surface dyslexia and surface dysgraphia: Treatment studies and their theoretical implications. *Cognitive Neuropsychology*, **13**, 277–315.

Weekes, B., Coltheart, M., and Gordon, E. (1997). Deep dyslexia and right hemisphere reading-regional blood flow study. *Aphasiology*, **11**, 1139–1158.

Woollams, A.M., Lambon Ralph, M.A., Plaut, D.C., and Patterson K. (2007). SD-squared: on the association between semantic dementia and surface dyslexia. *Psychological Review*, **114**, 316–339.

Chapter 17

Neuropsychological assessment and rehabilitation of writing disorders

Pélagie M. Beeson and Steven Z. Rapcsak

1 Introduction

Written language provides a means to transform speech into durable, static visual representations, allowing communication of specific thoughts and ideas to transcend time and place. As literate adults, we tend to take for granted our ability to receive and transmit written messages, but this skill requires the integrated function of cognitive, linguistic, and sensorimotor processes that are vulnerable to the effects of acquired brain damage. The goal of neuropsychological assessment of writing is to examine the status of the component processes necessary to support written communication. An understanding of the nature and degree of impairment to specific processes, as well as the availability of residual abilities, provides guidance for the design and implementation of a behavioral rehabilitation plan that is appropriate for a given individual. In this chapter, we provide an overview of the cognitive processes that support writing and a description of the major acquired agraphia syndromes, followed by a review of evidence-based treatment approaches for these writing impairments.

2 A cognitive model of writing

The cognitive-linguistic and sensorimotor processes necessary for writing single words are specified in Figure 17.1.

2.1 Central processes engaged during written language production

- Semantic system: knowledge of word meanings stored in long-term memory.
- Orthographic lexicon: memory store of learned spellings.
- Phonological lexicon: memory store of sound-based representations for familiar words.
- Graphemes: single letters or letter combinations that represent a single sound (i.e., phoneme) of a language.
- Phonemes: the smallest meaningful units of sound in a language.

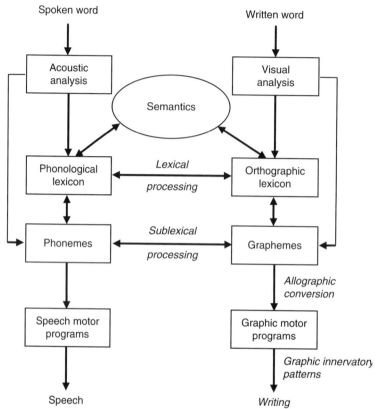

Fig. 17.1 A dual-route model of written language processing indicating lexical (whole-word) and sublexical (phoneme-grapheme conversion) spelling routes.

2.2 **Peripheral writing processes**

- Allographic conversion: the process by which abstract orthographic representations are converted into appropriate physical letter shapes.
- Graphic motor programs: spatio-temporal codes for writing movements which contain information about the sequence, position, direction, and relative size of the strokes necessary to create different letters.
- Graphic innervatory patterns: motor commands to specific muscle effector systems involved in the production of handwriting.

2.3 **Lexical-semantic and sublexical spelling routes**

According to the dual-route model of written language processing that will provide the framework for our discussion (see Figure 17.1), orthographic information is processed in parallel by both lexical and sublexical procedures that operate in an interactive manner. Access to the orthographic lexicon via the semantic system, either directly or with concurrent input from the phonological lexicon, is referred to as the lexical-semantic spelling route. This is the most common manner of spelling familiar words. Spelling can also be assembled in a sublexical (or non-lexical) manner on the basis of sound-letter correspondence rules (Ellis 1993; Rapcsak and Beeson 2002; Tainturier and Rapp 2001). Using the sublexical route, plausible spellings can be generated for both words and nonwords by the conversion of phonemes to graphemes as depicted in Figure 17.1. Assembled spellings are likely to reflect common sound-spelling correspondences, so that irregularly spelled words with exceptional phoneme-grapheme mappings might be regularized (for example, "tough" might be spelled as *tuff*). The sublexical route can provide an important compensatory spelling strategy when the lexical-semantic spelling route is impaired. This route is also critical for spelling pronounceable nonwords (e.g., *chulf*) that do not exist in the orthographic lexicon.

Spellings generated by the lexical-semantic and sublexical spelling routes are held in short term storage while they are converted into output for handwriting (or typing or oral spelling). This working memory system for orthographic information is referred to as the graphemic buffer, and it serves as an interface between central spelling processes and the peripheral procedures that support the production of handwriting. Peripheral writing procedures are accomplished through a series of hierarchically organized stages that include allographic conversion, motor programming, and the generation of graphic innervatory patterns.

3 Clinical assessment of spelling and writing

The initial goal of writing assessment is to determine whether an individual can meet their daily needs for written language production. Writing abilities should be considered relative to premorbid language skills. When agraphia is evident, careful assessment should be performed to determine the functional integrity of the various processing components involved in writing.

A variety of tasks can be used to sample writing performance, and the comparative performance across tasks allows for the relative isolation of the damaged components (see Table 17.1). Conceptually mediated writing can be sampled by asking the patient to compose a written narrative on a specific topic or using picture description tasks from standardized tests, such as the *Western Aphasia Battery* (*WAB*; Kertesz 1982) or the *Boston Diagnostic Aphasia Examination* (*BDAE*; Goodglass 2001). Written narratives require grammatical and syntactic knowledge, as well as higher level conceptual organization. Written naming can be assessed by using pictured stimuli or objects from standardized tests, such as the *WAB*, *BDAE*, the *Boston Naming Test* (*BNT*; Kaplan *et al.* 2001) or the *Psycholinguistic Assessments of Language Processing in Aphasia* (*PALPA*; Kay *et al.* 1992). Writing single words to dictation allows examination of various linguistic variables known to affect spelling performance including word length, orthographic regularity, word frequency, concreteness, grammatical class, morphological complexity, and lexical status (word vs. nonword). Word lists controlled for such variables are available in published tests like the *PALPA* (Kay *et al.* 1992) or in the literature (e.g., the Johns Hopkins Dyslexia

Table 17.1 Tasks used for the assessment of spelling. Check marks indicate those processes or representations that are necessary to accomplish the various tasks. (See discussion in text.)

Tasks	Lexical-semantic processes			Sublexical processes	Central-peripheral interface	Peripheral spelling processes		
	Syntax/ Grammar rules	Semantic representation	Orthographic representation	Phoneme-grapheme conversion	Graphemic buffer	Allographic conversion	Graphic Motor programs	Letter Name selection
Conceptual								
Written narrative or picture description	√	√	√		√	√	√	
Written Naming		√	√		√	√	√	
Dictation								
Writing to Dictation		√	√		√	√	√	
Writing Homophones		√	√		√	√	√	
Typing or Anagram Spelling			√		√			
Oral Spelling			√		√			√
Writing Nonwords				√	√	√	√	
Copy								
Case Conversion						√	√	
Direct Copy							√	

Table 17.2 Summary of the primary features of various central agraphia syndromes

Central agraphia syndrome	Effect						
	Word length short>long	Spelling regularity reg>irreg	Word freq HF>LF	Concrete con>abstr	Word class cont>func	Inability to spell nonwords	Characteristic errors
Lexical (or Surface) Agraphia		√	√				phonologically plausible misspellings; homophone confusions
Phonological/ Deep Dysgraphia			√	√	√	√	phonologically implausible errors; functor substitutions; morphological errors; semantic errors (deep dysgraphia)
Graphemic Buffer Agraphia	√						letter omissions, substitutions, additions, transpositions

√ = significant effect; Reg = regular spelling; Irreg = irregular spelling; HF = high frequency words; LF = low frequency words; Concrete = concreteness; Con = concrete; Abstr = abstract words; Cont = content words; Func = functors.

and Dysgraphia Batteries; Goodman and Caramazza 1984/2001). Certain linguistic features and characteristic error types are associated with damage to particular spelling processes and may result in specific agraphia syndromes (Table 17.2).

3.1 Central processing components assessed by various writing tasks

♦ *Semantic processing* is necessary for the composition of written narratives, written naming, and spelling words that sound the same but have different meanings (i.e., homophones, such as *bear – bare*). Although semantic activation typically occurs when words are spelled to dictation, these tasks may be accomplished by transcoding directly between corresponding representations in the phonological and orthographic lexica (and also by phoneme-grapheme conversion), therefore bypassing semantics.

♦ *Activation of orthographic representations* is necessary to support spelling of familiar words regardless of output modality (i.e., written spelling, oral spelling, typing, or spelling with anagram letters).

♦ *Sublexical spelling procedures* rely on knowledge of phoneme-grapheme correspondence rules. These skills can be tested directly with the spelling of pronounceable nonwords (e.g. *merber*) that do not have representations in the orthographic lexicon.

- The *graphemic buffer* holds orthographic information in short term memory as sequential letters are written, typed, or spelled aloud. The capacity of the graphemic buffer is examined by spelling words of increasing length.

3.2 Assessment of peripheral writing processes

Peripheral writing processes serve to transcode abstract orthographic representations into actual letter shapes. These abilities can be examined using any of the writing tasks shown in Table 17.1. Performance on these tasks may be compared to oral spelling, typing, and spelling by arrangement of letters (i.e., anagrams) in order to identify potential dissociations between the various output modalities.

- *Allographic conversion* refers to the ability to assign each grapheme to the appropriate physical letter shape. This ability can be assessed by asking patients to transcribe letters from upper to lower case and vice versa, or to copy words in a different case or style (e.g., print vs. cursive).

- *Graphic motor programs and graphic innervatory patterns* control the motor execution of handwriting movements affecting the overall legibility, size, and morphology of handwriting. Poor control of movement speed, force, and amplitude may be readily apparent as the patient is observed in the act of writing. Peripheral writing processes may also be examined by asking the patient to copy words or single letters. Keep in mind that copying may be accomplished without activation of the orthographic lexicon, letter shape selection, or graphic motor programs if it is performed in a manner that is more like drawing a picture than writing.

3.3 Comparison of writing abilities with related language and motor skills

Writing abilities should be contrasted with performance on other language comprehension and production tasks and relative to the performance of other skilled limb movements.

- Examine *single-word auditory comprehension* (point to picture in response to spoken word). Impairment will negatively affect performance on writing to dictation tasks.

- Examine *single-word reading comprehension* (match written word to picture) and the ability to recognize correctly spelled real words versus pseudowords, such as *flig* (visual lexical decision task). Poor word recognition abilities will impair the ability to detect spelling errors.

- Examine *reading aloud* to determine whether written words provide access to appropriate entries in the phonological lexicon. Good oral reading skills may provide strategies for self-detection of spelling errors.

- Examine *spoken picture naming* and compare it to written naming of the same items to identify modality-specific impairments of lexical retrieval.

- Examine *limb praxis* for tasks other than handwriting using an apraxia screening test or praxis subtests from comprehensive aphasia batteries, such as the *WAB* or *BDAE*.

4 Principles of agraphia classification and treatment

The assessment of impaired and preserved writing processes should allow for the determination of whether a patient's performance fits the diagnostic criteria for a specific agraphia syndrome.

4.1 Acquired disorders of writing can be subdivided into central and peripheral types.

- *Central agraphia syndromes* reflect damage to the lexical-semantic or sublexical spelling routes, or the graphemic buffer, and result in similar impairments across different modalities of output (e.g., written spelling, oral spelling, typing). Central agraphia syndromes include lexical (or surface) agraphia, phonological agraphia, deep agraphia, and graphemic buffer agraphia (Table 17.2) (Ellis 1988; Rapcsak and Beeson 2000; 2002; Roeltgen 1993).

- *Peripheral agraphia syndromes* reflect damage to writing processes that are distal to the graphemic buffer. Dysfunction primarily affects the selection or production of letters in handwriting. These syndromes include allographic disorders, apraxic agraphia, and non-apraxic disorders of neuromuscular execution (Table 17.3) (Rapcsak 1997; Rapcsak and Beeson 2000; 2002).

Individual agraphia syndromes and appropriate treatment approaches are detailed in Sections 5–10. The presumed neuroanatomical correlates of these syndromes are drawn from careful examination of lesions in patients with well-defined agraphia profiles (Henry *et al.* 2007; Hillis and Rapp 2004; Rapcsak and Beeson 2002; 2004; Roeltgen 1993).

Table 17.3 Summary of the primary features of various peripheral agraphia syndromes.

Peripheral agraphia syndrome	Distinctive features		
	Impairment	Spared abilities	Characteristic errors
Allographic Disorders	Inability to generate or select correct letter shapes in handwriting	oral spelling	Substitution of physically similar letter forms; case mixing errors. May be specific to case (upper vs. lower) or style (print vs. cursive)
Apraxic Agraphia	Poor letter formation not attributable to allographic disorder, sensorimotor, cerebellar, or extrapyramidal dysfunction	oral spelling, typing, spelling with anagram letters	Gross errors of letter morphology, spatial distortions, stroke insertions and deletions. Writing may be completely illegible
Nonapraxic Disorders of Motor Function	Defective regulation of movement force, speed, and amplitude in handwriting	oral spelling, spelling with anagram letters (typing may be impaired due to disordered motor function)	Micrographia (Parkinson's disease); disjointed and irregular writing movements (cerebellar disorders)

When an individual's agraphia profile does not conform to a recognized agraphia syndrome, it can be characterized by a description of the status of impaired and preserved processes.

4.2 Treatment principles and supporting evidence

A review of the literature yields about 45 empirical studies of treatment for acquired impairments of spelling and writing in adults. One randomized controlled trial conducted with a diverse group of 94 individuals with aphasia (and alexia and agraphia) showed that patients who received treatment for spoken and written language made significantly greater improvement in writing than patients who did not receive treatment (Wertz *et al.* 1986). In addition, several group studies demonstrated a therapeutic effect of behavioral treatment for written spelling (Schechter *et al.* 1985; Schwartz *et al.* 1974; Sugishita *et al.* 1993), and words typed on a keyboard (Deloche *et al.* 1992; Katz and Nagy 1984; Pizzamiglio and Roberts 1967). The majority of the writing treatment studies are controlled single-subject experiments (including 1 to 8 participants) that examine the effects of specific treatment approaches on well-described writing impairments. To date, these studies provide the clearest evidence regarding the influence of treatment on specific cognitive processes for spelling and writing (cf. Beeson and Hillis 2001; Beeson and Rapcsak 2002; 2006; Behrmann and Byng 1992; Carlomagno *et al.* 1994; Luzzatti *et al.* 2000; Patterson, 1994).

Agraphia treatment may target central or peripheral components of the writing process. Treatments for central agraphias may be directed toward the lexical-semantic or sublexical spelling routes, or the interaction between these complementary spelling procedures. Lexical-semantic treatments focus on strengthening specific orthographic word forms and their links to meaning, whereas sublexical treatments focus on the links between phonology and orthography (i.e., sound-letter correspondences). Treatments for peripheral agraphias are designed to improve the selection and implementation of graphic motor programs for handwriting. In general, treatments are designed to strengthen damaged processing components and to take advantage of residual abilities. Treatment examples are described below relative to specific agraphia profiles. For a more detailed description of agraphia treatment procedures, see Beeson (2004) or Beeson and Henry (2008).

5 Lexical agraphia (also called surface agraphia)

Lexical agraphia is a central agraphia syndrome that results from damage to the lexical-semantic spelling route. It is characterized by the loss or unavailability of word-specific spelling knowledge so that patients are forced to rely on spelling by a sublexical strategy (i.e., phoneme-to-grapheme conversion) and they tend to spell words as they sound. Relative to the processes depicted in Figure 17.1, lexical agraphia results from damage to the orthographic lexicon and/or the semantic system.

5.1 Distinctive features

Spelling accuracy is strongly influenced by orthographic regularity in that regular words (e.g., *chart*) and nonwords (e.g., *floke*) are spelled better than words with irregular spellings (e.g., *choir*). This profile is shown in Figure 17.2 reflecting the average perform-ance of a group of 8 individuals with lexical agraphia (Rapcsak and Beeson 2004). Attempts to spell irregular words often result in effortful, deliberate attempts to assemble spelling on the basis of sound-to-spelling relationships, and result in phonologically plausible errors, such as *tomb* written as *toom* (see examples in Figure 17.2). Low frequency irregu-lar words are especially vulnerable to error. In addition, the loss of semantic influence on spelling creates difficulties in writing homophonic words that cannot be spelled correctly without reference to the word's meaning (e.g. *dear – deer*).

a. Lexical agraphia spelling profile

b. Example lesion associated with lexical agraphia

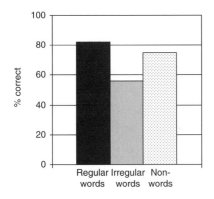

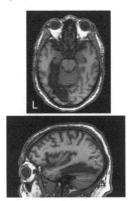

c. Writing to dictation examples (irregular words and nonwords)

chef *Shef* grest *grest*

broom *Brume* mofer *Mofer*

choir *Quire* smode *Smode*

d. Writing to dictation (after treatment)

*Tung (Tongue)** *Clorine (Chlorine)**

Fig. 17.2 a. Spelling profile of a group of individuals with damage to left temporo-occipital regions resulting in lexical agraphia characterized by greater difficulty spelling irregular words relative to regular words and nonwords (from Rapcsak & Beeson, 2004). b. Left inferior tempo-ro-occipital damage in an individual with lexical agraphia. c. Phonologically plausible spelling errors made on irregularly spelled words and correct spelling of nonwords by an individual with lexical agraphia. d. Example of self-detection and correction of spelling errors in an individual with lexical agraphia.

5.2 **Locus of neurological damage**

Lexical agraphia is typically seen following focal damage to left extrasylvian temporo-parieto-occipital regions, as shown in Figure 17.2. The syndrome has also been described in patients with damage to these cortical regions due to neurodegenerative disorders such as Alzheimer's disease (Rapcsak *et al.* 1989; Croisile 1995; Hughes *et al.* 1997; Lambert *et al.* 2007) and semantic dementia (Graham *et al.* 2000).

5.3 **Treatment**

Treatment for lexical agraphia may be directed toward improving the spelling of irregular words and homophones by strengthening word-specific links between the semantic system and the orthographic output lexicon. Another approach involves maximizing the interactive use of residual lexical and sublexical knowledge.

5.3.1 Strengthening interactive use of sublexical and lexical knowledge

- *Goal.* To promote interactive use of residual orthographic and sublexical (i.e., phoneme-grapheme conversion) knowledge.
- *Task example(s).* Using a problem-solving approach, patients are trained to self-detect and correct spelling errors. Individuals with lexical agraphia often have partial word-form knowledge, as well as relative preservation of sublexical spelling abilities that allow them to assemble plausible spellings for difficult words. Interactive treatment procedures guide patients to self-evaluate assembled spellings relative to their residual orthographic knowledge, and then to self-detect and correct errors. An electronic speller that is sensitive to phonologically plausible errors, such as the Franklin Spelling Ace® can be used to check spelling. Such a device offers alternative spellings on the basis of phonological plausibility, allowing patients to select from several written choices.
- *Expectation.* Although this approach involves a compensatory strategy for spelling that is supported by an external aid (the electronic speller), treatment also results in improved spelling accuracy that is not specific to particular words, and improved ability to resolve spelling difficulties (Beeson *et al.* 2000).

5.3.2 Strengthening lexical-semantic spelling abilities

- *Goal.* To strengthen specific orthographic representations for writing and their links to semantic meaning.
- *Task example(s).* Hierarchically ordered tasks with progressively increasing demands on spelling knowledge can be used to strengthen spelling of specific words. Such tasks include, for example, the arrangement of component letters (i.e., anagram task), direct copying of the target word, and delayed copying (after 10–15 second delays) of target words. A critical component of these treatment protocols is repeated, corrected spelling of the targeted words. The re-training of orthography should take place in the presence of pictured stimuli or in response to semantic information about the word,

so that the link between semantics and restored orthographic representations is also strengthened. To emphasize the semantic meaning of written word forms, some researchers have used words with embedded drawings to evoke imagery associated with the target words (de Partz *et al.* 1992).

The direct training of homophone pairs (e.g., *red* vs. *read*) may be approached using word-to-picture matching tasks with corrective feedback stressing the orthographic and semantic differences between words in each pair (Behrmann 1987). These tasks are typically supplemented by repeated copying and writing to dictation of target words, and homework may include looking up target words in the dictionary and copying the spelling and definitions as a means to strengthen links between spelling and meaning.

- *Expectation.* Spelling for targeted words improves, but may have limited generalization to untrained words (Carlomagno *et al.* 1994; de Partz *et al.* 1992; Hillis and Caramazza 1987; Weekes and Coltheart, 1996). However, generalized improvement in spelling irregular words has been shown to result if self-detection and correction of errors improves (Behrmann 1987). Patients with lexical agraphia may be able to abandon sublexical spelling strategies as representations in the orthographic lexicon are restored. Other patients may combine partially spared (or recovered) orthographic knowledge with sublexical procedures to actively resolve spelling difficulties (Beeson *et al.* 2000).

6 Phonological agraphia and deep agraphia

Phonological agraphia and deep agraphia are central agraphia syndromes attributable to dysfunction of the sublexical spelling route. In both syndromes, spelling is accomplished primarily via a lexical-semantic strategy and patients have difficulty spelling nonwords. This profile of markedly impaired nonword spelling relative to real word spelling is shown in Figure 17.3a. In mild cases of phonological agraphia, the spelling of familiar words (both regular and irregular) is relatively spared; however, in most instances the decreased input from phonology to orthography results in reduced spelling accuracy for real words as well (see Figure 17.3). Within the framework of the cognitive model presented in Figure 17.1, phonological and deep agraphia result from damage to sublexical processing (phoneme-grapheme conversion), and deep agraphia reflects additional damage to semantics or the links between semantics and the orthographic lexicon.

6.1 Distinctive features

In both phonological and deep agraphia, spelling accuracy is influenced by lexical-semantic variables (concreteness, word class, and frequency), consistent with reliance on a lexical-semantic strategy. Individuals with deep agraphia also produce semantic errors (e.g. *boy – girl*, and see examples in Figure 17.3), indicating additional impairment of the lexical-semantic spelling route. Other spelling errors may include morphological errors

a. Phonological agraphia spelling profile

b. Example lesion associated phonological agraphia

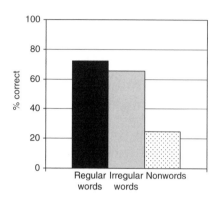

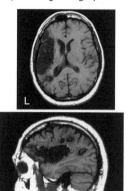

c. Writing to dictation examples (irregular words and nonwords)

colonel   *Colonel*   dusp   *druffs*

yacht   *yacht*   grest   *groese*

blood   *blood*   ked   *theun*

d. Writing to dictation by individual with large left hemisphere lesion shown on the right

shove   *push*

grab   *caught*

Fig. 17.3 a. Spelling profile from a group of individuals with left perisylvian damage and phonological agraphia showing greater difficulty with nonword spelling relative to regular and irregular words (from Henry, Beeson, Stark, & Rapcsak, 2007). b. Left perisylvian damage in an individual with phonological agraphia. c. Spelling examples from an individual with phonological agraphia showing preserved spelling for irregular words and markedly impaired spelling of nonwords. d. Semantic errors characteristic of deep agraphia made by patient with large left perisylvian lesion.

a. Global agraphia spelling profile

b. Example lesion associated with global agraphia

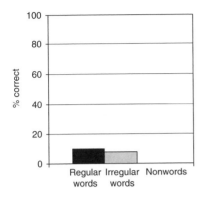

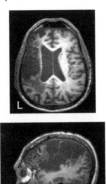

c. Writing to dictation examples (words and nonwords)

stop	58pt	flig	Fome
pillow	Pow	hoach	Home
doubt	Do.	snite	Sine

d. Writing to dictation after treatment for specific words.

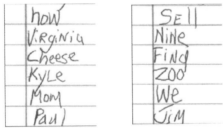

Fig. 17.4 a. Characteristic spelling profile of an individual with global agraphia showing limited residual spelling knowledge for real words and nonwords. b. Large left perisylvian lesion resulting in Broca's aphasia and global agraphia. c. Limited residual spelling knowledge for words and nonwords in patient shown in figure b. d. Spelling of trained words following lexical treatment (in same individual).

(*walked – walking*), functor substitutions (*while – into*), and substitution of unrelated words (*table – shoe*). As in any of the central agraphia syndromes, patients may recall only some of the letters of the target word.

Phonological and deep agraphia have been conceptualized as representing endpoints along a continuum of increasingly severe phonological and lexical-semantic spelling deficits (Rapcsak and Beeson 2000; 2002). Consistent with this view, mild phonological agraphia may have limited clinical significance, whereas deep agraphia typically is associated with severe limitations in written communication. The severity continuum can be extended to include global agraphia in which there is little to no residual ability to write words (see Figure 17.4.).

6.2 Locus of neurological damage

Phonological and deep agraphia are associated with damage to the perisylvian language areas including Broca's area, Wernicke's area, and the supramarginal gyrus (see Figure 17.3). Deep agraphia in patients with extensive left-hemisphere lesions may reflect reliance on the right hemisphere for writing (Rapcsak *et al.* 1991). Global agraphia is also associated with extensive left hemisphere lesions, which may be indistinguishable from those associated with deep agraphia (see Figure 17.4).

6.3 Treatment

Treatment for phonological or deep agraphia may be directed toward improving the availability and use of sublexical spelling procedures. In deep agraphia, additional treatment is required to restore the dysfunctional lexical-semantic spelling route in order to eliminate semantic errors. Similarly, treatment for individuals with global agraphia may be directed toward sublexical or lexical-semantic spelling routes, or both (Greenwald 2004).

6.3.1 Strengthening sublexical spelling abilities

- *Goal.* To re-establish phoneme-grapheme conversion skills so that lexical-semantic spelling procedures are supported by phonological input, and to allow reliance on sublexical spelling procedures as needed. Strengthening of the sublexical spelling route may also help constrain the output of the unstable lexical-semantic spelling route thus reducing the potential for semantic errors in deep dysgraphia. Partial orthographic information derived by the application of sound-to-letter correspondences can also serve to cue the retrieval of word-specific spellings from the orthographic output lexicon.

- *Task example(s).* Sound-to-letter correspondences may be trained directly using structured drill and corrective feedback procedures. This treatment may also require specific training of phonological segmentation of the syllables and individual sounds of words, as well as sound blending skills to assist in self-evaluation of assembled spellings. It is often necessary to establish a corpus of key words (also called "relay words") that can be used to derive orthography from phonology. For example, if the patient is able to say and spell the word *baby* then this will be used as the 'key word' to derive 'b' when spelling other words. Key words may include proper or common nouns that are preserved for a given individual, and are used to retrieve the spelling of consonants and vowels. Retrieval of the first letter or two of a word may serve to cue retrieval of word-specific spellings and to block semantic errors in writing. Given that sound-to-letter correspondences for consonants are more predictable (i.e., less variable) than for vowels, it is best to begin with the establishment of key words for consonants (see suggested sequence in Beeson and Henry, 2008).

◆ *Expectation.* The retraining of sound-letter correspondences typically improves the spelling of regular words, as well as single-word reading (Luzzatti *et al.* 2000). Using a lexical relay strategy, patients have been able to derive the spelling of untrained words, or to cue the recall of orthographic representations (Carlomagno and Parlato 1989; Hatfield 1983; Hillis Trupe 1986; Hillis and Caramazza 1991; 1994). The establishment of key words to derive sound-to-letter correspondences may be a tedious process, however daily homework may be implemented to accomplish the goal efficiently. Self-correction of phonologically plausible spellings may be trained using electronic devices such as a portable computer that provides synthesized speech for communication (Hillis Trupe 1986), or an electronic spell checker that offers possible correct spellings (Beeson *et al.* 2000).

6.3.2 Strengthening (and improving access to) orthographic representations

◆ *Goal.* To strengthen memory for specific orthographic representations, and to strengthen the link between semantic and orthographic representations in patients who make semantic errors as a result of faulty transmission of information between semantics and orthography.

◆ *Task example(s).* A cueing hierarchy for written naming of pictured stimuli may include tasks such as arrangement of component letters (i.e., anagram task) combined with direct and delayed copying of target words (referred to as Anagram and Copy Treatment, or ACT; Beeson 1999; 2004). Lexical treatment may focus exclusively on the repeated copying and recall of targeted words (referred to as Copy and Recall Treatment, or CART; Beeson 1999; 2004). These procedures should include corrective feedback to retrain or stabilize the association between concepts and written words, and to strengthen word-specific spellings. A relatively small set of words (about 5) should be trained to mastery, with additional groups of words subsequently targeted for treatment. When semantic errors arise, corrective feedback may be provided to highlight the distinctive features of the target in contrast to other members of the semantic category. For example, if 'apple' is written for 'orange' the distinguishing features of color would be highlighted for the two semantically related words. Thus, treatment tasks are directed toward semantic specification.

◆ *Expectation.* Improved written naming of targeted items (Aliminosa *et al.* 1993; Beeson 1999; Beeson *et al.* 2002; Hillis 1989; Rapp and Kane 2002). Generalization to untrained items in the same semantic category may also occur when semantic representations are strengthened in addition to reinforcing functional links between semantics and orthographic lexicon (Hillis 1990). Such generalization is not likely in severely agraphic individuals for whom orthographic representations are degraded to the extent that they must be rebuilt one word at a time. However, even globally agraphic individuals can relearn the spellings of specific words, as shown in Figure 17.4d, and single-word writing can provide a much-needed communication modality for individuals with severe impairments of spoken language (Beeson *et al.* 2003; Clausen and Beeson 2003; Robson *et al.* 2001).

The lexical-semantic treatment can also be combined with phonological treatment so that sound-letter correspondences are re-trained in the context of specific regular words targeted for treatment. Such treatment has been shown to result in generalization to spelling of other regular words in some individuals (Kiran 2005). Lexical spelling treatment can also be paired with spoken repetition of target words, which results in improved spoken naming as well as written naming in some individuals (Beeson and Egnor 2006). Another variation of lexical treatment involves training target sentences rather than isolated words; this approach has potential value for communication via email (Greenwald 2004).

7 Graphemic buffer agraphia

Graphemic buffer agraphia reflects impairment of the ability to retain orthographic representations in short-term memory as the appropriate graphic motor programs are selected and implemented. Damage to the graphemic buffer leads to abnormally rapid decay of information relevant to the serial order and identity of stored graphemes. Relative to Figure 17.1, the graphemic buffer is conceptualized as the maintenance of activated graphemes generated by lexical or sublexical spelling routes.

7.1 Distinctive features

Spelling accuracy is notably affected by word length because each additional grapheme increases the demand on limited storage capacity. This word-length effect is shown in Figure 17.5. Spelling is not significantly influenced by lexical status (words vs. nonwords), lexical-semantic features (concreteness, word class, frequency), or orthographic regularity (see Table 17.2). Dysfunction of the buffer results in loss of the information regarding serial order and identity of graphemes leading to letter substitutions, additions, deletions, and transpositions (e.g., *flower – florew*; see examples in Figure 17.5). These errors are observed in all spelling tasks and across all modalities of output (handwriting, typing, oral spelling). Individuals with graphemic buffer agraphia may have relatively good spelling for words up to about four letters, but have increasing difficulty with longer words.

7.2 Locus of neurological damage

Lesion sites in patients with graphemic buffer agraphia have been variable and include left fronto-parietal networks that are implicated in working memory functions (see example lesion in Figure 17.5).

7.3 Treatment

Although it is not clear whether the graphemic buffer itself can be restored, several successful treatments have been documented that reduce spelling errors associated with graphemic buffer agraphia.

7.3.1 Lexical treatment for graphemic buffer impairment

- ◆ *Goal.* To strengthen specific orthographic representations so they are less subject to decay and to develop strategies to compensate for the limited short-term memory for orthographic information.

a. Graphemic buffer agraphia profile before treatment (left) and after treatment (right).

b. Example lesion associated with graphemic buffer agraphia.

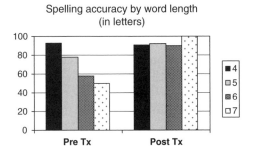

Spelling accuracy by word length (in letters)

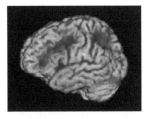

c. Writing to dictation examples in graphemic buffer agraphia (before treatment).

column → colu

member → memer

decent → decett

angry → angya

Fig. 17.5 a. Characteristic spelling profile of an individual with graphemic buffer agraphia showing decreasing accuracy as word length increases (left), and showing improved spelling performance and loss of word-length effect following spelling treatment. b. Surface rendering of cortical damage to frontal and parietal lobes in the individual whose spelling performance is shown in a. c. Example spelling errors from this individual with graphemic buffer agraphia.

- *Task example(s).* Lexical spelling treatments that serve to strengthen orthographic representations, such as ACT and CART (described above), are also appropriate for treatment of graphemic buffer agraphia. Another approach involves the segmentation of long words into shorter units that can be retained in the graphemic buffer. For example, long words that contain embedded words, such as pencil or basement, are selected as target words in order to train the segmentation of words into smaller units. The lexical sub-segments (i.e. embedded words) are underlined as the words are presented for study. Delayed copying of the target word is used to test recall of spelling using the segmentation strategy. Homework involves studying and copying the segmented words.

    Individuals with graphemic buffer impairment also benefit from training to improve their ability to self-detect and correct spelling errors. A search strategy should be used to detect errors, with each word sounded out as it is written to call attention to phonologically implausible misspellings.

- *Expectation.* Improved spelling of words targeted for treatment, so that the word-length effect is diminished (Cardell and Chenery 1999; Hillis 1989; Raymer *et al.* 2003). Ideally, treatment effects generalize to untrained words, confirming improved capacity of the graphemic buffer to maintain the activation of orthographic representations (Rapp and Kane 2002; Rapp 2005; Raymer *et al.* 2003). This effect is demonstrated by the pre-post treatment profile for the patient shown in Figure 17.5 (Ramage *et al.* 1998). Spelling improvement is also likely to generalize to untrained words if self-detection and correction of spelling errors is enhanced (Hillis and Caramazza 1987; Sage and Ellis 2006). Improvement for the spelling of long words that contain embedded short words has been documented for words trained using a segmentation strategy (de Partz, 1995).

8 Allographic writing impairment

Allographic disorders are peripheral writing impairments that reflect the breakdown of procedures by which orthographic representations are mapped onto letter-specific graphic motor programs (see Figure 17.1).

8.1 Distinctive features

Allographic disorders are characterized by an inability to activate or select letter shapes appropriate for orthographic representations held in the graphemic buffer. Patients may have selective difficulty in writing upper- or lower-case letters, or they may produce case-mixing errors (e.g., tAblE). Other patients produce well-formed letter substitution errors that may or may not bear physical similarity to the target (see examples in Figure 17.6a). Allographic disorders are typically observed in the presence of preserved oral spelling.

8.2 Locus of neurological damage

Allographic disorders are usually associated with damage to the left temporo-parieto-occipital region (Rapcsak and Beeson 2002).

8.3 Treatment for allographic disorders

- *Goal.* To improve letter selection and implementation of letter shape, or to develop compensatory strategies to overcome the allographic impairment.
- *Task example(s).* An alphabet card may be used to assist the patient when a model is needed for letter shapes, but treatment may be necessary to achieve effective use of this strategy. If oral spelling is preserved, self-dictation may provide a means to monitor letter selection and promote self-correction of errors. Repeated copying of target words followed by writing the word from memory, and case conversion tasks (e.g., transcoding words written in upper case into words written in lower case) also may be used to strengthen allographic conversion.
- *Expectation.* Use of the self-dictation strategy to prevent and self-correct errors has the potential to support generalized improvement in letter selection (Pound 1996). Repeated copying of target words may result in item-specific improvements, but has the potential for generalized improvement as allographic skills are strengthened.

9 **Apraxic agraphia**

Apraxic agraphia is a peripheral writing impairment caused by damage to graphic motor programs (see Figure 17.1), or it may reflect an inability to translate information contained in these programs into specific motor commands.

9.1 **Distinctive features**

Apraxic agraphia is characterized by poor letter formation that cannot be attributed to sensorimotor (i.e., weakness, deafferentation), basal ganglia (i.e., tremor, rigidity) or cerebellar (i.e., ataxia, dysmetria) dysfunction affecting the writing limb. Errors of letter shape include spatial distortions, stroke additions or deletions, frequently resulting in production of illegible handwriting (see example in Figure 17.6b). Oral spelling is typically preserved and, in some cases, typing remains intact.

9.2 **Locus of neurological damage**

In right-handers, apraxic agraphia is associated with damage to a left-hemisphere cortical network dedicated to the motor programming of handwriting movements. The major functional components of this neural network include posterior-superior parietal cortex

a. Allographic errors on single-letter case conversion task (convert upper to lowercase) and single-word copying task.

R H   though

K K   HROUGF

E O

b. Apraxic agraphia shown on a single-word copying task.

KNIFE

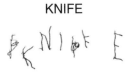

c. Micrographia shown on self-generated sentence composition.

Your blouse is black.

Fig. 17.6 a. Letter selection errors (allographic dysgraphia) following damage to left temporo-parietal cortex due to stroke. b. Apraxic agraphia associated with focal cortical atrophy affecting left superior parietal cortex. c. Micrographia associated with Parkinson disease.

(i.e., the region of the intraparietal sulcus), dorsolateral premotor cortex, and the supplementary motor area (SMA). Callosal lesions in right-handers may be accompanied by unilateral apraxic agraphia of the left hand.

9.3 Treatment for apraxic agraphia

Treatments for apraxic agraphia have not been well documented in the literature, so rehabilitation may be considered on a trial basis. When central spelling processes are intact, it may be possible to circumvent handwriting difficulties by using a keyboard for written communication.

- *Goal.* To re-establish the ability to control hand movements necessary to write letters and words.
- *Task example(s).* When copying skills are relatively preserved, treatment should include repeated direct and delayed copying tasks to re-establish the ability to write letters and words. A task hierarchy should initially include deliberate and feedback-dependent writing to regain graphomotor control, with repeated productions to improve the automaticity of motor execution.
- *Expectation.* Limited evidence of improvement in apraxic agraphia is available. Several sessions of trial therapy should provide an indication of a patient's responsiveness to treatment.

10 Writing disorders due to impaired neuromuscular execution

Damage to motor systems involved in generating graphic innervatory patterns results in defective control of writing force, speed, and amplitude.

10.1 Distinctive features

Writing disorders due to impaired neuromuscular execution reflect the specific underlying disease or locus of damage. In the case of Parkinson's disease, reduced force and amplitude of movements of the hand result in micrographia (see example in Figure 17.6c). In patients with cerebellar dysfunction, movements of the pen may be disjointed and erratic. Patients with hemiparesis often have weakness and spasticity of the hand and limb that markedly impairs their ability to write with the preferred hand.

10.2 Locus of neurological damage

Breakdown of graphomotor control in these neurological conditions suggests that the basal ganglia and the cerebellum, working in concert with dorsolateral premotor cortex and the SMA, are critically involved in the selection and implementation of kinematic parameters for writing movements.

10.3 Treatment

Although there are a variety of causes for impaired graphomotor control, there are relatively few rehabilitation reports. Successful rehabilitation strategies have been demonstrated for some patients with micrographia, and some with hemiparetic writing.

10.3.1 Treatment for micrographia

◆ *Goal.* To increase graphomotor control and thus improve legibility of handwriting.

◆ *Task examples(s).* An increase in letter size may be accomplished by the provision of parallel lines or a template to facilitate the re-calibration of the range and force of movements for writing. Another approach to facilitate increased amplitude of the motor movements for writing in Parkinson disease involves training to self-monitor by thinking "WRITE BIG" (Farley *et al.* 2006). This cognitive approach is analogous (and can be combined with) a voice treatment for Parkinson disease that involves a recalibration of speech effort by training individuals to "THINK LOUD" (Farley *et al.* 2008; Volume 24, pp. 99–114; Ramig *et al.* 2001).

◆ *Expectation.* Improved letter formation is expected with provision of external cues (Oliveira *et al.* 1997). Maintenance of increased letter size is dependent upon establishing adequate self-monitoring abilities so that adjustments are made as legibility declines.

10.3.2 Hemiparetic writing

Writing with the nondominant hand can be mastered with practice, however, several investigators have reported on the use of various prosthetic devices to support the paralyzed right hand during writing.

◆ *Goal.* To learn to write with the paretic dominant hand using a prosthesis.

◆ *Task example(s).* Using a custom-made splint with wheels that allows easy movement across the writing surface, the patient learns to move the affixed pen to form letters.

◆ *Expectation.* Some researchers have found that writing produced with the aided hemiparetic right hand proves to be linguistically superior to that written with the nondominant left hand (Brown *et al.* 1983; Leischner 1983; Lorch 1995).

11 Treatment schedule

11.1 Initiation of treatment

The majority of empirical studies document improved spelling and writing following agraphia treatment initiated long after onset of the neurological damage, suggesting that there is not a "critical period" for the implementation of treatment.

11.2 Frequency of treatment

Reviews of the agraphia treatment literature reveal considerable variability in the frequency of treatment sessions that resulted in improved writing. Treatment schedules range from twice daily to once a week or even biweekly; however, daily practice is often incorporated in the treatment plan and appears to be important for bringing about enduring changes in writing. Therefore, regardless of the frequency of clinical treatment sessions, appropriate daily homework should accompany writing treatment protocols whenever possible.

11.3 **Response to treatment**

The likelihood that a patient will respond to a given treatment is based on several factors including the severity of the deficit, the status of the impaired and residual abilities, the nature of the neurological illness, as well as the patient's motivation. In some cases, patients who appear to have similar functional deficits may respond differently to the same treatment. A patient's response to treatment may further clarify the nature of the writing impairment, and subsequently prompt modification of procedures, determination of the next stage of treatment, or indicate that treatment should be terminated.

12 **Functional impact of treatment**

This chapter has focused on the nature and treatment of the cognitive and sensorimotor processes necessary for written communication. It is important to emphasize that the assessment and treatment of individuals with spoken and written language impairment should be tailored so that the functional needs of the person with agraphia are taken into account. In a clinical context, the selection of skills and specific lexical representations that will be the focus of treatment should be individualized and determined jointly with the patient (see Panton and Marshall 2007, for a recent example). In other words, treatment planning and implementation should be guided by a strong understanding of the cognitive neuropsychology of the impairment, but should also be influenced by the needs, desires, and goals of the individual. Ultimately, the rehabilitation of writing should lead to enhanced communication skills and an improved quality of life.

Acknowledgement

This work was supported by RO1DC007646 and RO1DC008286 from the National Institute on Deafness and other Communication Disorders. The authors thank Sarah Andersen for her assistance in the preparation of this manuscript.

Recommended reading

Beeson PM and Henry ML (2008). Comprehension and production of written words. In R Chapey, ed. *Language intervention strategies in adult aphasia* (5th ed.), pp. 654–688. Lippincott, Williams, and Wilkins, Baltimore, MD.

Beeson PM and Rapcsak SZ (2002). Clinical diagnosis and treatment of spelling disorders. In AE Hillis, ed. *Handbook on adult language disorders: Integrating cognitive neuropsychology, neurology, and rehabilitation*, pp. 101–120. Psychology Press, Philadelphia.

Rapcsak SZ and Beeson PM (2002). Neuroanatomical correlates of spelling and writing. In AE Hillis, ed. *The handbook of adult language disorders: Integrating cognitive neuropsychology, neurology, and rehabilitation*, pp. 71–99. Psychology Press, Philadelphia.

Selective references

Aliminosa D, McCloskey M, Goodman-Schulman R, and Sokol SM (1993). Remediation of acquired dysgraphia as a technique for testing interpretations of deficits. *Aphasiology*, 7(1), 55–69.

Beeson PM (1999). Treating acquired writing impairment: Strengthening graphemic representations. *Aphasiology*, 13(9), 767–785.

Beeson PM (2004). Remediation of written language. *Topics in stroke rehabilitation*, *11*(1), 37–48.

Beeson PM and Egnor H (2006). Combining treatment for written and spoken naming. *Journal of the International Neuropsychological Society*, *12*(6), 816–827.

Beeson PM and Henry M (2008). Comprehension and production of written words. In R Chapey, ed. *Language intervention strategies in aphasia and related neurogenic communication disorders* (5th ed.), 654–688. Lippincott, Williams and Wilkins, Baltimore, MD.

Beeson PM and Hillis AE (2001). Comprehension and production of written words. In R Chapey, ed. *Language intervention strategies in aphasia and related neurogenic communication disorders* (4th ed.), pp. 572–604. Lippincott, Williams and Wilkins, Baltimore, MD.

Beeson PM, Hirsh F, and Rewega MA (2002). Successful single-writing treatment: Experimental analysis of four cases. *Aphasiology*, *16*, 473–491.

Beeson PM and Rapcsak SZ (2002). Clinical diagnosis and treatment of spelling disorders. In AE Hillis, ed. *Handbook on adult language disorders: Integrating cognitive neuropsychology, neurology, and rehabilitation*, pp. 101–120. Psychology Press, Philadelphia.

Beeson PM and Rapcsak SZ (2006). Treatment of alexia and agraphia. In JH Noseworthy, ed. *Neurological therapeutics: Principles and practice* (2nd ed.), pp. 3045–3060. Martin Dunitz, London.

Beeson PM, Rewega MA, Vail S, and Rapcsak SZ (2000). Problem-solving approach to agraphia treatment: Interactive use of lexical and sublexical spelling routes. *Aphasiology*, *14*(5), 551–565.

Beeson PM, Rising K, and Volk J (2003). Writing treatment for severe aphasia: Who benefits? *Journal of speech, language, and hearing research*, *46*(5), 1038–1060.

Behrmann M (1987). The rites of righting writing: Homophone remediation in acquired dysgraphia. *Cognitive Neuropsychology*, *4*(3), 365–384.

Behrmann M and Byng S (1992). A cognitive approach to the neurorehabilitation of acquired language disorders. In D I Margolin, ed. *Cognitive neuropsychology in clinical practice*, pp. 327–350. Oxford University Press, New York.

Brown JW, Leader BJ, and Blum CS (1983). Hemiplegic writing in severe aphasia. *Brain and language*, *19*(2), 204–215.

Cardell EA and Chenery HJ (1999). A cognitive neuropsychological approach to the assessment and remediation of acquired dysgraphia. *Language Testing*, *16*(3), 353–388.

Carlomagno S, Iavarone A, and Colombo A (1994). Cognitive approaches to writing rehabilitation: From single case to group studies. In MJ Riddoch and GW Humphreys, eds. *Cognitive neuropsychology and cognitive rehabilitation*, pp. 485–502. Lawrence Erlbaum Associates, Hillsdale, NJ.

Carlomagno S and Parlato V (1989). Writing rehabilitation in brain-damaged adult aphasics: A cognitive approach. In X Seron **and** G Deloche, eds. *Cognitive approaches in neuropsychological rehabilitation*, pp. 175–209. Lawrence Erlbaum Associates, Hillsdale, NJ.

Clausen N and Beeson PM (2003). Conversational use of writing in severe aphasia: A group treatment approach. *Aphasiology*, *17*(6), 625–644.

Croisile B, Carmoi T, Adeleine P, and Trillet M (1995). Spelling in Alzheimer's disease. *Behavioral Neurology*, *8*, 135–143.

de Partz MP (1995). Deficit of the graphemic buffer: Effects of a written lexical segmentation strategy. *Neuropsychological Rehabilitation*, *5*(1), 129–147.

de Partz MP, Seron X, and Van der Linden M (1992). Re-education of a surface dysgraphia with a visual imagery strategy. *Cognitive Neuropsychology*, *9*(5), 369–401.

Deloche G, Ferrand I, Metz-Lutz MN, *et al.* (1992). Confrontation naming rehabilitation in aphasics: A computerised written technique. *Neuropsychological Rehabilitation*, *2*(2), 117–124.

Ellis AW (1988). Normal writing processes and peripheral acquired dysgraphias. *Language and Cognitive Processes*, *3*(2), 99–127.

Ellis AW (1993). *Reading, writing and dyslexia: A cognitive analysis* (2nd ed.). Lawrence Erlbaum Associates, Hillsdale, NJ.

Farley BG, Derosa S, Koshland GF, Fox CM, and Van Gemmert AWA (2006). Training generalized amplitude across motor systems (training BIG and LOUD) transfers to an untrained handwriting task in early Parkinson disease [Abstract]. *Program no. 655.13, Society for Neuroscience, Atlanta, GA.*

Farley BG, Fox CM, Ramig LO, and McFarland D (in press). Intensive amplitude-specific therapeutic approaches for Parkinson disease: Toward a neuroplasticity-principled rehabilitation model. *Topics in Geriatric Rehabilitation.*

Goodglass H (2001). *Boston diagnostic aphasia examination* (3rd ed.). Lippincott, Williams, and Wilkins, Philadelphia.

Goodman RA and Caramazza A (1984). The Johns Hopkins University dyslexia and dysgraphia batteries. Published in Beeson PM and Hillis AE (2001). Comprehension and production of written words. In R Chapey, ed. *Language intervention strategies in adult aphasia* (4th ed.), 572–604. Lippincott, Williams and Wilkins, Baltimore, MD.

Graham NL, Patterson K, and Hodges JR (2000). The impact of semantic memory impairment on spelling: Evidence from semantic dementia. *Neuropsychologia*, 38(2), 143–163.

Greenwald M (2004). "Blocking" lexical competitors in severe global agraphia: A treatment of reading and spelling. *Neurocase*, 10(2), 156–174.

Hatfield FM (1983). Aspects of acquired dysgraphia and implications for re-education. In C Code and DJ Muller, eds. *Aphasia therapy*. Edward Arnold, London.

Henry ML, Beeson, PM, Stark, AJ, and Rapcsak SZ (2007). The role of left perisylvian cortical regions in spelling. *Brain and language*, 100(1), 44–52.

Hillis Trupe AE (1986). Effectiveness of retraining phoneme to grapheme conversion. In RH Brookshire, ed. *Clinical aphasiology*, pp. 163–171. BRK Publishers, Minneapolis, MN.

Hillis AE (1989). Efficacy and generalization of treatment for aphasic naming errors. *Archives of Physical Medicine and Rehabilitation*, 70(8), 632–636.

Hillis AE (1990). Effects of separate treatments for distinct impairments within the naming process. *Clinical Aphasiology*, 19, 255–265.

Hillis AE and Caramazza A (1987). Model-driven treatment of dysgraphia. In RH Brookshire, ed. *Clinical aphasiology*, pp. 84–105. BRK Publishers, Minneapolis, MN.

Hillis AE and Caramazza A (1991). Mechanisms for accessing lexical representations for output: Evidence from a category-specific semantic deficit. *Brain and language*, 40(1), 106–144.

Hillis AE and Caramazza A (1994). Theories of lexical processing and rehabilitation of lexical deficits. In MJ Riddoch and GW Humphreys, eds. *Cognitive neuropsychology and cognitive rehabilitation*, pp. 449–484. Lawrence Erlbaum Assoicates, Hillsdale, NJ.

Hillis AE and Rapp B. (2004). Cognitive and neural substrates of written language comprehension and production. In MS Gazzaniga, ed. *The cognitive neurosciences III*, pp. 775–787. MIT Press, Cambridge, MA.

Hughes JC, Graham N, Patterson K, and Hodges JR (1997). Dysgraphia in mild dementia of the Alzheimer's type. *Neuropsychologia*, 35(4), 533–545.

Kaplan E, Goodglass H, and Weintraub S (2001). *Boston naming test* (2nd ed.). Lippincott, Williams, and Wilkins, Philadelphia.

Katz, R and Nagy V (1984). An intelligent computer-based spelling task for chronic aphasic patients. In RH Brookshire, ed. *Clinical aphasiology: Conference proceedings*, pp. 159–165. BRK Publishers, Minneapolis, MN.

Kay J, Lesser R, and Coltheart M (1992). *PALPA: Psycholinguistic assessments of language processing in aphasia*. Lawrence Erlbaum Associates Ltd, East Sussex, England.

Kertesz A (1982). *Western aphasia battery (WAB)*. The Psychological Corporation, San Antonio, TX.

Kiran S (2005). Training phoneme to grapheme conversion for patients with written and oral production deficits: A model-based approach. *Aphasiology*, *19*(1), 53–76.

Lambert J, Giffard B, Nore F, de la Sayette V, Pasquier F, and Eustache F (2007). Central and peripheral agraphia in Alzheimer's disease: from the case of August D. to a cognitive neuropsychology approach. *Cortex*, *43*(7), 935–951.

Leischner A (1983). Side differences in writing to dictation of aphasics with agraphia: A graphic disconnection syndrome. *Brain and language*, *18*(1), 1–19.

Lorch MP (1995). Laterality and rehabilitation: Differences in left and right hand productions in aphasic agraphic hemiplegics. *Aphasiology*, *9*(3), 257–271.

Luzzatti C, Colombo C, Frustaci M, and Vitolo F (2000). Rehabilitation of spelling along the sub-word-level routine. *Neuropsychological Rehabilitation*, *10*(3), 249–278.

Oliveira RM, Gurd JM, Nixon P, Marshall JC, and Passingham RE (1997). Micrographia in parkinson's disease: The effect of providing external cues. *British medical journal*, *63*(4), 429–433.

Panton A and Marshall J (2007). Improving spelling and everyday writing after a CVA: A single-case therapy study. *Aphasiology*, *21*(1), 1–20.

Patterson K (1994). Reading, writing, and rehabilitation: A reckoning. In MJ Riddoch and GW Humphreys, eds. *Cognitive neuropsychology and cognitive rehabilitation*, pp. 425–448. Lawrence Eralbaum Associates, Hilsdale, NJ.

Pizzamiglio L and Roberts MM (1967). Writing in aphasia: A learning study. *Cortex*, *3*, 250–257.

Pound C (1996). Writing remediation using preserved oral spelling: A case for separate output buffers. *Aphasiology*, *10*(3), 283–296.

Ramage A, Beeson PM, and Rapcsak SZ (1998). Dissociation between oral and written spelling: Clinical characteristics and possible mechanisms [Abstract]. *Presentation at the Clinical Aphasiology Conference, Ashville, NC, June,*

Ramig LO, Sapir S, Fox C, and Countryman S (2001). Changes in vocal loudness following intensive voice treatment (LSVT) in individuals with Parkinson's disease: A comparison with untreated patients and normal age-matched controls. *Movement disorders*, *16*(1), 79–83.

Rapcsak SZ (1997). Disorders of writing. In LJG Rothi and KM Heilman, eds. *Apraxia: The neuropsychology of action*, pp. 149–172. Psychology Press, Hove, England UK.

Rapcsak SZ, Arthur SA, Bliklen DA, and Rubens AB (1989). Lexical agraphia in Alzheimer's disease. *Archives of Neurology*, *46*(1), 935–951.

Rapcsak SZ, Beeson PM, and Rubens AB (1991). Writing with the right hemisphere. *Brain and language*, *41*(4), 510–530.

Rapcsak SZ and Beeson PM (2000). Agraphia. In LJG Rothi, BA Crosson, and S Nadeau, eds. *Aphasia and language: Theory and practice*, pp. 184–220. Guilford, New York.

Rapcsak SZ and Beeson PM (2002). Neuroanatomical correlates of spelling and writing. In AE Hillis, ed. *The handbook of adult language disorders: Integrating cognitive neuropsychology, neurology, and rehabilitation*. Psychology Press, Philadelphia.

Rapcsak SZ and Beeson PM (2004). The role of left posterior inferior temporal cortex in spelling. *Neurology*, *62*(12), 2221–2229.

Rapp B (2005). The relationship between treatment outcomes and the underlying cognitive deficit: Evidence from the remediation of acquired dysgraphia. *Aphasiology*, *19*(10), 994–1008.

Rapp B and Kane A (2002). Remediation of deficits affecting different components of the spelling process. *Aphasiology*, *16*(4), 439–454.

Raymer A, Cudworth C, and Haley M (2003). Spelling treatment for an individual with dysgraphia: Analysis of generalisation to untrained words. *Aphasiology*, *17*(6), 607–624.

Robson J, Marshall J, Chiat S, and Pring T (2001). Enhancing communication in jargon aphasia: a small group study of writing therapy. *International Journal of Language and Communication Disorders*, *36*(4), 471–488.

Roeltgen DP (1993). Agraphia. In KM Heilman and E Valenstein, eds. *Clinical neuropsychology* (3rd ed.), pp. 63–89. Oxford University Press, New York.

Sage K and Ellis AW (2006). Using orthographic neighbours to treat a case of graphemic buffer disorder. *Aphasiology, 20*(9), 851–870.

Schechter I, Bar-Israel J, Ben-Nun Y, and Bergman M (1985). The phonemic analysis as a treatment method in dysgraphic aphasic patients. *Scandinavian journal of rehabilitation medicine. Supplement, 12,* 80–83.

Schwartz L, Nemeroff S, and Reiss M (1974). An investigation of writing therapy for the adult aphasic: The word level. *Cortex, 10*(3), 278–283.

Sugishita M, Seki K, Kabe S, and Yunoki K (1993). A material-control single-case study of the efficacy of treatment for written and oral naming difficulties. *Neuropsychologia, 31*(6), 559–569.

Tainturier MJ and Rapp B (2001). The spelling process. In B Rapp, ed. *The handbook of cognitive neuropsychology: What deficits reveal about the human mind.* Psychology Press, Philadelphia.

Weekes B and Coltheart M (1996). Surface Dyslexia and Surface Dysgraphia: Treatment Studies and Their Theoretical Implications. *Cognitive Neuropsychology, 13*(2), 277–315.

Wertz RT, Weiss DG, Aten JL, *et al.* (1986). Comparison of clinic, home, and deferred language treatment for aphasia. A Veterans Administration cooperative study. *Archives of Neurology, 43*(7), 653–658.

Chapter 18

Assessment of executive function

Paul W. Burgess

1 Introduction

Executive function is probably the newest of the fields of neuropsychology. Although observations of patients showing symptoms of executive dysfunction have existed for over 150 years, and experimental investigation for at least half of that time, the area has only really become the focus of very widespread investigation in the last 20 years or so. And, since the translation of scientific findings into clinically useful techniques occurs relatively slowly, it is only recently that the experimental findings are being translated into procedures for clinical use. As a consequence, the practising clinician should take special care to follow the latest developments in this fast-moving field.

This chapter does not provide an exhaustive description of all the various tests of executive function available to the neuropsychologist since excellent summaries appear elsewhere (e.g. Lezak 1995; Spreen and Strauss 1998; Alderman and Burgess 2002). Instead, while we do briefly describe some of the most commonly used tests, the principal aim is to outline the philosophy of the assessment procedure, so that the reader can know what to look for, decide which tests to use, and understand the issues surrounding the possible choices of assessment procedure. This information is much harder to come by.

1.1 What are executive functions?

At the most basic level, executive functions are the abilities that enable a person to establish new behaviour patterns and ways of thinking, and to introspect upon them. This is required most in unfamiliar situations, where one doesn't know what to do, or in situations where established ways of behaving are no longer useful or appropriate. As such, the term 'executive function' refers to a whole range of adaptive abilities such as creative and abstract thought, introspection, and all the processes that enable a person to analyse what they want, how they might get it (i.e. form a plan, based often on recollections of past experience), and then carry that plan out. It is also widely accepted that executive functions play a critical part in complex social behaviour, such as understanding how others see us, being tactful, or deceitful. Therefore, there is probably no activity beyond the most routinized and practised ones that does not to some extent involve 'executive processing'. It is not clear, however, how much overlap there is between the processes underlying these various abilities. Identifying the processes and working out how they may relate to each other is the current focus of much exciting research, but we are just in the early stages.

These abilities are collectively referred to as 'executive functions' because it is believed that the region of the brain that supports them (the frontal lobes) operates in a 'supervisory' (Shallice 1988) or 'executive' (Pribram 1973) capacity over the rest of the brain. For many researchers, 'executive function' is synonymous with 'frontal lobe function'. However, the latter term is of little use to the practising clinician for two reasons.

- ◆ What is important clinically is the function that is impaired rather than the brain region that is damaged.

- ◆ Recent advances in cognitive neuroscience show that, whilst the frontal lobes play an important part in executive functions such as planning and organization of behaviour, the frontal lobe contribution is just one part of a wider network of brain involvement.

In the 1980s there was a move away from discussing 'frontal lobe function' towards use of the terms 'executive function' and 'dysexecutive symptoms' (to describe executive function impairments) in order to reflect this more function-oriented focus.

1.2 Symptoms of executive dysfunction

The 20 most commonly reported symptoms of executive dysfunction are shown in Table 18.1. This is by no means an exhaustive list, however, and there are also many other, generally less frequently encountered dysexecutive symptoms (e.g. utilization behaviour, alien hand sign).

Recent evidence suggests that at least some executive abilities may be impaired in neurological patients when others are not. The term 'dysexecutive syndrome', which is commonly used as shorthand to refer to executive function impairments, can therefore be misleading since it suggests that symptoms are invariably seen together. This is not the case. However, it is equally true to say that in normal clinical practice it is less common to see people with isolated problems than with clusters of them. There are probably two main reasons.

- ◆ Even apparently quite localized brain dysfunction is unlikely to affect only one brain system and, because of the highly interconnected nature of the brain, dysfunction in one region in any case can probably cause disruptions in others.

- ◆ Some researchers contend that there are some executive processes that are used in many situations (e.g. Duncan *et al.* 2000), e.g. those that govern attention and arousal, as well as others that are required in more specific situations, e.g. those requiring multitasking (Burgess *et al.* 2000).

1.3 The impact of executive dysfunction on everyday life

Even apparently quite mild deficits of executive function can have a devastating impact upon an individual's effectiveness in everyday life and their relationships with others. A key reason for this is the attributions that observers make about the causes of the behaviour they see. Many dysexecutive symptoms mimic exaggerated versions of behaviour that are sometimes seen in healthy people and therefore can easily be misunderstood.

Table 18.1 Frequency of 20 of the most common symptoms of executive dysfunction (adapted from Burgess and Robertson, 2002)

Symptom	Percentage reporting problem	
	Patients	Carers
Poor abstract thinking	17	21
Impulsivity	22	22
Confabulation	5	5
Planning	16	48
Euphoria	14	28
Poor temporal sequencing	18	25
Lack of insight	17	39
Apathy	20	27
Disinhibition (social)	15	23
Variable motivation	13	15
Shallow affect	14	23
Aggression	12	25
Lack of concern	9	26
Perseveration	17	26
Restlessness	25	28
Can't inhibit responses	11	21
Know–do dissociation	13	21
Distractibility	32	42
Poor decision-making	26	38
Unconcern for social rules	13	38

Take, for example, confabulation. All ordinary, healthy people at some time or another tell lies. This is a common event. So when a patient says something that is quite obviously untrue, it is easy for observers to assume that the patient is deliberately lying. Of course, this is not the case. Confabulation is caused by a problem with the cognitive control processes that govern recollection, leading to memories and thoughts becoming jumbled up with each other (see Burgess and Shallice 1996*b*). The patient can't help it. However, if one doesn't know this and has not seen confabulation before (as most spouses or relatives of neurological patients will not have), it is easy to make this mistake, and get irritated with the patient for 'lying' or 'making things up'. The same point can be made about many of the dysexecutive symptoms shown in Table 18.1. Especially difficult to live with are the social changes such as lack of concern or increased aggressive reactions to troublesome situations. Relatives or partners might quite justifiably claim that these 'personality changes' mean that the patient 'is no longer the person she/he used to be'.

The non-social changes can also be a severe handicap, especially in the work situation. A good example is those patients who show relatively isolated multitasking deficits.

These people may still be extremely intellectually gifted, with little or no (retrospective) memory, language, or other problems, and some are even very competent on most tests of executive function. However, for all reported cases in the literature, their return to work has been tragically unsuccessful, with employers complaining of tardiness and disorganization (see Burgess 2000 for review). Common complaints from the employers of these cases are that the patient starts many jobs but never completes any of them, and/or shows no awareness of the relative priorities of different jobs, treating the most trivial (e.g. the sticky tape needs replacing) as equally pressing as the most important (e.g. delivering an important letter to the company chairman). It is simply very difficult to work with someone who shows these sorts of symptoms—certainly more so in many contexts—than with a more predictable and obvious handicap (e.g. a language or visual impairment) for which compensatory methods exist and that can be readily understood by co-workers.

A further complication of executive dysfunction is that the associated problems are exactly the kinds of problems that interfere with learning new ways of behaving, or prevent patients from benefiting from therapy aimed at ameliorating other sorts of problems (e.g. physiotherapy). For this reason, combined with the typical lack of insight that accompanies these symptoms, dysexecutive problems present a real challenge for rehabilitation. (For further information see Burgess and Robertson, 2002.)

1.4 Prognosis for executive deficits

One of the reasons why the functions of the frontal lobes were described by a leading researcher over 30 years ago as a 'riddle' was that some apparently severe symptoms could resolve well in time, whereas other apparently milder problems could persist. This is just as true today: symptoms such as confabulation typically (but not always) resolve quite well on their own within a few weeks or months, but others (e.g. multitasking problems) when they persist beyond the initial stage of medical trauma are often best considered permanent handicaps requiring intervention before improvement will occur. We still do not understand why this should be the case, and this is an underresearched area. The wise clinician will freely admit this lack of knowledge to relatives, carers, or the patients themselves. There should be no embarrassment in not knowing when there is nothing to know. Freely admitting that no one knows the answer has the advantage of removing the temptation to speculate whilst also avoiding seeming obscure or evasive.

2 Choosing the assessment approach

The ideal assessment would obviously attempt to assess all of the symptoms shown in Table 18.1, plus the less common signs of executive dysfunction (e.g. utilization behaviour, alien hand sign, subtle attentional changes). However, this is impractical in most clinical settings, and formal assessment measures do not yet exist for many of the symptoms. Moreover, relatively little is known about what many of the tests shown to be sensitive to frontal lobe lesions are actually measuring in these cases. (This is a theoretical problem that is far more complex than it seems at first.) One is left therefore with five choices of how to proceed:

- *Time*. Administer the greatest number of tests possible in the available time.
- *Psychometrics*. Base your choice of measures on test-based factors such as ease of use and cost, psychometric validity, how widely the tests are used, how often they have been used with a particular client group, etc.
- *Expectation*. Base assessment on what you expect to find, given knowledge of the medical history and/or previous assessments.
- *Observation*. Base assessment on symptoms already observed by carers or relatives.
- *Theory*. Adopt a particular theoretical stance and choose the tests that make most the sense according to it.

These methods are of different merit. Remarkably, perhaps, none is entirely meritless and, in practice, most experienced clinicians develop their own assessment procedure based on a personal weighting of these methods. In principle, this is appropriate. Too often, however, this choice has merely evolved haphazardly over time. Instead, the choice should be made deliberately and with good justification. If the same battery of tests is given to all clients, this choice should be reviewed regularly. The clinician should always be able to clearly articulate and defend the reasons behind his/her choice of procedures.

In practice, I have observed a further method of determining the assessment procedure: to just use whichever tests are most familiar and/or everyone else is using. This method might in some circumstances be most appropriate for students, but it would be dubious indeed for a qualified clinician, and this method will be considered no further.

Let us consider the legitimate approaches in turn.

2.1 Method 1. Time

This is not as unjustifiable as it might at first seem, for two reasons.

- As mentioned above, we know little about many of the traditional tests of executive function (e.g. Wisconsin Card Sorting Test, Stroop Test) or what they measure.
- The ecological validity of these tests (i.e. the extent to which they are indicators of real-world impairment) has not yet been clearly established. (It does, however, seem at present that the more modern tests designed to be more like real-life activities are often—but not always—better in this respect.)

Thus one solution to this problem is just to give as many tests as one can in the available time, in the hope of covering as many possible functions/situations as possible. The disadvantages of this approach are the following.

- As the number of tests administered rises, so does the likelihood of a false-positive result (unless the clinician statistically corrects for the number of tests administered, which is uncommon).

◆ Unless the clinician has at least some hypothesis about what he/she is measuring, it is difficult to know what might be usefully concluded from a task failure. Clinically, it is rarely sufficient to just baldly state 'this person failed this test', without further interpretation.

2.2 Method 2. Psychometrics

All people involved in the administration of psychometric tests should have at least some basic grounding in psychometric theory. This allows them to understand the relative merits of the measurement aspects of different tests, and to select accordingly. In particular, there may be times when some aspect of the psychometric dynamic of relative tests might strongly influence the clinician's choice, e.g. where parallel forms are required, where there is to be repeated testing using the same measure, or where various different people may make assessments on the same person.

In general, however, it is harder in the field of executive function to use psychometric values (e.g. test–retest and interrater reliability; interitem consistency, etc.) as a guide to test choice. This is because the tests are often measuring abilities such as response to novelty or strategy formation. These can subvert the theory behind traditional psychometrics, and render the values a poor guide to a test's actual clinical utility (see Burgess 1997 for more detail). In addition, there is another problem that is applicable to the use of most psychometric tests with pathological populations. This is that the construct validity of a task (i.e. the extent to which you are measuring what you intend to measure) alters with level of performance. Overall, these matters present a highly complex theoretical problem for someone trying to base their choice of assessment procedure upon psychometric values, especially when they are derived from the performance of a different population than the one you intend to test (e.g. healthy control subjects). In summary, *all other things being equal*, one should choose the test with the best psychometric validity. However, all other things are unlikely to often be equal.

2.3 Method 3. Expectation

If we knew more about what executive tests measure, this would probably be the most frequently appropriate single method. For success it does, however, rely upon at least four variables:

◆ The quality of the information, case history, or previous assessment that you have received.

◆ Your knowledge of the test's performance in different populations.

◆ How the test is affected by a variety of background variables (e.g. education, culture, age, etc.).

◆ The ecological validity of the task (i.e. how strongly you can make a prediction that your test measures the function that was observed to be impaired elsewhere).

This method therefore requires a high degree of knowledge and clinical judgement. This requirement should decrease as our knowledge of the performance of the tests and what they measure increases.

2.4 Method 4. Observation

Although the examinee should always be asked about the symptoms they notice since it is important to assess the patient's degree of insight and knowledge about their condition, it is unwise to base your assessment upon this report. Self-report of dysexecutive difficulties is notoriously inaccurate (e.g. Burgess and Robertson 2002). However, the reports of carers, relatives, or other people who know the examinee well can be very useful indeed, and should always be sought if possible.

The best witnesses are usually those who knew the person premorbidly, since *change* in behaviour is usually more instructive than comparisons of current behaviour with some population norm. This is important for executive function assessment since the behaviours under examination are often at the extreme of the range of behaviours that might be observed occasionally in the normal population. This is one of the important ways in which executive function assessment differs from assessment of other functions in neuropsychology. In, say, language assessment, or assessment of visuospatial skills, pathological symptoms (e.g. jargon aphasia, neglect) are rarely or never seen in the healthy normal population. However, many of the symptoms of executive dysfunction are seen occasionally in the healthy population, albeit perhaps under special circumstances, and in a milder form (e.g. confabulation (Burgess and Shallice 1996*b*), impulsivity, disinhibition). Since, therefore, it is often the extremity (i.e. severity, frequency) of the behavioural sign rather than its type that is at issue, it is important if possible to have an observer 'baseline' with which to compare current behaviour.

Once the clinician has collected the observations, however, he/she is faced with the challenge of interpreting them for the purposes of the examination procedure. There is no substitute for experience and knowledge in this respect. The job is made easier by some of the newer assessment procedures that are more like real-world situations, since one can ask the observer about situations in which the examinee experiences problems and then choose the closest test situations. However, for experienced examiners, more experimentally derived procedures also have their merits.

- Often the theory of how they work is more developed.
- They may be more specific in what they measure.
- The link with damage to certain brain regions may be more direct.

These factors can add up to a strong advantage if you have a clear idea what it is that you are looking for and have experience in interpreting the observations of others.

2.5 Method 5. Theory

All assessment and treatment has to start with some theory of what it is that is being studied, even if this is very basic. The assessment implications of all theories of executive function cannot be covered here. However a few of the leading ones will be selected as examples.

2.5.1 Single-process theories

These hold that damage to a single process or system is responsible for a number of different dysexecutive symptoms. An example is the theory of Cohen (e.g. Cohen *et al.* 1990). This holds that prefrontal cortex is used to represent 'context information', which is the 'information necessary to mediate an appropriate behavioural response' (Cohen *et al.* 1998, p. 196). Two functions of the prefrontal cortex may be effected by this system—active memory and behavioural inhibition—with both functions reflecting the operation of the context layer under different task conditions. Under the conditions of response competition the context module plays an inhibitory role by supporting the processing of task relevant information. But, when there is a delay until the execution of a response, the context module plays a role in memory by maintaining that information over time.

Following this theory, clinical assessment would include tests of response suppression (e.g. Hayling Test, Stroop) plus tests with a 'working memory' component (e.g. Wisconsin Card Sorting Test (WCST), Cambridge Neuropsychological Test Automated Battery (CANTAB) spatial working memory test).

2.5.2 Construct-led theories

Construct-led theories are those that propose a construct (i.e. a theoretical ability) such as 'working memory' or 'fluid intelligence' as a key function of the frontal lobe executive system.

Working memory theories Two leading theorists in this area are Petrides and Goldman-Rakic.

- Petrides believes that the mid-dorsolateral prefrontal region (areas 9 and 46) supports a brain system 'in which information can be held on-line for monitoring and manipulation of stimuli' (Petrides 1998, p. 106). The mid-ventrolateral region, however, is used in explicit encoding and retrieval of information. Obvious suggested tests are therefore Petrides and Milner's (1982) Self-Ordered Pointing Test, and other memory tests that particularly stress explicit encoding and retrieval (e.g. recall of complex figures such as the Rey figure; recall of short stories or word lists).

- Goldman-Rakic's position is different in that she believes that the various different frontal lobe regions all perform a similar role in working memory, but that each processes a different type of information (Goldman-Rakic 1995). She suggests that dysfunction of this system can cause a variety of deficits on e.g. verbal fluency and Stroop tasks due to an inability to use working memory to initiate the correct response.

Duncan's theory of '*g*' (e.g. Duncan *et al.* 1995, 2000) Duncan suggests that the principal purpose of the frontal executive system is to support a single function that is used in many situations, called 'fluid intelligence' or Spearman's g. Of the commercially available tests, he believes Cattell's Culture-Fair Test and (by implication from his studies) the Six Element Test of the Behavioural Assessment of the Dysexecutive Syndrome (BADS) measure this function.

2.5.3 Multiple-process theories

These propose that the frontal lobe executive system consists of a number of components that typically work together in everyday actions.

Fuster's temporal integration framework (Fuster 1997) This holds that the frontal lobe executive system performs three functions:

- working memory;
- set attainment;
- inhibition.

Suggested tasks are, therefore, WCST or CANTAB working memory tests, Brixton Test, Hayling Test, or Stroop.

Stuss's anterior attentional functions (e.g. Stuss *et al.* 1995; Stuss and Alexander 2000) The focus of Stuss *et al.*'s theoretical approach is attention. They propose seven different attentional functions. The closest clinical test is probably the Test of Everyday Attention (TEA).

Shallice's supervisory attentional system (e.g. Norman and Shallice 1986; Shallice 1988; Shallice and Burgess 1991*a,b*, 1996; Burgess *et al.* 2000) This is one of the longest established and best known theories. In this model, the frontal lobes support a cognitive system known as the supervisory attentional system (SAS). This plays a part in at least eight different processes, each of which may be impaired in isolation:

- working memory;
- monitoring;
- rejection of schema;
- spontaneous schema generation;
- adoption of processing mode;
- goal-setting;
- delayed intention marker realization;
- episodic memory retrieval.

On these grounds, and as the result of a study that examined the relationship between symptoms in everyday life and executive test performance, Burgess *et al.* (1998) recommend that *at the very least* an assessment of a dysexecutive patient should include the following.

- A general measure of inhibitory abilities (e.g. Hayling Test; however this function is probably also measured to varying degrees by many other tests, e.g. verbal fluency, Trail-Making).
- Measures of executive memory abilities both in the short-term (i.e. working memory tests) and long-term (i.e. accuracy of episodic recollection). Suggested tests would be WCST; Brixton Test; story, figure, and word list recall; and also observation of real-life ability to recollect events accurately.

- A measure of multitasking ability, e.g. Six Element Test from the BADS; Multiple Errands Test (Shallice and Burgess 1991*a*; Burgess *et al.* 1996*b*, 2000; Alderman *et al.* in press).

However, Burgess *et al.* (1998) make two further points.

- Neuropsychological tests of executive function do not measure well many of the emotional changes that can be part of the dysexecutive syndrome (e.g. euphoria, apathy). The formal tests need therefore to be supplemented by more general observation, preferably using a structured or semistructured interview, perhaps based around a symptom checklist or questionnaire such as the Dysexecutive Questionnaire (DEX; Burgess *et al.* 1996*a*) from the BADS test battery.

- Since many impairments can be seen in isolation, a true assessment will be as comprehensive as possible—the list above could be considered only as a basic screening assessment. For instance, one might also wish to supplement it routinely with measures of planning (e.g. Zoo-Map test of the BADS; abstract reasoning and judgement (e.g. proverb interpretation, cognitive estimates, or similar); initiation (e.g. Hayling Test section 1); problem-solving and strategy formation (e.g. Action Program and Key Search tests from the BADS); rule attainment and following (e.g. Brixton Test).

2.5.4 Single-symptom theories

These are theories of specific symptoms, such as confabulation (e.g. Burgess and Shallice 1996*b*; Burgess and McNeil 1999) or multitasking deficits (e.g. Burgess *et al.* 2000). In general, however, there are not tests specifically marketed to measure single symptoms. Clinicians therefore typically just make observations, or copy an experimental method.

3 Types of executive function test

The perfect test for most clinical applications would probably have the following characteristics (in addition to those that would be desirable in any psychometric test):

- perfect, and known correspondence to everyday life impairment;
- strong proven link to operation of one particular brain region or system;
- well understood psychometric dynamics;
- comprehensive theory as to what the test measures.

However as can be inferred from the discussions above, there is currently no test that could be said to have all these characteristics. Take for instance, probably the best-known executive test: the Wisconsin Card Sorting Task (WCST). This test was not originally designed for use with neurological patients (Berg 1948). Impairment of dorsolateral prefrontal lesioned patients was first demonstrated by Milner (1963), but there are few replications of this finding (see Stuss *et al.* 2000 for possible explanations). More positively, there is some early evidence about its relationship with everyday life impairments (Burgess *et al.* 1998), and there are various theories about what the test measures.

Similarly, the Stroop test, although widely used for the assessment of executive functions in neurological patients, was not designed with this purpose in mind. Moreover, in my opinion there is only one convincing demonstration of its sensitivity to frontal lesions (Perret 1974), and one convincing failure to replicate (Shallice 1982). There is disagreement about what the test measures (see MacLeod 1991), although there are some theories that have been made relevant to the assessment of executive functions, as outlined above. Moreover, there is little information that would allow one to predict from test impairment what deficits in real life might be expected.

Some of these shortcomings no doubt stem from the fact that the procedures were not designed with neuropsychological assessment in mind. In recognition of this situation, there have recently been tests invented for this specific purpose (e.g. BADS battery, Hayling and Brixton tests, CANTAB battery). Due to their newness, these tests have not, of course, yet been thoroughly put to the test of time (although there has been considerable work using the CANTAB in different populations), and it is possible that they will turn out not to fulfil the criteria above in any greater fashion than the older tests. However they do start with the advantage of being purpose-built.

3.1 Specificity and sensitivity

The *specificity* of a task refers to the degree to which a test measures the particular process or function of interest compared with other processes or functions that are not intended to be measured. The *sensitivity* of a task in this context refers to the degree to which any cognitive impairment can cause impairment on the task. There is some evidence that the different executive tasks differ greatly along these dimensions. For instance, the Cognitive Estimates Test does not seem to be particularly sensitive to any kind of neurological dysfunction *per se* (Burgess *et al.* 1998), but it does show consistent correlations with specific symptoms (e.g. fantastic confabulation), which suggests that it has good specificity. By contrast, the WCST appears to be more generally sensitive to cognitive decline, as well as to dysexecutive problems (e.g. Stuss *et al.* 2000). There is not room here for a discussion of the specificity and sensitivity of every test. However the clinician should consider matching the test to the clinical question under consideration. Using the current examples, for instance, the Cognitive Estimates test is probably not the best choice as a general screening measure for dysexecutive problems. However, its ecological validity is excellent and, if the clinical question instead concerns whether a patient has a specific executive problem rather than more general cognitive dysfunction, then the test is well suited to that application.

In many clinical settings the ideal test would have a combination of both characteristics, i.e.:

- sensitivity to a range of executive problems;
- relative insensitivity to non-executive cognitive impairments.

This compromise is generally closest in those tests that have been shown to be impaired in group studies of frontally lesioned patients compared with patients whose lesions were elsewhere in the brain (e.g. Hayling and Brixton Tests, Burgess and Shallice 1996*a,c*, 1997).

Some tests appear to be both locally specific and more generally sensitive. For instance, impairment on the Six Element Test (a test of multitasking ability; see below) has been demonstrated in neurological patients with frontal lobe lesions who show no impairment on other executive function tests (e.g. Shallice and Burgess 1991a). However, this type of test is also more generally sensitive to executive (and to a lesser extent non-executive) impairments (Burgess *et al.* 2000). This combination of characteristics can make a test particularly useful in a wide range of settings. However, once a patient has failed a task, it generally requires that one should consider performances on other tasks in its interpretation (using this example, for instance, to find out whether the locus of the problem is a pure multitasking failure or, for instance, a more basic memory problem that prevents the examinee from learning the task rules).

3.2 **Summary**

Assessment of executive functions is probably the most technically and theoretically complex aspect of neuropsychological assessment. Executive test scores should always be administered in the context of a wider neuropsychological assessment since executive test performance can be affected by dysfunction in other cognitive systems (e.g. memory, etc.). The clinician's choice of tests and procedure should be made with careful consideration of the factors outlined above and, if not made on a case-by-case basis, they should be reviewed regularly.

Executive function as a subject area is one of the newest and fastest developing in neuropsychology, and there are still many gaps in our knowledge. However, since even relatively mild executive dysfunction has repeatedly been shown to greatly affect the long-term outcome of rehabilitation and recovery, any neuropsychological assessment is not complete without at least a basic evaluation of executive function abilities. New procedures and tests are appearing at a rapid rate. The assessment professional would therefore be wise to be circumspect when interpreting executive test scores, and make every attempt to benefit from the latest developments in the area as they appear.

4 **Description of some key tests**

There are many tests of executive function. A brief description of a few of the most commonly used is given in Sections 4.1–4.11. However, lack of inclusion in this list should not be seen as a failure of endorsement. There are a number of tests (e.g. the Test of Everyday Attention; Rey Complex Figure Recall) that could be seen as falling under the heading of 'executive function' but that have not been included since they also fall under other topic areas (e.g. attention, memory). There are also other methods that combine tests or aspects of them to increase specificity or sensitivity (e.g. the Frontal Lobe Score, see Ettlin *et al.* 2000; Wildgruber *et al.* 2000) and are worthy of consideration. Excellent summaries of the range of executive tests can be found in Lezak (1995) and Spreen and Strauss (1998) and, where publisher information etc. is not given below, it can be found in these texts. It should be borne in mind that dysexecutive problems demonstrate themselves as impairment on a wide range of neuropsychological tests, not just those specifically aimed at measuring 'executive function', so the *manner* of failure on a test can also be instructive.

4.1 Behavioural Assessment of the Dysexecutive Syndrome (BADS)

- *Original reference.* Wilson *et al.* (1998). Commercially available from various distributors worldwide. For details contact the Thames Valley Test Company, 7–9 The Green, Flempton, Suffolk, IP28 6EL UK. (tvtc@msn.com)

- *Test description.* The BADS is a test battery aimed at predicting everyday difficulties arising from the dysexecutive syndrome. It contains six tests (and a questionnaire (the DEX) that has two versions, one to be filled in by the patient and one by an independent rater, which can be used as the basis for a semistructured interview). The six different tests (Rule Shift, Action Program, Key Search, Temporal Judgement, Zoo-Map, and Six Elements Test) are designed to have high ecological validity, and scores from the tests can be combined to give an overall executive function measure that can be compared with measures of cognitive functioning.

4.2 Cambridge Neuropsychological Test Automated Battery (CANTAB)

- *Original reference.* Robbins *et al.* (1994).

- *Test description.* A computerized battery of 13 tests that evaluate more than executive functions alone. However, it contains two tests that are particularly oriented towards executive function assessment: ID/ED Shift and the Stockings of Cambridge test, which are developments of the WCST and Tower of London (Shallice 1982) tests, respectively.

4.3 Cognitive estimates test

- *Original reference.* Shallice and Evans (1978).

- *Test description.* Patients are asked 15 questions about everyday magnitudes where no rote knowledge or routine method seems available. Axelrod and Millis (1994) issued a shorter version (10 questions) adapted to the North-American population.

- *Scoring method.* Answers rated as normal, quite extreme, extreme, and very extreme according to how much they vary from the estimates of a control group.

4.4 Hayling and Brixton tests

- *Original references*
  — Hayling: Burgess and Shallice (1996*c*).
  — Brixton: Burgess and Shallice (1996*a*). Commercially available from various distributors worldwide; for details contact the Thames Valley Test Company, 7–9 The Green, Flempton, Suffolk, IP28 6EL UK. (tvtc@msn.com)

◆ *Test description.*

— Hayling: Patients have to complete 30 sentences from which the last word was omitted. In the first half (initiation condition), they complete the sentences with a word that makes sense. In the second half (inhibition condition) they have to supply a word that makes no sense in the context of the sentence (e.g. 'London is a very busy *banana*').

— Brixton: A nonverbal test of set attainment and rule detection. The patient is shown a 56-page stimulus book, one page at a time. All pages contain 10 circles in the same basic array (see Fig. 18.1(a)). Only one circle is filled on each page and the patient has to predict where the next filled position will be, based on what they have seen in the previous pages.

◆ *Scoring method.*

— Hayling: Sum of all response latencies for part 1; sum of all response latencies and error score for part 2.

— Brixton: Total number of errors (maximum is 54).

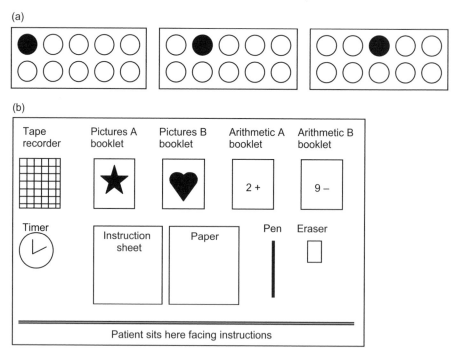

Figure 18.1 (a) Sample sequence from the Brixton Test. Here one might reasonably expect the filled circle to be at number 4 on the next page (on the testing booklet, circles are numbered from 1 to 10 on each array to make it easier to refer to their position). (b) Materials used for the Six Elements Test.

4.5 **Multiple Errands Test (MET)**

♦ *Original reference.* Shallice and Burgess (1991*a*).

♦ *Test description.* The test with probably the most obvious ecological validity in current use, this is a formalized version of a shopping task. It is conducted in a real shopping centre or mall, so a specific version has to be adapted to the local circumstances available to the clinician. There is also a version that can be carried out in most hospital environments (Knight *et al.* 2002). Appears to be highly sensitive both to brain damage in general, and to specific dysexecutive problems. Details of how to set up the test for your own local environment can be obtained from: Dr Nick Alderman, Consultant Clinical Neuropsychologist, Kemsley Brain Injury Rehabilitation Centre, St. Andrew's Hospital, Billing Road, Northampton, NN1 5DG, UK. (See also Alderman *et al.* 2003.)

♦ *Scoring method.* A number of different types of error are collected: rule-breaks; social rule-breaks; interpretation failures; inefficiencies; task failures.

4.6 **Proverbs test**

♦ *Original reference.* Gorham (1956).

♦ *Test description.* Patients are asked to recognize and interpret a certain number of proverbs (e.g. 'Rome wasn't built in a day') in two different ways. In the first part, they must provide free verbal interpretations of each proverb. In the second part, they must choose one out of four possible answers provided for each proverb.

♦ *Scoring method.* Free verbal interpretations are scored on a 3-point scale according to their degree of 'concreteness'. In the multiple-choice test, there is only one correct response for each proverb (the other three are either wrong, partial, or concrete).

4.7 **Six Elements Test (SET)**

♦ *Original reference.* Shallice and Burgess (1991*a*).

♦ *Test description.* A modified version of this multitasking test for general clinical use (Burgess *et al.* 1996*b*) is commercially available as part of the BADS battery (see Section 4.1). Additionally, there are other versions of this test that have recently been developed by groups in Cambridge and Toronto, plus more extensive versions by the original authors (Burgess *et al.* 2000). Patients have 10 minutes to do three tasks (dictation, arithmetic, and picture naming; see Fig. 18.1(b)). Each task has two parts, called A and B. The two parts of each task cannot be carried out one after the other (for instance, dictation A immediately followed by dictation B, or vice versa). There are more items in the six tasks than can possibly be completed in the time allowed, so the aim is to do a bit of each part of each task within the 10 minutes and thus patients have to plan their time accordingly. The original, and some later versions also use weightings for certain items which gives them particular significance, but this is not used in the most widely used BADS subtest version of the SET.

- *Scoring method.* In the BADS version, a profile score is calculated from the number of tasks attempted minus the number of tasks where rule breaks were made. A further point is deducted if the maximum time on any one task is more than 271 seconds.

4.8 Stroop test

- *Original reference.* Stroop (1935).
- *Test description.* In the Victoria version, patients are presented with three cards, each with a different stimulus: 24 coloured dots where one is asked to name their colour; 24 common words where one has to name the colour of the ink in which the words are printed; and 24 colour names, where the task is again to name the colour of the ink. There are other versions, for instance, using an additional card on which words are printed in black ink. Another version includes only two cards, both with colour names printed in different colour inks (first card, names are read; second card, the ink colour is named).
- *Scoring method.* For each card, the time to complete the task and the number of errors are recorded. The amount of time required for the interference card (name ink colour) is typically compared to the amount of time required in the other conditions(s).

4.9 Trail making test

- *Original reference.* Originally, the test was one of the Performance subtests of the US Army Individual Test Battery, published in 1944. Earliest use with neurological patients: Armitage (1946).
- *Test description.* In part A, examinees draw lines to connect consecutively numbered circles from 1 to 25 on a sheet of paper. Part B follows the same principle but this time the lines drawn must connect consecutively numbered and lettered circles (also 25 circles) by alternating between the two types of sequences (see Fig. 18.2(a)). There are various forms of this test.
- *Scoring method.* There is a separate score for Part A and Part B, which is the amount of seconds taken to complete each task.

4.9 Verbal fluency test

- *Original reference.* Thurstone (1938).
- *Test description.* Patients are asked to say as many words as they can, beginning with the letters F, A, and S (usually 1 minute per letter). They are asked not to give proper nouns or alternative forms of the same word (e.g. 'made' and 'making'). There are many alternate versions: written; semantic categories (e.g. animals); different letters.
- *Scoring method.* Total number of correct words; number of correct words for each letter.

4.11 Wisconsin card sorting test

- *Original reference.* Milner (1963). (Originally invented by Berg 1948.)
- *Test description.* The patients sort 128 response cards under four stimulus cards according to colour, form, and number (see Fig. 18.2(b)). The aim is to work out the

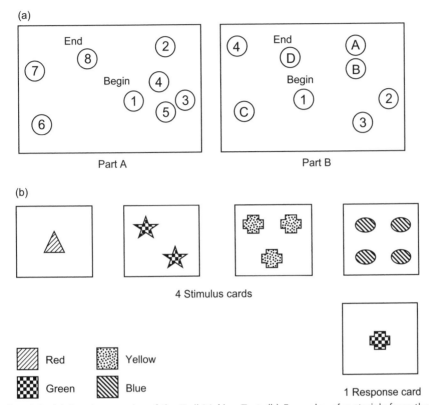

Fig. 18.2 (a) Practice samples of the Trail Making Test. (b) Examples of materials from the Wisconsin Card Sorting Test.

sorting category according to feedback from the examiner. Nelson (1976) introduced a shorter version with 48 cards, quicker shifts, and more feedback to the examinee.

- *Scoring method*. Number of categories achieved; total number of errors; nonperseverative errors; perseverative errors (definitions vary).

Acknowledgements

Paul Burgess is supported by Wellcome Trust grant ref: 049241/Z/96/Z/WRE/HA/JAT. I am grateful to Laure Coates, who gave valuable help with this manuscript.

Selective references

Alderman, N. and Burgess, P.W. (2002). Assessment and rehabilitation of the dysexecutive syndrome. In *Handbook of neurological rehabilitation*, 2nd edn (ed. R. Greenwood, T.M. McMillan, M.P. Barnes, and C.D. Ward). Psychology Press, Hove, East Sussex.

Alderman, N, Burgess, P.W., Knight, C., and Henman, C. (2003). Ecological validity of a simplified version of the multiple errands shopping test. *J. Int. Neuropsychol. Soc.* 9, 31–44.

Armitage, S.G. (1946). An analysis of certain psychological tests used for the evaluation of brain injury. *Psychol. Monogr.* **60**, 91–6.

Axelrod, B.N. and Millis, S.R. (1994). Preliminary standardisation of the Cognitive Estimation Test. *Assessment.* **1**, 269–74.

Berg, E.A. (1948). A simple objective technique for measuring flexibility in thinking. *J. Gen. Psychol.* **39**, 15–22.

Burgess, P.W. (1997). Theory and methodology in executive function research. In *Methodology of frontal and executive function* (ed. P. Rabbitt), pp. 81–116. Psychology Press, Hove, East Sussex.

Burgess, P.W. (2000). Strategy application disorder: the role of the frontal lobes in human multitasking. *Psychol. Res.* **63**, 279–88.

Burgess, P.W. and McNeil, J.E. (1999). Content-specific confabulation. *Cortex.* **35**, 163–82.

Burgess, P.W. and Robertson, I.H. (2002). Principles of the rehabilitation of executive function. In *Principles of frontal lobe function* (ed. D.T. Stuss and R. Knight), pp. 557–72, Oxford University Press, Oxford.

Burgess, P.W. and Shallice, T. (1996a). Bizarre responses, rule detection and frontal lobe lesions. *Cortex.* **32**, 241–60.

Burgess, P.W. and Shallice, T. (1996b). Confabulation and the control of recollection. *Memory.* **4**, 359–411.

Burgess, P.W. and Shallice, T. (1996c). Response suppression, initiation and strategy use following frontal lobe lesion. *Neuropsychologia.* **34**, 263–76.

Burgess, P.W. and Shallice, T. (1997). *The Hayling and Brixton Tests.* Thames Valley Test Company, Flempton.

Burgess, P.W., Alderman, N., Emslie, H., Evans, J.J., and Wilson, B.A. (1996a). The dysexecutive questionnaire. In *Behavioural assessment of the dysexecutive syndrome* (ed. B.A. Wilson, N. Alderman, P.W. Burgess, H. Emslie, and J.J. Evans). Thames Valley Test Company, Bury St. Edmunds.

Burgess, P.W., Alderman, N., Emslie, H., Evans, J.J., Wilson, B.A., and Shallice, T. (1996b). The simplified six element test. In *Behavioural assessment of the dysexecutive syndrome* (ed. B.A. Wilson, N. Alderman, P.W. Burgess, H. Emslie, and J.J. Evans). Thames Valley Test Company, Bury St. Edmunds.

Burgess, P.W., Alderman, N., Evans, J., Emslie, H., and Wilson, B.A. (1998). The ecological validity of tests of executive function. *J. Int. Neuropsychol. Soc.* **4**, 547–58.

Burgess, P.W., Veitch, E., Costello, A., and Shallice, T. (2000). The cognitive and neuroanatomical correlates of multitasking. *Neuropsychologia.* **38**, 848–63.

Cohen, J.D., Dunbar, K., and McClelland, J.L. (1990). On the control of automatic processes: a parallel distributed processing account of the Stroop effect. *Psychol. Rev.* **97**, 332–61.

Cohen, L.D., Braver, T.S., and O'Reilly, R.C. (1998). A computational approach to prefrontal cortex, cognitive control, and schizophrenia: recent developments and current challenges. In *The prefrontal cortex: executive and cognitive functions* (ed. A.C. Roberts, T.W. Robbins, and L. Weiskrantz), pp. 195–200. Oxford University Press, Oxford.

Duncan, J., Burgess, P.W., and Emslie, H. (1995). Fluid intelligence after frontal lobe lesions. *Neuropsychologia.* **33**, 261–8.

Duncan, J., Seitz, R. J., Kolodny, J., Bor, D., Herzog, H., Ahmed, A., Newell, F.N., and Emslie, H. (2000). A neural basis for intelligence. *Science.* **289**, 457–60.

Ettlin, T.M., Kischka, U., Beckson, M., Gaggiotti, M., Rauchfleisch, U., and Benson, D.F. (2000). The frontal lobe score: part II: construction of a mental status of frontal systems. *Clin. Rehabil.* **14**, 260–71.

Fuster, J.M. (1997). *The prefrontal cortex: anatomy, physiology and neuropsychology of the frontal lobe*, 3rd edn. Lippincott-Raven, Philadelphia.

Goldman-Rakic, P.S. (1995). Architecture of the prefrontal cortex and the central executive. *Ann. NY Acad. Sci.* **769**, 212–20.

Gorham, D.R. (1956). A Proverbs Test for clinical and experimental use. *Psychol. Rep.* **1**, 1–12.

Knight, C., Alderman, N., and Burgess, P.W. (2002). Development of a simplified version of the multiple errands test for use in hospital settings. *Neuropsychological Rehabilitation.* **12**, 231–55.

Lezak, M.D. (1995). *Neuropsychological assessment*, 3rd edn. Oxford: Oxford University Press, Oxford.

MacLeod, C.M. (1991). Half a century of research on the Stroop effect: an integrative review. *Psychol. Bull.* **109**, 163–203.

Milner, B. (1963). Effects of different brain lesions on card sorting. *Arch. Neurol.* **9**, 100–10.

Nelson, H.E. (1976). A modified card sorting test sensitive to frontal lobe defects. *Cortex.* **12**, 313–24.

Norman, D.A. and Shallice, T. (1986). Attention to action: willed and automatic control of behaviour. In *Consciousness and Self*-regulation, Vol. 4 (ed. R.J. Davidson, G.E. Schwartz, and D. Shapiro). Plenum Press, New York.

Perret, E. (1974). The left frontal lobe in man and the suppression of habitual responses in verbal categorical behaviour. *Neuropsychologia.* **12**, 323–30.

Petrides, M. (1994). Frontal lobes and working memory: evidence from investigations of the effects of cortical excisions in nonhuman primates. In *Handbook of neuropsychology*, Vol. 9 (ed. F. Boller and J. Grafman), pp. 59–82. Elsevier, Amsterdam.

Petrides, M. (1998). Specialized systems for the processing of mnemonic information within the primate frontal cortex. In *The prefrontal cortex: executive and cognitive functions* (ed. A.C. Roberts, T.W. Robbins, and L. Weiskrantz), pp. 103–16. Oxford University Press, Oxford.

Petrides, M. and Milner, B. (1982). Deficits on subject-ordered tasks after frontal- and temporal-lobe lesions in man. *Neuropsychologia.* **20**, 249–62.

Pribram, K.H. (1973). The primate frontal cortex—executive of the brain. In *Psychophysiology of the frontal lobes* (ed. K.H. Pribram and A.R. Luria), pp. 293–314. Academic Press, New York.

Robbins, T.W., James, M., Owen, A.M., Lange, K.W., Lees, A.J., Leigh, P.N., Marsden, C.D., Quinn, N.P., and Summers, B.A. (1994). CANTAB: a factor analytic study of a large sample of normal elderly volunteers. *Dementia.* **5**, 266–81.

Shallice, T. (1982). Specific impairments of planning. *Phil. Trans. R. Soc. London B* **298**, 199–209.

Shallice, T. (1988). *From neuropsychology to mental structure.* Cambridge University Press, New York.

Shallice, T. and Burgess, P.W. (1991*a*). Deficits in strategy application following frontal lobe damage in man. *Brain.* **114**, 727–41.

Shallice, T. and Burgess, P.W. (1991*b*). Higher-order cognitive impairments and frontal lobe lesions in man. In *Frontal lobe function and dysfunction* (ed. H.S. Levin, H.M. Eisenberg, and A.L. Benton), pp. 125–38. Oxford University Press, New York.

Shallice, T. and Burgess, P. W. (1996). The domain of supervisory processes and the temporal organisation of behaviour. *Phil. Trans. R. Soc. London B* **351**, 1405–12.

Shallice, T. and Evans, M. (1978). The involvement of the frontal lobes in cognitive estimation. *Cortex.* **14**, 294–303.

Spreen, O. and Strauss, E. (1998). *A compendium of neuropsychological tests*, 2nd edn. Oxford University Press, Oxford.

Stroop, J.R. (1935). Studies of interference in serial verbal reaction. *J. Exp. Psychol.* **18**, 643–62.

Stuss, D.T. and Alexander, M.P. (2000). Executive functions and the frontal lobes: a conceptual view. *Psychol. Res.* **63**, 289–98.

Stuss, D.T., Shallice, T., Alexander, M.P., and Picton, T.W. (1995). A mulitidisciplinary approach to anterior attentional functions. *Ann. NY Acad. Sci.* **769**, 191–211.

Stuss, D.T., Toth, J.P., Franchi, D., Alexander, M.P., Tipper, S., and Craik, F.I.M. (1999). Dissociation of attentional processes in patients with focal frontal and posterior lesions. *Neuropsychologia*. 37, 1005–27.

Stuss, D.T., Levine, B., Alexander, M.P., Hong, J., Palumbo, C., Hamer, L., Murphy, K.J., and Izukawa, D. (2000). Wisconsin Card Sorting Test performance in patients with focal frontal and posterior brain damage: effects of lesion location and test structure on separable cognitive processes. *Neuropsychologia*. 38, 388–402.

Thurstone, L.L. (1938). *Primary mental abilities*. Chicago University Press, Chicago.

Wildgruber, D., Kischka, U., Fassbender, K., and Ettlin, T.M. (2000). The frontal lobe score: part II: evaluation of its clinical utility. *Clin. Rehabil.* 14, 272–8.

Wilson, B.A., Alderman, N., Burgess, P.W., Emslie, H., and Evans, J.J. (1996). *Behavioural Assessment of the Dysexecutive Syndrome (BADS)*. Thames Valley Test Company, Bury St. Edmunds.

Wilson, B.A., Evans, J.J., Emslie, H., Alderman, N., and Burgess, P. (1998). The development of an ecologically valid test for assessing patiets with a dysexecutive syndrome. *Neuropsychol. Rehabil.* 8(3), 213–28.

Chapter 19

The natural recovery and treatment of executive disorders

Andrew D. Worthington

1 Introduction

Consider a typical household at breakfast time and it becomes easy to appreciate the organisational or executive skills that we normally take for granted. To prepare breakfast one needs to decide what to eat, to search for the relevant food items; recall how to boil an egg, make toast, or fry bacon, and carry out the steps in sequence so that everything is cooked safely and is ready to eat at the same time. During this activity other aspects of the environment are very likely being monitored too: keeping a check on the time; perhaps listening to the television news, while simultaneously trying to stop the children squabbling and ensuring they are ready for school; mentally preparing for an important meeting at work; or trying to anticipate whether you will have time visit the bank in your lunch break. As if this were not complex enough, a barrage of irrelevant stimuli assault the senses – an advertisement on the radio, a stray dog barking at the postman, a neighbour trying to start their car. All this information is processed, evaluated and then discarded or accommodated within on-going behaviour. The ability to carry out such naturalistic activities successfully requires the co-ordinated and regulated implementation of many cognitive operations, especially those which have come to be associated with the term executive functioning. These include skills such as goal setting, planning, action initiation, self-monitoring and behavioural inhibition. Disruption to any of these underlying processes as a result of brain injury produces characteristically impaired performance on many complex tasks that are fundamental to daily living.

Consequently treatment of executive functioning may be, not only the most important part of an individual's rehabilitation, but also the most difficult, affecting the highest levels of cognitive ability, awareness and self-regulation. If intervention is undertaken successfully a person's life may be transformed in a manner more familiar to transplant surgeons than to psychologists. Effective treatment of severe executive disorder can enable a person to sustain a degree of employment, leisure activity and family integrity previously inaccessible to them. In contrast, persistent dysexecutive problems may render an otherwise intelligent individual unable to undertake even the most rudimentary of everyday activities.

For practitioners, three facts make rehabilitation of executive skills particularly problematic:

◆ The manifestations of executive dysfunction are diverse, affecting cognition, mood and behaviour;

◆ The problems are not readily encapsulated in the manner of traditional psychological assessment;

◆ There is no consensus regarding a conceptual or methodological approach to either investigation or treatment.

Effective rehabilitation depends on the therapist's skill in overcoming these fundamental difficulties. This chapter is intended to assist by providing an overview of the context and content of the management of executive dysfunction. Traditional approaches to this field tend to be structured in terms of intervention type such as restorative versus compensation techniques (Sohlberg *et al.*1993; Evans, 2001). By contrast, this chapter is organised around a basic conceptual framework of normal executive functioning, and disorders that occur at each stage of the processing continuum are addressed in turn. This is not a 'cookbook' approach to treatment, and its coverage is certainly not exhaustive, but the reader will find that this structure permits systematic discussion of practical intervention strategies for each of the most common executive dysfunctions. Repetition of interventions is limited to cross-references. The chapter has been organised pragmatically to help clinicians who are typically faced with problems and want to know what methods are available to manage the difficulties presented.

2 Natural recovery of executive disorders

Disorders of executive functioning are amongst the most persistent sequelae of brain injury. Paradoxically they are often difficult to identify in hospital due to the presence of ward routine, the limited behavioural demands on patients and the usual absence of skilled observers. Furthermore, when they are apparent, executive disorders often exclude people from rehabilitation, leading to overly pessimistic prognoses. Finally, the manifestations of executive dysfunction are typically misunderstood in the community, with the result that many people fall by the wayside or come to the attention of psychiatric or forensic services. Many of the personality changes that follow serious brain damage are attributable to disorders of executive functioning, and it is these changes, rather than physical or specific cognitive deficits, which cause long-term breakdown of relationships and status. The true severity of executive dysfunction may be apparent only after formal rehabilitation has ended and a person has returned home or back to work. However, significant improvements in everyday functioning can be made, even several years after the original injury, largely through compensatory interventions.

Clinicians should be aware of factors that influence prognosis. Important positive signs are:

◆ Brain injury occurring as an adult rather than as a child.

◆ Single incident brain injury without complications.

- Circumscribed rather than diffuse cerebral involvement.
- Motivation to participate in treatment. *(NB. this is not the same as motivation to go home or return to work, which can be counter-productive).*
- Awareness of problems in thinking or personality.
- Absence of severe behaviour disorders.
- No previous history of alcohol or substance abuse.
- No premorbid psychiatric history.
- Supportive social and family circumstances.

Investigating rehabilitation potential for executive disorders

- Establish the organic basis for an executive disorder, then considering non-organic confounding factors.
- Certain neuropathology is especially likely to cause executive disorders: traumatic brain injury, herpes simplex encephalitis, aneurysms of the anterior communicating artery, certain tumours, dementia of fronto-temporal type, subcortical infarcts involving the thalamus, basal ganglia or internal capsule.
- Severe executive dysfunction in everyday life can occur in the absence of structural frontal lobe pathology on an MRI scan.
- Basal skull fractures / cerebellar lesions may be associated with significant executive deficits.
- Behaviour at home or work is a better index of executive problems than behaviour in hospital or formal assessment in a consulting room.
- Listen to what friends and family members say – give them permission to report changes in personality or behaviour.

3 A conceptual basis for the treatment of executive dysfunction

Clinicians can be forgiven for feeling that the burgeoning literature on executive functions and 'frontal lobology' is abstruse and bewildering. Even so, when faced with multiple executive problems a simple framework is helpful in structuring treatment interventions, as diverse disorders of cognition and behaviour may be manifestations of the same underlying deficits. Below is a rudimentary but robust framework for clinicians. The role of action schemas is central to this model. An action schema is a representation of basic action, which, when arranged in hierarchical fashion with lower-level motor acts and higher-level organisational processes, forms part of the executive system for governing behaviour. For example, in the model below, planning occurs at the level of assembly of action schemas relevant to a task.

A three-stage framework for prioritising deficits for treatment

Cognitive process at work	Behavioural manifestation
I Schema assembly	**Disorders of goal articulation and planning** *formulating intentions, clarifying goals, planning and anticipation*
II Schema activation	**Disorders of initiation and sequencing** *aspontaneity, action sequencing, prospective remembering*
III Schema regulation	**Disorders of inhibition and control** *Utilisation behaviour, impulsiveness, perseveration, disinhibition, aggression*
	Disorders of monitoring and evaluation *attention and awareness, reasoning, judgment, decision making, problem solving, confabulation*

A wide range of action and behaviour disorders can be encompassed within this simple scheme. Effective intervention requires identification of the level of dysfunction. Therefore clinicians should consider how well a person can carry out each of the following key stages in turn:

◆ Generating an intent to act (goal articulation) and formulating a plan.

◆ Activating the plan and implementing the action to achieve the desired goal.

◆ Monitoring progression towards the goal and regulating behaviour accordingly.

We turn now to consider rehabilitation methods. Most techniques can be considered to conform to one of three broad types, loosely based on putative mechanisms of effectiveness, as illustrated. However such taxonomies are mostly intuitive, atheoretical, and not mutually exclusive (Worthington, 2005). In preference therefore this chapter reviews intervention methods in terms of their utility for disorders at each of the above stages.

A broad taxonomy of intervention types

Environmental modification
Essentially a compensatory means of therapeutic intervention - changing the physical or social setting and modifying the contingencies of reward. (eg. changing layout of a room, using notebooks, diaries, pagers). Much under-rated, often unfairly regarded as the therapist's last ditch option. Consider using for: (a) deficits in initial goal setting, or in task execution, (b) in situations of stimulus overload/competition, (c) context-driven behavioural deficits, in the presence of other cognitive impairment.

A broad taxonomy of intervention types *(continued)*

Cognitive remediation techniques

Tasks aimed at restoring impaired cognitive processes - repetitive practice of a specific (sometimes rather contrived) task. Intervention delivered on structured exercises in set treatment sessions. Some promising results in the treatment of attentional deficits, but yet to demonstrate wider utility for executive problems (generalisability of treatment gains is poor). Be sceptical of interventions claiming to restore underlying cognitive processes (eg. memory process training, organisational skills training, problem solving therapy).

Specific skills training

Variety of methods from cognitive and behavioural psychology intended to teach people how to perform very specific everyday activities. Often used in conjunction with environmental modifications to good effect. Includes training of metacognitive skills (eg. monitoring, evaluation, feedback and awareness). Not limited to classroom activities, can be employed in real life settings. Most of the active interventions in this chapter conform to some kind of skills training approach.

4 Interventions for deficits in the creation of action plans

4.1 Impairments of planning and goal formulation

Difficulty in formulating intentions or clear objectives before starting a task. Caused by inability to devise an appropriate action plan - commonly occurs with complex multi-stage tasks (Shallice, 1982). The clinician should *educate* (reiterate the importance of planning to eventual outcome) and *moderate* (consider changes in routine or the task environment). Some apparent planning impairments are in reality, impulsive behaviours, which respond to self-instructional or verbal mediation interventions (eg. Cicerone and Wood, 1987). Poor planning may be improved by generating an appropriate action script by asking people to verbally rehearse what is required for a task (Zalla *et al.*, 2001) or cueing autobiographical memories (Hewitt *et al.*, 2006). Task-based checklists can also provide an explicit framework for developing plans (Burke *et al.*, 1991). For complex deficits of strategic planning, consider training programmes with an early emphasis on goal articulation and planning (see *Goal Management Training*, stages 1–3; and *Problem Solving Therapy* below). Alternatively, where time constraints are important, *Time Pressure Management* (TPM) training (Fasotti *et al.*, 2000) offers a problem-solving framework which can be linked to self-instruction to help individuals plan more effectively.

4.2 Degradation of everyday action schema

Problems in carrying out everyday routine activities; this is not really an executive deficit but manifests as one. It is caused by the breakdown of conceptual knowledge or 'schema assemblies' (Schwartz *et al.*, 1991) for well-established actions – may manifest as part of an ideational or frontal apraxia. It may be associated with semantic impairments. Treatment as for *action disorganisation* (below): Ensure a good understanding of the task objectives and operations before commencing action. Follow this with on-line assistance (verbal prompts, physical cues) as necessary.

5 Interventions for deficits in the activation and implementation of everyday action schema

Deficits in activating intentions or initiating behaviour cause poverty of action, an extremely debilitating condition. Manifestations may vary.

5.1 Aspontaneity

A marked reduction in spontaneous purposeful activity; this must be distinguished from the neurological conditions of abulia and akinesia, and the neuropsychiatric syndromes of apathy and depression. Environmental cues and verbal prompts are often ineffective because the problem is not one of goal clarity but represents a difficulty putting plans into action. Solutions are as follows:

1 Modify the environment to increase the salience of antecedent stimuli and reduce the significance of irrelevant stimuli (see *discrimination training* below);

2 self-prompting schedules can also be beneficial (Burke *et al.*, 1991) but only if linked to clear rewards for the individual. Too often intervention fails because the person has no desire to engage in particular activities.

3 Pharmacological agents may help (eg. dopamine agonists).

5.2 Action disorganisation

Problems with common everyday tasks (eg. making a cup of tea); this is not a pure executive disorder, but is caused by disruption to the procedural knowledge base for over-learned actions (such as brushing one's teeth), rendering the activity dependent on inadequate executive control.

Intervention should ensure conditions are optimal for action schema activation, and include procedures to improve behavioural regulatory functions, to ensure efficient operation of the relevant action schema once activated. Treatment options include:

1 environmental simplification to minimise off-task errors;

2 provide a visual sequence of correct action stages to be followed;

3 use behavioural techniques: where a desired response does not occur spontaneously such an action can be developed using the technique of shaping, which involves positively reinforcing successive approximations to the desired behaviour. Chaining techniques are recommended if the primary problem is in action sequencing;

4 use verbal self-regulation methods.

Clinicians usually select whatever seems likely to work, and then modify accordingly (see Wilson, 1999).

5.3 **Prospective remembering**

The inability to carry out an intention to act at some future time; this is commonly associated with other executive deficits, but not necessarily with other memory problems. It
needs to be distinguished from initiation disorder (see *aspontaneity* above) and impairments of retrospective memory, as memory for the intent to act may be preserved.
Therapeutically, internal memory strategies have limited success. Likewise, the use of
spaced retrieval methods (increasing the time lag between encoding and execution of
intentions) has been disappointing (Sohlberg *et al.*, 1992). Instead, external cueing systems should be considered (individualised checklists are a good example). As long as the
person can use the technology electronic aids can be effective such as a pager (Evans *et al.*
1998; Emslie *et al.*, 2004) or SMS text message (Pijnenborg *et al.*, 2007). A text message
that says 'Stop' may be sufficient to re-focus attention (Fish *et al.*, 2007). If severe anterograde memory problems are also present, start with a very basic task and simple cues (eg.
prompt with telephone calls). Gradually a self-cueing programme can be devised using a
combination of checklists and external prompts to use the checklists, in order to develop
a simple routine of action initiation. Many people develop their own idiosyncratic methods. These should be respected, but may be improved.

6 **Interventions for deficits in the regulation of behaviour**

For goal-oriented behaviour to be adaptive in the real world it has to be efficiently regulated. The majority of cognitive and behavioural disorders that characterise the dysexecutive syndrome arise from disturbance to regulatory control mechanisms. These comprise
fundamental processes of attention and awareness, judgment and inhibition.

6.1 **Disorders of inhibition**

Disorders of inhibition arise principally from a deficiency of executive control over lower-
level action schemas, leading to unmodulated contention scheduling (see Chapter 18).
The manifestations of impaired inhibitory control are varied. In some cases one observes
a failure to exercise a socially-acceptable degree of self-restraint in translating thoughts or
feelings into action. In other instances, behaviour is clearly driven by external stimuli
without any apparent cognitive mediation. Treatment of the most common manifestations is as follows:

6.1.1 Utilisation behaviour

A non-planned and irrelevant response to an object that often interferes with an existing
activity; it is caused by automatic activation of an action schema, usually triggered by a
specific object, resulting in behaviour that may be socially unacceptable (drinking from
someone's cup, answering their telephone). It is important to distinguish utilisation
behaviour from a simple frontal grasp reflex (objects do not have to be within immediate
grasping range to elicit utilisation behaviour) and 'alien hand'. Verbal prompting does
not usually help, as awareness may be preserved. Modifying the environmental triggers
offers a partial solution, though the problem often resolves spontaneously.

6.1.2 Distractibility

Responding to external stimuli (noise, people) at the expense of current activity; this is essentially a deficit in attentional control, allowing attention to be captured by task-irrelevant events. Can produce severe disability in everyday life, but is amenable to treatment with cognitive and behavioural techniques. [See *Discrimination Training* below and also Chapter 5 on Attention]. Intermittent cues, such as periodic auditory alerts (Manly *et al.*, 2002), may help re-focus attention to the task at hand.

6.1.3 Impulsiveness

A tendency to act without pre-planning or thinking through the consequences; this is caused by inadequate executive control over behaviour - unconstrained contention scheduling. It is commonly associated with other signs of dysregulation including mood.

The consequences of impulsive behaviour can be ameliorated to a degree by removing temptation, a simple but effective strategy at times. In treating impulsiveness itself, practical (and perhaps ethical) constraints prevent more widespread use of counter-conditioning methods, massed practice or paradoxical intention. Consequential learning methods can be used, where there is some incentive for demonstrating self-restraint. In practice this is better tied to a concurrent verbal task to capture attention (eg. counting 1–5 and then carrying out the action). A personal favourite is the cue word "WAIT!" – short, clear and effective in interrupting action. It is also an acronym for 'What Alternative Is There?' which can be incorporated into a self-instructional programme.

6.1.4 Perseveration

A repetitive pattern of action that is no longer relevant to the situation. Even if an action is triggered appropriately, there comes a time when it is redundant due to changes in circumstances (eg. a goal has been achieved). Inability to change action schema accordingly leads to inefficient, often highly inappropriate, behaviour.

The clinician should establish whether the behaviour is exclusively organically-driven (*frontal perseveration*) or has been learned (*habitual behaviour*). Awareness may be preserved and the problem may improve within six to twelve months after brain injury.

Training a person to use self-statements during perseverative acts can reduce the problem. There is some evidence that massed practice or 'cognitive over-learning' is effective in reducing verbal perseverative behaviour (Alderman and Ward, 1991). Repetitive habitual behaviour needs a functional analysis, followed by appropriate cognitive-behavioural treatment to address the environmental contingencies helping to maintain the behaviour. In this way Matthey (1996) reduced perseverative behaviour, but effects did not generalise to the home environment, presumably because the external contingencies at home were different from the treatment environment. This problem could be minimised if the therapy specifically included the discharge environment as a legitimate treatment arena.

6.1.5 Disinhibition

This is acting or speaking in a manner which contravenes acceptable social conduct.

Disinhibited behaviour can take many forms, from mild over-familiarity with strangers to acts of sexual indecency. Situations may vary and the first step in treatment is to conduct comprehensive assessment of the circumstances of the behaviour. Although organically-derived, the behaviour is often exacerbated or sustained by reactions from others. Therefore investigation should encompass social context, including antecedents and consequences, as the key to successful treatment. Amelioration has typically been based on principles of behaviour modification, including time-out from positive reinforcement (Wood, 1990), though attention constraints associated with dysexecutive impairment may interfere with conditioning.

Intervention should therefore be immediate, providing a direct feedback (usually a specific verbal response). For individuals with adequate memory, additional delayed feedback (up to 1 hour later) encourages reflection on behaviour and provides opportunity to rehearse alternative responses (thus developing a more acceptable action schema). Here verbal mediation methods can help towards the development of a self-management approach (Wood and Worthington, 2001).

Example of a verbal mediation dialogue

How are you this morning?
Fed up, I missed my breakfast

What happened at breakfast?
I had an argument with Jason, because he was staring at me

Why do you think he did that?
I don't know, maybe he was trying to annoy me. He was doing it on purpose

How did that make you feel?
I got angry, he was doing it on purpose to annoy me

What did you do then?
I started shouting and calling him names

What happened next?
He shouted back...we just kept shouting, until we got told to leave the dining room

What else could you have done?
I could have carried on eating my breakfast and ignored him

How do you think Jason would have reacted then?
He would have got fed up as I was ignoring him

Would that have been better for you too?
Yeah, because he's just a loser, but I would have had my breakfast

So if you feel Jason is trying to wind you up at breakfast tomorrow, what will you do?
I'll take no notice, and carry on

6.1.6 Aggression

Aggression can be verbal or physical, towards objects or persons, including self-directed anger, and has many causes. It is often an attempt to intimidate rather than harm. Inability to articulate goals, solve problems or communicate intentions can lead to frustrations and, if unchecked, to aggression. It is important to differentiate this from irritability and episodic dyscontrol. Remember also that aggression is a normal response to certain situations, but after frontal brain injury impaired behavioural control mechanisms mean that it becomes a default response in many situations. Once triggered, aggression may not be constrained by normal regulatory processes. There are several approaches to treatment. Pharmacological intervention is usually necessary in severe cases, and can augment psychological methods. Medication alone is not a long-term solution. Modification of the environment can help reduce trigger events, but this is rarely adequate. The objective of treatment is usually to restore a degree of self-control. This can be done using behavioural methods alone, such as cost-response techniques which link the anti-social behaviour to a meaningful sanction (eg. failure to earn privileges). Some understanding of response-consequence relationships is necessary for learning, so ensure learning intervals are brief where cognition is severely disturbed. Alderman and Burgess (1994) recommended cost-response techniques as especially useful in such cases.

For higher-functioning individuals cognitive-behavioural methods can be used, either in a self-instructional programme or a problem-solving anger management intervention (Medd and Tate, 2000). In all cases the aim is to encourage the activation (consciously or otherwise) of an incompatible, more acceptable action schema in response to identifiable trigger stimuli. *Caveat*: change on self-report measures of anger is not the same as spontaneous use of anger management strategies in everyday life, and generalisation of treatment effects is problematic, especially after group interventions.

6.2 Disorders of evaluation and judgment

The inability to make sensible decisions or express sound judgments is a cardinal feature of executive dysfunction. In extreme cases, otherwise intelligent individuals mix with bad company, frit away their savings on fruitless ventures, and generally go through life from one mishap to another, unless supervision is imposed. In such cases the matter of competency to manage one's affairs becomes important. In many other instances the deficiencies are subtle and may only be apparent some time after rehabilitation has ended.

6.2.1 Impairments of judgment and decision making

First, establish whether impaired judgment is a specific or more general defect. For example, poor road safety judgment may be secondary to subtle perceptual deficits. Commonly, generalised impairments of judgment are accompanied by diminished self-awareness.

The type of intervention depends on the likely underlying problem. Inability to select a single course of action from plausible options can produce impairments in both judgment and decision making, or may even result in deficits of initiation. Therefore it is important to distinguish between difficulty in making just about *any* kind of decision from a tendency to make poor decisions. The former need interventions aimed at clarifying the issues and generating solutions, whereas the latter requires focus on the process of comparative evaluations and anticipated consequences. Strategies used in training problem solving (see next section) are valid in both cases.

6.2.2 Impairments of reasoning and problem solving

Reasoning and problem solving are two high-level skills which are often compromised as part of a dysexecutive presentation, but often the full magnitude of the deficits is only evident on real-life tasks (Shallice and Burgess,1991; Goel *et al.*, 1997; Goel and Grafman, 2000). Unfortunately, treatment for such deficits is still largely classroom–based (see Evans, 2001). One comprehensive programme is *Problem Solving Training*, or PST (von Cramon *et al.*, 1991; von Cramon and Matthes-von Cramon, 1992). The essence of the treatment is to train persons in key aspects of problem solving. This kind of mental discipline training can improve performance on problem solving exercises within a few weeks. However, the real difficulty is that patients with executive disorders can acquire knowledge and skills but may nevertheless fail to apply this spontaneously outside the treatment environment. Evidence to date suggests that effort would be better spent improving use of such skills in specific everyday environments (von Cramon and Matthes-von Cramon, 1994).

A related approach is employed in *Goal Management Training*. This is really another form of verbal mediation training intended to improve self-regulation, but with an abstract set of principles that can be applied across situations. This method can improve performance of everyday tasks (Levine *et al.*, 2000), but, as with PST, it is not clear whether all the components are really necessary, and some stages may be more relevant than others for particular deficits.

Stages in Problem Solving Therapy

1 Problem formulation (defining the task objective)
2 Generation of solutions (brainstorming)
3 Deciding on a solution (weighing-up the options)
4 Verifying the outcome (recognising errors, correcting mistakes)

Steps to Goal Management Training

1 Problem orientation
2 Problem definition (specifying the goal)
3 Listing (breakdown goals into relevant stages - subgoals)
4 Learning (encoding and retention of steps)
5 Monitoring (comparing outcome with intention)

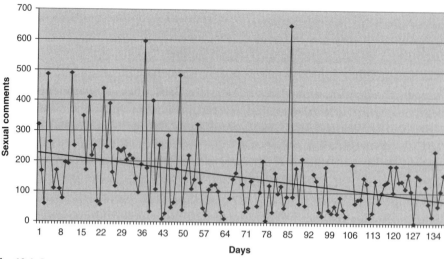

Fig. 19.1 Response-cost programme in progress for verbal sexual disinhibition.

6.3 Impairments of self-monitoring

6.3.1 Self-awareness of behaviour

Many behavioural interventions work successfully without specifically recruiting self-awareness. Other methods however explicitly target awareness as an integral aspect of the rehabilitative process. Disruption to the normal feedback mechanism linking conscious intentions with the external world results in an inability to monitor one's behaviour and its effect on others. This is why social disinhibition does not improve with experience alone. This is usually treated by response-consequence methods, for example, by linking this with subtle social reinforcement, explicit feedback or tangible reward. Fig. 19.1 is a snapshot of the gradual reduction in sexual comments taking place during a social reinforcement cost-response programme for a 40 year-old man with very severe traumatic brain injury.

A self-instruction programme

A self-instructional programme was employed to good effect with a 29 year-old woman two years after her severe head injury. She could take up to three hours to get washed and dressed in the morning as a result of severe distractibility and obsessive behaviour. A programme was devised during which a support worker read out specific action prompts. These were repeated by the client as she performed the actions. These statements gradually came to act as internal prompts, improving her attention to task and increasing her speed to wash and dress to half an hour. Fig. 19.2 shows the mean number of daily verbal prompts in a two week baseline period and for four weeks following withdrawal of the self-instructional programme.

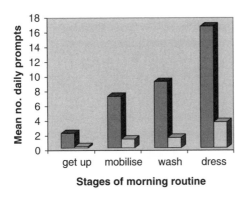

Fig. 19.2 Self-instructional programme for washing and dressing.

To promote generalisation of gains clinicians should remember to include graded exposure to successively more challenging stimuli or situations. Self-instructional or self-management approaches have been under-used in brain injury. True, many cognitive skills packages (eg GMT) and behaviour modification techniques invoke an appeal to self-awareness and thereby to self-monitoring. But, few deal specifically with this crucial aspect of executive disorder.

An exception is *Self-monitoring Training* (SMT) reported by Alderman (*et al.*, 1995) to reduce to the frequency of inappropriate utterances. This multi-stage programme is really a hybrid for improving self-awareness in combination with a procedure for reinforcing successively lower frequencies of target behaviour (DRL), although DRL methods can be effective without such self-monitoring (Knight *et al.*, 2002). Personal experience suggests that increased self-awareness can be achieved within a few weeks, at most, but does not necessarily generalise to changes in behaviour.

Fig. 19.3 shows how this method was effective in reducing a range of disinhibited verbal behaviours in a young woman following herpes simplex encephalitis, first reported by Worthington (2005). The technique is recommended for high frequency problems, and can be enhanced by self-completion of a daily record or diary (Burke *et al.*, 1991). In many cases however the problem is not one of self-evaluation, but an inability to divide attention between the task in hand and other pressures. In this case intervention should focus on the temporal aspect of the task (see *Time Pressure Management*, above).

6.3.2 Confabulation from memory

Confabulation is the production of false memories following brain injury, which the person confuses for, and cannot distinguish from, veridical recollection. It is generally associated with frontal-subcortical damage, and is considered to result from deficient executive control over memory retrieval – (ie. faulty verification procedures). Improvement often occurs spontaneously, and there are few treatment studies. However Dayus and van den Broek (2000) successfully employed self-monitoring training to reduce debilitating delusional confabulations.

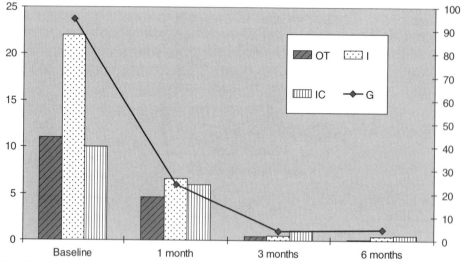

Fig. 19.3 Self-monitoring programme with generalisation of behaviour across settings. Key: I = interruptions; IC = inappropriate comments; OT = off the topic comments; G = generalisation probe (second axis) reprinted with permission.

Components of self-monitoring training

1 Baseline assessment of frequency of target behaviour

2 Spontaneous (ie. unprompted) self-monitoring of target behaviour

3 Prompted self-monitoring, with assistance of therapist

4 Independent self-monitoring (with reward contingent on achieving a pre-determined level of agreement in frequency ratings between therapist and client)

5 Independent self-monitoring and reduction of target behaviour (delivery of reward contingent upon graded reduction in frequency of target behaviour)

7 Issues in the treatment of executive disorders

7.1 Evaluating clinical efficacy

Well-designed rehabilitation studies for executive skills are a rare breed. The so-called dysexecutive syndrome encompasses a wide range of deficits, some presenting as behaviour problems, some manifesting as higher cognitive impairments. Treatment efficacy has to be evaluated for specific subtypes of executive disorder, indicating whether the behaviour or the underlying the cognitive processes are the focus of intervention. Evidence of effectiveness is limited to small group studies or single cases. While many of these seem to show good results (and clinical experience would support this), it is difficult to infer who benefits from which interventions. Comprehensive treatment packages may contain much redundant material and need to be examined in detail. In this light, studies comparing different interventions (eg. Alderman and Burgess, 1994) are particularly instructive.

7.2 The role of attention and self-awareness

Recruitment of attention is critical to improving many high-level executive skills, but attention is often impaired in conjunction with executive processes. Brain injury can also cause disorders of awareness and prevent use of attentional resources in regulating behaviour. This is why techniques based solely on positive reinforcement may be ineffective in modifying behaviour in the context of a dysexecutive syndrome. Rehabilitation can be focussed on the attention deficit or the behavioural manifestation - the clinician must decide.

In terms of self-regulatory disorders, attention per se is rarely the focus of intervention, but treatment does involve techniques for modifying attention to what is therapeutically important. This is the basis of *discriminative attention training* that underpins much of the learning process in rehabilitation. Treatment methods, involving either environmental modification or manipulation of consequences of actions, focus on alternative or incompatible reactions to a situation. This allows selective reinforcement by therapists for certain actions and thereby increases the likelihood of the desired behaviours recurring. Such discriminative reinforcement techniques were reviewed by Wood (1990). Attentional re-directing is also integral to cognitive-behavioural approaches to improving social and functional skills, and is central to the development of self-monitoring programmes. Clinicians should establish first whether there is a significant attentional contribution to an executive disorder, as this is often the key to successful treatment. For a comprehensive review of attention disorders and remediation, the reader should refer to the chapter on attentional disorders in this volume.

7.3 Designing effective interventions for executive disorders

The principles of sound clinical practice apply to rehabilitation of executive dysfunction. Thus budding therapists need to:

- Carry out assessment of both spared and impaired abilities (ie. a reliable baseline).
- Decide on priorities for treatment.
- Agree specific operational goals with family, client and therapy team.
- Devise a clear explicit intervention, based on a hypothesis of the nature of the executive dysfunction.

In addition, rehabilitation of executive deficits requires close attention to the following aspects of treatment design:

- Consider the conceptual basis for a deficit in order to rationalise choice of intervention strategy.
- Select practical tasks as targets for intervention.
- Avoid tasks reliant on regurgitation of old knowledge.
- Avoid highly constrained tasks where responsibility for correcting performance rests solely with therapist.
- Breakdown intervention into discrete stages.

- Consider most-to-least-prompts and spaced retrieval (using errorless learning principles).
- Deliver treatment in different settings to facilitate generalisation.
- Start with a simple analogue but work towards increasing complexity of treatment environment.
- Assess similar non-treated tasks to investigate generalisation of skills to related tasks.
- Assess non-treated domains of cognitive functioning to control for natural recovery.

The treatment of executive dysfunction is one of the least understood and most complex areas of brain injury rehabilitation. It is not sufficient to show improvements on a task with practice; to be effective an intervention must also address the problem of spontaneous application and self-evaluation of skills once acquired. The therapeutic techniques described are largely in their infancy, there is much we still have to learn about optimal methods for improving self-regulation (Muraven and Baumeister, 2000). Nevertheless, if intervention is undertaken sensitively and rationally, executive functioning can be improved to the extent that real change can be effected in quality of life.

Selective references

Alderman, N. and Ward, A. (1991). Behavioural treatment of the dysexecutive syndrome: reduction of repetitive speech using response cost and cognitive overlearning. *Neuropsychological Rehabilitation*, **1**, 65–80.

Alderman, N. and Burgess, P.W. (2001). Assessment and rehabilitation of the dysexecutive syndrome. In R. Greenwod, T.M. McMillan, M.P. Barnes, and C.D. Ward, (Eds.). *Handbook of Neurological Rehabilitation* (2nd edition) Psychology Press, Hove.

Alderman, N. and Burgess, P. (1994). A comparison of treatment methods for behaviour disorer following herpes simplex encephalitis. *Neuropsychological Rehabilitation*, **4**, 31–48.

Alderman, N., Fry, R.K. and Youngson, H.A. (1995). Improvement of self-monitoring skills, reduction of behaviour disturbance and the dysexecutive syndrome: comparison of response cost and a new programme of Self-Management Training. *Neuropsychological Rehabilitation*, **5**, 193–221.

Ashley, M.J., Krych, D.K., Persel, C.S. and Persel, C.H. (1995). *Working with behaviour disorders. Strategies for traumatic brain injury rehabilitation*. Communication Skill Builders (Psychological Corporation), San Antonio.

Burke, W.H., Zenicus, A.H., Wesolowski, M.D. and Doubleday, F. (1991). Improving executive function disorders in brain injured clients. *Brain Injury*, **5**, 241–252.

Cicerone, K.D. and Wood, J.C. (1987). Planning disorder after closed head injury: a case study. *Archives of Physical Medicine and Rehabilitation*, **68**, 111–115.

Cramon, D.Y. von, Matthes-von Cramon, G. and Mai, N. (1991). Problem solving deficits inbrain injured patients: a therapeutic approach. *Neuropsychological Rehabilitation*, **1**, 45–64.

Cramon von, D.Y. and Matthes-von Cramon, G. (1992). Reflections on the treatment of brain-injured patients suffering from problem solving disorders. *Neuropsychological Rehabilitation*, **2**, 207–229.

Cramon von, D.Y. and Matthes von Cramon, G. (1994). Back to work with a chronic dysexecutive syndrome? (a case study). *Neuropsychological Rehabilitation*, **4**, 399–417.

Dayus, B. and van den Broek, M.D. (2000). Treatment of stable delusional confabulations using self-monitoring training. *Neuropsychological Rehabilitation*, **10**, 415–427.

Emslie, H., Wilson, B.A, Quirk, K., Evans, J.J, Watson, P. (2004). Using a paging system in the rehabilitation of encephalitic patients. *Neuropsychological Rehabilitation*, **17**, 567–581.

Evans, J.J., Emslie, H. and Wilson, B.A. (1998). External cueing systems in the rehabilitation of executive impairments of action. *Journal of the International Neuropsychological Society*, **4**, 399–408.

Evans, J.J. (2001). Rehabilitation of the dysexecutive syndrome. In *Neurobehavioural Disability and Social Handicap Following Traumatic Brain Injury* (ed. R.Ll. Wood, and T.M. McMillan). pp. 209–227 Psychology Press, Hove.

Fasotti, L., Kovacs, F., Eling, P.A.T.M and Brouwer, W.H. (2000). Time pressure management as a compensatory strategy training after closed head injury. *Neuropsychological Rehabilitation*, **10**, 47–65.

Fish, J., Evans, J.J, Nimmo, M., Martin, E., Kersel, D., Bateman, A., Wilson, B. A, Manly, T. (2007). Rehabilitation of executive dysfunction following brain injury: 'Content-free' cueing improves everyday prospective memory performance. *Neuropsychologia*, **45**, 1318–1330.

Goel, V, and Grafman, J. (2000). Role of the right prefrontal cortex in ill-structured planning. *Cognitive Neuropsychology*, **17**, 415–436.

Goel, V., Grafman, J., Tajik, J., Gana, S. and Danto, D. (1997). A study of the performance of patients with frontal lobe lesions in a financial planning task. *Brain*, **120**, 1805–1822.

Hewitt, J., Evans, J.J., Dritschel, B. (2006). Theory driven rehabilitation of executive functioning: improving planning skills in people with traumatic brain injury through the use of an autobiographical episodic memory cueing procedure. *Neuropsychologia*, **44**, 1468–1474.

Knight, C.A., Rutterford, N.A., Alderman, N., Swan, L.J. (2002). Is accurate self-monitoring necessary for people with acquired neurological problems to benefit from the use of differential reinforcement methods? *Brain Injury*, **16**, 75–87.

Levine, B., Robertson, I.H., Clare, L., Carter, G., Hong, J., Wilson, B., Duncan, J. and Stuss, DT. (2000). Rehabilitation of executive functioning: an experimental-clinical validation of Goal Management Training. *Journal of the International Neuropsychological Society*, **6**, 299–312.

Manly, T., Hawkins, K., Evans, J., Woldt, K., Robertson, I.H. (2002). Rehabilitation of executive function: facilitation of effective goal management on complex tasks using periodic auditory alerts. *Neuropsychologia*, **40**, 271–281.

Matthey, S. (1996). Modification of perseverative behaviour in an adult with anoxic brain damage. *Brain Injury*, **3**, 219–227.

Medd, J. and Tate, R.L. (2000). Evaluation of an Anger management therapy programme following acquired brain injury: a preliminary study. *Neuropsychological Rehabilitation*, **10**, 185–201.

Muraven, M. and Baumeister, R.F. (2000). Self-regulation and depletion of limited resources: does self-control resemble a muscle? *Psychological Bulletin*, **126**, 247–259.

Pijnenborg, G.H.M., Withaar, F.K., Evans, J.J., van den Bosch, R.J., Brouwer, W.H. (2007). SMS text messages as a prosthetic aid in the cognitive rehabilitation of schizophrenia. *Rehabilitation Psychology*, **52**, 236–240.

Schwartz, M.F., Reed, E.S., Montgomery, M.W., Palmer, C. and Mayer, NH. (1991). The quantitative description of action organisation after brain damage: a case study. *Cognitive Neuropsychology*, **8**, 381–414.

Shallice, T. (1982). Specific impairments of planning. *Philosophical Transactions of the Royal Society of London* B. **298**, 199–209.

Shallice, T. and Burgess, P.W. (1991). Deficits in strategy application following frontal lobe lesions in man. *Brain*, **114**, 727–741.

Sohlberg, M.M., Mateer, C.A. and Stuss, D.T. (1993). Contemporary approaches to the management of executive control dysfunction. *Journal of Head Trauma Rehabilitation*, **8**, 45–58.

Sohlberg, M.M., White, O., Evans, E. and Mateer, C. (1992). An investigation into the effects of prospective memory training. *Brain Injury*, **6**, 139–154.

Wilson, B.A. (1999). *Case Studies in Neuropsychological Rehabilitation*. Oxford University Press, New York.

Wood, R.Ll. (1990). Conditioning procedures in brain injury rehabilitation. In *Neurobehavioural Sequelae of Traumatic Brain Injury* (ed. R. Ll. Wood). pp. 153–174. Taylor & Francis, London.

Wood, R.Ll. and Worthington, A.D. (2001). Neurobehavioral rehabilitation in practice. In *Neurobehavioural Disability and Social Handicap Following Traumatic Brain Injury*. (ed. R.Ll. Wood, and T.M. McMillan) pp. 133–155. Psychology Press, Hove.

Worthington, A. (2005). Rehabilitation of executive deficits: effective treatment of related disabilities. In: P.W. Halligan, and D.T. Wade, (Eds.). *Effectiveness of Rehabilitation of Cognitive Deficits*, New York: Oxford University Press, 257–267.

Zalla, T., Plassiart, C., Pillon, B., Grafman, J. and Sirigu, A. (2001). Action planning in a virtual context after prefrontal cortex damage. *Neuropsychologia*, **39**, 759–770.

Chapter 20

The neuropsychological assessment and treatment of disorders of voluntary movement

Georg Goldenberg

1 Introduction

Neuropsychology is concerned with 'higher order' rather than 'elementary' disorders of movement. The theoretical model underlying such a distinction is questionable but it is useful for delimiting a collection of disorders which deviate from other motor symptoms of brain damage by marked dissociations between normal and abnormal motor acts of the same body part. One class of such disorders is characterized by incorrect or awkward movements which differ from 'elementary' motor disorders in that the same movements which give rise to errors in one condition can successfully be performed in other conditions and success or failure depend on non-motor factors. Such factors may be the visual control of the movements, its communicative meaning, or its relationship to tools and objects. Another class of higher order motor problems is constituted by well executed and apparently purposeful movements which do not conform to the subject's intentions. Table 20.1 gives an overview of disturbances fullfilling these criteria.

2 Incorrect and awkward movements

They can occur on one or both sides of the body. Kinaesthetic ataxia affects the hand and optic ataxia affects the visual field contralateral to the lesion. Face apraxia and limb apraxia are bilateral disorders resulting from unilateral, mainly left sided, lesions. Callosal apraxia disturbs movements of the left sided extremities.

2.1 Kinaesthetic ataxia (parietal hand)

Patients need vision to compensate for insufficient processing of kinaesthetic afferences. Shaping of the hand for grasp and manipulations is clumsy and needs visual attention. When out of visual control, the arm may involuntarily change its position but it does not unintentionally perform goal directed action. Kinaesthetic ataxia is a very disabling condition. The need for visual control renders the hand unusable for manipulation of objects in daily living because patients must concentrate their attention on the affected hand rather than on the external actions they want to accomplish.

Table 20.1 Higher level motor disorders resulting from hemisphere damage*

Incorrect and awkward movements		Movement out of voluntary control	
contralesional	bilateral	contralesional	bilateral
Kinaesthetic ataxia	Face apraxia	Grasping & groping	Motor perseverations
Optic Ataxia	Limb apraxia	anarchic hand	Imitation behaviour
			Utilization behaviour
Parietal lesions		Frontal lesions	

* Callosal apraxia is not considered in this table

- *Clinical diagnosis*:
    - Note involuntary displacement of the arm when attention is directed elsewhere.
    - Palpation of objects given for stereognosis is awkward and when the patient is prevented from seeing the hand the object may slip out of the hand.
    - Ask blindfolded patient to replicate with the sound arm a passively induced position of the affected arm: they cannot do so because they lack kinaesthetic information.
- *Lesion*. Anterior parietal lobe (Freund, 1987), lateral thalamus, or fibre tracts connecting these structures.
- *Therapy*. Explaining the mechanisms of the disorder and the importance of visual feedback can alleviate the patient's distress and help them to develop compensatory strategies in daily living. Occupational therapy can train performance of simple unimanual actions, like drinking or eating. Success remains contingent on allocation of attention to the affected hand. Integration of its movements into swift bimanual actions is rarely achieved.

2.2 Optic ataxia

Patients are unable to exploit visual information for exact guidance of goal-directed motor action of their hands. Inaccuracy and hesitancy of reaching to visually presented objects (e.g. the finger of the examiner) contrast with fast and accurate reaching to parts of their own body (e.g. the tip of the nose or the finger of the other hand). Experimentally it has been demonstrated that accuracy of visual reaching improves when a delay is interpolated between visual presentation and start of the movement (Rossetti *et al.*, 2005). Optic ataxia is more severe in the periphery of the affected visual hemi-field than in foveal vision. If optic guidance of eye movements is preserved, patients can compensate for optic ataxia by making a saccade to fixate a peripheral target and then reach it in the centre of the visual field. Optic ataxia affects reaching with either hand, but is sometimes more severe for the contralateral hand.

Bilateral lesions can cause optic ataxia of the whole visual field. Because of the proximity of responsible lesions, bilateral optic ataxia can be associated with Balint's Syndrome (see Chapter 11). Left sided optic ataxia can be associated with hemi-neglect, but most patients with hemi-neglect reach accurately to targets on the neglected side once they have noticed them.

The ecological significance of optic ataxia depends on whether it is uni- or bilateral and whether reaching in central fixation is preserved. If only reaching in the periphery of one visual field is inaccurate, the impact on everyday functioning is moderate.

- *Clinical diagnosis*
  - Sit opposite the patient and ask the patient to fixate on your eyes (as in confrontation perimetry). Raise a finger or a small object (e.g. a pencil) to different locations and ask the patient to touch it with their index finger.
  - To document preserved non-visual pointing ask the patient to touch their nose or fingers of the other hand.
- *Lesion*. Superior parietal lobe and parieto-occipital junction (Karnath & Perenin, 2005).
- *Therapy*. If visual fixation is preserved, the strategy of self-cueing by visual fixation (see above) can be trained.

2.3 Face apraxia

Patients have difficulties in performing facial or oral movements on command, although very similar movements are carried out spontaneously. For example, a patient may be unable to move the tongue into one cheek on command, but can perform the same movement when cleaning the mouth from remainders of a meal. Face apraxia may be associated with contralesional facial paralysis but can also be demonstrated on the ipsilesional side of the face. Face apraxia is rarely noted by the patients themselves and has no impact on life outside the testing situation. It may, however, constitute an obstacle for speech therapy in patients with LBD and apraxia of speech.

- *Clinical diagnosis:* To avoid confusion with problems of language comprehension, movements are tested in imitation. Table 20.2 provides a list of items arranged by difficulty (Bizzozero *et al.*, 2000).
- *Lesion*: Face apraxia can result from lesions of either hemisphere, but tends to be more persistent and more severe after left brain damage (LBD) than right brain damage (RBD). In LBD patients it is predominantly caused by inferior frontal and precentral lesions (Raade *et al.*, 1991).
- *Therapy:* Face apraxia per se does not need therapy.

2.4 Limb apraxia (see box)

Patients commit errors on performing some kinds of motor actions even when using the hand ipsilateral to the lesion which shows completely normal skill on other kinds of actions. The affected domains of action are imitation of gestures, performance of meaningful gestures, and use of tools and objects which can be further subdivided into the use of single tools or tool-objects pairs, and multi-step actions with several objects.

2.4.1 Imitation of gestures

Patients understand the request to imitate (if they do not, apraxia cannot be diagnosed) and try to provide a gesture resembling the demonstration, but the resulting posture is

Table 20.2 Items for testing facial apraxia

A Lower face
B Easy
Open your mouth
Show your teeth
Blow
B Medium
Make a clip-clop noise with your tongue
Push the tip of your tongue against the inside of your left cheek
Move your jaw to the right (and from right to left) three times
B Difficult
Puff out your right cheek
Push out your lower teeth (prognathism)
Push your tongue against the inside of your lower lip
A Upper face
Wrinkle your forehead
Wrinkle your nose
Blink your right eye (tight)

Easy, medium, and difficult refer to the ease with which normals perform these gestures. All upper face items are medium to difficult. Performance should be considered pathological if the patient produces random and amorphous movements, if response is preceded by additional, unsolicited movements, or if the required movement is incomplete or not performed at all. Items are from (Bizzozero *et al.*, 2000) in which a complete list is given together with normative data.

Bizzozero, I., Costato, D., Della Sala, S., Papagno, C., Spinnler, H., and Venneri, A. (2000). Upper and lower face apraxia: role of right hemisphere. Brain, **123**, 2213–2230.

Box 20.1 Classification of apraxia

There is a traditional distinction between three forms of limb apraxia:

- Ideational
- Ideomotor
- Limb-kinetic

This classification goes back to a hierarchical model of motor control proposed by Liepmann about 100 years ago. Liepmann thought that patients with ideational apraxia could not generate the idea or, respectively, the mental image of the intended action, whereas ideomotor apraxia disrupts the transformation of this idea into appropriate motor commands. Limb-kinetic apraxia should result from loss of 'motor engrams' which each hemisphere possesses and which direct overlearned routine actions of the opposite hand.

It is difficult to define clinical criteria that unequivocally distinguish between these variants of apraxia. Consequently, they have received very different interpretations. The theoretical model underlying the classification does not accord well with current knowledge of the physiology of motor control. There are thus no convincing reasons for retaining the historical classification.

spatially wrong. The movement to the final position may be hesitant and searching, but there are patients who attain the wrong position by a quick and confident movement. The problem concerns the definition of the target posture rather than its motor execution, and patients also commit errors when asked to replicate the gestures on a mannikin, or to match photographs of the same gestures performed by different persons seen from different angles. Imitation of meaningful gestures may be preserved, as patients may be able to recognize the meaning of the gesture and reproduce it without actually copying the shape of the gesture.

Disturbed imitation of gestures is a very impressive and easily demonstrable symptom of high theoretical interest, but as imitation is rarely required outside the testing situation it has little ecological significance. However, disturbed imitation may be an obstacle for efficient therapy of other motor impairments in physical and occupational therapy.

Clinical diagnosis It is preferable to test meaningless gestures as they provide an uncontaminated indication of the ability to imitate the shape of gestures. The examiner sits opposite the patient and demonstrates the gestures 'like a mirror' using the right hand for left hand imitation and vice versa. Patients should always use the hand ipsilateral to the lesion. The patient is allowed to start imitation only immediately after demonstration. Figure 20.1 shows 10 hand postures and 10 finger postures for which norms are available (Goldenberg, 1996).

Lesion LBD disturbs imitation of hand postures more than finger postures. RBD affects imitation of finger postures but spares hand postures. Imitation of foot postures can be deficient in both LBD and RBD. Within the left hemisphere, disturbed imitation of hand postures is linked to inferior parietal, and disturbed imitation of finger postures to inferior frontal and precentral lesions (Goldenberg & Karnath, 2006).

Therapy As it does not affect the patient's independence in daily living, disturbed imitation would not by itself justify therapeutic intervention. It may, however, be useful to train imitation of hand and finger postures as a prerequisite to acquiring the use of meaningful gestures to compensate for aphasia.

2.4.2 Meaningful gestures

Patients are unable to demonstrate meaningful gestures on command. Such gestures may either have a conventionally agreed, more or less arbitrary, meaning like 'somebody is nuts', 'military salute', or 'okay', or they may indicate objects by miming their use. Outside the testing situation the deficit can be observed when aphasic patients try to express themselves in spite of severe language impairment. They either do not employ gestures at all or produce amorphous, stereotypic, or incomprehensible gestures. Because it restricts the range of possible compensation for the language deficit, this manifestation of apraxia has ecological significance.

Clinical diagnosis Usually, diagnosis concentrates on miming of object use, because aphasic patients may not understand the verbal label of gestures with conventional meaning, whereas comprehension of the object name can be facilitated by showing either the object (e.g. a hammer, a key, a screwdriver) or a picture of it. Even with this help, understanding

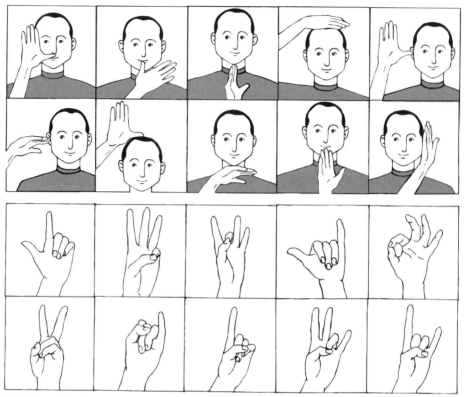

Fig. 20.1 10 hand postures and 10 finger postures for testing imitation of meaningless gestures. Two points are given for correct imitation on first trial, and 1 point for correct imitation on second trial, scores of 18 for hand postures and 16 for finger postures are borderline and scores below these values are pathological (Goldenberg, 1996). Illustration from (Goldenberg et al., 2001).

the instruction may be problematic. The demand to demonstrate the movements associated with object use without actually handling the object, taxes not only speech comprehension but also 'abstract attitude' which is frequently compromised in patients with aphasia. A diagnosis of apraxia should be made only if patients respond to the presentation of the object with a movement of the hand which can be clearly distinguished from spontaneous 'baton' movements accompanying attempts of verbal expression. A further difficulty is posed by the great variability of gesture performance in normal subjects. For example, the replacement of the absent object by the hand ('body part as object': e.g. brushing teeth with the index rather than demonstrating the manipulation of a toothbrush) is a strategy frequently employed to indicate an absent object when the verbal label is lacking (e.g. when trying to buy a toothbrush in a country the language of which you cannot speak). There are, however, errors which unequivocally indicate apraxia:

◆ Perseveration of a more or less amorphic movement (e.g. a circling movement above the table or repeated hitting of the fist against one's chest)

- Pointing to the location where the object should be applied (e.g. pointing to the mouth for a toothbrush or to the table for a pencil)
- Searching movements of the hand and fingers which eventually result in a recognizable pantomime ('conduite d'approche')

Lesion Apraxia for meaningful gestures is a symptom of LBD. It is virtually always associated with aphasia, but the severity of apraxia may differ from that of language impairment. Within the left hemisphere, lesions of inferior frontal lobe and underlying white matter are crucial. Contrary to a widely held belief, parietal lesions do not interfere with pantomime of tool use (Goldenberg *et al.*, 2007). This independence is corroborated by observation of patients in whom parietal lesion causes "visuo-imitative apraxia". These patients have severe difficulties with imitation of meaningless gestures (particularly hand postures) but perform pantomime of tool use and other meaningful gestures to command flawlessly.

Therapy In patients with severe expressive language problems it may be worth while to train gesturing as an alternative channel for communication. Training must take into account the loss of 'abstract attitude' and behavioural flexibility which frequently accompany severe aphasia. Thus a first step in the training is to familiarize patients with the possibility of using gestures for replacing speech. A second step is the training of specific gestures. Rarely do patients generalize to create and use gestures which have not been explicitly trained. Even for trained gestures, use outside the therapeutic setting may fail because patients persist in fruitless attempts at verbal expression rather than spontaneously changing to an alternative means of communication (Purdy & Koch, 2006). It is therefore advisable to concentrate on gestures which are important for everyday communication (e.g. I am hungry or tired, I need to go to the toilet etc), and to instruct the patients' partners to encourage use of gesture when verbal communication fails.

2.4.3 Use of single tools and objects

Use of single familiar tools and objects can fail for two reasons. Patients may have lost knowledge about the purpose of the tool and the prototypical manner of its use. For example, they may use a toothbrush for cleaning their jacket, because they have lost knowledge about the special purpose of toothbrushes. Conversely, they may know the purpose of the tool but be unable to adapt their actions to the constraints and affordances of the mechanical interaction between tool and object. For example, they press a knife into a loaf without a sawing movement, because they pursue the aim of dividing the loaf but cannot adapt the manner of cutting to the resistance of the loaf.

Clinical diagnosis

- Present familiar, easy to use, objects like a padlock with a key, a hammer and a nail, a comb, or a pair of binoculars and ask patients to use them. For examining hemiplegic patients objects must be prepared for one-handed use (e.g., provide a wooden block with a hole in which the nail to be hammered can be fixed).
- Examine one-handed tool use with the non-dominant left hand in several control persons to obtain an estimation of normal clumsiness of the non-dominant hand.

You will see that it is not difficult to distinguish apraxic errors made by the left hand of patients with right sided hemiplegia from normal variations of manual skill.

- Record errors and try to classify them according to whether they betray preserved knowledge about the usual purpose of the tool.

Lesion In patients with circumscribed brain lesions (e.g. from vascular accidents), misuse of familiar objects is due to left brain lesions, associated with aphasia and other manifestations of apraxia (Goldenberg & Hagmann, 1998). Lesions involve the parietal lobe but are rarely restricted to it.

Loss of knowledge about the purpose and prototypical use of tools in combination with preserved ability to infer possible functions has been documented in patients with bilateral temporal lobe lesions (e.g. from Herpes Simplex Encephalitis or Semantic Dementia) (Hodges *et al.*, 2000).

Therapy Training the application of single tools and objects, forms part of the therapy of multi-step activities of daily living (see 2.4.4).

2.4.4 Multi step actions with several tools and objects ("naturalistic action")

In daily life the use of the single tool is frequently embedded in a chain of actions involving several tools and objects and aiming at a superordinate goal transgressing and modulating the purposes of each single action step. Proper sequencing of actions and maintenance of the ultimate goal puts demands on memory and attention which can lead to errors even in patients who have no problems with use of single tools. In patients who already have problems with single tools and objects, the additional cognitive demands of multi-step planning may unmask misuse of single tools which did not appear during isolated testing.

Clinical diagnosis A task which can easily be administered at the examiner's desktop is to provide a sheet of paper, a perforator, and a folder, and to ask the patient to punch the paper and insert it into the folder. Preparation of coffee or a meal and performance of technical tasks can be observed in occupational therapy.

Lesions Errors and action slips in chains of actions with multiple tools and objects have been documented in patients with LBD, RBD, frontal, or diffuse brain damage (Rumiati, 2005). Although systematic studies failed to find significant differences between the error rates of these patient groups, clinical experience suggests that the most severe and persistent problems occur in patients with LBD and aphasia who also have apraxia for use of single tools and objects.

Therapy Patients can relearn use of tools and objects and even performance of complex chains of actions by training, but it is questionable whether improvement on trained activities generalizes to non-trained activities (Goldenberg *et al.*, 2001; Geusgens *et al.*, 2006). Possibly the flexibility of transposing therapeutic gains to other tasks and other circumstances depends on the presence and severity of other accompanying neuropsychological problems. In patients with severe aphasia as well as apraxia for use of single tools and objects, therapy success may remain restricted not only to the task but even to the exemplars of tools and objects used in therapy. Presumably, the most enduring way to enhance the independence of such patients, is to train them within their permanent environment, on tasks which they want to perform every day.

2.5 Callosal apraxia

Callosal disconnection deprives the right hemisphere from left hemisphere competence and renders the left hand apraxic. Like bilateral apraxia from LBD, left hand apraxia from callosal disconnection affects imitation, performance of meaningful gestures and object use. Disturbed object use may be restricted to objects not normally used by the right hand (e.g. knife, but not fork). Because natural lesions destroying the corpus callosum frequently encroach on neighbouring mesial frontal regions, callosal apraxia can be associated with disorders of voluntary control of motor actions such as motor neglect, grasping and groping, or anarchic hand (see below). On the other hand, destruction of callosal fibres is rarely absolute. Particularly when there is no additional mesial frontal lobe damage, imitation and object use by the left hand may recover due to enhanced employment of remaining callosal fibres or of ipsilateral motor pathways. (Goldenberg *et al.*, 2001).

Clinical diagnosis The hallmark of callosal apraxia is a discrepancy between apraxia of the left hand, and normal praxis of the right hand. In addition, there are signs of sensory-motor, sensory-verbal, and verbal-motor disconnection:

♦ Blindfolded patients cannot indicate the location of touch on their left hand either verbally or by pointing with their right hand, although they can point to the location with their left thumb.

♦ They cannot name objects put into their left hand, although the left hand palpates them skilfully.

♦ They cannot move single fingers of their left hand on verbal command although they can do so on imitation (note that imitation of finger postures depends less on the left hemisphere than does imitation of hand postures).

Lesion Callosal apraxia is contingent upon destruction of the middle portion of the corpus callosum.

Therapy Callosal apraxia is a fascinating syndrome of questionable ecological validity. Patients will rarely feel handicapped by the inability of their left hand to perform meaningful gestures on command. However, the insufficiency of callosal transfer of sensorimotor information may impede swift bimanual coordination, and this may be worth a trial of occupational therapy.

3 Disturbed voluntary control of motor actions

The affected limbs either do not spontaneously participate in an intended action (motor neglect) or do perform actions which are not intended (all other syndromes). Non-performance of intended actions, and performance of non-intended actions are not mutually exclusive.

3.1 Motor neglect

Patients need extra voluntary effort to make the affected limbs comply with their intentions. The limb is not used spontaneously although force and coordination are preserved. In severe cases the affected limb may appear to be completely paralyzed, although it may be raised and moved readily on command. Motor neglect becomes worse when attention is distracted. Thus patients with mild paresis of a leg who can safely stand and walk, may fall when attention is directed towards a simultaneous manual activity or external distractor. Simultaneous movement of the opposite limbs may also increase motor neglect, particularly if it is asymmetric.

If there has initially been paresis of an affected limb, it may be difficult to distinguish motor neglect from 'learned non-use': patients may have formed a habit of preferentially using the unaffected limb even for tasks which could easily be accomplished with the affected limb. Motor neglect is a disabling condition as it prevents normal use of the affected limb. Even very mild forms of motor neglect can be disastrous when combined with hemiparesis. Patients who have partly recovered from paresis and are able to stand and walk may neglect the affected limb when distracted and consequently fall and hurt themselves.

- *Clinical diagnosis*: Observe spontaneous motor behaviour and compare it with explicit testing of motor function. Place an object (e.g. a glass) in different locations on a table before the patient and ask them to grasp it. They will use the non-affected hand even if the glass is placed on the affected side.

- *Lesion:* Extended lesions including the parietal lobes can cause motor neglect together with perceptual and representational neglect, but frontal or deep lesions can cause pure motor neglect. Predominance of right sided lesions is less conspicuous for motor than for sensory and representational neglect (Siekierka-Kleiser *et al.*, 2006).

- *Therapy*: Frequent reminders to use the contralesional limbs are integrated in physio and occupational therapy. It is questionable whether therapies aimed at alleviating visuo-spatial neglect (see Chapter 6) have an effect on accompanying motor neglect.

3.2 Grasping and groping

When getting in touch with an object, the affected hand grasps it. It may also grope for visually perceived objects located in its proximity and grasp them. Few patients are able to suppress the grasp reaction by an effort of will. The majority have to interfere with their sound hand to loosen the grasp. They may sit on their hand or permanently place an object into it to prevent it from grasping external objects. Groping and grasping are embarassing and compromise the use of the affected hand.

- *Clinical diagnosis*:
  — Move your finger or a comparable object (e.g. handle of reflex hammer) over palm exerting some pressure on skin. If the patient grasps, advise them not to do so and repeat the manoeuvre.

— To elicit groping, move an object (e.g. reflex hammer) close to the patient's hand and withdraw it slowly if the hand moves towards it. If the hand follows the object, advise the patient not to do so, and repeat.

- *Lesion:* Medial face of superior frontal lobe (cingulate gyrus and supplementary motor area). Unilateral lesions of either side can cause bilateral grasping (De Renzi & Barbieri, 1992).

- *Therapy:* Spontaneous recovery is frequent, particularly when the lesion is unilateral. In collaboration with the patient, therapists may try to devise strategies which enhance the voluntary control of the afflicted hand.

3.3 Anarchic hand

One hand performs complex movements which are goal-directed and well executed but unintended. These unwanted movements cannot be voluntarily interrupted and may interfere with desired actions carried out by the other hand. Most of the unwanted actions are composed of seizing and pulling objects (e.g. pulling away a sheet on which the other hand is writing). Patients never deny that the hand is part of their own body but may accuse it of being disobedient and having a will of its own.

In the literature the term "alien hand" is frequently used synonymously with anarchic hand, although originally it referred to the failure to recognize one's own hand when placed into the other hand out of sight (Brion & Jedynak, 1972).

- *Clinical diagnosis*: Relies on complaints of patients and observation of spontaneous behaviour of the hand.

- *Lesion*: Anarchic hand can result from mesial superior frontal lobe lesion of the opposite hemisphere. In this case it may be associated with forced grasping or motor neglect (Marchetti & Della Sala, 1998). It has, however, also been observed following thalamic lesions with sensory loss of the afflicted hand which might be considered as a variant of kinaesthetic ataxia (Coulthard *et al.*, 2007). When lesions encroach on callosal fibres, anarchic hand can be associated with callosal apraxia of the left hand, but there are cases of right-sided anarchic hand as well.

- *Therapy*: The unwanted actions of the anarchic hand can be very embarrassing and a severe handicap for bimanual actions in activities of daily life such as dressing or eating. Experimental approaches to improving coordination, train rhythmic switching of objects between hands, or use of a mirror for enhancing visual control of the disobedient hand. Some success has been seen during training session but it rarely carries over to daily living (Brainin *et al.*, 2008).

3.4 Motor perseverations

Patients continue a motor action although its original purpose has been attained. For example, they may continue to peel all the oranges in a basket after they have peeled one for eating, or they may be unable to stop tooth brushing, or washing and spend hours in the bathroom. Patients may experience perseveration of actions as compulsive and against their own intentions, or they may justify them by ostensible motives (e.g. hygienic reasons for perseverative washing).

- *Clinical diagnosis*: Rests mainly on history taking and observation of the patient. In examination motor perseveration can be provoked by asking patients to draw a series of figures each consisting of three consecutive loops. Patients will increase the number of loops.

- *Lesion*: Uni- or bilateral lesions of superior mesial frontal lobe, similar to grasp reaction with which it may be associated. Persistent and severe motor perseverations are likely due to large bilateral frontal lesions or additional diffuse brain damage.

- *Therapy*: If motor perseverations do not recover spontaneously and constitute an obstacle for activities of daily living, strategies for interrupting them may be explored.

3.5 Utilization behaviour

Patients use objects which happen to be within their grasp in a way which is appropriate to the object but not to the situation. For example, they may take glasses which the examiner has laid down and put them on their nose, or they may take a stamp and repeatedly press it on a sheet of paper. If occurring outside the test situation, utilization behaviour may be socially disturbing.

- *Clinical diagnosis*: Care must be taken to distinguish utilization behaviour from enhanced suggestibility of brain damaged patients. If, for example, the examiner interrupts testing and puts objects on the table without commenting on their purpose and waits for the patient's reaction (L'hermitte, 1983), patients may understand this to be a non-verbal invitation to use the objects. It is therefore preferable to have attractive objects (e.g. glasses, matchbox, cigarettes, a pack of cards, a filled bottle and a glass.) already placed on the periphery of the table when the patient enters the room, then to engage the patient in unrelated conversation or testing, and observe their spontaneous behaviour (Shallice *et al.*, 1989).

- *Lesion*: Large, bilateral mesial frontal lesions. Lesions must be associated with some diffuse brain damage to give rise to utilization behaviour.

- *Therapy*: Methods from behavioural therapy may help to reduce socially embarrassing utilization behaviour.

3.6 Imitation behaviour

Although not requested to do so, patients imitate gestures and actions of the examiner or other persons. For example, patients may take off their glasses when the examiner does so or repeat back questions rather than answering them. An explicit command not to imitate can stop imitation but introduction of a pause is sufficient for reappearance of imitation. When asked why they imitated patients are puzzled and say nothing or they claim that they thought this was the implicit request made by the examiner (De Renzi *et al.*, 1996).

Like utilization behaviour, imitation behaviour may cause irritation when occurring outside the testing situation.

- *Clinical diagnosis*: Rests mainly on observation of spontaneous behaviour during conversation and testing. Avoidance of non-verbal requests to imitate can be very difficult when gestures are introduced explicitly for provoking imitation behaviour.

- *Lesions and therapy*: As in utilization behaviour

3.7 Voluntary motor control and social demands

The classification of utilization and imitation behaviour as disorders of voluntary control of movement can be called into doubt. The particular actions are wrong only with respect to the specific demands of the testing situation. The subtlety of their deviance from appropriate behaviour is highlighted by the fact that the very same actions – utilization of objects and imitation of gestures – are explicitly asked for when the examiner is interested in testing for apraxia (which may happen in the same session!). The observation that normal controls never utilize objects or imitate under the same conditions proves that they can easily understand such subtle distinctions, whereas patients with frontal lobe damage cannot. It is, however, questionable whether this failure should be classified as a disorder of motor control or as a manifestation of the effects of frontal lobe damage on comprehension and observance of social demands.

Selective references

Bizzozero, I., Costato, D., Della Sala, S., Papagno, C., Spinnler, H., and Venneri, A. (2000). Upper and lower face apraxia: role of the right hemisphere. *Brain*, **123**, 2213–2230.

Brainin, M., Seiser, A., and Matz, K. (2008). The mirror world of motor inhibition: The alien hand syndrome in chronic stroke. *Journal of Neurology, Neurosurgery, and Psychiatry*, **79**, 246–252.

Brion, S. and Jedynak, C. P. (1972). Troubles de transfert interhémisphérique (callosal disconnection). A propos de trois observations de tumeurs du corps calleux. Le signe de la main étrangère. *Revue Neurologique*, **126**, 257–266.

Coulthard, E., Rudd, A., Playford, E. D., and Husain, M. (2007). Alien limb following posterior cerebral artery stroke: failure to recognize internally generated movements? Movement Disorders, **22**, 1498–1502.

De Renzi, E. and Barbieri, C. (1992). The incidence of the grasp reflex following hemispheric lesions and its relation to frontal damage. *Brain*, **115**, 293–313.

De Renzi, E., Cavalleri, F., and Facchini, S. (1996). Imitation and utilisation behaviour. *Journal of Neurology, Neurosurgery, and Psychiatry*, **61**, 396–400.

Freund, H. J. (1987). Abnormalities of motor behavior after cortical lesions in humans. In V.B. Mountcastle, F. Plum, & S. R. Geiger (Eds.), *Handbook of Physiology Section 1: The Nervous System Volume 5: Higher Functions of the Brain Part 2* (pp. 763–810). Bethesda Maryland: American Physiological Society.

Geusgens, C., van Heugten, C. M., Donkervoort, M., van den Ende, E., Jolles, J., and van den Heuvel, W. (2006). Transferf of training effects in stroke patients with apraxia: An exploratory study. *Neuropsychological Rehabilitation*, **16**, 213–229.

Goldenberg, G. (1996). Defective imitation of gestures in patients with damage in the left or right hemisphere. *Journal of Neurology, Neurosurgery, and Psychiatry*, **61**, 176–180.

Goldenberg, G., Daumüller, M., and Hagmann, S. (2001). Assessment and therapy of complex ADL in apraxia. *Neuropsychological Rehabilitation*, **11**, 147–168.

Goldenberg, G. and Hagmann, S. (1998). Tool use and mechanical problem solving in apraxia. *Neuropsychologia*, **36**, 581–589.

Goldenberg, G., Hermsdörfer, J., Glindemann, R., Rorden, C., and Karnath, H. O. (2007). Pantomime of tool use depends on integrity of left inferior frontal cortex. *Cerebral Cortex*, **17**, 2769–2776.

Goldenberg, G., Hermsdörfer, J., and Laimgruber, K. (2001). Imitation of gestures by disconnected hemispheres. *Neuropsychologia*, **39**, 1432–1443.

Goldenberg, G. and Karnath, H. O. (2006). The neural basis of imitation is body part specific. *Journal of Neuroscience*, **26**, 6282–6287.

Hodges, J. R., Bozeat, S., Lambon Ralph, M. A., Patterson, K., and Spatt, J. (2000). The role of conceptual knowledge in object use - evidence from semantic dementia. *Brain*, **123**, 1913–1925.

Karnath, H. O. and Perenin, M. T. (2005). Cortical control of visually guided reaching: Evidence from patients with optic ataxia. *Cerebral Cortex*, **15**, 1561–1569.

Lhermitte, F. (1983). "Utilization behaviour" and its relation to lesions of the frontal lobes. *Brain*, **106**, 237–255.

Marchetti, C. and Della-Sala, S. (1998). Disentangling the alien and anarchic hand. *Cognitive Neuropsychiatry*, **3**, 191–207.

Purdy, M. and Koch, A. (2006). Prediction of strategy usage by adults with aphasia. *Aphasiology*, **20**, 337–348.

Raade, A. S., Rothi, L. J. G., and Heilman, K. M. (1991). The relationship between buccofacial and limb apraxia. *Brain and Cognition*, **16**, 130–146.

Rossetti, Y., Revol, P., McIntosh, R., Pisella, L., Rode, G., Danckert, J. *et al.* (2005). Visually guided reaching: bilateral posterior parietal lesions cause a switch from fast visuomotor to slow cognitive control. *Neuropsychologia*, **43**, 162–177.

Rumiati, R. I. (2005). Right, left, or both? Brain hemispheres and apraxia of naturalistic actions. *Trends in Cognitive Sciences*, **9**, 167–169.

Shallice, T., Burgess, P. W., Schon, F., and Baxter, D. M. (1989). The origins of utilization behaviour. *Brain*, **112**, 1587–1598.

Siekierka-Kleiser, E. M., Kleiser, R., Wohlschläger, A. M., Freund, H. J., and Seitz, R. J. (2006). Quantitative assessment of recovery from motor hemineglect in acute stroke patients. *Cerebrovascular. Diseases*, **21**, 307–314.

Chapter 21

The neuropsychology of acquired calculation disorders

Marinella Cappelletti and Lisa Cipolotti

1 Acalculia

Acalculia is an acquired disorder of number processing and calculation skills following cerebral damage (Henschen, 1919). The inability to use numbers can be very incapacitating as it interferes with several everyday activities such as shopping, using bank accounts and telephones (Butterworth, 1999; Dehaene, 1997). Acalculia is not a unitary disorder and can take a variety of different forms: patients may present with impairments in number processing, in calculation or both. The incidence of acalculia in patients with left hemisphere lesions has been estimated between 16% and 28%, and 90% of patients at the early stage of Alzheimer disease present with acalculia (Carlomagno *et al.*, 1999). Knowing the incidence of acalculia and its impact on everyday life has helped to improve assessment techniques and it has recently promoted the development of rehabilitation programs. In this chapter, we will:

1 present the basic components of the number and calculation system;

2 discuss cases of selective impairment of number processing and calculation;

3 discuss cases of selective preservation of number processing and calculation;

4 briefly outline the brain localization of number and calculation disorders;

5 propose some guidelines for the assessment and rehabilitation of acalculia in neurological patients.

2 The basic components of number and calculation processing

2.1 Number comprehension and production

Number comprehension usually refers to the ability to generate a semantic representation of numbers. This commonly refers to the quantity associated with numbers, for instance '21' indicates the numerosity of 21. The representation of quantity is thought to be abstract in nature (Dehaene and Cohen, 1997; McCloskey *et al.*, 1990 but see Cohen Kadosh *et al.*, 2005). The quantity expressed by numbers is often processed when comparing numbers, for instance when deciding which of two products is the most expensive. In doing so, we are usually faster and more accurate when two numbers (or two prices) are further apart, e.g. £1.20 and £2.55, relative to when they are close to each other, e.g. £1.20 and £1.15. This phenomenon is referred to as the 'distance effect' (Moyer and Landauer, 1967). Impairments in processing numerical quantity may result in a 'reverse distance effect', which indicates that the time needed to process numbers increases as the numerical distance between them increases (e.g. Delazer and Butterworth, 1995). This is because the quantity associated with numbers can not be accessed automatically and other strategies, for instance counting, have to be used instead. Besides indicating quantities, numbers can also have a 'nominal' function, for instance '21' may also indicate a house or a bus number or the age of consent (Butterworth, 1999; Dehaene, 1997).

Number production refers to the process of converting a numeral's semantic representation into an output format. The most commonly used formats are the Arabic, e.g. '21' and the verbal, e.g. 'twenty-one'. The production of a number in one of these formats is based on input and output processes. For instance, reading Arabic numerals is based first on visually identifying the string of digits, second on translating this string of digits into a sequence of words according to a set of rules, and third on producing an oral or written output. This transformation of numbers from one format to another is usually referred to as *'transcoding'* (Dehaene and Cohen, 1995; Deloche and Seron, 1982; McCloskey *et al.*, 1986).

2.2 Calculation

Processing oral and written arithmetical operations require a set of specific and independent processes including:

(i) The processing of arithmetical symbols (i.e. +, ×, −, ÷)

(ii) The retrieval of arithmetical facts, defined as a vocabulary of 'number combinations', such as '3 + 3 = 6' or '3 × 3 = 9'.

(iii) The execution of calculation procedures consisting of the specific algorithms required to solve multi-digit calculations, for instance carrying (e.g. in '234 + 159') and borrowing (e.g. in '234 − 159') procedures.

(iv) Arithmetic conceptual knowledge, namely the understanding of the principles underlying arithmetical facts and procedures (e.g. the principle of commutativity, such as a + b = b + a).

3 Selective impairment of number processing and calculation

Neurological patients may present with specific impairments in the processing of numbers, in calculation, or in both. Table 21.1 provides an overview of the range of potential deficits which can be observed in acalculic patients. Here we will describe the impairments of:

1 number transcoding;

2 quantity processing;

3 calculation, which in turn may consist of impairments in processing arithmetical signs, simple facts, procedures, or arithmetical conceptual knowledge.

Table 21.1 Overview of the potential disorders of (A) number processing and (B) calculation (right column)

A. Disorders of number processing	
Disorders of number production affecting	lexical processing
	syntactical processing
Disorders of number comprehension affecting	cardinal number meaning
	sequence number meaning
B. Disorders of calculation affecting processing of	
	arithmetical symbol processing
	arithmetical fact retrieval
	calculation procedures
	conceptual knowledge

3.1 Impairments of number production

Studies have described patients with disorders in number production have primarily focussed on reading and writing numbers (e.g. Cipolotti *et al.*, 1995; Deloche and Seron, 1982; McCloskey *et al.*, 1986; 1990; Sokol and McCloskey, 1988). Some of these studies have looked at the errors made by patients when reading or writing numbers. This permitted the identification of two major cognitive mechanisms within number transcoding: the syntactic, and the lexical number processes.

Syntactic processes involve the specification of the relationship among the elements of the number, e.g. number class, i.e. to read aloud 600, one needs to retrieve the correct number class {hundred}. Syntactic errors are errors which occur when the wrong number class is selected (e.g. stimulus: '5', response: 'fifty' or stimulus: 'two thousand and thirty eight', response: '2000308'). For example, patient SF's syntactic errors occurred in reading aloud Arabic numerals and could best be classified as 'quantity-shift' errors (e.g. 207 → 'two thousand and seven'; 80 → 'eight') (Cipolotti, 1995).

Lexical processes involve the specification of individual elements in the numeral, for instance to read aloud 600, has to be retrieved once the correct class {hundred} has been identified the correct element {6}. Lexical errors involve the incorrect production of one or more of the individual elements in a numeral (stimulus: '29', response: 'forty-nine'). Patient HY's errors in reading aloud Arabic numerals were mainly lexical, for instance he read number '5' as 'seven' and '29' as 'forty-nine' (Sokol *et al.*, 1991).

Other studies have demonstrated that transcoding skills can be independent from other numerical abilities. For example, patient HY was impaired in reading aloud Arabic numerals (McCloskey *et al.*, 1986). When attempting to read aloud an Arabic numeral, he often made mistakes such as reading number '5' as 'seven', and '29' as 'forty-nine'. In contrast, results from a series of number comprehension tasks showed that patient HY was unimpaired in comprehending Arabic numerals. Thus, his impaired performance in reading aloud Arabic numerals reflected his impairment in number transcoding rather than a deficit in comprehending the Arabic stimuli.

This pattern of performance has also been shown by other patients (e.g. Cipolotti and Butterworth, 1995), and the opposite performance, (i.e. poor performance in calculation and preserved transcoding has also been documented) (e.g. Cipolotti and Butterworth, 1995; Sokol *et al.*, 1991). This suggests that transcoding skills are distinct from other numerical abilities.

A frequent type of error in writing numbers to dictation or from a written input has been referred to as 'intrusion errors'. These consist of reproducing part of the input code when formulating the output one. This type of error has been described in patients with dementia of the Alzheimer type as well as in those with focal brain lesions (Della Sala *et al.*, 2000; Thioux *et al.*, 1999). According to Thioux and colleagues (1999), three different types of intrusion errors can be distinguished.

- The first consists of producing a numerical output in the same format as the source one, has been called 'complete lexical shift error' or 'perseveration'. For example when the Arabic numeral '75' is written as '75' instead of as the number word 'seventy five', (or conversely the 'seventy five' written as the number word 'seventy five' instead of as the numeral '75').

- The second type of intrusion error is called 'partial lexical shifting', and occurs when only one part of the input is transposed onto the output, (e.g. the Arabic numeral '75' written as 'seventy5').

- Thirdly, 'intra lexical shift' errors consist of writing a numeral in a mixture of verbal and Arabic formats, for example, the Arabic numeral '70' written as '7ty'.

Some authors explained these errors in terms of the combination of impaired transcoding mechanisms on the one hand, and impaired inhibitory processes on the other (Thioux *et al.*, 1999). Other authors have suggested that perseveration and intrusion errors are attentional in nature and originate from a unique impairment in selective attentional capacities (Macoir *et al.*, 2002).

3.2 Impairments of number comprehension

A few studies have reported patients with a basic failure of understanding and processing the quantity indicated by numbers (Cipolotti *et al.*, 1991; Dehaene and Cohen, 1997; Delazer and Benke, 1997; Delazer and Butterworth 1997; Lemer *et al.*, 2003; Noel and Seron, 1993; Polk *et al.*, 2001). For example, patient NR showed impairment in understanding Arabic numerals (Noël and Seron, 1993). Thus, she could no longer point to the larger of two Arabic numerals (e.g. 345 vs 785 or 265 vs 237). Moreover, she lost the ability to match spoken number names to the corresponding Arabic numeral. A profoundly acalculic patients (CG) presented with an unusual pattern of performance (Cipolotti *et al.*, 1991). Although she had retained the ability to process abstract quantities, she lost the meaning of all numbers above 4. For example, she was unable to say how many days were in a week or which was larger, 5 or 10. Her deficit was so pervasive that it seriously limited her activities of daily living, for instance, CG was unable to do her own shopping, deal with money, make phone calls, use a calendar, or read the time, although her intellectual skills, language, memory and visuospatial abilities were largely preserved.

Recent studies have focused on quantity processing in neglect patients. Two of these studies have shown that neglect patients can correctly indicate the larger or smaller of two numbers (Cappelletti and Cipolotti, 2006; Vuilleumier *et al.*, 2004). The patients' performance in number comparison indicated that even the numerical stimuli appearing in the neglected hemifield could be processed even when not reported (Cappelletti and Cipolotti, 2006). Moreover neglect patients are typically slower to process numbers which are located to the left of '5', (i.e. '4') relative to numbers located to its right (i.e. '6'), suggesting that their number impairment is consistent with their spacial impairment (Vuilleumier *et al.*, 2004).

Thus, the idea that the spatial impairments in neglect may affect numerical processing has recently been explored in studies, specifically, which tested whether neglect may affect the mental 'number line'; a metaphor used to represent numbers as oriented from smaller to larger (Dehaene *et al.*, 1993). One way to test the integrity of a mental number line is with the bisection task. This consists of orally presenting two numbers, (e.g. '1' and '5') and asking which number falls in the middle. Neglect patients typically select a number which is larger than the middle one, for instance they say that '4' and not '3' is mid-way between '1' and '5' (Cappelletti *et al.*, 2007a; Doricchi *et al.*, 2005; Zorzi *et al.*, 2002). This pattern of performance mirrors the classical leftward bias which neglect patients show in bisecting physical lines, although their performance also seems to depend on the line orientation of the physical and numerical lines (Cappelletti *et al.*, 2007).

3.3 Impairments of calculation

Each of the different cognitive processes involved in calculation (i.e. processing arithmetic symbols, facts, procedures and conceptual knowledge), appear to be functionally independent as well as differentially susceptible to brain damage. Examples of selective impairments in such components of calculation are described below.

3.3.1 Disorders of arithmetic symbol processing

Very few patients with selective impairment in understanding arithmetic symbols have been reported (e.g. Ferro and Botelho, 1980; Laiacona and Lunghi, 1997). For example, Laiacona and Lunghi (1997) investigated a patient who misnamed and misidentified the arithmetic signs and performed written arithmetic operations according to this misidentification, for instance the patient systematically added up instead of multiplying (See Fig. 21.1a). This deficit however, was not specific to arithmetic symbols, but was part of a more general impairment in processing also non-arithmetic symbols such as punctuation marks.

a) Performance of patient EB, with a selective impairment in arithmetical symbol processing (Laiacona and Lunghi, 1997). Specifically, the patient systematically plussed the times.

```
        48                    59
    ×   67                ×   29
    ─────                 ─────
       115                   88
```

Fig. 21.1a Disorders of arithmetric processing symbols.

3.3.2 Disorders of arithmetic fact retrieval

Several patients have been documented with selective impairments of arithmetic fact retrieval. Typically, these patients have severe difficulties in performing very simple single-digit addition, subtraction, multiplication and division. They produce many errors such as '5 + 7' = '13 roughly' (e.g. Dehaene and Cohen, 1991), and their response times are abnormally slow (e.g. >2 seconds). An error classification has been proposed by McCloskey *et al.*, (1991c). Errors can be classed as *operand errors*, if the incorrect answer is the correct answer to a computation that shares one of the operands (e.g. 6×5 = 25); as *operation errors*, if the incorrect answer constitutes a correct answer to another computation involving the same operands, but a different operation (e.g. 3×4 = 12); as *table errors*, if the incorrect answer represents the product of two different single digit numbers (e.g. 4×4 = 25); and as *non table errors*, if the incorrect answer is neither an operand, a table or an operation error (e.g. 9 x 8 = 52). Patients who make these errors often show intact knowledge of arithmetical principles and procedures. Typically, they are able to retrieve and apply the appropriate arithmetic steps required to solve complex arithmetic problems and they are able to define arithmetic operations (e.g. Delazer and Benke, 1997; Sokol *et al.*, 1991; Warrington, 1982). For this type of patient everyday activities such as checking their change or their bank statements pose great difficulties.

Impairment of arithmetic facts can also manifest in a highly selective manner. Selectively preserved and impaired arithmetic facts have been reported according to specific types of operation. For example, patients have been documented with selective impairments or selective preservations of multiplication (e.g. Dehaene and Cohen, 1997; McCloskey *et al.*, 1991b; Grafman *et al.*, 1989; Delazer and Benke, 1997), and subtraction facts (e.g. Dagenbach and McCloskey, 1992; Pesenti *et al.*, 1994; McNeil and Warrington, 1994; Lampl *et al.*, 1994; Dehaene and Cohen, 1997). Selective impairments of addition and division have also been reported. Cipolotti and de Lacy Costello (1995) described a patient who could no longer solve '4 ÷ 2', while being able to solve '27×26'. Van Harskamp and Cipolotti (2001) described a patient with selective addition impairment who could no longer add 2 + 3, but was still able to solve 13 − 6 and 8×9.

3.3.3 Disorders of calculation procedures

There have only been a few reports of patients with selective impairment of calculation procedures. Girelli and Delazer (1996) described patient MT, who systematically subtracted the smaller number from the larger one, irrespective of whether the larger was at the top or the bottom line (see Fig. 21.1b). His impairment in solving multi-digit

b) Performance of patient MT with a calculation procedure impairment. He showed 'Smaller from Larger' subtraction bugs (Girelli and Delazer, 1996).

$$
\begin{array}{r}
923 \\
-\ 644 \\
\hline
321
\end{array}
\qquad
\begin{array}{r}
171 \\
-\ 48 \\
\hline
127
\end{array}
$$

Fig. 21.1b Disorders of arithmetric processing symbols.

subtractions was attributed to a defective knowledge of calculation procedures. This deficit was selective for subtraction, as the patient was able to correctly carry out multi-digit addition problems involving the carry over procedure (such as $78 + 26$).

Other impairments in the use of calculation procedures may consist of misaligning the digit in multi-digit operations, of errors using carrying procedures in addition problems, or of not applying the problem-specific procedure in the correct order. For example, in multi-digit multiplications this consists of multiply digits in the upper number starting from the rightmost, by digits in the bottom number starting from the rightmost etc. (e.g. Benson and Weir, 1972; Grana *et al.*, 2006; Sokol *et al.*, 1991; Sokol and McCloskey, 1991).

3.3.4 Disorders of arithmetic conceptual knowledge

Delazer and Benke (1997) described a patient (JG) who had lost arithmetical conceptual knowledge, which is defined as 'An understanding of arithmetical operations and laws pertaining to these operations' (Hittmair-Delazer *et al.*, 1994, p. 117). JG could retrieve multiplication tables from memory despite severe problems in all tasks requiring conceptual knowledge. The patient could correctly calculate '3×3,' but did not know that '3×3' equals '$3 + 3 + 3$'. The patient was encouraged to use any 'back-up strategies', such as counting on fingers for simple addition problems. Usually this strategy is adopted spontaneously by patients with impairments in arithmetic fact retrieval. However, JG never succeeded in representing problems with her fingers (Delazer and Benke, 1997, p.705). She did not apply even very basic principles such as commutativity in multiplication (i.e. $4 \times 12 = 12 \times 4$), and she was unable to recognize that multiplication can be transformed into repeated addition ($4 \times 12 = 12 + 12 + 12 + 12$).

The opposite side of the dissociation, namely intact conceptual knowledge with impaired fact retrieval, has been reported in two single-case studies (Hittmair-Delazer *et al.*, 1994, 1995). The first study described a patient who demonstrated excellent conceptual knowledge despite a severe acalculia. For example, when presented with arithmetic operations such as 8x6, he adopted the following strategy $8 \times 10 = 80$; $80:2 = 40$; $40+8=48$ (see Fig. 21.1c). Another patient who was no longer able to solve simple elementary arithmetic such as $2 + 3$, showed excellent understanding and use of abstract equations such as $(b \times a)$: $(a \times b)=1$ and $(cd + ed):d= c + e$ (Hittmair-Delazer *et al.*, 1994). Similarly, a semantic dementia patient demonstrated well preserved understanding of arithmetic concepts despite the loss of arithmetic facts (Cappelletti *et al.*, 2005). He spontaneously developed strategies which allowed him to perform computations when he could not access simple facts or use canonical procedures (e.g. using multiple additions

c) Performance of patient BE with impaired arithmetical fact retrieval but preserved conceptual knowledge. When asked to perform arithmetical problems such as 8x6, he adopted the strategy below (Hittmair-Delazer et al, 1994)

$$8 \times 10 = 80; 80 : 2 = 40; 40 + 8 = 48$$

Fig. 21.1c Disorders of arithmetric processing symbols.

d) An example of IH's performance in solving a multidigit multiplication operation (Cappelletti et al., 2005). Number 531 was decomposed into the subparts 1, 30, and 500. Numbers in squared brackets indicate the main steps in performing the operation. Step [1] is 27x1. Steps [2] to [4] show how 327x30 was obtained. Step [2] is 327x5; [3] is 327x10 and [4] is 327x30; [5] is 327x100 obtained through multiple additions; [6] is 327x500, again obtained through multiple additions. Finally, [7] is (327×500)+(327×30)+(327×1). The final result is correct.

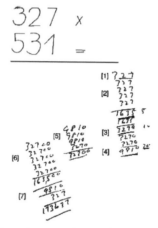

Fig. 21.1d Disorders of arithmetric processing symbols.

to solve a multiplication problem, see Fig. 21.1d). These cases demonstrate that conceptual knowledge is a functionally independent component of calculation.

4 Selective preservation of number processing and calculation

It is now well established that numerical and calculation abilities can be largely independent from other cognitive abilities, such as general intellectual skills (e.g. Remond-Besuchet *et al.*, 1999), language (e.g. Rossor *et al.*, 1995; Thioux *et al.*, 1998), short-term memory (e.g. Butterworth *et al.*, 1995), and semantic knowledge (e.g. Cappelletti *et al.*, 2001; Crutch and Warrington, 2004). For example, a patient with semantic dementia (IH) presented with severe impairment in understanding the meaning of words and the use of objects, but was nevertheless able to understand numerical concepts and to perform arithmetical operations (Cappelletti *et al.*, 2001), even in the later stages of illness (Cappelletti *et al.*, 2005). This suggests that a patient's understanding of arithmetical concepts may remain preserved despite severe inability to process the meanings of words and objects. A similar pattern of performance on numerical and calculation tasks has been reported in other semantic dementia patients (e.g. Crutch and Warrington, 2002), suggesting that knowledge of verbal concepts can be independent.

5 Localisation of brain lesions in number and calculation disorders

An overview of group and single case studies has indicated that numerical skills may have discrete and independent brain substrates (Cipolotti and van Harskamp, 2001). The majority of patients with number production and/or number comprehension impairments have left posterior lesions, often involving the parietal lobe. Similarly, the majority of patients with arithmetical fact retrieval impairments had lesions mainly implicating the left parietal lobe. This is also the case for the majority of patients with impairment of arithmetic fact retrieval for specific types of operations. In particular, patients with impairments of multiplication or subtraction typically have lesions encroaching on the left parietal lobule.

The neuropsychological evidence indicating the involvement of the parietal lobe in numerical processing has been corroborated by neuroimaging studies (e.g. Cappelletti *et al.*, 2009; Dehaene *et al.*, 1999, 2003; Pesenti *et al.*, 2000), and by studies using transcranial magnetic stimulation (TMS, e.g. Andres *et al.*, 2005; Cappelletti *et al.*, 2007b). However, it is important to note that not all parietal lesions result in numerical impairments. For instance, only about 20% of patients with left parietal lesions show numerical deficits (e.g. Jackson and Warrington, 1986). Moreover, most patients with right parietal lesions show preserved comprehension of core numerical concepts (e.g. Cappelletti and Cipolotti, 2006; Cappelletti *et al.*, 2007; Cohen *et al.*, 2007; but c.f. Rosselli and Ardilla, 1989; Langdon and Warrington, 1997 for a different pattern of results). Similarly, not all numerical impairments are due to parietal lesions. For instance, deficits in arithmetical procedures have been reported in patients with more anterior lesions (e.g. Grana *et al.*, 2006). Future research will help to clarify the extent to which parietal regions are critical for number and calculation processing, and elucidate the role of the left and the right parietal lobes in these processes.

6 Assessment and rehabilitation of acalculia

6.1 Diagnosis and assessment tools

The diagnosis of acalculia relies on the establishment of appropriate tools to detect the presence of number processing and/or of calculation impairment in subjects with intact premorbid calculation skills. The diagnosis of pure acalculia needs to exclude that numeracy skills are not a secondary consequence of other cognitive deficits such as language, attention, and visuospatial functions.

Formal assessment of the patient's numeracy skills requires detailed evaluation of number processing and calculation abilities. Number processing can be assessed using number reading, writing to dictation, and repetition tasks. Numerical stimuli can be presented as either Arabic numerals (e.g. 8), written (*eight*) or spoken number names ('eight'). Patients can be simply asked to read, write or repeat the numeral presented. Comprehension of number quantity is usually assessed with magnitude comparison tasks, whereby patients are asked to indicate the larger of two numbers (e.g. which is bigger: 6 or 9?).

Another test of number comprehension is the number composition task in which subjects have to compose the value of a given number using poker chips which range in value from 1 to 500. The ability to subitize is another way to test comprehension of number quantity. Subitizing is the ability to rapidly indicate the number of items contained in a small set (usually up to 4 or 5). Larger sets of objects require additional processing, such as counting. Patients' subitizing can be tested by presenting them with displays containing items which vary in number and position. Patients can simply be asked to report the number of items contained in each display. Intact quantity processing is expected to correspond to the ability to rapidly and correctly indicate the numerosity of the set; the time required to produce an answer is expected to increase with the number of items presented with a sharp increase after number 4 or 5. This is because enumeration over four items is slow, more error-prone, and thought to require counting (e.g. Trick and Pylyshyn, 1993, Sathian *et al.*, 1999).

Calculation skills can be assessed with tasks exploring knowledge of arithmetical signs, arithmetical facts, and arithmetical procedures. To evaluate the ability to process arithmetical signs, patients are usually required to read, point to and write, the arithmetical signs. To test the ability to retrieve simple arithmetical facts, patients are asked to compute orally presented single-digit arithmetical calculations (e.g. $4+2$, 3×4 or $5-2$). The access to arithmetical procedures is usually assessed by performing multi-digit calculation, such as $294+12=306$, either in the written or in the oral modality. Both response hires and accuracy should be recorded.

Error analysis, although usually not included in standardised tests, adds useful extra information to the assessment, in so far as it can provide further details about the nature of the impairment. Thus, when patients have problems in reading and writing numerals, a common analysis of errors is the distinction between lexical or syntactical errors. When patients have problems in the retrieval of arithmetical facts, it is useful to distinguish between operand errors, operation errors, table errors, and non-table errors.

6.2 Natural recovery from acalculia

Although acalculia is a frequent disorder in left-brain damaged patients, relatively little is known about its prognosis. Only one study has investigated the natural evolution of acalculia in patients with left hemisphere vascular lesions (Caporali *et al.*, 2000). This study indicates that some patients recover completely in the first months post-stroke even without specific rehabilitation. Apparently, this improvement can also present in severely acalculic patients. This would suggest that initial severity of acalculia may not significantly influence recovery.

The authors suggest that recovery might be due to the resolution of the diachises in the first months after stroke (3-6 months post-onset). However, besides this more general and 'passive' recovery, the authors suggest that a more specialised functional reorganisation might play a role several months post onset (>7 months). This suggestion would account for the fact that some patients continued to improve even several months after stroke although it is not clear whether the recovery was specific for acalculia. In fact, most patients also improve in other cognitive domains, such as language.

6.3 Rehabilitation of number processing and calculation skills

The high frequency and disabling consequences of acalculia underline the importance of developing remediation techniques and intervention for arithmetical disorders. A complete and detailed assessment of the patient's numerical processing and calculation skills is essential to understanding the nature of numeracy impairment and will continue the basis for designing suitable rehabiliation programs (Girelli and Seron, 2001). According to the specific type of acalculia, different kinds of rehabilitative intervention may be required. Thus, a detailed assessment of a patient's number processing and calculation skills will constitute the basis for designing suitable rehabilitation programmes. For example, a patient may show a highly selective impairment in the retrieval of simple multiplication facts. However, he/she may still be able to perform simple addition and subtraction. The re-acquisition of multiplication facts may then be facilitated by the use of back-up strategies based on addition (e.g. counting-on procedure: $3 \times 6 = 6 + 6 + 6$).

Recent reviews (e.g. Girelli and Seron, 2001; Lochy et al., in press) have shown that very few studies have been devoted to the rehabilitation of numerical skills. These few studies concentrated on the rehabilitation of number transcoding deficits (e.g. Deloche et al., 1989; Sullivan et al., 1996), arithmetical fact retrieval (e.g. Domahs, 2003, 2007; Girelli et al., 1996, 2002; Hittmair-Delazer et al., 1994; Whetstone, 1998), and the development of strategies for solving problems (Fasotti et al., 1992).

6.3.1 Rehabilitation of transcoding skills

The rehabilitation of transcoding skills has concentrated on the ability to translate numerical stimuli into different codes (e.g. 'four' → 4). As an example we will discuss an interesting rehabilitation programme implemented by Deloche and colleagues. (1989). They treated a patient with selective and very severe difficulties in the production of written verbal numerals from Arabic numerals (i.e. 7001 → *seven thousand zero one*). This deficit was very severe. Indeed, the patient showed a 45% error rate. His errors were mostly syntactic (e.g. 114 → one hundred ten four). Deloche *et al.*'s rehabilitation programme consisted of re-teaching a set of explicit transcoding rules using a step-by-step procedure. They used highly specific exercises which targeted a single transcoding rule. There were several facilitation procedures (e.g. colour cues, vocabulary panels) to help the patient with his learning process. For example, they rehabilitated the patient's ability to transcode a 2-digit Arabic numeral such as *73* into the corresponding written number word *seventy-three*, by explicitly stating the rule 'transcode the left digit by a ten name and the right digit by a unit name'. During training a vocabulary panel with two coloured columns was placed in front of him. The red part of the vocabulary panel contained the TENS names (ten, twenty, thirty etc up to ninety), and the blue part contained the UNIT names (one, two, etc up to nine). After 25 training sessions of 30 to 60 minutes each, the patient's performance was close to ceiling. Interestingly, the long-term effects of the treatment were reassessed 7 months post-training. Only a very small increase in error rate relative to post-training evaluation was reported (6%). Overall, the patient continued to perform better than before training.

6.3.2 Rehabilitation of arithmetical facts

Rehabilitation of arithmetical fact retrieval consists primarily of attempts to re-teach 'lost' arithmetical knowledge via extensive practice. The underlying assumption is that practice may 're-create' or 're-strengthen' lost associations between problems and answers. Thus, for example, two patients (TL and ZA) with specific impairment of multiplication fact retrieval underwent twice-weekly training sessions over a period of eight weeks (Girelli et al., 1996). During the training session the arithmetical problems were presented in written form and simultaneously read aloud by the examiner. The patients were asked to answer, either verbally whilst pointing to the number on a table, or by writing the Arabic numeral. Errors were always corrected immediately. Patient TL relearned the answers as 'labels', by reciting one operand's table (e.g. $4 \times 3 = 4, 8, 12,$). Patient ZA relearned the answers as serial additions (e.g. $4 \times 3 = 3 + 3 + 3 = 12$).

At the end of the session, both patients improved considerably and showed stable recovery at one month follow-up. Strikingly, after treatment, their overall error rate dropped to 10% (from pre-treatment error rates of 91% (TL), and 81% (ZA)). Not only did the error rates decrease dramatically over the course of remediation in both patients, but the nature of the errors also changed. This change in error patterns was interpreted as being due to different strategies used by the two patients in relearning their facts. As described above, patient TL relied on the recitation of Nx1 forward until she could access the solution to the problem. Patient ZA relied on the strategy of repeated addition of the second operand. Thus, back-up strategies may certainly play a facilitative role in the re-acquisition of simple arithmetic. Similar training programs for the rehabilitation of arithmetical fact impairment have been adopted in other cases as well (e.g. Hittmair-Delazer et al.,1994; Whetstone, 1998).

The conventional 'drill' approach to rehabilitation of arithmetical facts can be lightened by simultaneous presentation of visual or auditory cues (Domahs et al., 2004, 2007). Another approach has been to rehabilitate arithmetic facts based on conceptual knowledge rather than extensive training. This method is based on inducing a meaningful re-organisation of arithmetical facts according to the principles underlying them, for instance the commutative law or decomposition using known facts, (i.e. 10s, ties and 2s) (Girelli et al., 2002).

Girelli and Seron (2001) also stressed the importance of minimising the opportunity to make mistakes, since repeated errors may strengthen the wrong associations between problems and answers. Moreover, the use of back-up strategies based on the principles underlying arithmetical facts such as the order-irrelevant principle (e.g. $8 \times 6 = 6 \times 8 = 48$), decomposition strategies (e.g. $4 \times 8 = 2 \times 8 + 2 \times 8 = 32$) or repeated addition of the second operand (e.g. $3 \times 5 = 5 + 5 + 5 = 15$) seem important in rehabilitation of arithmetical facts.

Overall, research has indicated that patients benefit significantly from training, and that improvement is retained over time (and in some cases, spontaneously generalises).

7 Conclusions

This review described acalculia as a heterogeneous disorder consisting of impairments in processing numbers, in calculation, or in both. Specific components of number and calculation have been presented in the context of both normal functioning and impaired performance following cerebral damage. This included disorders in transcoding processing, quantity processing, calculation, and their sub-components. Cases of selective preservation of number processing have also been analysed. This review also offered a short outline of lesions' localization with respect to number and calculation disorders, and indicated the parietal areas most relevant for numeracy and its impairments.

Finally, we have proposed some guidelines for the assessment of acalculia and discussed some of the rehabilitation programmes for acalculia in neurological patients. These programmes have indicated the importance of systematic intervention in acalculia, but have also shown that there are several important aspects of numerical skills for which no specific interventions have been developed. Future studies are needed to create treatments for different numeracy impairments and to test whether these treatments generalise to real-life situations; the purpose of any rehabilitation programme.

Acknowledgments

This work was supported by a grant from the Wellcome Trust and the Royal Society Dorothy Nod glan fellowship(MC).

Selective references

Andres, M., Seron, X. and Olivier, E (2005). Hemispheric lateralization of number comparison. *Cognitive Brain Research*, **25**, 283–90.

Benson, D. F. and Weir, W.F. (1972). Acalculia: acquired anarithmetia. *Cortex*, **8**, 465–472.

Butterworth B. (1999). The Mathematical Brain. London: Macmillan.

Butterworth, B., Cipolotti, L. and Warrington, E.K. (1995). Short-term memory impairments and arithmetical ability. *Quarterly Journal of Experimental Psychology*, **49A**, 251–262.

Caporali, A., Burgio, F. and Basso, A. (2000). The natural course of acalculia in left-brain-damaged patients. *Neurological Science*, **21**, 143–149.

Cappelletti, M., Butterworth, B. and Kopelman, M. (2001). Spared numerical abilities in a case of semantic dementia. *Neuropsychologia*, **39**, 1224–39.

Cappelletti, M., Morton, J., Kopelman, M. and Butterworth, B. (2005). The progressive loss of numerical knowledge in a semantic dementia patient: A follow-up study. *Cognitive Neuropsychology*, **22**, 771–793.

Cappelletti, M. and Cipolotti, L. (2006). Unconscious processing of Arabic numerals in unilateral neglect. *Neuropsychologia*, **44**, 10, 1999–2006.

Cappelletti, M., Freeman, E.D. and Cipolotti, L. (2007a). The middle house or the middle floor: bisecting horizontal and vertical mental number lines in neglect, *Neuropsychologia*, **45**, 2989–3000.

Cappelletti, M., Barth, H., Fregni, F., Pascual Leone, A. and Spelke, E. (2007b). rTMS over the left and the right intraparietal sulcus disrupts discrete and continuous quantity processing. *Experimental Brain Research*, **179**, 631–642.

Carlomagno, S., Iaverone, A., Nolfe, G., Bourene, G., Martin, C. and Deloche, G. (1999). Dyscalculia in the early stages of Alzheimer's disease. *Acta Neuropsychologica Scandinavia*, **3**, 166–174.

Cipolotti, L., Butterworth, B. and Denes, G. (1991). A specific deficit for numbers in case of dense acalculia. *Brain*, **114**, 2619–2637.

Cipolotti, L. (1995). Multiple routes for reading words, why not numbers? Evidence from a case of Arabic numeral dyslexia. *Cognitive Neuropsychology*, **12**, 313–342.

Cipolotti, L., Warrington, E. and Butterworth, B. (1995). Selective impairment in manipulating Arabic numerals. *Cortex*, **31**, 73–86.

Cipolotti, L. and Butterworth, B. (1995). Toward a multiroute model of number processing: Impaired number transcoding with preserved calculation skills: *Journal of Experimental Psychology: General*, **124** (4), 375–390.

Cipolotti, L. and De Lacy Costello, A. (1995). Selective impairment for simple division. *Cortex*, **31**, 33–449.

Cipolotti L. and van Harskamp N.J. (2001). Disturbances of number processing and calculation. In *Handbook of Neuropsychology* (ed. F. Boller **and** J. Grafman), pp 305–331. Amsterdam-New York: Elsevier.

Cohen, Kadosh, R., Henik, A., Rubinstein, O., Mohr, H., Dori, H., Van de ven, V., Zorzi, M., Goebel, R., and Linden, D. (2005). Are Numbers Special? The Comparison Systems of the Human Brain Investigated by fMRI. *Neuropsychologia*, **43**, 1238–1248.

Cohen, L., Wilson, A.J., Izard, V. and Dehaene, S. (2007). Acalculia and Gerstmann's Syndrome. In: *Cognitive and Behavioral Neurology of Stroke*; Eds: O Godefroy & J Bogousslavsky. Cambridge University Press.

Crutch, S.J. and Warrington, E.K. (2002). Preserved calculation skills in a case of semantic dementia. *Cortex*, **38**, 389–399.

Dagenbach, D. and McCloskey, M. (1992). The organisation of Arithmetical Facts in Memory: Evidence from a Brain-Damaged Patient. *Brain and Cognition*, **20**, 345–366.

Dehaene, S. and Cohen, L (1991). Two mental calculation systems: A case study of severe acalculia with preserved approximation. *Neuropsychologia*, **29**, 1045–1074.

Dehaene, S., Bossini, S. and Giraux, P. (1993). The mental representation of parity and number magnitude. *Journal of Experimental Psychology: Human, Memory, and Cognition*, **21**, 314–326.

Dehaene, S. and Cohen, L. (1994). Dissociable Mechanisms of Subitizing and Counting: Neuropsychological Evidence from Simultanagnosic Patients. *Journal of Experimental Psychology: Human Perception and Performance* **29** (5), 958–975.

Dehaene, S. and Cohen, L. (1995). Towards an anatomical and functional model of number processing. *Mathematical Cognition*, **1**, 83–120.

Dehaene, S., Tzourio, N., Frak, V., Raynaud, L., Cohen, L., Mehler, J. and Mazoyer, B. (1996). Cerebral activations during number multiplication and comparison: a PET study. *Neuropsychologia*, **34**, 1097–1106.

Dehaene S. (1997). *The Number Sense: How the Mind Creates Mathematics*. New York: Oxford University Press.

Dehaene, S. and Cohen, L. (1997). Cerebral pathways for calculation: double dissociation between rote verbal and quantitative knowledge of arithmetic. *Cortex*, **33**, 219–250.

Dehaene, S., Spelke, E., Pinel, P., Stanescu, R. and Tsivkin, S. (1999). Sources of mathematical thinking: Behavioral and brain-imaging evidence. *Science*, **284**, 970–974.

Dehaene, S., Piazza, M., Pinel, P. and Cohen, L. (2003). Three parietal circuits for number processing. *Cognitive Neuropsychology*, **20**, 487–506.

Delazer, M. and Benke, T. (1997). Arithmetic facts without meaning. *Cortex*, **33**, 697–710.

Delazer, M. and Butterworth, B. (1997). A dissociation of number meanings. *Cognitive Neuropsychology*, **14**, 613–636.

Delazer, M., Girelli, L., Grana A. and Domahs, F. (2003). Number processing and calculation-Normative data from healthy adults, *Clinical Neuropsychology* 17, 3, 331–350.

Della Sala, S., Gentileschi, V., Gray, C. and Spinnler, H. (2000). Intrusion errors in numerical transcoding by Alzheimer patients. *Neuropsychologia*, **38**, 768–777.

Deloche, G. and Seron, X. (1982). From one to 1: An analysis of a transcoding process by means of neuropsychological data. *Cognition*, **12**, 119–149.

Deloche, G., Seron, X. and Ferrand, I. (1989). Re-education of Number transcoding mechanisms: A procedural approach. In *Cognitive Approaches in Neuropsychological Rehabilitation*. (Eds. X. Seron and S. Deloche), pp. 249–287. Hillsdale, NJ: Lawrence Erlbaum.

Deloche, G., Seron, X., Larroque, C., Magnien, C., Metz-Lutz, M.N., Noel, M.N., Riva, I., Dordain M., Schils, J.P., Ferrand, I., Baeta, E., Basso, A., Cipolotti L., Claros-Salinas, D., Gaillard, F., Goldenberg, G., Howard, D., Mazzuchi, A., Stachowiack F., Tzavaras, A., Vendrell, J., Bergego, C. and Pradat-Diehl, P. (1994). Calculation and number processing: Assessment battery; role of demographic factors. *Journal of Clinical and Experimental Neuropsychology*, **16**, 195–208.

Deloche, G., Hannequin, D., Carlomagno, S., Agniel, A., Dordain, M., Pasquir, F., Pellat, J., Dennis, P., Desi, M., Beauchamp, D., Metz-Lutz, M.N., Cesaro, P. and Seron, X. (1995). Calculation and number processing in mild Alzheimer's disease. *Journal of Clinical and Experimental Neuropsychology*, **17**, 634–639.

Deloche, G., Dellatolas, G., Vendrell, J. and Bergego, C. (1996). Calculation and number processing: Neuropsychological assessment and daily life difficulties. *Journal of the International Neuropsychological Society*, **2**, 177–180.

Domahs, F., Bartha, L., Delazer, M. (2003). Rehabilitation of arithmetic abilities: Different intervention strategies for multiplication. *Brain and Language*, **87**, 165–166.

Domahs, F., Zamarian, L., Delazer, M. (2007). Sound arithmetic: Auditory cues in the rehabilitation of impaired fact retrieval. *Neuropsychological Rehabilitation*, **1**, 49–64.

Doricchi, F., Guariglia, P., Gasparini, M., Tomaiuolo, F. (2005). Dissociation between physical and mental number line bisection in right hemisphere brain damage. *Nature Neuroscience*, **8**, 12, 1663–1666.

Fasotti, L., Bremer, J.J.C.B., Eling, P.A.T.M. (1992). Influence of improved test encoding on arithmetical word problem solving after frontal lobe damage. *Neuropsychological Rehabilitation*, **2**, 3–20.

Ferro, J.M., and Botelho, M.A.S. (1980). Alexia for arithmetical signs: a cause of disturbed calculation. *Cortex*, **16**, 175–180.

Girelli, L. and Delazer, M. (1996). Subtraction bugs in an acalculic patient. *Cortex*, **32**, 547–555.

Girelli, L., Delazer, M., Semenza, C. and Denes, G. (1996). The representation of arithmetical facts: Evidence from two rehabilitation studies. *Cortex*, **32**, 49–66.

Girelli, L. and Seron, X (2001). Rehabilitation of number processing and calculation skills. *Aphasiology*, **15** (7), 695–712.

Girelli, L., Bartha, L., Delazer, M. (2002). Strategic learning in the rehabilitation of semantic knowledge. *Neuropsychological Rehabilitation*, **12**, 41–61.

Grafman, J., Kampen, D., Rosenberg, J., Salazar, A. and Boller, F. (1989b). Calculation abilities in a patient with a virtual left hemispherectomy. *Behavioural Neurology*, **2**, 183–194.

Granà, A., Hofer, R., Semenza, C. (2006). Acalculia from a right hemisphere lesion Dealing with 'where' in multiplication procedures. *Neuropsychologia* 44, 2972–2986.

Henschen, SE. (1919). Uber Sprach-Musik-und Rechenmechanismen und ihre Lokalisationen im Grosshirn. *Zeitschrift fur die gesamte Neurologie und Psychiatrie*, **52**, 273–98.

Hittmair-Delazer, M., Semenza, C. and Denes, G. (1994). Concepts and facts in calculation. *Brain*, **117**, 715–728.

Hittmair-Delazer, M., Sailer, U. and Benke, T. (1995). Impaired arithmetic facts but intact conceptual knowledge - A single case study of dyscalculia. *Cortex*, **31**, 139–148.

Jackson, M. and Warrington, E.K (1986). Arithmetic skills in patients with unilateral cerebral lesions. *Cortex*, **22**, 611–620.

Laiacona, M. and Lunghi, A. (1997). A case of concomitant impairment of operational signs and punctuation marks. *Neuropsychologia*, **35**, 325–332.

Lampl, Y., Eshel, Y., Gilad, R. and Sarova-Pinhas, I. (1994). Selective acalculia with sparing of the subtraction process in a patient with left parieto-temporal haemorrhage. *Neurology*, **44**, 1759–1761.

Langdon, D.W., Warrington, EK. (1997). The abstraction of numerical relations: a role for the right hemisphere in arithmetic? *Journal of the International Neuropsychological Society*, **3**, 260–268.

Lemer, C., Dehaene, S., Spelke, E., Cohen, L. (2003). Approximate quantities and exact number words: Dissociable systems. *Neuropsychologia*, **41**, 1942–1958.

Lochy, A., Domahs, F, Delazer, M. Rehabilitation of acquired calculation and number processing disorders. In: Campbell J, editor. *The Handbook of Mathematical Cognition*, in press.

Macoir, J., Audet, T., Lecomte, S. Delisle, J. (2002). From 'Cinquante-Six' to '5quante-Six': The origin of intrusion errors in a patient with probable Alzheimer disease. *Cognitive Neuropsychology*, **19**, 579–601.

McCloskey, M., Sokol, S.M. and Goodman, R.A. (1986). Cognitive processes in verbal-number production: Inferences from the performance of brain-damaged subjects. *Journal of Experimental Psychology General*, **115**(4), 307–330.

McCloskey, M., Sokol, S.M., Goodman-Schulman, R.A. and Caramazza, A. (1990). Cognitive representations and processes in number production: Evidence from cases of acquired dyscalculia. In *Advances in cognitive neuropsychology and neurolinguistics*. (ed. A. Caramazza), pp. 1–32, New Jersey: Lawrence Erlbaum.

McCloskey, M., Aliminosa, D. and Macaruso, P. (1991a). Theory-based assessment of acquired dyscalculia. *Brain and Cognition*, **17**, 285–308.

McCloskey, M., Aliminosa, D. and Sokol, S.M. (1991b). Facts, rules and procedures in normal calculation: Evidence from multiple single-patient studies of impaired arithmetic fact retrieval. *Brain and Cognition*, **17**, 154–203.

McCloskey, M., Harley, W. and Sokol, S.M. (1991c). Models of arithmetic fact retrieval: An evaluation in light of findings from normal and brain-damaged subjects. *Journal of Experimental Psychology: Learning, Memory and Cognition*, **17**, 377–397.

McNeil, J. and Warrington, E.K. (1994). A dissociation between addition and subtraction with written calculation. *Neuropsychologia*, **32**, 717–728.

Miceli G. and Capasso, R. (1999). Calculation and number processing. In *Handbook of Clinical and Experimental Neuropsychology* (Eds G. Denes **and** L. Pizzamiglio.), pp. 583–612. Hove, UK, Psychology Press.

Moyer, R.S. and Landauer, T.K. (1967). Time required for judgements of numerical inequality. *Nature*, **215**, 1519–20.

Noël, M.P. and Seron, X (1993). Arabic number reading deficit: A single case study. *Cognitive Neuropsychology*, **10**, 317–339.

Noël, M.P. (2001). Numerical Cognition. In *The Handbook of Cognitive Neuropsychology: what deficits reveal about the human mind*. (ed B.Rapp), pp 495–518, Taylor and Francis, Psychology press.

Pesenti, M., Seron, X. and Van Der Linden, M. (1994). Selective impairment as evidence for mental organisation of arithmetical facts: BB, a case of preserved subtraction? *Cortex*, **30**, 661–671.

Pesenti, M., Thioux, M., Seron, X. and De Volder, A. (2000). Neuroanatomical substrates of Arabic number processing, numerical comparison, and simple addition: A PET study. *Journal of cognitive neuroscience*, **12** (3), 461–479.

Polk, T., Reed, C., Keenan, J., Hogard, P., Anderson, C.A. (2001). A dissociation between symbolic number knowledge and analogue magnitude information. *Brain & Cognition*, **47**, 545–563.

Remond-Besuchet, C., Noël, M.P., Seron, X., Thioux, M., Brun, M. and Aspe, X. (1999). Selective preservation of exceptional arithmetical knowledge in a demented patient. *Mathematical Cognition*, **5** (1), 41–63.

Rosselli, M., Ardila, A. (1989). Calculation deficits in patients with right and left hemisphere damage. *Neuropsychologia*, **27**, 607–617.

Rossor, M.N., Warrington, E.K. and Cipolotti, L. (1995). The isolation of calculation skills. *Journal of Neurology*, **242**, 78–81.

Sathian, K., Simon, T. J., Peterson S, Patel, G.A., Hoffman, J.M., and Grafton, S.T. (1999). Neural evidence linking visual object enumeration and attention. *Journal of Cognitive Neuroscience* **11**(1), 36–51.

Sokol, S.M. and McCloskey, M. (1988). Levels of representation in verbal number production. *Applied Psycholinguistics*, **9**, 267–281.

Sokol, S.M., McCloskey, M., Cohen, N.J.and Aliminosa, D. (1991). Cognitive representations and processes in arithmetic: Inferences from the performance of brain-damaged subjects. *Journal of Experimental Psychology: Learning, Memory and Cognition*,17(3), 355–376.

Sullivan, K.S., Macaruso, P. and Sokol, S.M. (1996). Remediation of Arabic numerals in numeral processing in a case of developmental dyscalculia. *Neuropsychological Rehabilitation*, **6**, 27–53.

Thioux, M., Pillon, A., Samson, D., de Partz, M.P., Noë,l M.P. and Seron, X. (1998). The isolation of numerals at the semantic level. *Neurocase*, **4**, 371–389.

Thioux, M., Ivanoiu, A., Turconi, E., Seron, X. (1999). Intrusion of the verbal code during the production of Arabic numerals: A single-case study in patient with probable Alzheimer Disease. *Cognitive Neuropsychology*, **16**, 749–773.

Trick, L. M. and Pylyshyn, Z. W. (1993). What enumeration studies can show us about spatial attention: evidence for limited capacity preattentive processes. *Journal of Experimental Psychology: Human Perception and Performance* **19**, (2), 331–351.

Van Harskamp, N.J. and Cipolotti, L. (2001). Selective impairments in addition, subtraction and multiplication: Implications for the organisation of arithmetical facts. *Cortex*, **37**, 363–388.

Vuilleumier, P., Ortigue, S., Brugger, P. (2004). The number space and neglect. *Cortex*, **40**, 399–410.

Warrington, E.K. (1982). The fractionation of arithmetical skills: A single study. *Quarterly Journal of Experimental Psychology*, **34**, 31–51.

Whetstone, T. (1998). The representation of arithmetic facts in memory: Results from retraining a brain-damaged patient. *Brain and Cognition*, **36**, 290–309.

Zorzi, M., Priftis, K., Umilta, C. (2002). Brain damage: neglect disrupts the mental number line. *Nature*, **417**, 138-9.

Chapter 22

The assessment and treatment of emotional disorders

Guido Gainotti

1 Introduction

The juxtaposition, in this and in most other books of neuropsychology, of emotional disorders and disorders of language, memory, attention, visuospatial exploration, etc. could implicitly suggest that a basic similarity exists among all these 'neuropsychological' disorders. This suggestion, however, is misleading from both the conceptual and the pathophysiological point of view. Conceptually, emotions cannot be placed under the same general heading as the above-mentioned cognitive functions. Pathophysiologically, the relationship between brain damage and clinical symptomatology is different in the cases of cognitive and of emotional disorders.

1.1 Emotion as a general 'adaptive system'

From the 'conceptual' point of view, language, memory, attention, etc. must be viewed as components of a general, phylogenetically advanced, adaptive system (the 'cognitive system'). Emotion, on the other hand, should be considered as a second (more primitive) general adaptive system, also composed of different functional subsystems. The adaptive nature of both the emotional and the cognitive system has been stressed by Oatley and Johnson-Laird (1987), who have claimed that, in order to face a partially unpredictable environment and to select the most appropriate response pattern, the organism makes use of two operative (the emotional and the cognitive) systems.

- The emotional system is considered as an automatic emergency system, based on processes involved in the quick appraisal of external events and the immediate activation of a small number of innate operative patterns. These action patterns correspond to a few basic emotions (e.g. fear, rage, joy, sadness, surprise and disgust) that reflect, at the level of interpersonal communication and of proness toward action, the most important interactive schemata for the human species.

- The cognitive system can be considered, in contrast, to be a powerful propositional adaptive system, based on the exhaustive computation of sensory data and on the selection of complex strategic plans, but one that requires much more time to carry out its adaptive function (see Gainotti 2000).

If we turn now to the different pathophysiology responsible for cognitive and emotional disorders resulting from brain injury, we can say that the relationship between brain damage and clinical symptomatology is immediate (and the functional defect closely related to the anatomical locus of lesion) in various kinds of cognitive disorders. This relation, however, is at least in part indirect (and the behavioural pattern only in part related to the anatomical locus of damage) in the case of emotional disorders.

1.2 Emotional reactions to the consequences of a brain damage

According to most theorists of emotions (e.g. Lazarus 1982), the process of emotional appraisal (or emotional evaluation) is a fundamental step of every kind of emotional reaction and consists of the subjective evaluation.

(a) of the personal significance of a situation or an event;

(b) of the capacity to cope adequately with this event.

Now, since a stroke, brain trauma or other cause of brain damage is an event that can have a tremendous personal meaning for the patient, a significant emotional reaction to the brain damage is to be expected, irrespective of the extent and of the anatomical location of the brain lesion.

2 Taxonomies of emotions and their underlying theoretical models

The theoretical debate between biologically and cognitively oriented authors about the nature of emotions has been dominated in recent years by a controversy on the relationships between emotion and cognition. On the one hand, authors such as Zajonc (1980), Panksepp (1982) and LeDoux (1996) have stressed the biological foundations of emotions, maintaining that emotion and cognition must be considered as independent systems. On the other hand, cognitively oriented authors, such as Lazarus (1982), Frijda (1986) and Scherer (2000) have argued that there are not two independent adaptive systems, but that cognition plays an integral in emotion. This controversy stems from the facts that human emotions are very complex, hierarchically organized phenomena (Gainotti 2001) and that the levels of emotions taken into account by biologically oriented and by cognitively oriented authors, can be very different.

- The biologically oriented authors, being interested in the brain-behaviour relationships, and drawing on Darwin's (1872/1965) seminal work on the survival value of the social aspects of emotions, focus their attention on the simplest aspects of emotion, as they appear in animals and in the early stages of human development.

- The cognitively oriented authors, attracted by the complexity of emotional phenomena, focus their attention on the subtleties of human interactions, consider the biological approach as inappropriate and reductionistic, and base their taxonomies of human emotions on various types of situational antecedents and of appraisal criteria (Scherer 2000).

Biologically oriented authors are therefore right in considering that, from the phylogenetic and from the functional points of view emotion and cognition constitute two partly independent adaptive systems, and are subserved by different brain structures. However, cognitively oriented theorists are also right in stressing the interaction that exists between the two systems and the integral role that cognition plays in functions of emotional appraisal.

Trying to construct a bridge between these two different, but not necessarily alternative positions, Leventhal (1974 and 1987) has proposed an ontogenetic model of emotions that implicitly acknowledges both the earlier autonomy and the later dependency of emotionsl on the cognitive system. In particular, Leventhal has proposed a model of human emotion based on three functional levels:

* The *sensori-motor level* consist of a set of innate expressive-motor programs, that are triggered automatically by certain stimuli and which include components of motor and autonomic activation, as well as subjective emotional feelings. During an individual's psychological development, expressive-motor programs are created through a process of linking conditioned learning to situations within the individual's experience - building an 'emotional schemata' for each person.

* The second schematic level consists of the units that make up the emotional schemata for each individual. These units determine spontaneous emotions as well as emotional feelings and these give each schemata the hallmarks of true emotion.

* The last stage of this model is the *conceptual level* where the individual does not store instances of concrete emotional experiences but draws on conscious declarative memory, abstract notions about emotions and social rules in order to express emotion.

More recently, Rolls (2005) has examined aspects of the Leventhal's hierarchical model and has explored in some detail how cognitive states can modulate emotions and, in turn, how emotions can influence both cognition and decision-making. The distinction between biologically grounded basic levels and the more complex psychologically oriented levels of emotions can allow us to understand why emotional disorders can result, in some cases, as a consequence of neurological factors and in other cases because of psychological or psychosocial factors (Gainotti, 1993).

3 Neurological, psychological and psychosocial factors causing disorders in brain-damaged patients

3.1 Neurological factors

Emotional disorders are due to neurological factors when they result from the encroachment of the lesion upon 'limbic' structures (such as the fronto-orbital cortex, the cingulate gyrus, the amygdala or the hypothalamus) specifically involved in various aspects of emotions (see Gainotti 2006 for a survey of this subject). A schematic representation of these structures, mapped on to a medial view of a cerebral hemisphere, is shown in Figure 22.1.

3.1.1 Emotional disorders as long-term sequelae of closed head injury

Of the various categories of diseases which can provoke brain damage, closed head injury is probably the one that shows the most direct link between structural brain lesions and emotional disorders. This is due to the fact that, in patients who report a typical road accident of the acceleration-deceleration type, the injury mostly involves the axial brain structures and the mesiobasal parts of the frontal and temporal lobes (Adams *et al.*, 1980). Particularly damaged are, therefore, are structures such as the fronto-orbital cortex, the

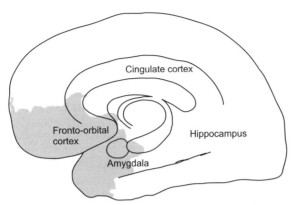

Fig. 22.1 A schematic representation of the fronto-orbital cortex, the cingulate gyrus, and the amygdala mapped on to a medial view of a cerebral hemisphere. The hatched parts of the figure indicate the brain structures usually damaged in patients with a severe closed head injury

anterior part of the cingulate gyrus and the amygdala (Fig. 22.1), which are critically involved in various aspects of emotional and motivational processes. The clinical counterpart of the preferential encroachment of the lesion upon these limbic structures is a prevalence of emotional and behavioural disorders (rather than of motor, sensory or aphasic disturbances) as the the long-term sequelae of severe head injury. These emotional disorders usually consist of:

(a) a severe apathetic syndrome, with a lack of emotional reaction to pleasant or unpleasant events and of goal-directed behaviours;

(b) a marked inability to keep under control socially unacceptable emotional reactions, such as aggressive outbursts when experiencing frustrating situations;

(c) less specific anxious or depressive reactions.

According to Mega & Cummings (1994) the apathetic syndrome and the disinhibition of emotional outbursts may be due to loss of function in different pathophysiological mechanisms within different parts of the frontal cortex. Here, apathy is seen as the result of disruptions in dopaminergic circuits (running from the mesencephalic ventral segmental areas to the frontal cortex), reducing motivated behaviour. In contract, disinhibition is seen as the result of a breakdown of control activity exerted by the fronto-orbital cortex on the amygdala.

From a theoretical point of view, the inability of patients with fronto-orbital lesions to assimilate external stimuli results from deficiencies s in the activation of the 'somatic markers' which converge in the ventro-medial frontal cortex. (For an examination of the autonomic emotional response within appropriate social and cognitive context and proprioceptive afferences associated with emotional consequences for personal decisions see Damasio (1994)). Results supporting these views have been reported by Bechara *et al.* (1997, 2000) using a gambling task, in which choices that yield high immediate gains are followed by higher future losses. Contrary to control subjects, who rapidly realized the need of changing their initial options, patients with ventro-medial frontal (FO) lesions were insensitive to future consequences and were primarily guided by immediate reward.

However, from a clinical point of view and irrespective of the nature of the underlying disorder, mental changes in patients with severe head injuries are extremely important. Not least, because they usually affect young or very young persons and are associated with important memory disorders and poor awareness of cognitive and behavioural disturbances. These mental changes hamper resumption of gainful employment and place a heavy burden upon family members, who must cope with the patient's childishness, impaired initiative, low tolerance of frustration, and impulsive or aggressive reactions.

3.2 Psychological factors

Emotional disorders due to psychological or psychodynamic (rather than to neurological) factors result from the process of appraisal:

- evaluating the personal significance that the consequences of the brain damage will have for the subject;
- evaluating his/her capacity to cope with these consequences.

A factor that critically contributes to the outcome of this (implicit or explicit) appraisal process is the awareness of the brain damage and of its consequences. When this awareness is full and painful, as in many patients with Broca's aphasia and a right-sided hemiplegia, the emotional response often consists of 'catastrophic reactions' following frustrating attempts at verbal expression and a more stable anxious-depressive disorder. When, in contrast, this awareness is poor (as in patients with a frontal lesion resulting from a traumatic brain injury, or in stroke patients with a right hemisphere lesion and a syndrome of neglect for the left half of the body and of extrapersonal space), then a lack of concern and an apathetic behaviour are usually observed.

It must be acknowledged, however, that the relationship between awareness of the disorder, the appraisal process and the emotional reaction is not necessarily one-way, simple or direct. According to Lambie and Marcel (2002), experience of emotion can take various forms and phenomenological knowledge can be distinguished from awareness. Marcel et al.(2004) have shown that anosognosia for hemiplegia is not a unitary phenomenon and that several factors underlie deficits in bodily awareness. Sometimes, the (apparent) unawareness of the functional defect and of the resulting disability ('anosognosia') can be considered to be a primitive form of coping mechanism, rather than as a factor influencing the appraisal process. In this case it seems preferable to use the term 'denial of illness', rather than the term 'unawareness of the disability', to mean that the patient is somehow aware of his/her disabilities, but is forced to verbally deny their existence.

3.2.1 Anosognosia of left-sided hemiplegia

The more impressive form of 'denial of illness' is often observed in patients who have sustained a massive stroke in the territory of the right middle cerebral artery but who verbally deny their left-sided hemiplegia or behave as if this side of their body is perfectly normal.

Patients exhibiting the syndrome of 'denial of left-sided hemiplegia' have been included in psychoanalytically oriented research studies (Kaplan-Solms and Solms, 2000;

Turnbull *et al.*, 2002) and the existence of a 'denial syndrome' due to general psychody-namic mechanisms and not resulting directly from brain damage is suggested by several lines of enquiry. One of these is that denial syndrome is often observed in life-threatening conditions, such as cancer or miocardial infarction where there is no evidence of brain damage.

Difficulty in determining whether an emotional behaviour is a consequence of a proc-ess of emotional appraisal or is, instead, due to a biologically determined factor that influ-ences the outcome of this process is frequently experienced in brain-damaged patients (see Orfei *et al.*, 2007). This problem raises important methodological problems (see Ownsworth and Clare, 2006) and may concern not only the awareness of the disease, but also other important aspects of emotional behaviour, such as a depressive mood or an apathetic state.

3.2.2 Post-stroke depression

The syndrome of major 'post-stroke depression'(PSD), that is observed in a high propor-tion (20-25%) of stroke patients, has been considered by Robinson *et al.* (1984, Robinson 2001) to be a biological consequence of stroke, resulting from disruption of monoamin-ergic pathways running from the brainstem to the cerebral cortex. These conclusions, however, have been criticized on methodological grounds by Gainotti *et al.* (1997), who have reanalyzed the question using a new instrument (the Post-Stroke Depression Rating Scale) specifically constructed to take account of symptoms and problems of stroke patients, and have shown that major PSD is phenomenologically different from 'endog-enous' forms of major depression. On the basis of these data, Gainotti and Marra (2005) conclude that PSD must be considered a motivated form of depression, provoked by the serious obstacles that the consequences of brain damage put in the way of the patient's attainment of personal goals. The emphasis on the personal/ subjective nature of emo-tional problems caused by brain damage underlies the weakness of the main objection of supporters of the 'neurological' model to the psychological interpretation of PSD, namely that since in some studies no significant association has been found between degree of disability and severity of PSD, no relationship should exist between psychological factors and PSD. The weakness of this argument consists in its assumption that a linear and objective relationship must exist between disability and emotional reaction. This assump-tion does not take into account the subjective nature of the process of emotional reaction. Emphasis on the subjective component implies that a motivated form of depression does not result from the objective consequences of brain damage, but from the personal sig-nificance that the subject attributes to these consequences, in terms of social roles and of personal goals.

3.3 Psychosocial factors

Emotional disorders can be due to psychosocial factors rather than to the the appraisal of the immediate consequences of brain damage, when they result from the long-term consequences of this event on the full range of activities, social roles and social relationships of the patient.

The most important of these social consequences is perhaps represented by the process of social isolation, which increases over time, extending from the patient to his or her family.

This process implies two major modifications in the patient's social network:

(1) a reduction in its size, as the number of people interacting with the patient progressively decreases;

(2) an increase of its intensity, since the only persons remaining in contact with the patient are those who are committed to a lasting relationship with them, (i.e. family members, closely related to each other) (Gainotti, 1993).

From an emotional point of view, the first modification leads patients to become apathetic, lonely and depressed, whereas the second modification usually leads to an increasing strain among the members of this isolated group, with development of feelings of resentment and hostility.

3.3.1 Circular interactions between patients and their families

It is important to note in this context that the circular interactions that can develop between patients and their families can, not supprisingly, have either a positive or a negative influence on the patient's own emotional attitude and, consequently, on the rehabilitation process and outcome. Thus, if close relatives are unable to tolerate the emotional problems of these patients and the associated role changes that the patients' disabilities introduce in the family system, then their negative attitude will further decrease the self-esteem of the patient and their motivation toward rehabilitation. If, on the other hand, family members warmly support their relatives and assume a realistically positive attitude toward their condition, then this positive attitude will be inculcated by the patient, restoring their self-esteem and increasing motivation toward rehabilitation.

4 The major types of emotional disorders following brain damage

As mentioned in previous sections, depression, anxiety, apathy and lack of control over disruptive emotional outbursts are among the most prevalent and clinically relevant forms of emotional disorders usually observed in brain-damaged patients. The prevalence of these disorders and their clinical characteristics are different, however, following different categories of brain damage and during different stages in the evolution of the same disease. The anatomical locus of lesion and the time elapsed from onset are very important determinants of this heterogeneity in the patterns of emotional behaviour shown by different clinical categories of brain-damaged patients.

In particular, the anatomical locus of lesion, which is the more powerful source of variance from this point of view, probably acts trough two main mechanisms:

(a) the encroachment of the lesion upon limbic structures (or neurochemical circuits) crucially involved emotional functions;

(b) the level of awareness of physical and cognitive disorders provoked by the lesion of different functional systems.

This Section we will analyze in some detail the emotional disorders corresponding to some important clusters of physical and cognitive disorders that are usually provoked by the encroachment of the lesion upon some well defined cortical areas. The aim of this description will be twofold:

(1) to illustrate how some of the most frequent emotional phenomena present clinically;

(2) to show that these different kinds of emotional reactions are mostly due to a different level of awareness of physical and cognitive disorders.

The emotional disorders that will be discussed here correspond to the early stages following infarcts affecting the territories of:

(a) the anterior branches of the left sylvian artery;

(b) the posterior branches of the same artery;

(c) the right middle cerebral artery.

4.1 The 'catastrophical reaction' of patients with Broca's aphasia

Lesions involve the inferior part of the left frontal lobe and the patient presents with a severe sensorimotor defect on the right side of the body, affecting hand and face. From the (cognitive) linguistic point of view, the most striking defect is severe Broca's aphasia, characterised by difficulty in engaging in any form of propositional speech, very low speech rate, effortful speech production, and inability to produce fluent and well formed verbal utterances, but relatively spared comprehension of oral and written language. The emotional counterpart of this cluster of motor and speech disorders is a marked tendency to 'catastrophical reactions' (i.e. to show increasing signs of anxiety and/or to suddenly burst into tears) because of frustrating and repeated attempts at verbal expression.

4.2 The anosognosic 'excitement' of patients with a severe Wernicke's aphasia.

Here, the vascular lesion encroaches upon the temporoparietal areas of the left hemisphere, involving the Wernicke's area, and produces a quite different pattern of sensorimotor, linguistic and emotional disturbances. -Sensorimotor disorders are absent or very mild, and usually only a partial visual defect for the right half space can be detected. The verbal production of these patients appears fluent, harmonious and well formed, but its meaning cannot be understood, since the most informative parts of speech (namely nouns and other content words) are affected by phonemic or semantic transformations, producing a quite incomprehensible jargon. Equally important (and, if possible, even more striking) are disorders of comprehension which hamper these patients' understanding not only of the content of verbal messages addressed to them, but also of the pathological nature of their own verbal production. The emotional behaviour of these subjects sharply contrasts with the catastrophical attitude of patients affected by a Broca's aphasia, since these patients usually appear unaware of their language disorders and appear overtalkative, excited and often even aggressive against people who appear not to understand their verbal messages.

4.3 The 'indifference reaction' of right-brain-damaged patients

This cluster of physical, cognitive and emotional disorders results from a focal brain lesion that affects the territory of the right sylvian artery, (particularly involving the right parietal lobe). From the physical point of view, these patients usually present with a severe left-sided hemiplegia and a marked deviation toward the right side of space of all the components of their body-orienting apparatus, (i.e. trunk, head and eyes). From the cognitive point of view, the most striking defect consists of a strong tendency to neglect the left half of the body and of extrapersonal space with an automatic capture of attention by stimuli rising on the right half space. Finally from the emotional point of view, these patients show a composite pattern of emotional disorders that can be grouped in three sets of emotional abnormalities.

- The first and most important set, 'emotional indifference', includes an apparent lack of appropriate concern for the disability and an attitude of indifference toward other kinds of emotionally laden events.

- The second set, labelled 'verbal disinhibition', consists of a tendency to joke in a fatuous ironic or sarcastic manner.

- The third set, includes the verbal denial of left-sided hemiplegia(considered in Section 3.2.1) and other phenomena that all suggest an implicit attitude of denial of illness. These last features often suggest feelings of rejection of the paralyzed limbs that are felt not to belong to the patient ('somatoparaphrenia') or described with expressions of hatred, couched in a grotesque or exaggerated language ('misoplegia').

4.4 Factors underlying the awareness of the disorder

From the pathophysiological viewpoint, one of the most important factors that can explain the of brain-damaged patients different patterns of emotional behavioural brain-damaged patients is the different extent of awareness of the defect following disruption of the functional systems subserved by these different anatomical regions. This awareness could in turn be related both to neurological and to psychological factors (Ownsworth and Clare, 2006). From the psychological point of view, the level of awareness of a defect could result from the amount of attention and of effort required by patients to overcome their functional defect. This could explain why patients with Broca's aphasia, being obliged to make a sustained conscious effort to mobilize their articulatory apparatus and to overcome their difficulties of speech production, are acutely aware of their communication difficulties, whereas patients with Wernicke's aphasia, having a fluent speech and a severe comprehension disorder, that do not allow them to monitor their meaningless utterances, are unaware of their language disorders. Analogously, right brain-damaged patients with a left sided hemiplegia and an ipsilateral neglect may be unable to automatically orient their attention toward the paralyzed limbs and this fact could explain the most important aspects of their emotional disturbances.

4.5 The stigma of language expression disorders

A final mechanism which can explain the various emotional behaviours of patients with differing lesions pertains to the varying meaning and psychosocial impacts which different kinds of cognitive and communication disorders can have for the patient. In particular, the high level of depression and of discouragement often show by left brain-damaged patients with expressive aphasia may be due to the feelings of inadequacy, embarassment and self-depreciation that communicative disorders provoke in these subjects. Several authors (e.g. Sarno and Gainotti, 1998) have noted that aphasic patients feel particularly stigmatized, and often report lowered self-esteem accompanied by feelings of shame as a consequence of their communication disorders.

Obviously, it is not possible to consider here the complex problem of the many other facets that emotional disorders can have following various categories of brain damage and during the various stages of evolution of the diseases. For simplicity sake, Table 22.1 summarises the most important points concerning the pathophysiology and prevalence of three broad categories of emotional disorders (anxiety and depression, apathy and poor control of disruptive emotional outbursts) following three important kinds of brain damage, namely stroke, closed head injury and Alzheimer's disease (see also Starkstein and Manes, 2001).

The data reported in Table 22.1 are relevant from both the epidemiological and the pathophysiological point of view. On one hand, they show that all these kinds of emotional disorders are widely, although unevenly distributed in different clinical forms of brain damage or in different stages of evolution of the same disease. On the other hand, they confirm that anxiety and depression are mostly due to psychological factors, whereas apathy and disruptive emotional outbursts usually result from properly neurological factors. The relationship between anxiety/depression and a painful realisation of the consequences of the disease is, in fact, present not only in stroke patients but also in closed

Table 22.1 Pathophysiology and prevalence of the most important kinds of emotional disorders in various categories of brain damage

Categories of brain damage	Stroke	Brain injury	Alzheimer's disease
Pathophysiology			
Anxiety and depression			
Psychological factors. 'Painful' awareness of the adverse effects of handicaps and disabilities on the patient's social role and personal goals	Very common (40–50%) in hospitalized patients and less common (20–30%) in community Settings	Rather uncommon in the earliest post-traumatic periods; tend to develop with the increased awareness of handicaps and disabilities	Rather common (40%) in the first stages of the disease; tend to disappear in later stages with the progression of dementia
Neurological factors? (major PSD). Disruption of monoaminergic pathways relaying the brainstem to the cerebral cortex	According to some authors more common after left than right hemisphere damage		
Apathy			
Neurological factors. Lesions encroaching upon the mesial parts of the frontal lobes, the anterior cingulate gyrus and the mesolimbichemisphere dopaminergic System	More common after right (20–25%) than left (10–15%) stroke	Very frequent and due to neurological factors in the earliest stages and to psychosocial factors in late periods	Very frequent (30–80%). Its frequency and severity increase with the progression of dementia
Psychological factors. Can result from the tendency to avoid the frustrations resulting from handicaps, disabilities, and communication disorders			
Lack of control over disruptive emotional outbursts			
Neurological factors. Lesions encroaching upon the orbitofrontal cortex and the fibres connecting these structures to the amygdala	Very uncommon	Very frequent after the earliest posttraumatic periods	Rather common in the most advanced stages of the disease progression

head injury or in dementia of the Alzheimer's type (DAT). However, in the last two categories of brain damage, these emotional disorders are only observed in the stage of evolution of the disease characterized by the highest level of awareness, namely in the earliest stages of DAT and in the late stages of brain injury. This is very different to the context in which disruptive emotional outbursts and apathetic disorders are usually observed.

- Disruptive emotional outbursts are mainly observed in patients with a severe traumatic injury of the fronto-orbital cortex (and in the most advanced stages of DAT).
- Apathetic disorders are particularly severe in patients with lesions encroaching upon the anteromesial parts of the frontal lobes, but are also observed in patients with an extensive infarct impinging upon the the right parietal region and in the advanced stages of DAT.

5 Assessment of emotional disorders following brain-damage

In recent years, behavioural and emotional disorders of brain-damaged patients have attracted more and more attention in the field of neurorehabilitation for two main reasons.

- These disorders constitute an important obstacle not only to the resumption of productive activities, but also to the rehabilitation process. They are indeed responsible for the lack of collaboration of the patient, which impedes the improvement of potentially treatable physical and cognitive defects.
- The fact that emotional and personality disorders are the consequence of brain damage is likely to be difficult to accept for family members (Lezak, 1978; Brooks et al., 1983, 1986). These disorders are, therefore, the factors that more frequently trigger the negative circular interactions between patients and their families briefly described in Section 3.3.1.

A careful assessment of emotional and behavioural disorders is, therefore, critical to the process of evaluation of the specific needs of each brain-damaged individual and is crucial when establishing comprehensive (holistic) rehabilitation programmes. Furthermore, the recent development of evidence-based rehabilitation medicine stresses the need for using a large array of standard psychometric instruments that could be appropriate to the assessment of emotional disorders of brain-damaged patients and that could, in turn, be used as outcome measures for various kinds and stages of neuropsychological rehabilitation (see Fleminger and Powell 1999). Obviously, the in-depth assessment required to understand individual problems and to establish personalized rehabilitation programs overlaps only in part with the standard psychometeric assessment required by the evidence-based rehabilitation medicine. Consequently, this chapter will only deal with two forms of evaluative processes:

- the personalized kind of assessment;
- the psychometric instruments currently used for a standard assessment of emotional disorders.

5.1 Personalized assessment of the significance of emotional disorders

The subjective, personalized assessment of the significance of emotional disorders consists of two main steps:

(a) distinguishing the neurological from the motivated (psychological or psychosocial) components of these disorders;

(b) delineating the main problems and psychosocial resources of the patient.

Snyder (1994) developed an interesting construct to clarify this problem. He defined the the construct of 'hopeful thinking' as a relatively enduring personality style that is based on self-referential beliefs about:

(a) the development of personally meaningful goals;

(b) finding ways (around obstacles) to achieve these goals;

(c) being motivated to implement these pathways.

'Hopeful thinking' is relevant to understanding the emotional functioning of stroke patients because of the importance of goals in their disability and recovery. Stroke patients who remain hopeful believe that they can both overcome the obstacles caused by the disability and attain their goals. They are likely, therefore, to be less depressed and actually achieve more goals than patients who are less hopeful. In his study Gum *et al.* (2006) confirmed that three months after a stroke, patients who are more hopeful were less likely to exhibit symptoms of depression and more likely to show higher levels of participation in general social activities.

5.2 The standard psychometric assessment of emotional disturbances

The standard psychometric assessment is much less relevant for the evaluation of individual problems and difficulties, but has the virtue of being more objective and quantitative. It is, therefore, much more reliable as a method of assessment for the negative effects that emotional disturbances can exert on the rehabilitation process. Important methodological objections have been raised the use of these psychometric measures of emotional and affective disorders. These will be considerd briefly and Table 22.2 summarises some of the instruments commonly used for the assessment of anxiety or depression, apathy and some disruptive behavioural disorders.

5.2.1 Methodologial objections

◆ One general problem for all of these scales, and in particular for those assessing anxious-depressive disorders, consists of the fact that they have usually been developed for psychiatric patients and that their transfer into the field of organic brain-damaged patients may produce misleading results. It is for this reason that some authors have developed instruments specifically constructed for well defined groups of brain-damaged patients, such as the already mentioned 'Post-Stroke Depression Rating Scale' (PSDRS), designed by Gainotti *et al.* (1997) to clarify the meaning of major depressive disorders frequently observed in stroke patients.

◆ A different, but equally important, problem can be recognised in the use of self-report instruments, such as the 'Beck Depression Inventory'(1961), the Zung Self-Rating Inventory' (Zung *et al.*, 1965), the 'Hospital Anxiety and Depression Scale' (Zigmond & Snait, 1983) or the 'Wimbledon Self-Report Scale' (Coughlan & Storey, 1988). Since patients with dementia or with severe brain injury may well be unaware not only of their physical problems, but also of their cognitive or emotional difficulties, the assessment based on the use of self-report scales must be considered quite unreliable.

Table 22.2 Main instruments used for the standard neuropsychological assessment of the most important kinds of emotional disorders

Anxiety	Hamilton Anxiety Scale (HAS: Hamilton, 1959)	Designed for psychiatric settings
	Hospital Anxiety and Depression Scale. See Balon (2007) for review	Self report instrument for detecting anxiety and depression in hospitalized medical and neurological patients
Depression	Hamilton Depression Rating Scale (HDRS; Hamilton, 1960)	Designed for psychiatric settings
	Post-stroke depression rating scale (PSDRS; Gainotti et al. 1997)	Clinician rated scale specifically constructed for stroke patients.
	Montgomery-Asberg Depression Rating Scale (MADRS; Montgomery & Asberg, 1979; Demyttenaere and De Fruyt (2003)	Psychiatric scale consisting of 9 reported and 1 observed items
	Wimbledon Self-report scale (WSRS; Coughlan e Storey, 1988)	Self report scale devised to assess mood in brain-damaged patients
Apathy	Apathy evaluation scale (AES; Marin et al., 1991) Glenn et al. (2002)	Self-informant and clinician rated versions of this scale have been developed
Disruptive behavioural disorders	Overt aggression Scale (OAS ; Yudowsky et al., 1986)	Designed to be rated by nursing staff in psychiatric setting, is also used in brain injury patients
General Neurobehavioural	Neurobehavioural Rating Scale (NRS ; Levin et al., 1987)	Sensitive to behavioural disorders related to frontal lobe injury
Rating Scales	Neuropsychiatric Inventory (NPI; Cummings et al., 1994) Sink et al. (2005)	Clinician rated instrument developed as an assessment tool for patients with dementia

6 Treatment of emotional and behavioural disorders in brain-damaged patients

The treatment of emotional disorders in brain-damaged patients is based on a large array of methods and techniques from the pharmacological treatment in the most severe emotional disorders, through behavioural management techniques used to modify inertia or disruptive patterns of social behaviour in patients with severe brain injury, to various kinds of group treatments and of individual psychotherapies.

6.1 Management of unawareness of deficits

Several studies, summarized by Ownsworth and Clare (2006), suggest that a lack of deficit awareness is often associated with poor rehabilitation outcome, However, the usefulness of treating these deficits remain a contested issue - primarily because patients with these deficits may develop harmful emotional distress very early in the adjustment process (Langer and Padrone, 1992; Ownsworth, 2005). In contrast, individuals with persistent unawareness of deficits are more at risk of long-term emotional disorders, due to their unrealistic expectations of recovery and inability to understand the reason for restrictions imposed upon them. In these cases, the need for therapeutic interventions seems very strong. Fleming and Ownsworth (2006), in their review of a range of awareness interventions in brain injury rehabilitation, makes an important distinction between intervention approaches for unawareness due to neurocognitive factors or psychological factors.

6.2 Cognitive behavioural therapy in the treatment of post-stroke depression

Lincoln *et al.* (1997) have considered the use of cognitive behavioural therapy (CBT) (which is effective in the treatment of late-life depression) in the treatment of PSD. In an initial study Lincoln *et al.*, (1997) implemented 10 sessions of CBT treatment over a 4-week baseline period and found that there was a tendency for improvement in the mood in some patients. However, in a second, randomized controlled trial, Lincoln and Flannaghan (2003) concluded that there were no significant differences between groups in patients' mood, independence, handicap or satisfaction with care.

6.3 Group treatment of emotional and behavioural disorders

Group treatment of emotional and behavioural disorders of patients with severe brain injury has several advantages:

(a) It increases the level of awareness of the patients' defects and capabilities, allowing them to check the adequacy of their current behaviour;

(b) It promotes interactions that, on one hand, increases the level of initiative and of personal involvement of patients and, on the other hand, improves their control over irritability, overt aggression or other disinhibited patterns of behaviour;

(c) It improves the level of participation to shared activities, favouring some degree of competition and, consequently, a more independent attitude.

6.4 Behavioural management techniques

Behavioural management techniques tend to induce an implicit learning of the suggested behavioural modifications by means of (classical or operant) conditioning methods. These techiques make use of positive and negative reinforcements to increase favourable changes (e.g. the development of intentional action schemata in patients with inertia or severe apathy) and to inhibit socially unacceptable emotional outbursts. Wood (1987) has suggested, for example, the systematic use of the 'time out' procedures (the complete suspension of every kind of reaction to the onset of undesirable behavioural patterns) since the patient implicitly learns from this unexpected lack of response that his pro-vocative behavioural patterns are unable to produce any effect on the external milieu.

6.5 The pharmacological treatment of emotional disorders

With respect to the pharmacological treatment of patients with severe forms of emotional disorders Table 22.3 indicate that several drugs are able to ameliorate the depressive disorders, apathy aand disruptive behavioural outbursts of brain-damaged patients. For example, Fleminger *et al.* (2003) and Deb and Crownshaw (2004) have provided system-atic reviews of the pharmacological treatment of agitation and aggression in people withn brain injury, Yury and Fisher (2007) have published a meta-analysis of the effectiveness of atypical antipsychotics for treatment of behavioural problems in people with dementia,

Table 22.3 Drugs used for the treatment of post-stroke depression, apathy and behavioural disorders of brain-damaged patients

Emotional Disorder	Therapeutic approach	Reference
Post-strokes depression	**Serotonine selective reuptake inhibitors** Citalopram Fluoxetine Sertraline	Andersen *et al.*, (1993) Gainotti *et al.*, (2001) Fruehwald *et al.*, (2003) Murray *et al.*, 2002 Hackett *et al.*, (2005)
	Other antidepressants Trazodone Nortriptyline	Reding *et al.*, (1986) Robinson *et al.*, (2000)
Apathy	**Dopaminergic drugs** Selegiline Bromocriptine Pergolide Modafinil	Newburn *et al.*, (2005) Campbell and Duffy (1997) Padala *et al.*, (2007)
	Stimulant drugs Methylphenidate	Marin *et al.*, (1995) Deb and Crownshaw (2004)
Aggression and other behavioural disorders	**Atypical antipsychotic medications** Clozapine Risperidone Quetiapine Beta Blockers	Perino *et al.*, (2001) McAllister and Ferrell (2002) Yury, C.A., Fisher, J.E. (2007) Tiihonen, (2009) Fleminger *et al.*, (2003) Deb and Crownshaw (2004)

and Hackett *et al.* (2005) have reviewed the effectiveness of antidepressants for the treatment and prevention of post-stroke depression.

In 2004, Given such strong data, the Committee for the Safety of Medicines (CSM) in the UK issued a warning that olanzapine and risperidone should not be given to elderly patients with dementia, because of an increased risk of stroke and Gill *et al.* (2007) have shown that there is an increased risk of death with conventional antipsychotics as opposed to atypical antipsychotics.

This does not imply, however, that purely biological methods are sufficient to treat, in the long term, the emotional problems and disorders of brain-damaged patients. Pharmacological treatments are necessary to improve the most severe emotional disorders of these patients and to re-establish a physiological process of emotional appraisal, but the emotional problems of these patients will lose their dramatic nature only when the outcome of this process will become more acceptable to them. From this point of view, it is probably correct to say that the rehabilitation process is the most powerful instrument that we can use to improve the long term the emotional equilibrium of these patients.

Selective References

Adams, J.H., Scott, G., Parker, L., Grham, D.I., and Doyle, D. (1980). Contusion index: a quantitative approach to cerebral contusions in head injury. *Neuropathology and Applied Neurobiology* 6, 319–324.

Andersen, G., Vestergaard, K., and Lauritzen, L. (1994). Effective treatment of post-stroke depression with the selective serotonin reuptake inhibitor citalopram. *Stroke* 25, 1099–1104.

Balon, R. (2007). Rating scales for anxiety/anxiety disordesrs. *Current Psychiatry Reports* 9, 271–7.

Bechara, A., Damasio, H., and Tranel, D. *et al.* (1997). Deciding advantageously before knowing the advantageous strategy. *Science* 275, 1293–1295.

Bechara, A., Tranel, D., and Damasco, H. (2000). Characterization of decision-making deficit of patients with ventromedial prefrontal cortex. *Brain* 123, 2189–2202.

Beck, A.T. (1961). An inventory for measuring depression. *Archives of General Psychiatry*, 4, 561–571.

Brooks, D.N., Campsie, L., Symington, C., Beattie, A., and McKinlay, W. (1986). The five years outcome of severe blunt herad injury: a relative's view. *Journal of Neurology, Neurosurgery and Psychiatry*, 49, 764–770.

Brooks, D.N., and McKinlay, W. (1983). Personality and behavioural change after severe blunt herad injury: a relative's view. *Journal of Neurology, Neurosurgery and Psychiatry*, 46, 336–344.

Campbell, J.J., and Duffy, J.D. (1997). Treatment strategies in amotivated patients. *Psychiatric Annals*, 27, 44–49.

Corrigan, J.D., Dickerson, J., Fisher, E, and Meyer, P. (1990). The Neurobehavioural Rating Scale: replication in an acute, inpatient rehabilitation setting. *Brain Injury*, 4, 215–222.

Coughlan, A.K., and Storey, P. (1988). The Wimbledon Self-Report Scale: emotional and mood appraisal. *Clinical Rehabilitation*, 2, 207–213.

Cummings, J.L. Mega, M. Gray, K. Rosenberg-Thompson, S. Carusi, D.A. and Gornbein, J. (1994). The Neuropsychiatric Inventory: Comprehensive assessment of psychopathology in dementia. *Neurology*, 44, 2308–2314.

Damasio, A.R. (1994). *Descartes' error: Emotion, research and the human brain*. Avon, New York.

Darwin, C. (1872). *The expression of emotions in man and animals*. Murray, London (reprinted University of Chicago Press, Chicago, 1965).

Deb, S., and Crownshaw, T. (2004). The role of pharmacotherapy in the management of behaviour disorders in traumatic brain injury patients. *Brain Injury* 18, 1–31.

Demyttenaere, K., and De Fruyt, J. (2003). Getting what you ask for: on the selectivity of depression rating scales. *Psychotherapy and Psychosomatics*, 72, 61–70.

Fleming J.M., and Ownsworth T. (2006). A review of awareness interventions in brain injury rehabilitation. *Neuropsychological Rehabilitation*, 16, 474–500.

Fleminger, S., Greenwood, R.J., Oliver, and D.L. (2003). Pharmacological management for agitation and aggression in people with acquired brain injury. *Cochrane Database of Systematic Reviews* (1): CD003299.

Fleminger, S. and Powell, J. (Eds.) (1999). *Evaluation of outcomes in brain injury rehabilitation*. Psychology Press, Hove, East Sussex.

Frijda, N. H. (1986). *The emotions*. Cambridge University Press, New York.

Fruehwald, S., Gatterbauer E., Rehak, P., and Baumhackl, U. (2003). Early fluoxetine treatment of post-stroke depression: a three months double-blind placebo-controlled study with an open-label long-term follow-up. *Journal of Neurology*, 250, 347–351.

Gainotti, G. (1993). Emotional and psychosocial problems after brain injury. *Neuropsychological Rehabilitation*, 3: 259-277.

Gainotti, G. (2000). Neuropsychological theories of Emotion. In *The Neuropsychology of Emotion* (ed. by C. Borod), pp. 214–236. Oxford University Press, New York.

Gainotti, G. (2001). Components and levels of emotion disrupted in patients with unilateral brain damage. In: *Emotional behaviour and its disorders*. (ed. by G. Gainotti), pp. 1–15. Handbook of Neuropsychology, 2nd Edition (ed. by F. Boller & J. Grafman) ,Vol 5. Elsevier, Amsterdam.

Gainotti G. (2006). Brain lesions and emotional disorders. *Future Neurology*, 1: 323–334.

Gainotti, G. Azzoni, A. Razzano, C. Lanzillotta, M. Marra, C. and Gasparini, F. (1997). The Post-Stroke Depression Rating Scale: a test specifically devised to investigate affective disorders of stroke patients. *Journal of Clinical and Experimental. Neuropsychology*, 19, 340–356.

Gainotti, G. Antonucci, G. Marra, C. and Paolucci, S. (2001). Relation between depression after stroke, antidepressant therapy, and functional recovery. *Journal of Neurology, Neurosurgery and Psychiatry*, 71, 258–261.

Gainotti G, and Marra C. (2005). Controversies on Post-Stroke Depression. In: *Focus on Stroke Research*. Brown SP(Ed.) Nova Science Publishers, New York 191–206.

Gill, S.S., Bronskill, S.E., Normand, S.L., Anderson, G.M., Sykora, K., Lam, K., Bell, C.M., Lee, P.E., Fischer, H.D., Herrmann, N., Gurwitz, J.H., and Rochon, P.A. (2007). Antipsychotic drug use and mortality in older adults with dementia. *Annals of Internal Medicine.* **146**, 775–86.

Glenn, M.B., Burke, D.T., O'Neil-Pirozzi, T, Goldstein, R., Jacob, L., and Kettell, J. (2002). Cutoff score on the apathy evaluation scale in subjects with traumatic brain injury. *Brain Injury* **16**, 509–16.

Gum, A., Snyder, C.R., and Duncan, P.W. (2006). Hopeful thinking, participation and depressive symptoms three months after stroke. *Psychology and Health*, **21**, 319–334.

Hackett, M.L., Anderson, C.S., and House, A.O. (2005). Management of depression after stroke. A systematic review of pharmacological therapies. *Stroke*, **36**, 1092–1103.

Hamilton, H. (1960). A rating scale for depression. *Journal of Neurology, Neurosurgery and Psychiatry.* **23**, 56–62.

Hamilton, M. (1959). The assessment of anxiety scales by rating. *British Journal of Medical Psychology*, **32**, 50–55.

Kaplan-Solms, K., and Solms, M. (2000). *Clinical studies in Neuro-Psychoanalysis: Introduction to a deep Neuropsychology*. London, Karnac.

Lambie, J.A., and Marcel, A.J. (2002) Consciousness and the varieties of emotion experience: a theoretical framework. *Psychological Review*, **109**, 219–59.

Langer, K.G., and Padrone, F.J. (1992). Psychotherapeutic treatment of awareness in acute rehabilitation of traumatic brain injury. *Neuropsychological Rehabilitation*, **2**, 59–70.

Lazarus, R.S. (1982). Thoughts on relations between emotion and cognition. *American Psychologist*, **37**, 1019–1024.

LeDoux, J. (1996). *The emotional brain*. Simon and Schuster, New York.

Leventhal, H. (1974) *Emotions: a basic problem for social psychology: classic and contemporary integrations*. McNally, Chicago.

Leventhal, H. (1987). A perceptual motor theory of emotion. In: *Advances in Experimental Social Psychology*. Berkowitz L (Ed.), Vol. 17, Academic Press, New York, 117–182.

Levin, H.S., High, W.M., and Goethe, K.E. *et al.* (1987). The Neurobehavioural Rating Scale: assessment of the behavioural sequelae of head injury by clinician. *Journal of Neurology, Neurosurgery and Psychiatry*, **50**, 183–193.

Lezak, M.D., (1978). Living with the characterogically altered brain injured patient. *Journal of Clinical Psychiatry*, **39**, 592–598.

Lincoln, N.B., and Flannaghan, T. (2003). Cognitive behavioural psychotherapy for depression following stroke. A randomized controlled trial. *Stroke*, **34**: 111–115.

Lincoln, N.B., Flannaghan, T., Sutcliffe, L., and Rother, L. (1997). Evaluation of cognitive behavioural treatment for depression after stroke a pilot study. *Clinical Rehabilitation*, **11**, 114–122.

Marcel, A, Tegnér, R, and Nimmo-Smith, I. (2004) Anosognosia for plegia: specificity, extension, partiality and disunity of bodily unawareness. *Cortex*, **40**, 19–40.

Marin, R.S. Biedrzycki, R.C. and Firinciogullori, S. (1991). Reliability and validity of the Apathy Evaluation Scale. *Psychiatry Research*, **38**, 143–162.

Martensson B., Gustavvson P., and Murray V. (in press) Symptom profile in post-stroke depression: major vs minor depression with reference to 'psychiatric' depression.

McAllister, T.W., and Ferrell, R.B. (2002). Evaluation and treatment of psychosis after traumatic brain injury. *NeuroRehabilitation* **17**, 357–368.

Mega M.S., and Cummings J.L. (1994). Frontal-subcortical circuits and neuropsychiatric disorders. *Journal of Neuropsychiatry and Clinical Neurosciences*, **6**, 358–370.

Montgomery, S.A., and Asberg M. (1979). A new depression scale designed to be sensitive to change. *British Journal of Psychiatry*, **134**, 382–389.

Murray, V., Von Arbin, M.,Varelius, R., Olsson, J.E., Terent, A., Samuelsson, M., Berggren, A.L., Landtblom, A.M., Asberg, M., Bartfai, A., Bengtsson, F., and Martensson B. (2002). Sertraline in post-stroke depression – a controlled study. *Stroke*, 33, 292.

Newburn, G., and Newburn, D. (2005). Selegiline in the management of apathy following traumatic brain injury *Brain Injury*, 19, 149–154.

Oatley, K. and Johnson-Laird, P. (1987). Toward a cognitive theory of emotions. *Cognition and Emotion*, 1, 29–50.

Orfei, M.D., Robinson, R.G., Prigatano G.P., Starkstein, S.E., Rush, N., Bria, P., Caltagirone, C., and Spalletta G. (2007) Anosognia for hemiplegia after stroke is a multifacet phenomenon: a systematic review of the literature. *Brain*130, 753–764.

Ownsworth, T. (2005). The impact of defensive denial upon adjustment following traumatic brain injury. *Neuropsychoanalysis*, 7, 83–94.

Ownsworth, T. and Clare, L. (2006). A critical review of the association between awareness deficits and rehabilitation outcome following acquired brain injury. *Clinical Psychology Review*, 26, 783–795.

Padala, P.R., Burke, W.J., and Bhatia, S.C. (2007). Modafinil therapy for apathy in an elderly patient. *Annals of Pharmacotherapy*. 41, 346–9.

Panksepp, J. (1982). Toward a general psychobiological theory of emotions. *Behavioral and Brain Science*, 5, 407–467.

Perino, C., Rago, R., Cicolin, A., and Torta, R. (2001). Mood and behavioural disorders following traumatic brain injury; clinical evaluation and pharmacological management. *Brain Injury*, 15, 139–148.

Robinson, R.G. (2001). The neuropsychiatry of stroke. In Miyoshi K, Shapiro CM, Gaviria M and Morita Y. (eds.) *Contemporary Neuropsychiatry*, pp. 116–127. Springer-Verlag, Tokyo.

Robinson, R.G. Kubos, K.L. Starr, L.B. Rao, K. and Price, T.R. (1984). Mood disorders in stroke patients: importance of lesion location. *Brain*, 107, 81–93.

Rolls E.T. (2005). *The brain and emotion*. Oxford University Press, New York.

Sarno, J.E., and Gainotti G. (1998). The psychological and social sequelae of aphasia. In: *Acquired Aphasia*. (ed by M. Taylor-Sarno), pp. 569–594. Academic Press, San Diego.

Scherer, K.R. (2000) Psychological models of emotion. In The Neuropsychology of Emotion (ed. by C. Borod), pp. I37–162. Oxford University Press, New York.

Sink, K.M., Holden, K.F., and Yaffe, K. (2005) Pharmacological treatment of neuropsychiatric symptoms of dementia: a review of the evidence. *JAMA*. 293, 596–608.

Snyder, C.R. (1994). *The psychology of hope: you can get there from here*. Free Press, New York.

Starkstein, S.E. and Manes F. (2001) Neural mechanisms of anxiety, depression and disinhibition. In: *Emotional behaviour and its disorders*. (ed. by G. Gainotti), pp. 263–284. Handbook of Neuropsychology, 2nd Edition (ed. by F. Boller & J. Grafman), Vol 5. Elsevier, Amsterdam.

Tiihonen, J. (2009). "11-year follow-up of mortality in patients with schizophrenia: a population-based cohort study (FIN11 study)". *The Lancet* 374: 620–627.

Turnbull, O.H., Jones, K., and Reed-Screen, J. (2002). Implicit awareness of deficit in anosognosia: An emotion-based account of denial of deficit. *Neuro*-Psychoanalysi 4, 69–86

Yudowsky, S.C. Silver, J.M. Jackson, W. Edicott, J. and Williams, D.W. (1986). The Overt Aggression Scale for the objective rating of verbal and physical aggression. *American Journal of Psychiatry*, 143, 35–39.

Yury, C.A., and Fisher, J.E. (2007). Meta-analysis of the effectiveness of atypical antipsychotics for the treatment of behavioural problems in persons with dementia. *Psychotherapy and psychosomatics* 76, 213–218.

Wood, R.L. (1987). *Brain injury rehabilitation. A neurobehavioral approach*. Croom Helm, London

Zajonc, R.B. (1980) Feeling and thinking: preferences need no inferences. *American Psychologist*, 2, 151–176.

Zung, W.W.K., Richards, C.B., and Short, M.F. (1965). Self-rating depression in an outpatient clinic: further validation of the SDS. *Archives of General Psychiatry*, 13, 508–515

Chapter 23

Assessment of anosognosia for motor impairments

Anne M. Aimola Davies, Rebekah C. White, and Martin Davies

1 Introduction

Patients with anosognosia fail to acknowledge their motor impairments. Anosognosia is usually assessed by means of a structured interview, beginning with questions about general health and moving to specific questions about the patient's motor impairment. A patient whose arm or leg is paralysed or weak following a stroke may deny the weakness in response to questions like 'Is there anything wrong with your arm or leg?' or 'Is your limb weak, paralysed, or numb?' (questions from Cutting, 1978; Nathanson, Bergman and Gordon, 1952; Starkstein, Federoff, Price, Leiguarda and Robinson, 1992), and may continue to deny the impairment even when it has been demonstrated. The examiner may ask the patient to raise both arms and then demonstrate to the patient that one arm is not raised as high as the other. Recognising that a patient has anosognosia may be relatively straightforward, for example, when the patient denies outright that there is anything the matter. In many patients, however, a full assessment will reveal a more complex profile.

In this chapter, we begin (Section 2) with a threefold distinction that organises our investigation of anosognosia — the distinction between *failure to experience* a motor impairment (*concurrent unawareness*), *failure to acknowledge* the impairment itself, and *failure to appreciate the consequences* of the impairment (Aimola Davies, Davies, Ogden, Smithson and White, 2009). Then, we review methods for the assessment of motor impairments and anosognosia for motor impairments (Section 3) including structured anosognosia interviews that have been published (Section 4). This literature review reveals considerable variation in the methods by which patients with anosognosia have been assessed. The development of a comprehensive and widely accepted procedure for assessing anosognosia for motor impairments would contribute to a better understanding of the many factors in anosognosia and might also lead to improvement in the clinical management of patients (Orfei, Caltagirone and Spalletta, 2009). We present a structured interview (Section 5) that offers a theoretically motivated and relatively comprehensive approach to the assessment of anosognosia for motor impairments.

2 **A threefold distinction**

Two ideas figure in the *Oxford English Dictionary* definition of anosognosia: 'unawareness of or failure to acknowledge one's hemiplegia or other disability'. *Unawareness* suggests a failure of experience (sensation and perception). *Failure to acknowledge* suggests a failure of judgement (belief and assertion). This important distinction is obscured if the term 'unawareness' is used interchangeably with 'anosognosia'. We regard anosognosia as a failure or pathology of belief: a mismatch between the patient's estimate of his or her abilities and the reality of the impairment. The patient believes that he or she does not have the impairment despite the fact that it is clearly present. This incorrect belief will be manifested in the patient's failure to acknowledge the impairment verbally in response to questions.

Consider a hypothetical case of a patient with hemiplegia following right-hemisphere stroke. When the patient intends to raise his left arm, proprioception and vision tell him that the arm is still hanging by his side. When the patient tries to raise his arm, a comparator within the motor control system detects a mismatch between the expected movement of the arm and what actually happens and the patient is alerted to his paralysis. If the patient directs his attention to the left side of his body, this only confirms that his left arm has not moved. This hypothetical patient has immediate experiences — concurrent awareness — of his motoric failure and these experiences may lead him to abandon long-held beliefs about his motor abilities. In contrast, patients with proprioceptive loss (Levine, 1990), or unilateral neglect (Vuilleumier, 2004), or with damage to the comparator in the motor control system (Gold, Adair, Jacobs and Heilman, 1994; Heilman, 1991; Heilman, Barrett and Adair, 1998), may not fully experience their motoric failures. They may even seem to experience motoric success — illusory limb movements (Frith, Blakemore and Wolpert, 2000; Feinberg, Roane and Ali, 2000; Levine, Calvanio and Rinn, 1991). Such patients, with concurrent unawareness of motoric failure, may be more likely to maintain long-held beliefs that are now incorrect — beliefs that overestimate their motor abilities.

It is plausible that concurrent unawareness often plays an important role in the aetiology of anosognosia. But the distinction between concurrent unawareness (a failure to experience motoric failures when they occur) and anosognosia (a failure of belief) is confirmed by thought experiments and empirical findings (Marcel, Tegnér and Nimmo-Smith, 2004). In principle, a patient with impaired proprioception might have no immediate bodily experience of failure to move a paralysed limb yet, on the basis of other evidence, the patient might still reach the correct belief about his or her paralysis (failure of experience without failure of belief). Conversely, a patient with intact proprioception might have vivid bodily experiences of failure to move a paralysed limb but, because the information is not consolidated into more lasting representations, the patient might fail to reach the correct belief about his or her paralysis (failure of belief without failure of experience).

Having an incorrect belief about the severity of an impairment itself is also distinct from having an incorrect belief about the seriousness of the consequences of the impairment for activities of daily living. House and Hodges (1988) present an example that is relevant to this second distinction. They describe an 89-year-old woman who suffered left-side paralysis following a right-hemisphere stroke. When she was examined six months after her stroke, she acknowledged that her left arm was weak, and weaker than her left leg. When it was demonstrated to her that her left arm was completely paralysed and her left leg nearly completely paralysed, she rated the strength of her left elbow and hand/wrist zero out of ten and her left hip, knee and ankle/foot two out of ten. But even while she acknowledged her motor impairments she failed to appreciate their consequences, 'she insisted that she could walk upstairs unaided if she were allowed to' (whereas, in reality, she was restricted to a wheelchair) (House and Hodges, 1988, p. 113). Marcel and colleagues (2004) also report several patients who acknowledged that their left arm was paralysed yet overestimated their ability to carry out bimanual tasks such as tying a knot, clapping hands, or shuffling cards. We might describe such patients as having anosognosia for the consequences of their motor impairment but not anosognosia for the impairment itself. They overestimate their ability to carry out activities of daily living even if they do not, strictly speaking, overestimate their motor abilities.

Thus, we reach the threefold distinction between *concurrent unawareness* of an impairment, *failure to acknowledge* the impairment itself, and *failure to appreciate the consequences* of the impairment for activities of daily living. The first is a failure of experience; the second and third are both failures of belief.

In cases of mild motor impairment, where patients have considerable residual movement in their impaired limbs, there is less room for overestimation of motor abilities. It may be difficult to classify such patients as having substantially incorrect beliefs about their motor abilities. Even mild motor impairments can, however, have serious consequences for activities of daily living such as walking, washing, dressing, grooming, and feeding. So patients who do not have complete hemiplegia may still have dramatically incorrect beliefs about their ability to carry out everyday activities. Assessment of anosognosia, considered as a pathology of belief, should investigate both failure to acknowledge the motor impairment itself and failure to appreciate its consequences. Assessment of the causes of anosognosia should extend to investigation of concurrent unawareness of motoric failure.

3 Assessment of motor impairments and anosognosia

Before one can assess whether a patient has anosognosia for motor impairments, it is necessary to establish that the patient does have a motor impairment. In fact, some researchers (e.g., Berti, Spinazzola, Pia and Rabuffetti, 2007) have argued that only patients with complete hemiplegia should be included in studies of anosognosia because, otherwise, the patient's belief that he or she can move the affected limbs is at least partly correct (see also Berti, Làdavas and Della Corte, 1996; Bisiach, Vallar, Perani, Papagno and Berti, 1986; for discussion, see Vallar and Ronchi, 2006, pp. 252–3).

3.1 Simple assessment of motor impairments and anosognosia

We now outline a procedure for establishing that the patient has a motor impairment. If the primary purpose is to identify patients with complete hemiplegia then a simple assessment of motor performance is sufficient. The examiner might, for example, ask the patient to raise the affected limb, or to maintain a raised position following passive elevation by the examiner. Three ordinal rating scales that can be used to assess patient performance are presented in Table 23.1: Medical Research Council (MRC) Scale (Guarantors of Brain, 2000), National Institute of Health (NIH) Stroke Scale (Brott, Adams, Olinger, Marler, Barsan, Biller *et al.*, 1989; Goldstein, Bertels and Davis, 1989; Lyden, Lu, Levine, Brott and Broderick, 2001), and the Bisiach Motor Impairment Scale (Bisiach *et al.*, 1986). Complete plegia corresponds to a score of 0 on the MRC Scale, 4 on the NIH scale, and 3 on the Bisiach scale. All three scales have been used in previous studies of anosognosia.

Alongside the Bisiach Motor Impairment Scale (see Table 23.1), Bisiach and colleagues (Bisiach *et al.*, 1986) introduced the Bisiach Anosognosia Scale. A four-point scale is used for assessment of anosognosia, ranging from 0 (no anosognosia) to 3 (severe anosognosia):

0 The disorder is spontaneously reported or mentioned by the patient following a general question about his complaints (no anosognosia)

1 The disorder is reported only following a specific question about the strength of the patient's affected limbs (mild anosognosia)

2 The disorder is acknowledged only after its demonstration through routine techniques of neurological examination (moderate anosognosia)

3 No acknowledgement of the disorder can be obtained (severe anosognosia).

The distinction between moderate and severe anosognosia depends on whether or not the patient acknowledges the disorder 'after its demonstration through routine techniques of neurological examination'. This demonstration would be provided by the assessment of motor impairments mentioned in the previous paragraph. In the case of a patient with a score of 3 for motor impairment of the left arm according to the Bisiach Motor Impairment Scale, the demonstration would be provided by the patient's raised arm falling to the bed surface within five seconds (see Table 23.1).

Many studies (including Bisiach *et al.*, 1986; see also Baier and Karnath, 2005; Berti, Bottini, Gandola, Pia, Smania, Stracciari *et al.*, 2005; Karnath, Baier and Nägele, 2005; Spalletta, Serra, Fadda, Ripa, Bria and Caltagirone, 2007) classify patients as having anosognosia only if they receive a score of 2 (moderate anosognosia) or 3 (severe anosognosia). In a recent study of 128 acute left- and right-hemisphere stroke patients, Baier and Karnath (2005) found that twelve patients (9%) had a score of 2 or 3 (moderate or severe anosognosia). They also found that sixteen of the seventeen patients with a score of 1 (mild anosognosia) spontaneously mentioned other neurological deficits or symptoms of stroke when asked a general question and immediately acknowledged their motor impairments when asked specifically about the strength of their limbs. Baier and Karnath proposed that these patients had no problem accepting their motor impairments but simply mentioned 'subjectively more prominent' symptoms (p. 361) in response to a general question. The authors therefore argued that patients with a score of 1 on Bisiach's Anosognosia Scale should not be classified as having anosognosia.

Table 23.1 Assessment of Motor Impairments

Scale	Instruction	Rating scale

Medical Research Council (MRC) Scale*	*Upper limb*: The patient abducts the upper arm against resistance. (Guarantors of Brain, 2000, Fig. 21).
	
	Lower limb: The patient lies on his or her back and flexes the thigh at the hip against resistance with the leg flexed at the knee and hip (Guarantors of Brain, 2000, Fig. 70).
		5. Normal power
		4. Active movement against gravity and resistance:
		  4+ strong resistance
		  4 moderate resistance
		  4 – slight resistance
		3. Active movement against gravity
		2. Active movement with gravity eliminated
		1. Flicker or trace of contraction
		0. No contraction

National Institute of Health (NIH) Stroke Scale	*Upper limb*: The arms are placed in the appropriate position: arms outstretched (palms down) at 90° if sitting, or at 45° if supine. Full effort is requested for 10 seconds. If consciousness or comprehension are abnormal, cue patient by actively lifting arms into position as request for effort is orally given. *Lower limb*: The leg is placed in the appropriate position: while supine, the patient is asked to maintain weaker leg at 30° for 5 seconds. If consciousness or comprehension are abnormal, cue patient by actively lifting the leg into position as request for effort is orally given.	0. No drift; arm holds 90° (or 45°) for full 10 seconds 1. Drift; arm holds 90° (or 45°) but drifts down before full 10 seconds; does not hit bed or other support 2. Some effort against gravity; arm cannot get to or maintain (if cued) 90°(or 45°), drifts down to bed but has some effort against gravity 3. No effort against gravity; arm falls 4. No movement of arm 0. No drift; leg holds 30° position for full 5 seconds 1. Drift; leg falls by the end of the 5-second period but does not hit bed 2. Some effort against gravity; leg falls to bed by 5 seconds, but has some effort against gravity 3. No effort against gravity; leg falls to bed immediately 4. No movement of leg
Bisiach Motor Impairment Scale	*Upper limb*: The supine patient is asked to hold the following position for 30 seconds: arm flexed at 45°, forearm extended and supinated, fingers abducted. *Lower limb*: The supine patient is asked to hold the following position for 30 seconds: thigh flexed at 90°, leg flexed at 90°.	0. No defects or minimal defects not scorable as 1 1. Appearance of at least one of the following signs: finger adduction, pronation of the forearm, lowering of limb without reaching bed surface within 15 seconds 2. Limb lowers and reaches bed surface within 15 seconds 3. Limb reaches bed surface within 5 seconds 0. No defects or minimal defects not scorable as 1 1. Lowering of limb without reaching bed surface within 15 seconds 2. Limb lowers and reaches bed surface within 15 seconds 3. Limb reaches bed surface within 5 seconds

* Medical Research Council Scale is different in two ways from the NIH Stroke Scale and the Bisiach Motor Impairment Scale: the assessment is for raising the limb (as opposed to maintaining a raised limb) and scoring is in the opposite direction, so that higher scores indicate better motor function.

This recent discussion of 'mild anosognosia' recalls an insightful and perhaps insufficiently recognised contribution to the field by Willanger, Danielsen and Ankerhus (1981). In their study, 55 patients admitted to hospital following right-hemisphere stroke were asked general questions about their stay in hospital and were also explicitly asked whether they could move their limbs. Patients who consistently reported their motor impairments 'were grouped as having adequate understanding of these symptoms' (p. 315). What is noteworthy is that patients who acknowledged their motor impairments only when they were specifically asked if they could move their limbs (fulfilling Bisiach's criterion for mild anosognosia) were not classified as having anosognosia.

Patients who did not report their motor impairments in this initial stage of questioning were asked to move their affected limb, and immediately afterwards were asked to reflect on their performance during their attempt to move the limb. Once their impairments had been demonstrated, eleven patients who 'admitted either that they could not move or had certain difficulties in moving the affected limb' (p. 316) were classified as having neglect of their motor impairments. They did not acknowledge their impairments in the initial stage of questioning, they acknowledged their impairments when they were demonstrated, but usually the acknowledgement was not lasting. These patients fulfilled Bisiach's criterion for moderate anosognosia. Fourteen patients who demonstrated 'obstinate denial of paresis even when the defect was concretely shown at least three times' (p. 316) were classified as having denial of their motor impairments. These patients fulfilled Bisiach's criterion for severe anosognosia. Thus, in total, 25 of 55 right-hemisphere stroke patients (45%) were classified as having neglect or denial of motor impairments (that is, moderate or severe anosognosia, a score of 2 or 3 on Bisiach's anosognosia scale).

3.2 Further assessment of motor impairments

The requirement of complete hemiplegia (score of 0 on the MRC Scale; see Table 23.1) will exclude patients who, despite retaining some movement of the affected limb (scores of 1 to 4 on the MRC Scale), overestimate their ability to move the limb (claiming, for example, that the affected limb is just as strong as the corresponding unaffected limb). In more inclusive studies of anosognosia for motor impairments, rather than only anosognosia for complete hemiplegia, a brief yet detailed motor assessment such as the Motricity Index (or the abridged version of the Medical Research Council Scale[1]) can be used to assess the degree of impairment across different body parts and movement types.

---

[1] The sixteen commonly tested upper and lower limb movements from the abridged version of the Medical Research Council Scale are listed below (Guarantors of Brain, 2000, p. 62). Five of these sixteen movements are included in the Motricity Index for Motor Impairment after Stroke.

   a) *Upper Limb Movements* (shoulder abduction; elbow flexion; elbow extension; radial wrist extension; finger extension; finger flexion; finger abduction);

   b) *Lower Limb Movements* (hip flexion; hip abduction; hip extension; knee flexion; knee extension; ankle dorsiflexion; ankle eversion; ankle plantar flexion; big toe extension).

The Motricity Index (MI) for Motor Impairment after Stroke (Demeurisse, Demol and Robaye, 1980) takes about five minutes to administer, and consists of six tests providing a rapid overall assessment of motor impairment:

1 Pinch grip using a 2.5 cm cube between the thumb and forefinger

2 Elbow flexion from 90° so that the arm touches the shoulder

3 Shoulder abduction moving the flexed elbow from off the chest

4 Ankle dorsiflexion with the foot in a plantar flexed position

5 Knee extension with the foot unsupported and the knee at 90°

6 Hip flexion with the hip bent at 90° moving the knee towards the chin.

Medical Research Council grades MRC 0 to MRC 5 are used to measure movement at each joint, and these six grades are then converted into weighted scores ranging from 0 (no movement) to 33 (normal power). Full guidelines for administration and scoring the Motricity Index are provided by Collin and Wade (1990, p. 57).[2] Patients receive an overall score from 0 (no motricity) to 100 (normal motricity) for the upper limb (Tests 1–3) and lower limb (Tests 4–6). As with the MRC scoring, these grades 'indicate strength on the basis of a patient's ability to activate a muscle group, to move a limb segment through a range of motion, and to resist the force of an examiner' (Bohannon, 1999, p. 59).

The Motricity Index has been shown to have excellent validity for both the upper and lower limb scales. Upper limb validity is supported by correlations with grip strength (Sunderland, Tinson, Bradley and Hewer, 1989), with dynamometer measures of muscle strength (Bohannon, 1999) and with other measures of arm function (e.g., Action Research Arm Test: Hsieh, Hsueh, Chiang and Lin, 1998; Rivermead Motor Assessment: Collin and Wade, 1990). Lower limb validity is supported by correlations with dynamometer measures of muscle strength (Cameron and Bohannon, 2000) and with other measures of leg function (e.g., Rivermead Motor Assessment: Collin and Wade, 1990).

---

[2] Scoring for Test 1:

   0 No movement

11 Beginnings of prehension (any movement of finger or thumb)

19 Able to grip the cube, but not hold it against gravity (examiner may need to lift wrist)

22 Able to grip and hold the cube against gravity, but not against a weak pull

26 Able to grip and hold the cube against a weak pull, but weaker than the other side

33 Normal pinch grip.

Scoring for Tests 2–6:

   0 No movement

   9 Palpable contraction in muscle, but no movement

14 Visible movement, but not full range and not against gravity

19 Full range of movement against gravity but not against resistance

25 Full movement against resistance, but weaker than the other side

33 Normal power.

3.3 Assessment of the consequences of motor impairments for activities of daily living

For a more comprehensive profile of a patient's motor impairments, encompassing the impairments themselves and their consequences, the examiner may wish to use a standard assessment of motor function, such as the Motricity Index, together with an assessment of fundamental mobility (e.g., Rivermead Mobility Index; Collen, Wade, Robb and Bradshaw, 1991) and a measure of functional independence (e.g., Barthel Activities of Daily Living Index; Collin, Wade, Davies and Horne, 1988; Mahoney and Barthel, 1965).[3] While the assessment of motor function provides quantitative information about muscle activation, range of movement and motor strength, the functional measures provide information about the impact of motor impairments on mobility and independence when the patient is engaged in activities of daily living. Together, these measures provide the basis for subsequent assessment of whether the patient acknowledges the impairment itself and appreciates the consequences of the impairment for activities of daily living.

The Rivermead Mobility Index (RMI) is a short, simple, clinically relevant and widely used outcome measure, which focuses on aspects of mobility that are fundamental 'activities that most people will undertake if they possibly can' (Wade, 1992, p. 77). The RMI takes about five minutes to administer, and consists of one direct observation (Question 5, below) and fourteen questions about the patient's ability to perform common daily movements:

1 Turning over in bed

2 From lying in bed to sitting on edge of bed

3 Sitting balance (on edge of bed without holding on for 10 seconds)

4 From sitting in chair to standing

5 *Observe* patient standing unsupported for 10 seconds (no aid and no support)

6 Transfer (from bed to chair and back without help)

7 Walking 10 metres inside (with an aid if needed but no standby help)

8 Flight of stairs (without help)

9 Walking outside (even ground, without help)

10 Walking 10 metres inside (with no aid or standby help)

11 Picking items off floor (walking 5 metres to the dropped item and back)

12 Walking outside (uneven ground, without help)

13 Bathing (in and out of bath or shower unsupervised)

14 Climbing up and down four steps (with no rail, but with an aid if needed)

15 Running or fast walking (10 metres in 4 seconds).

---

[3] Recommended versions of each measure – Motricity Index, Rivermead Mobility Index and Barthel Activities of Daily Living Index – can also be found in *Measurement in neurological rehabilitation* (Wade, 1992).

Patients receive a score from 0 to 15, with higher scores indicating better mobility. The RMI has been shown to be reliable and sensitive to change during hospital rehabilitation and it is a valid measure of functional status, both before and after rehabilitation programmes (Antonucci, Aprile and Paolucci, 2002; Chen, Hsieh, Lo, Liaw, Chen and Lin, 2007; Green, Forster and Young, 2001). Good validity has been demonstrated in correlations with other validated measures (e.g., Motricity Index for the Lower Limb, Trunk Control Test and Functional Independence Measure: Franchignoni, Tesio, Benevolo and Ottonello, 2003).

The Barthel Activities of Daily Living (ADL) Index (Collin et al., 1988; Mahoney and Barthel, 1965) is probably the most widely used instrument for measuring functional independence following stroke, and for most patients the ten questions take only five minutes to complete:

1 Control bowels

2 Control bladder

3 Grooming (personal care with implement provided: face, hair, teeth, shave)

4 Toilet use (reach toilet, handle clothes, clean self)

5 Feeding (food provided within reach but not cut up)

6 Transfer (from bed to chair and back)

7 Mobility (with aid e.g., stick; in wheelchair must negotiate corners/doors unaided)

8 Dressing (selecting clothes and using buttons, zips, laces)

9 Stairs (ascending and descending)

10 Bathing self (bath or shower, unsupervised and unaided).

A scale ranging from 0 to 20 in one-point increments is commonly used, as it has been argued that Mahoney and Barthel's original scoring (with a scale ranging from 0 to 100 in five-point increments) may give an exaggerated impression of accuracy (Collin et al., 1988; Wade and Hewer, 1987). For each item, the patient is rated as either independent (1, 2, or 3 points, depending on the item), able to perform the given task with help (0, 1, or 2 points, depending on the item), or cannot meet the criteria for a higher score (0 points). A maximum score of 20 (or 100 in the original scoring system) means that the patient is functionally independent (but not necessarily that the patient has normal mobility). Full guidelines for administration and scoring of the Barthel ADL Index, using the 20-point scale, are provided by Collin and colleagues (1988). Reliability and validity of the Barthel ADL Index as a measure of disability have been established in a number of studies (Collin et al., 1988; Green et al., 2001; Wade and Collin, 1988; Wade and Hewer, 1987).

3.4 Assessment of anosognosia for the consequences of motor impairments

Collin and colleagues (1988) also investigated four methods of obtaining information for the Barthel ADL Index:

(a) asking for information from:

    — (1) the patient (or a relative) or

— (2) a nurse who had worked with the patient for at least one shift,

(b) direct observation of the patient, who was tested either by:

— (3) a trained nurse or

— (4) an occupational therapist.

The findings obtained by the four methods were comparable, and the authors state 'the method of obtaining the information does not appear to be important, but allowance needs to be made for confused patients if self-reporting is used' (p. 62). They found that method (1) was slightly less reliable, in that the patient's (or relative's) report was the most likely not to agree with the other three methods.

These findings lead us to implement a dual scoring system when administering the Barthel ADL Index (and also the Rivermead Mobility Index). Specifically, the system separates a score based on *self*-report (that is, by the patient) from a score based on report by a nurse who had worked with the patient for at least one shift. On this dual scoring system, the nurse's report provides a quick and reliable measure of the patient's mobility and independence, while comparison with the patient's self-report reveals the extent to which the patient fails to appreciate the consequences of his or her motor impairments for activities of daily living.

Summary: A simple assessment of motor impairments using the MRC Scale, the NIH Stroke Scale, or the Bisiach Motor Impairment Scale can be combined with a simple assessment of anosognosia for motor impairments using Bisiach's Anosognosia Scale. A diagnosis of anosognosia would be based on a score of 2 (moderate anosognosia) or 3 (severe anosognosia) on Bisiach's Anosognosia Scale. A more comprehensive assessment of motor impairments and their consequences (using, for example, the Motricity Index, the Rivermead Mobility Index, and the Barthel ADL Index) invites a more nuanced assessment of anosognosia for motor impairments and, with a dual scoring system for the functional measures, allows an initial assessment of anosognosia for the consequences of motor impairments. A diagnosis of anosognosia would be based on a substantial difference between the patient's self-report and the report by a nurse who had worked with the patient for at least one shift.

4 Assessment of anosognosia: structured interviews

A structured interview can provide important information concerning the patient's beliefs—whether the patient acknowledges his or her motor impairments and whether the patient appreciates the consequences of those impairments for activities of daily living. Table 23.2 lists the questions used in nine structured interviews for which the assessment protocol has been published. The table reveals the overlap amongst these interviews, and the manner in which later protocols have built on earlier ones. For example, the interviews presented by Nathanson and colleagues (1952), Cutting (1978) and Starkstein and colleagues (1992) include five questions in common, two general questions about the reasons for the patient's hospitalisation and three questions about the patient's motor impairments (see columns 1, 2, and 4 of Table 23.2A and 23.2B).

Table 23.2 Questions from Nine Structured Interviews for the Assessment of Anosognosia

	Nathanson et al. (1952)	Cutting (1978)	Anderson and Tranel (1989)	Starkstein et al. (1992)	Berti et al. (1996)	Maeshima et al. (1997)	Feinberg et al. (2000)	Marcel et al. (2004)	Spinazzola et al. (2008)
A. General Questions:									
Where are we?					√				√
Do you have any trouble?						√			
Why are you here? or Why are you in the hospital? or Why are you now in the hospital?	√	√	√	√	√	√		√	√
What is the matter with you? or What is wrong with you?	√	√	√	√				√	
Is there anything wrong with you?									√
If primary reason for hospitalisation is not explicitly described, Examiner asks: Did you have a stroke?			√						
B. Acknowledgement of Motor Impairments:									
Are you paralysed?						√			
How do your arms (legs) work? Can you move them normally? Both of them?			√						
Can you move your arms or legs?						√			
Examiner indicates paralysed limb: Can you move this hand or foot?						√			
Is there anything wrong with it [limb]? or Is there anything wrong with your arm or leg?	√	√		√					
Examiner either points to or raises the affected limb: Is there anything wrong with it?	√								
Can you move it [limb]? Raise it?	√								

Question			
Is your limb weak, paralysed, or numb? How does your limb feel?		√	
Examiner holds up affected limb: What is this?	√	√	
Can you lift it [arm]? You clearly have some problem with this?	√	√	
Examiner asks patient to raise both arms: Can't you see that the two arms are not at the same level?		√	
How well do your arms and legs work?			√
Can you move your arms (legs) normally? Both of them?			√
Is either of your arms (legs) weak? This one, that one?			√
Do you have weakness anywhere?			√
Is your arm causing you any problems?			√
Does it [arm] feel normal?			√
Can you use it [arm] as well as you used to?			√
Are you fearful about losing your ability to use your arm?			√
The doctors tell me that there is some paralysis of your arm. Do you agree?			√
Examiner lifts and drops patient's affected arm, first in contralateral hemispace, then in ipsilateral hemispace: It seems there is some weakness. Do you agree?			√
Take your right arm, and use it to lift your left arm. Is there any weakness of your left arm?			√
How is your left arm (leg)? Can you move it?		√	
If patient says he/she cannot move arm, Examiner asks: Why can you not move your left arm?		√	√

√ Researchers who used the question(s) indicated.

(continued)

Table 23.2 (continued) Questions from Nine Structured Interviews for the Assessment of Anosognosia

	Nathanson et al. (1952)	Cutting (1978)	Anderson and Tranel (1989)	Starkstein et al. (1992)	Berti et al. (1996)	Maeshima et al. (1997)	Feinberg et al. (2000)	Marcel et al. (2004)	Spinazzola et al. (2008)
If patient verbally denies left upper limb motor impairment, Examiner asks: Please, touch my hand with your left hand. Have you done it? Why have you not done it? Are you sure? It is very strange because I have not seen your hand touching my hand.					√				
C. Appreciation of the Consequences of Motor Impairments:									
How do you think you did on these tests today?			√						
Based on how you are doing now, do you think you will be able to return to your normal activities in the next several weeks?			√						
In your current state, do you have any problems with daily activities (e.g., eating, dressing, washing, getting about)?								√	
Patient asked whether he or she can perform a range of 'analytic' movements (e.g., put left hand on left shoulder, straighten knee).									√
Patient asked to estimate his or her capacity to perform unimanual, bimanual and bipedal tasks.					√			√	√
Third-person estimate: Patient asked to estimate examiner's capacity to perform unimanual, bimanual and bipedal tasks if the examiner were in the patient's present state.					√			√	

Can you walk without any problem?

Post-performance estimate: Patient asked to re-estimate capacity to perform unimanual, bimanual and bipedal tasks (after attempt has been made to perform these tasks). √

D. Anosognosic Phenomena:

Is it a nuisance? How much trouble does it cause you? What caused it? √

Do you ever feel that it doesn't belong? Do you feel that it belongs to someone else? √

Do you feel the arm is strange or odd? √

Has your arm or leg felt strange in any way? √

Have you had any other strange sensations? √

Do you dislike the arm? Do you hate it? √

Do you have strong feelings about it? √

Do you ever call it names? √

Do you ever feel it moves without your moving it yourself? √

How is the other arm? √

Do you ever feel a strange arm lying beside you separate from the real arm? √

√ Researchers who used the question(s) indicated.

It is important to notice that, although most researchers ask patients whether they are able to move or raise their limbs, the researcher may or may not ask the patient actually to attempt the movement. Questions that do involve a request for the patient to move an affected limb, and consequently provide a demonstration of the patient's impairment, allow the examiner to distinguish moderate from severe anosognosia (Bisiach *et al.*, 1986) or, equivalently, mere neglect of motor impairments from full denial of motor impairments (Willanger *et al.*, 1981).

Some structured interviews investigate the patient's appreciation of the consequences of motor impairments for activities of daily living (see Table 23.2C). Patients who correctly acknowledge their motor impairments may still fail to appreciate the consequences of those motor impairments and so they may overestimate their ability to carry out everyday activities. In the structured interview of Marcel and colleagues (2004), patients are specifically asked whether they have problems with everyday activities of eating, dressing, washing, and getting about. Since patients with motor impairments may develop strategies for accomplishing these tasks, denial of problems with these everyday activities does not, by itself, amount to unequivocal evidence of anosognosia.

A more sensitive method of detecting anosognosia for the consequences of motor impairments is to ask patients about their capacity to perform bimanual and bipedal tasks (Nimmo-Smith, Marcel and Tegnér, 2005), that is, tasks that involve both sides of the body. This approach has been used by Berti and colleagues (1996), Marcel and colleagues (2004) and Spinazzola and colleagues (Spinazzola, Pia, Folegatti, Marchetti and Berti, 2008).

However, the patient's answers to questions about tasks that are assumed to be bimanual or bipedal may still not provide an accurate assessment of whether the patient appreciates his or her limitations. It is strongly recommended that the examiner should ask patients to demonstrate, or at least describe how they would execute, any bimanual or bipedal tasks that they claim to be able to perform. Recently, we assessed a gentleman with complete right-side hemiplegia. When asked whether he could attach a handkerchief to a ring by tying a knot, he responded 'yes' and promptly carried out the task — antecedently classified as bimanual — using his left hand only. The patient's affirmative answer to our initial question whether he could perform the task might have led us to assume that he was overestimating his abilities and had anosognosia for the consequences of his motor impairments. (The 'tie a knot' question is a good predictor of consistent overestimation of bimanual abilities; Nimmo-Smith *et al.*, 2005.) Only by asking the patient actually to perform the action did we discover that, having acknowledged his impairments and appreciated their consequences, he had developed impressive skills for managing so-called bimanual tasks with his unaffected left hand.

Patients who, in response to questions, overestimate their abilities may nevertheless display some partial or implicit knowledge of their limitations. For example, patients may make an accurate estimate of the abilities of another impaired person, even while acknowledging that the other person's condition is similar to their own (House and Hodges, 1988).

Marcel and colleagues (2004) investigated this phenomenon by asking questions about bimanual and bipedal tasks in two forms. For example: 'In your present state, how well can you tie a knot?' (first-person form) versus 'If I were in your present state, how well would I be able to tie a knot?' (third-person form).[4] Marcel and colleagues (2004) found that some patients following right-hemisphere stroke gave higher estimates in response to the first-person form of questions than in response to the third-person form (for discussion, see Vallar and Ronchi, 2006, p. 249). Using a similar protocol, Berti and colleagues (1996) did not find differences in patients' responses to the two forms of the questions.

The final section of the table (see Table 23.2D) lists questions on *anosognosic phenomena*, defined as unusual beliefs or experiences relating to the affected limbs. These questions are for the most part taken from Cutting (1978), who assessed a wide range of phenomena involving the contralesional arm, such as beliefs about non-belonging of the arm, including attribution of the arm to another person (somatoparaphrenia) and experiences of a third arm protruding from the patient's own body (supernumerary phantom limb). The structured interview of Marcel and colleagues (2004) also includes questions along these lines.

4.1 Occurrence rates for anosognosia

There are substantial differences in reported occurrence rates for anosognosia (number of patients with anosognosia divided by study population). Table 23.3 presents the occurrence rates for those studies that did not use presence (or absence) of anosognosia, or related pathologies such as unilateral neglect, as a selection criterion. As can be seen from the table, the method of assessment of anosognosia varies widely across the studies (column 1). This variation may contribute to the differences in reported occurrence rates. Some studies include both left- and right-hemisphere stroke patients while other studies include only left-hemisphere or only right-hemisphere patients (column 3). These differences in study population may impact on occurrence rates, as may time since stroke (column 4) and the level of motor impairment that is required for entry to the study (column 5). In addition, as discussed in Section 3.1, reported occurrence rates may depend heavily on the decision whether to classify patients with a score of 1 on Bisiach's Anosognosia Scale as having anosognosia (Baier and Karnath, 2005).

---

[4] The questions actually used by Marcel and colleagues (2004, p. 24) were rather more complicated than this. First-person form: 'In your present state how well, compared with your normal ability, can you tie a knot? If you can do it as well as usual, say "ten". If you cannot do it at all, say "nought".' Third-person form: 'If I were in your present state, how well would I be able to tie a knot, compared with my usual ability? If I could do it as well as usual, say "ten". If I could not do it at all, say "nought".'

Table 23.3 Occurrence Rates for Anosognosia in Patients with Left- or Right-Hemisphere Lesions

Method of assessment	Published report	Study population	Time since stroke	Level of motor impairment	Occurrence rates for anosognosia: % (number assessed)		
					Left hemisphere	Right hemisphere	Left and right hemisphere
Nathanson et al. (1952)	Nathanson et al. (1952)	100 (95 stroke) consecutive patients with hemiplegia; 76 assessed for anosognosia.	1 day to several years.	Complete hemiplegia.	23.08% (39)	51.35% (37)	36.84% (76)
Cutting (1978)	Cutting (1978)	100 (96 stroke) patients with hemiplegia over 2-year period in a General Hospital; 70 assessed for anosognosia.	Within 8 days.	4-point scale: slight, moderate, severe, total.	13.64% (22)	58.33% (48)	44.29% (70)
	Stone et al. (1993)	171 consecutive stroke patients; 116 assessed for anosognosia.	2–3 days.	Not selected by motor impairment.	5.36% (56)	28.33% (60)	17.24% (116)
Willanger et al. (1981)	Willanger et al. (1981)	55 consecutive RH-stroke patients over a 3-year period.	Not specified.	Paresis graded as: slight-moderate or marked-severe.		45.45% (55)*	
Hier et al. (1983)	Hier et al. (1983)	41 RH-stroke patients assessed consecutively by Stroke Service.	Within 7 days.	6-point scale: 0 (no movement) to 5 (normal strength).		36.59% (41)	

Study	Patients	Time of assessment	Motor impairment				
Bisiach et al. (1986)	97 RH patients; 36 with complete hemiplegia assessed for anosognosia.	Within 37 days.	Severe motor impairment.			33.33% (36)*	
Pederson et al. (1996)	566 consecutive unselected stroke patients.	Within first week.	Not selected by motor impairment.	9%	36%		20.85% (566)
Azouvi et al. (2002)	206 consecutive RH patients with first-ever stroke.	Average 11.1 weeks.	4-point scale: 0 (no deficit) to 3 (severe hemiplegia).		17% (206)		
Beis et al. (2004)	89 consecutive LH-stroke patients from 19 Centres; 78 assessed for anosognosia.	Average 10.8 weeks.	3-point scale: 0 (no deficit) to 2 (severe hemiplegia).	6.41% (78)			
Baier and Karnath (2005)	128 consecutive stroke patients with hemiparesis or hemiplegia.	Up to 15 days.	6-point scale: 0 (no movement) to 5 (normal movement).				Total: 22.66% (128) Moderate or severe: 9.38% (128)*
Spalletta et al. (2007)	50 consecutive RH-stroke inpatients.	Within 3 months.	Not selected by motor impairment.		26% (50)*		
Baier and Karnath (2008)	79 RH-stroke patients with left hemiparesis or hemiplegia.	Within 10 days.	6-point scale: 0 (no movement) to 5 (normal movement).		15.19% (79)*		

(continued)

Table 23.3 (*continued*) Occurrence Rates for Anosognosia in Patients with Left- or Right-Hemisphere Lesions

Method of assessment	Published report	Study population	Time since stroke	Level of motor impairment	Occurrence rates for anosognosia: % (number assessed)		
					Left hemisphere	Right hemisphere	Left and right hemisphere
Anderson and Tranel (1989)	Anderson and Tranel (1989)	32 stroke patients referred for neuropsychological assessment; 18 with dense hemiparesis assessed for anosognosia.	3–25 days.	Dense hemiparesis.			27.77% (18)
	Wagner and Cushman (1994)	108 consecutive stroke patients from two acute Neurorehabilitation Centres.	Average 4.9 weeks.	Not selected by motor impairment.			18.1% (108)
	Hartman-Maeir et al. (2001)	60 patients with first-ever stroke; 46 with severe motor deficit of arm assessed for anosognosia.	4–8 weeks.	Severe.	23.53% (17)	27.59% (29)	26.09% (46)
Starkstein et al. (1992)	Starkstein et al. (1992)	80 stroke patients selected from 96 consecutive admissions.	Approximately 1 week.	Not selected by motor impairment.			Total: 33.75% (80) Moderate or severe: 23.75% (80)*
	Appelros et al. (2002)	377 stroke patients recruited from Örebro, Sweden over 12 months; 276 assessed for anosognosia.	1–4 days.	Not selected by motor impairment.			Total: 17.39% (276) Moderate or severe: 11.96% (276)*

Study	Sample	Time	Motor deficit	Occurrence rate		
Berti et al. (1996)	34 chronic stoke patients from Geriatrics, selected by RH damage and complete hemiplegia.	Average 60 days.	Complete hemiplegia.	26.47% (34)		
Maeshima et al. (1997)	50 patients with RH cerebral haemorrhage.	Within 30 days.	Severe or moderate-mild.	24% (50)		
Marcel et al. (2004)	64 stroke patients recruited from seven hospitals, selected by hemiplegia.	Average 79.1 days (LH) 55.7 days (RH).	Severe motor deficit in at least one limb.	Arm: 0% (22) Leg: 9.09% (22) ADL: 13.64% (22)	Arm: 28.57% (42) Leg: 29.27% (41) ADL: 52.38% (42)	Arm: 18.75% (64) Leg: 22.22% (63) ADL: 39.06% (64)
Cocchini et al. (2009)	33 LH-stroke patients with motor impairments; 30 patients selected as per reliable responses on the Visual Analogue Test.	Average 73.8 days.	4-point scale: 0 (normal motor performance) to 3 (complete hemiplegia).	40% (30)		

LH = Left Hemisphere; RH = Right Hemisphere; ADL = Activities of Daily Living.

* Moderate or severe anosognosia: The patient did not acknowledge his or her deficits until these were demonstrated (moderate) or never acknowledged the deficits (severe).

5 A comprehensive assessment of anosognosia for motor impairments

A new structured interview for the assessment of anosognosia for motor impairments is presented at the end of this chapter. The approach is theoretically motivated and relatively comprehensive. The assessment incorporates items from the interviews presented in Table 23.2 as well as items that build on earlier protocols. Any assessment of anosognosia depends on a prior assessment of the patient's motor impairments and their consequences and so the structured interview is to be used alongside assessments of motor impairments and their functional consequences, such as the Motricity Index, the Rivermead Mobility Index, and the Barthel Activities of Daily Living Index (Section 3). A full investigation of anosognosia must also include assessments of factors that may play a role in its aetiology such as unilateral neglect, 'a notable suspect in anosognosia' (Vuilleumier, 2004, p. 10), and other factors that may impact on recovery and rehabilitation.

The new structured interview is made up of four modules. The first module does not involve any request for the patient actually to perform tasks using the affected limbs. It includes questions about the primary reason for hospitalisation (Q1), about the patient's acknowledgement of motor impairments (Q2), and about the patient's appreciation of the consequences of his or her motor impairments for activities of daily living (Q3). It also investigates anosognosic phenomena (Q4). Although questions about these phenomena have not been incorporated into most structured interviews, we believe that they may prove useful for assessment and rehabilitation, since patients are unlikely to mention these unusual beliefs and experiences spontaneously.

Thereafter, the structure of the assessment is dictated by the threefold distinction (explained in Section 2 of this chapter) between concurrent unawareness of an impairment, failure to acknowledge the impairment itself, and failure to appreciate the consequences of the impairment for activities of daily living. Thus, the second module investigates whether the patient is concurrently aware of motoric failures of the affected arm or leg. With vision precluded, the patient is requested, for the first time, to move his or her limbs (Q5). If the patient is seated, he or she is requested to raise each arm, and then both arms, to shoulder level and to raise each leg by extending it at the knee. If the patient is supine, he or she is requested to raise each arm, and then both arms, and each leg from the bed surface, to a position indicated by the examiner.

It is not the primary purpose of this second module to investigate the patient's beliefs as to whether he or she is really able to move the affected limbs. Still less is it intended to challenge the patient's beliefs by providing evidence of failure. Instead, the purpose of the module is to provide information about the patient's proprioceptive experience as he or she tries to move the affected limbs; that is, information about the patient's bodily awareness or unawareness of motoric failures when they occur.[5] This is theoretically important because concurrent

---

[5] The second module builds on a protocol used by Marcel and colleagues (2004). In their study, as part of an assessment of motor function and separately from the main anosognosia interview, patients were

unawareness of motor impairments may be a factor in failure to acknowledge those impairments. It is only at the end of the module, and only if the patient has reported feeling as if he or she succeeded in moving the affected limbs (illusory limb movements), that the examiner asks whether the patient believes that the limbs really moved. The patient's beliefs about whether he or she can move the affected limbs are the focus of the next module.

As we have seen, one of the key aspects of the assessments of anosognosia by Willanger and colleagues (1981) and Bisiach and colleagues (1986) is that the patient's impairment is demonstrated and the patient is given the opportunity to reflect on this evidence of failure and to acknowledge his or her motor impairments. This allows us to distinguish between moderate and severe anosognosia. The third module investigates whether the patient acknowledges his or her motor impairments, both before (prior belief) and after (posterior belief) an impairment is demonstrated (Q6, raise the limb, and Q7, maintain the limb in a raised position). In order that the evidence of failure should be maximally available to the patient, vision is permitted. All questions are first asked concerning the unaffected limb. This allows the examiner to check that the patient understands the task and also provides a control condition against which responses to questions about the affected limb can be compared.

The fourth module investigates whether the patient appreciates the consequences of motor impairments for activities of daily living. One of the key points in Section 4 of this chapter is that an investigation of anosognosia for the consequences of motor impairments should include asking the patient to perform, or at least describe how they would perform, various tasks. In this module, first-person and third-person forms of questions about unimanual, bimanual, and bipedal tasks are used (Q8) and the patient is asked to rate his or her abilities both before (prior belief) and after (posterior belief) actually trying to perform an action (Q9). Some of the actions involve interaction with objects and so the subsequent position of the objects provides clear evidence of success or failure of the attempt.

By testing the patient's belief revision, the third and fourth modules assess whether the patient makes appropriate use of available evidence of his or her limitations. Thus, the second, third, and fourth modules together could, in principle, go beyond detecting anosognosia for motor impairments and provide the beginnings of an explanation of some cases of anosognosia. The explanation would be of a familiar two-factor kind in which impairment of immediate bodily experience of motoric failure, and cognitive impairments that obstruct the appropriate use of available evidence to update beliefs, would

---

asked to raise each limb with vision precluded and their performance was rated objectively using the MRC scale (Table 23.1). As soon as the assessment of motor function was complete, 'patients were asked how much they had been able to move each arm and each leg' (p. 23). In making this post-performance evaluation, patients had to rely on 'immediate episodic experience' provided by proprioception, since they were blindfolded and no other feedback was given (p. 32). To the extent that patients gave an unrealistically high evaluation of their performance in trying to move their affected limbs, they were judged to be concurrently unaware of their motoric failure.

both play a role (Aimola Davies and Davies, 2009; Aimola Davies *et al.*, 2009; Davies, Aimola Davies and Coltheart, 2005; Levine, 1990; Levine *et al.*, 1991). As Vuilleumier says (2004, p. 11): 'any neurological dysfunction susceptible to alter the phenomenal experience of a defect might provide the ground out of which anosognosia can develop when permissive cognitive factors are also present'.

6 Conclusion

A theoretical framework for this chapter is provided by the threefold distinction between concurrent unawareness of an impairment, failure to acknowledge the impairment itself, and failure to appreciate the consequences of the impairment for activities of daily living (Section 2). A simple assessment of anosognosia for motor impairments can be carried out at the same time as a routine assessment of motor impairments. An initial assessment of anosognosia for the consequences of motor impairments can be obtained by using a dual scoring system with functional measures of mobility and independence. A more comprehensive assessment of motor impairments and their consequences invites a correspondingly more nuanced assessment of anosognosia (Section 3).

We began this chapter with the proposal that a comprehensive and widely accepted procedure for assessing anosognosia for motor impairments would contribute to a better understanding of the many factors in anosognosia and might also lead to improvement in the clinical management of patients. Building on published structured interviews (Section 4) and other protocols, we have presented a theoretically motivated and relatively comprehensive instrument for assessing anosognosia (Section 5). We hope that this new structured interview will contribute to our understanding of the occurrence, aetiology, time course, and treatment of anosognosia and that this will lead, in turn, to improved recovery and rehabilitation for patients.

References

Aimola Davies, A. M. and Davies, M. (2009). Explaining pathologies of belief. In M. R. Broome and L. Bortolotti (Eds.), *Psychiatry as cognitive neuroscience: Philosophical perspectives* (pp. 285–323). Oxford: Oxford University Press.

Aimola Davies, A. M., Davies, M., Ogden, J. A., Smithson, M. and White, R. C. (2009). Cognitive and motivational factors in anosognosia. In T. J. Bayne and J. Fernández (Eds.), *Delusions and self-deception: Affective and motivational influences on belief formation* (pp. 187–225). Hove, East Sussex: Psychology Press.

Anderson, S. W. and Tranel, D. (1989). Awareness of disease states following cerebral infarction, dementia, and head trauma: Standardized assessment. *The Clinical Neuropsychologist, 3*, 327–339.

Antonucci, G., Aprile, T. and Paolucci, S. (2002). Rasch analysis of the Rivermead Mobility Index: A study using mobility measures of first-stroke inpatients. *Archives of Physical Medicine and Rehabilitation, 83*, 1442–1449.

Appelros, P., Karlsson, G. M., Seiger, Å. and Nydevik, I. (2002). Neglect and anosognosia after first-ever stroke: Incidence and relationship to impairment and disability. *Journal of Rehabilitative Medicine, 34*, 215–220.

Azouvi, P., Samuel, C., Louis-Dreyfus, A., Bernati, T., Bartolomeo, P., Beis, J.-M. *et al.* (2002). Sensitivity of clinical and behavioural tests of spatial neglect after right hemisphere stroke. *Journal of Neurology, Neurosurgery, and Psychiatry, 73*, 160–166.

Baier, B. and Karnath, H.-O. (2005). Incidence and diagnosis of anosognosia for hemiparesis revisited. *Journal of Neurology, Neurosurgery, and Psychiatry, 76*, 358–361.

Baier, B. and Karnath, H.-O. (2008). Tight link between our sense of limb ownership and self-awareness of actions. *Stroke, 39*, 486–488.

Beis, J. M., Keller, C., Morin, N., Bartolomeo, P., Bernati, T., Chokron, S. *et al.* (2004). Right spatial neglect after left hemisphere stroke: Qualitative and quantitative study. *Neurology, 9*, 1600–1605.

Berti, A., Làdavas, E. and Della Corte, M. (1996). Anosognosia for hemiplegia, neglect dyslexia, and drawing neglect: Clinical findings and theoretical considerations. *Journal of the International Neuropsychological Society, 2*, 426–440.

Berti, A., Bottini, G., Gandola, M., Pia, L., Smania, N., Stracciari, A. *et al.* (2005). Shared cortical anatomy for motor awareness and motor control. *Science, 309*, 488–491.

Berti, A., Spinazzola, L., Pia, L. and Rabuffetti, M. (2007). Motor awareness and motor intention in anosognosia for hemiplegia. In P. Haggard, Y. Rossetti and M. Kawato (Eds.), *Sensorimotor foundations of higher cognition (Attention and Performance XXII)* (pp. 163-181). Oxford: Oxford University Press.

Bisiach, E., Vallar, G., Perani, D., Papagno, C. and Berti, A. (1986). Unawareness of disease following lesions of the right hemisphere: Anosognosia for hemiplegia and anosognosia for hemianopia. *Neuropsychologia, 24*, 471–482.

Bohannon, R. W. (1999). Motricity Index scores are valid indicators of paretic upper extremity strength following stroke. *Journal of Physical Therapy Science, 11*, 59–61.

Brott, T., Adams, H. P., Olinger, C. P., Marler, J. R., Barsan, W. G., Biller, J. *et al.* (1989). Measurements of acute cerebral infarction: A clinical examination scale. *Stroke, 20*, 864–870.

Cameron, D. and Bohannon, R. W. (2000). Criterion validity of lower extremity Motricity Index scores. *Clinical Rehabilitation, 14*, 208–211.

Chen, H.-M., Hsieh, C.-L., Lo, S. K., Liaw, L.-J., Chen, S.-M. and Lin, J.-H. (2007). The test-retest reliability of 2 mobility performance tests in patients with chronic stroke. *Neurorehabilitation and Neural Repair, 21*, 347–352.

Cocchini, G., Beschin, N., Cameron, A., Fotopoulou, A. and Della Sala, S. (2009). Anosognosia for motor impairment following left brain damage. *Neuropsychology, 23*, 223–230.

Collen, F. M., Wade, D. T., Robb, G. F. and Bradshaw, C. M. (1991). The Rivermead Mobility Index: A further development of the Rivermead Motor Assessment. *International Disability Studies, 13*, 50–54.

Collin, C. and Wade, D. (1990). Assessing motor impairment after stroke: A pilot reliability study. *Journal of Neurology, Neurosurgery, and Psychiatry, 53*, 576–579.

Collin, C., Wade, D. T., Davies, S. and Horne, V. (1988). The Barthel ADL Index: A reliability study. *International Disability Studies, 10*, 61–63.

Cutting, J. (1978). Study of anosognosia. *Journal of Neurology, Neurosurgery, and Psychiatry, 41*, 548–555.

Davies, M., Aimola Davies, A. M. and Coltheart, M. (2005). Anosognosia and the two-factor theory of delusions. *Mind and Language, 20*, 209–236.

Demeurisse, G., Demol, O. and Robaye, E. (1980). Motor evaluation in vascular hemiplegia. *European Neurology, 19*, 382–389.

Feinberg, T. E., Roane, D. M. and Ali, J. (2000). Illusory limb movements in anosognosia for hemiplegia. *Journal of Neurology, Neurosurgery, and Psychiatry, 68*, 511–513.

Franchignoni, F., Tesio, L., Benevolo, E. and Ottonello, M. (2003). Psychometric properties of the Rivermead Mobility Index in Italian stroke rehabilitation inpatients. *Clinical Rehabilitation, 17*, 273–282.

Frith, C. D., Blakemore, S.-J. and Wolpert, D. M. (2000). Abnormalities in the awareness and control of action. *Philosophical Transactions of the Royal Society of London B, 355*, 1771–1788.

Gold, M., Adair, J. C., Jacobs, D. H. and Heilman, K. M. (1994). Anosognsosia for hemiplegia: An electrophysiologic investigation of the feed-forward hypothesis. *Neurology, 44,* 1804–1808.

Goldstein, L. B., Bertels, C. and Davis, J. N. (1989). Interrater reliability of the NIH Stroke Scale. *Archives of Neurology, 46,* 660–662.

Green, J., Forster, A. and Young, J. (2001). A test-retest reliability study of the Barthel Index, the Rivermead Mobility Index, the Nottingham Extended Activities of Daily Living Scale and the Frenchay Activities Index in stroke patients. *Disability and Rehabilitation, 23,* 670–676.

Guarantors of Brain (2000). *Aids to the examination of the peripheral nervous system* (4th ed.). Edinburgh: W. B. Saunders.

Hartman-Maeir, A., Soroker, N. and Katz, N. (2001). Anosognosia for hemiplegia in stroke rehabilitation. *Neurorehabilitation and Neural Repair, 15,* 213–222.

Heilman, K. M. (1991). Anosognosia: Possible neuropsychological mechanisms. In G. P. Prigatano and D. L. Schacter (Eds.), *Awareness of deficit after brain injury* (pp. 53-62). New York: Oxford University Press.

Heilman, K. M., Barrett, A. M. and Adair, J. C. (1998). Possible mechanisms of anosognosia: A defect in self-awareness. *Philosophical Transactions of the Royal Society of London B, 353,* 1903–1909.

Hier, D. B., Mondlock, J. and Caplan, L. R. (1983). Behavioral abnormalities after right hemisphere stroke. *Neurology, 33,* 337–344.

House, A. and Hodges, J. (1988). Persistent denial of handicap after infarction of the right basal ganglia: A case study. *Journal of Neurology, Neurosurgery, and Psychiatry, 51,* 112–115.

Hsieh, C.-L., Hsueh, I.-P., Chiang, F.-M. and Lin, P.-H. (1998). Inter-rater reliability and validity of the action research arm test in stroke patients. *Age and Ageing, 27,* 107–113.

Karnath, H.-O., Baier, B. and Nägele, T. (2005). Awareness of the functioning of one's own limbs mediated by the insular cortex? *The Journal of Neuroscience, 25,* 7134–7138.

Levine, D. N. (1990). Unawareness of visual and sensorimotor defects: A hypothesis. *Brain and Cognition, 13,* 233–281.

Levine, D. N., Calvanio, R. and Rinn, W. E. (1991). The pathogenesis of anosognosia for hemiplegia. *Neurology, 41,* 1771–1781.

Lyden, P. D., Lu, M., Levine, S. R., Brott, T. G. and Broderick, J. (2001). A modified national institutes of health stroke scale for use in stroke clinical trials: Preliminary reliability and validity. *Stroke, 32,* 1310–1317.

Maeshima, S., Dohi, N., Funahashi, K., Nakai, K., Itakura, T. and Komai, N. (1997). Rehabilitation of patients with anosognosia for hemiplegia due to intracerebral haemorrhage. *Brain Injury, 11,* 691–697.

Mahoney, F. I. and Barthel, D. W. (1965). Functional evaluation: The Barthel Index. *Maryland State Medical Journal, 14,* 61–65.

Marcel, A. J., Tegnér, R. and Nimmo-Smith, I. (2004). Anosognosia for plegia: Specificity, extension, partiality and disunity of bodily unawareness. *Cortex, 40,* 19–40.

Nathanson, M., Bergman, P. S. and Gordon, G. G. (1952). Denial of illness: Its occurrence in one hundred consecutive cases of hemiplegia. *Archives of Neurology and Psychiatry, 68,* 380–387.

Nimmo-Smith, I., Marcel, A. J. and Tegnér, R. (2005). A diagnostic test of unawareness of bilateral motor task abilities in anosognosia for hemiplegia. *Journal of Neurology, Neurosurgery, and Psychiatry, 76,* 1167–1169.

Orfei, M. D., Caltagirone, C. and Spalletta, G. (2009). The evaluation of anosognosia in stroke patients. *Cerebrovascular Diseases, 27,* 280–289.

Pedersen, P. M., Jørgensen, H. S., Nakayama, H., Raaschou, H. O. and Olsen, T. S. (1996). Frequency, determinants, and consequences of anosognosia in acute stroke. *Journal of Neurologic Rehabilitation, 10,* 243–250.

Spalletta, G., Serra, L., Fadda, L., Ripa, A., Bria, P. and Caltagirone, C. (2007). Unawareness of motor impairment and emotions in right hemisphere stroke: A preliminary investigation. *International Journal of Geriatric Psychiatry*, **22**, 1241–1246.

Spinazzola, L., Pia, L., Folegatti, A., Marchetti, C. and Berti, A. (2008). Modular structure of awareness for sensorimotor disorders: Evidence from anosognosia for hemiplegia and anosognosia for hemianaesthesia. *Neuropsychologia*, **46**, 915–926.

Starkstein, S. E., Federoff, J. P., Price, T. R., Leiguarda, R. C. and Robinson, R. G. (1992). Anosognosia in patients with cerebrovascular lesions. A study of causative factors. *Stroke*, **23**, 1446–1453.

Stone, S. P., Halligan, P. W. and Greenwood, R. J. (1993). Selection of acute stroke patients for treatment of visual neglect. *Journal of Neurology, Neurosurgery, and Psychiatry*, **56**, 463–466.

Sunderland, A., Tinson, D. J., Bradley, L. and Hewer, R. L. (1989). Arm function after stroke. An evaluation of grip strength as a measure of recovery and a prognostic indicator. *Journal of Neurology, Neurosurgery, and Psychiatry*, **52**, 1267–1272.

Vallar, G. and Ronchi, R. (2006). Anosognosia for motor and sensory deficits after unilateral brain damage: A review. *Restorative Neurology and Neuroscience*, **24**, 247–257.

Vuilleumier, P. (2004). Anosognosia: The neurology of beliefs and uncertainties. *Cortex*, **40**, 9–17.

Wade, D. T. (1992). *Measurement in neurological rehabilitation*. Oxford: Oxford University Press.

Wade, D. T. and Collin, C. (1988). The Barthel ADL Index: A standard measure of physical disability? *International Disability Studies*, **10**, 64–67.

Wade, D. T. and Hewer, R. L. (1987). Functional abilities after stroke: Measurement, natural history and prognosis. *Journal of Neurology, Neurosurgery, and Psychiatry*, **50**, 177–182.

Wagner, M. T. and Cushman, L. A. (1994). Neuroanatomic and neuropsychological predictors of unawareness of cognitive deficit in the vascular population. *Archives of Clinical Neuropsychology*, **9**, 57–69.

Willanger, R., Danielsen, U. T. and Ankerhus, J. (1981). Denial and neglect of hemiparesis in right-sided apoplectic lesions. *Acta Neurologica Scandinavica*, **64**, 310–326.

Table 23.4 Structured Interview: Anosognosia for Motor Impairments

Question			Score (Circle as appropriate)	Patient's Responses
Q1. Does the patient acknowledge he or she has had a stroke?	A	Where are we?	0: Patient describes primary reason for hospitalisation	
	B	Why are you here? Why are you in the hospital?	1: Patient admits primary reason for hospitalisation but only following question, 'Did you have a stroke?'	
	C	What is the matter with you?	2: Patient explicitly denies primary reason for hospitalisation	
		Examiner asks QD if patient does not describe primary reason for hospitalisation.		
	D	Did you have a stroke?		
Q2. Does the patient acknowledge motor impairments of the arm or leg?	A	Is there anything wrong with your arms?	0: Patient describes significant motor impairment	
	B	Do you have a problem moving your right arm?	1: Patient acknowledges impairment but only following question, 'Do you have a problem moving your left arm?'	
	C	Do you have a problem moving your left arm?	2: Patient denies any motor impairment	
		Examiner asks QD only if the patient answers 'yes' to QB or QC.		
	D	Why can't you move your arm?		
	E	Is there anything wrong with your legs?	0: Patient describes significant motor impairment	
	F	Do you have a problem moving your right leg?	1: Patient acknowledges impairment but only following question, 'Do you have a problem moving your left leg?'	
	G	Do you have a problem moving your left leg?	2: Patient denies any motor impairment	
		Examiner asks QH only if the patient answers 'yes' to QF or QG.		
	H	Why can't you move your leg?		
Q3. Does the patient appreciate the consequences of motor impairments for activities of daily living?	A	Do you have any problems with daily activities?	0: Realistic / 1: Unrealistic	
	B	Do you have any problems with eating?	0: Realistic / 1: Unrealistic	
	C	Do you have any problems with dressing?	0: Realistic / 1: Unrealistic	
	D	Do you have any problems with washing?	0: Realistic / 1: Unrealistic	
	E	Do you have any problems with getting around?	0: Realistic / 1: Unrealistic	
	F	*Examiner includes activities the patient is able to perform without problems. For example: Do you have any problems with watching TV?*	0: Realistic / 1: Unrealistic	
Q4. Does the patient have any unusual beliefs or experiences relating to the affected limbs?	A	Patients sometimes feel as if their arm or leg does not belong to them. Have you experienced this feeling? *If patient responds 'yes', then ask:* Do you feel as if your arm or leg belongs to someone else?	0: Absent / 1: Present	*Somatoparaphrenia*
	B	Patients sometimes feel as if their arm or leg moves unexpectedly, and is not under their control. Do you ever feel as if your arm or leg moves without you moving it yourself?	0: Absent / 1: Present	*Alien Movements*
	C	Do you ever feel as if your arm or leg moves even when others tell you it has not moved?	0: Absent / 1: Present	*Illusory Limb Movements*
	D	Do you ever feel as if your arm or leg moves even when you can see that it is still?	0: Absent / 1: Present	*Illusory Limb Movements*
	E	Patients sometimes feel as if they have a third limb. Do you ever feel as if you have a third arm or leg?	0: Absent / 1: Present	*Supernumerary Phantom Limb*
	F	Patients sometimes refer to their arm or leg as if it were another person. For example, they give the limb its own name. Are there particular names that you use when referring to your arm or leg?	0: Absent / 1: Present	*Personification*

Instructions

Q5. With vision precluded, is the patient concurrently aware of motoric failures of the arm or leg?

Vision Precluded: Raise a) unaffected arm, b) affected arm, c) both arms together. *Examiner test unaffected arm first, before affected arm or both arms together, to ensure patient understands task.*

Step 1. Movement. *Examiner point to patient's arm:* I am going to ask you to close your eyes and try to raise your arm(s) to shoulder level and try to raise your arm and tell me when it feels as if it reaches shoulder level. I will ask you about your experience, what it felt like. Please CLOSE your eyes now. When I say 'start', try to raise your arm and tell me when it feels as if it reaches shoulder level. OK, start. *Examiner start stopwatch.*
Examiner prompt patient if patient does not indicate it feels as if arm has reached shoulder level. Examiner: Does it feel as if your arm has reached shoulder level? (Yes/No) *Examiner record:*
(i) Movement of limb? (Yes/No), (ii) Patient's Performance (score on MRC scale, 0–5; see Table 23.1);
(iii) Time arm takes to reach shoulder level (seconds); (iv) Time patient reports it feels as if arm reaches shoulder level (seconds).

Step 2. Experience. *The following questions are about the patient's experience (what they felt), not the patient's beliefs about what really happened.*
(i) *Examiner:* Did it feel to you as if your arm was rising? *Examiner record:* Feeling of Movement? (Yes/No)
If patient responds 'yes', Examiner: Did it feel as if your arm rose just a little or all the way to shoulder level? *Examiner record verbatim:* Patient's Description of Experience
(ii) *Examiner:* I would like you to rate the feeling of raising your arm, from 0 to 10.
0 means it felt as if your arm did not rise at all; 5 means it felt as if your arm rose halfway to shoulder level; 10 means it felt as if your arm rose all the way to shoulder level.
Examiner prompt patient if there is no response to previous question: How would you rate the feeling of raising your arm? *Examiner record:* Patient's Rating of Experience. (0–10)
(iii) *Examiner record your assessment of whether the patient's experience was veridical or illusory:* Examiner's Assessment. (Veridical/Illusory)

Vision Precluded: Raise a) unaffected leg, b) affected leg. *Examiner test unaffected leg first, before affected leg, to ensure patient understands task.*

Step 1. Movement. *Examiner point to patient's leg:* I am going to ask you to close your eyes and try to raise your leg like this for 10 seconds. I will ask you about your experience, what it felt like. Please CLOSE your eyes now. When I say 'start', try to raise your leg and tell me when it feels as if it reaches (position). OK, start. *Examiner start stopwatch.*
Examiner prompt patient if patient does not indicate it feels as if leg has reached position. Examiner: Does it feel as if your leg has reached (position)? (Yes/No) *Examiner record:*
(i) Movement of limb? (Yes/No); (ii) Patient's Performance (score on MRC scale, 0–5; see Table 23.1);
(iii) Time leg takes to reach position (seconds); (iv) Time patient reports it feels as if leg reaches position (seconds).

Step 2. Experience. *The following questions are about the patient's experience (what they felt), not the patient's beliefs about what really happened.*
(i) *Examiner:* Did it feel to you as if your leg was rising? *Examiner record:* Feeling of Movement? (Yes/No)
If patient responds 'yes', Examiner: Did it feel as if your leg rose just a little or all the way to (position)? *Examiner record verbatim:* Patient's Description of Experience
(ii) *Examiner:* I would like you to rate the feeling of raising your leg, from 0 to 10.
0 means it felt as if your leg did not rise at all; 5 means it felt as if your leg rose halfway; 10 means it felt as if your leg rose all the way.
Examiner prompt patient if there is no response to previous question: How would you rate the feeling of raising your leg? *Examiner record:* Patient's Rating of Experience. (0–10)
(iii) *Examiner record your assessment of whether the patient's experience was veridical or illusory:* Examiner's Assessment. (Veridical/Illusory)

Step 3. Post-Performance Evaluation. *Examiner ask the following questions ONLY if patient has reported illusory experience of movement in Step 2. Examiner ask questions for ONLY one example.*
(i) *Examiner:* Just now, you said it felt to you as if this arm/leg was moving when you tried to move it. Do you believe that, when it felt as if it was moving, it really did move? *Examiner record:* Patient's Assessment. (Yes/No)
(ii) *Examiner:* I would like you to rate how much your arm/leg really moved, from 0 to 10. 0 means it did not rise at all; 5 means it rose halfway; 10 means it rose all the way. *Examiner record:* Patient's Rating of Movement. (0–10)

Limb(s) Tested	Step 1. Movement				Step 2. Experience			Step 3. Post-Performance Evaluation (ONLY one)	
	(i) Movement of Limb?	(ii) Patient's Performance (0–5)	(iii) Time to Position (seconds)	(iv) Time to Patient's Report (seconds)	(i) Feeling of Movement?	(ii) Patient's Rating of Experience (0–10)	(iii) Examiner's Assessment	(i) Patient's Assessment	(ii) Patient's Rating of Movement (0–10)
Unaffected Arm	Yes/No	0/1/3/5			Yes/No		0: Veridical 1: Illusory		
Affected Arm	Yes/No	0/1/3/5			Yes/No		0: Veridical 1: Illusory	Yes/No	
Both Arms: Left Both Arms: Right	Yes/No Yes/No	0/1/3/5 0/1/3/5	Affected arm only	Affected arm only	Affected arm only Yes/No	Affected arm only	0: Veridical 1: Illusory	Affected arm only Yes/No	Affected arm only
Unaffected Leg	Yes/No	0/1/3/5			Yes/No		0: Veridical 1: Illusory		
Affected Leg	Yes/No	0/1/3/5			Yes/No		0: Veridical 1: Illusory	Yes/No	

(continued)

Table 23.4 (*continued*) Structured Interview: Anosognosia for Motor Impairments

Instructions

Q6. Does the patient acknowledge movement impairments of the arm or leg?

and

Does the patient revise his or her beliefs after evidence of the impairment is provided?

Vision Permitted: Raise a) unaffected arm, b) affected arm, c) both arms together. *Examiner test unaffected arm first, before affected arm or both arms together, to ensure patient understands task.*

Step 1. Prior Belief. *Examiner:* Look at your arm(s). I am going to ask you to try to raise your arm(s) to shoulder level like this for 10 seconds. I would like you to rate how well you can do this, from 0 to 10. 0 means you cannot raise your arm at all; 5 means you can raise your arm halfway to shoulder level; 10 means you can raise your arm all the way to shoulder level. *Examiner record:* Patient's Rating of Ability to raise arm to shoulder level. (0–10)

Step 2. Movement. *Examiner point to patient's arm:* When I say 'start', try to raise your arm and tell me when it reaches shoulder level. OK, start. *Examiner start stopwatch. Examiner prompt patient if patient moves arm but does not indicate it has reached shoulder level. Examiner:* Has your arm reached shoulder level? (Yes/No) *Examiner record:*
(i) Movement of limb? (Yes/No); (ii) Patient's Performance (score on MRC scale, 0–5; see Table 23.1);
(iii) Time arm takes to reach shoulder level (seconds); (iv) Time patient reports arm reaches shoulder level (seconds).

Step 3. Prior Belief. *Based on patient's performance in Step 2, Examiner record your assessment of whether the patient's prior belief was realistic or unrealistic:* Examiner's Assessment (Realistic/Unrealistic)

Step 4. Post-Performance Evaluation. *Examiner:* How did that go? How well were you able to raise your arm? *Examiner record verbatim:* Patient's Post-Performance Evaluation
(i) *Examiner:* I would like you to rate how well you were able to raise your arm, from 0 to 10. 0 means your arm did not rise at all; 5 means your arm rose halfway to shoulder level; 10 means your arm rose all the way to shoulder level. *Examiner prompt patient if there is no response to previous question:* How would you rate how well you were able to raise your arm? *Examiner record:* Patient's Rating of Movement (0–10)
(ii) *Examiner record your assessment of whether the patient's post-performance evaluation is accurate or inaccurate:* Examiner's Assessment (Accurate/Inaccurate)

Step 5. Posterior Belief. *Examiner:* If I asked you again to raise your arm, do you think you could? (Yes/No) I would like you once again to rate how well you can raise your arm, from 0 to 10. *Examiner use rating Scale from Step 1.*
(i) *Examiner record:* Patient's Rating of Ability to raise arm to shoulder level (0–10); (ii) *Examiner record your assessment of whether the patient's posterior belief is realistic or unrealistic:* Examiner's Assessment (Realistic/Unrealistic)

Vision Permitted: Raise a) unaffected leg, b) affected leg. *Examiner test unaffected leg first, before affected leg, to ensure patient understands task.*

Step 1. Prior Belief. *Examiner:* Look at your leg. I am going to ask you to try to raise your leg like this for 10 seconds. I would like you to rate how well you can do this, from 0 to 10. 0 means you cannot raise your leg at all; 5 means you can raise your leg halfway to (position); 10 means you can raise your leg all the way to (position). *Examiner record:* Patient's Rating of Ability to raise leg to position. (0–10)

Step 2. Movement. *Examiner point to patient's leg:* When I say 'start', try to raise your leg and tell me when it reaches (position). OK, start. *Examiner start stopwatch. Examiner prompt patient if patient moves leg but does not indicate it has reached position. Examiner:* Has your leg reached (position)? (Yes/No) *Examiner record:*
(i) Movement of limb? (Yes/No); (ii) Patient's Performance (score on MRC scale, 0–5; see Table 23.1);
(iii) Time leg takes to reach position (seconds); (iv) Time patient reports leg reaches position (seconds).

Step 3. Prior Belief. *Based on patient's performance in Step 2, Examiner record your assessment of whether the patient's prior belief was realistic or unrealistic:* Examiner's Assessment (Realistic/Unrealistic)

Step 4. Post-Performance Evaluation. *Examiner:* How did that go? How well were you able to raise your leg? *Examiner record verbatim:* Patient's Post-Performance Evaluation
(i) *Examiner:* I would like you to rate how well you were able to raise your leg, from 0 to 10. 0 means your leg did not rise at all; 5 means your leg rose halfway; 10 means your leg rose all the way. *Examiner prompt patient if there is no response to previous question:* How would you rate how well you were able to raise your leg, do you think you could? (Yes/No) *Examiner record:* Patient's Rating of Movement (0–10)
(ii) *Examiner record your assessment of whether the patient's post-performance evaluation is accurate or inaccurate:* Examiner's Assessment (Accurate/Inaccurate)

Step 5. Posterior Belief. *Examiner:* If I asked you again to raise your leg, do you think you could? (Yes/No) I would like you once again to rate how well you can raise your leg, from 0 to 10. *Examiner use rating Scale from Step 1.*
(i) *Examiner record:* Patient's Rating of Ability to raise leg to shoulder level (0–10); (ii) *Examiner record your assessment of whether the patient's posterior belief is realistic or unrealistic:* Examiner's Assessment (Realistic/Unrealistic)

Limb(s) Tested	Step 1. Prior Belief — Patient's Rating of Ability (0–10) (i)	Step 2. Movement — Movement of Limb? (i)	Patient's Performance (0–5) (ii)	Time to Position (seconds) (iii)	Time to Patient's Report (seconds) (iv)	Step 3. Prior Belief — Examiner's Assessment	Step 4. Post-Performance Evaluation — Patient's Rating of Movement (0–10) (i)	Examiner's Assessment (ii)	Step 5. Posterior Belief — Patient's Rating of Ability (0–10) (i)	Examiner's Assessment (ii)
Unaffected Arm		Yes/No	0/1/2/3/4/5			0: Realistic / 1: Unrealistic		0: Accurate / 1: Inaccurate		0: Realistic / 1: Unrealistic
Affected Arm		Yes/No	0/1/2/3/4/5			0: Realistic / 1: Unrealistic		0: Accurate / 1: Inaccurate		0: Realistic / 1: Unrealistic
Both Arms: Left		Yes/No	0/1/2/3/4/5	Affected arm only	Affected arm only	0: Realistic / 1: Unrealistic		0: Accurate / 1: Inaccurate		0: Realistic / 1: Unrealistic
Both Arms: Right		Yes/No	0/1/2/3/4/5							
Unaffected Leg		Yes/No	0/1/2/3/4/5			0: Realistic / 1: Unrealistic		0: Accurate / 1: Inaccurate		0: Realistic / 1: Unrealistic
Affected Leg		Yes/No	0/1/2/3/4/5			0: Realistic / 1: Unrealistic		0: Accurate / 1: Inaccurate		0: Realistic / 1: Unrealistic

Instructions

Q7. Does the patient acknowledge maintenance impairments of the arm or leg?

and

Does the patient revise his or her beliefs after evidence of the impairment is provided?

Vision Permitted: Maintain Raised a) unaffected arm, b) affected arm, c) both arms together. *Examiner test unaffected arm first, before affected arm or both arms together, to ensure patient understands task.*

Step 1. Prior Belief. *Examiner:* Look at your arm(s). I will help you raise your arm to shoulder level. I am going to ask you to hold it like this for 30 seconds. I would like you to rate how well you can do this, from 0 to 10. 0 means you cannot maintain the position at all and your arm will return to the pillow straightaway; 5 means your arm will slowly drift down; 10 means you can hold the position for the full 30 seconds. *Examiner record:* Patient's Rating of Ability to maintain arm at shoulder level. (0–10)

Step 2. Maintenance. *Examiner point to patient's arm:* When I say 'start', try to maintain your arm at shoulder level for 30 seconds, and tell me if it returns to the pillow. OK, start. *Examiner start stopwatch. Examiner prompt patient if arm falls but patient does not indicate it has returned to the pillow. Examiner:* Has your arm returned to the pillow? (Yes/No) *Examiner record:*
(i) Maintenance of Position? (Yes/No); (ii) Patient's Performance (score on NIH scale, 0–4; see Table 23.1);
(iii) Time arm returns to pillow (seconds); (iv) Time patient reports arm returns to pillow (seconds)

Step 3. Prior Belief. *Based on patient's performance in Step 2, Examiner record your assessment of whether the patient's prior belief was realistic or unrealistic:* Examiner's Assessment. (Realistic/Unrealistic)

Step 4. Post-Performance Evaluation. *Examiner:* How did that go? How well were you able to maintain your arm in the raised position, from 0 to 10.
(i) *Examiner:* I would like you to rate how well you were able to maintain your arm in the raised position, from 0 to 10. 0 means your arm returned to the pillow straightaway; 5 means your arm slowly drifted down; 10 means you held the position for the full 30 seconds. *Examiner record:* Patient's Rating of Maintenance. (0–10)
(ii) *Examiner record your assessment of whether the patient's post-performance evaluation is accurate or inaccurate:* Examiner's Assessment. (Accurate/Inaccurate)

Step 5. Posterior Belief. *Examiner:* If I asked you again to maintain your arm at shoulder level for 30 seconds, do you think you could? (Yes/No)
I would like you once again to rate how well you can maintain the position, from 0 to 10. *Examiner use rating Scale from Table 1.*
(i) *Examiner record:* Patient's Rating of Ability to maintain arm at shoulder level (0–10); (ii) *Examiner record your assessment of whether the patient's posterior belief is realistic or unrealistic:* Examiner's Assessment. (Realistic/Unrealistic)

Vision Permitted: Maintain Raised a) unaffected leg, b) affected leg. *Examiner test unaffected leg first, before affected leg, to ensure patient understands task.*

Step 1. Prior Belief. *Examiner:* Look at your leg. I will help you raise your leg. I am going to ask you to hold it there like this for 30 seconds. I would like you to rate how well you can do this, from 0 to 10. 0 means you cannot maintain the position at all and your leg will return to the floor/bed straightaway; 5 means your leg will slowly drift down; 10 means you can hold the position for the full 30 seconds. *Examiner record:* Patient's Rating of Ability to maintain leg in raised position. (0–10)

Step 2. Maintenance. *Examiner point to patient's leg:* When I say 'start', try to maintain your leg in the raised position for 30 seconds, and tell me if it returns to the floor/bed. OK, start. *Examiner start stopwatch. Examiner prompt patient if leg falls but patient does not indicate it has returned to floor/bed. Examiner:* Has your leg returned to the floor/bed? (Yes/No) *Examiner record:*
(i) Maintenance of Position? (Yes/No); (ii) Patient's Performance (score on NIH scale, 0–4; see Table 23.1);
(iii) Time leg returns to floor/bed (seconds); (iv) Time patient reports leg returns to floor/bed (seconds)

Step 3. Prior Belief. *Based on patient's performance in Step 2, Examiner record your assessment of whether the patient's prior belief was realistic or unrealistic:* Examiner's Assessment. (Realistic/Unrealistic)

Step 4. Post-Performance Evaluation. *Examiner:* How did that go? How well were you were able to maintain your leg in the raised position? *Examiner record verbatim:* Patient's Post-Performance Evaluation
(i) *Examiner:* I would like you to rate how well you were able to maintain your leg in the raised position, from 0 to 10. 0 means your leg returned to the floor/bed straightaway; 5 means your leg slowly drifted down; 10 means you held the position for the full 30 seconds. *Examiner record:* Patient's Rating of Maintenance. (0–10)
(ii) *Examiner record your assessment of whether the patient's post-performance evaluation is accurate or inaccurate:* Examiner's Assessment. (Accurate/Inaccurate)

Step 5. Posterior Belief. *Examiner:* If I asked you again to maintain your leg in the raised position for 30 seconds, do you think you could? (Yes/No)
I would like you once again to rate how well you can maintain the position, from 0 to 10. *Examiner use rating Scale from Table 1.*
(i) *Examiner record:* Patient's Rating of Ability to maintain leg in raised position (0–10); (ii) *Examiner record your assessment of whether the patient's posterior belief is realistic or unrealistic:* Examiner's Assessment. (Realistic/Unrealistic)

| Limb(s) Tested | Step 1. Prior Belief | Step 2. Maintenance | | | | Step 3. Prior Belief | Step 4. Post-Performance Evaluation | | Step 5. Posterior Belief | |
| | Patient's Rating of Ability (0–10) | Maintenance of Position? | Patient's Performance (0–4) | Time to Return (seconds) | Time to Patient's Report (seconds) | Examiner's Assessment | Patient's Rating of Maintenance (0–10) | Examiner's Assessment | Patient's Rating of Ability (0–10) | Examiner's Assessment |
		(i)	(ii)	(iii)	(iv)		(i)	(ii)	(i)	(ii)
Unaffected Arm		Yes/No	0/1/2/3/4			0: Realistic 1: Unrealistic		0: Accurate 1: Inaccurate		0: Realistic 1: Unrealistic
Affected Arm		Yes/No	0/1/2/3/4			0: Realistic 1: Unrealistic		0: Accurate 1: Inaccurate		0: Realistic 1: Unrealistic
Both Arms: Left Both Arms: Right		Yes/No Yes/No	0/1/2/3/4 0/1/2/3/4	Affected arm only	Affected arm only	0: Realistic 1: Unrealistic		0: Accurate 1: Inaccurate		0: Realistic 1: Unrealistic
Unaffected Leg		Yes/No	0/1/2/3/4			0: Realistic 1: Unrealistic		0: Accurate 1: Inaccurate		0: Realistic 1: Unrealistic
Affected Leg		Yes/No	0/1/2/3/4			0: Realistic 1: Unrealistic		0: Accurate 1: Inaccurate		0: Realistic 1: Unrealistic

(continued)

Table 23.4 (*continued*) Structured Interview: Anosognosia for Motor Impairments

	Instructions
Q8. Does the patient appreciate the consequences of motor impairments for his or her ability to perform everyday actions? *and* Does the patient give different assessments of his or her abilities from first-person and third-person perspectives?	**Step 1. First-Person Perspective.** *Examiner*: I am going to read you a list of actions. For each action, I would like you to rate how well you, in your present condition, can perform it, from 0 to 10. <u>0 means</u> you cannot perform the action at all; <u>10 means</u> you can perform the action well – as well as always.* For each action, *Examiner*: In your present condition, how well can you… (e.g., drink from a glass using your right hand)? *Examiner prompt patient if there is no response to previous question*: How would you rate how well you can… (e.g., drink from a glass using your right hand)? *Examiner record*: <u>First-Person Rating of ability to perform action.</u> (0–10) **Step 2. Third-Person Perspective.** *Examiner*: I am going to read you the same list of actions again. This time I would like you to rate how well another person, in the same condition as you are now, could perform the action, from 0 to 10. <u>0 means</u> he/she could not perform the action at all; <u>10 means</u> he/she could perform the action well.* For each action, *Examiner*: If another person was in the same condition as you are now, how well could he/she… (e.g., drink from a glass using his/her right hand)? *Examiner prompt patient if there is no response to previous question*: How would you rate how well he/she could… (e.g., drink from a glass using his/her right hand)? *Examiner record*: <u>Third-Person Rating of ability to perform action.</u> (0–10) **Step 3. Explanation**. *Examiner ask the following question ONLY for actions involving the affected limb with a first-person rating of 5 or more in Step 1.* For each action, *Examiner*: Just now, you gave a rating of X for your ability to… (e.g., drink from a glass using your left hand). Please describe to me <u>how</u> you would do that. *Examiner record verbatim*: <u>Patient's Explanation and code the response.</u> N: No explanation; R: Reasonable; U: Unaware; B: Bizarre.**

	Actions: Unimanual, Bimanual and Bipedal		Step 1. First-Person Perspective First-Person Rating (0–10)	Step 2. Third-Person Perspective Third-Person Rating (0–10)	Step 3. Explanation Patient's explanation of how he or she would perform action
A	Drink from a glass using your right hand.	(U)			N R U B
B	Drink from a glass using your left hand.	(U)			N R U B
C	Comb your hair using your right hand.	(U)			N R U B
D	Comb your hair using your left hand.	(U)			N R U B
E	Brush your teeth using your right hand.	(U)			N R U B
F	Brush your teeth using your left hand.	(U)			N R U B
G	Clap your hands.	(B)			N R U B
H	Tie a knot.	(B)			N R U B
I	Shuffle cards.	(B)			N R U B
J	Unscrew a bottle.	(B)			N R U B
K	Climb the stairs.	(Bp)			N R U B
L	Jump.	(Bp)			N R U B
M	Walk.	(Bp)			N R U B
N	Stand.	(Bp)			N R U B

*Whenever possible, present a visual scale indicating 0 (cannot perform the action at all) to 10 (can perform the action as well as always).

**N: No explanation (patient remains silent or cannot explain); R: Reasonable (reasonable response, even if inadequate); U: Unaware (response is irrelevant or implausible); B: Bizarre (response explicitly states or entails use of affected limb).

Instructions

(continued)

Q9. Does the patient revise beliefs about his or her abilities after attempting to perform an action?

Step 1. Prior Belief. *Examiner ask patient these questions for ALL actions before proceeding to Step 2.*
Examiner: I am going to read you a new list of actions. For each action, I would like you to rate how well you can perform it, from 0 to 10.
0 means you cannot perform the action at all; 10 means you can perform the action as well as always. *
For each action, Examiner: How well can you... (e.g., raise your right arm)? If patient is asked to interact with Examiner or with an object, Examiner position your own hands or the object as appropriate.
Examiner prompt patient if there is no response to previous question: How would you rate how well you can... (e.g., raise your right arm)? Examiner record: Patient's Rating of Ability to perform action. (0–10)

Step 2. Performance and Post-Performance Evaluation. *Examiner ask patient these questions for ALL actions before proceeding to Step 3.*
(i) Examiner: I am going to ask you to try to perform each action on the list I just read you. After you try the action, I will ask you to rate your performance.
When I say 'start', try to... (e.g., raise your right arm). OK, start. Examiner record: Patient's Performance *(score 0 to 10).*
(ii) Based on patient's performance, Examiner record your assessment of whether the patient's prior belief was realistic or unrealistic: Examiner's Assessment *(Realistic/Unrealistic)*
(iii) Examiner: How did that go? I would like you to rate how well you were able to... (e.g., raise your right arm), from 0 to 10.
0 means you could not perform the action at all; 10 means you could perform the action as well as always. * Examiner record:* Patient's Rating of Performance. *(0–10)*
(iv) Examiner record your assessment of whether the patient's post-performance evaluation is accurate or inaccurate: Examiner's Assessment. *(Accurate/Inaccurate)*
(v) For questions G–L, Q and R, if patient's post-performance evaluation is inaccurate, Examiner ask follow-up question and record: Patient's Object Belief. *(Yes/No)*

Step 3. Posterior Belief. *Examiner ask patient these questions only after Step 2 has been completed for ALL actions.*
(i) Examiner: I am going to ask you again to rate how well you can perform each action on the list, from 0 to 10.
0 means you cannot perform the action at all; 10 means you can perform the action as well as always. *
For each action, Examiner: How well can you... (e.g., raise your right arm)? If patient is asked to interact with Examiner or with an object, Examiner position your own hands or the object as appropriate.
Examiner prompt patient if there is no response to previous question: How would you rate how well you can... (e.g., raise your right arm)? Examiner record: Patient's Rating of Ability to perform action. (0–10)
(ii) Examiner record your assessment of whether the patient's posterior belief is realistic or unrealistic: Examiner's Assessment. *(Realistic/Unrealistic)*

	Action	Step 1. Prior Belief (i) Patient's Rating of Ability (0–10)	Step 2. Performance and Post-Performance Evaluation (i) Patient's Performance (0–10)	(ii) Examiner's Assessment	(iii) Patient's Rating of Performance (0–10)	(iv) Examiner's Assessment	(v) Patient's Object Belief?	Step 3. Posterior Belief (i) Patient's Rating of Ability (0–10)	(ii) Examiner's Assessment
A	Raise your right arm.			0: Realistic 1: Unrealistic		0: Accurate 1: Inaccurate			0: Realistic 1: Unrealistic
B	Raise your left arm.			0: Realistic 1: Unrealistic		0: Accurate 1: Inaccurate			0: Realistic 1: Unrealistic
C	Raise both arms together.			0: Realistic 1: Unrealistic		0: Accurate 1: Inaccurate			0: Realistic 1: Unrealistic
D	Use your right hand to touch my left hand.			0: Realistic 1: Unrealistic		0: Accurate 1: Inaccurate			0: Realistic 1: Unrealistic
E	Use your left hand to touch my right hand.			0: Realistic 1: Unrealistic		0: Accurate 1: Inaccurate			0: Realistic 1: Unrealistic
F	Touch my hands, your right hand to my left hand and your left hand to my right hand.			0: Realistic 1: Unrealistic		0: Accurate 1: Inaccurate			0: Realistic 1: Unrealistic
G	*Examiner hold handkerchief in left hand:* Use your right hand to take this handkerchief from my hand. (Q: Are you holding the handkerchief?)			0: Realistic 1: Unrealistic		0: Accurate 1: Inaccurate	Yes/No		0: Realistic 1: Unrealistic
H	*Examiner hold handkerchief in right hand:* Use your left hand to take this handkerchief from my hand. (Q: Are you holding the handkerchief?)			0: Realistic 1: Unrealistic		0: Accurate 1: Inaccurate	Yes/No		0: Realistic 1: Unrealistic
I	*Examiner hold two handkerchiefs:* Use both hands to take these handkerchiefs from me, one with your right hand and the other with your left hand. (Q: Are you holding both handkerchiefs?)			0: Realistic 1: Unrealistic		0: Accurate 1: Inaccurate	Yes/No		0: Realistic 1: Unrealistic

*Whenever possible, present a visual scale indicating 0 (cannot perform the action at all) to 10 (can perform the action as well as always).

Table 23.4 (*continued*) Structured Interview: Anosognosia for Motor Impairments

Q9. (continued) Does the patient revise beliefs about his or her abilities after attempting to perform an action?		Step 1. Prior Belief	Step 2. Performance and Post-Performance Evaluation					Step 3. Posterior Belief	
Action		(i) Patient's Rating of Ability (0–10)	(i) Patient's Performance (0–10)	(ii) Examiner's Assessment	(iii) Patient's Rating of Performance (0–10)	(iv) Examiner's Assessment	(v) Patient's Object Belief?	(i) Patient's Rating of Ability (0–10)	(ii) Examiner's Assessment
J	*Examiner hold handkerchief and ring:* Use your right hand to thread this handkerchief through the ring. (Q: Is the handkerchief through the ring?)			0: Realistic 1: Unrealistic		0: Accurate 1: Inaccurate	Yes/No		0: Realistic 1: Unrealistic
K	*Examiner hold handkerchief and ring:* Use your left hand to thread this handkerchief through the ring. (Q: Is the handkerchief through the ring?)			0: Realistic 1: Unrealistic		0: Accurate 1: Inaccurate	Yes/No		0: Realistic 1: Unrealistic
L	*Examiner hold handkerchief and ring:* Use both hands to attach this handkerchief to the ring by tying a knot. (Q: Is the handkerchief tied on the ring?)			0: Realistic 1: Unrealistic		0: Accurate 1: Inaccurate	Yes/No		0: Realistic 1: Unrealistic
M	Raise your right foot.			0: Realistic 1: Unrealistic		0: Accurate 1: Inaccurate			0: Realistic 1: Unrealistic
N	Raise your left foot.			0: Realistic 1: Unrealistic		0: Accurate 1: Inaccurate			0: Realistic 1: Unrealistic
O	*Examiner hold your left hand 20 cm from patient's right foot:* Use your right foot to touch my left hand.			0: Realistic 1: Unrealistic		0: Accurate 1: Inaccurate			0: Realistic 1: Unrealistic
P	*Examiner hold your right hand 20 cm from patient's left foot:* Use your left foot to touch my right hand.			0: Realistic 1: Unrealistic		0: Accurate 1: Inaccurate			0: Realistic 1: Unrealistic
Q	*Examiner place a ball 20 cm from patient's right foot:* Use your right foot to push this ball towards me. (Q: Did the ball move?)			0: Realistic 1: Unrealistic		0: Accurate 1: Inaccurate	Yes/No		0: Realistic 1: Unrealistic
R	*Examiner place a ball 20 cm from patient's left foot:* Use your left foot to push this ball towards me. (Q: Did the ball move?)			0: Realistic 1: Unrealistic		0: Accurate 1: Inaccurate	Yes/No		0: Realistic 1: Unrealistic

*Whenever possible, present a visual scale indicating 0 (cannot perform the action at all) to 10 (can perform the action as well as always).

Part 4

Developmental and paediatric neuropsychology

Treatment and rehabilitation of paediatric/developmental neuropsychological disorders

Stephen Whitfield

1 The role of the paediatric neuropsychologist

The role of the paediatric neuropsychologist differs from that of clinical neuropsychologists working with adults both in terms of: (1) the perspective adopted, i.e. that the child is a growing individual so that a developmental view must be adopted when considering the results of clinical assessment and implementing treatment programmes, and (2) the context within which treatment/rehabilitation takes place. In terms of context, the paediatric neuropsychologist is generally much more involved in multidisciplinary working with health, social services, and education personnel than would be the case when working with adults. Treatment is also frequently carried out by others and in non-health (particularly educational) environments.

In the area of intervention/treatment the paediatric neuropsychologist contributes in an advisory, monitoring, and/or therapeutic role.

- The advisory role will include educating and informing the child (where appropriate and practicable), parents, therapists, teachers, and peers of the nature of the child's condition or injury and its likely impact upon his/her development and future education/occupation.

- Monitoring will include the evaluation of any intellectual or behavioural changes brought about by a disorder or injury and its clinical (e.g. radiation treatment) or pharmacological management (e.g. antiepileptic medication side-effects).

- The therapeutic role will include the management/treatment of behaviour disorders, memory complaints, emotional and adjustment problems, etc.

The psychological approaches used will include neurobehavioural and cognitive-behavioural methods; application of psychometric, developmental, and observational assessment techniques; rehabilitation methodology; and counselling. Contexts for interventions will include all aspects of the child's environment including home, school/college (or work), and leisure situations.

2 Specific issues in paediatric treatment and rehabilitation

2.1 Neuroplasticity

For children predictive factors would be the extent of damage (the more localized the damage, the greater the chance of a plastic response) and age at time of injury. Theoretically, plastic reorganization should be more easily achieved in the younger (under 2 years) brain where less development has taken place. Animal studies have shown some evidence to support this view, but it is not supported by research with human infants. Consequently, the process is either not a spontaneous one or it has critical periods during which injury will not stimulate neuronal modification. If the latter is true, the evidence so far suggests that the least favourable time for a plastic response is probably the period from the end of gestation to the first month of life, while the most favourable period is the age band of 1 to 2 years. At present neural transplantation has no role in childhood disorders.

2.2 Localization, lateralization, and modularity

Traditional approaches to adult neuropsychological assessment have emphasized localization or lateralization of cognitive functioning. This view has never been appropriate in young children where abnormal cerebral development or acquired injury could interrupt the establishment of localized or lateralized functions.

The view of cognitive abilities that emphasizes 'modularized' skills is more appropriate to the mature brain of adults. Cognitive—developmental views see a generalized and interdependent progression in skills throughout childhood, which explains the different patterns of deficit seen in adults and children following similar insults (see Section 3). The most important aspect of the paediatric neuropsychologist's approach is to relate neuropsychological observations to the developmental stage of the child.

2.3 Recovery

In the earliest stages of recovery the regular monitoring of the extent of postinjury confusion and disorientation is essential to ensure that therapeutic interventions with cognitive requirements are matched to orientation level.

- There is no UK-derived assessment for children. One can modify the Children's Orientation and Amnesia Test (Ewing-Cobbs *et al.* 1990).
- Questions relating to orientation to person, place, and time are most commonly used, with return of orientation usually occurring in this same order.

2.4 Rehabilitation

There is no evidence that rehabilitation efforts during the early stages of recovery alter its course or that sensory stimulation reduces the depth or duration of coma. However, physical health can deteriorate without appropriate medical and nursing support during this time. Children are also prone to the development of maladaptive behaviours during this period, which require management to prevent them entering the child's behavioural repertoire. A hospital or rehabilitation setting may prevent all the above.

Rehabilitation is distinct from recovery (the spontaneous process of return of pre-injury skills) and habilitation (the passive adaptation of environments to disabilities). The aim of rehabilitation is to reduce the 'mismatch between the skills a person possesses and the actual demands of the environment' (Dixon and Bäckman 1999). Its methodology is to use 'restorative' or 'compensatory/adaptive' strategies. This distinction is of less value in children as early insult denies many early learning experiences that the 'restorative' approach would utilize in rehabilitating adults. Consequently, the 'compensatory/adaptive' approach has primacy in younger children.

Restoration focuses upon reducing disability, whereas compensation and adaptation focus upon the reduction of handicap (World Health Organization 1980). The differences in these approaches can be summarized as follows.

- Restorative approaches are based upon recovering a lost skill.
- Compensation approaches aim to revive and/or modify a latent skill or develop a new skill to substitute for the lost one.
- Adaptation focuses upon modifying environments to reduce the mismatch between skills and demands or on altering the parents', teachers', and child's expectations to meet the changed circumstances.

Restorative and compensatory approaches are appropriate to higher levels of meta-awareness; adaptation to the lowest levels. As orientation returns, the strategies used will need to be adapted to incorporate the former as well as the latter.

2.5 Adjustment

2.5.1 Adjustment to a developmental disorder

A child with a developmental disorder may have little difficulty in adjusting to the neuropsychological consequences of the disorder as he or she will have always lived with it and will not have a model of 'normality'. The difficulty lies in trying to alert others to view the world from the child's perspective. This may not only yield empathic understanding of 'oddities' in the child's behaviour, but may also be useful in generating creative behavioural management solutions.

2.5.2 Adjustment to an acquired brain injury

Conversely, a child with an acquired brain injury in the later stages of recovery may feel a sense of loss for those things that he or she was able to do prior to the injury, but cannot do postinjury. This not infrequently leads to anxiety, frustration, and depression that can manifest themselves as oppositionality and aggression. Behavioural management will not be successful without addressing the underlying emotional adjustment issues involved.

Sharing with older children and their parents the rehabilitation team's analysis of their predicament and prognosis together with their full involvement in rehabilitation programme goal-setting can, in appropriate cases, be highly efficacious in reducing these feelings and moving forward the process of adjustment. After a period in which the child and parents have largely been recipients of medical treatment, they can find this emphasis on involvement empowering. However, such an approach is dependent upon an adequate degree of self-awareness, which may not be present in the early stages of recovery, in severe attentional or executive disorders, or where the child has been left with significant generalized learning difficulties. The same criteria would apply to those children who might benefit from cognitive-behavioural therapy.

2.5.3 Adjustment for parents and families

Parental adjustment encompasses a whole range of emotions including fear, detachment, helplessness, denial, anger, anxiety, depression, and guilt. Information, though needed by parents, may not be heard or may be rejected if given at the wrong time. Anger directed at professional staff, or even the child, is evidence of poor adjustment at that time, but not necessarily of poor overall adjustment.

Families have resources that they have to allocate to deal with life events with each member contributing their share to the collective whole. Multiple demands on these resources decrease that which can be devoted to any particular situation. Continuous demands, as produced by the long-term care of a family member, deplete the resources of the entire family. The additional demands of poverty, divorce, work pressures, young children, elderly parents, etc. draw even further on these finite resources.

Parents do not experience their child as a collection of cognitive abilities, but as a functioning individual within a social and personal historical context. Adjustment will be facilitated if the paediatric neuropsychologist does not describe the child's deficits, but integrates findings into an explanation of the neurological disorder in the context of the child's world and his or her past and future.

3 Neuropsychological dysfunction

Disturbance to central nervous system (CNS) development in the prenatal period primarily results in structural abnormalities (e.g. dysplasias, spina bifida, agenesis of the corpus callosum). Postnatal interruptions affect the elaboration of connections within the brain, processes that continue into early adolescence. The nature and severity of the insult determine, as for adults, outcome in a dose-response fashion. However, in children, the developmental stage attained at the time of insult/onset interacts with the nature of the insult to produce a complex pattern of deficits, unlike the more proscribed impairments found in adults.

Childhood CNS disorders are more likely to have a generalized effect (traumatic brain injury, infections, etc.). Focal disorders (tumour, stroke) are relatively rare. Consequently, specific impairments such as apraxias and aphasias are less common, while attention, memory, and executive disorders are most prevalent (see box below).

NEUROPATHOLOGICAL DISORDERS | 475

Functional impairments associated with specific conditions

Perceptual and spatial disorders

- Turner's syndrome
  - — Impairments in visual Gestalt perception and integrative spatial construction
  - — Most significant in children with karyotype 45XO
- William's syndrome
  - — Problems with drawing, copying, and block design
  - — Attention to detail rather than overall picture

Memory disorders

- Epilepsy
  - — Memory problems primarily associated with temporal lobe epilepsy (TLE) due to close anatomical association with hippocampus
  - — Lateralized impairments to verbal and nonverbal memory associated in some studies with side of TLE focus

Language disorders

- Auditory agnosia in Landau–Kleffner syndrome
- Pragmatic disorders in autism and Asperger's syndrome

Executive disorders

- Autism
- Phenylketonuria
- Gilles de la Tourette's syndrome
- Treatment of acute lymphoblastic leukaemia
- Turner's syndrome

---

4 Neuropathological disorders

4.1 Acquired brain injury

The types of acquired brain injuries are summarized in the box below.

4.1.1 Prognosis

The extent of cognitive sequelae and subsequent prognosis for intellectual recovery are dependent upon the nature and severity of the injury and the age at time of injury.

Suitable indices of severity of injury are the depth and duration of coma and length of posttraumatic amnesia (PTA).

Types of acquired brain injury

Traumatic

- Road traffic accidents (RTA) result in a combination of focal and diffuse injury
- Falls
- Non-accidental injury
  - Cause of the majority of severe head injuries in children under 1 year, 10% of injuries in the under-fives. 50% will have permanent cognitive sequelae
  - High incidence of repeated assaults/damage
  - Higher incidence during teenage years probably as a result of parent–child conflicts
- Projectile injury

Hypoxic–ischaemic

- Near drowning
- Neonatal hypoxia—most commonly problems with labour and delivery.
- Anaesthetic accidents
- Prolonged status epilepticus
- Cerebrovascular accidents

Other medical

- CNS infections
- Tumours and their treatment
- Acute encephalopathies
- Metabolic disorders

- *Depth of coma* is most commonly assessed by the Glasgow Coma Scale (Jennett and Teasdale, pp. 258–63) or the paediatric version (Simpson *et al.* 1991). The lower the score, the poorer the prognosis for recovery.

- *Duration of coma*. Less than 20 minutes, mild; 20 minutes to 6 hours, moderate; 6–48 hours, severe; over 48 hours, very severe.

- *Length of PTA*. Under 60 minutes, mild; 1–24 hours, moderate; 1–7 days, severe; 1–4 weeks, very severe; over 4 weeks, extremely severe.

PTA is more difficult to assess in children as they may become confused between actual memories and information provided by parents/visitors.

The 'nature' of the injury relates to primary brain damage (whether focal, diffuse, or both) combined with results of any secondary factors (oedema, raised intracranial pressure, hypoxic/ischaemic injury, haematoma).

Contrary to the Kennard principle (commonly interpreted as 'if you are going to have brain damage, have it early'), experimental and clinical work now indicates that injuries sustained at a young age, before the brain has had time to mature, lead to greater cognitive sequelae than those occurring in the adult years (Johnson and Rose 1996). Functional deficits may not be obvious until the area of the brain concerned begins to mature. For the prefrontal lobes this happens between about 8 and 15 years. These delayed effects are sometimes referred to as 'sleeper' phenomena.

4.1.2 Cognitive sequelae

The most common cognitive sequelae to an acquired head injury are impairments to orientation and attention, memory (in children this includes access to long-term memory, which will be less well developed than in adults), new learning, and executive skills.

4.1.3 Behavioural sequelae

These are present in 30% of children with mild to severe traumatic brain injury (TBI) and 73% of children with multiple functional impairments. They occur most commonly after frontal and temporal lobe damage. They arise in part from cognitive impairments such as poor insight into their own behaviour and poor application of environmental feedback.

Disinhibition presents severe problems of social acceptability, which can be aided by a set of rules to apply in common settings, e.g. do not shout out in class. This approach is only successful if memory skills have returned to a level that permits its retention. Behavioural contracts can be successful with less severe cases.

4.1.4 The rehabilitation of neuropsychological functions

Cognitive rehabilitation This consists of the application of strategies (largely behavioural) to improve cognitive and affective functioning following acquired brain injury. The methodology tends to be split between direct training of cognitive processes and functional skills training. The evidence is that functionally based cognitive rehabilitation in everyday life settings is more successful than rehabilitation exercises detached from the child's normal living environment. Success appears to be independent of the particular method used.

Attention training There is no solid research basis that proves the effectiveness of retraining approaches.

Memory rehabilitation The effectiveness of retraining has not been proven. Compensatory aids are useful in improving function. The use of external memory aids to assist recall is only successful if the child remembers that they have a problem with their memory! Without this they go unused. Thus, they are more useful for those with mild rather than severe problems. The use of aids has to be built up with frequent reminders in 'real-life' situations. Similar considerations apply to the use of internal (verbal mnemonics) aids.

As procedural memory is frequently retained when explicit memory is impaired, this is often incorporated into compensatory strategies, e.g. inclusion of pre-injury procedural learning into new behaviours that are repeatedly practised using errorless learning approaches.

Rehabilitation of executive functions There has been some success in training for specific tasks, e.g. self-organization skills. Compensatory aids, e.g. diaries, electronic organizers, copies of school timetables, home–school books, picture sequences, etc., completed under guidance can be useful in training these skills. However, only limited generalization is seen in the training of problem-solving skills.

4.1.5 Neurobehavioural management

On emergence from coma, restlessness, wandering, and destructiveness occur. Acute phase problems with behaviour usually resolve with reduction in PTA. However, environmental control is important with avoidance of high-level stimulation, minimalization of staff changes, uncluttered treatment areas, acoustically quiet environments, etc.

In the early post-acute phase, whilst orientation is poor, memory is thrown back upon procedural learning rather than the more explicit systems. If not prevented, errors become established that are not open to correction using cognitively based interventions. In particular, this makes the child prone to the development of maladaptive behaviours and requires preventive management emphasizing errorless learning approaches. This stage may continue for months if the child's recovery is slow.

While cognitive difficulties persist (orientation, attention, and memory in particular), the use of contingency management will prove less effective than antecedent control techniques in the treatment of behavioural excess or deficit.

Focal impairments to the frontal lobes in the teenage years generally lead to one of two behavioural phenotypes manifesting as:

- irritability, anxiety, obsessionality, false euphoria, over sexualized behaviour, poor social responses, increased risk-taking behaviour (though unimpaired social or moral reasoning), and poor self-monitoring. The fundamental problem appears to be one of failure to inhibit responses.

- apathy, poor initiation, failure to maintain activity, and pseudo-depression.

Both groups benefit from a structured approach with a regular timetable, clear rules, and contingencies. Behavioural approaches are helpful. Management based upon reasoning, dependent as it is upon the ability to self-reflect, is seldom effective. It is preferable to create overlearned responses to simple everyday situations that utilize the tendency towards stimulus-driven behaviour. This approach is of proven effectiveness. Such an approach will allow basic anger management techniques to be trained with well-oriented children.

The psychosocial environment of the child during recovery is an important additional source of behavioural difficulties. Parental reactions to the child's injury may lead to overprotection, overindulgence, loss of confidence, guilt, anger, stress, anxiety or depression, all of which can have an effect upon behaviour. Social factors of peer rejection, loss of status (academic or sporting), and social isolation may add to this.

Neuropsychiatric disorders appearing after TBI include the following.

- *Disorders of thought and perception.* Their manifestations are aggression, agitation, conduct disorders, or disinhibition. Their neuropathology is still unclear. Paediatric neuropsychiatric evaluation is required.

- *Disorders of mood and affect.* The head-injured child is vulnerable to emotional and psychiatric disorders (double the vulnerability of peers at 2 years post-injury) emerging as lowered self-esteem and depression linked to poor adaptive skills. Daily variation is common and can be investigated by a paediatric neuropsychologist through standard behavioural recording. However, one should be aware that problems might arise from cyclical neuropsychiatric disturbance as well as environmental stimuli or contingencies.

4.1.6 Rehabilitation settings

The majority of children with an acquired brain injury will have early post-acute rehabilitation provided within their local community following discharge from hospital. A planning conference to coordinate professional inputs and resources will generally take place within 1 or 2 weeks of discharge. A key worker is generally identified to act as a case manager, though this should not be confused with head injury case management services, usually appointed following the settlement of a claim for compensation. Though postacute head injury teams exist in some health authorities, they seldom consist of staff dedicated to this role. In consequence, the head-injured child has to compete for resources with other children. Alternatively, some areas will use staff from adult head injury services to provide services. This is problematic in that staff may have little experience or knowledge of childhood disorders, child development, or paediatric interventions.

A small number of children, usually with more severe and complex needs, will be catered for within specialist paediatric head injury facilities.

The role of the paediatric neuropsychologist in rehabilitation is to provide a framework within which other therapeutic interventions may take place. He or she should ensure that the cognitive demands placed upon the child are within their present level of cognitive functioning, while bearing in mind that this will alter as the process of recovery takes place.

4.1.7 Education

Unlike adults who may become unemployed following head injury, there is a statutory duty to educate all children whatever their degree of disability. This means that the educational system has a central role to play in the rehabilitation of head-injured children, as schools will be the principal environments to which the children will return. Advice given to teachers should be precisely geared to the individual child rather than general based upon a particular syndrome or condition. The latter will reflect too great a variability across children to allow the teacher to formulate specific educational programmes for the child.

Unfortunately, few local education authorities have specific policies on providing for the educational needs of brain-injured children. The situation in the UK has several disadvantages.

- The system established in England and Wales (with minor variations in Scotland and Northern Ireland) for the drawing up of statements of special educational needs embodies a view of static educational needs. This model is unsuited to the situation of head-injured children who have (at least during the early postacute phase and not uncommonly during later 'spurts' in recovery) frequently changing needs. Though the review system for such statements can be utilized to accommodate changes, the time period for implementing changes can be protracted.

- There is a danger that the recovering child will have a placement suited to their apparent level of cognitive functioning at the time of assessment, but increasingly inappropriate as recovery takes place.

- If physical needs are significant, placements may be offered based on the location of resources such as physio- and occupational therapy, nursing, etc., rather than based upon the appropriateness of educational environment.

The paediatric neuropsychologist must have a role as an advocate for the child in seeking appropriate provision.

4.1.8 Family needs

The early stages of postacute recovery are important ones in beginning the process of adjustment to the changed circumstances of the child. Adjustment is an essential step to the success of rehabilitation.

- Parents may become 'stuck' and become focused upon the physical aspects of recovery (will she be able to walk?) when cognitive recovery may be the more important determinant of successful rehabilitation.

- Information is critical to parental adjustment and the paediatric neuropsychologist is best placed within a multidisciplinary team to objectively outline (after comprehensive assessment) what has happened to their child's brain and what the cognitive prognosis is likely to be.

- The paediatric neuropsychologist has an importance similar to that of other key figures in the child's world, e.g. teachers, classmates, friends on the social side, social workers, educational psychologists, and solicitors.

- Siblings frequently get left out whilst the focus is on the injured child. They too will suffer shock and sometimes guilt at their resentment of the attention being given to their brother or sister. Embarrassment at the reaction of friends can lead to anger and frustration. Counselling and play therapy can assist adjustment.

4.2 Brain tumours

Sixty per cent are astrocytomas or gliomas; 20–25% primitive neuroectodermal tumours. Neuropsychological sequelae include problems with:

- fine-motor coordination;
- perceptual–motor skills;
- visual constructional abilities;
- memory.

In turn these lead to decrements in IQ. The functional consequences are in academic and vocational skills. Memory problems can affect daily living and self-care.

However, these sequelae seem principally to be a consequence of radio- and, to a lesser degree, chemotherapy treatments, not of surgery. Age at diagnosis and treatment and the type and location of the tumour are also important factors in long-term outcome.

Academic difficulties should be anticipated and teachers informed in order to adjust expectations in the classroom. Neuropsychologists have a role as information providers and interpreters and in the monitoring of post-treatment changes.

4.3 **Epilepsy**

The distribution of IQ in children with epilepsy is close to that of the general population. However, some epilepsy syndromes are associated with specific cognitive sequelae.

- Moderate to severe learning difficulties are observed in the majority of children with Lennox–Gastaut and West's syndrome.

- There are many other abnormalities of brain development or acquired disorders that include epilepsy in their symptomatology. These would include: developmental disorders, e.g. tuberous sclerosis and Angelman syndrome; CNS infections; acquired brain injuries; metabolic disorders; Rett syndrome; and neurofibromatosis.

- Epilepsy is a co-symptom of severe learning difficulties (9–31%), autism (11–35%), and cerebral palsy (18–35%).

Other factors associated with cognitive or functional problems in epilepsy are the following.

- Intellectual decline in epilepsy (not associated with other underlying conditions) is usually associated with antiepileptic drug (AED) toxicity.

- A history of status epilepticus is associated with decreased functioning.

- Children with early onset to their seizure disorder, poor response to anticonvulsant medication, and mixed seizure types tend to perform more poorly on IQ measures. However, these factors could disguise a common factor in the existence of pre-existing neurological impairments prior to seizure onset.

- Specific impairments likely to be associated with epilepsy are poor sustained attention and reduced short-term memory performance. A confounding factor again is AED toxicity.

- Subclinical electrical activity of even brief duration can produce educational difficulties referred to as transitory cognitive impairments (TCI). The mediating factor here is most probably disruption to attention.

- Some studies suggest that left temporal lobe epilepsy is associated with decreased performance on verbal memory tasks and right temporal lobe epilepsy related to reduced visual memory function. Others suggest bilateral memory impairments.

- Hippocampal damage from frequent seizures is associated with decreased new learning.

Despite a near-normal distribution in IQ, children with epilepsy are more at risk of educational underachievement. This is not yet understood, but is *not* associated with seizure type, duration, severity, or AED used in treatment. Self-esteem and emotional variables such as locus of control appear important.

Behavioural and psychiatric problems are also more prevalent in children with epilepsy. There is no specific symptomatology. Difficulties arise from a combination of neurological (brain damage, seizure activity in areas of brain associated with affective functioning, variations in neurotransmitter function) and psychosocial factors (lowered self-esteem, externalized locus of control, stigmatization, lowered expectations, reactions to parental overprotection, and lack of independence). The degree of neuropsychological dysfunction predicts behavioural and neuropsychiatric dysfunction, i.e. brain dysfunction not epilepsy is causative. AED treatment is also a factor with phenobarbitone associated with the most difficulties and carbamazepine and sodium valproate with the least, but dosage and multiple drug therapy are also important factors. It is important to include assessment and treatment of affective and behavioural functioning in management.

The paediatric neuropsychologist's role is as part of a multidisciplinary approach addressing medical treatment, educational management, and emotional and social adjustment—specifically, the monitoring of cognitive and behavioural change and the provision of information and management advice to the child, his/her parents, and teachers.

4.4 Hydrocephalus

Hydrocephalus is a secondary condition arising from a number of primary disorders. It is the primary disorder that is the dominant factor in outcome. It is associated in all aetiological groups with:

- gross and fine motor problems and visuomotor and spatial difficulties;
- greater impairment to language content than to structure (particularly in children with shunts);
- list-learning problems—results in regard to other aspects of memory are unclear other than that children with shunted hydrocephalus perform more poorly than other groups.
- problems with focused attention;
- deficits in executive skills where children with shunted hydrocephalus require an increased number of trials to reach the correct answers in problem-solving tasks;
- behavioural difficulties—children with shunted hydrocephalus have higher rates of behaviour disorder than those without.

Functional difficulties are apparent in school work (associated with visuospatial, executive, and learning problems) and everyday living (language, attention, and behaviour) The paediatric neuropsychologist's role is in the interpretation of cognitive and behavioural findings and in the provision of information and management advice appropriate to the needs of the referred child.

4.5 Meningitis

This is an infectious disease involving inflammation of the meningeal membrane with either a viral or bacterial cause. The latter is more likely to lead to disability. Of children with early childhood bacterial meningitis, 40% suffer additional acute neurological problems (sensory impairments, hydrocephalus, seizures, etc.), but only 20% of those who survive have persistent difficulties. In addition, many have cognitive, behavioural, and educational sequelae. The pattern of these is diverse covering motor, perceptual, language, attentional, and executive skills. Overall IQ is probably little affected.

The pattern and extent of deficits is thought to be dependent upon the age at the time of infection, time since insult, and developmental stage at time of assessment.

- Age at the time of infection is significant in that that pre-infection learning is retained, but new learning is significantly impaired.
- During the time following the insult compensation may have taken place, which will in turn influence the deficit observed.
- The developmental stage at time of assessment determines the expectations of the child's abilities at that stage and thus helps determine the extent of the deficits.

Initially, gross motor problems dominate; subsequently fine motor problems. Perceptual and language difficulties occur during the primary years, while, in the secondary phase, impairments to higher-order language and executive skills are most frequently reported.

Once again, the picture is of a multifactorial process affecting outcome with psychosocial and environmental issues important contributory factors. This would suggest that rehabilitative efforts could have significant benefits in this condition. The paediatric neuropsychologist's role is to inform parents and educators of the implications of observed deficits and to formulate suitable management approaches to behaviour and adaptive learning. The changing pattern of deficits suggests the need for neuropsychological oversight throughout childhood.

4.6 Metabolic and neurodegenerative disorders

These disorders arise from built-in errors of metabolism leading to a build-up of neuro-toxins and consequent neurodegeneration. Cognitive deterioration is often difficult to detect in children due to the active interaction between normal development and the degenerative process. The earlier the onset, the more difficult this becomes with the lack of a clear premorbid period of 'normal' development. Decline in IQ can be misleading as it may represent a failure to maintain a rate of intellectual growth in keeping with one's peers, a period of 'plateaued development', or a 'real' loss of skills.

Initial identification of any decline should be by developmental history taking and educational reports (nursery, primary, and secondary) combined with cognitive assessment. Monitoring should be by periodic assessments combined with educational reports specifically asking if the child is keeping up with peers or has lost skills.

- Lost skills should be identified to ensure that their absence is not solely situation-specific or that they have not been subsumed into more complex behaviours.
- Educationalists may fear that a child is declining when they may simply not be keeping up with their peers—thus there is no absolute decline, only a relative one. Comparison of raw scores rather than scaled scores on normative tests will reveal the true state of affairs.

The pattern of decline observed is dependent on the periods between assessments. The shorter the period, the more obvious the continuing development of the child alongside the degenerative process. Longer periods give greater emphasis to the decline.

Childhood neurodegenerative diseases largely affect white rather than grey matter and consequently are enhanced by the factor of age at onset as it relates to the degree of both myelination and intellectual development that has already taken place. The specific neuropsychological and consequent functional sequelae of these multitudinous disorders are dependent upon the precise condition (see Shapiro and Balthazor 2000).

The paediatric neuropsychologist has a central role in the interpretation of this information, the provision of feedback to medical colleagues, and the support of parents and teachers coming to terms with a progressive intellectual decline in childhood.

4.7 Neurofibromatosis

Type one neurofibromatosis has known cognitive and behavioural sequelae; type two does not. The sequelae associated with type one are as follows.

◆ Mean IQ is lowered and mild-to-moderate learning difficulties are slightly more common than in the general population. About half of patients have reduced academic attainments.

◆ The range of neuropsychological impairments observed in different individuals includes attention deficits, speech and language difficulties, difficulties in visuospatial processing, and motor coordination problems. There is no specific neuropsychological profile.

◆ The increased presence of tumours (15–50% of cases) and their treatment may lead to further cognitive sequelae.

Educational provision should be matched to the individual's difficulties. There are no specialist approaches specific to neurofibromatosis type one or two. The extent of emotional problems appears to be related to the degree of physical disfigurement. Behavioural difficulties centre around attention deficits, hyperactivity, impulsivity, and distractability.

5 Neurodevelopmental disorders

5.1 Attention deficit hyperactivity disorders (ADHDs)

These are characterized by a triad of inattention, overactivity, and impulsivity. They can occur with or without 'hard' neurological signs. Symptoms persist into adolescence in two out of three cases. The problems associated with ADHD include:

◆ poor educational attainments;

◆ peer/friendship difficulties;

◆ conflict with parents;

◆ (in adolescence) engagement in high-risk behaviours—one in three has conduct disorder in adolescence.

These problems can result in reduced self-esteem and sometimes depression. The prognosis is poorer in the presence of a comorbid conduct disorder.

In carefully selected children stimulant medication can show significant benefits on attentional tasks and in everyday functioning. A multiple treatment approach would include:

- information provision;
- use of stimulant medication;
- family and school management advice;
- self-instructional training;
- (in some cases) dietary monitoring.

This approach improves long-term treatment efficacy.

The child clinical or paediatric neuropsychologist's role is the following.

- Diagnosis of children with the disorder. In particular, diagnosis must be based on the persistence of symptoms across settings. ADHDs are usually identified through use of structured questionnaires such as the Achenbach Child Behaviour Checklists (Achenbach 1991).
- On-going monitoring of cognitive and behavioural changes using measures of focused and sustained attention and behavioural observation schedules such as those by Conners (1996).
- Provision of information, behavioural management advice, and self-control training to be used as adjunctive therapy with medication.

5.2 Specific learning difficulties (SpLDs)

This term is applied by educators to a number of 'disorders' (reading, writing, arithmetic, and spelling) having some similarities in symptomatology to conditions seen in persons with an acquired brain injury. The nature of the underlying pathologies and their relationships to observed neuropsychological impairments continue to be investigated (Hynd and Hiemenz 1997), but these are considered to be 'necessary, but not sufficient' elements for the manifestation of the condition with significant contributions from environmental and pedagogical factors.

There is a range of proven educational approaches in use by specialist teachers working in this field selected according to a child's particular pattern of strengths and weaknesses. The paediatric neuropsychologist would be best advised to seek referral to such local services.

5.3 Nonverbal learning disability (NVLD)

NVLD is a postulated condition of multiple aetiology including neuropathological disorders. Its characteristics are:

- bilateral tactile–perceptual difficulties particularly affecting the left side;
- impaired visual recognition and discrimination;
- problems with visuospatial organization;

♦ bilateral psychomotor coordination difficulties, again more marked on the left side;

♦ problems with managing novel information.

Auditory–verbal processing is preserved as are simple motor skills, auditory perception, rote learning, selective and sustained attention for auditory–verbal information, basic expressive and receptive language, reading, and spelling. Rourke (1989) outlines a wide range of secondary and tertiary neuropsychological, academic, and socioemotional deficits arising from NVLD.

The model is specifically a cognitive–developmental one linking neurological impairment to neuropsychological deficit by way of the 'white-matter hypothesis' that emphasizes the need for integrity of white matter function for normal child development. Rourke reasons that in the right hemisphere white matter is important for development and maintenance of function; in the left hemisphere it is only important for development. Consequently, the right hemisphere is seen as particularly reliant upon cerebral integrity in order to continue functioning effectively. As one would expect from a cognitive–developmental model, the implication is that the degree of white matter damage, the nature of the lesion, and the developmental stage at the time of cerebral insult determine symptom severity.

There is no proven treatment for the condition. Management is through utilization of language-based strengths at home and in school. Visually based information needs to be supported with verbal description. Large tasks need to be broken down into smaller, more easily assimilated steps. Abstract material requires discussion and verbal labelling of concepts. There is limited evaluation of the success of such interventions.

Selective references

Achenbach, T. (1991). *Integrative guide for the 1991 Child Behaviour Checklist/4–18, YSR and TRF profiles*. University of Vermont Department of Psychiatry, Burlington, Vermont.

Anderson, V., Northam, E., Hendy, J., and Wrennall, J. (2001). *Developmental neuropsychology: a clinical approach*. Psychology Press, Hove, East Sussex.

Conners, C. (1996). *Conners Abbreviated Symptom Questionnaire*. Psychological Assessment Resources, Odessa, Florida.

Dixon, R.A. and Bäckman, L. (1999). Principles of compensation in neurorehabilitation. In *Cognitive rehabilitation* (ed. D.T. Stuss, G. Winocur, and I.H. Robertson), pp. 59–72. Cambridge University Press, Cambridge.

Ewing-Cobbs, L., Levin, H.S., Fletcher, J.M., Miner, M.E., and Eisenberg, H.M. (1990). The Children's Orientation and Amnesia Test: relationship to severity of acute head injury and to recovery of memory. *Neurosurgery* 27, 683–91.

Hynd, G.W. and Hiemenz, J.R. (1997). Dyslexia and gyral morphology variation. In *Dyslexia: biology, cognition and intervention* (ed. C. Hulme and M. Snowling), pp. 38–58. Whurr Publishers Ltd, London.

Jennett, B. and Teasdale, G. (1981). *The management of head injuries*. F.A. Davis and Co., Philadelphia.

Johnson, D. and Rose, D. (1996). *Brain injury in childhood—is younger better?*, Disability Awareness No. 13. Disability Management Research Group, Astley Ainslie Hospital, Edinburgh.

Rourke, B.P. (1989). *Nonverbal learning disabilities*. Guilford Press, New York.

Shapiro, E. and Balthazor, M. (2000). Metabolic and neurodegenerative disorders. In *Pediatric neuropsychology: research, theory and practice* (ed. K.O. Yeates, M.D. Ris, and H.G. Taylor), pp. 171–205. Guilford Press, New York.

Simpson, D.A., Cockington, R.A., Hanieh, A., Raftos, J., and Reilly, P.L. (1991). Head injuries in infants and young children: the value of a paediatric coma scale. *Child's Nerv. Syst.* 7, 183–90.

Temple. C. (1997). *Developmental Cognitive Neuropsychology*. Psychology Press, Hove, East Sussex.

World Health Organisation (WHO) (1980). International classification of impairments, disabilities and handicaps. WHO, Geneva.

Yeates, K.O., Ris, M.D., and Taylor H.G. (eds.) (2000). *Pediatric neuropsychology: research, theory and practice*. Guilford Press, New York.

Part 5

Neuropharmacology

Chapter 25

Neuropsychopharmacology

Chris M. Bradshaw

1 Introduction

An understanding of the principles of neuropsychopharmacology is important for the
practising clinical neuropsychologist because a large proportion of neurological and psychiatric patients receive medication that can affect higher functions, both for good and
for ill.

Improved understanding of the cellular mechanisms underlying the therapeutic and
adverse effects of psychoactive drugs has shed considerable light on the neural bases of
normal and abnormal neuropsychological function. As yet, however, there are no validated pharmacological treatments for specific neuropsychological dysfunctions (dysm-
nesias, dysphasias, etc.). Rational pharmacotherapy (i.e treatment based on the actions of
drugs on known pathological processes) exists for some neurological conditions (e.g.
Parkinson's disease, some forms of epilepsy), but the utility of nearly all the drugs that are
currently used to treat 'functional' psychiatric disorders has been discovered by fortui-
tous clinical observation.

Establishing the efficacy of drug treatment in psychiatry poses significant problems due
to the complex and variable symptatology and time-courses of the disorders, imperfect
measuring instruments, and the frequently weak effects of the drugs in question, which
are often confounded by side effects (see Section 5). A readable critique of the design of
controlled clinical trials, their advantages and pitfalls, is provided by Harrison-Read and
Tyrer (2004).

2 Synaptic transmission in the central nervous system

2.1 General principles

Chemical synaptic transmission involves the following steps:

- *Precursor accumulation*. Precursors of transmitters are often amino-acids that are
  present in the circulating blood. They are actively transported into neurones by a
  membrane 'pump'.

- *Transmitter synthesis*. Precursor molecules are converted into transmitter molecules
  by a sequence of enzyme-catalysed reactions.

- *Storage*. Transmitter molecules may be retained within vesicles in presynaptic terminals by a membrane 'pump'.

- *Release.* Ejection of transmitter molecules from the synaptic terminal is triggerred by the passage of an action potential along the axon, causing depolarization of the terminal membrane. Channels in the terminal membrane are opened, permitting influx of calcium ions, which cause the vesicles to discharge their contents into the synaptic cleft.

- *Receptor stimulation.* The binding of a transmitter molecule to a receptor initiates a sequence of events culmination in a change in the electrical excitability of the post-synaptic cell (see Section 2.3).

- *Inactivation.* Transmitter molecules may be removed from their site of action by the action of enzymes on the pre- and postsynaptic membranes, or by transport into presynaptic terminals (re-uptake). After re-uptake, transmitter molecules may be re-stored in vesicles or destroyed by enzymes.

2.2 **Neurotransmitters and neuromodulators**

2.2.1 Glutamate

Glutamate is an amino-acid that mediates excitatory transmission in many central path-ways. Corticofugal glutamatergic neurones are believed to play a key role in cognitive functions subserved by 'cortico-striatal loops'. Excessive release of glutamate may cause over-excitation of postsynaptic neurones, which may die as a consequence (*excitotoxicity*). This may account for neuronal loss in the area surrounding a cerebral infarct, and for neuronal loss in convulsive seizure disorders.

2.1.2 γ-Aminobutyric acid

γ-Aminobutyric acid (GABA) is the principal inhibitory amino-acid transmitter in supraspinal pathways. The inhibitory efferent pathways from the basal ganglia and the cerebellum are GABAergic, and GABA also mediates the inhibitory effects of intracortical neurones. Suppression of GABAergic transmission can lead to convulsions.

2.2.3 Acetylcholine

Acetylcholine is the transmitter at skeletal neuromuscular junctions, parasympathetic (and some sympathetic) effector junctions, and all autonomic ganglia. It mediates both excitatory and inhibitory effects in the central nervous system. It is synthesised from choline by the enzyme choline acetyltransferase. Synaptically released acetylcholine is metabolized by acetylcholinesterase located on pre-and postsynaptic membranes. Cholinergic interneurones oppose the influence of dopamine in the basal ganglia, and manipulation of cholinergic function is an important strategy in the management of Parkinson's disease and drug-induced parkinsonism (see below). Cholinergic neurones in the basal forebrain project to the hippocampus and neocortex; degeneration of these neurones is thought to underlie some of the cognitive deficits of Alzheimer's disease.

2.2.4 Dopamine

Dopamine is a catecholamine synthesised from the amino-acid tyrosine. Tyrosine hydroxylase converts tyrosine to L-DOPA, which is converted to dopamine by the action of aromatic amino-acid decarboxylase. Synaptically released dopamine is inactivated by re-uptake into presynaptic terminals followed by re-storage or degradation by mono-amine oxidase (MAO). The cell bodies of dopaminergic neurones reside in circumscribed nuclei in the brainstem, their unmyelinated fibres projecting to many parts of the neu-raxis. The three principal dopaminergic pathways are:

- the *nigrostriatal pathway* (substantia nigra → corpus striatum), whose degeneration underlies the pathophysiology of Parkinson's disease;
- the *mesolimbic/mesocortical pathway* (midbrain ventral tegmental area → limbic struc-tures and cerebral cortex), hyperfunction of which has been postulated to occur in schizophrenia;
- the *tuberoinfundibular pathway* (hypothalamus → pituitary stalk), which regulates the secretion of some adenohypophyseal hormones.

2.2.5 Noradrenaline (norepinephrine)

Noradrenaline is a catecholamine that is synthesised from tyrosine via the intermediate compounds L-DOPA and dopamine. Synaptically released noradrenaline is inactivated by re-uptake into terminals followed by re-storage or degradation by MAO. Noradrenaline is the transmitter at most sympathetic effector junctions. The cell bodies of central noradrenergic neurones reside in nuclei in the pons and medulla, their axons projecting to most parts of the neuraxis. Noradrenergic pathways include:

- the *dorsal noradrenergic bundle* (coeruleocortical pathway: locus coeruleus → neocor-tex and hippocampus);
- the *ventral noradrenergic bundle* (tegmental nuclei → hypothalamus);
- *descending noradrenergic pathways* (tegmental nuclei → spinal cord and medullary autonomic nuclei).

Central noradrenergic transmission may contribute to the 'fine tuning' of some higher functions (e.g. improving the signal/noise ratio in some sensory pathways) and the main-tenance of arousal. Central noradrenergic dysfunction may be involved in some anxiety states.

2.2.6 5-Hydroxytryptamine (5-HT, serotonin)

5-HT is an indolamine synthesised from tryptophan via the intermediate precursor 5-hydroxytryptophan. Synaptically released 5-HT is inactivated by re-uptake into termi-nals followed by re-storage or degradation by MAO. The cell bodies of 5-HTergic neu-rones reside in the raphe nuclei of the brainstem, their axons projecting to most parts of the neuraxis. 5-HTergic pathways include:

- ascending pathways from the dorsal and median raphe nuclei;
- descending raphe-spinal pathways.

The projections from the dorsal and median raphe nuclei show considerable overlap. However the median nucleus provides most of the 5-HTergic afferents to the hippocam-pus, while the dorsal nucleus provides most of the input to the striatum. 5-HTergic dys-function has been proposed as a pathophysiological factor in depressive illness, obsessive-compulsive disorder and anxiety disorders. There is evidence for 5-HTergic hypofunction in some impulse-control disorders.

2.2.7 Histamine

Histamine is a monoamine. It plays an important role in the control of acid secretion in the stomach. Its presence in the brain has been known for some time, but its neurotransmitter role has only recently been established. Histaminergic neurones in the tubero-mammillary nucleus of the hypothalamus project to the cerebral cortex. They are believed to play an important role in the maintenance of wakefulness.

2.2.9 Neuropeptides

Neuropeptides are large molecules, made up of sequences of amino-acids. Many 'families' of neuropeptides have been identified (e.g. hypothalamic hormone-releasing and release-inhibiting factors, tachykinins, opioid peptides). In some cases they are *co-localized* with 'classical' neurotransmitters, and act at specific receptors on pre- and postsynaptic membranes. One of the postulated roles of neuropeptides is to modulate the action of co-localized 'classical' transmitters. Neuropeptites have been implicated in pain transmission (substance P), anxiety (cholecystokinin) and the rewarding effects of drugs of abuse (enkephalin) (Hökfelt *et al.* 2000; Leonard 2004). The orexins, two peptides expressed by groups of neurones in the lateral and dorsomedial hypothalamus, have been implicated in arousal mechanisms and feeding. Orexinergic neurones of the lateral hypothalamus, which project to the ventral tegmental area (the origin of the mesolimbic/mesocortical dopaminergic pathway), may help to regulate the 'reward value' of both food and drug reinforcers (Harris and Aston-Jones 2006).

2.3 Receptors

There are two main receptor 'superfamilies', distinguished by the effector mechanisms to which they are coupled:

- *ionotropic (ion-channel-coupled) receptors*, in which the transmitter (or drug) molecule binds directly to a site on an ion channel and thereby regulates the movement of ions in or out of the postsynaptic cell;
- *metabotropic (G-protein-coupled) receptors*, in which binding of the transmitter or drug molecule initiates a cascade of events within the postsynaptic cell, culminating in a change in the permeability of the membrane to particular ionic species.

Ionotropic receptors mediate rapid changes in electrical excitability, whereas metabotropic receptors mediate slower responses. In the case of metabotropic receptors, attachment of the transmitter molecule to the binding site alters the state of a protein in the postsynaptic membrane ('G-protein'), which in turn alters the activity of an enzyme. Two principal enzymes are associated with metabotropic receptors:

- *adenylyl cyclase*, which converts adenosine triphosphate (ATP) to cyclic adenosine monophosphate (cyclic AMP);
- *phospholipase-C*, which converts phosphatidylinositol to inositol trisphosphate and diacylglycerol.

The products of these reactions are called *second messengers* (in distinction from the neurotransmitter, the 'first messenger'); they activate a protein kinase that regulates ion channel opening. A transmitter may act at many types of receptor coupled to different effector mechanisms, giving scope for a great variety of postsynaptic effects (Table 25.1).

2.4 Regulation of neurotransmitter function

Many neurones regulate their own function via *autoreceptors* (receptors on the membrane of a neurone which respond to that neurone's own transmitters). *Somatodendritic autoreceptors* reside on the cell bodies and dendrites, and *terminal autoreceptors* on the

Table 25.1 The major central nervous system transmitters and some of their receptors

Transmitter	Receptor	Type[a]	Effector[b]	Function
Glutamate	AMPA	IR	Na^+/K^+ channels	postsynaptic excitation
	Kainate	IR	Na^+/K^+ channels	postsynaptic excitation
	NMDA	IR	$Ca^{2+}/Na^+/K^+$ channels	postsynaptic excitation
	mGlu group I	MR	PL (↑)	postsynaptic excitation
	mGlu groups II, III	MR	AC (↓)	postsynaptic excitation
GABA	$GABA_A$	IR	Cl^- channel	postsynaptic inhibition
	$GABA_B$	MR	?	postsynaptic inhibition
Acetylcholine	Nicotinic	IR	$Ca^{2+}/Na^+/K^+$ channels	postsynaptic excitation
	muscarinic M_1	MR	PL (↑)	postsynaptic excitation
	muscarinic M_2	MR	AC (↓)	postsynaptic excitation/inhibition (?)
	muscarinic M_3	MR	PL (↑)	postsynaptic excitation
	muscarinic M_4	MR	AC (↓)	postsynaptic excitation/inhibition (?)
Dopamine	D_1	MR	AC (↑)	postsynaptic inhibition (?)
	D_2	MR	AC (↓)	postsynaptic excitation/inhibition (?), somatodendritic autoreceptor
	D_3	MR	?	postsynaptic excitation/inhibition (?), somatodendritic autoreceptor
	D_4	MR	?	postsynaptic excitation/inhibition (?)
Noradrenaline	α_1-adrenoceptor	MR	PL (↑)	postsynaptic excitation
	α_2-adrenoceptor	MR	AC (↓), K^+/Ca^{2+} channels	somatodendritic autoreceptors
	β_1-adrenoceptor	MR	AC (↑)	postsynaptic inhibition
	β_2-adrenoceptor	MR	AC (↑)	non-neuronal (glial, vascular) responses

(continued)

Table 25.1 (*continued*) The major central nervous system transmitters and some of their receptors

Transmitter	Receptor	Type[a]	Effector[b]	Function
5-HT	5-HT_{1A}	MR	AC ($\downarrow$)	somatodendritic autoreceptor, postsynaptic inhibition (?)
	$5\text{-HT}_{1B/D}$	MR	AC ($\downarrow$)	terminal autoreceptor, postsynaptic inhibition (?)
	5-HT_{2A}	MR	PL ($\uparrow$)	postsynaptic excitation/inhibition (?)
	5-HT_{2C}	MR	PL ($\uparrow$)	postsynaptic excitation/inhibition (?)
	5-HT_3	IR	Na^+/K^+ channels	postsynaptic excitation
	5-HT_4	MR	AC ($\uparrow$)	postsynaptic excitation/inhibition (?)
	5-HT_5	MR	AC ($\downarrow$)	?
	5-HT_6	MR	AC ($\uparrow$)	?
	5-HT_7	MR	AC ($\uparrow$)	?

[a]*receptor types:* IR, ionotropic receptor; MR, metabotropic receptor.

[b]*effectors:* AC, adenylyl cyclase system; PL, phospholipase-C system.

$\uparrow$ and $\downarrow$ indicate stimulation or inhibition, respectively.

Note that the list is not exhaustive, and that the functions mediated by many of the receptors are poorly understood.

presynaptic terminals. Autoreceptors usually serve a negative feedback role, receptor stimulation resulting in suppression of neuronal activity.

Neurotransmitter function is also regulated by *receptor adaptation*. Excessive receptor stimulation leads to a decrease in the number of available receptors (down-regulation), with a consequent loss of sensitivity to the transmitter and other agonists (desensitization). Conversely, low levels of receptor stimulation (e.g. following atrophy of afferent fibres) result in homeostatic receptor proliferation (up-regulation), with consequent enhancement of sensitivity.

3 **Pharmacodynamic principles**

The attachment of transmitters and other drugs to receptor molecules is determined by the laws of reversible chemical reactions. The *affinity* of a drug (D) for a receptor (R) is defined by the ratio of the rate constants for the formation and dissolution of a drug–receptor complex (DR). In the absence of any complicating biological processes, the concentration of DR is hyperbolically related to the drug concentration:

$$[DR] = \frac{R_t \cdot [D]}{K_D \cdot [D]}$$

where R_t is the total number of receptors, and K_D, the equilibrium dissociation constant, is the reciprocal of the affinity. This *concentration-binding relation* has a sigmoidal form when concentration is plotted on a logarithmic scale (Fig. 25.1(a)). In a living system, the magnitude of the biological response evoked by an agonist is related to concentration of occupied receptors [DR]. However the nature of this relationship can be

highly complex. In addition to the affinity constant and the size of the receptor population, empirical dose-response relations depend upon a host of other factors, including
limitations on the response capacity of the effector (biological 'ceiling'), limtations on the
ability of the agonist to elicit a full response ('instrinsic activity'), and factors unrelated to
receptor, such as drug inactivation mechanisms (e.g. uptake and enzymatic degradation)
and biological 'barriers' that impede access of the drug molecules to the receptor sites.

Transmitters and drugs that stimulate receptors and evoke physiological responses are
referred to as *agonists*. *Antagonists* evoke no response of their own but prevent the action

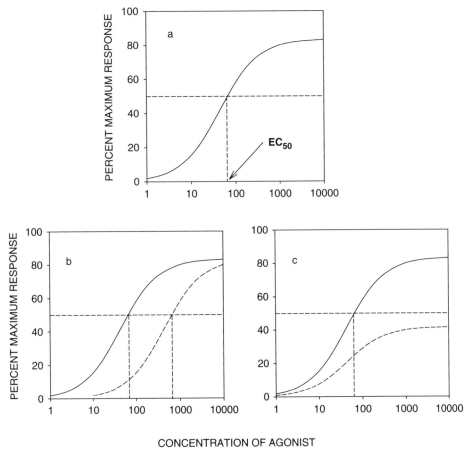

CONCENTRATION OF AGONIST

Fig. 25.1 Pharmacological concentration-response curves. (a) Relation between response
(expressed as a percentage of the maximum response) and concentration of an agonist (note
logarithmic scale). The concentration corresponding to the half-maximal response (EC_{50}) is indicated by the arrow. (b) Effect of a competitive antagonist. The concentration-response curve for
the agonist alone is shown by the continuous line, and the curve for the agonist in the presence
of a fixed concentration of the antagonist by the broken line. Note the parallel displacement of
the curve by the antagonist. (c) Effect of a non-competitive antagonist (conventions as in (b)).
Note that the antagonist depresses the maximum response without displacing the curve to the
right. (See text for details.)

of agonists. Different forms of drug antagonism are possible. In *competitive antagonism* the agonist and antagonist compete for access to the same receptor site. Competitive antagonism is *surmountable*, because increasing the concentration of the agonist results in displacement of antagonist molecules from the receptors. The dose-response curve is displaced to the right without any change in the maximum response (Fig. 25.1(b)). In *non-competitive antagonism* the antagonist impedes the production of the biological response but does not prevent the agonist from binding to its receptor. In this case, the maximum of the dose-response curve is reduced, but the curve is not displaced to the right (Fig. 25.1(c)). *Partial agonists* are agonists with low intrinsic activity.

4 Pharmacokinetic principles

The magnitude of a drug's effect is related to its concentration at its site of action. For centrally acting drugs, this is not directly measurable, and plasma concentration provides the only practical index of tissue concentration. This is satisfactory for drugs that gain easy access to the brain. However, many drugs enter the brain with difficulty, because of the blood-brain barrier (see Section 4.4).

4.1 Absorption, distribution and elimination

The single-dose kinetics of a drug describe the rise in plasma concentration as the drug is absorbed into the circulation, and the subsequent fall in concentration as the drug is distributed to the tissues and eliminated by metabolism and/or excretion (Fig. 25.2(a)). The rate of elimination of a drug relative to its concentration in the plasma is known as *clearance*. The clearance of most drugs is fairly constant over a wide range of concentrations; i.e. a constant fraction of the total amount of drug present in the plasma is eliminated per unit time (*first-order kinetics*). The *plasma half-life* ($t_{1/2}$) is the time taken for the plasma concentration to fall by 50%. Active metabolism of a drug may result in a short $t_{1/2}$. However this does not necessarily imply a short duration of action; for example, the benzodiazepine flurazepam has a $t_{1/2}$ of about 2 hours, but its effects are prolonged due to the production of an active metabolite, desalkylflurazepam, whose $t_{1/2}$ is about 30-100 hours.

The rate of absorption is influenced by the route of administration. The most common routes are:

◆ *intravenous (i.v.)* infusion, which results in a very rapid rise in concentration because the obstacles to absorption posed by lipid membranes in the gut and the capillaries are bypassed;

◆ *intramuscular (i.m.)* injection, which results in somewhat slower absorption into the circulation;

◆ *oral (per os, p.o.)* administration, which results in the slowest absorption, and is also less reliable than parenteral routes because the rate of absorption may be affected by such factors as the presence of food in the stomach. An orally administered drug, having been absorbed into the circulation, is first transported to the liver via the hepatic portal vein. Liver enzymes may destroy a substantial proportion of the absorbed drug (*first-pass metabolism*).

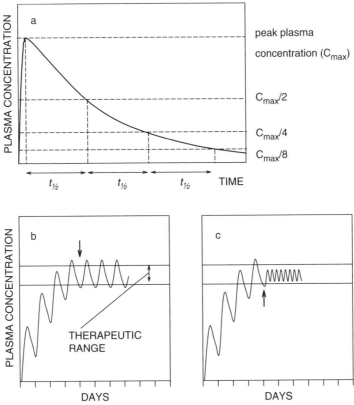

Fig. 25.2 (a) Single-dose kinetics. Ordinate, plasma concentration of the drug; abscissa, time measured from the time of administration. Note that plasma concentration falls to half its peak level in one half-life ($t_{1/2}$). A further half-life results in a further halving of plasma concentration, and so on. (b) Change in plasma concentration following repeated dosing at intervals of approximately $t_{1/2}$. The therapeutic range is indicated by the horizontal lines. Steady-state mean plasma concentration is attained after approximately 4 half-lives (indicated by the arrow). Note that the peaks and troughs of the steady-state concentration may fall outside the therapeutic range. (c) Administration of smaller doses more frequently (indicated by the arrow) results in smaller fluctuations in plasma concentration. (See text for details.)

4.2 Multiple dosing and steady-state concentration

To produce a sustained effect, a drug must be continuously present in the body in an adequate concentration. The purpose of repeated dosing is to maintain the concentration within the therapeutic range. If the drug concentration is not allowed to fall to zero between doses, mean plasma concentration rises progressively with repeated dosing, eventually approaching a steady state (Fig. 25.2(b)). However, in the case of a drug with a narrow therapeutic range, the inter-dose fluctuations in concentration may result in unacceptable side-effects soon after a dose and therapeutically insufficient concentrations before the next dose is administered. One solution to this problem is to give smaller doses more frequently (Fig. 25.2(c)); however this may place an unbearable burden of inconvenience on the patient. More satisfactory alternatives are available for some drugs in the form of sustained-release or depot preparations.

4.3 Sustained-release and depot preparation

Sustained-release preparations provide a gradual release of the drug from particles during their passage through the gut. They allow once-daily dosing rather than the three or four doses per day that may be needed with conventional oral preparations. Depot preparations provide a slow release from an oily vehicle administered by deep intramuscular injection; injections given at 2- or 4-week intervals may be used in place of multiple daily oral doses.

4.4 Blood-brain barrier (BBB)

This is a property of capillaries in the cerebral circulation that prevents passage of fat-insoluble molecules into the brain tissue.

4.5 Drug interactions

The presence of one drug in the body may alter the effect of another drug. There are two main types of interaction:

* *pharmacodynamic interactions*, e.g. drugs A and B competing for the same receptor site, as in competitive antagonism (see Section 3);
* *pharmacokinetic interactions*, e.g. drug A altering the activity of an enzyme that metabolizes drug B.

5 Therapeutic effects and side-effects

Most centrally acting drugs have multiple effects. However, different concentrations of a drug may be needed to exert its desired (therapeutic) effect and undesired effects (side-effects). The *therapeutic range* is the concentration range in which therapeutic effects are obtained without intolerable side-effects. The *therapeutic index* is the ratio of the maximum tolerated concentration to the minimum effective concentration.

5.1 Cognitive side-effects

Cognitive side-effects of psychoactive drugs are readily quantifiable in placebo-controlled single-dose laboratory experiments, but are difficult to pin down in clinical settings. Many psychiatric and neurological conditions are associated with cognitive dysfunction which may be mistaken for side-effects of the drug. Side-effects seen in single-dose studies may be poor predictors of side-effects in chronic treatment; some side-effects dissipate during continuous treatment, whereas other emerge only after months of regular treatment.

In most cases, cognitive side-effects of psychoactive drugs are not specific to particular classes of drug, although strongly sedative drugs and drugs that affect extrapyramidal functions have especially pronounced effects on test performance that requires fine movement or rapid responding. Memory test performance tends to be more vulnerable than linguistic or visuospatial performance. Although cognitive side-effects do complicate the interpretation of neuropsychometric data, it should be remembered that psychiatric symptoms (mood disturbance, psychosis) may distort test results to an even greater degree than the drug used to treat them.

5.2 Drug withdrawal

Adverse effects are sometimes seen in drug withdrawal. During continued use, *tolerance* may occur to the therapeutic and/or side-effects of the drug. This may arise from:

- a change in tissue sensitivity (*neuroadaptation, pharmacodynamic tolerance*); and/or
- a change in the rate of elimination of the drug (*pharmacokinetic tolerance*).

After drug withdrawal there may be a rebound of physiological processes that have been suppressed by the drug, and reversal of tolerance that may have developed during chronic treatment. An example of the former is the occurrence of seizures on rapid withdrawal of a drug with anticonvulsant properties. An example of the latter is the fatal overdose that may occur when an opiate addict takes his 'usual' dose after a period of abstinence.

6 Classes of centrally acting drugs

6.1 Antipsychotics

Antipsychotics (neuroleptics) are currently classified as (i) *conventional* or *typical* and (ii) *atypical*, on the basis of their pharmacological profiles.

6.1.1 Conventional antipsychotics

These include the chemical classes:

- *phenothiazines* (e.g. chlorpromazine, trifluperazine, thioridazine);
- *thiaxanthines* (e.g. flupenthixol, clopenthixol);
- *butyrophenones* (e.g. haloperidol, droperidol);
- *diphenylbutylpiperidines* (e.g. pimozide);
- *substituted benzamides* (e.g. sulpiride).

Mode of action Conventional antipsychotics are D_2 dopamine receptor antagonists. This fact is one of the cornerstones of the dopamine theory of schizophrenia (see Kapur *et al.* 2000). D_2 receptors mediate postsynaptic effects of dopamine in the three major dopaminergic pathways. Blockade of D_2 receptors in the neocortex and limbic structures (mesolimbic/mesocortical projection) probably underlies the therapeutic action of conventional antipsychotics, whereas blockade of D_2 receptors in the striatum (nigrastriatal projection) and pituitary stalk (tuberinfundibular pathway) is responsible for many of their side-effects (see below). These drugs differ widely in therapeutic potency. The average prescribed daily dose correlates highly with affinity for D_2 receptors (Seeman *et al.* 1976).

Receptor cloning techniques have revealed a 'family' of D_2-like receptors (D_2, D_3, D_4) with different regional distributions. D_3 and D_4 receptors are more abundant in the limbic system and neocortex than in the striatum. Conventional antipsychotics have somewhat higher affinity for D_2 than for D_3 and D_4 receptors. At therapeutic doses, conventional antipsychotics occupy 65-80% of D_2 receptors (Kapur *et al.* 2000).

Therapeutic uses Conventional antipsychotics are effective in managing acute psychotic episodes and as maintenance therapy for relapse prevention in chronic schizophrenia. They are better able to ameliorate positive psychotic symptoms (hallucinations, delusions) than negative symptoms (avolition, anhedonia, poverty of thought). They are also used to suppress manic excitement, and (in combination with antidepressants) to treat psychotic depression.

Pharmacokinetics Conventional antipsychotics are well absorbed following oral or parenteral administration, peak plasma concentration being attained 1-4 hours after oral administration. The $t_{1/2}$ of most typical antipsychotics is between 10 and 30 hours. They undergo first-pass metabolism. Hepatic metabolism of some drugs (e.g. chlorpromazine) increases during chronic treatment (*enzyme induction*), resulting in falling plasma concentration. Treatment with depot preparations may require months to attain steady-state plasma levels, and the drug may be detected months after discontinuation.

Side-effects Conventional antipsychotics, particularly high-potency butyrophenones, are liable to induce extrapyramidal side-effects (EPSs: akathisia, dystonia and 'parkinsonian' symptoms – rigidity, bradykinesia and tremor). EPSs probably arise from dopamine receptor blockade in the striatum. They are treated by co-administration of centrally-acting anticholinergic drugs (e.g. benztropine), which may correct the imbalance of dopaminergic and cholinergic influences on striatal function occasioned by D_2 receptor blockade. Phenothiazines have some anticholinergic action and are therefore less liable to induce EPSs than butyrophenones. About 10% of patients undergoing chronic treatment with conventional antipsychotics experience a delayed side-effect, *tardive dyskinesia* (involuntary orofacial movements and choreoathetoid movements of the extremities). Patients suffering from Lewy-body dementia show greatly enhanced sensitivity to the EPS-inducing effects of antipsychotics (Ballard *et al.* 1998).

Single acute doses of conventional antipsychotics reduce vigilance and impair psychomotor performance. In patients undergoing chronic treatment, it is difficult to disentangle the effects of the drug from the effects of the illness. Cognitive performance may actually improve as a result of antipsychotic medication, relative to the impairment seen in the unmedicated state (King and Waddington, 2004).

These drugs increase prolactin secretion due to D_2 receptor antagonism in the tuberoinfundibular system. In sensitive males this may cause impotence and galactorrhoea.

A rare, idiosyncratic, life-threatening side-effect is the *neuroleptic malignant syndrome*, characterized by fever, muscular rigidity, autonomic instability and coma.

6.1.2 Atypical antipsychotics

These include clozapine, risperidone, quetiapine, olanzapine, amisulpiride, aripiprazole and sertindole.

Mode of action These drugs have lower affinity for D_2 receptors than conventional antipsychotics. Clozapine has high affinity for many receptors (D_3 and D_4 receptors, 5-HT$_{2A}$,

5-HT$_{2C}$ and 5-HT$_{1A}$ receptors, muscarinic cholinoceptors, α_1- and α_2- adrenoceptors, H$_1$ histamine receptors), making it difficult to attribute its therapeutic efficacy to any one mechanism. Most other atypical antipsychotics share clozapine's high affinity for 5-HT$_2$ receptors. It has been suggested that dual antagonism of dopamine and 5-HT receptors may underlie the therapeutic effect of these drugs (Meltzer 1995). Some writers, however, argue that since affinity for dopamine receptors is a common feature of most, if not all, atypical antipsychotics, dopamine receptor blockade offers the most parsimonious account of all antipsychotic action (Kapur et al. 2000). One (controversial) explanation for the low incidence of EPSs induced by atypical antipsychotics (see below) is that these drugs may have a higher affinity for dopamine receptors in limbic structures than in the dorsal striatum ('limbic selectivity'), resulting in effective symptom control without concomitant disruption of extrapyramidal motor control.

Therapeutic uses Atypical antipsychotics are generally as effective as the conventional antipsychotics in treating positive psychotic symptoms. Good symptom control may be achieved in some patients whose illness is refractory to conventional antipsychotics. There is a growing body of evidence that negative schizophrenic symptoms respond more favourably to atypical antipsychotics, which are notoriously refractory to conventional antipsychotics (Burton, 2006).

Pharmacokinetics Clozapine, olanzapine and quetipine are rapidly absorbed from the gut and undergo first-pass metabolism. Their $t_{1/2}$ values are 7 (quetiapine), 15 (clozapine) and 30 (olanzapine) hours. Olanzapine can be given once daily, but twice-daily dosing is recommended for the others. Risperidone is now available as a depot injection preparation.

Side-effects Atypical antipsychotics are less liable to induce EPSs than conventional antipsychotics, possibly due to their relatively low affinity for D$_2$ receptors in the striatum (see above). Clozapine produces a potentially life-threatening blood disorder, agranulocytosis, in 1-2% of patients. Its use is therefore restricted to patients whose symptoms do not respond well to other antipsychotics, and regular blood counts are implemented during treatment. Other adverse effects of clozapine include sedation, nocturnal hypersalivation, and anticholinergic effects (blurred vision, urinary retention, constipation). Other atypical antipsychotics that have lower affinity for muscarinic cholinoceptors are less liable to induce anticholinergic side-effects. Olanzapine and risperidone have been associated with increased risk of stroke in elderly patients.

6.2 Antidepressants and mood-stabilizing drugs

Two major classes of antidepressants are:

• *monoamine oxidase inhibitors (MAOIs)*;

• *monoamine uptake inhibitors.*

   A few drugs with clinical antidepressant efficacy do not fit into either category (see Szabadi and Bradshaw (2004). The most widely prescribed mood stabilizer is lithium. Carbamazepine, valproate and lamotrigine also have mood-stabilizing properties (see Section 6.4).

6.2.1 MAOIs

Mode of action MAOIs block the enzyme MAO that normally destroys monoamine transmitters within presynaptic terminals. This increases the availability of the transmitter, and thus increases postsynaptic receptor stimulation. MAO exists in two forms, A and B. In the brain, noradrenaline and 5-HT are deaminated mainly by MAO-A, and dopamine by MAO-B. The traditional MAOIs, phenylzine, tranylcypromine and isocarboxasid, block both forms irreversibly. Clorgyline is selective for MAO-A and deprenyl for MAO-B. Deprenyl is not an effective antidepressant, suggesting that dopaminergic mechanisms do not play a major role in depressive illness. Unlike the aforementioned MAOIs, moclobemide is a reversible inhibitor of MAO-A (RIMA). Reversible MAO-A inhibition conveys some advantage in terms of safety (see 'Side-effects', this section).

When administered chronically, MAOIs induce downregulation of central 5-HT_2 and 5-HT_{1A} receptors and β-adrenoceptors. The functional significance of this is controversial. The overall effect of chronic MAOI treatment on monoaminergic transmission is mainly facilitatory, as receptor downregulation merely attenuates the increased postsynaptic receptor stimulation caused by increased transmitter availability (Blier *et al.* 1991).

Therapeutic uses MAOIs are seldom the first choice of antidepressant due to their potential for adverse effects (see below). They are useful in some anxiety disorders (panic disorder, post-traumatic disorder, social phobia) (Krishnan 1998).

Pharmacokinetics MAOIs are rapidly absorbed. They undergo extensive first-pass metabolism, and have short half-lives (Mallinger and Smith 1991).

Side-effects Orthostatic hypotension is a common-side effect. MAOIs potentiate the effects of sympathomimetic amines, including tyramine (a constituent of some foods, e.g. cheese) and amphetamines, and may induce hypertensive crises. RIMAs are safer in this respect, because high concentrations of sympathomimetic amines are able to displace the RIMA from the MAO molecule, allowing effective metabolism of the amines. MAOIs are never combined with selective serotonin reuptake inhibitors (SSRIs) as this can result in the potentially lethal *serotonin syndrome* (agitation, autonomic instability, progressing to convulsions and coma).

6.2.2 Monoamine uptake inhibitors

Mode of action Re-uptake into presynaptic terminals is the principal inactivation mechanism for monoamine transmitters. Uptake blockade therefore potentiates monoaminergic transmission. Chronic administration of uptake inhibitors results in downregulation of β-adrenoceptors, α_2-adrenoceptors, 5-HT_2 receptors and presynaptic 5-HT_{1A} receptors. These changes may reflect homeostatic adaptation to increased postsynaptic stimulation. Electrophysiological evidence indicates that monoaminergic transmission continues to be enhanced during chronic treatment with uptake inhibitors (Blier *et al.* 1991).

Monoamine uptake inhibitors are classified as:

- *tricyclic antidepressants (TCAs)* include imipramine, desipramine, amitriptyline dosulepin [previously, dothiepin], clomipramine, lofepramine, nortriptyline and trimipramine.

They inhibit both noradrenaline and 5-HT uptake, and block muscarinic cholinoceptors and α_1-adrenoceptors.

- *selective serotonin re-uptake inhibitors (SSRIs)* include fluoxetine, fluvoxamine, paroxetine, sertraline, citalopram and escitalopram. These drugs specifically block 5-HT uptake;
- *selective noradrenaline re-uptake inhibitors (NARIs)* include maprotiline and reboxetine;
- *serotonin-noradrenaline re-uptake inhibitors (SNRIs)* include venlafaxine and duloxetine. They block the uptake of both noradrenaline and 5-HT, but lack the anticholinergic and adrenolytic effects of TCAs.

Therapeutic uses TCAs are effective treatments for moderate/severe depressive illness. However, SSRIs, and more recently NARIs and SNRIs, have become more popular because they have fewer side-effects and are safer in overdose than TCAs. It should be recognised, however, that a favourable response to treatment is not the same as complete remission of symptoms. In double-blind trials, only about 40% of patients attain full remission of depressive symptoms (Trivedi *et al.* 2006), and the remission rate in general clinical practice may be even lower (Israel 2006). Augmentation treatment may be helpful in difficult cases; the use of lithium and thyroid hormone is supported by evidence from controlled clinical trials (DeBattista 2006).

TCAs and SSRIs are prescribed at low dose levels for chronic pain. SSRIs are prescribed for panic disorder, obsessive-compulsive disorder and impulse-control disorders (den Boer *et al.* 2000).

Pharmacokinetics TCAs are readily absorbed from the gut. They have relatively long half-lives (8-36 hours), allowing once-daily dosing. SSRIs are also eliminated slowly and are therefore suitable for once-daily dosing. Fluoxetine has a particularly long $t_{1/2}$ (85 hours) and its active metabolite even longer; it is recommended that 5 weeks be allowed for effective 'washout' before replacement with potentially interactive drugs (e.g. MAOIs). Venlafaxine and its active metabolite have shorter half-lives (4-10 hours); venlafaxine is usually given in divided doses or as an extended-release preparation.

Side-effects The affinity of TCAs for muscarinic cholinoceptors accounts for the cluster of side-effects (anticholinergic side-effects) brought about by suppression of parasympathetically mediated functions: dry mouth, constipation, blurred vision, urinary hesitancy/retention and erectile impotence. Tachycardia may reflect both anticholinergic action and peripheral noradrenaline uptake blockade, and postural hypotension may reflect β-adrenoceptor blockade. Increased sweating probably reflects central noradrenaline uptake blockade, as peripheral muscarinic receptor blockade would be expected to supress sweating. TCAs are notoriously sedative, which may reflect blockade of central α_1-adrenoceptors and H_1 histamine receptors. TCAs may cause cognitive dysfunction, especially memory impairment, which may reflect central cholinoceptor blockade.

SSRIs have fewer side-effects and a wider therapeutic range than SSRIs (Szabadi and Bradshaw 2004). In combination with MAOIs they can cause the serotonin syndrome (see above). Sexual dysfunction, a common complaint, is attributable to central 5-HT potentiation. Nausea is common, but usually disappears during continued use. Although early reports of increased risk of suicide in patients treated with SSRIs have not been substantiated (Warshaw and Keller, 1996), close monitoring of suicidal or hostile ideation is recommended, particularly at the beginning of treatment of after a dosage change.

NARIs and SNRIs have the expected side-effect profile of drugs that potentiate central and peripheral noradrenergic transmission, including mild hypertension and increased alertness.

6.2.3 Other antidepressant drugs

For a review of the pharmacology of the following compounds, see Szabadi and Bradshaw (2004).

- Mirtazepine is a presynaptic α_2-adrenoceptor antagonist. Blockade of these receptors is proposed to enhance central noradrenergic and 5-HTergic transmission. The drug has some sedative effect but lacks the antimuscarinic effects of TCAs.

- Trazodone is a weak 5-HT uptake inhibitor. It has antagonistic action at α_1- and α_2-adrenoceptors.

- Mianserin has some noradrenaline uptake inhibiting action and is a potent antagonist at α_2-adrenoceptors.

- Tryptophan, the precursor of 5-HT, is occasionally used as an adjunct to standard antidepressant therapy in refractory depresion.

6.2.4 Lithium

Mode of action Lithium is administered as a salt (lithium carbonate or lithium citrate), in which lithium exists as a monovalent cation. It can replace other cations in ion transport systems, allowing it to enter neurones and blood cells. It has numerous effects on monoaminergic transmission, including facilitation of tryptophan uptake, increased 5-HT and noradrenaline release, prevention of postsynaptic dopamine receptor supersensitivity, and inhibition of the cyclic AMP and phosphoinositol second messenger systems. The relationship between these effects and clinical mood stabilization is uncertain (Lenox and Manji 1998).

Therapeutic uses Lithium is the first-line treatment for manic-depressive illness. Because of the high relapse rate of this disorder, continued treatment over a period of years is recommended (see Goodwin and Young 2003). Lithium can augment the effects of TCAs and SSRIs in treating refractory depression. It has also been advocated in the management of impulsive agression (Kavoussi and Coccaro 1998).

Pharmacokinetics Lithium is rapidly absorbed from the gut and has a $t_{1/2}$ of about 20 hours. Because of its low therapeutic index (see below), divided doses are recommended in the early stages of treatment in order to avoid toxic side-effects.

Side-effects Lithium has a low therapeutic index, and regular monitoring of serum concentration is standard practice. Serum concentrations of 0.4–1.0 mEq l^{-1} are cited as the therapeutic range, but there is considerable variation between individuals. The signs of lithium toxicity are vomiting, diarrhoea, coarse tremor, ataxia, dysarthria, agitation or lassitude, and cognitive impairment. Untreated, lithium toxicity can progress to seizures and coma. Within the therapeutic range many patients experience side-effects, including memory problems, thirst, polyuria and fine tremor. There are few objective data about the cognitive side-effects of lithium, although in this writer's experience memory impairment and general reduction of mental acuity are not uncommon in patients treated with lithium.

6.3 Anxiolytics and hypnotics

Barbiturates are no longer used as anxiolytics or sedatives. Benzodiazepines, β-adrenoceptor antagonists and 5-HT$_{1A}$ receptor agonists are considered here. Antidepressants are also used to treat some anxiety disorders (see Section 6.2). Pregabalin is finding increasing popularity as an anxiolytic for medium- or long-term use (see Section 6.4).

6.3.1 Benzodiazepines

Mode of action Benzodiazepines bind to specific sites on the GABA$_A$ receptor-ionophore complex. GABA's inhibitory action is mediated by the opening of Cl$^-$ channels in postsynaptic membranes. Benzodiazepines have no effect of their own on the Cl$^-$ channel, but potentiate GABA's channel-opening action. This action of benzodiazepines differs from that of barbiturates which act directly on the ionophore to promote Cl$^-$ influx (Haefely 1990). The sites within the brain where benzodiazepines' GABA-potentiating action gives rise to their anxiolytic, sedative and anticonvulsant actions remain elusive. The GABA$_A$ receptor-ionophore complex comprises several 'subunits', different forms of which are differentially expressed in different brain regions. This offers the hope of developing benzodiazepine-like drugs that may target specific regions and thereby exert more selective therapeutic effects.

Therapeutic uses Benzodiazepines are effective in relieving the symptoms of generalized anxiety disorder. Their popularity waned in the 1980s when problems of dependence were first recognized. However more recent studies have generally failed to find compelling evidence for addiction to benzodiazepines in routine clinical use (Miller *et al.* 1995). In the UK they are recommended for prescription for limited periods only (2-4 weeks) in severe anxiety. In longer-term treatment their effectiveness is equalled by SSRIs, venlafaxine and pregabalin (Hidalgo *et al*, 2007). Benzodiazepines are also used as night-time sedatives, as anticonvulsants, in alcohol withdrawal (to reduce distress and prevent seizures), and as intravenous anaesthetics for minor surgery.

Pharmacokinetics A range of benzodiazepines is available with pharmacokinetic profiles to suit their different uses. An ideal hypnotic has a rapid onset of action, and should not produce a 'hangover' the following day. Temazepam, which is rapidly absorbed and has a $t_{1/2}$ of about 8 hours, is appropriate for this purpose. Patients with generalized anxiety disorder require sustained anxiolysis, such as that afforded by the long $t_{1/2}$ of diazepam. Diazepam's slow elimination is also advantageous in the management of withdrawal from alcohol or other benzodiazepines.

Side-effects Benzodiazepines are among the safest centrally acting drugs when taken in overdose. Their principal side-effect is sedation, resulting in impairment psychomotor performance and slow information processing. Higher doses induce dysarthria and ataxia. Antergrade amnesia may follow intravenous administration (Cooper 2004).

6.3.2 β-adrenoceptor antagonists

Mode of action These drugs (e.g. propranolol) block the effects of noradrenaline mediated by β-adrenoceptors, including tachycardia and tremor. By preventing these somatic manifestations of anxiety they may break the 'vicious cycle' of physiological and psychological responses that is postulated by some theories of anxiety (Granville-Grossman and Turner, 1966).

Therapeutic uses β-adrenoceptor antagonists suppress somatic anxiety symptoms (excluding sweating and xerostomia, which are cholinoceptor- and α-adrenoceptor-mediated). They are helpful in managing situational anxiety, for example in performing artists or public speakers. They are not useful for patients whose subjective anxiety is not accompanied by β-adrenoceptor-mediated somatic symptoms.

Pharmacokinetics Propranolol's $t_{1/2}$ is about 4 hours. A slow-release preparation is available.

Side-effects β-adrenoceptor blockade can induce hypotension and dizziness, and may provoke asthma attacks in susceptible individuals. Lethargy is the most common central side-effect.

6.3.3 5-HT$_{1A}$ receptor antagonists

Mode of action Buspirone (the only drug of this class available for prescription) is an antagonist at somatodendritic 5-HT$_{1A}$ autoreceptors and a partial agonist at postsynaptic 5-HT$_{1A}$ receptors; it also blocks dopamine receptors. Under conditions of 5-HTergic hypofunction (which is postulated to occur in anxiety states), buspirone's net effect is to promote 5-HTergic function.

Therapeutic uses Buspirone is mainly used in generalized anxiety disorder, although it may also have some antidepressant potential (den Boer *et al.* 2000). Unlike the benzodiazepines, the onset of buspirone's anxiolytic action is usually delayed by about two weeks.

Pharmacokinetics Buspirone undergoes first-pass metabolism and has a short $t_{1/2}$, but its major metabolite, 1-PP, is eliminated more slowly from the brain.

Side-effects Buspirone is much less sedative than the benzodiazepines. Adverse effects on cognition are seldom encountered. Nausea is the most commonly reported side-effect.

6.4 Antiepileptic drugs (anticonvulsants)

Mode of action The pathophysiological basis of all epileptic seizures is assumed to be the abnormal synchronous discharge of neurones. All antiepileptic drugs share the ability to suppress neuronal excitability, either by enhancing inhibitory neurotransmission or by suppressing excitatory transmission (see Table 25.2). For reviews of current developments in antiepileptic medication, see Löscher and Schmidt (2006) and Rogawski (2006).

Table 25.2 Commonly prescribed antiepileptic drugs and their putative mechanisms of action

Drug	Indication	Neuronal effect	Probable mechanism
First-line treatments			
carbamazepine	all seizures except absences	reduces excitation	inhibition of voltage-/use-dependent Na$^+$ channels
phenytoin	all seizures	reduces excitation	inhibition of voltage-/use-dependent Na$^+$ channels
valproate	all seizures	reduces excitation	inhibition of voltage-/use-dependent Na$^+$ channels
ethosuximide	absence seizures	reduces excitation	inhibition of voltage-dependent Ca^{2+} channels
lamotrigine	all seizures	reduces excitation	inhibition of voltage-/use-dependent Na$^+$ channels
topiramate	mainly partial seizures	reduces excitation	blockade of AMPA glutamate receptors, inhibition of Na$^+$ channels
oxcarbazepine	complex partial seizures with or without generalization	reduces excitation	inhibition of voltage-/use-dependent Na$^+$ channels
Adjunctive treatments			
gabapentin	partial seizures with or without generalization	reduces excitation	reduction of vesicular transmitter release
pregabalin	partial seizures with or without generalization	reduces excitation	reduction of vesicular transmitter release
levetiracetam	partial seizures with or without generalization	reduces excitation	reduction of vesicular transmitter release
phenobarbitone, primidone	generalized seizures	increase inhibition	facilitation of Cl$^-$ channel opening
tiagabine	complex partial seizures	increases inhibition	inhibits GABA uptake
vigabatrin	complex partial seizures	increases inhibition	blockade of GABA catabolism by GABA transaminase
zonisamide	complex partial seizures	reduces excitation	inhibition of voltage-/use-dependent Na$^+$ channels and Ca^{2+} channels
clobazam, clonazepam, midazolam	all seizures, status epilepticus	increase inhibition	potentiation of GABA-induced Cl$^-$ channel opening

Therapeutic uses Although monotherapy is always desirable, combination therapy is often necessary to produce adequate seizure control. The main first-line options are as follows:

♦ *carbamazepine* is effective in primary convulsive generalized seizures (tonic-clonic seizures – grand mal) and complex partial seizures, but not in primary absence seizures (petit mal).

- *phenytoin*, although effective in both convulsive and complex partial seizures, is seldom used as a first-line treatment because of its unfortunate pharmacokinetics and side-effect profile (see below);
- *valproate* is effective in most forms of epilepsy, and is widely prescribed for complex partial seizures (with and without secondary generalization) and absence epilepsy;
- *ethosuximide* is especially effective in absence seizures;
- *lamotrigine* and *topiramate* are used to treat generalized and complex partial seizures;
- *oxcarbazepine* is prescribed for complex partial seizures with or without secondary generalization.

The following drugs are more commonly prescribed as adjuncts to first-line drugs, or as alternative monotherapies when first-line treatments have failed to produce adequate seizure control:

- *gabapentin* and *pregabalin* are used in complex partial seizures with or without secondary generalization;
- *levetiracetam* is also used for treating complex partial seizures, occasionally as a monotherapy;
- the barbiturates *phenobarbitone* and *primidone* are rarely used except in highly refractory epilepsy, because of their cognitive side effects;
- *tiagabine, vigabatrin* and *zonisamide* are used as an adjunctive treatments in complex partial seizures;
- the benzodiazepines *clobazam* and *clonazepam* are sometimes used as adjunctive treatments in refractory epilepsy. *Diazepam,* administered intravenously or per rectum, is used to arrest status epilepticus; *midazolam* is available as a buccal preparation for this purpose.

In addition to their use in the treatment of epilepsy, carbamazepine and valproate are used as mood stabilizers and in the management of impulsive aggression. Pregabalin is used in the management of neuropathic pain, and as an anxiolytic. According to a recent meta-analysis, pregabalin may be more effective than benzodiazepines and SSRIs in generalized anxiety disorder (Hidalgo *et al.*, 2007).

Pharmacokinetics

- *Phenytoin* Unlike other antiepileptics, phenytoin's pharmacokinetics are non-linear (zero-order kinetics); i.e. metabolism of phenytoin is saturable at therapeutic concentrations, resulting in a decline in clearance and a rise in $t_{1/2}$ with increasing doses. Since small changes in dose can produce large changes in plasma concentration of phenytoin, regular monitoring of plasma concentration is essential;
- *Carbamazepine* is slowly absorbed following oral administration, and has a $t_{1/2}$ of about 10 hours;
- *Valproate* is rapidly absorbed and has a $t_{1/2}$ of about 15 hours;
- *Ethosuximide's* absorption is also rapid, but its $t_{1/2}$ is >30 hours;

With the exception of *tiagabine, pregabalin* and *gabapentin*, which have short half-lives (6 hours), most of the newer antiepileptics have $t_{1/2}$s >8 hours, and are suitable for twice-daily administration.

A major problem in prescribing anitepileptics is pharmacokinetic interaction (e.g. one drug altering the metabolism of another):

- Carbamazepine enhances the metabolism of (and therefore reduces plasma levels of) phenytoin and valproate;
- Valproate inhibits the metabolism of phenobarbitone and lamotrigine;
- Vigabatrin, levetiracetam and gabapentin are relatively free of pharmacokinetic interactions (Elwes and Binnie, 1996).

Side-effects

- *Phenytoin* has a low therapeutic index. Acute toxic effects include cerebellar and vestibular dysfunction (ataxia, intention tremor, nystagmus, imbalance). Hirsutism and thickening of the gums are troublesome long-term side-effects.
- *Carbamazepine* and *valproate* can induce liver dysfunction, which necessitates immediate discontinuation of treatment.

All antiepileptics can induce sedation and cognitive impairment. *Barbiturates, benzodiazepines, phenytoin* and *topiramate* are especially culpable. However, *valproate* and *carbamazepine* may also adversely affect cognition at therapeutic plasma concentrations (Kalvainen *et al.* 1996). *Lamotrigine, gabapentin* and *vigabatrin* may be less sedative than other antiepileptics. There have been reports of confusion, aggression and psychosis with *lamotrigine* and *vigabatrin*; *levetiracetam* may also induce irritability and aggression. Visual field defects have been associated with *vigabatrin*. Skin reactions are troublesome side-effects of *carbamazepine* and *lamotrigine*.

6.5 **Antiparkinsonian drugs**

The main symptoms of Parkinson's disease (PD), rigidity, bradykinesia and tremor, arise from atrophy of the brainstem catecholaminergic nuclei. Atrophy of the dopaminergic nigrostriatal pathway results in >90% loss of dopamine from the striatum in advanced PD. Conventional antipsychotics, which block D_2 dopamine receptors, induce EPSs which include some features of PD (drug-induced parkinsonism). Drug treatment of PD aims to:

1 restore dopaminergic function, or

2 restore the balance of dopaminergic/cholinergic function in the basal ganglia.

Treatment of drug-induced parkinsonism is discussed in Section 6.1.

6.5.1 L-DOPA and other 'dopamine-enhancing' drugs

Mode of action L-DOPA is converted into dopamine by L-aromatic amino-acid decarbolylase, an enzyme that is present in both 5-HTergic and catecholaminergic neurones. *Amantadine* releases dopamine and blocks dopamine uptake. *Bromocriptine, cabergoline, lisuride, pergolide, pramipexole, ropinirole* and *rotigotine* are postsynaptic D_2 receptor agonists.

Selegiline is an MAO-B inhibitor. All these drugs are assumed to promote dopaminergic function in the striatum.

Therapeutic uses L-DOPA is the most effective treatment for PD. Other 'dopamine-enhancing' drugs may be used as monotherapies in the early stages of the disease, and are often prescribed as adjuncts to L-DOPA therapy in more advanced disease. Dopamine-enhancing therapy is generally unsuccessful in counteracting drug-induced parkinsonism, presumably because high concentrations are needed to displace the antagonist from receptor sites. *Bromocriptine* is useful in treating hyperprolactinaemia (e.g. due to pituitary tumours), because prolactin secretion is regulated by the dopaminergic tuberoinfundibular pathway.

Pharmacokinetics L-DOPA is rapidly absorbed from the gut. However, more than 90% of the administered dose is metabolized by peripheral L-aromatic amino-acid decarboxylase. This problem is overcome by administering an inhibitor of this enzyme (e.g. carbidopa) together with L-DOPA. This prevents the conversion of L-DOPA to dopamine in the periphery, but, as carbidopa cannot cross the BBB, the therapeutically useful metabolism of L-DOPA in the brain is not affected.

Most of the dopamine receptor agonists have relatively short half-lives, and twice- or thrice-daily dosing is needed. *Rotigotine* is available as a slow-release skin patch preparation.

Side-effects Nausea is troublesome early in L-DOPA therapy. Dyskinesias constitute a more serious problem for about 50% of patients during prolonged treatment. Behavioural side-effects include mood disturbance (depression or mania), insomnia, delirium and, occasionally, psychosis. Hypersexuality may result from limbic/hypothalamic dopaminergic hyperfunction. The *on/off effect* refers to episodes of relapse into akinesia and rigidity which occur with increasing frequency during prolonged L-DOPA therapy. D_2 receptor agonists are useful in managing 'off' periods.

6.5.2 Anticholinergic drugs

Mode of action *Procyclidine, benztropine* and related drugs block muscarinic cholinoceptors. By suppressing cholinergic function in the striatum they may restore the dopaminergic/cholinergic balance that is disturbed by dopamine insufficiency in PD.

Therapeutic uses They are used in the initial stages of PD, and in cases where dopamine-enhancing treatments produce intolerable side-effects. They are routinely used to treat drug-induced parkinsonism and other EPSs (see Section 6.1).

Pharmacokinetics They are well absorbed following oral administration. Treatment is usually by divided doses; intramuscular injection is used for rapid relief of dystonias.

Side-effects Peripheral anticholinergic effects are common. Sedation may occur. In view of the putative role of the central cholinergic pathways in cognition, cognitive impairment might be expected; however, there do not appear to be any data on the long-term neuropsychological effects of these drugs. Dependence/abuse is a problem in some patients.

6.6 **Psychostimulants**

Mode of action *Cocaine* and *amphetamine* enhance catecholaminergic neurotransmission: cocaine inhibits uptake, whereas amphetamine releases catecholamines (it also has some uptake-blocking and MAO-inhibiting actions). Dopamine potentiation in the mesolimbic pathway probably underlies the euphoriant/reinforcing effects. Noradrenaline potentiation in the periphery accounts for many of the adverse effects. The precise mode of action of *methylphenidate, atomoxetine* and *modafinil* remains controversial, although potentiation of catecholaminergic function is probably involved. It has been proposed that modafinil enhances central noradrenergic function by facilitating transmission in the 'mesocoerulear' dopaminergic pathway from the ventral tegmental area to the locus coeruleus (Hou et al. 2005; Szabadi 2006).

Therapeutic uses Historically, amphetamine was used as an antidepressant and anorectic. Its alerting effect, exploited by pilots and radar operators in World War II, is the basis of its use in narcolepsy. This application has been largely supplanted by modafinil, which lacks amphetamine's propensity for abuse. Modafinil is also used to counteract fatigue in various conditions including PD, multiple sclerosis and fibromyalgia (US Modafinil in Narcolepsy Multicentre Study Group 2000). Amphetamine's use in attention-deficit hyperactivy disorder has been largely usurped by the less dependence-prone methylphenidate and atomoxetine.

Pharmacokinetics Amphetamine is rapidly absorbed from the gut, and has a $t_{1/2}$ of about 10 hours. Intravenous infusion produces a very rapid onset of action ('rush'). Cocaine is well absorbed via the nasal mucosa ('snorting') and alveolar surface (smoking). Inhalation of the aesosol of particles produced by heating cocaine base ('crack') produces a very rapid rise to peak plasma concentration, resulting in an intense subjective effect. The $t_{1/2}$ of cocaine is about one hour. Modafinil is readily absorbed from the gut, reaching a peak plasma concentration after about 2-4 hours. It is metabolized in the liver and its elimination half-life is about 15 hours.

Side effects The vigilance-enhancing effects of small doses of amphetamine represent the peak of a Yerkes-Dodson 'inverted-U' function; higher doses produce disorganization of cognitive performance and a disadvantageous speed/accuracy tradeoff. Psychotoxic effects of psychostimulants include anorexia, anxiety, hallucinations, paranoid ideation and behavioural stereotypies. Peripheral adverse effects, reflecting noradrenergic potentiation, include tachycardia, hypertension, tremor and pupil dilatation (mydriasis). *Tolerance* to the psychostimulants may be partly pharmacokinetic (facilitated elimination). *Sensitization* ('reverse tolerance') to repeated doses occurs in some users, possibly reflecting enhanced dopaminergic function. The *withdrawal syndrome* includes fatigue, somnolence, dysphoria, anhedonia and hyperphagia. The side-effects of modafinil, methylphenidate and atomoxetine are qualitatively similar to those of amphetamine, but are much less severe. In general, these drugs are relatively well tolerated in therapeutically useful doses.

6.7 **Opiates**

Mode of action Morphine, diamorphine (heroin) and related drugs are agonists at opioid receptors (μ-, δ- and κ-receptors). Their action is blocked by opioid antagonists (e.g. naloxone). Stimulation of μ-receptors in the brain and κ-receptors in the spinal cord mediates their analgesic effects. Stimulation of μ-receptors in the mesolimbic dopaminergic pathway probably underlies their euphoriant/reinforcing effects.

Therapeutic uses Opiates are the most effective treatment available for acute pain due to tissue damage and the pain of cancer. They are less effective in relieving neuropathic pain and 'chronic pain'. Opiates are occasionally used to suppress cough and to produce a firmer stool following ileostomy or colostomy.

Pharmacokinetics Opiates are well absorbed from the gut, but undergo extensive first-pass metabolism, Parenteral administration is commonly used both therapeutically and illicitly. Morphine's $t_{1/2}$ is about 2 hours. As its therapeutic index is quite low, continuous infusion is sometimes employed in order to maintain a stable plasma concentration in the management of intolerable pain. Methadone, which is used in replacement therapy for opiate addiction, has a $t_{1/2}$ of 12-16 hours.

Side-effects Respiratory depression, nausea, vomiting and constipation are significant adverse effects during therapeutic use. Central side-effects include euphoria, sedation and pupil constriction (miosis). Delirium/hallucinosis occurs occasionally; this has been attributed to σ-receptor stimulation. Pharmacodynamic *tolerance* develops to the eur-phoriant and analgesic effects. The *withdrawal syndrome* includes restlessness, craving, anxiety, mydriasis, lacrimation and piloerection ('gooseflesh').

6.8 **Hallucinogens and other drugs affecting perception**

These drugs include:

- 'indoleamine-like' hallucinogens (e.g. lysergic acid diethylamide [LSD], psilocybin);
- 'catecholamine-like' hallucinogens (e.g. mescaline, methylenedioxy-methamphetamine [MDMA, 'ecstasy']);
- dissociative anaesthetics (e.g. ketamine, phencyclidine [PCP]);
- cannabinoids (e.g. Δ^9-tetrahydrocannabinol [THC] – the principal active ingredient of cannabis resin).

Mode of action LSD and related drugs have both agonist and antagonist actions at 5-HT receptors; their principal action is thought to be stimulation of somatodendritic 5-HT$_{1A}$ autoreceptors. Mescaline and related drugs combine sympathomimetic ('amphetamine-like') action with LSD-like effects; facilitation of dopaminergic/noradrenergic mechanisms contribute to their mode of action. MDMA releases 5-HT and has a selective neurotoxic effect on 5-HTergic neurones. PCP binds to specific sites (*sigma receptors*) within the ionophore linked to glutamate (*N*-methyl-D-aspartate, NMDA) receptors; it thus interferes with glutamatergic transmission mediated by these receptors. THC binds to specific metabotropic receptors (*cannabinoid receptors*). The relationship between these actions and the perceptual and cognitive effects of these drugs is unknown.

Therapeutic uses Mescaline- and LSD-like drugs have no legitimate therapeutic use. Ketamine is used as an analgesic/anaesthetic. THC (in the form of cannabis) is used illegally not only for recreational purposes, but also as an anxiolytic and, notably by some multiple sclerosis sufferers, as an alalgesic. THC has anti-nauseant and anti-emetic effects which have been used to counteract the side-effects of cancer chemotherapy.

Pharmacokinetics Mescaline- and LSD-like drugs are well absorbed from the gut. Their half-lives are in the range of 3-6 hours. However, depending on the dose, the psychological effects may last for 24 hours or more. PCP's $t_{1/2}$ can be as long as 3 days, but in treating overdose victims, excretion can be facilitated by acidification of the urine. Ketamine is administered intravenously as an anaesthetic; its $t_{1/2}$ is about 3 hours. THC, which is usually self-administered by inhaling the smoke of cannabis resin, has an elimination $t_{1/2}$ of about 30 hours; however, its metabolites are eliminated much more slowly, and can be detected in the plasma and urine weeks after cannabis use.

Psychological and somatic effects These drugs alter perception in all modalities. Enhanced subjective sensory acuity, perceptual distortion and illusions are more common than frank hallucinosis. LSD- and mescaline-like drugs have little effect on arousal, whereas PCP and ketamine induce drowsiness. THC in modest recreational doses impairs attention and information-processing performance. Mood is affected somewhat unpredictably by all drugs in this class; eurphoria may give way to dysphoria and outright panic within a single 'trip'.

Mescaline and related drugs induce emesis, probably by an action on the chemosensitive 'trigger-zone' in the brainstem. Tachycardia and mydriasis reflect the sympathomimetic effects of these drugs (see above).

Long-term effects of habitual use of hallucinogens are controversial. Delayed 'flashbacks' are sometimes reported by LSD users; these may reflect persistent, rather than episodic, perceptual disturbance (Abraham *et al.* 1996). MDMA's neurotoxic effects may be irreversible. Regular use of THC may lead to an 'amotivational syndrome' and sexual dysfunction. However there is little evidence that this is not fully reversible following discontinuation (Leonard 2004). PCP, administered chronically to animals, produces a range of cognitive and motivational deficits that has been proposed as a veridical model of the negative symptom profile of schizophrenia.

The tar from cannabis resin is more carcinogenic than that from tobacco.

6.9 Drug treatment of Alzheimer's-type dementia

6.9.1 Cholinergic enhancement treatments

The major neuropathological features of Alzheimer's disease (AD) are:

◆ extracellular *plaques* containing β-amyloid protein;

◆ intraneuronal *neurofibrillary tangles*;

◆ *neuronal loss.*

Among the most severely affected pathways are the cholinergic projections from the basal forebrain to the hippocampus and neoocortex, atrophy of which has been held responsible for the cognitive decline in AD (Whitehouse 1998). A number of treatments have been developed with the aim of boosting cholinergic function and thereby slowing down or reversing the dementing process. It is fair to say that the outcome of this endeavour has, so far, been somewhat disappointing. There are currently three drugs of this class licenced in the UK for the treatment of 'moderate' AD: *donepezil, rivastigmine* and *gallantamine*.

Mode of action Donepezil and gallantamine are reversible competitive inhibitors of acetylcholinesterase, the enzyme that curtails the postsynaptic action of acetylcholine. Gallamantine is also an allosteric modulator of nicotinic cholinoceptors. Rivastigmine is a reversible non-competitive acetylcholinesterase inhibitor.

Therapeutic uses Anticholinesterases are used to treat mild-to-moderate AD. There have been some reports that patients suffering from Lewy-body dementia respond well to these drugs, perhaps better than patients with AD. Anticholinesterases may also be useful in vascular dementia (Roman 2004). However, they are not generally regarded as useful in frontotemporal lobar degeneration. The evidence for the clinical efficacy of these drugs has been controversial, and has been the source of heated public debate (Pelosi et al. 2006). Recent reviews and commentaries generally give them credit for producing modest clinical benefit in terms of slowing the progression of cognitive decline and deterioration of activities of daily living (Hogan *et al.* 2007; Lemstra *et al.* 2007).

Pharmacokinetics Donepezil has a $t_{1/2}$ of 70-100 hours, allowing once-daily dosing. Gallantamine's $t_{1/2}$ is about 10 hours; it is usually given twice daily. Rivastigmine has a very short $t_{1/2}$ (1 hour), but acetylcholinesterase inhibition lasts for about 10 hours, making it suitable for twice-daily dosing. All three drugs undergo metabolism in the liver.

Side-effects All three drugs are prone to inducing nausea, vomiting, diarrhoea, anorexia and fatigue. Gradually increasing doses are recommended.

6.9.2 Memantine

Mode of action Memantine is a non-competitive blocker of NMDA glutamate receptor-regulated ion channels. It is assumed that, by reducing glutamate-induced excitation, memantine exerts a 'neuroprotective' effect – preventing neuronal death due to excitotoxicity (Johnson and Kotermanski 2006)

Therapeutic uses Memantine is used to treat 'moderate-to-severe' AD.

Pharmacokinetics The elimination half-life of memantine is about 60 hours. Nevertheless, twice-daily treatment is usual.

Side-effects Memantine is generally well tolerated, constipation, drowsiness, dizziness and headache being the most commonly reported adverse effects.

Acknowledgement

I am grateful to my colleague Professor E. Szabadi for helpful discussions and practical suggestions for improving an earlier version of this chapter.

Selective references

Abraham, H.D., Aldridge, A.M., and Gogia, P. (1996). The psychopharmacology of hallucinogens. *Neuropsychopharmacology.* **14**, 285–298.

Ballard, C.G., Grace, J., McKeith, I.G., and Holmes, C. (1998). Neuroleptic sensitivity in dementia with Lewy bodies and Alzheimer's disease. *Lancet.* **351**, 1032–1033.

Blier, P., de Montigny, C., and Chaput, Y. (1991). A role for the serotonin system in the mechanism of action of antidepressant treatments: preclinical evidence. *J. Clin. Psychiat.* **51**, 4–15.

Burton, S. (2006). Symptom domains of schizophrenia: the role of atypical antipsychotic drugs. *J. Psychopharmac.* **20** suppl., 6–19.

Cooper S.J. (2004). Anxiolytics, sedatives and hypnotics. In *Seminars in clinical psychopharmacology*, 2nd edn., ed. King, D.J. pp 141–177. Gaskell, London.

DeBattista, C. (2006). Augmentation and combination strategies for depression. *J. Psychopharmac.* **20** suppl., 11–18.

den Boer, J.A., Bosker, F.J., and Slapp, B.R. (2000). Serotonergic drugs in the treatment of depressive and anxiety disorders. *Human Psychopharmac.* **15**, 315–336.

Elwes, R.D.C. and Binnie, C.D. (1996). Clinical pharmacokinetics of newer antiepileptic drugs. *Clin. Pharmacokin.* **30**, 403–415.

Goodwin, G.M. and Young, A.H. (2003). The British Association for Psychopharmacology guidelines for treatment of bipolar disorder: a summary. *J. Psychopharmac.* **17** suppl., 3–6.

Granville-Grossman, K.L. and Turner, P. (1966). The effects of propranolol on anxiety. *Lancet.* i, 788–790.

Haefely, W. (1990). The GABA$_A$-benzodiazepine receptor: biology and pharmacology. In *Handbook of anxiety, Vol. 3: The neurobiology of anxiety*, ed. Burrows, G.D., Roth, M., and Noyes, R. pp 165–188. Elsevier, Amsterdam.

Harris, G.C. and Aston-Jones, G. (2006). Arousal and reward: a dichotomy in orexin function. *Trends in Neurosciences.* **29**, 571–577.

Harrison-Read and Tyrer (2004). The clinical principles underlying drug treatment in psychiatric practice. In *Seminars in clinical psychopharmacology*, 2nd edn., ed. King, D.J. pp 92–138. Gaskell, London.

Hidalgo, R.B., Tupler, L.A., and Davidson, J.R.T. (2007). An effect-size analysis of pharmacologic treatments for generalized anxiety disorder. *J Psychopharmac.* **21**, 864–872.

Hogan, D.B., Bailey, P., Carswell, A., Clarke, B., Cohen, C., Forbes, D., Man-Son-Hing, M., Lanctôt, Morgan, D., and Thorpe, L. (2007). Management of mild to moderate Alzheimer's disease and dementia. *Alzheimer's and Dementia.* **3**, 355–384.

Hökfelt, T., Broberger, C., Xu, Z.-Q.D., Sergeyev, V., Ubunk, R., and, Diez, M. (2000). Neuropeptides – an overview. *Neuropharmacology.* **39**, 1337–1356.

Hou, R.H., Freeman, C., Langley, R.W., Szabadi, E., and Bradshaw, C.M. (2005). Does modafinil activate the locus coeruleus in man? Comparison of modafinil and clonidine on arousal and autonomic functions in human volunteers. *Psychopharmac.* **184**, 537–549.

Israel, J.A. (2006). Remission in depression: definition and initial treatment approaches. *J. Psychopharmac.* **20** suppl., 5–10.

Johnson, J.W. and Kotermanski, S.E. (2006). Mechanism of action of memantine. *Curr. Opin. Pharmac.* **6**, 61–67.

Kapur, S., Zipursky, R., Jones, C., Remington, G., and Houle, S. (2000). Relationship between dopamine D_2 occupancy, clinical response, and side-effects: a double-blind PET study of first-episode schizophrenia. *Am. J. Psychiat.* **157**, 514–520.

Kalvainen, R., Aika, M., and Riekkinen, P.J. (1996). Cognitive adverse of antiepileptic drugs. *CNS Drugs.* **5**, 358–368.

Kavoussi, R. and Coccaro, E.F. (1998). Psychopharmacological treatment of impulsive aggression. In *Neurobiology and clinical views on aggression and impulsivity*, ed. Maes, M. **and** Coccaro, E.F. pp 197–211. Wiley, New York.

King D.J. and Waddington, J.L. (2004). Antipsychotic drugs and the treatment of schizophrenia. In *Seminars in clinical psychopharmacology*, 2nd edn., ed. King, D.J. pp 316–380. Gaskell, London.

Krishnan, K.R.R. (1998). Monoamine oxidase inhibitors. In *Textbook of psychopharmacology*, 2nd edn., ed. Schatzberg, A.F. **and** Nemeroff, C.B., pp 239–249. American Psychiatric Press, New York.

Lemstra, A.F., Richard, E., and van Gool, W.A. (2007). Cholinesterase inhibitors in dementia: yes, no, or maybe? *Age and Ageing.* **36**, 625–627.

Lenox, R.H. and Manji, H.K. (1998). Lithium. In *Textbook of psychopharmacology*, 2nd edn., ed. Schatzberg, A.F. **and** Nemeroff, C.B., pp 379–430. American Psychiatric Press, New York.

Leonard B.E. (2004). Pharmacological aspects of drugs of misuse. In *Seminars in clinical psychopharmacology*, 2nd edn., ed. King, D.J. pp 485–528. Gaskell, London.

Löscher, W. and Schmidt, D. (2006). New horizons in antiepileptic drugs: innovative strategies. *Epilepsy Research.* **69**, 183–272.

Mallinger, A.G. and Smith, E. (1991). Pharmacokinetic of monoamine oxidase inhibitors. *Psychopharmacol. Bull.* **17**, 155–160.

Meltzer, H.Y. (1995). Role of serotonin in the action of atypical antipsychotic drugs. *Clin. Neurosci.* **3**, 64–75.

Miller, N.S., Gold, M.S., and Stennie, K. (1995). Benzodiazepines: the dissociation of addiction from pharmacological dependence/withdrawal. *Psychiat. Annals*, **25**, 149–152.

Pelosi, A.J., McNulty, S.V., and Jackson, G.A. (2006). Role of cholinesterase inhibitors in dementia care needs rethinking. *Br. Med. J.* **333**, 491–493.

Rogawski, M.A. (2006). Diverse mechanisms of antiepileptic drugs in the development pipeline. *Epilepsy Research.* **69**, 273–294.

Román, G.C. (2004). Facts, myths, and controversies in vascular dementia. *J. Neurol. Sci.* **226**, 49–52.

Seeman, P., Lee, T., Cha-Wong, M., *et al.* (1976). Antipsychotic drug dose and neuroleptic/dopamine receptors. *Nature.* **261**, 717–719.

Szabadi E. (2006). Drugs for sleep disorders: mechanisms and therapeutic prospects. *Br. J. Clin. Pharmac.* **61**, 761–766.

Szabadi, E. and Bradshaw, C.M. (2004). Affective disorders: 1. Antidepressants. In *Seminars in clinical psychopharmacology*, 2nd edn., ed. King, D.J. pp 178–243. Gaskell, London.

Trivedi, M.H., Rush, A.J., Wisniewski, S.R., *et al.* (2006). Evaluation of outcomes with citalopram for depression using measurement-based care in STAR*D; implications for clinical research and practice. *Am. J. Psychiat.* **163**, 28–40.

US Modafinil in Narcolepsy Multicentre Study Group (2000). Randomized trial of modafinil as a treatment for the excessive daytime somnolence of narcolepsy. *Neurology.* **54**, 1166–1175.

Warshaw, M.G. and Keller, M.B. (1996). The relationship between fluoxetine use and suicidal behavior in 654 subjects with anxiety disorders. *J. Clin. Psychiat.* **57**, 158–166.

Whitehouse, P.J. (1998). The cholinergic deficit in Alzheimer's disease. *J. Clin. Psychiat.* **59** suppl., 19–22.

Part 6

Underlying medical disorders

Chapter 26

The neuropsychology of vascular disorders

Clive Skilbeck

1 Introduction

The term 'vascular disorders' covers a range of conditions, including cerebrovascular disease (e.g., stroke, vascular dementia) and specific blood vessel problems, such as aneurysm with associated sub-arachnoid haemorrhage (SAH), or arteriovenous malformation (AVM). An apparently discrete event, such as stroke, is often associated with a prior history of transient ischaemic attacks (TIAs) and pre-existing risk factors (eg, hypertension). There have been recent major advances in the characterisation of vascular disorders, including development of the concept of mild cognitive impairment (MCI) from cerebrovascular disease and a greater understanding of precursor/risk conditions for stroke or vascular dementia.

Due to the wide range of conditions subsumed under 'vascular disorders', there are a number of roles for the clinical neuropsychologist. These range from early screening to identify possible cognitive changes from pre-stroke vascular problems in people apparently functioning "normally" (e.g., SVD – small vessel disease), through an involvement at the acute, diagnostic, stage (for example, in evaluating cognitive functioning early in the course of a vascular dementia), to an extended participation in the rehabilitation process following stroke. In assessment terms, the clinical neuropsychologist may be monitoring the cognitive abilities of a patient with hypertension, or SVD, over a prolonged period, be charting the process of recovery after neurosurgery in SAH, or be providing data on the rate and extent of cognitive decline in vascular dementia. Increasingly, clinical neuropsychologists are active in the rehabilitation process, offering interventions both for the cognitive deficits they have documented and for psychological problems such as anxiety and depression that accompany vascular disorders.

2 Pre-stroke conditions

2.1 Hypertension

2.1.1 Definition

Raised blood pressure: high systolic pressure is a major risk factor for stroke (hypertension has been estimated as the cause of intracerebral haemorrhages in 25%-94% of cases; Allen *et al.* 1988).

2.1.2 Diagnosis

Unfortunately, hypertension often appears virtually symptom-free for a considerable period of time and so the most efficient method for its detection is routine screening. In recent years there has been research interest in investigating the cognitive functioning of those who are non-symptomatic, or pre-symptomatic, as indicated below.

2.1.3 Neuropsychological presentation

People aged 70 years or older who are hypertensive (but have not suffered stroke) will show a wide range of cognitive difficulties, including a variety of memory and learning deficits, compared with people of the same age who have normal blood pressure. Similarly, high blood pressure in patients at age 50 years has been shown to correlate with the cognitive deficits noted (using the neuropsychological tasks of digit span, trail making, and verbal fluency) in these same patients when they were tested approximately 20 years later (Kilander *et al.* 2000). There is evidence that the longer the period of uncontrolled hypertension, the more marked is the resulting cognitive impairment (eg, Dufouil *et al.* 2001). Very strong evidence of the link between hypertension and cognitive impairment was provided by Li *et al.* (2007) in their very large (n=2,356) prospective community study of hypertension. These authors noted a highly significant relationship between high systolic blood pressure or borderline-high diastolic blood pressure and the subsequent development of dementia, compared with participants showing normal systolic and diastolic blood pressure. These findings held for those aged 65–74 years, but not for older people.

Recent research interest has included the examination of vascular indicators in 'normal' (i.e., non-symptomatic, or pre-symptomatic) people. For example, Waldstein *et al.*(2005) tested 101 older adults (aged 53–84 years), reporting that the subgroup with undiagnosed high blood pressure showed cognitive deficits involving visuo-spatial memory (Wechsler Memory Scale), motor speed, and manual dexterity (Grooved Pegboard). As was expected, the subgroup with diagnosed and poorly controlled blood pressure displayed more severe deficits, including visuomotor speed (Trails A).

2.1.4 Psychosocial aspects

These are minor in the absence of significant adverse physical effects upon the patient. Similarly, patient compliance with the medication regimen and recommended lifestyle changes can be problematic when no short-term threat to health is obvious.

2.1.5 Treatment & outcome

If blood pressure is raised during mid-life, then there is a greater risk of cognitive impairment in late-life (Kivipelto *et al.* 2001). A significant reduction in the probability of subsequent stroke or vascular dementia is achieved when hypertension has been successfully treated and blood pressure is reduced and controlled. However, blood pressure reduction in hypertensive patients needs to be at a controlled rate: if the reduction is too rapid, patients risk white matter damage with associated attentional deficits. There is evidence that providing biofeedback training to control heart rate variability is effective in reducing hypertension, and that it can be used to reduce anti-hypertensive medication dosage.

Given the increasing aged profile of the population in many countries, coupled with increasing longevity, there is great interest in the possible beneficial effects of treating hypertension in elderly patients: one current study involves 16 countries and patients aged at least 80 years, in a randomised, double-blind, placebo-controlled trial (Peters *et al.* 2006). There is also a role for the clinical neuropsychologist in providing advice to hypertensive patients who wish to reduce their risk of stroke by stopping smoking and adopting a healthier diet and lifestyle. The identification of early/mild cognitive impairment may help to persuade patients to better adhere to medical advice. Issues of cognitive rehabilitation are dealt with under the 'Stroke' section, below.

2.2 Hypotension

2.2.1 Definition

Low blood pressure.

2.2.2 Diagnosis

Patients often complain of light headedness, dizziness, or weakness accompanying sudden postural change. The diagnosis can usually be confirmed by noting a significant drop in blood pressure on moving from sitting to standing.

2.2.3 Neuropsychological presentation

Low blood pressure is associated with cognitive impairment in those aged 80 years and above (Nilsson *et al.* 2007), although Wharton *et al.* (2006) also demonstrated such a significant association, involving poorer visuospatial ability, in healthy young adults. There is very recent evidence that the adverse effects of chronic hypotension upon cognitive functioning can be treated pharmacologically: Duschek *et al.* (2007a,b) noted gains in visual processing using Vernum.

2.3 Cerebral Small Vessel Disease (SVD)

2.3.1 Definition

A narrowing of penetrating arterioles which supply the deep white matter of the brain, leading to gradual ischaemic damage. It is a major cause of Vascular Dementia (VaD; see below).

2.3.2 Diagnosis

Lesions in the white matter identified using MRI. McManus and Stott (2005) provided a comprehensive review.

2.3.3 Neuropsychological presentation

If detected and assessed early, then mild general cognitive difficulties are expected similar to those observed with TIAs. A number of studies suggest that executive dysfunction is the early, prominent cognitive feature of the disease. If initial assessment is undertaken only after a first stroke, then greater cognitive deficit is observed, the pattern being determined by the site of the stroke. A stepwise progression of the disease usually occurs, resulting in dementia for approximately 50% of patients. Given the importance of SVD, O'Sullivan *et al.* (2005) investigated possible cognitive screening instruments for its identification. Although Mini-Mental State Examination (MMSE) total scores were significantly lower in SVD patients compared with normal age-matched controls, the authors noted that a brief (< 20 minutes) executive test battery, comprising Trails A & B, letter fluency (FAS), WAIS-R Digits Backwards, and WAIS-R Digit Symbol was superior to the MMSE in correctly assigning participants to 'Normal' or 'SVD' groups. Such identification should aid early identification and intervention of patients at risk of subsequent VaD or stroke. The importance of the executive function findings were supported by Prins *et al.* (2005), in a large prospective Dutch study involving repeat testing of over 800 participants prior to the development of SVD. These authors also noted a significant reduction in information processing speed in those patients who developed SVD.

Patients showing Mild Cognitive Impairment (MCI) with vascular disease show greater impairments than MCI patients without vascular disease on tests of speed and attention, visuospatial function, and executive function. As might be predicted, those MCI patients with a pre-existing stroke or multiple cognitive deficits are significantly more likely to progress to VaD.

2.3.4 Psychosocial aspects

Mood problems are noted in 20% of SVD patients.

2.3.5 Treatment & outcome

As knowledge of SVD increases, the indications for early treatment with acetyl cholinesterase inhibitors to slow the progression of cognitive deficits strengthen.

2.4 SVD: CADASIL (Cerebral Autosomal Dominant Arteriopathy with Subcortical Infarcts and Leuoencephalopathy)

2.4.1 Definition

This rare genetic variant of SVD produces cerebrovascular problems in early adulthood or middle age (Vikelis *et al.* 2006).

2.4.2 Diagnosis

In approximately 75% of cases, the disease presents as TIAs or young stroke, with migraine also being a frequent (40%) presenting symptom. MRI examination reveals subcortical white matter lesions, with cerebral hypointense (lacunar) lesions and microhaemorrhages. The number and size of the lacunar lesions relates significantly to the severity of the cognitive impairment observed (MMSE), and to the level of physical disability as assessed using the modified Rankin Scale and the Barthel Index (Viswanathan *et al.* 2007).

2.4.3 Neuropsychological presentation

The cognitive natural history of CADASIL is that of VaD, although progression begins at an earlier age. A very rare study (Harris and Filley 2001) involved case studies across three generations of one family, noting a range of cognitive deficits with relatively well preserved language functions.

2.4.4 Psychosocial aspects

Depression is a presenting symptom in approximately 10% of patients and with a prevalence of mood disorder of about 30%. Frequent coping problems are to be expected, given the disease's relatively early onset, its predictable progression, and the lack of any effective treatment.

2.4.5 Treatment & outcome

Currently, there is no proven effective treatment for CADASIL, although anti-hypertensive medication may slow the rate of progression. Disease progression is faster in men, although the reasons for this are not clear (a role for sex hormones has been suggested). For most patients the picture is one of deteriorating cognitive and physical functions. For example, more than 50% will be unable to walk unaided after the age of 60 years. The prognosis is poorer for men, in terms of psychological intervention. In addition to addressing any mood disorder in the patient, which should include family support, given the genetic basis of CADASIL any intervention may need to be episodic over a prolonged period.

2.5 Transient Ischaemic Attacks (TIAs)

2.5.1 Definition

As the name suggests, TIAs are temporary (lasting less than 24 hours) neurological deficits arising from an ischaemic episode.

2.5.2 Diagnosis

This is made on clinical grounds and in the light of the patient's history.

2.5.3 Neuropsychological presentation

Given that TIAs usually occur against a history of a generally deteriorating cerebrovascular supply, a wide range of cognitive deficits may be observed. There is evidence that severity of cognitive impairment correlates significantly with the patient's longest TIA episode. Early adverse cognitive effects from TIA include a slowed speed of information processing (e.g., reduced WAIS-III Digit Symbol age-scale score) and new learning (e.g., relatively poor Rey Auditory Verbal Learning Test scores).

2.5.4 Psychosocial aspects

These are usually relatively minor, but expressed anxiety by the patient can be utilised to reinforce adherence to medical advice. If TIAs persist they are likely to acquire occupational relevance, as job performance suffers with developing cognitive impairment.

2.5.5 Treatment & outcome

One of the reasons why TIAs are important is because they carry an annual 10% risk of subsequent stroke for the patient. Hart *et al.* (2001) found that a simple four-item questionnaire on TIA was an excellent predictor of subsequent stroke in a study involving over 15,000 participants and a 20-year follow-up. For the large majority of patients aspirin or short-term anticoagulation therapy is recommended. In a national UK five-year study (Gibbs *et al.* 2001) results indicated that the prescription of antiplatelet and anticoagulant agents significantly reduced the subsequent occurrence of stroke. Pharmacological treatment of TIA may also reduce the probability of developing vascular dementia (Bos *et al.*2007). In cases where major stenosis (narrowing) of the carotid artery is noted, referral for carotid endarterectomy surgery may be appropriate although an uncertain cognitive prognosis may be the result (Lunn *et al.* 1999). The issue of cognitive rehabilitation is dealt with under the 'Stroke' section, below.

3 Stroke

3.1 Definition

Stroke is a disruption of the vascular supply to the brain, of rapid onset with neurological symptoms persisting longer than 24 hours, caused by haemorrhage from an artery or from its occlusion through progressive narrowing of the vessel (athetosclerosis) or a blockage (embolism). Haemorrhage accounts for only about 10%-15% of strokes and is particularly associated with coma, neck stiffness and vomiting.

3.2 Risk factors

These include age, cardiac disease, TIAs (see above), hypertension (see above), and Diabetes Melitus (Allen *et al.* 1989). For example, from age 60 years the risk of suffering a stroke doubles each decade. Smoking is a risk factor for those under 65 years old, as is gender (30% higher risk in men).

3.3 Diagnosis

Initially, the diagnosis of stroke is usually a clinical decision, based upon medical exami-nation and symptoms, although it may be confirmed by a subsequent CT or MRI scan.

3.4 Neuropsychological presentation

This is extremely variable – impairment in any cognitive ability can be observed, depend-ing upon the site of the stroke and its severity. The length of the period of cerebrov-ascular disease pre-stroke will also influence the cognitive picture. Motor deficits in the limbs contralateral to the side of stroke may be acquired, in severe cases constituting hemiplegia. When the stroke involves the hemisphere in which the patient's primary language centres are located, aphasic problems often result. The 'classic' cognitive distur-bance in right hemisphere stroke is perceptual deficit, particularly left-sided neglect: the patient behaves as if the left side of visual space does not exist. They are unaware of it and so neglect in-coming information from this side. For example, this lack of awareness can lead to the patient bumping into/falling over furniture on their left side and (in severe cases) ignoring food on the left-hand side of their plate during meals. Although most of the early reports of this disorder stressed the right hemisphere-left visual space relationship, right side neglect following left hemisphere stroke is now well recognised (although occurring less frequently, and less severely). The visual impairment demonstrated is *perceptual* - the deficit occurs at the cortical level, in the presence of adequate primary sensory and motor input from peripheral receptors (it is not merely the consequence of a visual field defect).

3.5 Neuropsychological examination

Again, the specific content of this will depend partly upon the site of stroke, although given the likelihood of significant pre-existing cerebrovascular disease a wide range of cognitive functions should be assessed. Skilbeck (1992) provided a general review of the assessment of cognitive functions in stroke. There are a number of reasons for carrying out a neuropsychological assessment, including the provision of prognostically useful information and the obtaining of a baseline against which to judge spontaneous recovery or the effectiveness of cognitive rehabilitation. It may also make a contribution towards the decision relating to the most appropriate post-acute care setting for the patient.

In the last few years the validity of reading tests traditionally used in estimating pre-morbid IQ has received much attention. In the absence of significant oral and/or written language impairment, the National Adult reading Test (NART; Nelson 1982) probably still offers the best estimation of premorbid intellectual level. However, recent research indicates that reading test estimators of pre-morbid IQ may be affected by cognitive impairment. Skilbeck *et al.* (2005), using the NART, concluded that mod/severe cognitive impairment led to too-low estimates of premorbid IQ. In a comparison study of the NART and WTAR (Wechsler Test of Adult Reading) in healthy Australians, Mathias *et al.* (2007a), noted that the NART was more accurate in its estimations of IQ. In another study, (Mathias *et al.* (2007b) she also found that the WTAR underestimated premorbid IQ in severe TBI. Similar findings of prediction underestimates have been noted with the WTAR in mild Alzheimer's Disease. (McFarlane *et al.* 2006).

The Wechsler Adult Intelligence Scale-III (WAIS-III; Wechsler 1997) is the most often used instrument to assess IQ, although obtaining a meaningful verbal IQ may be impossible if the stroke involves the language-dominant hemisphere and produces significant dysphasia. Similarly, marked manual motor deficit as a consequence of stroke often renders the WAIS-III inappropriate for the assessment of performance IQ. When either marked language or motor impairment is apparent post-stroke, then Raven's Matrices can be particularly useful in assessing intellectual level, as it only requires either a simple pointing, or a minimal verbal, response and time to respond is not included in scoring the test. A number of versions of this test are available, to cover a wide age range (Raven 1977).

Examination of perceptual functions may employ a number of instruments. The most appropriate include assessment for unilateral visual neglect, given that the reported rate of this disorder after right hemisphere stroke is very high (up to 85% immediately and approximately 40% at least one week after stroke). Examples are the Rivermead Perceptual Assessment Battery (RPAB; Whiting *et al.* 1985) and the Behavioural Inattention Test (BIT; Wilson *et al.* 1987). The RPAB has been shown to be useful in predicting patients' functional outcome at discharge from rehabilitation (Donnelly, 2002). Star Cancellation tasks, such as that offered by the BIT have been shown to be amongst the best predictors of functional outcome after stroke, and the BIT is often used as an outcome measure by which to judge the efficacy of a treatment intervention (e.g., Shindo *et al.*, 2007). The BIT was specifically devised to test for visual neglect, as was the Balloons Test (Edgeworth *et al.* 1998). The latter not only assesses unilateral visual neglect, but also allows computation of an index of general visual inattention. It comprises two subtests. Subtest A incorporates the phenomenon of perceptual 'Pop-out', providing a measure in which the attentional processing demands for serial search are minimal. Subtest B requires effortful serial search, thereby requiring a much greater attentional resource. Patients showing unilateral visual neglect are significantly more impaired on subtest B than subtest A. Whilst subtest A scores do not differ in healthy older adults and dementia, the latter show subtest B scores which are significantly lower (Lincoln *et al.* 2006).

Even very simple, brief testing, such as asking the patient to draw a clock face or a daisy, can also elicit contralateral visual neglect. When attempting to write in the numbers around the clock face, the right hemisphere stroke patient with neglect tends to ignore its left side, resulting in all of the numbers being crammed into the right-hand side (between positions '12' and '6'). When drawing a daisy the same patient will usually omit the petals on the left side of the flower or produce only rudimentary versions of them. An excellent and comprehensive consideration of the clinical and theoretical aspects of unilateral neglect phenomena was provided by Robertson and Marshall (1993).

3.6 Assessing memory

Assessment of memory functioning after stroke can involve a number of approaches, from brief screening instruments through to test batteries. While memory screening tests often show a number of disadvantages, including poor/no data on their reliability and validity, some provide useful clinical information.

- The Mini-Mental State Examination (MMSE; Folstein *et al.* 1975) remains amongst the most useful. The MMSE offers only a brief screen, with scores <24/30 usually being interpreted as indicating cognitive impairment.

- The Rivermead Behavioural Memory Test (Wilson *et al.* 1989) is a particularly appropriate test of everyday memory functioning, often used in assessing stroke patients and their progress through rehabilitation.

- Examples of batteries for memory examination are the BIRT Memory and Information Processing Battery (BMIPB; Oddy *et al.* 2007), a revision and extension of the Adult memory and Information Processing Battery (AMIPB; Coughlan & Hollows 1985), and the Wechsler Memory Scale-III (WMS-III; Wechsler 1998). The BMIPB has a number of advantages, including its inclusion of three parallel forms which allows repeat testing to assess the progression of cerebrovascular disease over time or recovery from stroke.

Studies suggest that approximately 20% of patients will be dysphasic at one month post-stroke, reducing slightly to about 15% by the six months follow-up. Information on disordered language is obtained from intellectual assessment, though specialised and comprehensive instruments such as the Boston Diagnostic Aphasia Examination and the Western Aphasia Battery may be employed by speech therapists or neuropsychologists working with stroke patients. Walker (1992) provided a very good overview of language dysfunction and its assessment.

3.7 Importance of cognitive deficits

Continuing cognitive impairment post-stroke has implications for a person's daily living activities. For example, someone with significant persisting memory difficulties may not remember to switch the cooker off after preparing food, may forget to buy needed food items when shopping, and may not recall 'phone messages. Post-stroke perceptual problems will often preclude the person from taking responsibility for personal self-care such as shaving, food preparation, or leaving the house unaccompanied. The assessment methods outlined above will help to form a judgement of the person's abilities and functional competence after stroke. A recent example study by Jehkonen *et al.* (2000) noted that the presence of visual neglect following right hemisphere stroke, identified using the BIT, was associated with poor real-life activities at follow-up 12 months post-stroke. A number of studies have shown significant correlations between scores on the RPAB and ADL performance, with some RPAB scores on admission to rehabilitation being good predictors of discharge home. Admission scores from memory tests and Raven's Coloured Matrices have also proved useful in predicting discharge from hospital and ADL competence. Even the brief cognitive screen offered by the MMSE, administered soon after stroke has been shown to predict later functional independence (Hama *et al.* 2007). In addition, the findings from cognitive assessment after stroke provide good predictors of subsequent driving ability (eg, Klavora, *et al.* 2000), which is an important finding given that older adults are at greater risk of causing a road traffic accident after stroke.

In addition, post-stroke cognitive problems can help in coming to an opinion regarding physical prognosis. Wang *et al.* (2000) found that cognitive impairment was a significant independent factor in predicting survival for at least two years post-stroke, and in a major review of relevant studies Anstey *et al.* (2006) noted a large number of studies reporting an association between post-stroke cognitive functioning and subsequent death.

3.8 Psychosocial aspects

A limited range of mood and quality of life instruments has been used with stroke patients and their relatives, including Hospital Anxiety and Depression Scales, Frenchay Activities Index, Beck Scales, Nottingham Health Profile and the Sickness Impact Profile (Skilbeck 1996; Ellis-Hill and Horn 2000). However, many studies have investigated depression following stroke, usually concluding that it is a frequent problem. In a rare population study, involving 850 patients, Wade *et al.* (1985) noted a 20% depression rate in both patients and their carers six months post-stroke, and there is evidence that the frequency of patient depression may rise as high as 33% by one year after stroke. In addition to its direct negative effects upon the individual stroke patient's well being, depression also has adverse effects upon cognitive functioning, producing 'dementia of depression'.

The question of the cause of this depression is unresolved, there being conflicting evidence to implicate the site and size of the stroke and the occurrence of cognitive sequelae. Recent research findings (Hama *et al.* 2007) suggest that affective aspects of depression are associated with left frontal stroke, whereas apathy is more often a result of bilateral stroke in the basal ganglia. Depression at three months post-stroke shows a similar prevalence and hemisphere link, and is associated with slower information processing, poor verbal memory, and a younger age group (Barker 2007). By three years post-stroke approximately 20% of patients are still depressed, their mood disorder being associated with poor functional independence. A high level of depression in carers is not surprising given the major physical, functional and cognitive impairments that many stroke patients are left with. The position of spouses as carers is made more difficult given that they are likely to be of similar age to their patient partner. Spouses of stroke patients provided with group CBT report improvements in their level of depression (Beck Depression Inventory) and quality of life (Wilz and Barskova 2007). Such early interventions are important, as improvements in psychological health and the prevention of medical problems in spouse caregivers are very important in enabling stroke patients with disabilities to live at home.

3.9 Treatment & outcome

One of the best predictors of death or long-term disability following stroke is urinary incontinence (Wang *et al.* 2001). In addition, Baird *et al.* (2001) found that recovery could be predicted from the extent of the ischaemic damage noted on MRI and a stroke scale score, these measures being obtained within 36 hours of the stroke. Medical treatment for stroke is limited. Vascular surgery to remove the blockage is not supported by research studies, and endarterectomy to prevent stroke may raise the mortality rate. However, recent research (Hillis *et al.* 2000) has demonstrated the role of hypoperfusion in determining acquired cognitive deficits in acute stroke. Reducing hypertension has also been shown to reduce the probability of recurrent stroke, and secondary prevention can also be assisted through the use of Aspirin and antiplatelet medication generally. Although the possible treatment of stroke using transplanted neuronal tissue has yet to investigated adequately, there are studies (for example, using basal ganglia stroke patients) reporting relevant research and arguing for the feasibility of this approach. In addition, there is now good evidence that a significant element in the spontaneous recovery of functioning post-stroke is associated with a complex pattern of brain reorganisation (Cramer and Bastings 2000). Research using Transcranial Magnetic Stimulation (TMS; Tropetto *et al.* 2000), in which magnetic pulses are delivered to the motor cortex and adjacent areas via the scalp surface, suggests that reorganisation of motor tissue post-stroke and functional gains can be enhanced using TMS. Rehabilitation after stroke is still primarily directed towards physical, rather than cognitive, functioning. In a major review of the relevant studies, Majid *et al.* (2000) concluded that there was insufficient evidence to decide whether or not cognitive rehabilitation of memory deficits following stroke is effective, although there is strong support from meta-analysis studies for rehabilitation effectiveness with a range of language and perceptual deficits. With regard to the latter, work by Robertson has demonstrated the therapeutic value of ipsilateral motor stimulation in treating unilateral visual neglect. Research has also demonstrated the successful, stable, transfer (generalisation) from rehabilitation unit to home of apraxia rehabilitation. Skilbeck (2000) provided a review of the range of strategies available to treat cognitive deficits in people suffering stroke, dividing them into internal and external approaches. The former aim to directly reduce the level of cognitive deficit using remedial training on the affected function (examples being the use of mnemonics with memory impairments and scanning training in visual neglect). External approaches concentrate upon the use of aids to ameliorate the effects of cognitive deficits, such as the employment of electronic diaries and 'reminder' systems. Older adults have been shown to cope surprisingly well with the involvement of PC and electronic aids in the re-training of, or compensation for, their cognitive impairments.

Mood disorder following stroke represents a major challenge for services. It is important in itself, although there is evidence that its successful resolution also carries the bonus of enhanced ADL gains (Chemerinski *et al.* 2001). Psychological intervention for post-stroke depression is under-researched, though the evidence suggests that CBT is the current treatment of choice. Recent examination of pharmacological approaches to treatment of depression after stroke, using double-blind studies, have supported the use of Nortryptyline and Fluoxetine, with some evidence that the former may be more effective in improving both cognitive abilities and ADL functioning as measured by the Functional Independence Measure (Robinson *et al.* 2000).

4 Vascular Dementia (VaD)

4.1 Definition

A generalised, significant reduction in cognitive functioning that is cerebrovascular in origin. The term 'vascular' dementia has tended to replace the traditional and more specific characterisation of 'multi-infarct' dementia.

4.2 Diagnosis

As with other dementias, the most frequent identification is carried out using the WAIS-III, comparing the IQ figures obtained with the predicted pre-morbid IQs for the patient generated using the NART. Significant discrepancies between the two methods of IQ estimation, favouring the pre-morbid figures, can lead to the label 'dementia'. In addition other neuropsychological test data, such as evidence that memory/learning abilities are significantly poorer than would be predicted from estimated premorbid cognitive level may also be used in the decision.

4.3 Neuropsychological presentation

In the most frequently observed dementia, namely Alzheimer's Disease, neuropsychological examination early in the condition frequently produces a characteristic profile of subtest results in which the age-scale scores for Vocabulary and Information within the Verbal scale will be higher than for Similarities and Digit Span. Similarly, within the Performance scale, the Picture Completion age-scale score is usually higher than the scores observed for Block Design and for Digit Symbol/Coding. Of course, the timing of the emergence of this pattern of subtest scores, and how marked it is, depends upon the stage of dementia when testing is undertaken and upon its speed of progression.

Whilst the above pattern of IQ subtest scores is also noted in VaD, its appearance is much more variable. This is because the development of vascular dementia is more idiosyncratic, the particular cognitive deficits emerging according to the location and number of infarcts of a significant size at the time of assessment. It may be worth distinguishing two versions of VaD, the first being this less predictable pattern of cognitive deficits that is dependent upon infarct location and number. The second is more generalised, producing an IQ subtest profile that is more predictable and similar to that noted in Alzheimer's Disease. Its basis is prolonged cerebrovascular disease, without major stroke, in which the gradual reduction of the blood supply to the cerebral cortex, principally through the narrowing of vessels, produces cognitive loss. Interestingly, one of the significant differences between Alzheimer's and VaD patients is the greater sleep disturbance seen in the latter.

4.4 Psychosocial aspects

Whilst in some ways the psychosocial issues raised in VaD are the same as those in Alzheimer's Disease, there are some differences. The principal amongst these is the question of insight. Frequently (and sometimes mercifully) in Alzheimer's Disease quite early in the progression of the illness patients lose insight into their condition and their failing cognitive and ADL abilities. This loss of insight occurs less often for patients with a vascular dementia, unless there is significant ischaemic damage to frontal areas. An understandably higher level of distress usually accompanies preservation of insight for the patient, and sometimes for relatives. As with Alzheimer's Disease, the general picture is one of progressive cognitive decline, which requires much of the coping responses of both patient and relatives. Commensurate with the preservation of insight, depression in VaD has been found to be resistant to treatment (Li *et al.* 2001). A comprehensive review of depression in vascular disorders has been provided by McDougall and Brayne 2007).

4.5 Treatment & outcome

The rate of cognitive decline is dependent upon perfusion decline. Risk factors that accelerate the latter include TIAs and hypertension, so the use of aspirin and/or anti-hypertensive agents is recommended. The effectiveness of antithrombotic/antiplatelet drugs in preventing VaD remains to be proved. Cognitive rehabilitation efforts are modelled on those referred to in stroke (above), although the realistic successful outcome may be one of slowing down, or temporarily ameliorating, the process of cognitive impairment, rather than arresting or reversing its effects. There is some evidence that recreational rehabilitation (e.g., dancing, board games) arrests cognitive decline in VaD patients, possibly by improving cortical blood flow.

5 Subarachnoid Haemorrhage (SAH)

5.1 Definition

The term 'haemorrhagic Stroke' is usually applied to bleeding into the substance of the brain, whereas SAH refers to a blood vessel rupturing and bleeding into the subarachnoid space. However, the separation of these two causes of cerebrovascular haemorrhage is not always clear cut. About 80% of SAHs arise from the rupture of an aneurysm (sac extruded from the wall of an artery). Aneurysms can vary widely in their shape and size, although the majority are small ('berry'). In approximately 15% of SAH no cause is found, with the remaining 5% of cases involving blood vessel malformations (arteriovenous malformations; AVM) or other causes.

Most aneurysms arise sporadically, although a familial link is identified in a minority of cases, and it is worth noting that SAH affects a younger population (average age 50–55 years) than 'stroke' and has a higher incidence in women (60%). The overall incidence in the general population is 1–2 per 10,000 per year (Deane *et al.* 1996).

5.2 Diagnosis

Patients often present to the Accident and Emergency Department of their local hospital complaining of severe headache of sudden onset, although in a minority of cases initial loss of consciousness occurs. Diagnosis of SAH is confirmed via CT scan and angiography.

5.3 Neuropsychological presentation

This varies widely, according to site of SAH and severity of the haemorrhage. 85% of aneurysms are found on the anterior cerebral artery distribution (Adams and Biller 1992). The next most common are middle cerebral artery aneurysms, with the posterior cerebral circulation having the lowest occurrence. As might be predicted, those patients with an SAH involving an anterior artery often show some changes in personality, with increased irritability. Research studies in the past have provided inconsistent evidence of severe memory deficits following anterior communicating artery (ACA) SAH and it may be that at one time the neurosurgical intervention to clip the aneurysm itself used to produce some additional damage (to small perforator blood vessels).

The pattern of neuropsychological impairments observed generally follows that expected from cerebral functional geography with, for example, left hemisphere aneurysms of the anterior or middle cerebral arterial supply producing deficits in verbal expression and verbal memory.

5.4 Psychosocial aspects

SAH often produces a very poor psychological (as opposed to cognitive) response. Depression of mood is frequently seen, with a minority seeking pharmacological treatment.

A key factor in post-SAH mood problems appears to be the unexpected nature of the event – for nearly all patients there are no warning signs of the impending haemorrhage, as far as they were aware they were healthy, and many are young or middle-aged. The psychological shock of the SAH, with its serious health implications and probable 'brain surgery', also results in marked anxiety in patients. In a number of ways, the picture presented by some patients is similar to that noted in Post-Traumatic Stress Disorder (Sheldrick *et al.* 2006).

5.5 **Treatment & outcome**

Except in the cases where the SAH is of unknown origin, specific treatment for the aneurysm will be undertaken. Most often this requires neurosurgical intervention to clip the aneurysm, thereby ablating it, sometimes with the additional procedure of wrapping the vessel for extra security. Successful surgically treatment provides a permanent solution. It is also sometimes possible to avoid surgical intervention completely by using a coil. In this procedure a coil is passed, via the cerebrovascular arterial supply, to the site of the aneurysm and into it. This results in clotting, which seals off the aneurysm. This procedure is only suitable for a minority of aneurysms (generally, small and narrow-necked). A coil intervention is associated with a better neuropsychological presentation and recovery, probably because neurosurgical intervention is not required and because coiling can only be used only with smaller (ie, less destructive) aneurysms.

Cognitive recovery at six months post-SAH provides a good guide to the final outcome although, unlike stroke, significant cognitive gains can be noted to at least the 12-month follow-up point. The occurrence of vasospasm or hydrocephalus following SAH are poor prognostic signs for the final cognitive recovery achieved by the patient. Whilst there are few longer-term outcome studies, the available research suggests that a majority of patients show some permanent cognitive impairment as a consequence of SAH (eg, Tidswell *et al.* 1995). One of the most difficult cognitive deficits to rehabilitate is apraxia. There is some evidence to suggest improvements are possible: in a recent small study involving four SAH participants (all being at least 10 months post-haemorrhage), Geusgens *et al.* (2007) noted significant gains in ADL skills which generalised to patients' homes and were stable over time.

Despite reassurances from neurosurgeon and neuropsychologist, a sizeable minority of patients harbour the belief that an SAH may happen again (which is only realistic in cases where a person has multiple aneurysms). This can result in patients post-SAH being very reluctant to leave their house at all, or only doing so if accompanied. An almost phobic anxiety about being away from their house or being in public places may result. Symptoms of depression and anxiety tend to remit over the first few months after the haemorrhage, although a significant mood disturbance may persist for 6–12 months post-SAH. For these patients, intervention by a clinical neuropsychologist is recommended. Longer-term psychological difficulties tend to result from either marked persisting cognitive deficit (usually involving memory and/or language functions) or from permanent personality change.

6 **Vascular surgery**

6.1 **Cardiovascular disease**

Cardiovscular disease is frequently associated with cognitive impairment. Whilst this cognitive impairment has often been shown to be a consequence of cardiovascular dysfunction, the value of cognitive deficits in predicting the subsequent development of cardiovascular disease in asymptomatic patients has only recently been investigated. In a very large prospective study involving more than 12,000 middle-aged people, none of whom had any history or evidence of heart disease at the time of assessment, Elkins *et al.* (2007) found that cognitive test scores (WAIS-R Digit Symbol, Benton FAS) predicted the subsequent development of cardiovascular disease (median follow-up time of 6.4 years).

6.2 **Cardiopulmonary bypass surgery**

Whilst the evidence is that cognitive impairments affecting attention and both verbal & visual memory occurs post-operatively, the use of a neuro-protective agent, such as Trasylol, during surgery, limits the subsequent observed cognitive deficits.

6.3 **Carotid revascularisation**

There have been mixed findings from the few studies which have specifically investigated the association between carotid stenosis (narrowing) and cognitive dysfunction. However, in a large Norwegian study (Mathiesen *et al.* 2004) cognitive impairment was noted in a group of 189 *asymptomatic* patients showing carotid stenosis. Early studies on revascularisation, focussing upon Carotid Endarterectomy, tended to find cognitive impairments following neurosurgery (or, at best, equivocal outcomes). However, a recent review of the field (Berman *et al.* 2007), involving 18 studies on carotid revascularisation, noted significant gains in most of the studies, with only 3 studies noting cognitive impairment after surgery. One of the studies in the latter category focussed on older patients (mean age: 72 years), and using the MMSE and Clock Tests and found a cognitive decline only in those patients with pre-surgical symptomatic Left Internal Carotid Artery (LICA) stenosis; asymptomatic LICA patients and those with Right Internal Carotid disease showed few post-operative cognitive problems (Bo, *et al.*, 2006). Research in this field is becoming increasingly specific, including into genetic factors, and it is now clear that the APOE-ε4 allele is a good predictor of cognitive impairment after Carotid Endarterectomy surgery.

6.4 **Coronary Bypass Graft Surgery (CABG)**

Research in this area usually finds a significant percentage of patients (50%–60%) showing post-operative cognitive impairment. Some studies have only noted cognitive decline long after the surgery. In terms of psychosocial outcome, poor pre-operative psychological functioning is the major psychological risk factor for poor psychological functioning, including mood, six months post-operatively (Oxlad *et al.*(2008). A recent study of women (>= 65 years) undergoing CABG surgery demonstrated the value of an intervention to manage post-operative symptoms, both in terms of physical activities and psychological well-being (Zimmermann *et al.* 2007). Preoperative psycho-education to help patients for surgery and its aftermath is highly recommended.

7 Summary

From the neuropsychological point of view, vascular disorders are best regarded as specific features of the general process of cerebrovascular disease. Early signs of this process are represented by persisting hypertension and TIA, which are associated with usually mild, though developing cognitive impairment, and Small Vessel Disease. Strokes are major events, involving physical, cognitive and psychosocial sequelae. The pattern of deficits noted is dependant upon the site and size of the lesion caused by the stroke. Significant coping and adjustment problems are caused for patient and carers by stroke, which are somewhat different for those presented to people suffering SAH. The latter often occurs in middle-aged, rather than older, adults and for these patients there is a need to judge their recovery against additional criteria, including those linked to employment. The term Vascular Dementia encompasses both the step-wise deterioration in functioning arising out of multi-infarct dementia and the more general progression of cognitive impairment produced by cerebrovascular disease. The role of the neuropsychologist continues to develop. The well-established contributions in the diagnostic process and the assessment of change include both the measurement of recovery (e.g., following stroke or vascular surgery) and the charting of disease progression (e.g., in vascular dementia). In addition, recent research findings point to an important role in the assessment/screening of pre-symptomatic/sub-clinical populations to identify important risk factors such hypertension and Small Vessel Disease. Such a role is extremely useful in facilitating early intervention.

Selective references

Anstey, J., Mack, A., and von Sanden, C. (2006). The relationship between cognition and mortality in patients with stroke, coronary heart disease, or cancer. *European Psychologist. Special Issue: Death and Cognition*, **11**, 182–195.

Baird, A.E., Dambrosia, J., Janket, S., Eichbaum, Q *et al.* (2001). A three-item scale for the early prediction of stroke recovery. *Lancet*, **357**(9274), 2095–9.

Barker-Collo, S. Depression and anxiety 3 months post stroke: prevalence and correlates. *Archives of Clinical Neuropsychology*, **22**, 519–531.

Berman, L., Pietrzak, R.H. and Mayes, L. (2007). Neurocognitive changes after carotid revascularization: A review of the current literature. *Journal of Psychosomatic Research*, **63**, 599–612.

Bo, M., Massaia, M., Speme, S., Cappa, G., *et al.* (2006). Risk of cognitive decline in older patients after Carotid Endarterectomy: An observational study. *Journal of the American Geriatrics Society*, **54**, 932–936.

Boggio, P.S., Nunes, A., Rigonatti, S.P., Nitsche, M.A., Pascual-Leone, A., and Fregni, F. (2007). Repeated sessions of non-invasive brain DC stimulation is associated with motor function improvement in stroke patients. *Restorative Neurology and Neuroscience*, **25**, 123–129.

Bos M.J., van Rijn M.J., Witteman J.C., Hofman A., Koudstaal P.J., Breteler M.M. (2007). Incidence and prognosis of transient neurological attacks. *Journal of the American Medical Association*, **298**, 2877–2885.

Chemerinski, E., Robinson, R.G., Arndt, S. and Kosier, J.T. (2001). The effect of remission of post-stroke depression on activities of daily living in a double-blind randomised treatment study. *Journal of Nervous and Mental Diseases*, **189**, 421–25.

Coughlan, A.K. and Hollows, S.E. (1985). *The adult memory and information processing battery.* St James' University Hospital, Leeds.

Cramer, S.C. and Bastings, G.P. (2000). Mapping clinically relevant plasticity after stroke. *Neuropharmacology*, **39**, 842–51.

Deane, M., Piggott, T. and Dearing, P. (1996). The value of the short form 36 score in the outcome assessment of subarachnoid haemorrhage. *British Journal of Neurosurgery*, **10**, 187–191.

Donnelly, S. (2002). The Rivermead Perceptual Assessment Battery: Can it predict functional performance?. *Australian Occupational Therapy Journal*, **49**, 71–81.

Dufouil, C., deKersaint, G.A., Besancon, L., Alperovitch, A., *et al.* (2001). Longitudinal study of blood pressure and white matter hyperintensities: the EVA MRI cohort. *Neurology*, **56**, 921–6.

Duschek, S., Hadjamu, M., and Schandry, R. (2007a). Enhancement of cerebral blood flow and cognitive performance following pharmacological blood pressure elevation in chronic hypotension. *Psychophysiology*, **44**, 145–153.

Duschek, S., Hadjamu, M., and Schandry, R. (2007b). Dissociation between cortical activation and cognitive performance under pharmacological blood pressure elevation in chronic hypotension. *Biological Psychology*, **75**, 277–285.

Edgeworth, J. A., Robertson, I. H. and McMillan, T. M. (1998). *Manual for the balloons test.* Thames Valley Test Company Limited, Bury St Edmunds.

Elkins, J., Knopman, D. S., Yaffe, K., Johnston, S. C. (2005). Cognitive function predicts first-time stroke and heart disease. *Neurology*, **64**, 1750–1755.

Ellis-Hill, C.S., and Horn, S. (2000). Change in identity and self-concept: A new theoretical approach to recovery following a stroke. *Clinical Rehabilitation*, **14**, 279–287.

Folstein, M. F., Folstein, S. E. and McHeugh, P. R. (1975). "Mini-mental state: a practical method for grading the cognitive state of outpatients for the clinician. *Journal of Psychiatric Research*, **12**, 189–98.

Gibbs, R.G., Newson, R., Lawrenson, R., Greenhalgh, R.M., and Davies, A.H. (2001). Diagnosis and initial management of stroke and transient ischaemic attack across UK health regions from 1992–1996: experience of a national primary care database. *Stroke*, **32**, 1085–90.

Geusgens, C.A.V., van Heugten, C.M., Cooijmans, P.J., Jolles, J. and van den Heuvel, W.J.A. (2007). Transfer effects of a cognitive strategy training for stroke patients with apraxia. *Journal of Clinical and Experimental Neuropsychology*, **29**, 831–841.

Hama, S. Yamashita, H., Shigenobu, M., Watanabe, A., Hiramoto, K, Kurisu, K. *et al.* (2007a). Depression or apathy and functional recovery after stroke. *International Journal of Geriatric Psychiatry*, **22**, 1046–1051.

Hama, S., Yamashita, H., Shigenobu, M., Watanabe, A., Kurisu, K., Yamawaki, S., *et al.* (2007b). Kitaoka, Tamotsu1Post-stroke affective of apathetic depression and lesion location: Left frontal lobe and bilateral basal ganglia. *European Archives of Psychiatry and Clinical Neuroscience*, **257**, 149–152.

Harris, J.G. and Filley, C.M. (2001). CADASIL: neuropsychological findings in three generations of an affected family. *Journal of the International Neuropsychological Society*, **7**, 768–774.

Hart, C.L., Hole, D.J. and Smith, G.D. (2001). The relation between questions indicating transient ischaemic attack and stroke in 20 years of follow-up in men and women in the renfrew/paisley study. *Journal of Epidemiological Community Health*, **55**, 653–6.

Hillis, A.E., Barker, P.B., Beauchamp, N.J., Gordon, B. and Wityk, R.J. (2000). MR perfusion imaging reveals regions of hypoperfusion associated with aphasia and neglect. *Neurology*, **55**, 782–8.

Jehkonen, M., Ahonen, J.P., Dastidar, P., Koivisto, A.M. *et al.* (2000). Visual neglect as a predictor of functional outcome one year after stroke. *Acta Neurologica Scandinavica*, **101**, 193–201.

Kilander, L., Nyman, H, Boberg, M. and Lithell, H. (2000). The association between low diastolic blood pressure in middle age and cognitive function in old age. *A population-based study. Age & Ageing*, **29**, 243–8.

Kivipelto, M., Helkala, E.L., Hanninen, T., Laakso, M.P. *et al.* (2001). Midlife vascular risk factors and late-life mild cognitive impairment: a population-based study. *Neurology*, **56**, 1683–89.

Klavora, P., Heslegrave, R.J. and Young, M. (2000). Driving skills in elderly persons with stroke: comparison of two new assessment options. *Archives of physical and medical rehabilitation*, **81**, 701–5.

Kondziolka, D., Wechsler, L., Goldstein, S. Meltzer, C. *et al.* (2000). Transplantation of cultured human neuronal cells for patients with stroke. *Neurology*, **55**, 565–9.

Li, G, Rhew, I.C., Shofer, J.B., Kukull, W.A., *et al.* (2007). Age-varying association between blood pressure and risk of dementia in those aged 65 and older: A community-based prospective cohort study. *Journal of the American Geriatrics Society*, **55**, 1161–1167.

Li, Y.S., Meyer, J.S. and Thornby, J. (2001). Longitudinal follow-up of depressive symptoms among normal versus cognitively impaired elderly. *International Journal of Geriatric Psychiatry*, **16**, 718–27.

Lincoln, N.B., Radford, K.A., Lee, E.,2 and Reay, A.C. (2006). The assessment of fitness to drive in people with dementia. *International Journal of Geriatric Psychiatry*, **21**, 1044–1051.

Lunn, S., Crawley, F., Harrison, M.J., Brown, M.M. and Newman, S.P. (1999). Impact of carotid endarterectomy upon cognitive functioning. A systematic review of the literature. *Cerebrovascular Disease*, **9**, 74–81.

McDougall, F. and Brayne, C. (2007). Systematic review of the depressive symptoms associated with vascular conditions. *Journal of Affective Disorders*, **104**, 25–35.

McFarlane J., Welch J. and Rodgers J. (2006). Severity of Alzheimer's disease and effect on premorbid measures of intelligence. *British Journal of Clinical Psychology*, **45**, 453–463.

McManus, J., and Stott, D. (2005). Small-vessel cerebrovascular disease in older people. *Reviews in Clinical Gerontology*, **15**, 207–217.

Majid, M. J., Lincoln, N. B. and Weyman, N. (2000). Cognitive rehabilitation for memory deficits following stroke. *Cochrane database systematic reviews 2000*, **3**: CD002293.

Mathias, J.L., Bowden S.C., and Barrett-Woodbridge, M. (2007). Accuracy of the Wechsler Test of Adult Reading (WTAR) and National Adult Reading Test (NART) when estimating IQ in a healthy Australian sample. *Australian Psychologist*, **42**, 49–56.

Mathias J.L., Bowden S.C., Bigler E.D., and Rosenfeld J.V. (2007). Is performance on the Wechsler test of adult reading affected by traumatic brain injury?. *British Journal of Clinical Psychology*, **46**, 457–466.

Nelson, H. (1982). *The national adult reading test.* NFER-Nelson, Windsor.

Nilsson S.E., Read S., Berg S., Johansson B., Mel ander. A., and Lindblad U. (2005). Low systolic blood pressure is associated with impaired cognitive function in the oldest old: longitudinal observations in a population-based sample 80 years and older. *Aging Clinical Experimental Research*, **19**, 41–47.

Oddy, M, Coughlan, A.K. and Crawford, J. (2007). The BIRT memory and information processing battery. BIRT; West Sussex, UK.

O'Sullivan, M, Morris, R.G. and Markus, H. S. (2005). Brief cognitive assessment for patients with cerebral small vessel disease. *Journal of Neurology, Neurosurgery & Psychiatry*, **76**, 1140–1145.

Oxlad, M., and Wade, T. (2008). Longitudinal risk factors for adverse psychological functioning six months after coronary artery bypass graft surgery. *Journal of Health Psychology*, **13**, 79–92.

Peters, R., Beckett, N., Nunes, M., Fletcher, A., Forette, F. and Bulpitt, C. (2006). A substudy protocol of the hypertension in the very elderly trial assessing cognitive decline and dementia incidence (hyvet-cog): an ongoing randomised, double-blind, placebo-controlled trial. *Drugs and Aging*, **23**, 83–92.

Prins, N.D., van Dijk, E.J., den Heijer, T, Vermeer, S.E., Jolles, J., Koudstaal, P.J., *et al.* (2005). Cerebral small-vessel disease and decline in information processing speed, executive function and memory. *Brain*, **128**, 2034–2041.

Raven, J.C. (1977). *Manuals for Raven's progressive and coloured matrices.* Lewis & Co, London.

Robertson, I. H. and Marshall, J. C. (eds). (1993). *Unilateral neglect: clinical and experimental studies.* LEA, Hove.

Robinson, R.G., Schultz, S.K., Castillo, C., Kopel, T *et al.* (2000). Nortryptyline versus fluoxetine in the treatment of depression and in short-term recovery after stroke: a placebo-controlled, double-blind, study. *American Journal of Psychiatry*, **157**, 351–9.

Sheldrick, R., Tarrier, N., Berry, E. and Kincey, J. (2006). Post-traumatic stress disorder and illness perceptions over time following myocardial infarction and subarachnoid haemorrhage. *British Journal of Health Psychology*, **11**, 387–400.

Shindo K., Sugiyama K., Huabao L., Nishijima K., Kondo T., and Izumi S. (2007). Long-term effect of low-frequency repetitive transcranial magnetic stimulation over the unaffected posterior parietal cortex in patients with unilateral spatial neglect. *Journal of Rehabilitation Medicine*, **38**, 65–7.

Skilbeck, C. E. (1996). Psychological aspects of stroke. In *Handbook of the clinical psychology of ageing* (ed R.T. Woods), pp. 283–301. Wiley, Chichester.

Skilbeck, C. E. (2000). Strategies for the rehabilitation of cognitive loss in late life due to stroke. In *Cognitive rehabilitation in old age* (eds R.D. Hill, L. Backman and A. S. Neely), pp. 270–290. Oxford University Press, New York.

Skilbeck, C.E., Allen, E.A., and Brechin, D. (2005). NART prediction and impairment in neurological patients. *Neuropsychological Rehabilitation*, **15**, 69–75.

Tidswell, P., Dias, P. S., Sagar, H. J. *et al.* (1995). Cognitive outcome after aneurysm rupture: relationship to aneurysm site and perioperative complications. *Neurology*, **45**, 875–82.

Trompetto, C., Assini, A., Buccolieri, A., Marchese, R. and Abbruzzese, G. (2000). Motor Recovery following stroke: a transcranial magnetic stimulation study. *Clinical Neurophysiology*, **111**, 1860–67.

Van Boxtel, M.P.J., Baars, L., and Jolles, J. (2007). Obesity, blood pressure and cognitive function. A reply to Waldstein and Katzel. *International Journal of Obesity*, **31**(7), Jul 2007, 1186.

Vikelis, M., Xifaras, M., Mitsikostas, D. (2006). *CADASIL: A short review of the literature and a description of the first family from Greece. Functional Neurology*, **21**, 77–82.

Viswanathan, A., Gschwendtner, A., Guichard, J.-P., Buffon, F., Cumurciuc, R., O'Sullivan, M. *et al.* (2007). Lacunar lesions are independently associated with disability and cognitive impairment in CADASIL. *Neurology*, **69**, 72–179.

Wade, D.T., Langton-Hewer, R., Skilbeck, C.E., Bainton, D. and Burns-Cox, C. (1985). Controlled trial of home-care service for acute stroke patients. *Lancet*, Feb, 323–6.

Waldstein, S.R., Brown, J.R.P., Maier, K.J., and Katzel, L.I. (2005). Diagnosis of Hypertension and high blood pressure levels negatively affect cognitive function in older adults. *Annals of Behavioral Medicine*, **29**(3), 174–180.

Walker, S. (1992). Assessment of language dysfunction. In *A handbook of neuropsychological assessment* (eds J. R. Crawford, D.M. Parker **and** W.W McKinlay), pp 177–221. LEA, Hove, UK.

Wang, S.L., Pan, W.H., Lee, M.C., Cheng, S.P. and Chang, M.C. (2000). Predictors of survival among elders suffering strokes in taiwan: observation from a nationally representative sample. *Stroke*, **31**, 2354–60.

Wang, Y., Lim, L.L., Levi, C., Heller, R.F. and Fischer, J. (2001). A prognostic index for 30-day mortality after stroke. *Journal of clinical epidemiology*, **54**, 766–73.

Wechsler, D. (1997). *Manual for the wechsler adult intelligence scale-*III. Psychological Corporation, New York.

Wechsler, D. (1997). *Manual for the wechsler memory scale-*III. Psychological Corporation, New York.

Wharton W., Hirshman E., Merritt P., Stangl B., Scanlin K., and Krieger L. (2006). Lower blood pressure correlates with poorer performance on visuospatial attention tasks in younger individuals. *Biological Psychology*, **73**, 227–234.

Whiting, S., Lincoln, N., Bhavnani, G. and Cockburn, J. (1985). *The Rivermead perceptual assessment battery: manual*. NFER-Nelson, Windsor.

Wilson, B., Cockburn, J. and Halligan, P. (1987). The behavioural inattention test: manual. Thames Valley Test Co, Fareham.

Wilz, G. and Barskova, T. (2007). Evaluation of a cognitive behavioral group intervention program for spouses of stroke patients. *Behaviour Research and Therapy*, **45**, 2508–2517.

Zimmerman, L., Barnason, S., Schulz, P., Nieveen, J., Miller, C.m., Hertzog, M. *et al.* (2007). The effects of a symptom management intervention on symptom evaluation, physical functioning, and physical activity for women after coronary artery bypass surgery. *Journal of Cardiovascular Nursing*, **22**, 493–500.

Further reading

Hill, R.D. and Backman, L. (eds) (2000). *Cognitive rehabilitation in old age*. Oxford University Press, New York.

Robinson, Robert G. (2006). The clinical neuropsychiatry of stroke: cognitive, behavioral, and emotional disorders after vascular brain injury (2nd Ed.). Cambridge University Press, Cambridge, UK.

Robertson, I.H. and Marshall, J.C. (eds) (1993). *Unilateral neglect: clinical and experimental studies*. LEA, Hove, UK.

Waldstein, S.R. and Elias, M.F. (eds) (2001). *Neuropsychology of cardiovascular disease*. LEA, New Jersey.

Chapter 27

Neuropsychological presentation and treatment of traumatic brain injury

Nigel S. King and Andy Tyerman

1 Introduction

1.1 Clinical neuropsychology and head injury

Clinical neuropsychologists play a vital role in assessment and treatment after head injury across acute, rehabilitation and community settings, drawing upon both specialist neuropsychological knowledge and general clinical training. The British Psychological Society (1989) identified a number of key functions for clinical neuropsychologists: carrying out detailed assessments of cognition, emotion, behaviour and social competence; devising and implementing training programmes; liaising with educational agencies/employers to advise on the resumption of educational/vocational life; providing and advising about long-term care; and facilitating personal, family and social adjustment (British Psychological Society, 1989). In a further report (British Psychological Society, 2005) key recommendations included the need for: a brain injury service network/care pathways; early assessment and treatment by specialist staff; specialist facilities for people with high physical dependence, severe challenging behaviour and for those who are minimally responsive; post-acute community rehabilitation service; and integration of brain injury and vocational rehabilitation services.

In the acute setting clinical neuropsychologists are usually based in regional neurosciences centres, working closely with neurosurgical and nursing staff during the acute admission. They will often see patients for more detailed assessment as out-patients at a 'post-acute' stage when the attention has shifted more towards cognitive and other psychological changes. Clinical neuropsychologists working in rehabilitation in the U.K. were based originally primarily within regional in-patient neurological rehabilitation centres or specialist units in the independent sector for the management of severe behavioural difficulties. However, they are now commonly based in generic physical disability teams, specialist community brain injury rehabilitation services and specialist centres for cognitive and vocational rehabilitation after brain injury.

1.2 Epidemiology

The annual incidence of hospital admission after head injury is estimated to be 229 per 100,000 in England: 356 per 100,000 for children (aged 0–15); 178 per 100,000 for adults (aged 16–75); and 384 per 100,000 for older adults (aged 75 and over) (Tennett, 2005). Whilst 75–85% of such injuries are mild in nature (Miller & Jones, 1985; Kraus & Nourjah, 1988), the incidence of moderate or severe TBI is estimated to be 25 per 100,000 (RCP/BSRM, 2003). The range of outcomes is huge, from complete recovery to persistent coma or death.

Serious disability from head injury occurs in an estimated 150 per 100,000 of the population in England and Wales (British Society of Rehabilitation Medicine, 1998), with an estimated 210 totally disabled and 1500 severely or profoundly disabled every year. One family in 300 is thought to have a member with persisting disability following a head injury (Lancet, 1983). A large proportion of head injury involves young males aged 18-25. Whilst rates vary with severity and geography, the most common causes of injury are road traffic accidents (RTAs), assaults, falls, occupational accidents and recreational accidents.

The disabilities associated with severe and very severe head injuries are extremely varied encompassing both physical disability (i.e. motor and sensory deficits) and psychological changes (e.g. cognitive impairment, altered emotional response and loss of behavioural control). These often impact not only on the injured person but also on the family and wider psychosocial networks. The vast majority of rehabilitation services are therefore targeted on the more severely injured.

1.3 Severity of head injury

The severity of a head injury is usually measured by: i) *depth of unconsciousness* -usually measured immediately after resuscitation, using the Glasgow Coma Scale (GCS) (Appendix 1); ii) *length of post traumatic amnesia (PTA)* - the period of time between receiving a head injury and regaining continuous day-to-day memory for events; iii). *length of unconsciousness* (i.e. GCS <9); and/or iv) *presence of neurological signs* (e.g. paresis, damage revealed by neuro-imaging techniques).

A widely accepted classification of severity is detailed in Table 27.1.

Table 27.1 Severity of head injury

Severity	Glasgow coma scale	Length of unconsciousness	Post-traumatic amnesia
Mild	13–15	<15 mins.	<1 hour
Moderate	9–12	15 mins.–6 hrs.	1–24 hours
Severe	3–8	>6 hrs.*	1–7 days
Very severe	N/a	*	1–4 weeks
Extremely severe	N/a	*	>4 weeks

*N.B. As many patients in extended coma are sedated and electively ventilated, it is often not possible to determine the duration of unconsciousness.

2 **Mild and moderate head injury**

2.1 **Pathophysiology**

For the majority of mild and moderately head injured patients there are no measurable pathophysiological changes. In some cases however temporary EEG abnormalities, reduced cerebral blood flow or temporary macroscopic lesions (revealed by CT or MRI) are present. These predominate in the frontal or temporal cortical areas and usually resolve within 3 months. Where apparently minor injuries are associated with neurologi-cal signs or complications, it is usually not appropriate to make a classification of 'mild' head injury. Such injuries should be classified according to the extent of neurological signs and/or complications.

2.2 **Clinical presentations and natural course**

Many with mild or moderate injuries experience few or no symptoms and make a full recovery within a few days. Approximately 50% will, however, experience post concus-sion symptoms (PCS)-headaches, dizziness, fatigue, irritability, poor concentration, nausea, sensitivity to light, sensitivity to noise, poor memory, sleep disturbance, tinnitus, slowed thinking, blurred/double vision, anxiety, depression, or frustration. These are caused by organic and/or psychological factors. For the majority, full recovery from PCS occurs within a few days to three months. However 6–8% have persisting PCS at and beyond 1 year post injury. Slow and/or incomplete recovery is associated with the following: >40 years old; pre-morbid psychopathology; previous head injury; pre-morbid alcohol/substance misuse; and female gender. When PCS do persist major psychosocial disabilities can result (King, 2003).

2.3 **Neuropsychological deficits**

The most common neuropsychological impairments following mild and moderate head injuries involve speed of information processing and divided attention (as measured by tests such as the Paced Auditory Serial Addition Task (PASAT) and Stroop Test). These types of impairments correlate well with severity of PCS and tend to mirror symptomatic recovery (i.e. recovery within three months of injury). Impairments in reaction time, verbal short term and long term memory (as measured by paragraph recall tests) and visuo-spatial short term and long term memory (as measured by figure recall tests) can also be present. These correlate less well with severity of PCS but also usually resolve within three months.

2.4 **Related emotional disorders**

The events which cause head injury are often precisely those where psychological trauma might also be expected. Post traumatic stress symptoms (PTS) are therefore quite com-mon and these often include phobic avoidance of situations where the injury occurred (e.g. driving). Whilst organic amnesia following head injury is thought to offer some protection against PTS the incidence of post traumatic stress disorder (PTSD) following RTA and mild head injury is similar to the equivalent non head injured population (20%). Frustration, depression and anxiety due to the psychosocial disabilities caused by persisting PCS are also common. A vicious cycle can easily develop where anxiety, depression or frustration exacerbates PCS and leads to reduced coping. This causes further distress and further exacerbation of PCS. They may also be exacerbated by uncertainty over the relative contribution of psychological and organic factors, particularly when symptoms persist and are of a chronic nature.

2.5 Treatment/Rehabilitation

Early assessment within 1–4 weeks of discharge is optimal and should include the following: assessment of the severity of head injury (e.g. by assessing the length of PTA); investigation of the extent and nature of PCS (e.g. using the Rivermead Post Concussion Symptoms Questionnaire); assessment of relevant premorbid factors (eg. neurological and psychological/psychiatric history); assessment of anxiety and depression symptoms (e.g. using the Hospital Anxiety & Depression Scale – HADS, Beck Depression Inventory – BDI; the Beck Anxiety Inventory - BAI); investigation of the extent and nature of any post traumatic stress symptoms (e.g. using the Revised Impact of Event Scale - IES); assessment of any co-morbid factors which might contribute to disabilities (eg. pain, orthopaedic injuries).

Intervention would normally focus on the provision of information, reassurance, education, support and regular monitoring of progress. The information should address: the normality of PCS; good prognosis; regulating and pacing activities in line with the severity of PCS (e.g. taking short breaks when PCS feel worse rather than trying to push on through until longer breaks become unavoidable); graduated return to work and premorbid activities; and education about the potential for developing the vicious cycle where stress and PCS becoming mutually exacerbating. The overall aim is to minimise the effects of anxiety, worry and stress on PCS by preventing the development of the vicious cycle. One single, hour long assessment and intervention session can be an effective intervention for the majority of cases (Wade *et al.* , 1998). Specialist psychological and medical interventions are appropriate for persisting problems with post-traumatic stress, headaches, dizziness, anxiety, depression, return to work difficulties, irritability, tinnitus or neuropsychological impairment.

When assessing and treating patients at later stages after their injury it is also important to investigate in some detail how their symptoms have developed over time (e.g., when symptoms were first noticed); whether any symptoms were present premorbidly; whether symptoms have improved, deteriorated, plateaued or remained constant over time. This will help in judging the relative contribution of organic and psychological factors in the sequelae presented. Interventions for those presenting with persisting post concussion symptoms should be preceded by the development of an individualised collaborative formulation of the patients' problems (King, 2003). This should focus on; i) helping the patient make sense of their symptoms, ii) aiding their understanding of the contributory factors involved in their problems and the interactions between them, and iii) the means by which their problems can be maximally ameliorated or managed.

For example a diagrammatic representation might be shared demonstrating how post concussion symptoms, post traumatic stress symptoms and orthopaedic pain symptoms may have become mutually exacerbating over time and led to reduced day to day coping, impoverished sleep, fatigue, increased anxieties/worries and the development of maladaptive cognitions like 'I'm going mad' or 'something wrong in my brain has been overlooked'. Component parts of the formulation might then be addressed in turn within the shared understanding of an agreed formulation.

2.6 Effectiveness

Studies evaluating the effectiveness of interventions for patients with mild and moderate head injuries are sparse. Randomised control trials in this area however have demonstrated that early intervention involving education, reassurance, support and monitoring of progress can reduce the incidence and severity of persisting post concussion symptoms. There is little hard evidence however to inform management guidelines when symptoms persist and become chronic. Later interventions are therefore mainly informed by experienced clinicians in the field rather than by empirical data.

3 Severe and very severe head injuries

There are two main types of severe injury - *open head injury and closed head injury.* Open head injury occurs when the skull and protective linings of the brain are damaged so that brain is exposed. Closed injury occurs when the skull and protective linings of the brain are not penetrated. The latter is by far the most common form of head injury in peace time.

3.1 Pathophysiology

There are two kinds of damage to the brain following severe forms of head injury-primary damage and secondary damage.

3.1.1 Primary damage

This includes diffuse white matter damage, contusion (bruising) and haemorrhage.

- Diffuse white matter damage is due to the widespread rupturing of axons caused mainly by the brain impacting against itself as it moves within the skull. This is usually the most prevalent form of damage.

- Contusion is usually most pronounced in the undersurfaces of the frontal and temporal poles where the shearing forces of the brain impacting upon the sharpest and most confined parts of skull are maximal. Contusion can also occur both under the direct point of impact of the injury and directly opposite it (contrecoup injury).

- Haemorrhage occurs when the blood vessels supplying oxygen to the brain are ruptured.

3.1.2 Secondary damage

This includes damage due to haematoma (collections of blood), cerebral haemorrhage leading to anoxic damage or death, sub-arachnoid haemorrhage, swelling, infection, hydrocephalus (build up of cerebro-spinal fluid) and hypoxic neural damage due to breathing difficulties or low blood pressure.

3.2 Clinical presentation and natural course

For the majority of severely injured patients improvement takes place slowly over months and years. It is usually best to use the word 'improvement' rather that 'recovery' after more severe injuries, as recovery implies complete restoration of function which may well not occur. Permanent cognitive impairments are probable with severe injuries, although for some they will be quite subtle and only evident under stress, in busy environments or on formal testing. Cognitive impairments are rarely absent after very severe injuries.

The rate and extent of recovery is impossible to predict early on and the process is not fully understood. It may involve the following: i) resolution of brain swelling and contusion, leading to restoration of neuronal efficiency; ii) disrupted neurotransmitters regaining some of their original efficiency; iii) damaged neurones repairing themselves/axonal sprouting; and possibly iv) some degree of neural plasticity for very widely distributed functions (e.g. language).

Typically the majority of recovery occurs in the first two years after injury such that significant difficulties evident at two years rarely resolve completely thereafter. However, further small amounts of natural recovery can occur up to and beyond five years for the more severe injuries. Adaptation to long-term disability is therefore an ongoing process and can result in improved function many years post-injury, especially when early rehabilitation has been limited.

3.3 Neuropsychological impairments

When physical disabilities (such as paresis, ataxia, dysarthria, dyspraxia or reduced motor speed) are present, they are often the main concern for the patient during the first months after injury. Cognitive impairments, however, tend to have greater impact on long term disability and handicap. These occur predominantly in the areas of attention, speed of information processing, explicit memory and executive functioning. They reflect the most common areas of damage in the frontal and temporal cortical areas and with diffuse axonal shearing.

3.3.1 Attention

Impairments in speed of information processing are one of the most common deficits following severe head injury. These are often evident on tests like the PASAT, BIRT Memory & Information Processing Battery (BMIPB), Stroop Test or Wechsler Adult Intelligence Scale III (WAIS-III) Digit Symbol Coding sub-test. They may also be evident on tests requiring speed (e.g. WAIS-III Performance sub-tests or Trail Making Test).

Specific deficits in divided, selective or sustained attention may be evident on tests like the Test of Everyday Attention, WAIS-III Picture Completion sub-test and Trail Making Test. Verbal active attention span is often impaired as evidenced by backward digit span deficits. Visuo-spatial attention span deficits may also be evident on tests like the Corsi Block Tapping Test. These deficits can cause reported problems with concentration, distractibility, tasks requiring more effort, memory, fatigue, irritability, reduced speed of thinking and increased error rates.

3.3.2 Memory

Short term and long term memory deficits are common for both verbal and visuo-spatial material. Verbal memory deficits are often indicated by impaired performance on paragraph recall tests and list learning tests (e.g. Wechsler Memory Scale III (WMS III) Paragraphs, WMS III Paired Associate Learning Test, BMIPB Story Recall and List Learning Tests). Visuo-spatial memory deficits are commonly indicated on measures like Figure Recall Tests (e.g. Rey Complex Figure, BMIPB Figure Recall). Remote memory and procedural/implicit memory functions are usually spared. Memory difficulties are therefore usually for new, explicit learning rather than from previously learned material, overlearned procedures and autobiographical memory. Some of the most commonly reported memory difficulties include not being able to remember conversations, appointments, reading material, peoples' names, new routes or where things have been put. The patient may also have been told that they repeat themselves a lot.

3.3.3 Executive

Executive impairment following severe head injury is common. It is not unusual however for there to be little such evidence on formal testing - neuropsychological assessment is by its very nature highly structured and is conducted in a distraction-free setting. Therefore, judgements on executive impairments must often be inferred from behavioural observations, qualitative aspects of test performance and reported observations by those close to the patient or other health care professionals. The patient's own reports are of the utmost importance but difficulties with insight can often mean that they, themselves are unaware of such deficits. Psychological denial of problems is a natural coping mechanism but can be mistaken for dysexecutive problems in some cases. Similarly, reports from those close to the patient may minimise difficulties due to their own psychological denial, in addition to the natural tendency to underplay the significance of difficulties early post-injury in the aftermath of major trauma.

Deficits in cognitive flexibility, mental set shifting and perseveration may be indicated on tests such as the Trail Making Test, Wisconsin Card Sorting Test, Stroop Test, Verbal Fluency Test or Card Sorting sub-test of the Behavioural Assessment of Dysexecutive Syndrome (BADS).

Verbal concept formation and verbal abstract thinking deficits may be evident on tests like the WAIS-III Similarities sub test and on proverbs tasks (e.g. from the WAIS-III Comprehension sub test). Planning and problem solving deficits may be evident on tests like the Six Elements, Zoo Search and Motor Action Program sub tests of the BADS and by the quality of performance on tests like the WAIS-III Block Design sub test and the copy task of figure recall tests.

Insight difficulties may be highlighted through large discrepancies between patient and others' reports of problems. Assessment of insight may be aided by separate administration of standard problem schedules with patients and family members as part of routine assessment. Specific questionnaires may also highlight cognitive, behavioural and emotional problems associated with executive impairments (e.g. Dex questionnaire from the BADS).

Observed problems in executive functioning might include difficulties with social regulation, fragmented speech, reduced abstract reasoning, fixed and concrete thinking, poor initiation, egocentricity, reduced creativity, tangential speech, reduced insight or difficulties with organising thoughts, decision-making, problem solving and in adapting to new situations.

3.3.4 Language

Pure language and dysphasic impairments following uncomplicated head injury are less common than attentional, memory and executive impairments. Indeed some language based tests are used as 'hold' measures to help estimate pre-morbid levels of intellectual functioning, due to their resistance to the effects of brain injury of a generalised nature (e.g. National Adult Reading Test, WAIS-III Vocabulary sub test). Problems with word finding, sentence construction paraphasias however are common language based impairments.

3.3.5 Visual perception

Visual perceptual impairments following uncomplicated head injury are rare. A small but significant proportion may have visuo-constructional difficulties but visual agnosias are not often seen. However patients may be slow in their processing of visual material.

A wide range of cognitive impairments are therefore seen after severe head injury. It can often be difficult to predict their specific impact upon an individual's life after head injury as such deficits typically form part of a complex interaction of cognitive and other disabilities. Management and resultant long-term impact of cognitive impairment is also mediated by level of insight, the use of compensatory strategies and the extent of concomitant behavioural and emotional difficulties.

3.3.6 Neuro-behavioural problems

An extensive array of behavioural change is often reported after severe head injury including increased irritability, disinhibition, impulsivity, emotional lability, mood swings and aggressive outbursts. Deficits in executive functioning (leading to lack of insight, egocentricity, poor social regulation and low initiation) often mean that a head injured patient's personality are seen as significantly changed, by both themselves and by others. In addition, problems arising from other impairments such as fatigue, low drive, frustration, irritability, reduced emotional and behavioural control, may lead to a very significant sense of changed personality. The wide range of behavioural changes observed, reflect the interaction of primary neurological damage and secondary psychological reactions to head injury and its effects.

3.4 Related emotional disorders

Short and long term emotional sequelae of severe head injury include the following:

i) post traumatic stress reactions (PTS) relating to the events which caused or followed the head injury (e.g. road traffic accidents, assaults etc). While unconsciousness and organic amnesia from severe injury can protect against PTS, this is not always the case. The prevalence of PTSD (3–6%), however, is almost certainly much less than in mild or moderate head injury.

ii) anger, frustration, depression and anxiety are common emotional responses to the disabilities that patients confront. For some this may be an early reaction to the trauma of neurological illness/injury, the loss of skills, roles and control over one's life, the slow pace of progress and the uncertain extent of future recovery. Reduced impulse control may also exacerbate the control of anger, irritability and aggression. However, early in rehabilitation, many may appear unconcerned about their predicament due to limited insight into the extent of cognitive and emotional/behavioural changes, together with unrealistic expectations of a full recovery.

iii) major distress in adjusting to and coming to terms with the losses and changes arising as a result of a head injury e.g. break up of relationships, inability to return to work, shattered aspirations and ambitions, changes in personality and sense of identity. These responses often develop over many years as changes and disabilities become emotionally 'accepted' by the patients as being permanent.

3.5 Social and family consequences

The complex array of disability after head injury often has far-reaching social consequences. Those with the most severe injuries may require assistance in daily living. This may include practical assistance in personal and domestic care for those with severe physical disability and guidance or supervision for those with marked cognitive or personality changes. Others may be independent in daily care but unable to travel independently, or need help from the family in making decisions or managing their financial affairs. Leisure pursuits are often compromised by motor, sensory and cognitive difficulties. Friendships and social opportunities often decline progressively over subsequent years. This may be due to a combination of loss of confidence, low mood, intolerance to noise or difficulty in contributing to conversations on the part of the patient, and embarrassment and unease on the part of others in response to unpredictable behaviour and loss of refinement in social skills.

Many people with severe head injury are unable to return to previous occupation due to a wide range of difficulties (BSRM/JCP/RCP, 2004). Reduced speed, poor concentration, unreliable memory, headaches and/or fatigue combine to render many uncompetitive in their work. Specific physical, sensory and/or cognitive difficulties (e.g. seizures, visual field loss, executive or communication difficulties) may restrict or preclude a return to occupations where such skills are vital. Executive difficulties may also limit awareness of restrictions and the effective use of coping strategies in the workplace. Emotional difficulties may reduce the capacity to cope with pressure or responsibility, irritability or frustration may cause difficulties in work relationships. Disinhibited or aggressive behaviour is rarely tolerated in the workplace. Difficulties may arise gradually after a seemingly successful initial return to work or later on moving to a new job.

The social impact for the patient is often paralleled by major impact upon the family. High levels of stress and distress for primary carers are common, tending to increase rather than decrease over time after very severe injuries. Couple relationships often become strained with increased discord and high rates of breakdown after more severe injuries. For couples who remain together, there is often a reduction in emotional intimacy and a lower frequency and satisfaction in sexual relations. Spouses may struggle to cope with competing needs of work, home, partner and children, whilst parents may find themselves locked into a long-term caring role for their adult children, with major concerns about the future. The impact on children and siblings can also be marked but tends to be more variable. Many families face far-reaching changes in roles and relationships and disruption to overall family functioning. As life revolves around the needs of the patient, so the occupational, leisure and social lives of family members often falters (cf. Oddy & Herbert, 2008).

3.6 **Treatment/Rehabilitation**

The focus of neuropsychological rehabilitation varies according to the nature and severity of injury, the patients' psychosocial context, the clinical setting (e.g. acute, post-acute or community) and time since injury. It is essentially a process by which creative and practical solutions are found to minimise the unique neuropsychological, emotional, social and vocational difficulties faced by the patient. The process emanates from, and is constantly informed by a thorough understanding of clinical neuropsychology in general and the specific cognitive strengths and weaknesses of the patient in particular. Neuropsychological understanding therefore provides both the bedrock and the framework for this approach. Early rehabilitation optimises outcome, but late rehabilitation can also improve function significantly. Two key principles underpin rehabilitation and these centre around the formation of effective therapeutic relationships and the development of insight and understanding: i) engaging and maintaining patient (and family) involvement with rehabilitation services by the provision of an emotionally supportive environment and relationships within which empathic expert help can be easily accessed and ii) increasing patients' (and their family's) understanding of head injury, their strengths and weaknesses and the means by which impairments may be best managed.

These principles become increasingly important as the patient moves beyond acute settings to post-acute and community settings where engagement with services may be impeded by poor insight, lack of understanding, psychological denial, emotional disorder or challenging behaviour.

There are at least four important aspects of the process of rehabilitation: i) engaging the patient (and their family) in the rehabilitation process; ii) facilitating the setting of realistic rehabilitation targets and goals; iii) facilitating the achievement of targets and goals via co-ordinated interventions; and iv) evaluating, reviewing and modifying targets and goals over time.

Successful engagement of a patient (and their family) is often linked intrinsically to the collaborative development of realistic targets and goals. It is common for the patient (and their family), initially, to have unrealistic expectations about the extent and pace of targets that are achievable (e.g. complete cognitive recovery or return to full time work within weeks of injury). These commonly need to be negotiated to allow for more time, a greater number of intervening targets or the inclusion of additional forms of support. Formal goal planning procedures may help this process, although there is no consistent evidence as yet that they affect outcomes (Levack *et al.* , 2005).

The principles which should guide the setting of goals and targets should include the following: i) the maintenance and development of appropriate levels of cognitive stimulation while avoiding cognitive overloading; ii) education and minimisation of the vicious cycle of cognitive impairments leading to reduced coping, leading to distress, leading to exacerbated cognitive impairments etc.; iii). the emphasis of cognitive rehabilitation through compensatory strategies and prostheses rather than through cognitive restoration and 'brain function therapy'(i.e. de-emphasising the analogy that the brain operates like a muscle and discouraging inappropriate attempts to train unaffected brain areas to take over damaged areas); iv) the provision of emotional support and specific psychological interventions for the emotional sequelae associated with head injuries for both the patient and their family; v) facilitating patients and families adjustment to changes in personality, identity and psychosocial functioning; and vi) liaison with education and vocational systems to advise on and plan return to previous work or education.

Co-ordination and review of interventions is essential so that there is continuous feedback between professionals, patient and family. This helps interventions to remain focused on mutually agreed goals and targets and goals to be refined and modified as the patient progresses and circumstances change.

The use of groups for cognitive rehabilitation, education and emotional support should not be underestimated. These allow peer support, sharing of cognitive and emotional coping responses and an opportunity to provide formal education in an efficient way. They can be a very powerful and supportive means for developing insight into impairments and for exploring ways of minimising disability.

Cognitive rehabilitation strategies which benefit patients with severe head injury are usually pragmatic in nature. Neuropsychological assessment, however, provides vital information for knowing what strategies should be attempted, what modifications might be beneficial, what might cause strategies to be unsuccessful, how to develop new strategies and what kind of advice and education is appropriate. The following list highlights frequent examples of management strategies for common areas of difficulty: general cognitive function; memory; executive function; behaviour difficulties; social skills. There is of course significant overlap between these areas.

3.6.1 General cognitive strategies

- *Developing habits, routines and over-learnt procedures* to:
  i) maximise the use of implicit and procedural memory functions;
  ii) provide structure; and
  iii) minimise cognitive load.
- *Developing a tidy living and working environment* where belongings are kept in the same, intuitively obvious, places and can easily be found. This helps to minimise demand on memory and problem solving skills and make maximum use of spared implicit memory.
- *Taking many small breaks when impairments become apparent* rather than 'pushing on' until forced to take a break due to 'cognitive overload'.
- *Rearranging working environments* to minimise background noise, 'busyness', unexpected events and time pressures. This helps to reduce restrictions arising from attentional deficits, slow speed of information processing and cognitive inflexibility.
- *Graduated return to premorbid activities and minimisation of non-essential activity* to reduce cognitive overload and fatigue. This maximises the chances of successful completion of activities.
- *Identifying specific times, or specific types of activity* where fatigue, irritability, anxiety or frustration occur and facilitating appropriate changes in these areas.
- *Training the patient to allow extra time* for tasks where temporal judgement or speed of information processing is reduced.
- Using a diary systematically as
  i) an aide-memoire,
  ii) a means of structuring time,
  iii) an orientation 'anchor',
  iv) an aid to overcoming initiation difficulties or
  v) a reminder of key messages, conclusions and 'self statements' from therapy.

3.6.2 Strategies for managing memory

- *Using a dictaphone/tape recorder* to record meetings, lectures, etc (i.e. as an aide-memoire).
- *Using a watch with an alarm or a paging device* as a cue to look in a diary, or perform particular tasks. (This may also increase immediate arousal levels sufficiently to overcome initiation impairments).

- *Systematically using written or photo journals* for episodic memory deficits (i.e. memory for events).
- *Using notes, calendars and lists* as external cues and reminders. These may also help with initiation difficulties.
- *Introduce a noticeboard or white board in a prominent place* in the home to prompt patients about specific actions, as well as daily/weekly schedules.
- *Systematising storage of household items with explicit labelling (e.g. colour coding)* (such strategies are especially important for safety of toxic substances for patients with visual agnosia).
- *Using errorless learning* when teaching new skills to minimise the need to 'unlearn' mistakes (i.e. prompting and cueing in such a way that no errors are made during a training process).
- *Developing internal memory strategies* via repetition, association, chunking, visualisation of verbal material, verbalisation of visual material; and/or maximising the relevance and depth of understanding (of material). It should be noted however that the degree of cognitive effort required for such 'internal' memory strategies often exceeds their utility for patients with memory and executive impairments. They can, however, be useful for specific tasks like remembering names of people or studying for an exam where external strategies are inappropriate.
- *Using principles from behavioural psychology* such as shaping, modelling, chaining, and contingent reinforcement, to maximise learning of new skills.

3.6.3 Strategies for executive difficulties

- *Providing problem solving skills training* to help develop an explicit and systematic approach to solving difficulties e.g.:
  - i) defining the problem to be overcome;
  - ii) generating different strategies to overcome problem;
  - iii) highlighting the pros and cons of each strategy;
  - iv) deciding the best strategy based on the pros and cons;
  - v) implementing the strategy; and
  - vi) evaluating the outcome.
- *Using an alarmed stopwatch* to help patients monitor the amount of time taken on given tasks to help planning and temporal judgement impairments.
- *Using self talk and self instruction (verbal mediation)* to help overcome initiation problems and to remind the patient of self statements for aiding social regulation.
- Breaking tasks down into their component steps with written instructions to reduce disabilities from planning deficits.
- *Introduce repeating routine/cycles* to reduce unnecessary decision-making (e.g. weekly menus; shopping lists, set times for visiting the gym etc.).

3.6.4 Strategies for behavioural management

- *Identifying a small range of people to provide behavioural feedback* to help modify inappropriate social behaviours. This should be done with careful and sensitive collaboration between the patient and those providing the feedback. (It is important to stress that the feedback should be immediate, concrete, supportive and constructive and aimed at very specific behaviours only).

- *Using a hand held counter* to aid the self monitoring of specified inappropriate social behaviours.

- *Using video feedback* to improve insight into specific inappropriate behaviours. As patients may be surprised or upset by being confronted visibly with inappropriate behaviours this should always:
    - i) be discussed and negotiated carefully with the patient;
    - ii) be undertaken in a controlled and supportive atmosphere; and
    - iii) be conducted with sufficient time allocated for debriefing immediately afterwards.

- *Using principles from behavioural psychology* to help shape, model and increase the frequency of appropriate social behaviours.

3.6.5 Strategies for social skills

- *Teaching conversation skills* for slowing, pacing and allowing 'thinking time' during interactions to help minimise word finding, sentence construction and concentration difficulties in conversation.

- *Teaching social skills* so that the patient is comfortable asking for things to be repeated during conversation when attention, memory or language deficits have caused them to lose track.

- *Encouraging others to use short sentences and high frequency words* and to allow enough time for the patient to reply to questions when word finding, attentional, receptive language or expressive language impairments are present.

- *Encouraging those close to patient to use closed, multiple choice type questions* rather than open ended questions where decision making and initiation of ideas is impaired.

3.6.6 Intervention for related emotional disorders

Psychological interventions for emotional disorders following head injury have largely been developed from the adult mental health field of clinical psychology and adapted to the specific challenges of this population. The most common forms of intervention include both individual and group therapies in the following areas: i) cognitive behavioural psychotherapy (CBT) with exposure and/or cognitive restructuring for post traumatic stress symptoms (with the possible adjunct of Serotonin Specific Re-uptake Inhibitor (SSRI) antidepressant medication following medical review); ii) CBT for anger management (with the possible adjunct of Carbamazepine or other mood stabilising medication); iii) CBT for anxiety and depression (with the possible adjunct of antidepressant medication); iv) anxiety management training and CBT for control of anxiety symptoms.

In utilising such interventions it is vital that the neuropsychological context and constraints are accommodated in the therapeutic process.

Alongside these types of interventions, there is a need for specialist 'neurorehabilitation counselling' to assist clients in their understanding and coping with the effects of head injury during the course of recovery. This is likely to involve provision of the following:

♦ general information and explanation about head injury; feedback about specific impairments; explanation of treatment rationale; negotiation of treatment goals; general advice and emotional support; promotion of insight, awareness and coping strategies; and progress review.

While the above list outlines some of the most commonly used interventions, it is in no way exhaustive. Also, it is essential that emotional disorders after head injury are addressed within the overall context of the head injury and patients' aspirations, hopes, social network and overall psychosocial circumstances. 'Atomising' their emotional experiences to a series of disorders or symptoms will not adequately address the complexity of emotional needs. Indeed, this principle must underpin all forms of rehabilitation for head injured patients.

3.6.7 Facilitating personal, vocational and family adjustment

Many persons with severe head injury face major challenges of adjustment as they are unable to resume their former work, family and social roles. The process of psychological adjustment is compounded by executive difficulties, especially lack of insight and reduced capacity for self-appraisal and problem solving, often combined with lack of emotional and behavioural control. Without specialist help many struggle to make the necessary adjustments to their residual disability and continue to strive for an unrealistic degree of recovery. Others make decisions which do not take due account of restrictions arising from head injury, leading to repeated failure, loss of confidence and self belief.

The need to support people with neurological conditions in making long-term psychological adjustments to altered personal, family and social circumstances is recognised in Quality Requirement 5 on 'Community Rehabilitation and Support' in the National Service Framework for Long-term Conditions (UK Department of Health, 2005). The National Clinical Guidelines on Rehabilitation following Acquired Brain Injury (RCP/ BSRM, 2003) include specific guidelines on individual and/or group neuropsychotherapeutic interventions to facilitate long-term psychological, family and social adjustment, including sexual relationships.

The provision of specialist 'neuropsychotherapy' requires the adaptation of standard psychotherapeutic techniques to take into account neuropsychological constraints of the person (cf. Tyerman & King, 2004). Our experience is that it is often possible to assist the person in moving from a position of denying, feeling controlled by (or of a sense of battling constantly with) one's disability and oneself, to a position of understanding and accommodation to disability and resultant personal and life changes sufficiently to deal constructively with their altered circumstances and move forward in their lives.

Return to education or employment represents for many a major decision, which can either facilitate positive adjustment or provoke a downward spiral of failure.

The National Service Framework for Long-term Conditions (UK Department of Health, 2005) includes a specific Quality Requirement on 'Vocational Rehabilitation'. This requires provision of:

- ◆ a coordinated multi-agency approach; routine identification of needs and vocational goals within local rehabilitation services; availability of specialist vocational rehabilitation programmes; and routine monitoring of vocational outcomes.

This is supported by guidelines on a co-ordinated inter-agency approach to vocational assessment and rehabilitation after brain injury (BSRM/JCP/RCP, 2004).

Those able to return to previous employment or training need a carefully managed process of return with advice and support in the workplace, close liaison with the employer (or tutor) and other agencies (e.g. Jobcentre Plus, Occupational Health), ongoing support and proactive review/follow-up (BSRM/JCP/RCP, 2004). For those unable to return to previous employment, a programme of specialist vocational rehabilitation may be required: to highlight vocational strengths and weaknesses; provided a graded return to alternative occupation; voluntary work trials to test out the viability of alternative occupations and refine coping strategies; assistance with job search/application and set up; and long-term supported placements with job coaching input as required (Tyerman *et al.* 2008).

It is vital to include the family as fully as possible in the process of rehabilitation. Close liaison with the family is essential both to obtain feedback about difficulties and progress in the home and to explain rehabilitation strategies, which can then be reinforced by family members. However, as set out in the National Service Framework for Long-term Conditions (UK Department of Health, 2005) family members need access to support both in their role as carer and in their own right. Family members may themselves need specialist advice and support in understanding and coping with the impact of severe head injury both upon themselves and the family as a whole. Kreutzer *et al.* (2002) for example, describe a brain injury family intervention commonly delivered through family, marital, individual or group therapy in combination with bibliotherapy. A wide range of family services is required to facilitate family adjustment including family education; individual and group family support; and specialist couple and family counselling.

3.6.8 Effectiveness

Studies evaluating the effectiveness of cognitive rehabilitation for patients with severe head injury are relatively sparse and frequently suffer from significant methodological constraints. There is some modest evidence that restorative techniques involving repeated practice of specific tasks in laboratory settings can be effective for improving some specific attention and language based functions. There is insufficient evidence, however, that any gains are generalised to everyday activities. Restorative strategies for other impairments have virtually no empirical support. In contrast, the current evidence suggests that compensatory strategies are effective in reducing everyday memory failures, minimising anxiety and increasing self-concept and quality of interpersonal relationships (Halligan and Wade, 2005). Behavioural approaches aimed at maximising skill acquisition and monitoring, including performance feedback and reinforcement, have also demonstrated their efficacy. It is these types of rehabilitation that generalise best to everyday life situations.

Cognitive rehabilitation programmes which have the strongest outcomes tend to be those combining early intervention, compensatory strategies and supported employment (Carney and Coudray, 2005). Our clinical experience is that neuropsychological interventions (including educational, cognitive, behavioural, psychotherapeutic and family components) are most effective when delivered as part of specialist inter-disciplinary brain injury rehabilitation programmes. There is evidence that multi-faceted post-acute rehabilitation programmes can significantly improve psycho-social outcome after severe head injury.

4 Summary and conclusions

Patients with head injury present with a complex interaction of cognitive, behavioural and emotional changes, which often exert a major impact upon their lives and the lives of their family.

After mild and moderate head injury cognitive impairments are usually of mild severity and temporary. Speed of information processing is most frequently affected but reaction time, short-term and long-term memory deficits are also common. Post-traumatic stress reactions are at least as prevalent as for those without head injury. Where post-concussion symptoms persist anxiety and depression are common reactions to the disabilities caused by these. Anxiety can also result from uncertainty over the relative contribution of psychological and organic factors to problems and the uncertainty of ultimate prognosis.

After severe head injury cognitive impairments are often wide spread, significant and permanent. They are most often in some or more of the following domains:

◆ speed of information processing; divided, selective and sustained attention; short-term and long-term memory; executive function; and expressive language (in terms of word finding and sentence construction).

Depression, anger, anxiety and frustration often result from the disabilities caused by severe head injury, while post-traumatic stress reactions are less prevalent than in mild/moderate injuries. Irritability, anger and aggression can be exacerbated by reduced impulse control. Difficulties in long-term adjustment are common, as are difficulties in marital, family and social relationships.

Specialist neuropsychological interventions are required across acute, post-acute and community settings if patients are to make and sustain their optimal recovery. For those with mild and moderate injury early brief assessment and intervention can help reduce further complications but individualised formulations are required when post concussion symptoms persist. Whilst patients with severe head injury often respond positively to rehabilitation and make marked improvement over a period of years, many are left with substantial psychological disability and associated social restrictions. Patients often struggle to maintain the full benefits of rehabilitation once active therapeutic involvement has been phased out, particularly those with executive difficulties. Even after long periods when patients have appeared settled, they may struggle to adapt to changes in work, family and social circumstances. As such, further intervention may be required from time to time throughout the whole of their life. Open door access to specialist rehabilitation and support is vital if patients and their families are to maintain optimal adjustment to the long-term effects of their injury.

Selective references

British Psychological Society (1989). *Services for adults patients with acquired brain injury.* Leicester: British Psychological Society.

British Psychological Society (2005). *Clinical Neuropsychology and Rehabilitation Services for Adults with Acquired Brain Injury.* Leicester: British Psychological Society - Division of Neuropsychology.

BSRM/JCP/RCP (2004). Vocational Assessment and Rehabilitation after Acquired Brain Injury. Inter-Agency Guidelines. (Edited by A Tyerman & MJ Meehan). *Inter-Agency Advisory Group on Vocational Rehabilitation after Brain Injury.* London: British Society of Rehabilitation Medicine, Jobcentre Plus and Royal College of Physicians.

British Society of Rehabilitation Medicine (1998). *Rehabilitation after traumatic brain injury.* A Working Party Report. London: British Society of Rehabilitation Medicine.

Carney N and Coudray H (2005). Cognitive rehabilitation outcomes for traumatic brain injury. In Halligan PW & Wade DT (eds). *Effectiveness of rehabilitation for cognitive deficits.* Oxford. Oxford University Press.

Department of Health (2005). *The National Service Framework for Long-term Conditions.* London: Department of Health. www.dh.gov.uk/longtermnsf.

Halligan P.W and Wade D.T (2005). *Effectiveness of rehabilitation for cognitive deficits.* Oxford. Oxford University Press.

King N.S (2003). The post concussion syndrome: clarity amid the controversy? *British Journal of Psychiatry,* **183,** 276–278.

Kraus J.F and Nourjah P (1988). The epidemiology of mild uncomplicated brain injury. *Trauma,* **28,** 1637–1643.

Kreutzer J.S., Kolakowsky-Hayner S.A., Demm S.R., and Meade M.A (2002). A structured approach to family intervention after brain injury. *Journal of Head Trauma Rehabilitation,* **17,** 349–367.

Lancet (1983). Caring for the disabled after head injury. *The Lancet,* II, 948–949.

Miller, J.D and Jones, P.A (1985). The work of a Regional Head Injury Service. *The Lancet,* May 18, 1141–1141.

Levack W.M.M., Taylor K., Siegert RJ., Dean S.G., McPherson K.M and Weatherall M (2005). Is goal planning in rehabilitation effective? A systematic review. *Clinical Rehabilitation,* **20,** 739–755.

Oddy M and Herbert C (2008). Brain injury and the family: A review. In A Tyerman & NS King (eds.). *Psychological approaches to rehabilitation after traumatic brain injury.* Oxford: BPS Blackwell.

RCP/BSRM (2003). *Rehabilitation following acquired brain injury: national clinical guidelines* (Turner-Stokes L, ed.). London: Royal College of Physicians/British Society of Rehabilitation Medicine

Tennett A (2005). Admission to hospital following head injury in England: Incidence and socio-economic determinants. *BioMedCentral Public Health* (March 2005), 5, 21.

Tyerman A and King N.S (2004). Interventions for psychological problems after brain injury. In LH. Goldstein & J. McNeil (eds.). *Clinical Neuropsychology. A Practical Guide to Assessment & Management for Clinicians.* Chichester: Wiley.

Tyerman A., Tyerman R., and Viney P (2008). Vocational rehabilitation programmes. In A. Tyerman & NS. King. (eds.). *Psychological approaches to rehabilitation after traumatic brain injury.* Oxford: BPS Blackwell.

Wade D.T., King, N.S., Wenden, F.S., Crawford, S., and Caldwell, F.E (1998). Routine follow-up after head injury: a second randomised controlled trial. *Journal of Neurology, Neurosurgery & Psychiatry,* **65**, 177–183.

Further reading

British Psychological Society (2005). *Clinical Neuropsychology and Rehabilitation Services for Adults with Acquired Brain Injury.* Leicester: British Psychological Society - Division of Neuropsychology.

BSRM/JCP/RCP (2004). Vocational Assessment and Rehabilitation after Acquired Brain Injury. Inter-Agency Guidelines. (Edited by A Tyerman & MJ Meehan). *Inter-Agency Advisory Group on Vocational Rehabilitation after Brain Injury.* London: British Society of Rehabilitation Medicine, Jobcentre Plus and Royal College of Physicians.

Halligan P.W and Wade D.T (eds) (2005). *Effectiveness of Rehabilitation for Cognitive Deficits.* Oxford. Oxford University Press.

King N.S (2003). The post concussion syndrome: clarity amid the controversy? *British Journal of Psychiatry,* **183**, 276–278.

Ponsford J., Sloan S., and Snow P (1995). *Traumatic brain injury: Rehabilitation for everyday adaptive living.* Hove: Lawrence Erlbaum Associates.

RCP/BSRM (2003). *Rehabilitation following acquired brain injury: national clinical guidelines* (Turner-Stokes L., ed.). London: Royal College of Physicans/British Society of Rehabilitation Medicine.

Rose, F.D and Johnson, D.A (1996). *Brain injury and after. Towards improved outcome.* John Wiley & Son, Chichester.

Tyerman A and King N.S (eds.). (2008) Psychological approaches to rehabilitation after traumatic brain injury. Oxford: BPS Blackwell.

Wade D.T., King N.S., Wenden F.S., Crawford S., and Caldwell F.E (1998). Routinefollow-up after head injury: a second randomised controlled trial. *Journal of Neurology, Neurosurgery & Psychiatry,* **65**, 177–183.

Wood R.L and McMillan T.M (2001). *Neurobehavioural disability and social handicap following traumatic brain injury.* Hove: Psychology Press.

APPENDIX 1 Glasgow coma scale

Sub-scale	Response	Score
Eye opening (score 0–4)	Opens eyes on his/her own	4
	Opens eyes when asked to do so in a loud voice	3
	Opens eyes to pain	2
	Does not open eyes	1
Verbal response (score 0–5)	Carries on a conversation correctly and tells examiner where he is, the year and month.	5
	Seems confused or disoriented	4
	Talks so the examiner can understand him/her but makes no sense	3
	Makes sounds that the examiner cannot understand	2
	Makes no noise	1
Motor response (score 0–6)	Follows simple commands	6
	Pulls examiner's hand away on painful stimuli	5
	Pulls a part of his body away on painful stimuli	4
	Flexes body appropriately to pain	3
	Decerebrate posture	2
	Has no motor response to pain	1
TOTAL SCORE		3–15

The neuropsychological presentation of Alzheimer's disease and other neurodegenerative disorders

Julie Snowden

1 Introduction

Alzheimer's disease and other neurodegenerative diseases that lead to progressive cognitive impairment are conventionally classified as 'the dementias'. Dementia is traditionally defined as a generalised impairment of intellect, the implication being that all aspects of mental function are uniformly impaired. A logical corollary is that the dementia associated with different disorders should be indistinguishable. This is far from the case. Degenerative diseases do not affect the brain in an undifferentiated manner. Rather, they have predilections for certain brain regions and show relative of sparing of others. In consequence, they are associated with distinct profiles of cognitive and behavioural change that can be identified with a high degree of accuracy. This chapter describes the neuropsychological presentations of the most common neurodegenerative disorders associated with cognitive change.

The disorders under consideration can be classed broadly in terms of the predominant topographical emphasis of pathological change (Table 28.1). Alzheimer's disease (AD), frontotemporal dementia (FTD) and its associated syndromes of semantic dementia and progressive aphasia result from degeneration principally of the neocortex. The salient presenting characteristic is alteration in mental function. Physical symptoms and signs are minimal or absent initially and typically emerge only late in the disease course.

By contrast, in conditions that fall within the category of 'movement disorders' the primary site of pathology is the basal ganglia. Physical symptoms and signs predominate and mental changes may be subsidiary or emerge later in the disease. Some disorders (e.g. dementia with Lewy bodies and corticobasal degeneration) may be characterised from the outset by a combination of cortical and subcortical features. Neuropsychological evaluation can aid recognition of each condition, but is particularly crucial in the cases of neocortical disorders, for which neurological examination provides few clues.

In the past, a common view was that accuracy of dementia diagnosis was unimportant. As there is no effective treatment - the argument went - provision of a precise diagnostic label has little value. This nihilistic view is beginning to change. The advent of novel therapies for disorders such as AD means that correct diagnosis is essential. Only then can therapies be targeted appropriately and their effects meaningfully evaluated. Basic science research, addressing causation and risk factors for disease, is critically dependent on accurate classification of patients' clinical phenotype. In clinical practice, the nature of patients' disorder can have profound implications for patients' management and for the advice offered to carers. Neuropsychologists have a vital role.

2 Alzheimer's disease (AD)

AD is the most common form of dementia. Its prevalence increases with age, although onset may occur in middle age and occasionally as early as the fourth decade of life. It is more common in women. The longer normal life span of women contributes to the higher female prevalence, although does not fully account for it. The course is insidiously progressive over about eight years. People with AD are typically physically well in the early stages, feature important in differential diagnosis. With progression parkinsonian signs of slowing and limb rigidity emerge and myoclonic jerking movements of the limbs. Nevertheless, physical problems are overshadowed by the momentous cognitive disturbance.

Table 28.1 Overview of neurodegenerative disorders associated with cognitive change

Disorder	Dominant site of pathology	Dominant impairment	Neuropsychological presentation
Alzheimer's disease	Medial temporal lobes Temporoparietal neocortex	Cognitive	Cognitive impairment, especially memory
Frontotemporal dementia	Frontal and anterior temporal lobes	Behavioural	Personality and behavioural change, executive impairment
Semantic dementia	Temporal neocortex, especially inferior and middle gyri	Cognitive	Loss of 'memory' for words and concepts. Impaired naming and word comprehension.
Progressive (non-fluent) aphasia	Left perisylvian cortex	Cognitive	Expressive language disorder
Dementia with Lewy bodies/Parkinson's disease dementia	Basal ganglia + neocortex	Mental + physical	Fluctuating mental state. Memory, perceptuospatial and executive impairments
Huntington's disease	Basal ganglia (striatum)	Mental + Physical	Psychomotor slowing, executive impairments
Motor neuron disease	Brain stem and motor cortex	Physical	Executive impairment
Progressive supranuclear palsy	Basal ganglia	Physical	Psychomotor slowing, executive impairments
Corticobasal degeneration	Basal ganglia + frontoparietal cortex	Physical	Ideomotor apraxia, executive impairments

There is not a single causal factor. In a minority of cases, AD is familial and shows an autosomal dominant mode of inheritance. Genes responsible for familial cases have been found on chromosomes 1,14 and 21. The presence of an e4 allele in the Apolipoprotein (APOE) gene is a known risk factor for AD. There are likely to be other genetic influences that increase susceptibility. The earliest pathological changes in AD are in medial temporal structures, and structural MR imaging shows atrophy of the hippocampi (Jack *et al.* 1999). On functional imaging (Jagust *et al.* 1988; Talbot *et al.* 1995) early changes are seen in temporoparietal cortex. Over the course of the disease structural and functional changes become more widespread. The characteristic histological appearances are of -A4 amyloid deposition, senile plaques consisting of degenerating neuronal processes and intra-neuronal neurofibrillary tangles, leading to the death of large cortical neurones. Detailed background information about AD can be found in Burns *et al.* (2005).

2.1 Cognition in AD

2.1.1 Memory

The earliest presenting symptom is typically of problems in memory (Welsh *et al.* 1991; Perry and Hodges 2000). Symptoms may include difficulty remembering appointments, impaired recall of recent events, repetitiveness in conversation and an increased tendency to mislay objects. Memory for the more remote past may appear to be better preserved, and patients 'live in the past'. Patients may themselves acknowledge memory problems although predictably (since they forget that they have asked the same question repeatedly), they often underplay the magnitude of the impairment. The disparity between relatives' and patients' account is of value in distinguishing AD from the memory complaints of the 'worried well'.

The history of memory problems is supported by findings of impaired performance on standard tests of episodic memory, such as list learning, story recall, face and object memory. Although performance may show some benefit from cueing and recognition memory procedures, performance is not typically restored to normal levels. Moreover, if memory is re-tested following a delay there is typically evidence of loss of information over time, suggesting that the problem is not simply one of initial attention/registration of information. Impairments are frequently demonstrable on both visual and verbal memory tasks. Nevertheless, impairment may be more marked in one modality, the visual-verbal disparity reflecting the greater emphasis of atrophy in the right or left medial temporal lobe.

2.1.2 Working memory and attention

Deficient immediate or 'working' memory may contribute to patients' impaired memory functioning. This is frequently manifest clinically by patients' tendency to lose train of thought. On testing patients may show a reduced digit span and require constant repetition of test instructions. The precise basis for 'working memory' deficits remains a subject of debate. Working memory deficits in early-stage AD have most commonly been attributed to a 'central executive' impairment (Baddeley *et al.* 1991) or to problems in divided attention (see Perry and Hodges 1999 for excellent review), by virtue of the fact that patients have difficulty coping with multiple tasks. The inference is that such executive/ attentional deficits reflect impaired frontal lobe function. Yet, at odds with this assumption is the characteristic finding on functional neuroimaging in early AD of changes in temporoparietal and not frontal regions. Moreover, an association has been demonstrated between working memory impairment and problems on posterior hemisphere (language and visuospatial) tasks (Stopford *et al.* 2007), suggesting that reduced storage capacity for phonological and spatial information may contribute substantially to patients' working memory difficulties. Recognition of the presence of problems in working memory is important. In some patients they occur in the absence of a severe classical amnesia. Such patients may have profound difficulty holding information in the immediate present, yet what information is assimilated is retained reasonably well over a delay.

2.1.3 Language

The most common language symptom in AD is a problem in word finding, which is often most pronounced for Proper nouns, such as recall of people's names. Conversational speech may become halting because of word retrieval difficulty, and sentences may be unfinished because of loss of train of thought. Occasional paraphasic errors may be noted, although phonological and semantic errors are rarely a prominent feature. Speech may develop a stuttering, festinant quality (logoclonia). Difficulties are not confined to spoken language. Patients frequently have difficulty in spelling, reading and writing as well as in calculation. Relatives may be dismayed to discover that patients can no longer produce their signature.

Word finding difficulties in AD are commonly ascribed to impaired semantic memory (Hodges *et al.* 1992a; Salmon *et al.* 1999). However, there is a need for caution in assuming that this is invariably the case. AD patients are frequently frustrated by their difficulty in word retrieval, suggesting that they have in mind words that they cannot retrieve. Moreover, in a factor analytic study of cognitive test performance in AD (Stopford *et al.* 2008) naming scores loaded on to a general language factor, which included measures of repetition and spelling that make no semantic demands, and not on to a factor comprising tasks ostensibly tapping semantic memory.

Understanding of language is typically relatively well preserved at a single word level. However, AD patients may have difficulty comprehending complex syntax and conversations involving multiple participants, a factor that may lead to a reticence to socialise. Appreciation that patients may become easily 'overloaded' is important in ensuring optimal communication.

2.1.4 Perception and spatial skills

A variety of symptoms may be indicators of perceptuospatial impairment, reflecting pathological involvement of parietal cortex. There may be reports of minor driving accidents, resulting from spatial misjudgement (e.g. driving too close to parked cars; veering across lanes, driving round a roundabout the wrong way). Patients may become lost, initially in unfamiliar and later familiar surroundings. Patients may have difficulty orienting clothing when dressing, and may put on garments back-to-front or inside out. They may have difficulty aligning cutlery when laying a table and folding clothes. They may be hesitant going up and down stairs, because of difficulty judging spatial depth. Severe spatial problems are manifest by disorientation within the home and a difficulty locating objects within the patients' visual fields. Frank perceptual impairments are usually relatively late features, and may include problems in recognising faces, including their own reflection in a mirror, and misidentification of objects.

Constructional tasks such as clock drawing and copying of simple line drawings are highly sensitive to spatial difficulties. The salient qualitative feature of performance is a breakdown in overall configuration and spatial relationship between elements. The Visual Object and Space Perception battery (VOSP) (Warrington and James 1991) is a valuable instrument in eliciting perceptual and spatial deficits. It makes minimal motor demands so allows spatial deficits to be identified independently of deficits in praxis, which may also contribute to patients' constructional problems. When shown an array of dots spatially impaired patients omit some dots while re-counting others. They have difficulty appreciating the three-dimensional nature of cubes and tend to count edges. They have difficulty identifying degraded perceptual stimuli and tend to respond on the basis of local features rather than global configuration.

2.1.5 Praxis

Manual skills such as symbolic gesture (e.g. waving) and manipulation of objects (e.g. folding clothes) may be compromised by spatial deficits. However, in some patients impairments in praxis far outweigh the degree of spatial impairment, and occasionally may be the dominant presenting feature of the disease (Green *et al.* 1995).

2.1.6 Executive Functions

AD patients commonly perform poorly on executive tasks, even when structural and functional imaging shows no evidence of frontal lobe pathology and patients' preserved social skills suggest an absence of "frontal" behaviour. It is important to keep in mind that executive tasks make multiple cognitive demands, so that performance failure might arise secondary to patients' problems in memory, language, perception, spatial appreciation or praxis (Thompson *et al.* 2005). Consideration of the qualitative nature of errors (perseverations, concrete responses, failures of mental set shifting) is crucial in interpreting the basis for executive test failures.

2.2 Behaviour and affect in AD

A striking feature of AD patients presenting to a diagnostic clinic is their preserved social façade. Patients' emotional warmth, social manner and facility in use of social platitudes in conversation frequently mask the magnitude of the underlying cognitive disorder. That is not to say that behavioural changes are totally absent. Relatives frequently report an increase in irritability, which is usually directed towards family members and may reflect frustration at failing cognitive powers and loss of functional independence. Patients may also be noted to be more anxious, low in mood, lacking in confidence and less gregarious than formerly, features that can also reasonably be interpreted as secondary to their emerging cognitive problems. Notwithstanding such alterations, gross character change is not a hallmark of early and middle-stage AD and patients are regarded as the 'same person' as before, albeit with acquired difficulties.

2.3 Phenotypic variation in AD

The prototypical picture of AD is of a constellation of cognitive difficulties, with memory impairment being a central feature. However, patients are not identical. Whereas some patients are densely amnesic, others show only mild inefficiencies in memory, despite more pervasive impairments in other cognitive domains. The prominence of language or visuospatial symptoms may differ. Aside from these general differences in weighting of symptoms there are some more striking phenotypic variations (Galton *et al.* 2000; Snowden *et al.* 2007a). Some patients present, not with symptoms of memory loss, but with a circumscribed disorder of language associated with asymmetric atrophy of the left hemisphere (aphasic presentation). Others may present with problems in 'vision', which may reflect impaired spatial skills (biparietal syndrome), or impaired visual perception (posterior cortical atrophy). Such patients have often consulted opticians and ophthamologists on the assumption that the problem is ocular. Occasionally, the dominant presenting feature is of difficulty in carrying out skilled actions (praxic presentation). These 'focal' presentations of AD are likely to represent extreme examples of the normal variation seen within the AD population (Snowden *et al.* 2007a; Stopford *et al.* 2008).

2.3.1 Factors influencing clinical phenotype

Age of onset influences presentation. Amnestic presentations, reflecting dominant medial temporal pathology, are most common in the elderly. Elderly patients are also more likely to exhibit 'frontal lobe' characteristics, although in many instances this is due to coincidental small vessel vascular disease affecting subcortical-frontal pathways. The presence of perceptuospatial impairment in the early stages of disease, reflecting involvement of temporoparietal cortex, is characteristic in patients presenting in their 50s and 60s. The APOE ε4 allele, an established risk factor for AD, appears specifically to influence the degree of amnesia (Snowden *et al.* 2007a).

2.4 Diagnostic criteria for AD

The most frequently used diagnostic criteria for AD in research studies remains the NINCDS-ADRDA criteria (McKhann *et al.* 1984). A diagnosis of probable AD requires the presence of impairments in memory and at least one other cognitive domain. Despite their continued use the criteria were intended, at their inception, to be provisional. They are limited for two main reasons. First, they lack specificity. They are sufficiently broad that many patients with disorders other than AD would fulfil AD criteria (Varma *et al.* 1999). Second, they are insensitive to early-stage disease. People with significant, yet relatively circumscribed memory deficits would be excluded, even though such patients might be expected to benefit most from anti-cholinesterase therapies.

Recognition of these limitations has prompted the development of a new set of AD criteria (Dubois *et al.* 2007), which focus exclusively on memory, reflecting the perceived importance of memory loss in AD. A diagnosis of probable AD is determined by historical reports of a gradual and progressive change in memory function together with demonstrations of significantly impaired episodic memory (encompassing recognition and cued recall as well as free recall) on neuropsychological testing. The memory loss should be supported by evidence of medial temporal lobe atrophy on structural imaging, a cerebrospinal fluid biomarker, functional imaging abnormalities or proven genetic mutation in the family.

These new criteria have the advantage of reducing the number of false positive diagnoses, so increasing specificity. Also, by acknowledging that the memory disorder may be an isolated symptom, the criteria are likely to be sensitive to earlier stage of disease. Their chief drawback is that they make the assumption that memory impairment is an invariable feature of AD and do not encompass other focal presentations of AD. It is important to keep in mind the fact that AD can present as a disorder of language, spatial function or "vision".

3 Frontotemporal lobar degeneration: frontotemporal dementia, progressive aphasia and semantic dementia

Frontotemporal lobar degeneration (FTLD) is an umbrella term for a collection of pathologically-linked clinical syndromes that result from circumscribed atrophy of the anterior hemispheres. These include frontotemporal dementia (FTD), a disorder of behaviour and executive function associated with bilateral atrophy of the frontal and anterior temporal lobes, progressive non-fluent aphasia (PNFA), a disorder of expressive language associated with left perisylvian atrophy, and semantic dementia (SD), a disorder of conceptual understanding associated with bilateral atrophy of the inferior and middle temporal cortices. Because of the psychological and anatomical specificity of these disorders they are frequently described under the rubric of 'focal dementias'. It is worth emphasising, however, that 'focal' does not necessarily imply 'less severe': the extent of tissue loss in the affected regions is typically greater in FTLD than in AD and overall brain weight at death is typically lower.

Unlike AD which increases in prevalence with advancing age the syndromes of FTLD present most commonly in the 50s and 60s and can present even earlier. Men and women are affected equally. A positive family history is present in approximately 40% of cases.

The disorders are insidiously progressive, and have an average total duration of about 8 years. There is, however, wide variation in time course, reflecting patients' physical state. Many patients remain physically well, parkinsonian signs emerging only late in the course. Such patients may survive for 10 or 15 years. By contrast, a minority of patients develop physical signs of motor neurone disease, leading to an attenuated course of 2-3 years.

The pathological changes underlying FTLD are not uniform, and can broadly be classified into two types. Some brains show transcortical gliosis with tau-reactive intraneuronal inclusions (Pick bodies) and sometimes swollen neurons (Pick cells). These cases would fulfil traditional pathological criteria for 'Pick's disease' and are now referred to as 'tau-positive' or 'Pick-type'. Other brains show microvacuolation, with intraneuronal inclusions that stain for ubiquitin, and are referred to as 'tau-negative, ubiquitin-positive' or FTLD-ubiquitinated (FTLD-U) type. FTD and PNFA can be associated with both histopathological types, whereas SD is typically associated with FTLD-U (Snowden *et al.* 2007b).

Just as the pathology underlying FTLD is not uniform, so too there appear to be different molecular substrates. Causal genetic defects have been identified on chromosome 17, in the *tau* gene in some familial cases of FTD and in the *progranulin* gene in cases of FTD and PNFA. These account collectively for less than half of all familial cases indicating that other faulty genes are yet to be discovered.

3.1 Behaviour in FTD

The dominant presenting feature of FTD is altered behaviour (Neary *et al.* 1988). Formerly responsible and conscientious individuals become disinhibited and socially inappropriate, they neglect self-care and personal responsibilities, and show a total lack of insight or concern into their altered mental state. Relatives report the patient to be radically altered in character and not the same person as before. Socially inappropriate behaviour may include infringements of social etiquette, such as ignoring visitors to the home or drinking wine from the bottle in a restaurant as well as more major violations of social norms, such as wandering naked, shoplifting and incontinence without concern.

There are three broad domains of behaviour that are particularly important in differentiating FTD from other common dementias (Bathgate *et al.* 2001): affect, repetitive behaviours/stereotypies and eating/oral behaviours. FTD patients no longer show the normal range of basic and social emotions. They are typically fatuous and puerile, or else emotionally blunted. They show a lack of sympathy, empathy or compassion towards others, and exhibit no signs of embarrassment at their socially inappropriate behaviour. An emotional response to a situation that is out-of-character may be the first signal that something is wrong: for example, an absence of grief reaction at the death of a loved one.

Repetitive behaviours in FTD range from simple motor mannerisms (e.g. repetitive humming, grunting, hand rubbing, clapping, foot tapping) to complex behavioural routines (e.g. wandering the same route, doing the same activity at the same time each day). There may be verbal stereotypies, such as saying a favoured word or phrase repeatedly. Some repetitive behaviours are environmentally driven. For example, patients may persistently read aloud notices or street signs, or hoard objects. Utilisation behaviour, which is occasionally seen, is an extreme form of environmental dependency: the patient carries out the action associated with an object (e.g. drinking from a cup; putting on glasses) even when that action is contextually inappropriate (e.g. the patient repeatedly picks up and drinks from a cup even though it is empty; the patient puts on the pair of glasses in front of him/her even though the glasses belong to the examiner).

FTD patients may eat excessively and cram food, leading to weight gain. Relatives may report that the patient would carry on eating if food was continually available, suggesting that excessive eating may in part be stimulus-driven. Often patients acquire a preference for sweet foods, and seek out sweets, chocolates and biscuits. Some patients show food fads, showing a preference for a particular brand of chocolate bar or biscuit. Hyperorality may include excessive drinking and smoking. An increase in alcohol consumption may raise the diagnostic question of an alcohol-related aetiology, although in the case of FTD the increase in alcohol intake is a symptom of the patient's disorder and not the cause. Attempts to eat inedible objects (Klüver-Bucy syndrome) may be present in late stage disease.

3.2 Cognition in FTD

3.2.1 Executive functions

FTD is predominantly a 'frontal' lobe disorder. In keeping with the distribution of atrophy, patients exhibit impairments in a range of frontal executive skills: abstraction, planning, organisation, attention and mental set switching. Performance is typically markedly impaired on standard rule-based tasks such as the Wisconsin card sorting, Weigls and Brixton spatial anticipation tests. Patients commonly show striking perseveration of one response pattern, and make no attempt to alter this pattern in the face of feedback that it is no longer correct. On verbal and design fluency tests they generate a paucity of items, and performance is characterised by response perseverations, concrete responses (e.g. naming their own dog instead of animal species) and rule violations (e.g. giving proper names when instructed not to do so). On picture sequencing tasks they may make minimal effort to alter the original ordering of items, and fail to notice logical anomalies. They typically perform poorly on tests of sustained and selective attention and response inhibition.

The prevailing qualitative characteristics of patients' cognitive performance are economy of mental effort, impulsivity of responding without checking, poor persistence, distractibility, concreteness of thought, perseveration of responses, and a general lack of concern for performance accuracy. These features colour patients' performance on tasks that extend well beyond the realm of executive function.

3.2.2 Language, perceptuospatial and constructional skills

In language, patients typically show reduced speech output, echolalia, perseveration, verbal stereotypies and ultimately mutism. On a standard confrontation naming test, although frank semantic errors may sometimes be present, low naming scores commonly reflect a high prevalence of perseverations or 'don't know' responses. On constructional tasks drawings may be poorly organised and show perseveration of strokes. On a simple spatial test such as counting an array of dots performance may be inaccurate because of patients' impulsive responding: if patients are asked to point to the dots they have no difficulty doing so (in contrast to spatially impaired AD patients), indicating that the low accuracy scores are not the result of primary problems in spatial localisation. The key message here is that it is important to take account of the qualitative characteristics of patients' performance in interpreting the nature of patients' deficits. There is not a one-to-one correspondence between a test and a function, and failure on 'posterior' hemisphere tests may arise for 'anterior' hemisphere reasons (Thompson *et al.* 2005).

3.2.3 Memory

FTD patients typically exhibit a characteristic "frontal" type of memory impairment. Performance is severely impaired on open-ended recall tests, yet improves on more constrained cued recall and multiple-choice recognition tests. Moreover, what information is assimilated is relatively well retained over a standard 20 or 30-minute delay, suggesting that the problem is one of registration rather than retention *per se*. Patients do not show the topographical memory loss that is so common in AD, evidenced by the fact that patients who wander often follow the same route without becoming lost. Qualitative characteristics of patients' memory performance are informative. Severely defective scores on a multiple-choice recognition test, when they occur, are typically associated with impulsive responding, overt distractibility, a high incidence of response perseverations (e.g. repeated selection of the right-hand item), or lack of adherence to goal (e.g. the patient selects the item he/she prefers rather than the one presented previously).

3.2.4 Social cognition and emotion recognition

Deficits can commonly be elicited on tests of social cognition (Lough *et al.* 2001; Snowden *et al.* 2003) and recognition of emotion (Keane *et al.* 2002). This domain is important because deficits may be elicited early in the disease course, at a time when performance on standard executive tests is relatively well preserved.

3.3 Phenotypic variation in FTD

In the initial stages of disease many FTD patients are fatuous and socially disinhibited and this gradually gives way to emotional blunting, apathy and inertia, reflecting spread of pathological change from orbitofrontal into dorsolateral frontal cortex. However, in some patients the presentation is, from the outset, of apathy and inertia, which may be mistaken for depression. Recognition of behavioural variation in FTD is important because it has a bearing on patients' cognition. Executive impairments on neuropsychological testing are most severe in patients with widespread frontal lobe pathology associated with an apathetic behavioural profile. Disinhibited patients in whom atrophy is more circumscribed may, at least in the early stages of disease, perform surprisingly well on standard tests of executive function, contrasting with the severe breakdown in social, interpersonal conduct.

3.4 Cognition in semantic dementia

3.4.1 Word meaning

Semantic dementia (Snowden *et al.* 1989; 1996; Hodges *et al.* 1992b) refers to a multimodal loss of conceptual knowledge. The initial presentation is most commonly of problems in word meaning. Patients have problems in naming and may make semantic category errors (e.g. "dog" for horse). They also have difficulty understanding words and may ask what individual words mean (e.g. Qu: "Would you like a banana?" Patient: "Banana. What's banana?"), a feature that is not notable in AD or any other neurodegenerative disorder. Non-semantic aspects of language are well preserved. Patients speak fluently and effortlessly, in grammatical sentences without phonological error. They do not struggle to retrieve words, since those words are no longer available to be retrieved, and indeed they may be frankly garrulous. Rather, there is simply a progressive reduction in the patient's range of vocabulary and repertoire of conversational topics. Patients use words over-inclusively (e.g. 'dog' to refer to all types of animal), and utterances have an increasingly stereotyped quality. In the later stages only a few stereotyped phrases remain and ultimately patients become mute. At no time does speech output have a non-fluent, effortful quality.

3.4.2 Non-verbal concepts

The semantic impairment is not confined to words. Patients develop difficulty recognising faces, objects, nonverbal environmental sounds, smells, tastes and tactile stimuli. It should be emphasised that the problem is not one of elementary perception. Patients have no difficulty carrying out perceptual matching and discrimination tasks in all modalities, and they can reproduce drawings of objects accurately indicating that they perceive them normally. The problem lies in attribution of meaning to sensory stimuli that are perceived normally.

3.4.3 Memory

The semantic impairment is frequently construed by both patients and their relatives as a problem in memory, and their presenting complaint is often that they 'do not remember things'. Not surprisingly, a misdiagnosis of AD is common. Important features in the history are, however, telling. If informants are asked to clarify the kind of things the patient cannot remember they describe problems specifically in semantic memory, such as difficulty remembering names of people and objects, difficulty recognising acquaintances. By contrast, patients' day-to-day event memory is well preserved. They find their way around without becoming lost, remember daily activities and keep track of time. They retain a degree of functional independence that would be unthinkable in a patient with a classical amnesia.

3.4.4 Cognitive assessment in semantic dementia

Patients' preserved speech fluency may convey the notion of a facility with language, which, at least in the early stages, masks the emerging semantic impairment. Neuropsychological assessment has a vital role to play. Whereas the semantic deficits may be barely apparent at clinical interview, performance on formal naming tests is typically dramatically impaired. Floor level scores on the demanding Graded Naming test are common. Assessment needs to include tests of word comprehension, which ideally should encompass biological categories (animals, fruits, vegetables) as well as inanimate objects. Forced choice word-picture tests are valuable because they can provide clear evidence of semantic breakdown (e.g. selection of a picture of a rhinoceros in response to the stimulus word 'duck'). Famous face and name recognition tests are also useful because of their sensitivity to disease. Whereas most patients in the early stages of AD recognise names such as Margaret Thatcher, Elvis Presley and Marilyn Monroe most semantic dementia patients do not. Patients with semantic dementia recognise names and faces of personal acquaintances better than those of famous people, whereas AD patients show no such disparity.

Formal memory tests may elicit impaired performance by virtue of their semantic demands. However, performance on picture recognition memory tests is typically well preserved. Moreover, although they may lose marks on place orientation questions because of a difficulty in naming, patients are typically very well oriented in time.

The Visual Object and Space Perception battery (Warrington and James 1991) is a valuable instrument in the identification of semantic dementia because it elicits a characteristic profile. Patients perform normally on spatial tests, contrasting with the spatial impairment typical of early onset AD. SD patients also perform generally well on perceptual subtests, except where these require recognition of identity. Failure is most pronounced on the Silhouettes subtest. Calculation performance can also help to differentiate SD from AD. Arithmetical skills are typically relatively preserved in SD, whereas they are impaired early in the course of AD.

3.5 Behaviour in semantic dementia

The semantic impairment is the defining feature of the disorder and the aspect that is most striking to the neuropsychologist. However, SD is also associated with alterations in behaviour and it is these changes that are often most troublesome to families. Patients become egocentric, reflecting their narrowed world view. They typically adhere to a rigid daily routine and show preoccupation with a narrowed range of interests which they pursue to excess. They may become time-bound and clockwatch constantly. They may restrict their diet to a narrow range of foods. There is some overlap with the behavioural changes of FTD. However, SD behaviours have a more compulsive quality (Snowden *et al.* 2001). Moreover, whereas FTD patients are typically inattentive and show a lack of engagement and persistence in activities, SD patients show a remarkable degree of focused attention and dogged persistence in their favoured pursuits.

3.6 Phenotypic variation in semantic dementia

Semantic dementia is perhaps the most homogeneous of all neurodegenerative disorders. Patients show predictable profiles of cognitive impairment and strikingly similar patterns of behavioural change. One identifiable difference between patients relates to hemispheric asymmetries. Patients with more left-sided temporal atrophy typically present with problems in naming and word comprehension whereas those with more right sided atrophy may present with problems in face recognition.

In 'pure' semantic dementia cases the atrophy is relatively confined to the temporal lobes. However, there are some patients in whom the atrophy encroaches into the frontal lobes. These patients show a mixed behavioural picture of FTD, combined with the semantic disturbance of SD. Such patients are more behaviourally disturbed than pure SD cases and show more obvious executive impairments.

3.7 Neuropsychological presentation of progressive non-fluent aphasia

Reports of primary progressive aphasia (Mesulam 1982, 2001; Tyrrell *et al.* 1990; Snowden *et al.* 1992) typically distinguish a fluent form, characterised by effortless output and problems in naming and word comprehension and a non-fluent form, characterised by marked problems in expressive language in the context of well preserved word comprehension. The former is likely to represent the precursor to semantic dementia: careful examination typically shows that the semantic impairment extends beyond the verbal domain. The non-fluent form (PNFA), by contrast, remains clinically and anatomically distinct from semantic dementia throughout the disease course.

3.7.1 Language

A prominent feature of most PNFA patients is anomia, which is characterised by a difficulty accessing words that remain within the patient's vocabulary. Unlike patients with semantic dementia, PNFA patients may exhibit a tip-of-the-tongue effect and show immense frustration, reflecting their awareness of the existence of the word that they cannot bring to mind. PNFA may be associated with effortful speech, agrammatism and phonological disturbances, and bear resemblance to Broca's aphasia. However, there is considerable heterogeneity within PNFA. Whereas phonological production errors are marked in some patients they are notable for their absence in others. Production is agrammatic in some patients but not in others. In some patients there are parallel difficulties in spoken and written language, whereas in other patients performance dissociates across modalities. In some patients 'non-fluency' reflects effortful production associated with speech apraxia, whereas in others there is no effort and the non-fluent quality of patients' speech output is a consequence of the magnitude of anomia. The latter distinction has anatomical and apparently also aetiological significance. The apraxic form of PNFA has been associated with neuroimaging changes predominantly in the left frontal regions, whereas the anomic form has been linked to extensive left perisylvian atrophy. The presence of speech apraxia is a strong predictor of tau histopathology, whereas its absence is a predictor of tau-negative, ubiquitin-positive histology.

3.7.2 Gesture

Even in patients without obvious speech apraxia, a difficulty in use of symbolic gesture may accompany patients' problems in spoken and written communication, preventing patients from compensating for their expressive language difficulties through nonverbal means. Effectively, patients become mute and all mediums of communication become lost. This predicament might intuitively be expected to lead to an increase in the patient's level of frustration. In reality, frustration and distress tend to diminish over the course of the disease, reflecting reduced insight due to spread of frontal lobe pathology.

3.7.3 Distinction from AD

PNFA is not always easy to distinguish from focal language presentations of AD, so that pathological series of patients with a clinical diagnosis of PNFA frequently include cases with AD pathology. Important features that typify non-Alzheimer PNFA include striking hemispheric asymmetry of atrophy and specificity in the nature of linguistic breakdown.

3.8 Diagnostic criteria for FTLD

Clinical and pathological diagnostic criteria published by the Lund and Manchester groups (1994) focused on the behavioural disorder of FTD. Subsequently published clinical criteria (Neary *et al.* 1998) extended to PNFA and SD, and provided more precise operational definitions of symptoms. They have been shown to have good sensitivity and specificity (Knopman *et al.* 2005). A simplified set of guidelines (McKhann *et al.* 2001) has also been introduced, aimed at the general physician, which subsumes PNFA, SD and FTD under the general umbrella of 'FTD' and refers to the overarching presenting feature as 'an early and progressive change in personality or language'. This definition inevitably excludes SD patients whose conceptual loss manifests as a disorder of face or object recognition, while including AD patients presenting with a circumscribed language disorder. Histopathological differences associated with FTD, PNFA and SD (Snowden *et al.* 2007), together with the very striking clinical differences and differing management needs of patients suggest that clinical distinctions should be maintained.

4 Dementia with Lewy bodies

The form of dementia most akin to AD, is dementia with Lewy bodies (DLB). This is a disorder principally (although not exclusively) of the elderly (McKeith *et al.* 2004), which shares clinical and pathological features with both Parkinson's disease and AD. The core defining features are cognitive impairment, together with mental fluctuations, visual hallucinations and parkinsonism. Recognition of the disorder is crucial for patients' optimal management. DLB patients frequently show sensitivity to traditional neuroleptic agents, which need to be avoided. On the other hand, DLB patients show greater benefit than AD patients from cholinesterase inhibitors, despite the fact that these therapies were originally designed for AD. Neuropsychological assessment can contribute substantially to the diagnosis.

4.1 Cognition in DLB

DLB patients, like those with AD, exhibit impairments in memory, language, visual perception, spatial, attention and executive functions. Comparative studies of the two disorders show that in DLB attentional deficits are particularly pronounced (e.g. Calderon *et al.* 2001). Perceptuospatial deficits are more marked in DLB than in AD whereas memory deficits are less severe (cf. Metzler-Baddeley 2007). Such *relative* quantitative differences are important and informative at a group level, but inevitably present ambiguities in the interpretation of data from individual patients. Qualitative features of patients' performance can provide valuable additional information that can improve accuracy of diagnosis (Doubleday *et al.* 2002). Qualitative differences between DLB and AD are summarised in Table 28.2, and described in more detail below.

4.2 Qualitative characteristics of DLB

4.2.1 Fluctuations and interference

A salient and striking characteristic of DLB patients is fluctuation in their mental state. The fluctuations are typically apparent to relatives who may describe the patient as having 'good days and bad days' and within a single day, periods of lucidity in which the patient appears 'back to his/her normal self' and periods of confusion during which the patient behaves and speaks irrationally. These fluctuations are reflected by variable performance on neuropsychological testing. Responses to questions may at one moment be entirely lucid and appropriate and at another moment incoherent and off the point. Sometimes a tenuous link can be detected between the wording of the question and the patient's response. For example, when requested to "point to the source of illumination in this room" the patient might respond by talking about Blackpool. There may also be interference from extraneous visual environmental stimuli. The patient might, for example, produce the entirely irrelevant response 'fire exit', because his/her gaze happens to fall on the Fire Exit notice in the room. Patients may be distracted too by irrelevant auditory stimuli, and ascribe personal relevance to extraneous sounds (e.g. a telephone ringing in a distant office: 'my daughter is calling me'; a noise outside the hospital consulting room: 'the cat's trying to get out'). In addition to intrusions arising from association of ideas and from environmental stimuli there is also characteristically evidence of interference within and across tests. Thus, elements of one short story may intrude into the recall of a second story; items from a picture arrangement test may intrude into the recall of a word list. Open-ended tasks such as story recall are of particular diagnostic value in the assessment of DLB because they provide the scope to elicit features that distinguish DLB from AD: confabulation (introduction of information not in the original story), misconstruction (incorrect juxtaposition and integration of story elements) and interference effects (within-task, across-task, induced from external environment or semantic association). Perseverations of verbal and motor responses are also more prominent in DLB than AD.

4.2.2 Hallucinations and perception

The core behavioural characteristic of DLB, other than mental fluctuation, is visual hallucinations. These are formed and most commonly consist of people or animals. The patient can typically provide a detailed vivid description of their appearance, including the colour and style of their clothing, and the activities in which they are engaged. They may

Table 28.2 Qualitative performance characteristics in DLB and AD

	DLB	AD
Performance consistency	May fluctuate over test session	Consistent over test session
Rate of performance	Slowed	Unremarkable
Conversational speech	Incoherent line of thought	Coherent, despite expressive difficulties
Distractibility	Distracted by irrelevant stimuli	Not overtly distractible
Interference	Within and between-test interference: intrusion errors	Minimal interference
Confabulation	Story recall may be confabulatory and misconstrued	Story recall poor but not confabulatory
Perseveration	Verbal and motor perseveration present	Minimal perseveration

be linked to a particular location (e.g. 'an old woman and little girl who sit on the sofa in the living room'), although they are not always static. Characteristically, the hallucinations are silent and non-threatening, so the patient accepts them with equanimity. Some apparent hallucinatory phenomena are more accurately classified as illusions since they have an identifiable perceptual substrate. For example, the patient might report seeing 'a monkey' in the pattern of a curtain, or 'a burglar trying to get in' in the swaying branches of the trees outside the window. It is of interest in this regard that patients often perform particularly poorly on perceptual sub-tests of the Visual Object and Space Perception battery and may over-interpret visual stimuli (e.g. a fragmented letter 'F': "a man riding a bicycle").

It is worthy of note, in relation to these misperceptions, that Capgras syndrome has also been reported in association with DLB (Baldwin *et al.* 1995). This is a form of delusion in which the patient believes a person, usually a close family member, to be an imposter. The patient concedes that the 'imposter' looks like the 'real' person (i.e. the patient's spouse), although may sometimes report subtle differences (e.g. 'he/she is about an inch taller'). Because of their entrenched belief, the patient may refer to their spouse in the third person when talking directly to him/her (e.g. 'he likes to play golf at weekends').

4.3 Phenotypic variation in DLB

The initial presentation and evolution of symptoms of DLB may vary. In some patients cognitive change is the earliest symptom and physical signs of parkinsonism emerge later. In other patients parkinsonism signs emerge first. The neuropsychological profile is identical in both types of patients (Doubleday *et al.* 2002).

4.4 Parkinson's disease dementia and DLB

Parkinson's disease is predominantly a movement disorder, characterised by tremor, physical slowing and rigidity. However, it is recognised that people with Parkinson's disease may develop cognitive problems during the disease course. In their mild form these may constitute mild inefficiencies in memory, reduced generation on fluency tasks and subtle difficulties on complex executive tests. However, cognitive changes may be of sufficient magnitude to acquire the label of Parkinson's disease dementia. This raises the important question of the relationship between DLB and the cognitive impairment of Parkinson's disease.

Early consensus criteria for DLB (McKeith *et al.* 1996) specified that for a diagnosis of DLB cognitive impairment should emerge prior to or within 12 months of the onset of extrapyramidal neurological signs. In cases where the clinical history of parkinsonism is longer than 12 months then a diagnosis of Parkinson's disease with dementia would be more appropriate. In reality, the 12 month cut-off is arbitrary, and the cognitive phenotype is identical regardless of whether the cognitive impairment emerges a few months or many years after the onset of parkinsonism. It is now generally accepted that DLB and Parkinson's disease dementia are the same disease.

4.5 Diagnostic criteria for DLB

Early consensus guidelines (McKeith *et al.* 1996) required for the diagnosis of DLB the presence of cognitive impairment, with prominent deficits in attention, frontal-subcortical skills and visuospatial ability, together with two of the following core features: fluctuating cognition, visual hallucinations and parkinsonism. These criteria yield acceptable specificity but suboptimal sensitivity, because at least two core features may not be present early in the course. A revised set of guidelines (McKeith *et al.* 2005) has attempted to improve sensitivity by introducing additional suggestive features, commonly present in DLB: a) REM sleep disorder, b) neuroleptic sensitivity and c) low dopamine transporter uptake in basal ganglia demonstrated on functional neuroimaging. It is suggested that a diagnosis of probable DLB can be made when at least one core feature and one additional feature is present. In neuropsychological practice, a diagnosis of DLB may be suspected, by virtue of the features of incoherence, misconstructions, perseverations and interference effects, prior to the frank development of all core symptoms.

5 Huntington's disease

Huntington's disease (HD) is a genetic disorder caused by a trinucleotide (CAG) repeat mutation in the *huntingtin* gene on chromosome 4. It is associated with autosomal dominant inheritance, each child of an affected parent having a 50% risk of inheriting the HD mutation and developing the disease. Onset of symptoms is typically around 40 years, although it may occur, rarely, both in childhood and in old age. The duration of illness to death is about 15 years, although there is a wide range. The cardinal features are involuntary (choreic and dystonic) movements, cognitive impairment and mood/behavioural changes (cf Bates *et al.* 2002 for comprehensive background to HD).

The writhing, involuntary movements of HD patients are the most visible sign of disease and their emergence typically provides the principle basis for making a clinical diagnosis and defining clinical onset. A genetic test is available that can be used to confirm the clinical diagnosis in patients showing symptoms and to offer pre-symptomatic testing for at-risk individuals. It might be presumed therefore that neuropsychology has little role. However, in HD it is the mental rather than physical changes that are often the most troublesome aspect of the disease and place greatest burden on families. Recognition of the nature of those changes is crucial for effective clinical management, as well as for providing appropriate cognitive and behavioural markers to assess efficacy of novel therapies.

5.1 Cognition in HD

The salient characteristics are psychomotor slowing, and impaired executive skills and memory (cf Craufurd and Snowden 2002). Patients show impoverished generation in verbal and design fluency tasks, poor sequencing, divided attention and mental set shifting. They typically make a high percentage of perseverative responses. Patients' behaviour in daily life is characterised by mental inefficiency and poor organisation. Despite the ubiquitous report of poor memory, patients do not exhibit a classical amnesia, as found in AD: HD patients are typically well oriented and can give an account of autobiographical events. Rather they show poor concentration and forgetfulness (e.g. forgetting to pick the children up from school, forgetting a boiling pan on the stove). On formal memory testing they show poor performance on open-ended recall tests, but benefit greatly when performance is assessed by cued recall and recognition techniques. The pattern of memory performance suggests failure in organisational aspects of memory, secondary to striato-frontal dysfunction. If information is structured for the patient then performance improves.

5.2 Mood and behaviour in HD

Common behavioural characteristics in HD include loss of initiative and drive, poor self care, emotional blunting, self-centredness, mental inflexibility, irritability, poor temper control and depressed mood (Craufurd and Snowden 2002). Apathy, like cognitive change, increases systematically over the course of the disease. Patients, if left to their own devices may stay in bed all day or watch television. Irritability tends to peak in the middle stages of the illness and then wanes. Depression has an increased prevalence in HD compared to the normal population but is unrelated to stage of disease.

5.3 Phenotypic variation in HD

An akinetic-rigid form of HD, as distinct from the typical choreic form, has been associated with juvenile onset of disease. In typical cases, there is some variation in the extent and characteristics of the movement disorder. Patients may vary too with respect to the degree of cognitive impairment. Typically, patients who have a late onset of disease exhibit milder cognitive impairment than those with early onset and show fewer behavioural problems.

6 Motor neurone disease

Motor neurone disease (MND) has traditionally been construed as a disease of the motor system, in which higher mental function is spared. This prevailing view has been challenged from two sources. First, a proportion of patients with established FTD develop, during the course of their illness, the physical signs of MND, suggesting a link between the two disorders (Neary et al. 1990). Second, close examination of patients attending MND clinics shows that a proportion develops cognitive impairment of varying degree. Deficits have been identified most commonly in the realm of executive functions, particularly on verbal fluency tasks (Abrahams et al. 2000). Some MND patients develop behavioural changes akin to those seen in FTD (Gibbons et al. 2008). In keeping with the cognitive and behavioural profiles, structural and functional imaging demonstrates abnormalities in the frontal lobes.

Current data point to a spectrum of change: at one extreme patients show no cognitive or behavioural impairment, whereas at the other extreme they fulfil criteria for FTD. The precise factors that determine patients' susceptibility to cognitive impairment remain to be determined.

7 Progressive supranuclear palsy

Progressive supranuclear palsy (PSP) is a basal ganglia disorder, the hallmark of which is a progressive reduction in voluntary eye movements, culminating in total ophthalmoplegia. Whereas patients with Parkinson's disease have a flexed posture those with PSP tend to hold their head in extension, and are prone to falling backwards. The pathological changes in PSP fall within the rubric of 'tauopathy', thus sharing a pathological link with FTD.

7.1 Cognition in PSP

PSP patients commonly show mental slowing, which may be most marked in the initiation of responses. They exhibit particular difficulties in open-ended tasks, requiring the active generation of information (e.g. verbal fluency; recall of story). By contrast, they perform relatively well when responses are constrained (e.g. confrontation naming, forced-choice recognition of story). They may also show impairments in sequencing and other executive tasks, The characteristic features of mental slowing and inefficiency, in the absence of frank 'cortical' features of aphasia, agnosia, spatial disorientation or apraxia has been referred to as a 'subcortical dementia' (Albert *et al.* 1976).

The cognitive profile in PSP shares commonalities with that of FTD, in keeping with disruption of striatal-frontal pathways. However, PSP patients do not typically show the gross character change, breakdown in social behaviour and lack of insight that is pathognomonic of FTD. Moreover, FTD patients are typically impulsive rather than slowed in their responses.

7.2 Phenotypic variation in PSP

Patients vary in the severity of cognitive impairment. In some patients cognitive change is mild and limited to slight slowing and inefficiencies, whereas in others there are very marked executive deficits, comparable to those found in FTD.

8 Corticobasal degeneration

Corticobasal degeneration (CBD), like PSP, falls within the rubric of 'Parkinson-plus' disorders. Patients show parkinsonian signs of akinesia and rigidity, resulting from pathological change in the basal ganglia, together with asymmetric limb apraxia, resulting from pathology in frontoparietal cortex. The pathological changes in CBD fall within the classification of 'tauopathy', providing a pathological link between CBD and both PSP and FTD.

8.1 Neuropsychological presentation of CBD

The striking abnormality in CBD is limb apraxia of the ideomotor type: the patient has the idea of the required action but cannot implement it effectively. Typically, both upper and lower limbs are affected, albeit to differential degree. Involvement is typically asymmetric, one side being affected more than the other. Buccofacial apraxia develops with progression of disease causing difficulty with speech. Patients are often insightful and initially frustrated by their profoundly disabling disorder. However, with disease progression patients develop increasing executive impairments associated with functional impairment of the frontal lobes, and insight and distress gradually diminish.

8.2 Phenotypic variation in CBD

The principle variation across patients is in the relative proportion of 'basal' and 'cortical' features. In the former, there is substantial limb rigidity and actions are slowed and reduced in amplitude but relatively accurate in terms of their spatial configuration, whereas in the latter configuration is impairment.

9 Management issues

The primary aim of this chapter has been to describe the neuropsychological characteristics of different neurodegenerative disorders, allowing those disorders to be recognised and differentiated from other disorders. An in-depth evaluation of management implications is beyond the scope of the chapter. Nevertheless, it is worth re-emphasising that provision of a correct diagnostic label is not merely an academic exercise. It can have considerable importance for patients and their families. Recognition that a specific 'disease' is the cause of patients' altered cognition or behaviour can aid considerably the process of adjustment. It can assuage relatives' feelings of guilt that they are to blame and eliminate beliefs that the patient's behaviour is wilful and therefore under his/her control.

Moreover, the particular characteristics of a patient's problems may reasonably lead to different and indeed even opposing forms of advice. For example, the family of an AD patient with a reduced immediate span might sensibly be advised to 'keep sentences short and simple' when conversing with the patient. Conversely, the family of a semantic dementia patient would be advised to 'provide a lot of context' in order to compensate for the patient's failure to understand individual nouns.

In the cases of neurological disorders that are associated with severe physical disability, the presence of alterations in cognition and/or behaviour may sometimes be ignored. Yet, recognition and acknowledgement of patients' mental status is crucial: to optimise patients' cooperation in physical and speech therapy; to involve patients and their relatives appropriately in clinical management decisions, and to provide support and advice to families who may have difficulty coping with patients' altered behaviour.

10 Theoretical considerations

The notion of dementia as a global, undifferentiated impairment of intellect is entrenched in the literature. Yet, the evidence against such a notion is overwhelming. Different neurodegenerative disorders lead to distinct and highly characteristic patterns of cognitive impairment and disorders can be differentiated with a high degree of accuracy on neuropsychological grounds. If dementia were 'global' then such differentiation should not be possible. Differences between patients are apparent not merely on sophisticated neuropsychological analysis, but are well recognised by nursing home carers and family members. For example, relatives of patients with frontotemporal or semantic dementia who attend an Alzheimer support group rapidly recognise that their relative 'is different' from the rest, even when they have not yet been formally diagnosed so are without preconceptions.

The development of neuropsychology, with its well validated assessment instruments, has undoubtedly contributed to improved recognition and understanding of the 'dementias'. Yet, it may unwittingly too have contributed to the notion of global impairment. If 'global' is defined as 'failure on tests that tap different areas of cognition' then most patients would fulfil those criteria. Yet, there is not a one-to-one correspondence between a test and a function, and patients may fail diverse tests for very circumscribed reasons, such as an impairment of attention due to frontal lobe damage. Clinical neuropsychologists need to bear in mind that 'posterior' hemisphere tests may be performed poorly for 'frontal' reasons and vice versa. Evaluation of patients' performance requires the analysis not only of overall test scores but also qualitative characteristics of performance failure.

The term 'focal' dementia has, in recent years, been adopted to refer to disorders such as FTD, in which there is very clear demarcation between areas that are atrophied and those that are not. It is worth re-iterating that the distinction between 'focal' and 'generalised' disorders is relative rather than absolute, since all disorders have some degree of anatomical selectivity. Moreover, 'focal' does not necessarily mean less severe. Atrophy in patients with forms of frontotemporal lobar degeneration is typically more profound than that found in AD patients, albeit more topographically circumscribed.

11 Conclusions

The notion of dementia as a global, undifferentiated impairment of intellect needs to be abandoned. It is more appropriate to regard the 'dementias' as representing constellations of deficits, which form distinct performance profiles, corresponding to the topographical distribution of degenerative change within the brain. Neuropsychological assessment can play a crucial role in characterising those distinct profiles, leading to improved clinical diagnosis and more person-centred management and care of patients and their families.

Selective references

Abrahams, S., Leigh, P.N., Harvey, A., Vythelingum, G.N., Grise, D., and Goldstein, L.H. (2000). Verbal fluency and executive dysfunction in amyotrophic lateral sclerosis. *Neuropsychologia* **38**, 734–47.

Albert, M.L., Feldman, R.G., and Willis, A.L. (1974). The 'subcortical dementia' of progressive supranuclear palsy. *J Neurol Neurosurg Psychiatry* **37**, 121–30.

Baddeley, A.D., Bressi, S., Della Sala, S., Logie, R., and Spinnler, H. (1991). The decline of working memory in AD. *Brain* **114**, 2521–42.

Baldwin, R.C., Snowden, J.S., and Mann, D.M.A. (1995). Delusional misidentification in association with cortical Lewy Body disease – a case report and overview of possible mechanisms. *Int J Geriatr Psychiatry* **10**, 893–8.

Bates, G., Harper, P., and Jones, L. (2002). Huntington's disease. 3rd edition. Oxford University Press, Oxford.

Bathgate, D., Snowden, J.S., Varma, A., Blackshaw, A., and Neary, D. (2001). Behaviour in fronto-temporal dementia: a comparison with Alzheimer's disease and vascular dementia. *Acta Neurologica Scandinavica* **103**, 367–78.

Burns, A., O'Brien, J., and Ames, D. (2005). Dementia. 3rd edition. Hodder Arnold, London.

Calderon, J., Perry, R.J., Erzinclioglu, S.W., Berrios, G.E., Dening, T.R., and Hodges, J.R. (2001). Perception, attention and working memory are disproportionately impaired in dementia with Lewy bodies compared with Alzheimer's disease. *J Neurol Neurosurg Psychiatry* **70**, 157–64.

Craufurd, D. and Snowden, J.S. (2002). Neuropsychological and neuropsychiatric aspects of Huntington's disease. In *Huntington's disease*, 3rd edition. (eds. G. Bates, P. Harper, and L. Jones), pp. 62–94. Oxford University Press, Oxford.

Doubleday, E.K., Snowden, J.S., Varma, A.R., and Neary, D. (2002). Qualitative performance characteristics differentiate dementia with Lewy bodies and Alzheimer's disease. *J Neurol Neurosurg Psychiatry* **72**, 602–7.

Dubois, B., Feldman, H.H., Jacova, C., DeKosky, S.T., Barberger-Gateau, P., Cummings, J., *et al.* (2007). Research criteria for the diagnosis of Alzheimer's disease: revising the NINCDS-ADRDA criteria. *Lancet Neurol* **6**, 734–46.

Galton, C.J., Patterson, K., Xuereb, J.H., and Hodges, J.R. (2000). Atypical and typical presentations of Alzheimer's disease: a clinical, neuropsychological, neuroimaging and pathological study of 13 cases. *Brain* **123**, 484–98.

Gibbons, Z.C., Richardson, A., Neary, D., and Snowden, J.S. (2008). Behaviour in amyotrophic lateral sclerosis. *Amyotroph Lat Sclerosis* in press.

Green, R.C., Goldstein, F.C., Mirra, S.S., Alazraki, N.P., Baxt, J.L., and Bakay, R.A. (1995). Slowly progressive apraxia in Alzheimer's disease. *J Neurol Neurosurg Psychiatry* **59**, 312–5.

Hodges, J.R, Salmon, D.P., and Butters, N. (1992a). Semantic memory impairment in Alzheimer's disease: failure of access or degraded knowledge? *Neuropsychologia* **30**, 301–14.

Hodges, J.R., Patterson, K., Oxbury, S., and Funnell, E. (1992b). Semantic dementia. Progressive fluent aphasia with temporal lobe atrophy. *Brain* **115**, 1783–806.

Jack, C.R., Petersen, R.C., Xu, Y.C., O'Brien, P.C., Smith, G.E., Ivnik, R.J. *et al.* (1999). Prediction of AD with MRI-based hippocampal volume in mild cognitive impairment. *Neurology* **52**, 1397–403.

Jagust, W.J., Friedland, R.P., Budinger, T.F., Koss, E., and Ober, B. (1988). Longitudinal studies of regional cerebral metabolism in Alzheimer's disease. *Neurology* **38**, 909–12.

Keane, J., Calder, A.J., Hodges, J.R., and Young, A.W. (2002). Face and emotion processing in frontal variant frontotemporal dementia. *Neuropsychologia* **40**, 655–65.

Knopman DS, Boeve BF, Parisi JE, Dickson DW, Smith GE, Ivnik RJ, *et al.* (2005). Antemortem diagnosis of frontotemporal lobar degeneration. *Ann Neurol* **57**, 480–8.

Lough, S., Gregory, C., and Hodges, J.R. (2001). Dissociation of social cognition and executive function in frontal variant frontotemporal dementia. *Neurocase* **7**, 123–30.

Lund and Manchester groups. (1994). Consensus Statement. Clinical and neuropathological criteria for frontotemporal dementia. *J Neurol Neurosurg Psychiatry* **4**, 416–8.

McKeith, I.G., Galasko, D., Kosaka, K., Perry, E.K., Dickson, D.W., Hansen, L.A., *et al.* (1996). Consensus guidelines for the clinical and pathologic diagnosis of dementia with Lewy bodies (DLB). *Neurology* **47**, 1113–24.

McKeith, I., Mintzer, J., Aarsland, D., Burn, D., Chiu, H., Cohen-Mansfield, J., *et al.* (2004). Dementia with Lewy bodies. *Lancet Neurol* **3**, 19–28.

McKeith, I.G., Dickson, D.W., Lowe, J., Emre, M., O'Brien, J.T., Feldman, H., *et al.* (2005). Diagnosis and management of dementia with Lewy bodies. *Neurology* **65**, 1863–72.

McKhann, G., Drachman, D.A., Folstein, M., Katzman, R., Price, D.L., and Stadlan, E.M. (1984). Clinical diagnosis of Alzheimer's disease – report of the NINCDS-ADRDA work group under the auspices of Department of Health and human Services Task force on Alzheimer's disease. *Neurology* **34**, 939–44.

McKhann, G.M., Albert, M.S., Grossman, M., Miller, B., Dickson, D., and Trojanowski JQ (2001). Clinical and pathological diagnosis of frontotemporal dementia. Report of the Work Group on frontotemporal dementia and Pick's disease. *Arch Neurol* **58**, 1803–9.

Mesulam, M-M. (1982). Slowly progressive aphasia without generalized dementia. *Ann Neurol* **11**, 592–8.

Mesulam, M-M (2001). Primary progressive aphasia. *Ann Neurol* **49**, 425–32.

Metzler-Baddeley, C. (2007). A review of cognitive impairments in dementia with Lewy bodies relative to Alzheimer's disease and Parkinson's disease with dementia. *Cortex* **43**, 583–600.

Neary, D., Snowden, J.S., Northen, B, and Goulding, P.J. (1988). Dementia of frontal lobe type. *J Neurol Neurosurg Psychiatry* **51**, 353–61.

Neary, D., Snowden, J.S., Mann, D.M.A., Northen, B., Goulding, P.J., and MacDermott, N. (1990). Frontal lobe dementia and motor neurone disease. *J Neurol Neurosurg Psychiatry* **53**, 23–32.

Neary, D., Snowden, J.S., Gustafson, L., Passant, U., Stuss, D., Black, S., et al. (1998). Frontotemporal lobar degeneration. A consensus on clinical diagnostic criteria. *Neurology* **51**, 1546–54.

Perry, R.J. and Hodges, J.R. (1999). Attention and executive deficits in Alzheimer's disease. A critical review. *Brain* **122**, 383–404.

Perry, R.J., and Hodges, J.R. (2000). Fate of patients with questionable (very mild) Alzheimer's disease: longitudinal profiles of individual subjects' decline. *Dement Geriatr Cog Disord* **11**, 342–9.

Salmon, D.P., Heindel, W.C., and Lange, K.L. (1999). Differential decline in word generation from phonemic and semantic categories during the course of Alzheimer's disease: implications for the integrity of semantic memory. *J Int Neuropsychol Soc* **5**, 692–703.

Snowden, J.S., Goulding, P.J., and Neary, D. (1989). Semantic dementia: a form of circumscribed cerebral atrophy. *Behav Neurol* **2**, 167–82.

Snowden, J.S., Neary, D., Mann, D.M.A., Goulding, P.J. and Testa, H.J. (1992). Progressive language disorder due to lobar atrophy. *Ann Neurol* **31**, 174–83.

Snowden, J.S., Neary, D., and Mann, D.M.A (1996). *Frontotemporal lobar degeneration: frontotemporal dementia, progressive aphasia and semantic dementia*. Churchill Livingstone, London.

Snowden, J.S., Bathgate, D., Varma, A., Blackshaw, A., Gibbons, Z.C. and Neary, D. (2001). Distinct behavioural profiles in frontotemporal dementia and semantic dementia. *J Neurol Neurosurg Psychiatry* **70**, 323–32.

Snowden, J.S., Gibbons, Z.C., Blackshaw, A., Doubleday, E., Thompson, J., Craufurd, D., et al. (2003). Social cognition in frontotemporal dementia and Huntington's disease. *Neuropsychologia* **41**, 688–701.

Snowden, J.S., Stopford, C., Julien, C., Thompson, J.C., Davidson, Y., Gibbons, L. et al. (2007a). Cognitive phenotypes in Alzheimer's disease and genetic risk. *Cortex, Special Issue on The Neuropsychology of Alzheimer's disease* **43**, 835–45.

Snowden, J.S., Neary, D., and Mann, D.M.A. (2007b). Frontotemporal lobar degeneration: clinical and pathological relationships. *Acta Neuropathologica* **114**, 31–8.

Stopford, C.L., Snowden, J.S., Thompson, J.C. and Neary, D. (2007). Distinct memory profiles in Alzheimer's disease. *Cortex (Special Issue on The Neuropsychology of Alzheimer's disease)* **43**, 846–57.

Stopford, C.L., Snowden, J.S., Thompson, J.C. and Neary, D. (2008). Variability in cognitive presentation of Alzheimer's disease. *Cortex* **44**, 185–95.

Talbot, P.R., Snowden, J.S., Lloyd, J.J., Neary, D. and Testa, H.J. (1995). The contribution of single photon emission tomography to the clinical differentiation of degenerative cortical brain disorders. *J Neurol* **242**, 579–86.

Thompson, J.C., Stopford, C.L., Snowden, J.S. and Neary, D. (2005). Qualitative neuropsychological performance characteristics in frontotemporal dementia and Alzheimer's disease. *J Neurol Neurosurg Psychiatry* **76**, 920–7.

Tyrrell, P.J., Warrington, E.K., Frackowiak, R.S.J. and Rossor, M.N. (1990). Heterogeneity in progressive aphasia due to focal cortical atrophy. A clinical and PET study. *Brain* **113**, 1321–36.

Varma, A.R., Snowden, J.S., Lloyd, J.J., Talbot, P.R., Mann, D.M.A., and Neary, D. (1999). Evaluation of the NINCDS-ADRDA criteria in the differentiation of Alzheimer's disease and frontotemporal dementia. *J Neurol Neurosurg Psychiatry* **66**, 184–8.

Warrington, E.K. and James, M. (1991). *Visual Object and Space Perception Battery (VOSP)*. Thames Valley Test Company, Bury St Edmunds.

Welsh, K.A., Butters, N., Hughes, J.P., Mohs, R.C., Heyman, A. (1991). Detection of abnormal memory decline in mild cases of Alzheimer's disease using CERAD neuropsychological measures. *Arch Neurol* **48**, 278–81.

Chapter 29

The neuropsychological presentation and treatment of demyelinating disorders

Peter A. Arnett and Amanda R. Rabinowitz

1 Introduction

By far the most commonly seen and studied demyelinating disorder in clinical neuropsychology is multiple sclerosis (MS). As such, most of this section will focus on MS. Other demyelinating disorders on which some neuropsychological data are available will be reviewed in a brief section at the end.

Clinical neuropsychologists play a pivotal role in assessment and treatment of MS patients. Prior to the advent of sensitive neuropsychological tests, when cognitive evaluations involving brief mental state examinations were primarily used, cognitive difficulties were thought to affect less than 5% of patients (Rao, 1986). Prevalence estimates with use of neuropsychological tests now range from 40-60% (see below). Because cognitive deficits in MS are associated with real-world functioning, neuropsychologists can first evaluate the extent to which tested difficulties displayed by patients may map onto real-world problems, then help patients make modifications to daily routines that allow them to circumvent cognitive difficulties they display. Neuropsychologists can also help identify and treat the depression that is so common, but often overlooked, in MS patients.

2 Pathophysiology of MS

MS is a demyelinating disease of the central nervous system whose cause is not yet fully explained, although it is thought to be related to an autoimmune process, a slow-acting virus or a delayed reaction to a common virus, or epigenetic factors interacting with the environment (ie. lack of vitamin D). One specific autoimmune process identified involves antibodies against antigens located on the myelin sheath that may infiltrate the blood-brain barrier and directly cause demyelination. Various pathophysiological processes may be involved in disease progression. Also, there is considerable variability among patients with regards to structural and immunologic disease features. These observations suggest that MS may be a series of syndromes, rather than a uniform disorder with a singular etiology and disease process (Noseworthy, Lucchinetti, Rodriguez, & Weinshenker, 2000).

The defining pathological feature of the disease is the demyelinated plaque - a lesion characterized by the loss of myelin, the relative preservation of axons, and the presence of astrocytic scars. Myelin is fatty tissue comprised of oligodendrocytic glial cells. Oligodendrocytes surround the neuronal axon and facilitate the propagation of action potentials. Multiple discrete plaques that are found at demyelinated sites are formed, in part, by proliferating astrocytes. Myelin sheaths within plaques are either destroyed or swollen and fragmented. Neural conduction facilitated by myelin because an intact nerve is enclosed in myelin sheaths separated by gaps from which the nerve impulse jumps. Affected areas thus interfere with or block neural transmission by limiting this process known as saltatory conduction. Axons and cell bodies of neurons often remain intact until late stage disease. Early symptoms of disease believed to be a result of the demyelination process. Remission of symptoms attributed to reduction of inflammatory edema and partial remyelination. As disease progresses, however, irreversible axonal injury may occur. Furthermore, oligodendrocyte progenitor pool exhaustion can inhibit remyelination. Remyelination much more likely to occur during acute phases and early in the disease process; minimal remyelination occurs with chronic lesions. These fluctuating disease processes may be responsible for chronic and progressive decline in functioning observed in many patients.

Size of plaques varies from about 1.0mm to several cm. Resulting symptoms typically reflect functions associated with affected areas. Plaques can occur in the brain or spinal cord. Location of plaques is highly variable between patients: Within the cerebrum, plaques near the lateral and 3rd ventricles are most common. Frontal lobes are the next most commonly affected, even when size of frontal lobes relative to rest of brain considered. Plaques in other major lobes of the brain are also frequently observed; additionally, plaques commonly seen in the optic nerves, chiasm, or tracts, as well as the corpus callosum, brain stem, and cerebellum. Majority of plaques (about 75%) are observed in white matter, but some occur in gray matter and in the juncture between gray and white matter. Some remyelination occurs with acute MS plaques.

2.1 Clinical presentation and natural course of MS

Likely acquired before puberty, but actual disease onset occurs in most (2/3rds) patients between ages 20 and 40. Onset before age 15 rare; late onset after age 40 is commonly characterized by quicker progression and greater morbidity. Average life expectancy following onset estimated at 30+ years, but variability is great.

Environmental contribution suggested by generally higher prevalence in temperate zones away from equator with prevalence decreasing near tropics towards equator. Highest prevalence rates (greater than 30 in 100,000) are in Northern Europe, Southern Australia, and middle latitude zones of North America. The 30-40% concordance in identical twins but only 1-13% in fraternal, suggests a genetic and/or epigenetic contribution. Risk in first-degree offspring of MS patients is only 5%, but 20-40 times greater than in general population. No increased risk in adopted children of patients with MS. Presence of HLA-DR2 allele significantly increases risk for MS; populations with greater incidence of this allele (such as Scotland) have greater risk of MS (Noseworthy, Lucchinetti, Rodriguez, & Weinshenker, 2000).

2.1.1 Symptoms

Common symptoms: Muscle weakness, urinary disturbance, and visual anomalies like diplopia, loss of visual acuity, blurry vision, and visual field defects. Fatigue, problems with balance, and paresthesias (usually numbness and tingling in the limbs, trunk, or face) are also common. Significant cognitive difficulties and problems with depression constitute very common symptoms as well. Most common symptoms at MS onset are muscle weakness, paresthesias, visual disturbances, and gait/balance problems. About 50% of patients require assistance walking within 15 years of disease onset (Noseworthy, Lucchinetti, Rodriguez, & Weinshenker, 2000). Mode of symptom onset is typically acute or subacute. Many MS symptoms are transient and unpredictable. For example, visual disturbances and paresthesias may last for seconds or hours. Because of the short-lived and sometimes bizarre nature of symptoms, it is not uncommon for patients in early stages before formal diagnosis to be labeled with hysteric/somatization disorders.

2.1.2 Diagnosis

Diagnosis of MS is clinical and laboratory based. Latest criteria involve various combinations of clinical and laboratory based evidence (McDonald *et al.*, 2001). Patients can get MS diagnosis from either discrete episodes or insidious progression. Regarding a diagnosis from discrete episodes, patients must have had at least one disease attack. If patients have had two or more attacks lasting at least 24 hours and separated in time (at least 30 days), combined with objective clinical evidence of two or more lesions, then that is sufficient for diagnosis. One attack can also lead to diagnosis if there is clinical evidence of at least two lesions, combined with the lesions being disseminated in time as demonstrated by MRI. Other combinations of attacks are also possible. MRI data are considered preferable to other paraclinical tests; however, additional tests can be used when clear-cut MRI findings are not present or atypical clinical presentations occur. Specifically, the presence of oligoclonal IgG bands in the cerebrospinal fluid (CSF) different from those in the serum, or elevated IgG, can be used. Additionally, Visual Evoked Potentials (VEPs) can be used to supplement the clinical examination to reveal evidence of additional lesions. Attacks, relapses, or exacerbations that imply new disease activity are common. Regarding insidious onset where discrete disease attacks are not present, positive CSF results involving presence of oligoclonal bands or raised IgG levels are necessary, combined with both abnormal VEP and various combinations of lesions disseminated in space. Furthermore, there must be MRI or abnormal VEP evidence that lesions are separated in space. Lastly, separation in time should be evident, as reflected by the onset of new MRI lesions or increased level of disability over the course of at least one year. McDonald and colleagues also lay out specific criteria for defining lesions detected on MRI as abnormal and characteristic of MS.

Several course types have been identified (Lublin & Reingold, 1996):

1 Relapsing-remitting (RR) - Most common and characterized by clearly defined disease relapses. Recovery can be full or with sequelae and residual deficit. Complete

remission following the initial episode of symptoms is common. Subsequent episodes are unpredictable, occurring weeks to years later. Symptoms associated with them remit less completely or not at all. Relapses are highly variable, lasting days to weeks, and more rarely, hours and months. No progression of disease between relapses. About 80% of MS patients have this type or secondary-progressive type. The RR and second-ary-progressive types are more common in females than males by about a 2:1 ratio.

2 Secondary-progressive (SP) - Next most common type: First characterized by RR course then progression. Relapses and remissions may or may not occur. Approximately 70% of RR proress into SP.

3 Primary-progressive - Next most common type: Unremitting disease progression from onset for most patients, but occasional stabilization and even improvement in functioning for others. No clear relapses. Prevalence is equivalent in males and females.

4 Progressive-relapsing - Least common type: Disease progression from onset. Acute relapses also occur from which patients may or may not fully recover. The term "chronic-progressive" formerly encompassed all progressive types.

Two severity outcome definitions also identified:

1 Benign - Patient remains fully functional 20 years post disease onset. This occurs in about 10% of patients.

2 Malignant - Rapidly progressing course leading to significant disability or death relatively soon after disease onset. Most patients fall in between these two extremes.

Several factors predict poor outcome including frequent relapses within first two years of onset, early motor and cerebellar findings, and male sex. Predictors of better outcome include female sex, predominantly sensory symptoms, and optic neuritis.

3 Neuropsychological deficits in MS

3.1 Prevalence of neuropsychological deficits

On average, about 45% of community based samples have been shown to have cognitive impairment (Jonsson et al., 2006; Rao, et al., 1991). Prevalence rates shown to be higher among clinic based samples, typically falling between 55% and 65% (Amato, Zipoli, & Portaccio, 2006). Most (about 80%) patients with deficits are relatively mildly affected. Global cognitive deficits uncommon, occurring in about 5-10% of patients (Longley, 2007). However, even mild cognitive problems in MS have been shown to relate to every-day activities (e.g., work, homemaking, personal care activities, social activities) (Higginson, Arnett, & Voss, 2000), including driving (Schultheis, Garay, & DeLuca, 2001), and even employment status (Benedict et al., 2005; Rao et al., 1991).

3.2 Nature of neuropsychological deficits

3.2.1 Intellectual functioning

This is affected significantly in about 20% of patients. Most patients score within a broad normal range.

3.2.2 Academic Skills

Little systematic research conducted on these in MS, but assumed to be intact in most patients.

3.2.3 Memory

One of the most commonly affected cognitive domains in MS. Problems encoding and/or retrieving both verbal and visual information are most common. It is typically manifested as immediate and delayed recall memory deficits on neuropsychological testing. About 30% of patients have substantial problems, another 30% have moderate problems, and the remaining 40% have mild or no problems with this type of memory (Brassington & Marsh, 1998). Working memory, the ability to maintain and manipulate information "on-line," also commonly impaired. Delayed recall deficits usually a function of deficient immediate recall, not forgetting. Learning curve across repeated trials is similar in slope to controls, but lower in magnitude. Percent retention, recognition, and incidental memory following a delay, and remote memory are usually intact. Clinically, memory problems often manifested as complaints of difficulty remembering conversations, appointments, work tasks, etc.

3.2.4 Attention & concentration/speeded information processing

One of the most commonly affected cognitive domains in MS. Difficult to separate speeded information processing from attentional functioning because the latter is necessary for performing any speeded cognitive task. Attention necessary in clinical evaluations to the possibility that memory problems in MS may, in part, be a function of deficits in these domains. MS patients show greatest difficulty on tasks requiring rapid and complex information processing, such as those requiring swift application of working memory operations, attentional switching, or rapid visual scanning. About 20-50% of MS patients have substantial difficulty with this cognitive domain, depending on the task used, with tasks like Oral Symbol Digit revealing more impairment than the PASAT (Benedict, Cookfair *et al.*, 2006). Such increased sensitivity may be due to the visual demands of the Symbol Digit, something that recent research has shown can compromise performance on the task in even MS patients with mild visual acuity problems (Bruce, Bruce, & Arnett, 2007). Simple attention span usually intact, but mild impairments sometimes found. Clinically, attention/speeded processing problems commonly manifested as difficulty tracking and keeping up with and focusing on details of conversations, work tasks, television programs, etc.

3.2.5 Verbal/linguistic deficits

Aphasias are rare in MS, but mild confrontation naming difficulties are sometimes seen. Deficits in verbal fluency are common. Important in clinical evaluations to determine if the latter deficits are associated with memory retrieval difficulties common to MS (Fischer *et al.*, 1994). Also, there is some evidence that the later parts of verbal fluency tasks are most sensitive to the fluency deficits in MS (Smith & Arnett, 2007). Because fluency tasks require rapid production of information, patients' poor performance on them may also be related to their speeded processing deficits. Additionally, slowed speech common to MS should be considered as possible contributor to patients' verbal fluency, as well as speeded attentional, deficits. 20-25% of patients have substantial problems on verbal fluency tasks (Rao, Leo, Bernardin, & Unverzagt, 1991), though some studies have reported impairment frequencies lower than 15% (Benedict, Cookfair *et al.*, 2006). Fluency problems may manifest clinically as word-finding problems impairing the flow of patients' conversations.

3.2.6 Visual-spatial deficits

About 10-20% of individuals with MS show substantial difficulty with higher-order visual-spatial skills involving angle matching or face recognition. Unclear whether higher order visual deficits are a function of primary visual disturbances involving blurred vision and diplopia (Bruce, Bruce, & Arnett, 2007; Rao, Leo, Bernardin, & Unverzagt, 1991). Clinical manifestations may involve accounts of running into things frequently while walking (e.g., doorways) or driving (e.g., curbs) because of visual miscalculations.

3.2.7 Executive skills

Executive skills are commonly affected in MS. Deficits in cognitive flexibility, concept-formation, verbal abstraction, problem-solving, and planning are found. 15-25% of individuals with MS show substantial difficulties in this cognitive domain. May manifest clinically as difficulty planning day-to-day activities (e.g., job tasks, meals, grocery shopping), verbal disinhibition and tangential speech, as well as problems organizing ideas and shifting appropriately from one topic to another in conversation.

3.3 Measurement of neuropsychological deficits

3.3.1 Brief screening batteries/repeatable batteries

An efficient way of approaching neuropsychological testing in MS is to conduct a brief screening evaluation to determine if further testing is warranted. MS patients impaired in one domain of cognitive functioning are not necessarily impaired in others (Rao *et al.*, 1991). Thus, neuropsychological assessments that evaluate major areas of cognitive functioning typically impaired in MS is critical because performance on a test in one domain provides little information about the likelihood of deficits in other domains.

Brief Repeatable Battery (BRB) Rao and colleagues have developed the Brief Repeatable Battery of Neuropsychological Tests in Multiple Sclerosis (Rao, and the Cognitive Function Study Group of the National Multiple Sclerosis Society, 1990) comprised of tests most sensitive to cognitive impairments typically seen in MS; most tests also include 15 alternate forms to allow for repeat testing. Battery includes six-trial version of the Verbal Selective Reminding Test, 10/36 Spatial Recall, Oral Symbol Digit Modalities Test, 2s and 3s Paced Auditory Serial Addition Test (PASAT), and Word List Generation (verbal fluency). Comprehensive norms for BRB can be found in Boringa *et al.* (2001). BRB takes 20-30 minutes to administer. Wechsler Test of Adult Reading (WTAR) (Psychological Corporation, 2001) also recommended and takes 5 minutes. Provides reliable and valid estimate of Full Scale WAIS-III IQ and has excellent norms. Adding the Chicago Multiscale Depression Inventory (CMDI) (Nyenhuis *et al.*, 1995), and Fatigue Severity Scale (FSS)

(Krupp *et al.*, 1988) also suggested. Together, the latter two measures take about 10 minutes and are self-administered, so could be completed in a waiting room before actual testing. Thus, in only 35-45 minutes of actual patient contact time, a reasonably comprehensive neuropsychological screen can be obtained and more extensive testing conducted if deficits are detected.

3.3.2 Minimal Assessment of Cognitive Functioning in MS (MACFIMS)

Developed by consensus from the meeting of a group of experts on neuropsychological functioning in MS (Benedict *et al.*, 2002). Somewhat longer than the BRB, taking approximately 90 minutes. The MACFIMS consists of the following five cognitive domains with tests measuring those domains listed in parentheses: Processing speed/working memory (Oral Symbol Digit Modalities Test, 2s and 3s PASAT), learning and memory (California Verbal Learning Test - 2nd Edition (CVLT-II) and Brief Visuospatial Memory Test – Revised (BVMT-R)), executive function (D-KEFS Sorting Test), visual-spatial processing (Judgment of Line Orientation), and word retrieval (Controlled Oral Word Association Test (COWAT)). In validation study, Benedict and colleagues (2006) found that nearly 60% of MS patients were impaired on at least two of these subtests. Caution required for PASAT use in lower functioning patients; can damage rapport because of their great difficulty performing. Poor performance on Arithmetic subtest of WRAT-4 (see below) may suggest that primary arithmetic calculation difficulties contribute to PASAT deficits.

The authors of MACFIMS also suggest including a number of additional measures to assess potential confounds. First, they recommended employing a culturally appropriate measure of premorbid ability on the first occasion a patient is seen. Several suggestions provided, with the North American Adult Reading Test (NAART) favored by most panel members.

Second, panel recommended that a measure of depression be routinely administered. The CMDI, a depression measure that includes mood, evaluative, and vegetative scales, was recommended as a screen for depression. Because of the overlap of MS disease symptoms and vegetative depression symptoms (e.g., fatigue, sleep disturbance, concentration difficulties, sexual dysfunction), CMDI allows clinician to evaluate whether total depression score is artificially elevated due to differential contribution of vegetative scale. The panel also suggested the possibility that the Beck Depression Inventory - Fast Screen (BDI – FS) be used, though this was recommended with caution since, at the time of this publication, the BDI – FS had not been validated on an MS sample, but since then it has (Benedict *et al.*, 2003). Consists of only 7 items and does not include any vegetative symptoms, thus it circumvents the potential vegetative depression symptom/MS disease symptom confound. Raw scores greater than 3 suggest further evaluation of depression is needed.

A third confound that the consensus authors suggested needed to be addressed were potential problems with vision. They recommended that a measure like the Rosenbaum Pocket Vision Screener could be used, and that a 20/50-70 threshold at 14 inches from the corrected eye was necessary because that was similar to the small print characters presented during neuropsychological testing.

Fourth, although most tests chosen involved a spoken response to circumvent fine motor writing deficits common to MS, the authors suggested that motor confounds that could potentially interfere with performance on the BVMT-R be addressed. They suggested using the copy portion of the BVMT-R administration, in addition to the 9-Hole Peg Test.

Related to motor functioning, the authors of the MACFIMS paper also suggested that a measure of rudimentary oral motor speed be included given that many of the recommended tests required a rapid spoken response. The task they recommended, the Maximum Repetition Rate of Syllables and Multisyllabic Combinations (MRRSMC), requires examinees to repeat the phonemes "pa" "ta" or "ka" as quickly as possible in one good breath lasting at least six seconds. A fourth trial requiring the repetition of the "pa-ta-ka" sequence is also administered. Number of syllables per second is the main scoring index. Given the frequency of dysarthria in MS, it was suggested that slowed speech might impair patients' performance on such tasks. At the time of the MACFIMS publication, no data were available on the MRRSMC. A recent publication examined this test in MS and controls and found that MS patients performed significantly slower on the task compared with controls (Arnett *et al.*, 2008). These authors also found that consideration of the MRRSMC task before comparing group differences on several standard neuropsychological tasks requiring a rapid oral motor response (e.g., COWAT, Animal Naming, Oral Symbol Digit, & PASAT) significantly reduced group differences with controls. Thus, the data suggested that a significant proportion of the variance in group differences between MS patients and controls on these standard neuropsychological tasks was due to the relatively slower speech of MS patients.

Finally, the authors suggested that fatigue be screened using the Fatigue Impact Scale. Although the authors acknowledged that the literature on the influence of fatigue on cognitive functioning in MS was mixed, they noted that fatigue may influence performance in some patients and also was known to influence other domains of quality of life in MS patients. A recent study has shown that the MACFIMS has excellent validity in detecting cognitive impairment in MS (Benedict *et al.*, 2006).

3.3.3 Comprehensive batteries

The MACFIMS provides a core battery from which a more comprehensive battery can be developed. In addition to this minimal battery, the following tests can be added if a more comprehensive evaluation is deemed clinical necessary.

Intellectual functioning Best measured using four-subtest (Vocabulary, Similarities, Matrix Reasoning, Block Design) form of WASI, which allows for derivation of reliable and valid Full Scale, Verbal, and Performance IQ estimates. Entire Wechsler Adult Intelligence Scale, 3rd Edition (WAIS-III) is not necessary in most cases. However, individual subtests are useful for measurement of specific functional areas and are highlighted below. Interpret Block Design cautiously because motor manipulation and visual demands required for it and many other WAIS-III Performance subtests make it difficult to use reliably and validly in MS patients with sensorimotor disturbance. Consider performance on 9-Hole Peg test mentioned above for assistance with interpretation.

Table 29.1 Recommended brief and comprehensive neuropsychological batteries for assessing Multiple Sclerosis patients

---

Brief Screening Battery (About 30 minutes)

Premorbid Intellectual Functioning
Wechsler Test of Adult Reading (WTAR)

Memory
Verbal Selective Reminding Test (6-Trial Version) with delayed recall and recognition
10/36 Spatial Recall with delayed recall and copy

Attention & Concentration/Speeded Information Processing
Symbol Digit Modalities Test (SDMT), Oral Version
Paced Auditory Serial Addition Test (PASAT), 2s and 3s versions

Verbal-Linguistic
Controlled Oral Word Association test (COWAT)

Affective/Emotional, Fatigue
Chicago Multiscale Depression Inventory (CMDI)
Fatigue Severity Scale

Mid-Length Battery (about 90 minutes)

Premorbid Intellectual Functioning
North American Adult Reading Test (NAART)

Memory
California Verbal Learning Test - 2nd Edition (CVLT-II)
Brief Visuospatial Memory Test – Revised (BVMT-R)

Attention & Concentration/Speeded Information Processing
Symbol Digit Modalities Test (SDMT), Oral Version
Paced Auditory Serial Addition Test (PASAT), 2s and 3s versions

Verbal-Linguistic
Controlled Oral Word Association test (COWAT)

Executive
D-KEFS Sorting Test

Visuospatial
Judgment of Line Orientation (JLO)

Affective/Emotional, Fatigue
Chicago Multiscale Depression Inventory (CMDI) or BDI – Fast Screen
Fatigue Impact Scale (FIS)

Sensorimotor
9-Hole Peg Test
Maximum Repetition Rate of Syllables and Multisyllabic Combinations (MRRSMC)
Rosenbaum Pocket Vision Screener

Standard Comprehensive Battery (About 3 hours)

Orientation
Information and Orientation subtest from Wechsler Memory Scale, 3rd Edition (WMS-III)

Intellectual Functioning
Four- subtest form of the Wechsler Abbreviated Scale of Intelligence (WASI)

Academic Functioning
Wide Range Achievement Test, 4th Edition (WRAT-4)

(continued)

Table 29.1 (*continued*) Recommended brief and comprehensive neuropsychological batteries for assessing Multiple Sclerosis patients

Memory
California Verbal Learning Test - 2nd Edition (CVLT-II)
Brief Visuospatial Memory Test – Revised (BVMT-R)
10/36 Spatial Recall with delayed recall and copy
Logical Memory subtests from WMS-III
Information subtest from Wechsler Adult Intelligence Scale, 3rd Edition (WAIS-III)

Attention & Concentration/Speeded Information Processing
Symbol Digit Modalities Test (SDMT), Oral Version
Paced Auditory Serial Addition Test (PASAT), 2s and 3s versions
Digit Span subtest from WMS-III
Spatial Span subtest from WMS-III
Letter-Number Sequencing subtest from WMS-III

Verbal-Linguistic
Controlled Oral Word Association test (COWAT)
Boston Naming Test

Executive
Tower subtest from Delis-Kaplan Executive Function System (D-KEFS)
Card Sorting subtest from D-KEFS, free-sorting condition only
Similarities subtest from WAIS-III

Visuospatial
Judgment of Line Orientation (JLO)

Affective/Emotional, Fatigue
Chicago Multiscale Depression Inventory (CMDI) or BDI – Fast Screen
Hospital Anxiety and Depression Scale (HADS)
Fatigue Impact Scale (FIS)

Sensorimotor
9-Hole Peg Test
Maximum Repetition Rate of Syllables and Multisyllabic Combinations (MRRSMC)
Rosenbaum Pocket Vision Screener

Disability
Multiple Sclerosis Functional Composite

Academic functioning Best evaluated using the Wide Range Achievement Test (WRAT-4), a battery that takes approximately 30-45 minutes to administer, and assesses reading, writing, and arithmetic skills. Significantly worse performance on subtests compared with Full Scale IQ can suggest possibility of a developmental learning disability contributing to pattern of cognitive test performance observed. Such a possibility should be explored in interview, as well, when discussing developmental history.

Memory The Logical Memory subtests (I & II) from the Wechsler Memory Scale - 3rd Edition (WMS-III) are a useful supplement to the memory tests suggested for the MACFIMS. The 10/36 Spatial Recall is also useful, as many patients have significant motor-writing difficulties and 10/36 tests visual memory without any drawing component. Remote memory screened by Information subtest of WAIS-III, orientation by Information and Orientation subtest from WMS-III.

Attention & concentration/speeded information processing In addition to PASAT and Oral Symbol Digit to assess this cognitive domain, Digit Span forward and Spatial Span forward from WMS-III most useful as measures of simple attention span. Letter-Number Sequencing, Spatial Span – Backward, and Digit Span – Backward subtests from WMS-III are recommended as measures of working memory relatively independent of speed.

Verbal/linguistic Confrontation naming may be assessed by Boston Naming Test, 2nd Edition, which is useful only as a screen for verbal function. In addition to the COWAT, semantic fluency (e.g., animal naming) can be useful. Significantly better animal naming than letter-word fluency can suggest that letter-word fluency problems are, in part, a function of semantic memory retrieval difficulties. Comprehensive review has suggested that semantic fluency is just as sensitive as letter-word fluency to verbal fluency problems in MS (Henry & Beatty, 2006), and can be more easily interpreted in non-English speakers (but base-line speaking rate needs to be measured, to rule out artifacts due to slowed articulation).

Executive Wisconsin Card Sorting Test (WCST) has traditionally been used to measure cognitive flexibility and concept formation in MS. However, a study by Beatty and colleagues (1996) suggested that the California Card Sorting Test (CCST) may be better because it allows for differentiation of perseverative responding and concept formation, unlike the WCST. It is important to note that MS patients tended to show impaired concept formation but not perseverative responding. The Delis-Kaplan Executive System battery (D-KEFS; (Delis *et al.*, 2001)) now includes a subtest analogous to CCST called the Card-Sorting Test that can be used and has excellent norms. Because of lengthy administration time, however, only administration of the free-sorting condition is recommended. The Tower Test from D-KEFS is recommended for measuring planning ability, and the Similarities subtest from WAIS-III is a good index of verbal abstraction.

3.4 Possible causes of cognitive deficits

Primary causes of cognitive deficits emanate from a direct consequence of location and extent of brain damage. Thus, cognitive problems caused by primary influences are generally not reversible. There is clear evidence that overall cognitive impairment is associated with total lesion damage in the brain (Rao *et al.*, 1989), gray matter hypointensities (Brass *et al.*, 2006), and especially atrophy (Benedict *et al.*, 2006). There is some evidence that frontal lobe lesions are associated with deficits on executive tasks like Wisconsin Card-Sorting Test (WCST). The association of lesions in other brain areas and specific cognitive deficits is less clear.

Secondary causes of cognitive impairment are a consequence of something associated with a disease such as depression, anxiety, or fatigue. Cognitive problems caused by these secondary influences are potentially reversible if the secondary influence is successfully treated. Relative to primary causes, less attention has been paid in the MS literature to these possible causes of cognitive dysfunction. Recent work shows that depression is associated with impairments in speeded attentional functioning, working memory, and executive functions, but this link is still controversial (Arnett, 2005; Landro *et al.*, 2004). There is little evidence that self-reported fatigue or anxiety are significantly associated with cognitive deficits in MS, but these associations are relatively infrequently examined to date. However, one study suggests that MS patients show greater decline in performance on cognitively demanding tasks over the course of an evaluation with other demanding cognitive tasks. This suggests the possiblity that there is greater susceptibility to cognitive fatigue during testing in MS (Krupp & Elkins, 2000), something that should be taken into consideration when ordering tests in a battery.

3.5 Relationship between cognitive deficits and illness variables

Kurtzke's Expanded Disability Status Scale (EDSS; (Kurtzke, 1983)) has been the most commonly used measure of disability in MS. Occasional studies have reported a relationship between EDSS scores and cognitive impairment, but the majority of studies have not found this. Because of problems with EDSS as a measure of disability, the Multiple Sclerosis Functional Composite (MSFC; (Fischer *et al.* 1999)) was developed. It assesses three clinical dimensions: Leg function/ambulation, arm/hand function, and cognitive function, and is now recommended for use in standard clinical evaluations.

Recent longitudinal work on cognitive decline in MS paints a variable picture. Most studies show relative stability over about a 3-4 year period (Longley, 2007). However, patients identified as cognitively impaired are the most likely to show cognitive decline (Kujala, Portin, & Ruutiainen, 1997), even over a relatively short period of time (e.g., three years). The most extensive longitudinal study to date (10 years) has shown that nearly 50% of MS patients unimpaired initially, remained so 10 years later (Amato *et al.*, 2001). These investigators also found, however, that whereas 26% of patients were mild/moderately impaired at baseline, 56% were impaired at the 10-year follow-up. Visual and verbal recall memory, verbal fluency, visuospatial function, processing speed, and verbal intelligence may be most susceptible to decline over an 8-10 year period (Achiron *et al.*, 2005; Bobholz & Rao, 2003; Piras *et al.*, 2003). Compared with relapsing-remitting patients, progressive patients show greater cognitive dysfunction; one study estimated that secondary-progressive patients had seven times greater risk of cognitive impairment than relapsing-remitting patients (Chelune *et al.*, 2004). Nonetheless, relapsing-remitting patients shown to be cognitively impaired relative to healthy matched controls even when they are in remission.

4 Related emotional disorders

4.1 Depression

Very common in MS with lifetime prevalence around 50% for major depression. Point prevalence rates vary between about 15-50%, depending on diagnostic approach. Studies using clinical interviews and diagnostic criteria report lower prevalence; those using cut-offs from self-report measures report higher. Accurate screening and diagnosis of depression is extremely important, given the increased risk of suicide in MS; the latter may be the cause of death in up to 15% of MS clinic patients (Chwastiak & Ehde, 2007).

Depression has been shown to be treatable through brief and even telephone-based cognitive-behavioral therapy (Mohr *et al.*, 2000), as well as group therapy. Also, cognitive-behavioral stress management training shown to reduce emotional distress in MS (Fischer *et al.*, 1994). Nonetheless, depression/distress historically undertreated in MS. Successful treatment of depression associated with greater adherence to immunotherapy.

There has been no consensus regarding the nature of depression in the MS literature. Some investigators have presented evidence that neurovegetative symptoms of depression are not valid indicators of depression because of their overlap with MS symptoms (e.g., sleep disturbance, fatigue, sexual dysfunction), while others have provided evidence to the contrary. This debate suggests caution is warranted in interpreting neurovegetative symptoms of depression as depression symptoms in any individual MS patient.

The cause of depression in MS unknown, but high levels of perceived stress, low levels of social support, and disease exacerbation/pharmacological treatment of shown to be associated with increased emotional distress. Depression is associated with reduced quality of life and employment of generally less effective (emotion-focused, avoidant) coping strategies in MS. Negative cognitive schema associated with depression, and these also may moderate the impact of pain (Bruce *et al.*, 2007) and stress (Beeney & Arnett, 2008) on depression in MS. Lesion burden, especially in temporal brain regions, associated with depression in MS, and may represent a neural substrate (Feinstein, 2004). Premorbid history of depression is no greater than in non-MS. However, patients with history of depression, before or after MS onset, may be at increased risk for future depressive and manic states.

4.2 Anxiety

Possibly more common than depression, but infrequently studied in MS. Data are limited, but point prevalence of clinically significant anxiety thought to be about 25% with lifetime prevalence estimates around 35% (Korostil & Feinstein, 2007). Lifetime prevalence of specific anxiety disorders has only been minimally studied, but most frequent include generalized anxiety disorder, followed by panic disorder, and then obsessive compulsive disorder. Cause of anxiety in MS unknown, but prominent in early stages of disease when diagnosis and prognosis most uncertain. Decline in distress associated with more definitive diagnostic statements by treatment professionals. Best predictors of anxiety disorders include being female, a co-morbid diagnosis of depression, and limited social support. Drinking to excess, higher social stress, and contemplation of suicide also associated with anxiety (Korostil & Feinstein, 2007). Comorbidity of anxiety and depression more associated with thoughts of self-harm, social dysfunction, and somatic complaints than either alone (Feinstein *et al.*, 1999). Limited existing research suggests that anxiety disorders are undetected and untreated in the majority of patients.

4.3 Other emotional disorders

Only other emotional disorder occurring with any significant frequency in MS is bipolar disorder. Point prevalence estimated at 0-2% and lifetime prevalence 13-16%. No published treatment studies of bipolar disorder in MS. Cause unknown. Pseudobulbar affect, a condition where patients laugh or cry out of proportion to any underlying emotion, occurs in some patients and is sometimes referred to as pathological laughing or crying (Chwastiak & Ehde, 2007). The cause is not well understood, but thought to represent some type of disconnection syndrome where there is a loss of brainstem inhibition of laughing and crying. It occurs in about 10% of patients.

4.4 Measurement of emotional disorders

There is no consensus on how depression is best measured in MS because of neurovegetative symptoms debate outlined above. However, CMDI recommended because it has been validated in MS and allows for breakdown of depression into mood, evaluative, and neurovegetative symptoms of depression in separate scales. Mood and evaluative scales are more likely to reflect depression in MS because they are not confounded with MS symptoms like neurovegetative scale. Nonetheless, neurovegetative symptoms may reflect depression in some patients, so should not be dismissed, just interpreted with caution. BDI – Fast Screen is also a useful screening tool that has been validated in MS. Clinical interview can be used to follow-up initial screening with CMDI, if necessary.

There is no consensus on how anxiety is best measured in MS, but the Hospital Anxiety and Depression Scale been shown to be useful (Feinstein *et al.*, 1999); a measure that takes only about 5 minutes to complete and can be followed up with clinical interview, if necessary. It is unclear how bipolar disorder is best measured in MS. Diagnostic interviews are the only reliable method reported to date.

5 Neuropsychological/cognitive rehabilitation in MS

Approaches to cognitive rehabilitation in MS have been suggested, but few have convincing empirical validation. Many early empirical studies of cognitive retraining interventions were characterized by small sample sizes, absence of control groups, and disappointing results in terms of their effect on cognitive functioning (Brassington & Marsh, 1998). However, more recent and well-designed studies have demonstrated positive initial results for some interventions. Given that many patients remain relatively stable cognitively over long periods of time, they may be more likely than patients with other neurological conditions to benefit from cognitive rehabilitation (Longley, 2007).

The story memory technique (SMT) is designed to train individuals to make use of imagery and context in order to improve learning. This intervention was investigated in a randomized clinical trial as a treatment for memory impairment in a group of MS patients with memory deficits. MS patients with moderate to severe impairments showed a significant improvement on the Selective Reminding Test compared with patients in the control condition. The treatment group also reported significant self-reported improvement in memory, suggesting that improved performance on the neuropsychological measure may be reflective of meaningful improvements in real life cognitive functioning (Chiaravalloti *et al.*, 2005; Krupp *et al.*, 2004).

Recent research on self-generated learning in MS patients has yielded promising results as well. Items generated by an individual are better remembered than items that are simply presented; this phenomenon is robust within the general population, and has been labeled the generation effect (Slamecka & Graf, 1978). Chiaravalloti and DeLuca (2002) demonstrated the generation effect in a sample of MS patients with mild to moderate memory impairment, reporting significantly better recall and recognition of self-generated stimuli compared with presented stimuli. These results were replicated and extended in a study by Basso and colleagues (2006). This study examined self-generated encoding for information related to activities of daily living - specifically names, appointments, and object locations. In a sample of MS patients with moderate to severe memory impairment, the investigators found significantly better memory for self-generated, compared with didactically presented, stimuli. The results of these two studies suggest that cognitive rehabilitation interventions based on self-generated learning could improve memory performance in MS patients. The findings reported by Basso and colleagues (2006) indicate that such an intervention may promote memory improvements that are relevant to real-life functioning.

Other interventions have focused on improving attentional functioning in MS patients. One study examined the efficacy of computer-aided retraining of memory and attention in a randomized, double-blind, controlled trial. The study treatment - a computer-assisted memory and attention retraining intervention - was compared with a control intervention - a visuo-constructional and visuo-motor coordination computer-assisted intervention. Although the results did not support superiority of the study treatment, in both groups about 45% of patients demonstrated significant improvement on measures of neuropsychological functioning (Solari et al., 2004). These results may suggest that computer-assisted cognitive intervention is helpful in MS patients, irrespective of specificity (Penner et al., 2006); however, as the authors acknowledge, improvements by all study participants could simply have been a function of practice effects.

Failure of some large well-designed studies to detect significant treatment effects of cognitive retraining interventions has suggested that cognitive rehabilitation may not be viable for MS patients. However, some have argued that certain methodological limitations are in part responsible for the disappointing findings to date. Chiaravalloti and colleagues (2005) suggest that future studies should focus on including only those patients who are selectively impaired in the cognitive domain targeted by the experimental intervention. This methodological consideration, in conjunction with some recent promising findings, suggests that cognitive retraining may be effective in some MS patients. However future work is needed to continue to develop effective treatments, and better identify patients who will respond to specific interventions.

The inconsistent findings in the literature regarding cognitive retraining have led some to suggest that pursuing compensatory strategies for MS patients may be more promising; however, cognitive retraining has not been sufficiently studied to rule out the possibility that it may work for some patients. Nonetheless, because compensatory strategies have been studied more extensively in other neurologic populations (e.g., traumatic brain injury) and been shown to be beneficial, it may be useful to apply them to MS patients (Fischer et al., 1994). These include strategies such as:

1 Using external aids (e.g., date books, wristwatches with alarms, electronic planners) for tracking and prompting for important information such as appointments, to-do lists, and medication times;

2 keeping things that must be remembered in one place; and

3 putting calendars in prominent locations and having family members use them so that the affected individual can track family and her/his own activities better.

Although also not systematically studied to date, making workplace modifications that involve things such as reducing distractions and minimizing requirements for speed in the work area might be especially beneficial to persons with MS who suffer from attentional and speeded processing difficulties. Also, because even MS patients with memory difficulties typically show learning with repetition, providing opportunities for recording important meetings, lectures, etc. for later review/rehearsal may be helpful to some patients. Given how common speeded processing difficulties are in MS, making changes in patients' day-to-day environments that allow for adequate time to process information may improve their accuracy in performing day-to-day cognitive tasks (Demaree *et al.*, 1999).

Some recent studies suggest that medications are a promising option for treating MS related cognitive impairment. An acetylcholinesterase inhibitor (donepezil) has been used to treat cognitive impairment in Alzheimer's disease. A recent study found that donepezil is also effective in improving memory performance on the Selective Reminding Test (SRT) in MS patients compared with placebo matched controls. This effect remained significant when controlling for physical disability, MS subtype, β-interferon use, gender, baseline SRT score, and other covariates (Christodoulou *et al.*, 2006).

Another study by Fischer and colleagues (2000) examined the efficacy of a β-interferon medication for improving cognitive functioning. 166 persons with relapsing forms of MS from the original double-blind, placebo-controlled trial of IFNβ-1a were compared at baseline then after two-year follow-up on a variety of neuropsychological tests. Compared with the placebo group, the IFNβ-1a group improved significantly more on the CVLT (trials 1-5 total), Tower of London, and Ruff Figural Fluency Test. Additionally, significantly fewer IFNβ-1a group patients showed sustained PASAT decline by treatment end. Because study sample restricted to patients with relapsing MS between ages 18-55 and very restricted range of EDSS scores (1-3.5), however, caution warranted in applying results to patients not meeting such criteria. Effect of depression treatment on neuropsychological functioning in MS has been studied systematically in only one study (Rodgers *et al.*, 1996). Significant improvement in performance on tests of word-list learning and verbal abstraction corresponded to significant reduction in depression in a cognitive therapy treatment group. Although characterized by non-random assignment of patients to treatment groups, non-clinically depressed patients, and relatively small n, results were promising and suggest that depression treatment (even in subclinical patients) could have beneficial cognitive effects in MS. Therefore, beyond improving the well being of individuals with MS and making them more likely to adhere to important disease-modifying medication regimens (see above), successful treatment of depression may improve patients' cognitive functioning in some domains.

6 Other considerations for MS

Sleep problems are common in MS, but poorly understood. High and debilitating levels of fatigue reported by MS patients appear likely to be related to sleep problems, disease severity, and depression (Strober & Arnett, 2005). Recommended that fatigue be briefly screened using FSS or examined in more detail using Fatigue Impact Scale (FIS) (Fisk *et al.*, 1994). The latter allows for evaluation of physical, social, and cognitive fatigue in separate scales. Cutoff score of 75 for total score recommended to identify those with significant functional limitations relating to fatigue. Providing breaks throughout testing day may help minimize possible impact of fatigue on test performance.

7 Other demyelinating diseases

Demyelinating diseases other than MS are comparatively rare, have been only minimally studied neuropsychologically, and are infrequently seen by clinical neuropsychologists. What follows is a brief discussion of two other demyelinating diseases.

7.1 Marchiafava-Bignami disease

This is characterized by focal demyelination in the medial zone of corpus callosum and most commonly associated with chronic alcoholism. Rare but well-documented cases have been reported in nonalcoholics. Degeneration of anterior and posterior commissures, centrum semiovale, middle cerebellar peduncles, subcortical white matter, and long association bundles also sometimes seen. Symptom onset is usually insidious and nonspecific with both focal and diffuse manifestations of cerebral disease common; acute presentations involving deteriorating speech, gait, orientation, and consciousness also seen. Psychiatric symptoms are frequently present including delusional states, paranoia, mania, and depression. Psychomotor slowing, apathy, and dysarthria also seen. Neuropsychologically, nonspecific dementia is most common. Callosal signs also characteristic. For example, patients may be able to name objects placed in one hand or presented to one visual field, but not in the other hand or field. Hemispheric disconnection signs also include unilateral apraxias and agraphias in the absence of aphasia, in addition to unilateral sensory (i.e., auditory, tactile, visual) simultaneous extinction. Alien hand syndrome is sometimes seen, most often on the left side or bilaterally.

7.2 Central Pontine Myelinolysis (CPM)

This involves destruction of the myelin sheaths in the central portion of the basis pontis, and is most often found in young to middle-aged adults. Myelinolytic lesions are not restricted to the brain stem and are observed in the cerebral cortex, thalamus, basal ganglia, subcortical white matter, amygdala, centrum semiovale, internal capsule, cerebellum, and corpus callosum. It is associated with chronic alcoholism and/or malnutrition in most cases, but also with liver, kidney, and brain disease and organ transplants. More recently it has been seen with AIDS, chemotherapy, and viral infections. Definitive causes are unknown, but rapid correction of hyponatremia is suspected. Acute symptoms include altered levels of consciousness, seizures, lethargy, mutism, pseudobulbar palsy, and quadriparesis. Course of disease can be rapid, with death ensuing within days or weeks of symptom onset, but more patients have survived acute phase of illness in recent years. Neuropsychological data to date are limited to case reports that indicate persistence of deficits beyond the acute stage involving global intelligence and reasoning, learning and memory, visual- and fine-motor speed, and attention and concentration. Confusional states most likely associated with underlying metabolic problem that causes CPM are not uncommon. Neuropsychiatric features including pressured and tangential speech, restlessness and agitation, and impaired insight and judgment have been reported as initial presenting symptoms of CPM.

Acknowledgements

Special thanks to our colleagues in the field Drs. Stephen Rao, Michael Basso, William Beatty, John DeLuca, Lauren Krupp, and David Mohr for their thoughts regarding the optimal battery of tests to be used for neuropsychological assessment of MS patients. We also express our gratitude to the MS participants and their significant others who have contributed their time in our studies to helping us to better understand the nature of multiple sclerosis.

Correspondence concerning this article should be addressed to: Peter Arnett, Psychology Department, Penn State University, 522 Moore Building, University Park, PA 16802-3105. Electronic mail: paa6@psu.edu.

Selective references

Achiron, A., Polliack, M., Rao, S. M., Barak, Y., Lavie, M., Appelboim, M., *et al.* (2005). Cognitive patterns and progression in multiple sclerosis: Construction and validation of percentile curves. *Journal of Neurology Neurosurgery and Psychiatry*, **76**, 744–749.

Amato, M. P., Ponziani, G., Siracusa, G., and Sorbi, S. (2001). Cognitive dysfunction in early-onset multiple sclerosis: A reappraisal after 10 years. *Archives of Neurology*, **58**, 1602–1606.

Amato, M. P., Zipoli, V., and Portaccio, E. (2006). Multiple sclerosis-related cognitive changes: a review of cross-sectional and longitudinal studies. *Journal of the Neurological Sciences*, **245**, 41–46.

Arnett, P. A. (2005). Longitudinal consistency of the relationship between depression symptoms and cognitive functioning in multiple sclerosis. *CNS Spectrums: The International Journal of Neuropsychiatric Medicine*, **10**, 372–382.

Arnett, P. A., Smith, M. M., Barwick, F. H., Benedict, R. H. B., and Ahlstrom, B. P. (2008). Oralmotor slowing in multiple sclerosis: Relationship to neuropsychological tasks requiring an oral response. *Journal of the International Neuropsychological Society*, **14**, 454–462.

Basso, M. R., Lowery, N., Ghormley, C., Combs, D., and Johnson, J. (2006). Self-generated learning in people with multiple sclerosis. *Journal of the International Neuropsychological Society*, **12**, 640–648.

Beatty, W. W., and Monson, N. (1996). Problem solving by patients with multiple sclerosis: Comparison of performance on the Wisconsin and California Card Sorting Test. *Journal of the International Neuropsychological Society*, **2**, 134–140.

Beeney, J. E., and Arnett, P. A. (2008). Stress and affective memory bias interact to predict depressive symptoms in multiple sclerosis. *Neuropsychology*, **22**, 118–126.

Benedict, R. H. B., Bruce, J. M., Dwyer, M. G., Abdelrahman, N., Hussein, S., Weinstock-Guttman, B., *et al.* (2006). Neocortical Atrophy, Third Ventricular Width, and Cognitive Dysfunction in Multiple Sclerosis. *Archives of Neurology*, **63**, 1301–1306.

Benedict, R. H. B., Cookfair, D., Gavett, R., Gunther, M., Munschauer, F., Garg, N., *et al.* (2006). Validity of the minimal assessment of cognitive function in multiple sclerosis (MACFIMS). *Journal of the International Neuropsychological Society*, **12**, 549–558.

Benedict, R. H. B., Fischer, J. S., Archibald, C. J., Arnett, P. A., Beatty, W. W., Bobholz, J., *et al.* (2002). Minimal neuropsychological assessment of MS patients: A consensus approach. *The Clinical Neuropsychologist*, **16**, 381–397.

Benedict, R. H. B., Fishman, I., McClellan, M. M., Bakshi, R., and Weinstock-Guttman, B. (2003). Validity of the Beck Depression Inventory-Fast Screen in multiple sclerosis. *Multiple Sclerosis*, **9**, 393–396.

Benedict, R. H. B., Wahlig, E., Bakshi, R., Fishman, I., Munschauer, F., Zivadinov, R., *et al.* (2005). Predicting quality of life in multiple sclerosis: accounting for physical disability, fatigue, cognition, mood disorder, personality, and behavior change. *Journal of the Neurological Sciences*, **231**, 29–34.

Bobholz, J., and Rao, S. (2003). Cognitive dysfunction in multiple sclerosis: a review of recent developments. *Current Opinion in Neurology*, **16**, 283–288.

Boringa, J. B., Lazeron, R. H. C., Reuling, I. E. W., Ader, H. J., Pfennings, L., Lindeboom, J., *et al.* (2001). The Brief Repeatable Battery of Neuropsychological Tests: Normative values allow application in multiple sclerosis clinical practice. *Multiple Sclerosis*, **7**, 263–267.

Brass, S. D., Benedict, R. H. B., Weinstock-Guttman, B., Munschauer, F., and Bakshi, R. (2006). Cognitive impairment is associated with subcortical magnetic resonance imaging grey matter T2 hypointensity in multiple sclerosis. *Multiple Sclerosis*, **12**, 437–444.

Brassington, J. C., and Marsh, N. V. (1998). Neuropsychological aspects of multiple sclerosis. *Neuropsychology Review*, **8**, 43–77.

Bruce, J. M., Bruce, A. S., and Arnett, P. A. (2007). Mild visual acuity disturbances are associated with performance on tests of complex visual attention in MS. *Journal of Clinical and Experimental Neuropsychology*, **13**, 544–548.

Bruce, J. M., Polen, D. M., and Arnett, P. A. (2007). Pain and affective memory biases interact to predict depressive symptoms in multiple sclerosis. *Multiple Sclerosis*, **13**, 58–66.

Chelune, G. J., Feisthamel, K., and Stone, L. (2004). Assessing the prevalence and relative risk of cognitive dysfunction in patients with multiple sclerosis. *Brain Impairment*, **5**(Suppl), 77.

Chiaravalloti, N. D., and DeLuca, J. (2002). Self-generation as a means of maximizing learning in multiple sclerosis: An application of the generation effect. *Archives of Physical Medicine and Rehabilitation*, **83**, 1070–1079.

Chiaravalloti, N. D., DeLuca, J., Moore, N. B., and Ricker, J. H. (2005). Treating learning impairments improves memory performance in multiple sclerosis: a randomized clinical trial. *Multiple Sclerosis*, **11**, 58–68.

Christodoulou, C., Melville, P., Scherl, W. F., MacAllister, W. S., Elkins, L. E., and Krupp, L. B. (2006). Effects of donepezil on memory and cognition in multiple sclerosis. *Journal of the Neurological Sciences*, **245**, 127–136.

Chwastiak, L. A., and Ehde, D. M. (2007). Psychiatric issues in multiple sclerosis. *Psychiatric Clinics of North America*, **30**, 803–817.

Corporation, T. P. (2001). *The Wechsler Test of Adult Reading (WTAR):Test Manual*. San Antonio, TX: The Psychological Corporation.

Delis, D. C., Kramer, J. H., and Kaplan, E. (2001). *Delis*-Kaplan *Executive Function Scale, Card Sorting Test*. San Antonio, TX: The Psychological Corporation.

Demaree, H. A., DeLuca, J., Gaudino, E. A., and Diamond, B. J. (1999). Speed of information processing as a key deficit in multiple sclerosis: implications for rehabilitation. *Journal of Neurology Neurosurgery and Psychiatry*, **67**, 661–663.

Feinstein, A. (2004). The neuropsychiatry of multiple sclerosis. *Canadian Journal of Psychiatry*, **49**, 157–163.

Feinstein, A., O'Connor, P., Gray, T., and Feinstein, K. (1999). The effects of anxiety on psychiatric morbidity in patients with multiple sclerosis. *Multiple Sclerosis*, **5**, 323–326.

Fischer, J. S., Foley, F. W., Aikens, J. E., Ericson, D. G., Rao, S. M., and Shindell, S. (1994). What do we *really* know about cognitive dysfunction, affective disorders, and stress in multiple sclerosis? A practitioner's guide. *Journal of Neurological Rehabilitation*, 8(3), 151–164.

Fischer, J. S., Priore, R. L., Jacobs, L. D., Cookfair, D. L., Rudick, R. A., Herndon, R. M., *et al.* (2000). Neuropsychological effects of interferon Beta-1a in relapsing multiple sclerosis. *Annals of Neurology*, 48, 885–892.

Fischer, J. S., Rudick, R. A., Cutter, G. A., and Reingold, S. C. (1999). The Multiple Sclerosis Functional Composite (MSFC): an integrated approach to MS clinical outcome assessment. *Multiple Sclerosis*, 3, 244–250.

Fisk, J. D., Pontefract, A., Ritvo, P. G., Archibald, C. J., and Murray, T. J. (1994). The impact of fatigue on patients with multiple sclerosis. *Canadian Journal of Neurological Sciences*, 21, 9–14.

Henry, J. D., and Beatty, W. W. (2006). Verbal fluency deficits in multiple sclerosis. *Neuropsychologia*, 44, 1166–1174.

Higginson, C. I., Arnett, P. A., and Voss, W. D. (2000). The ecological validity of clinical tests of memory and attention in multiple sclerosis. *Archives of Clinical Neuropsychology*, 15, 185–204.

Jonsson, A., Andresen, J., Storr, L., Tscherning, T., Sorensen, P. S., and Ravnborg, M. (2006). Cognitive impairment in newly diagnosed multiple sclerosis patients: A 4-year follow-up study. *Journal of the Neurological Sciences*, 245, 77–85.

Korostil, M., and Feinstein, A. (2007). Anxiety disorders and their clinical correlates in multiple sclerosis patients. *Multiple Sclerosis*, 13, 67–72.

Krupp, L. B., Alvarez, L. A., LaRocca, N. G., and Scheinberg, L. C. (1988). Fatigue in multiple sclerosis. *Archives of Neurology*, 45, 435–438.

Krupp, L. B., Christodoulou, C., Melville, P., Scherl, W. F., MacAllister, W. S., and Elkins, L. E. (2004). Donepezil improved memory in multiple sclerosis in a randomized clinical trial. *Neurology*, 63, 1579–1585.

Krupp, L. B., and Elkins, L. E. (2000). Fatigue and declines in cognitive functioning in multiple sclerosis. *Neurology*, 55, 934–939.

Kujala, P., Portin, R., and Ruutiainen, J. (1997). The progress of cognitive decline in multiple sclerosis: A controlled 3-year follow-up. *Brain*, 120, 289–297.

Kurtzke, J. F. (1983). Rating neurologic impairment in multiple sclerosis: an expanded disability status scale (EDSS). *Neurology*, 33, 1444–1452.

Landro, N. I., Celius, E. G., and Sletvold, H. (2004). Depressive symptoms account for deficient information processing speed but not for impaired working memory in early phase multiple sclerosis (MS). *Journal of the Neurological Sciences*, 217, 211–216.

Longley, W. A. (2007). Multiple sclerosis-related dementia: Relatively rare and often misunderstood. *Clinical practice -: Current opinion*, 8, 154–167.

Lublin, F. D., and Reingold, S. C. (1996). Defining the clinical course of multiple sclerosis: Results of an international survey. *Neurology*, 46, 907–911.

McDonald, W. I., Compston, A., Edan, G., Goodkin, D., Hartung, H.-P., Lublin, F. D., *et al.* (2001). Recommended diagnostic criteria for multiple sclerosis: Guidelines from the international panel on the diagnosis of multiple sclerosis. *Annals of Neurology*, 50, 121–127.

Mohr, D.C. Van Der Wende, J., Dwyer, P., and Dick, L.P. (2000). Telephone-administered cognitive-behavioural therapy for the treatment of depressive symptoms in multiple sclerosis. *Journal of Consulting and Clinical Psychology*, 68, 356–61.

Noseworthy, J. H., Lucchinetti, C., Rodriguez, M., and Weinshenker, B. G. (2000). Multiple Sclerosis. *New England Journal of Medicine*, 343, 938–952.

Nyenhuis, D. L., Rao, S. M., Ph.D., Zajecka, J., M.D., Luchetta, T., Bernardin, L., and Garron, D. (1995). Mood disturbance versus other symptoms of depression in multiple sclerosis. *Journal of the International Neuropsychological Society*, 1, 291–296.

Penner, I.-K., Kappos, L., Rausch, M., Opwis, K., and Radu, E. W. (2006). Therapy-induced plasticity of cognitive functions in MS patients: Insights from fMRI. *Journal of Physiology - Paris*, **99**, 455–462.

Piras, M. R., Magnano, I., Canu, E. D. G., Paulus, K. S., Satta, W. M., Soddu, A., *et al.* (2003). Longitudinal study of cognitive dysfunction in multiple sclerosis: neuropsychological, neuroradiological, and neurophysiological findings. *Journal of Neurology Neurosurgery and Psychiatry*, **74**, 878–885.

Rao, S. M. (1986). Neuropsychology of multiple sclerosis: a critical review. *Journal of Clinical and Experimental Neuropsychology*, **8**, 503–542.

Rao, S. M., and the Cognitive Function Study Group of the National Multiple Sclerosis Society. (1990). *Manual for the Brief Repeatable Battery of Neuropsychological Tests in Multiple Sclerosis*. New York: National Multiple Sclerosis Society.

Rao, S. M., Leo, G. J., Bernardin, L., and Unverzagt, F. (1991). Cognitive dysfunction in multiple sclerosis. 1. Frequency, patterns, and prediction. *Neurology*, **41**, 685–691.

Rao, S. M., Leo, G. J., Ellington, L., Nauertz, T., Bernardin, L., and Unverzagt, F. (1991). Cognitive dysfunction in multiple sclerosis. II. Impact on employment and social functioning. *Neurology*, **41**, 692–696.

Rao, S. M., Leo, G. J., Haughton, V. M., St.Aubin-Faubert, P., and Bernardin, L. (1989). Correlation of magnetic resonance imaging with neuropsychological testing in multiple sclerosis. *Neurology*, **39**, 161–166.

Rodgers, D., Khoo, K., MacEachen, M., Oven, M., and Beatty, W. W. (1996). Cognitive therapy for multiple sclerosis: A preliminary study. *Alternative Therapies*, **2**, 70–74.

Schultheis, M. T., Garay, E., and DeLuca, J. (2001). The influence of cognitive impairment on driving performance in multiple sclerosis. *Neurology*, **56**, 1089–1084.

Slamecka, N. J., and Graf, P. (1978). The generation effect: Delineation of a phenomenon. *Journal of Experimental Psychology: Human Learning and Memory*, **4**, 592–604.

Smith, M. M., and Arnett, P. A. (2007). Dysarthria Predicts Poorer Performance on Cognitive Tasks Requiring a Speeded Oral Response in an MS Population. *Journal of Clinical and Experimental Neuropsychology*, **29**, 804–812.

Solari, A., Motta, A., Mendozzi, L., Pucci, E., Forni, M., Mancardi, G., *et al.* (2004). Computer-aided retraining of memory and attention in people with multiple sclerosis: a randomized, double-blind controlled trial. *Journal of the Neurological Sciences*, **222**, 99–104.

Strober, L. B., and Arnett, P. A. (2005). An examination of four models predicting fatigue in multiple sclerosis. *Archives of Clinical Neuropsychology*, **20**, 631–646.

Chapter 30

The neuropsychology of endocrine disorders

David M. Erlanger, Geoffrey Tremont and
Jennifer Duncan Davis

1 Introduction

A basic understanding of how endocrine dysfunction affects the central nervous system is important for a majority of cases referred for assessment by clinical neuropsychologists. Beyond playing a role in assessment and management in more obvious scenarios, such as pituitary adenoma and Graves' disease, increasing attention is being paid to the role of neuropsychology in assessment and management of cognitive dysfunction due to illnesses with direct or indirect effects on the endocrine system and, secondarily, the central nervous system. Alternatively endocrine dysfunction can result from a primary neurologic insult or condition. In addition, patients referred for routine assessment of traumatic brain injury, attention deficit/hyperactivity disorder, or neurodegenerative disorder may have significant histories of thyroid dysfunction, diabetes, and other common endocrine conditions with known effects on the brain and cognitive function. In all such cases, neuropsychologists should be prepared to integrate their understanding of these factors into their clinical interview and the interpretation of their objective neuropsychological test findings.

Regardless of the referral question, clinical neuropsychologists have expertise in understanding how cognitive problems play out in real life situations at work and at home. Problems with the endocrine system can have discrete, often remediable, effects on motor function, learning, or even emotional functions. Monitoring and intervention in such cases by means of periodic assessment has the potential to lead to more cost-effective healthcare and improved quality of life (Ryan and Hendrickson, 1998).

1.1 Guidelines for assessment of metabolic history

Critical issues to keep in mind:

◆ Because patients may not be aware of the relevance of information, they may neglect to mention an illness with no obvious association with cognition. Therefore, neuropsychologists should carefully review medical records or ask detailed questions about medical history.

◆ Even though many treatments for some chronic clinical syndromes are provided in an outpatient setting, clinicians should be careful to include a thorough inpatient *and* outpatient medical history in their interview.

♦ Because chronic syndromes can be stable and well-controlled for years, history should extend to the initial onset of symptoms, regardless of how remote.

♦ Age may be an important consideration. Generally, perinatal and/or early childhood onset increases the possible relevance of such history to current cognitive dysfunction. Older adult onset of endocrine disorders may involve atypical symptoms. Also, because of the associated reductions in levels of metabolic and endocrine function, an aging brain may be more vulnerable and may be less responsive to intervention.

♦ Psychiatric and emotional disturbances can be associated, either directly or indirectly, with endocrine dysregulation. By obtaining a detailed history of psychiatric symptom onset, clinicians can examine these relationships.

Obtaining an accurate history of metabolic imbalance may be a complex undertaking. Determining the date of onset is frequently ambiguous. Because the endocrine system and metabolism in general is subject to degeneration due to age, subclinical syndromes may exist for years before being identified, which may be associated with poorer response to therapeutic intervention. Also, because multiple systems may be affected, presenting symptoms may be physiological, psychiatric, cognitive, or a combination. As a result, misdiagnosis is common, even in overt disease. Psychiatric symptoms, in particular, frequently accompany the insidious onset of symptoms in most syndromes entailing dysregulation of the endocrine system. Physiological symptoms secondary to autonomic system dysfunction such as weight gain or sexual dysfunction, similarly, may be useful indicators of the onset of illness retrospectively.

Once diagnosed, stabilization may entail ongoing consultation because (not infrequently), treatment of a hypofunctional system may result in hyperfunction of that same system (or vice-versa), resulting in an ongoing process of adjustment. Therefore in addition to noting the duration of the illness, severity should be ascertained according to the patient's individual history of metabolic control. Adolescent males with Type I diabetes, for example, typically have more difficulty maintaining stable glucose levels due to lifestyle factors. Even remote periods of poor control may be worthy of consideration. Of even greater importance, episodes associated with extreme hormonal imbalance and acute metabolic crises such as hypoglycemic shock are particularly relevant. A single such event may produce persistent symptoms, including cognitive sequelae.

Finally, metabolic control for the several days preceding neuropsychological assessment as well as on the day of the evaluation may affect neuropsychological test performance. This may be due to a direct effect of a hypometabolic condition on performance, or to a secondary effect of a psychiatric symptom such as anxiety or depression on the patient's interaction with the examiner and the test materials.

1.2 Guidelines for assessment

♦ With few exceptions, neuroendocrine dysregulation results in worsening of cognitive functions due to disruptions in neurochemical messages in a manner both generalized and focal. The cognitive domains of attention, memory, and psychomotor speed are most commonly affected, although the effects are often subtle. As such, it is important to use very sensitive measures of cognitive efficiency and working memory.

◆ Even in the context of minimal or no objective cognitive deficits, subjective cognitive and health complaints associated with endocrine dysfunction are common and can impact daily functioning and quality of life. Thus, it is important to include self-report measures of these domains in assessments.

◆ Because relatively subtle differences may be clinically meaningful, IQ data will be useful to determine relative decreases from an individual's expected level of performance.

◆ Because follow-up may be of interest for individuals receiving a treatment intervention such as hormone replacement therapy, neuropsychological instruments may be chosen based on the availability of alternate forms for repeat assessment.

◆ Because of the frequent comorbidity of psychiatric symptoms, the use of mood inventories and mental status evaluations will facilitate assessment and allow for recovery to be monitored multidimensionally (Erlanger *et al.*, 1999).

1.3 Principles of endocrine system operation

The endocrine system produces its effects on bodily and mental functions by means of various hormones secreted by specific endocrine glands and transmitted via the bloodstream to proximate or remote sites. Table 30.1 lists the endocrine glands and hormones with particular relevance to cognitive functioning. Metabolic control of hormone levels is maintained by feedback loops or *axes* of related hormones. For example, the hypothalamic-pituitary-thyroid axis, or HPT axis, is comprised of Thyrotropic Releasing Hormone (TRH), a hormone manufactured in the hypothalamus that induces the pituitary gland to produce Thyroid Stimulating Hormone (TSH), which stimulates the Thyroid gland to produce Triiodothyronine (T_3) and Thyroxine (T_4), the principle Thyroid hormones. These in turn provide feedback both directly and indirectly to the hypothalamus, thus regulating stable thyroid hormone levels. Disruption can occur at any location along the axis. It is in this way, for instance, that a pituitary tumor can affect thyroid functioning.

Individual hormones may perform a number of roles and have multiple types of receptors located throughout the body, including the brain. Two general categories of actions have been described. Those that affect the developing brain are known as *organizational* effects. For instance, congenital hypothyroidism can produce permanent functional and structural changes by altering the pattern of thyroid receptors present in the brain substrate. *Activational* effects on the other hand, are the result of a chemical being present at any given moment. Like any chemical substance, a given hormone's activational effects on behavior are due not only to the identity, dose, and duration of the hormone, but also to the brain substrate upon which it acts.

1.3.1 The hypothalamus

The hypothalamus is the principal autonomic center of the brain, acting on the sympathetic and parasympathetic nervous systems to maintain homeostasis and to prepare the

Table 30.1 Principal endocrine glands and hormones

Anterior pituitary gland

Growth Hormone causes growth of most bodily tissues and cells.
Prolactin promotes breast development and milk secretion.
Follicle-Stimulating Hormone is involved in reproductive and gonadal functioning.
Luteinizing Hormone causes ovulation in females and stimulates the gonads in both sexes.
Adrenocorticotropin stimulates the adrenal cortex to secrete adrenocortical hormones.
Thyroid Stimulating Hormone causes the release of thyroid hormones by the thyroid gland.

Posterior pituitary gland

Vasopressin causes the kidneys to retain water and regulates blood vessels.
Oxytocin facilitates childbirth and lactation.

Thyroid gland

Thyroxine and Triiodothyronine regulate the chemical processes in cells.
Calcitonin causes the deposit of calcium in bones.

Adrenal cortex

Cortisol contributes to the control of proteins, carbohydrates and fats.
Aldosterone regulates levels of sodium and potassium.

Pancreas

Insulin promotes the storage of glucose into cells.
Glucagon promotes the release of glucose into the bloodstream.

Testes

Testosterone causes growth of male sex organs and secondary sex characteristics.

Ovaries

Estrogen causes growth of female sex organs and secondary sex characteristics.
Progesterone nurtures the developing fetus and causes development of milk apparatus.

Pineal gland

Melatonin regulates circadian rhythms and aspects of sexual behavior.

Parathyroid gland

Parathormone controls calcium ion concentrations in extracellular fluid.

body to deal with emergencies. In addition, the hypothalamus is an integral component of the limbic system, mediating drives for hunger and thirst, sexual activity, and aggression. Finally, the hypothalamus directly regulates the vast majority of endocrine functions, largely by means of its regulatory effect on the pituitary gland.

1.3.2 The pituitary gland

Immediately juxtaposed to the hypothalamus is the pituitary gland, or *hypophysis*. Known as the master endocrine gland, the pituitary affects the body's overall metabolism, the nervous system, and many aspects of behavior both through the direct effect of its hormones and secondarily through its effects on other endocrine glands. Pituitary hormones are secreted primarily under stimulation by hormones generated in the hypothalamus, and are modulated by means of feedback loops and various neurotransmitter mechanisms.

The anterior pituitary secretes a number of hormones vital to the body's metabolic function and capacity to deal with stress. Known as *trophic* hormones, these substances act to stimulate their target organs at distances from the pituitary. Chief among these are Growth Hormone (GH), Adrenocorticotropin Hormone (ACTH), Thyroid Stimulating Hormone (TSH), the gonadotropins known as Follicle Stimulating Hormone (FSH) and Luteinizing Hormone (LH), and Prolactin.

2 Principal syndromes of the neuroendocrine system

Cognition and Generalized Dysfunction of the Neuroendocrine System

Cognitive dysfunction secondary to irregular hypothalamic or pituitary operation may be due to a number of causes including trauma, vascular disease, and neoplasm. As would be expected given their role as the principal mediators of the autonomic nervous system, the resulting symptoms can produce an array of autonomic dysregulation. Symptoms may include temperature dysregulation, obesity, aphagia, hypersomnia and sexual dystrophy. Affective symptoms of fear and rage may also ensue.

Commonly, hypothalamic dysfunction may result from compression secondary to a pituitary adenoma or craniopharyngioma. Macroadenomas (>10 mm) frequently come to medical attention due to their prominent mass effect, producing symptoms such as headache and visual abnormalities. Symptoms may result from either *hyper*secretion of a hormone as a result of the tumor and/or *hypo*secretion of other hormones secondary to the tumor's mass effect on the pituitary gland and hypothalamus. Hormonal declines due to mass effect follow a pattern: Hyposecretion of Growth Hormone (GH) precedes that of Lutenizing Hormone (LH) and Follicle Stimulating Hormone (FSH), which precedes Thyroid Stimulating Hormone (TSH), which precedes Adrenocorticotropin Hormone (ACTH). Cognitive deficits including amnesia and executive dysfunction have been noted following surgery and hormone replacement therapy (Grattan-Smith *et al.*, 1992; Peace *et al.*, 1997). However, these cognitive symptoms appear to be due to multiple factors such as surgical sequelae, pre- and postsurgical hormonal imbalance, tumor size, secondary hydrocephalus and radiotherapy. Indeed, some patients with craniopharyngiomas manifest physiological changes such as extreme weight gain and visual disturbance to such an extent neuropsychological test data may be difficult to interpret clearly.

The primary empty sella syndrome refers to a flattening or shrinkage of the sella turcica, which is the bony structure that houses the pituitary gland. As a result, the gland is compressed and difficult to view on neuroimaging. The syndrome is most common in women who are overweight or have high blood pressure and is typically an incidental finding on neuroimaging. In most cases, the pituitary gland is normal in function. When symptomatic, patients may complain of low libido, impotence, lack of menstruation, and visual changes. A secondary empty sella syndrome describes compression or shrinkage of the pituitary gland secondary to injury, tumor, or radiation and is associated with hypopituitarism.

In adults, a generalized hypopituitarism syndrome may result from pronounced age-related changes in multiple hormone systems including the gonadal, thyroid, pancreatic, and adrenal axes (Lamberts *et al.*, 1997). Patients experience a range of symptoms such as decreased energy, loss of libido and depressed mood and/or increased irritability. Women may experience irregular menses or amenorrhea and men may experience impotence and fertility problems.

3 Disorders involving the thyroid hormones

The thyroid hormones T_3 and T_4 result from iodine processed in the presence of thyroid stimulating hormone (TSH), a product of the anterior pituitary gland. Although the primary action of thyroid hormones is typically described as the stimulation of heat production, their influence on metabolic processes throughout the organs and tissues is significant. Dysregulation of thyroid functioning is therefore a frequent concomitant of systemic illness. The hormones and their receptors are widely distributed throughout the brain, affecting adrenergic function, striatal dopaminergic activity, and levels of substance P and serotonin.

3.1 Thyrotoxicosis and Graves' disease

An excessive presence of thyroid hormone is referred to as thyrotoxicosis (low TSH, elevated T_4). When associated with diffuse goiter, ophthalmopathy, and dermopathy due to an autoimmune disorder, hyperthyroidism is referred to as Graves' disease.

+ Patients with Graves' disease, the most common cause of thyrotoxicosis/hyperthyroidism, typically present with symptoms similar to a generalized anxiety disorder: nervousness, poor concentration, apprehension, restlessness, and emotional lability.

+ Other symptoms include heat intolerance, increased sweating, weight loss, muscle weakness, fatigue with dysomnia, and—in women—changes in menstrual flow. Increased metabolic rates may produce tachycardia autonomic tremor.

+ Incidence is approximately 0.3 per 1,000 in the United States. The condition peaks during the third and fourth decades of life and is seven to ten times more common in women than in men. The explanation for this gender difference and for the underlying cause of the disease is unknown.

+ Delayed diagnosis and misdiagnosis as a psychiatric condition is common.

3.1.1 Psychiatric symptoms

Although prominent psychiatric symptoms have been noted since the earliest descriptions by Parry (1825) and Graves (1835), researchers have generally found that psychiatric symptom presentations are understated. Whybrow *et al.* (1969), for instance, found MMPI profiles in thyrotoxic patients to be somewhat elevated, but inconsistent with hypomania. MacCrimmon *et al.* (1979) similarly found nonsignificant elevations on a number of MMPI scales (hypochondriasis, depression, hysteria, psychasthenia, and schizophrenia). Although a number of researchers have found that psychiatric symptoms largely resolve when patients are treated with beta-adrenergic antagonists (Trzepacz *et al.*, 1988) and/or are returned to a euthyroid state (e.g., Vogel *et al.*, 2007), in Stern *et al.*'s

(1996) survey, 33.1% of respondents reported being prescribed psychotropic medication following diagnosis and treatment of Graves' disease even though only 7.7% of the sample reported any premorbid history of psychotropic medication. In addition to any direct effects of altered thyroid hormones on mood, individuals with Graves' disease also report reductions in health-related quality of life and can experience psychiatric conditions related to coping with their illness (Watt *et al.*, 2007).

3.1.2 Neuropsychological symptoms

In the thyrotoxic state, many studies have found that patients manifest worsened performances on tests of attention, concentration, memory and fine motor speed (e.g., Tremont *et al.*, 2003; Trzepacz *et al.*, 1988). However, there are some conflicting findings revealing little impact of thyrotoxicosis on cognitive skills (e.g., Vogel *et al.*, 2007). Methodological and sampling factors may account for the differences. Many of the findings are consistent the presence of thyroid hormones acting on the noradregenergic system to affect attention with dose correlating as an inverted U-shaped curve. Thus, Schlote *et al.* (1992) also found impaired psychomotor speed in overt but not subclinical cases. However, it is plausible that the effects are due to a more general disruption of the brain's thyroid economy as well. Such would help account for reports of poor performances on tests of conceptual thinking and organization. In contrast to generally improved psychiatric symptoms, there are a number of reports of ongoing worsened performance on neuropsychological tests of attention, fine motor speed, and memory long after a euthyroid state has been established (Perrild *et al.*, 1986; Trzepacz *et al.*, 1988; Bommer *et al.*, 1990). One possible explanation of persisting cognitive changes may be that an autoimmune component of the disease is directed at the brain.

Although relatively rare in older adults, hyperthyroidism in elderly individuals often presents with fewer overt symptoms or with apathy and decreased motivation as the prominent symptoms (Trivalle *et al.*, 1996). There is also evidence of dementia associated with hyperthyroidism that reverses following achievement of euthyroidism (Fukui, 2001). Hyperthyroidism in children is quite rare, but can have a significant impact on growth and behavior.

3.2 Congenital hypothyroidism

Children born with congenital hypothyroidism (CH) are typically identified at birth. In the USA, whites are affected at a substantially higher rate than African-Americans (1:5,000 vs. 1:32,000). Due to the infant brain's vulnerability to the organizational effects of a lack of thyroid hormone, those who do not receive replacement therapy are at high risk for developing severe motor and sensory impairments, as well as mental retardation. Even in children receiving early intervention, however, meta-analysis demonstrates a relatively small but significant trend toward lower IQ ($\approx$ 6.3 points) and poorer motor skills in treated CH children (Derksen-Lubsen, 1996). Lower intellectual function is even seen when comparing children with CH treated early after newborn screening to their siblings (Rovet, 2005). Earlier and optimal treatment, appear to be two important variables for long-term outcome of intellectual and motor functioning. The earlier the treatment, the better outcome for overall intellectual functioning 7 years following birth, even when comparing groups receiving treatment at less than 15 days compared to greater than 3 weeks after birth (Boileau *et al.*, 2004). Similarly, the more rapidly serum thyroid hormones normalize following treatment, the better the outcome in overall intellectual functioning several years later (Oerbeck *et al.*, 2003; Salerno *et al.*, 2002). Untreated congenital hypothyroidism leads to a syndrome known as Cretinism, characterized by mental retardation, deaf mutism, short stature, and myxedema—a puffiness in the face, hands and feet due to the infiltration of the tissues with mucopolyscacharides. In geographic areas with iodine deficient diets, the severity of deficits correlates with the extent of the deficiency (Aghini-Lombardi *et al.*, 1995; Sankar *et al.*, 1994).

3.3 Adult hypothyroidism

Primary hypothyroidism (elevated TSH, low T4) in adults has an incidence approximately one-eighth that of hyperthyroidism. Hypothyroidism may also result from Hashimoto's thyroiditis, a condition similar to Graves' disease, in which the thyroid gland at first enlarges and subsequently atrophies. Autoimmunity is the underlying etiology of thyroid disease in Hashimoto's thyroiditis. Another frequent cause is secondary to thyroid replacement therapy for Graves' disease.

- Clinical symptoms of hypothyroidism include intolerance to cold, puffy face, coarse, dry skin and hair, fatigue and somnolence, muscular sluggishness, bradycardia and reduced cardiac output, weight gain, development of a husky voice, constipation, ematous body tissue and arteriosclerosis.

- There is a significant gender bias, being four to seven times more common in females than males.

- The prevalence of hypothyroidism steadily increases with age, with subclinical hypothyroidism manifesting as lethargy and dysphoria, although these symptoms appear to resolve with treatment.

- Myopathies and delayed tendon reflexes may be evident on neurologic exam.

- Depression is frequently a presenting symptom, and misdiagnosis as a psychiatric condition is common.

3.3.1 Psychiatric symptoms

The most typical presenting picture is that of a depressed patient: dysphoria, apathy, fatigue, diminished libido, motor and psychomotor retardation, and even suicidal ideation. MMPI profiles of individuals are characteristic of other depressed populations, with elevated Depressed and reduced Mania scales. With thyroid replacement therapy, remission of psychiatric symptoms is common.

3.3.2 Neuropsychological symptoms

Classically, severe hypothyroidism or 'Myxedema Madness' is considered a 'reversible dementia' with treatment by thyroid replacement therapy. However, variables mediating the extent of recovery following treatment are still being investigated. In extreme cases, coma can result from severe, prolonged hypothyroidism. Impairment in cognition has been noted in hypothyroidal patients since Gull's (1874) initial description.

Bradyphrenia, increased response latencies, poor concentration and memory are typical presenting symptoms (Burmeister *et al.*, 2001; Hall, 1983; Denicoff *et al.*, 1990; Whybrow *et al.*, 1969). There is a surprising lack of investigations into severe hypothyroidism despite its relative prevalence. A number of studies have identified cognitive deficits on tests of mental status, psychomotor speed, memory, semantic fluency, concentration, and design fluency during the acute stage. Treatment studies are equivocal with regard to reversibility of cognitive symptoms (cf. Davis and Tremont, 2006). Serum thyroid levels may take up to three months to normalize, and there is no consistent pattern of recovery of cognitive symptoms following treatment, nor prospective, objective research studies to clearly address reversibility of cognitive and/or psychiatric symptoms in overt hypothyroidism. Also, two published case studies (Menemeier *et al.*, 1993; Leentjens and Kappers, 1995) found that replacement therapy did not reverse cognitive deficits, but may have prevented further deterioration. These and other studies suggest that duration of thyroid dysfunction is an important factor, although such duration would have to be extreme because healthy individuals have up to a 100-day reserve available.

Controlled and uncontrolled treatment studies have focused on mild, or subclinical, hypothyroidism and generally show modest improvements in cognition and mood (Cooper *et al.*, 1984; Nyström *et al.*, 1988; Osterweil *et al.*, 1992; Monzani *et al.*, 1993; Jaeschke *et al.*, 1996; Baldini *et al.*, 1997; del Ser Quijano *et al.*, 2000; Meier *et al.*, 2001; Bono *et al.*, 2004; Gulseren *et al.*, 2006; Miller *et al.*, 2006). A few studies, however, have produced negative treatment results or lack of significant improvement on a number of cognitive tests following stabilization of thyroid levels (Osterweil *et al.*, 1992; Jorde *et al.*, 2006), suggesting deficits in effortful attention may persist.

3.4 **Hypothyroidism in the older adult**

There is evidence that age may increase vulnerability to the effects of hypothyroidism on cognitive functioning. The mechanism for this is unclear, though it is likely that the brain relies to a greater extent on hormone levels during aging and is more sensitive to changes in thyroid function (cf. Davis *et al.*, 2003; Loosen, 1992). In an analysis of 2781 cases of hypothyroidism, only one case of reversible dementia secondary to hypothyroidism was identified (Clarnette and Patterson, 1994). Despite the lack of complete reversibility, it appears that aspects of cognition respond to treatment (Haupt and Kurtz, 1993) across the lifespan. More recent data also indicates that mild thyroid failure may place an individual at greater risk for future dementia (Ganguli *et al.*, 1996; Volpato *et al.*, 2002).

4 **Diabetes mellitus**

Diabetes Mellitus is a term applied to certain disorders that result in chronic elevations in blood glucose levels or *hyperglycemia*.

- Type I Diabetes: In the United Sates, approximately 500,000 persons have been diagnosed with juvenile-onset insulin-dependent diabetes mellitus (IDDM), also known as Type I diabetes with most children diagnosed in their early teens. In these individuals, beta cells within the pancreas are destroyed, curtailing the body's supply of insulin. Treatment is by means of intramuscular injection of insulin, with the primary goal of therapy being the maintenance of metabolic control by avoiding both hyperglycemic and hypoglycemic states.

- Type II Diabetes: Non-insulin-dependent diabetes (NIDDM), or Type II diabetes, is characterized by an insidious onset of symptoms due to hyposecretion of insulin and/or insulin resistance. Type II diabetes typically occurs in adulthood with the prevalence increasing with age so that approximately 20% of the population over 65 years of age is affected (Winograd, 1990). Of recent concern is the emergence of childhood type II diabetes associated with the increasing rates of obesity in childhood. For a majority of adults and children diagnosed with NIDDM, metabolic control is frequently achieved through a combination of diet and/or oral hypoglycemic agents.

4.1 Psychiatric symptoms

Both Type I and Type II diabetes may be accompanied by symptoms of depression, anxiety, and, infrequently, mania. More severe psychiatric symptoms are correlated with poorer compliance to therapeutic regimes and more severe course, although no clear cause-effect model has been established. Stressors include factors associated with living with chronic disease such as stress and concern with dietary regimen. Chronic pain associated with neuropathy is also present for a sizable subset of diabetics. Importantly, depression may exacerbate current cognitive deficits associated with the disease (Watari *et al.*, 2006).

4.2 Neuropsychological symptoms

4.2.1 Type I diabetes

Cognitive deficits due to diabetes have been the subject of many investigations. For Type I patients, age of onset has been shown to be related to cognitive deficits with impairments in visuospatial tasks in patients afflicted before the age of four. This is likely due to higher rates of hypoglycemic seizures and the increased vulnerability of the developing brain, particularly the process of myelination (Ryan, 1988). Cognitive outcome also appears to be related to presence and duration of hypoglycemia as well as hyperglycemic episodes around the time of puberty (Desrocher and Rovet, 2004). Cognitive problems have been identified in motor strength, visuospatial functioning, attention, memory, and aspects of executive functioning, but the pattern of cognitive deficits and prognosis are complex and closely associated with disease variables. There is limited evidence for any long-term, significant declines in cognitive function in patients with type I diabetes, even in those with recurrent hypoglycemia (Jacobson *et al.*, 2007).

In adult Type I diabetics, medical complications due to macro- and microvascular damage are common, increasing diabetics' risk for stroke, heart attack, retinopathy and end-stage renal disease. Peripheral neuropathies with the potential to affect ADLs and IADLs are common as are paresthesias and/or painful sensations in the distal limbs. Cognitively, this increased risk of stroke results in increased rates of vascular dementia in diabetics (McCall, 1992). Long histories of poorly controlled glucose levels are associated with the vascular complications noted above, the peripheral neuropathies being most immediately pertinent to performance on neuropsychological tests entailing a psycho-motor speed component. Poorly controlled glucose levels have also been associated with reduced mental flexibility, poor conceptual reasoning, and inefficient information processing.

4.2.2 Type II diabetes

Ironically, neurocognitive deficits in Type II diabetics may be somewhat more pronounced—particularly in regard to memory function—despite these patients' shorter histories. Ryan and Williams (1993) hypothesized an age by hyperglycemia interaction to account for these findings, noting that the aging brain has been found to be increasingly vulnerable to mnestic dysfunction in other patient groups (e.g., alcoholics). This notion is supported by neuroimaging findings in which type II diabetics have been shown to have greater deep white matter disease and cortical atrophy than type I diabetics with a longer history of illness (Brands *et al.*, 2007). Cognitive deficits are typically mild and likely in the domains of verbal memory, processing speed, and executive functioning (Awad *et al.*, 2004). Moreover as with Type I diabetes, history of metabolic control has been found to be key to understanding who is most vulnerable (Assisi *et al.*, 1996). Research has shown that improved metabolic control may improve cognitive functions in both Type I and Type II diabetics.

Type II diabetes is also a risk factor for Alzheimer's disease (Ott *et al.*, 1999). The mechanism underlying this risk is unclear, but may be related to the effects of peripheral insulinemia on amyloid clearance from the brain (Selkoe, 2000). Recent attention is being paid to the role of insulin in Alzheimer's disease, and the possibility of neuronal insulin resistance reflecting a type III diabetes (de la Monte and Wands, 2005). As such, obtaining a history of blood glucose control and/or type II diabetes in the clinical inter-view is important and may be a possible prognostic indicator for conversion in patients with mild cognitive impairment (Luchsinger *et al.*, 2007; Williamson *et al.*, 2007).

5 Disorders involving the reproductive hormones

In concert with chromosomal factors, the reproductive hormones are responsible for sexually dimorphic characteristics in behavior, affect, and cognition. Through their influ-ence on sexual differentiation during key developmental phases, the reproductive hor-mones play an important organizational role in neuronal development, with women's brains having, on average, a larger corpus callosum and planum temporale. These differ-ences correlate with women generally out-performing men on certain verbal tasks and having lower rates of language disorders such as dyslexia. In contrast, men display relative strengths in quantitative and visuospatial skills, particularly mental rotation (Maccoby and Jacklin, 1974; Halpern, 1992). Importantly, differences between groups of men and women on such cognitive tests are far smaller than the variability within each gender group. Nevertheless, individuals affected by disorders marked by excessive or diminished levels of reproductive hormones during key developmental periods manifest behaviors and characteristics determined by permanent structural changes in brain morphology. Due to the effects of physiological differences on an individual's self-concept, resultant syndromes may require some period of social and emotional adjustment in adolescence or later. Reproductive hormones may also play an activational role in producing transient changes in cognitive function in both healthy and afflicted individuals. However, these changes appear to be relatively minor and may depend to an extent on pre-existing organizational pathways for their effects.

5.1 Genetic, perinatal, and environmental abnormalities

5.1.1 Klinefelter's syndrome

Klinefelter's syndrome results from the presence of an additional X chromosome in the male. The syndrome is characterized by delayed maturation, hypogonadism and infertility, gynecomastia, and androgen deficiency. Individuals manifest relative strengths in visuospatial abilities, and may rely more on the right hemisphere for processing both verbal and nonverbal information. Although lowered IQ has been found in a number of studies, this does not always appear to be the case (Netley and Rovet, 1984). Recent findings in adults provide evidence of three cognitive subtypes: 1) individuals with left hemisphere dysfunction, including VIQ<PIQ and language impairment; 2) individuals with right hemisphere dysfunction, including PIQ<VIQ, visuospatial deficits, and left-sided manual dexterity problems; 3) mild bilateral dysfunction, including VIQ=PIQ and executive dysfunction (Boone *et al.*, 2001). Interestingly, age is associated with lower PIQ scores suggesting an older age of onset in right hemisphere dysfunction in the PIQ<VIQ subtype. Mechanisms for subtypes are complex, but likely reflect varying responses to low levels of androgens and/or corresponding increases in estradiols.

5.1.2 Turner's syndrome

Turner's syndrome is due to a single X chromosome in females, resulting in short stature, webbing of the neck, and sexual infantilism. A number of deficiencies in brain structure have been identified, including decreased hippocampal, thalamic, caudate and lenticular nuclei volumes, and decreased right temporal evoked potentials. Cognitively, individuals with Turner's syndrome manifest relative weaknesses in visuospatial ability and nonverbal memory, consistent with right hemisphere dysfunction (Schucard *et al.*, 1994; cf Rovet, 2004). Although most verbal skills are intact, individuals with Turner's syndrome can show reduced fluency, poor articulation, and difficulties with language syntax (Temple, 2002). Motor clumsiness, attentional problems and executive dysfunction are also commonly associated with the syndrome. Many of the visuospatial and constructional deficits continue into adulthood, although improvements can be seen in motor planning and perceptual judgment (Romans *et al.*, 1998). Psychosocial problems can include low self esteem, social awkwardness, and face processing deficits (Rovet, 2004).

5.1.3 Congenital adrenal hyperplasia

Excessive levels of androgens are associated with congenital adrenal hyperplasia (CAH), an endocrine disorder beginning in the early prenatal environment. The condition is typically detected at birth and androgen levels are normalized. Clinically, CAH females manifest masculinization of the genitalia and clitoral hypertrophy. In males, an enlarged phallus typically results. CAH can be further divided into two subtypes:

1 salt wasters who experience high level prenatal androgen exposure and severe episodes of hyponatremia and hypotension; and

2 simple virilizers who only experience high level prenatal androgen exposure.

In understanding the effects of androgens on the developing brain, researchers have focused on CAH females since identifying the effects of excessive androgens in CAH males is by definition a difficult proposition. It has been hypothesized that overexposure to androgen also has masculinizing effects on brain development, resulting in enhanced spatial skills and increased incidence of left-handedness.

Research by Resnick *et al.* (1986) utilizing a sample of adolescent CAH females revealed selectively better performance on tests of mental rotation and hidden figures, compared to unaffected siblings. Similarly, Hampson *et al.* (1998) found an advantage in spatial capacity among pre-adolescent CAH females on a mental rotation test. Curiously, the researchers found that CAH boys scored significantly lower than control boys on a test of spatial relations, suggesting that overexposure to androgens may have a demasculinizing effect on males. Kelso *et al.* (2000) found a higher incidence of left-handers among CAH individuals and more frequent pattern of PIQ>VIQ. Other studies have not found these masculinizing effects in females for either spatial skills or handedness (Malouf *et al.*, 2006). Reasons for these contradictory findings may reflect methodological variability or sample bias or could be a result of mixing subgroups or males and females. Johannsen *et al.* (2006) found that individuals who were found to be salt wasters had lower IQs than simple virilizers. Despite higher IQ among simple virilizers, there is evidence of increased likelihood of language-based disorders (i.e., learning disabilities) in this group compared to salt wasters (Nass and Baker, 1991).

5.1.4 Androgen insensitivity

Patients with Androgen Insensitivity (AI) are genetic males who produce androgens but manifest partial to total insensitivity of androgen receptors. Depending on the degree of insensitivity they are born either with external female genitalia (and no female reproductive organs)–total AI–and are raised as girls, or ambiguous genitalia–partial AI–and are raised as either girls or boys. AI patients typically demonstrate a VIQ-PIQ discrepancy with decreased PIQ (Imperato-McGinley *et al.*, 1991). However, lower PIQ subtest scores in these individuals may be due to either visuospatial deficits or attentional factors on speeded tests.

5.1.5 Idiopathic hypogonadodtropic hypogonadism

At puberty, some males manifest a deficiency of gonadropic releasing factor (GnRF), resulting in smaller testes and decreased levels of androgens. Consistent with the organizational effects of androgens on the brain, IHH males have impaired visuospatial abilities and intact verbal skills (Hier and Crowley, 1982).

5.2 Gonadal hormones influence on adult behavior

5.2.1 Androgens

Behaviorally, androgens have been associated with sexual drive and increased aggression in both genders. However, because aggressive encounters alter testosterone levels, no clear cause/effect relationship between the two variables has been established. Males receiving testosterone replacement therapy report enhanced well-being and increased energy. However, testosterone in males is converted or *aromatized* into estrogens, obscuring the interpretation of these phenomena.

Optimal levels of androgens in both genders are necessary for normal visuospatial functioning. Moreover, androgens appear to have an activational effect on spatial abilities in females. However, high levels of testosterone in males have been associated with decreased spatial ability, suggesting a sex by hormone interaction (Gouchie and Kimura, 1991). These capacities are best measured by means of route learning tasks and mental rotation tasks, although gross PIQ-VIQ discrepancies may also be evident. There is support from the animal literature for enhanced spatial ability in males. In a number of non-human species, spatial-navigational ability is sexually differentiated, with males learning to utilize routes more efficiently (Beatty, 1984). Further, male mice castrated at birth exhibit reduced spatial efficiency in adulthood relative to controls (Williams *et al.*, 1990).

Aging is generally associated with progressive decline in testosterone in males, although it may vary based on physical health and other lifestyle factors. Consistent relationships have been found between testosterone levels (especially free testosterone) and cognitive functioning in older men, suggesting that lower levels of testosterone could lead to dementia or Alzheimer's disease (e.g., Yeap *et al.*, 2007). In fact, men with Alzheimer's disease have lower testosterone levels than age-matched controls (Hogervost *et al.*, 2004). Whether higher levels of testosterone are associated with a lower risk for Alzheimer's disease remains unclear given conflicting findings (Moffat *et al.*, 2004; Geerlings *et al.*, 2006). There also appears to be an interaction between testosterone levels and apoliproprotein ε4 allele, in which high levels of testosterone are associated with poor cognitive peformance in ε4-positive individuals and good cognitive functioning in non-carriers (Burkardt *et al.*, 2006). Finally, it remains uncertain whether testosterone supplementation can improve cognitive abilities, again because of several conflicting findings (Cherrier *et al.*, 2005; Lu *et al.*, 2006).

5.2.2 Estrogens and progesterone

Emotional changes have been associated with normal variation in ovarian hormones as well as with pre-menstrual syndrome (PMS), a cyclical disorder with depressive/mood-related and somatic symptoms occurring during the luteal phase of the menstrual cycle (Schmidt *et al.*, 1998). Cognitively, increased verbal ability and decreased spatial ability have been identified during the high estrogen phases, suggesting that estrogen may differentially affect hemispheric functioning. Despite clinical reports, there has been little empirical support for variation in memory functioning according to the menstrual cycle that cannot be accounted for by the co-occurrence of mood symptoms. Furthermore, there is no clear association between endogenous estrogen levels and cognition prior to, during, or after menopause (Herlitz *et al.*, 2007), despite the fact that women experiencing menopause often have memory complaints.

In post-menopausal women, hormone replacement therapy (HRT) has been utilized for many years due to its association with reduced risk of stroke, heart disease, vascular dementia, and osteoporosis. ERT may be contraindicated for some women, however, especially those with a family history of breast cancer (cf. Colditz *et al.*, 1995). The Women's Health Initiative, a very large longitudinal study to objectively address the risks and benefits for hormone replacement therapy on women's health, was stopped in 2002 due to increased incidence of breast cancer and cardiovascular disease (Writing Group for the Women's Health Initiative Investigators, 2002). As such, the utility of HRT for reducing health risks remains somewhat controversial and may be age dependent. Risk for coronary artery disease seems far less in women under the age of 60 who begin HRT closer to the onset of menopause (Rossouw *et al.*, 2007).

The effects of HRT on cognition have yielded conflicting results. Some reports have shown that HRT and ERT have a beneficial effect on verbal and nonverbal memory in younger women. Short-term, cognitive advantages in ERT may be due to enhanced activation of frontal lobe functioning, which could account for improved performance on cognitive measures in general, as well as on memory specifically via associated executive functions (Berman *et al.*, 1997; Joffe *et al.*, 2006). Interestingly, the effects of HRT on cognition may be age dependent with early initiation of HRT around the time of menopause being beneficial and later initiation could have a detrimental effect on cognition (MacLennan *et al.*, 2006; Rapp *et al.*, 2003). A review of randomized placebo-controlled trials concluded that there is minimal evidence to support cognitive enhancement with HRT or estrogen replacement therapy (ERT) in postmenopausal women (Hogervost *et al.*, 2002), but clearly other factors need to be considered, such as the timing of when HRT was initiated and for how long.

5.2.3 Estrogen and Alzheimer's disease

A potential role for female reproductive hormones in Alzheimer's Disease (AD) is suggested by the disease's greater prevalence among women than men, even after adjusting for differences in life expectancy (Jorm *et al.*, 1987). Likewise, several studies have found that women with AD perform worse than men with AD on various verbal tasks (Henderson and Buckwalter, 1994; Ripich *et al.*, 1995), despite a premorbid advantage on such tasks favoring women. A number of other clinical and experimental findings including body weight, neurophysiological processes and genetic mechanisms further support the relevance of estrogen to AD (cf. Henderson, 1997). Historically, ERT has been utilized in the treatment of women with Alzheimer's Disease for many years. However, trials of ERT to improve cognition and slow cognitive decline in women with Alzheimer's disease have been negative with only modest, positive short-term effects on memory (Hogervorst *et al.*, 2002).

The possible role of ERT in reducing an individual's risk for developing AD has also been investigated. Several retrospective studies found a reduced risk factor for dementia in women receiving ERT (Birge, 1994; Henderson *et al.*, 1994; Mortel and Meyer, 1995). Similarly, prospective epidemiological studies have also suggested a significant reduction—more than 50% in some studies—in risk for AD in women receiving ERT (Henderson *et al.*, 1994; Paganini-Hill and Henderson, 1994; Morrison *et al.*, 1996; Kawas *et al.*, 1997; Tang *et al.*, 1996; Yaffe *et al.*, 1998). However, very large controlled studies have failed to support the results seen in clinical observation or smaller cross-sectional studies. There is even recent evidence that women 65 years of age and older taking combination hormone therapy had twice the rate of dementia, including Alzheimer's disease, compared to placebo, and combined therapy did not protect against mild cognitive impairment (Shumaker *et al.*, 2003). Taken together, the beneficial effect for the use of hormone replacement therapy in treating the cognitive effects of Alzheimer's disease and reducing the risk of developing Alzheimer's disease appear minimal.

6 Disorders involving the adrenal hormones

The adrenal glands are located at the superior poles of the kidneys. Each gland is divided into two distinct portions:

- the adrenal medulla, which secretes the hormones epinephrine and norepinephrine and is functionally related to the sympathetic nervous system, and the adrenal cortex, which secretes the hormones known as corticosteroids, of which cortisol is of principle interest in regard to cognitive functions.

Another adrenal hormone, dehydroepiandrosterone (DHEA), has recently been studied for its possible effects on mood and memory and is discussed below. The adrenal glands also produce small amounts of certain androgens.

6.1 Cortisol

The hypothalamic-pituitary-adrenal axis is an integral component of the body's reactions to physiologic stressors. Cortisol acts to increase blood glucose concentrations, which in turn mobilizes available energy stores, and helps the body to maintain homeostasis through its regulatory effects on protein, carbohydrate, and lipid metabolism. The axis is controlled by a feedback loop as follows: Corticotropin releasing hormone (CRH) is produced by hypothalamic neurons both according to a circadian pattern and in response to physiologic stress. CRH regulates the release of adrenocorticotropin hormone (ACTH) from the pituitary. ACTH stimulates the adrenal glands, which in turn produce cortisol. Cortisol completes the feedback loop by its effect on the hypothalamus and other structures.

In normal subjects, administration of exogenous glucocorticoids may produce euphoria, hyperactivity, and increased appetite, leading to dependence and abuse. Short- and long-term administration of corticosteroids has been shown to produce mild impairments in verbal memory, although it is unclear if the dysfunction is due to disruption of attentional factors, memory processes or both. However, mild increases in psychomotor speed and verbal fluency have also been reported, possibly due to a hyperactivation effect (Naber et al., 1996). Elevated cortisol levels are also seen in individuals diagnosed with major depression, in whom memory and attention problems are frequently observed. However, elevations in serum cortisol cannot solely account for these cognitive problems.

6.1.1 Hypercortisolism

Cushing's syndrome refers to the clinical manifestation of increased concentrations of cortisol due to any number of disorders.

- *Cushing's syndrome* may be the result of a pituitary adenoma, a primary adrenal tumor, ectopic production of ACTH by a carcinoma of the lung or, frequently, the long-term treatment of a variety of diseases with exogenous cortisol such as cortisone or prednisone.

- When cortisol evelations are secondary to a pituitary adenoma, the condition is known as *Cushing's disease*. Onset typically occurs between the ages of 20–40, but has also been reported in infants and elderly patients. Unlike Cushing's syndrome, females are eight times more likely than males to develop Cushing's disease.

- Typical features associated with hypercortisolism include truncal obesity, plethoric (full) facies, hirsutism and baldness, osteoporosis, impotence or amenorrhea, hypertension, and generalized muscular weakness.

Psychiatric symptoms Psychiatric symptoms are present in more than half of all cases of hypercortisolism and may include depression, anxiety, irritability, affective lability, decreased libido, and psychosis (i.e., 'steroid psychosis'). Because psychiatric symptoms may be the initial indications of Cushing's syndrome, dexamethasone-suppression testing is frequently used as a screening tool. However, as noted above, patients with major depression may have elevated cortisol levels with no evidence of endocrinopathy.

Neuropsychological symptoms A wide array of cognitive functions may be affected in more than two-thirds of all patients with Cushing's syndrome, including deficits in attention, memory, and executive functions (Starkman et al., 1999, 2003). Both medial prefrontal cortex and hippocampus have been implicated as dysfunctional in Cushing's syndrome/disease because of their high concentrations of glucocorticoid receptors. In fact, hippocampal volumes decrease during the active phase of the illness and increase following stabilization of cortisol levels and show a relationship to memory performance (Starkman et al., 2003; Hook et al., 2007). Normalization of ACTH and cortisol levels is accompanied by a significant cognitive recovery for these patients, although there may be a delayed recovery in older individuals (Hook et al., 2007).

Chronic elevations in cortisol in the elderly have been associated with deficits in explicit memory and selective attention (Lupien *et al.*, 1994). Hippocampal atrophy has been associated with both chronic and short-term elevations in cortisol in patients with Alzheimer's disease, depression, post traumatic stress disorder (Davis *et al.*, 1986; Bremner *et al.*, 1995), consistent with the presence of concentrations of corticosterone receptors in the hippocampus (Ruel and DeKloet, 1985; Campbell *et al.*, 2004).

6.1.2 Hypocortisolism

Addison's disease, a rare autoimmune disorder, accounts for approximately 75% of all cases of primary adrenocortical insufficiency. Insufficient production of cortisol results in increased levels of ACTH due to decreased feedback to the hypothalamus and anterior pituitary. Etiology is typically an autoimmune adrenalitis due to tuberculosis, malignancy, sarcoidosis, or infection but may also result from bilateral adrenal hemorrhage after sepsis, trauma, surgery, or burns. Hypocortisolism may also result secondary to pituitary or hypothalamic dysfunction, resulting in diminished CRH and/or ACTH. Clinical features of hypocortisolism include pigmentation of the skin and mucous membranes, nausea, vomiting, weight loss, muscle weakness, fatigue, and dizziness. Psychiatric symptoms include depression, confusion, apathy, anhedonia, psychosis, paranoia, schizophrenic behaviors, and self-mutilation.

Neuropsychological sequelae of Addison's disease have been the subject of few studies. Reports document confusion and severe problems with short-term memory and attention in the acute stage, with improved cognition following treatment with adrenal replacement therapy. At present, it is unclear whether the psychiatric and cognitive symptoms are due to diminished cortisol, or increased CRH and ACTH acting on the central nervous system.

6.2 Dehydroepiandrosterone

The biological role of dehydroepiandrosterone (DHEA) and its sulfate (DHEA-S) have recently been the subject of numerous investigations due to their decrease with normal aging and correlation with age-related immune system decline (Thoman and Weigle, 1989). Epidemiological data has demonstrated an association between low circulating DHEA and cardiovascular morbidity in males (Barrett-Connor *et al.*, 1986) and breast cancer in females (Helzlsouer *et al.*, 1992). DHEA and DHEA-S are also thought to affect behavior and cognition by mediating GABA receptors and by acting as a GABA antagonist, respectively.

In healthy subjects, DHEA appears to enhance general well-being, manifested as increased energy, deeper sleep, improved mood, greater relaxation and better stress-handling capacity. Although some benefit in mnestic functions has been shown in depressed patients receiving DHEA, this has not been demonstrated in healthy populations, including age-related cognitive impairment in the elderly (Grimley Evans *et al.*, 2006). Despite reduced DHEA levels in Alzheimer's disease, DHEA-S levels do not correlate with cognitive impairment (Bo *et al.*, 2006), and placebo-controlled trials of DHEA

in patients with Alzheimer's disease have not significantly improved cognitive performance or overall ratings of change severity (Wolkowitz *et al.*, 2003).

7 Melatonin

The pineal gland is known by many as Descartes' hypothetical 'seat of the soul' and for its
phyloanatomical history as a remnant of a 'third eye' in the posterior portion of the head
in lower animals. In addition to its possible role in the seasonal regulation of human
sexual behavior and its role in regulating body temperature, the pineal gland has received
scrutiny because of its synthesis of the hormone melatonin.

Melatonin is secreted cyclically, with low levels associated with daylight, and increases
peaking toward midnight and then gradually returning to baseline by morning. Exogenous
melatonin is currently sold as a treatment for jet lag, due to its ability to re-set the body's
circadian rhythms, and to induce sleepiness. Several studies have found significant variation in cognitive functioning, particularly in reaction time tasks. However, there is no
evidence that circulating melatonin has a direct effect on cognitive functioning. Instead,
cognitive weaknesses appear to be due to reduced speed of information processing secondary to melatonin's hypothermic properties. Trials of melatonin for sleep disturbance
(Singer *et al.*, 2003) and cognitive impairment in Alzheimer's disease (cf. Jansen *et al.*,
2006) have been negative.

7.1 Growth hormone

There has been recent interest in the use of human growth hormone (GH) to potentially
stave off the effects of aging on the body and on cognition. For individuals with GH deficiency, GH replacement significantly improves cognition, especially in attention and
memory (Falletti *et al.*, 2006). Similarly, children with GH deficiency have notable cognitive deficits that improve with replacement therapy (Vander Reijden-Lakeman *et al.*,
1997). The use of GH in healthy individuals is quite controversial and is associated with
negative physical effects, including soft tissue edema, arthralgias, carpal tunnel syndrome,
and gynecomastia. There are also concerns about negative effects on glucose tolerance
and possible increased risk of cancer. Despite these effects, most studies have shown
improved cognition in healthy older adults after a trial of GH or GH-releasing hormone
(e.g., Deijen *et al.*, 1998; Vitiello *et al.*, 2006). Whether GH is a safe and effective anti-
aging therapy or a treatment for geriatric cognitive disorders, remains to be seen.

8 Summary

Hormones act on the brain and nervous system in general to produce an array of physiological, psychiatric, affective, and cognitive sequelae. In many instances, the resulting
symptoms may be mild, but they can have a pronounced impact on daily functioning,
quality of life, and perception of cognitive ability. Neuropsychologists are well prepared
to assess and interpret these multidimensional findings, given the comprehensive
and detailed nature of the exams. Neuropsychological assessment of neuroendocrine
dysfunction is a relatively new area of research. Consequently, no 'gold standards' have

been established regarding which instruments should be used in research and clinical applications. It is recommended that exams are comprehensive, including a broad range of cognitive measures, psychiatric instruments, and self report measures of cognitive complaints and daily functioning. The purpose of neuropsychological evaluation in endocrine disorders may vary somewhat based on age at presentation. For children, the evaluation may be geared toward developmental issues and establish overall intellectual and academic functioning. The evaluation will also focus on generating recommendations for school and related academic activities. For adults, differential diagnosis may be more salient, and the emphasis placed on establishing the contribution of psychiatric and other factors on cognitive abilities. For older adults, differential diagnosis is also important, particularly as it related to degenerative dementias. Table 30.2 presents cognitive domains and areas of emphasis for the different age groups. Examples of tests are provided as a guide, although clinicians may opt for different measures of the same domains. For ready reference, Table 30.3 summarizes the principal characteristics and cognitive findings relevant to neuropsychological assessment and the neuroendocrine system. Where known, response to intervention is indicated.

Table 30.2 Proposed areas to assess during neuropsychological evaluation based on different ages

	Child/Developmental	Adult	Older adult
Primary cognitive domains to assess			
Intellectual	Full IQ testing (note verbal- performance differences; Wechsler Intelligence Scale for Children – IV)	Abbreviated IQ (Wechsler Abbreviated Scale of Intelligence)	Abbreviated IQ WASI
Academic	Comprehensive (Woodcock-Johnson-III, Wechsler Individual Achievement Test II)	N/A	N/A
Attention	Sustained, Speed of Processing, multiple measures (Continuous Performance Test, Trail Making Test)	Information Processing and Psychomotor Speed (Paced Auditory Serial Addition Test, Trail Making Test A)	Information Processing and Psychomotor Speed (Digit Symbol, Trail Making Test B)
Executive Functions	Abstract Reasoning, Problem-Solving, Set Shifting, Inhibition (Dellis-Kaplan Executive Function System Wisconsin Card Sorting Test)	Abstract Reasoning, Problem-Solving, Set Shifting, Inhibition (Wisconsin Card Sorting Test, Trail Making Test-B, Stroop)	Abstract Reasoning, Problem-Solving, Set Shifting, Inhibition (Similarities, Trail Making Test -B)

(continued)

Table 30.2 *(continued)* Proposed areas to assess during neuropsychological evaluation based on different ages

	Child/Developmental	Adult	Older adult
Language	Fluency, articulation (Controlled Oral Word Association; Clinical Evaluation of Language Fundamentals –IV)	Screen (Controlled Oral Word Association)	Fluency, Naming (Controlled Oral Word Association, Boston Naming Test)
Visuospatial	Perceptual, construction, visuomotor integration (Beery-Buktenica Developmental Test of Visual-Motor Integration)	Construction (Rey-Osterrieth Complex Figure, Block Design)	Construction (Rey-Osterrieth Complex Figure, Block Design, Clock Drawing Test)
Motor/Sensory	Handedness	Fine Motor Skills (Grooved Pegboard)	Fine Motor Skills(Grooved Pegboard)
Learning and Memory	Comprehensive assessment of memory processes (encoding, retrieval, verbal, visual)(Wide Range Assessment of Memory and Learning, Children's Memory Scale)	Comprehensive assessment of memory processes (encoding, retrieval, verbal, visual) (Wechsler Memory Scale-III, California Verbal Learning Test - II)	Comprehensive assessment of memory processes (encoding, retrieval, verbal, visual) (Wechsler Memory Scale-III, Hopkins Verbal Learning Test - Revised)
Personality/ Behavior	Behavior checklists, parent and teacher report (Connors Behavior Checklist, Behavior Assessment System for Children-2)	Personality testing and mood questionnaires (Minnesota Multiphasic Personality Inventory – II, Beck Depression Inventory-II, State Trait Anxiety Inventory)	Mood questionnaires (Beck Depression Inventory-II, State-Trait Anxiety Inventory, Cornell Scale for Depression in Dementia)
Daily Functioning	Adaptive functioning (Vineland Adaptive Behavior Scales – II)	Quality of Life	Activities of Daily Living, Quality of Life (Lawton Brody ADLs)

Table 30.3 Reference summary of neuroendocrine effects on behavior and cognition

Hormone/Condition	Primary Hormonal Axis	Primary Axial Hormones	Aging Effects?	Psychological Features	Principal Cognitive Findings	Permanency of Deficits?
Androgens (Congenital Adrenal Hyperplasia, Androgen Insufficiency)	Hypothalamic-Pituitary-Gonadal	GnRH, LH, FSH, T, E$_2$, Progesterone	Gradual Decline in Males	Libido, Aggression	**Inverted U-Shaped Curve with Visuospatial in Males; Improved Visuospatial in Females**	Improvement with Replacement Therapy
Ovarian Hormones	Hypothalamic-Pituitary-Gonadal	GnRH, LH, FSH, T, E$_2$, Progesterone	Rapid Decline in Females	Depression, Anxiety	**E2 with Verbal Fluency; Verbal Memory;** Attention; Visual Memory; Executive Functions	Equivocal – Both Improvement and Declines Depending on Age of Initiation of Replacement Therapy
Hyperthyroidsim (Graves' Disease)	Hypothalamic-Pituitary-Thyroid	TRH, TSH, T$_3$, T$_4$	Decline	Anxiety, Hypomania	**Fine Motor; Attention;** Memory	Improvement with Beta-Adrenergic Blockers and Suppression Therapy
Hypothyroidism (Congenital Hypothyroidism)	Hypothalamic-Pituitary-Thyroid	TRH, TSH, T$_3$, T$_4$	Decline	Depressive Symptoms	**General Cognition; Attention; Learning; Psychomotor Speed**	Improvement in Depression; Limited Improvement in Cognition, Especially of Attention
Hypercortisolism (Cushing's Disease/ Syndrome)	Hypothalamic-Pituitary-Adrenal	CRH, ACTH, Cortisol	Possible Increase	Anxiety, Psychosis, Hypomania	**Memory; Attention**	Limited Improvement, Especially of Memory
Hypocortisolism (Addison's Disease)	Hypothalamic-Pituitary-Adrenal	CRH, ACTH, Cortisol	Possible Increase	Depression, Poor Motivation	**General Attention and Motivation**	Improvement with Suppression Therapy

(continued)

Table 30.3 (continued) Reference summary of neuroendocrine effects on behavior and cognition

Hormone/Condition	Primary Hormonal Axis	Primary Axial Hormones	Aging Effects?	Psychological Features	Principal Cognitive Findings	Permanency of Deficits?
DHEA	NA	DHEA, DHEAS	Decline	DHEA: Depression DHEA-S: Anxiety	**General Cognition;** Memory	Improvement with Replacement Therapy
Type I Diabetes (IDDM)	NA	Insulin, Glucagon, Somatostatin	Decline in Insulin	Anxiety	**Psychomotor Speed; Inefficient Processing; Visuospatial; Executive Functions;** Memory	Improvement with Replacement Therapy
Type II Diabetes (NIDDM)	NA	Insulin, Glucagon, Somatostatin	Decline in Insulin	Anxiety	**Psychomotor Speed; Inefficient Processing; Memory**	Improvement except for Memory
Melatonin	NA	Melatonin	None	NA	Reduced Speed of Information Processing	NA
Growth Hormone	Somatotrophic	GH, GHRH	Decline	Depression, Anxiety	**Memory, Attention**	Improvement with Replacement Therapy

*Normal Type indicates Inconsistent or Unreplicated Findings

Bold Type indicates Strong Findings

Selective references

Awad, N., Gagnon, M., and Messier, C. (2004). The relationship between impaired glucose tolerance, type 2 diabetes, and cognitive function. *Journal of Clinical and Experimental Neuropsychology*, **26**, 1044–1080.

Aghini-Lombardi, F.A., Pinchera, A., Anonangeli, L., *et al.* (1995). Mild iodine deficiency during fetal/neonatal life and neuropsychological impairment in Tuscany. *Journal of Endocrinological Investigation*, **18**, 57–62.

Assisi, A., Alimenti, M., Maceli, F., Di Pietro, S., Lalloni, G., and Montera, P. (1996). Diabetes and cognitive function: Preliminary studies. *Archives of Gerontology and Geriatrics (Suppl 5)*, 229–232.

Baldini, I.M., Wita, A., Mauri, M.C., *et al.* (1997). Psychopathological and cognitive features in subclinical hypothyroidism. *Progress in Neuro-Psychopharmacology and Biological Psychiatry*, **21**, 925–935.

Barrett-Connor, E., Khaw, K., and Yen, S.S.C. (1986). A prospective study of DS, mortality and cardiovascular disease. *New England Journal of Medicine*, **315**, 1519–1524.

Beatty, W.W. (1984). Hormonal organization of sex differences in play fighting and spatial behavior. *Progress in Brain Research*, **61**, 315–329.

Berman, F.B., Schmidt, P.J., Rubinow, D.R., *et al.* (1997). Modulation of congition-specific cortical activity by gonadal steroids: A positron-emission tomography study in women. *Proceedings of the National Academy of Sciences, USA*, **93**, 8836–8841.

Birge, S.J. (1994). The role of estrogen deficiency in the aging central nervous system. In R.A. Lobo (ed.), *Treatment of the postmenopausal woman: Basic and clinical aspects*. New York: Raven Press, pp. 153–157.

Bo, M., Massaia, M, Zanella, P., Cappa, G., Ferrario, E., Rainero, I., Arvat, E., Giordano, R., and Molaschi, M. (2006). Dehydroepiandrosterone sulfate (DHEA-S) and Alzheimer's dementia in older subjects. *International Journal of Geriatric Psychiatry*, **21**, 1065–1070.

Boileau, P., Bain, P., Rives, S., and Toublance, J.E. (2004). Earlier onset of treatment or increment in LT4 dose in screened congenital hypothyroidism: which is themore important factor for IQ at 7 years? *Hormone Research*, **61**, 228–33.

Bommer, M., Eversmann, T., Pickardt, R., Leohnardt, A., and Naber, D. (1990). Psychopathological and neuropsychological symptoms in patients with subclinical and remitted hyperthyroidism. *Klinische Wochenschrift*, **68**, 552–8.

Bono, G., Fancellu, R., Blandini,F., Santoro, G., and Mauri, M. (2004). Cognitive and affective status in mild hypothyroidism and interactions with L-thyroxine treatment. *Acta Neurologica Scandinavica*, **110**, 59–66.

Boone, K.B., Swerdloff, R.S., Miller, B.L., Geschwind, D.H., Razani, J., Lee, A., Gaw Gonzalo, I, Haddal, A., Rankin, K., Lu, P. and Paul, L. (2001). Neuropsychological profiles of adults with Klinefelter's syndrome. *Journal of the International Neuropsychological Society*, 7, 446–456.

Brands, A.M., Biessels, G.J., Kappelle, L.J., de Haan, E.H., de Valk, H.W., Algra, A., Kessels, R.P., and Utrecht Diabetic Encephalopathy Study Group. (2007). Cognitive functioning and brain MRI in patients with type 1 and type 2 diabetes mellitus: a comparative study. *Dementia and Geriatric Cognitive Disorders*, **23**, 343–350.

Bremner, J.D., Randall, P., Scott, T.M., *et al.* (1995). MRI-based measurement of hippocampal volume inpatients with combat-related posttraumatic stress disorder. *American Journal of Psychiatry*, **152**, 973–981.

Burkhardt, M.S., Foster, J.K., Clarnette, R.M., Chubb, S.A., Bruce, D.G., Drummond, P.D., Martins, R.N., and Yeap, B.B. (2006). Interaction between testosterone and epsilon 4 status on cognition in healthy older men. *Journal of Clinical Endocrinology and Metabolism*, **91**, 1168–1172.

Burmeister, L.A., Ganguli, M., Dodge, H.H., Toczek, T., DeKosky, S.T., and Nebes, R.D. (2001). Hypothyroidism and cognition: preliminary evidence for a specific defect in memory. *Thyroid*, **11**, 1177–1185.

Campbell, S. Marriott, M., Nahmias, C., and MacQueen, G.M. (2004). Lower hippocampal volume in patients suffering from depression: A meta-analysis. *American Journal of Psychiatry*, **161**, 598–607.

Cherrier, M.M., Matsumoto, A.M., Amory, J.K.,Asthana, S., Bremmer, W., Peskind, E.R., Raskind, E.R., and Craft, S. (2005). The role of aromatization in testosterone supplementation effects on cognition in older men. *Neurology*, **64**, 290–296.

Clarnette, R.M. and Patterson, C.J. (1994). Hypothyroidism: Does treatment cure dementia? *Journal of Geriatric Psychiatry and Neurology*, **6**, 23–27.

Colditz, G.A., Hankinson, S.E., Hunter, D.J., *et al.* (1995). The use of estrogens, and progestins and the risk of breast cancer in postmenopausal women. *New England Journal of Medicine*, **332**, 1589–1593.

Cooper DS, Halpern R, Wood LC, *et al.* (1984). L-thyroxine therapy in subclinical hypothyroidism: A double-blind, placebo-controlled trial. (1984). *Annals of Internal Medicine*, **101**, 18–24.

Davis, J.D., Stern, R.A., and Flashman, L. (2003). Cognitive and neuropsychiatric aspects of subclinical hypothyroidism: Significance in the elderly. *Current Psychiatry Reports*, 5, 384–90.

Davis, J.D. and Tremont, G. (2007). Neuropsychatric aspects of hypothyroidism and treatment reversibility. *Minerva Endocrinologica*, **32**, 49–65.

Davis, K.L, Davis, B.M., Greenwald, B.S., *et al.*, (1986). Cortisol and Alzheimer's disease. I. Basal studies. *American Journal of Psychiatry*, **143**, 300–305.

Deijen, J.B., deBoer, H., and van der Veen, E.A. (1998). Cognitive changes during growth hormone replacement in adult men. *Psychoneuroendocrinology*, **21**, 313–322.

de la Monte, S.M. and Wands, J.R. (2005). Review of insulin and insulin-like growth factor expression, signaling, and malfunction in the central nervous system: relevance to Alzheimer's disease. *Journal of Alzheimer's Disease*, 7, 45–61.

del Ser Quijano, T., Delgado, C., Martinez Espinosa, S., and Vazquez, C. (2000). Cognitive deficiency in mild hypothyroidism. *Neurologia*, **15**, 193–198.

Denicoff, K.D., Joffe, R.T., Lakshmanan, M.C., Robbins, J., and Rubinow, D.R. (1990). Neuropsychiatric manifestations of altered thyroid state. *American Journal of Psychiatry*, **147**, 94–9.

Derksen-Lubsen, G. (1996). Neuropsychologic development in early treated congenital hypothyroidism: Analysis of literature data. *Pediatric Research*, **39**, 561–566.

Desrocher, M. and Rovet, J. (2004). Neurocognitive correlates of type 1 diabetes mellitus in childhood. *Child Neuropsychology*, **10**, 36–52.

Erlanger, D.M., Kutner, K.C., and Jacobs, A.R. (1999). Hormones and cognition; Current concepts and issues in neuropsychology. *Neuropsychology Review*, 9, 175–207. (Review Article)

Falleti, M.G., MAruff, P, Burman, P., and Harris, A. (2006). The effects of growth hormone (GH) deficiency and GH replacement on cognitive performance in adults: A meta-analysis of the current literature. *Psychoneuroendocrinology*, **31**, 681–691.

Fukui, T., Hasegawa, Y., and Takenaka, H. (2001). Hyperthyroidism dementia: Clinicoradiological findings and response to treatment. *Journal of Neurological Sciences*, **184**, 81–88.

Ganguli, M., Burmeister, L.A., Seaberg, E.C., Belle, S., and DeKosky, S.T. (1996). Association between dementia and elevated TSH: a community-based study. *Biological Psychiatry*, **40**, 714–725.

Geerlings, M.I., Strozyk, D., Masaki, K., Remaley, A.T., Petrovitch, H., Ross, G.W., White, L.R., and Launer, L.J. (2006). Endogenous sex hormones, cognitive decline, and future dementia in old men. *Annals of Neurology*, **60**, 346–355.

Gouchie, C. and Kimura, D. (1991). The relationship between testosterone levels and cognitive ability patterns. *Psychoneuroendocrinology*, **16**, 323–334.

Grattan-Smith, P.J., Morris, J.G.L., Shores, E.A., Bachelor, J., and Sparks, R.S., (1992). Neuropsychological abnormalities in patients with pituitary tumors. *Acta Neurologica Scandinavica*, **86**, 626–631.

Grimley Evans, J., Malouf, R., Huppert, F., and van Niekerk, J.K. (2006). Dehydroepiandrosterone (DHEA) supplementation for cognitive function in healthy elderly people. *Cochrane Database of Systematic Reviews*, 4, CD006221.

Gull, W.W. (1873). On a cretinoid state supervening in adult life in women. *Transactions of the Medical Society of London*, **21**, 298–300.

Gulseren, S., Gulseren, L., Hekimsoy, Z., Cetinay, P., Ozen, C., Tokatlioglu, B. (2006). Depression, anxiety, health-related quality of life, and disability in patients with overt and subclinical thyroid dysfunction. *Archives of Medical Research*, **37**, 133–9.

Hall R.C. (1983). Psychiatric effects of thyroid hormone disturbance. *Psychosomatics*, **24**, 7–11.

Halpern, D.F. (1992). *Sex differences in cognitive abilities* (2nd ed.). Hillsdale, NJ: Erlbaum.

Hampson, E., Rovet, J.F., and Altmann, D. (1998). Spatial reasoning in children with congenital adrenal hyperplasia due to 21-hydroxylase deficiency. *Developmental Neuropsychology*, **13**, 299–320.

Haupt, M. and Kurz, A. (1993). Reversibility of dementia in hypothyroidism. *Journal of Neurology*, **240**, 333–35.

Helzlsouer, K.J., Gordon, G.B., Alberg, A., Bush, T.L., and Comstock, G.W. (1992). Relationship of prediagnositic serum levels of DHEA and DS to the risk of developing premenopausal breast cancer. *Cancer Research*, **52**, 1–4.

Henderson, V.W. (1997). Epidemiology of estrogen replacement therapy and Alzheimer's disease. *Neurology*, **48** (Suppl 7), S27-S35.

Henderson, V.W., and Buckwalter, J.G. (1994). Cognitive deficits of men and women with Alzheimer's disease. *Neurology*, **44**, 90–96.

Henderson, V.W., Paganini-Hill, A., Emanuel, C.K., *et al.* (1994). Estrogen replacement therapy in older woman: Comparisons between Alzheimer's disease cases and on-demented control subjects. *Archives of Neurology*, **51**, 896–900.

Herlitz, A., Thilers, P., Habib, and R. (2007). Endogenous estrogen is not associated with cognitive performance before, during, or after menopause. *Menopause*, **14**, 425–431.

Hier, D.B. and Crowley, W.F. (1982). Spatial ability in androgen-deficient men. *New England Journal of Medicine*, **306**, 1202–1205.

Hogervost, E., Bandelow, S., Combrink, M., and Smith, A.D. (2004). Low free testosterone is an independent risk factor for Alzheimer's disease. *Experimental Gerontology*, **39**, 1633–1639.

Hogervorst, E., Yafe, K., Richards, M., and Huppert, F. (2002). Hormone replacement therapy to maintain cognitive function in women with dementia. *Cochrane Database Systematic Review*, 3, CD003122.

Hook, J.N., Giordani, B., Schteingardt, D.E., Guire, K., Giles, J., Ryan, K., Gebarski, S.S., Langenecker, S.A., and Starkman, M.N. (2007). Patterns of cognitive change over time and relationship to age following successful treatment of Cushing's disease. *Journal of the International Neuropsychological Society*, **13**, 21–29.

Imperato-McGinley, J., Pichardo, M., Gautier, T., Voyer, D., and Bryden, M.P. (1991). Cognitive abilities in androgen-insensitive subjects: Comparison with control males and females from the same kindred. *Clinical Endocrinology*, **34**, 341–347.

Jacobson, A.M., Musen, G., Ryan, C.M., Silvers, N., Clearly, P., Waberski, B., Burwood, A., Weinger, K., Bayless, M., Dahms, W., and Harth, J. (2007). Diabetes Control and Complications Trial/Epidemiology of Diabetes Interventions and Complications Study Research Group. *New England Journal of Medicine*, **356**, 1842–1852.

Jaeschke, R., Guyatt, G., and Gerstein, H., *et al.* (1996). Does treatment with L-thyroxine influence health status in middle-aged and older adults with subclinical hypothyroidism? *Journal of General Internal Medicine*, **11**, 744–749.

Jansen, S.L., Forbes, D.A., Duncan, V., and Morgan, D.G. (2006). Melatonin for cognitive impairment. *Cochrane Database Systematic Review*, **25**, CD003802.

Joffe, H., Hall, J.E., Gurber, S., Sarmiento, I.A., Cohen, L.S., Yurgelun-Todd, D., and Martin, K.A. (2006). Estrogen therapy selectivey enhances prefrontal cognitive processes: a randomized, double-blind, placebo-controlled study with functional magnetic resonance imaging in perimenopausal and recently postmenopausal women. *Menopause*, **13**, 411–422.

Johannsen, T.H., Ripa, C.P.L., Reinisch, J.M., Schwartz, M., Mortensen, E.L., and Main, K.M. (2006). Impaired cognitive function in women with congenital adrenal hyperplasia. *The Journal of Clinical Endocrinology and Metabolism*, **91**, 1376–1381.

Jorde R., Waterloo K., Storhaug H., Nyrnes A. Sundsfjord J., and Jenssen TG. (2006). Neuropsychological function and symptoms in subjects with subclinical hypothyroidism and the effect of thyroxine treatment. *Journal of Clinical Endocrinology and Metabolism*, **91**, 145–53.

Jorm, A.F., Korten, A.E., and Henderson, A.S. (1987). The prevalence of dementia: A quantitative integration of the literature. *Acta Psychiatrica Scandinavia*, **76**, 475–479.

Kawas, C., Resnick, S., Morrison, A., *et al.* (1997). A prospective study of estrogen replacement therapy and the risk of developing Alzheimer's disease: The Baltimore Longitudinal study of Aging. *Neurology*, **48**, 1517–1521.

Kelso, W.M., Nicholls, M.E.R., Warne, G.L., and Zacharin, M. (2000). Cerebral lateralization and cognitive functioning in patients with congenital adrenal hyperplasia. *Neuropsychology*, **14**, 370–378.

Lamberts, S.W.J., van den Beld, A.W., and van der Lely, A. (1997). The endocrinology of aging. *Science*, **278**, 419–424.

Leentjens, A. F.G. and Kappers, E.J. (1995). Persistent cognitive defects after corrected hypothyroidism. *Psychopathology*, **28**, 235–237.

Luchsinger, J.A., Reitz, C., Patel, B., Tang, M-X, Manly, J.J., and Mayeaux, R. (2007). Relation of diabetes to mild cognitive impairment. *Archives of Neurology*, **64**, 570–575.

Loosen P.T. (1992). Effects of thyroid hormones on central nervous system in aging. *Psychoneuroendocrinology*, **17**, 355–74.

Lu, P.H., Masterman, D.A., Mulnard, R., Cotman, C., Miller, B., Yaffe, K., Reback, E., Porter, V., Swerloff, R., and Cummings, J.L. (2006). Effects of testosterone on cognition and mood in male patients with mild Alzheimer's disease and healthy elderly men. *Archives of Neurology*, **63**, 177–185.

Lupien, S., Lecours, A.R., Lussier, I., *et al.*, (1994). Basal cortisol levels and cognitive deficits in human aging. *The Journal of Neuroscience*, **14**, 2893–2903.

Maccoby, E.E., and Jacklin, C.N. (1974). *The psychology of sex differences*. Stanford: Stanford University Press.

MacCrimmon, D.J. Wallace, J.E., Goldberg, W.M., and Streiner, D.L. (1979). Emotional disturbance and cognitive deficits in hyperthyroidism. *Psychosomatic Medicine*, **41**, 331.

MacLennan, A.H., Henderson, V.W., Paine, B.J., Mathias, J., Ramsay, E.N., Ryan, P., Stocks, N.P., and Taylor, A.W. (2006). Hormone therapy, timing of initiation, and cognition in women aged older than 60 years: the REMEMBER pilot study. *Menopause*, **13**, 28–36.

Malouf, M.A., Migeon, C.J., Carson, K.A., Petrucci, L., and Wisniewski, A.B. (2006). Cognitive outcome in adult women affected by congenital adrenal hyperplasia due to 21-hydroylase deficiency. *Hormone Research*, **65**, 142–150.

McCall, A.L. (1992). The impact of diabetes on the CNS. *Diabetes*, **41**, 557–570.

Meier, C., Staub, J.J., Roth, C.B., *et al.* (2001). TSH-controlled L-thyroxine therapy reduces cholesterol levels and clinical symptoms in subclincal hypothyroidism: a double blind, placebo-controlled trial (Basel Thyroid Study). *Journal of Clinical Endocrinology and Metabolism*, **86**, 4860–4866.

Mennemeier, M., Garner, R.D., and Heilman, K.M. (1993). Memory, mood and measurement in hypothyroidism. *Journal of Clinical and Experimental Neuropsychology*, **15** (5), 822–831.

Miller, K.J., Parsons. T.D., Whybrow, P.C., van Herle, K., Rasgon, N., Martinez, D., *et al.* (2006). Memory improvement with treatment of hypothyroidism. *International Journal of Neuroscience*, **116**, 895–906.

Moffat, S.D., Zonderman, A.B., Metter, E.J., Kawas, C., Blackman, M.R., Harman, S.M., and Resnick, S.M. (2004). Free testosterone and risk for Alzheimer's disease in older men. *Neurology*, **62**, 866–871.

Monzani, R., Del Guerra, P., Caraccio, N., *et al.* (1993). Subclinical hypothyroidism: Neurobehavioral features and beneficial effect of L-thyroxine treatment. *Clinical Investigator*, **71**, 367–371.

Morrison, A., Resnick, S., Corrada, M., Zonderman, A., and Kawas, C. (1996). A prospective study of estrogen replacement therapy and the risk of developing Alzheimer's disease in the Baltimore Longitudinal Study of Aging. *Neurology*, **46**, A435–436.

Mortel, K.F. and Meyer, J.S. (1995). Lack of postmenopausal estrogen replacement therapy and the risk of dementia. *Journal of Neuropsychiatry and Clinical Neuroscience*, 7, 334–337.

Naber, D., Sand, P., and Heigl (1996). Psychopathological and neuropsychological effects of 8-days' corticosteroid treatment. A prospective study. *Psychoneuroendocrinology*, **21**, 25–31.

Nass, R. and Baker, S. (1991). Learning disabilities in children with congenital adrenal hyperplasia. *Journal of Child Neurology*, **6**, 306–12.

Netley, C. and Rovet, J. (1984). Hemispheric lateralization in 47, XXY Klinefelter's syndrome boys. *Brain and Cognition*, **3**, 10–18.

Nyström, E, Caidahl, K, Fager, G, *et al.* (1988). A double-blind cross-over 12-month study of L-thyroxine treatment of women with "subclinical" hypothryoidism. *Clinical Endocrinology*, **29**, 63–76.

Oerbeck, B., Sundet, K., Kase, B.F., and Heyerdahl, S. (2003). Congenital hypothyroidism: influence of disease severity and L-thyroxine treatment on intellectual, motor, and school-associated outcomes in young adults. *Pediatrics*, **112**, 923–930.

Osterweil, D., Syndulko, K., Cohen, S.N., Pettler-Jennings, P.D., Hershman, J.M., Cummings, J.L., Tourtellotte, W.W., and Solomon, D.H. (1992). Cognitive function in non-demented older adults with hypothyroidism. *Journal of the American Geriatric Society*, **40**, 325–335.

Ott, A., Stolk, R.P., van Harkskamp, F., Pols, H.A., Hofman, A., and Breteler, M.M. (1999). Diabetes mellitus and the risk of dementia: the Roterdam Study. *Neurology*, **53**, 1937–1942.

Paganini-Hill, A. and Henderson, V.W. (1994). Estrogen deficiency and risk of Alzheimer's disease in women. *American Journal of Epidemiology*, **140**, 256–261.

Peace, K.A., Orme, S.M., Thompson, A.R., Padayatt, S., Ellis, A.W., and Belchetz, P.E. (1997). Cognitive dysfunction in patients treated for pituitary tumours. *Journal of Clinical and Experimental Neuropsychology*, **19**, 1–6.

Perrild, H., Hansen, J.M., Arnung, K., Olsen, P.Z., and Danielsen, U. (1986). Intellectual impairment after hyperthyroidism. *Acta Endocrinologica*, **112**, 185–191.

Rapp, S.R., Espeland, M.A., Shumaker, S.A., Henderson, V.W., Burnner, R.L., Manson, J.E., Gass, M.L., Stefanick, M.L., Lane, D.S., Hays, J., Johnson, K.C., Coker, L.H., Dailey, M., Bowen, D., and Women's Health Initiative Investigators. (2003). Effect of estrogen plus progestin on global cognitive function in postmenopausal women: the Women's Health Initiative Memory Study: a randomized controlled trial. *Journal of the American Medical Association*, **28**, 2663–72.

Resnick, S.M. Berenbaum, S.A., Gottesman, I, and Bouchard, T.J. (1986). Early hormonal influences on cognitive functioning in congenital adrenal hyperplasia. *Developmental Psychology*, **12**, 524–533.

Ripich, D.N., Petril, S.A., Whitehouse, P.J. and Ziol, E.W. (1995). Gender differences in language of AD patients: A longitudinal study. *Neurology*, **45**, 299–302.

Romans, S.M., Stefanatos, G., Roeltgen, D.P., Kushner, H., and Ross, J.L. (1998). Transition to yound adulthood in Ulrich-Turner syndrome: Neurodevelopmental changes. *American Journal of Medical Genetics*, **79**, 1401–147.

Rossouw, J.E., Prentice, R.L., Manson, J.E., Wu, L., Barad, D., Barnabei, V.M., Ko, M., LaCroix, A.Z., Margolis, K.L., and Stefanick, M.L. (2007). Postmenopausal hormone therapy and risk of cardiovascular disease by age and years since menopause. *Journal of the American Medical Association*, **297**, 1465–1477.

Rovet, J.F. (2004). Turner syndrome: A review of hormonal and genetic influences on neuropsychological functioning. *Child Neuropsychology*, **10**, 262–279.

Rovet J.F. (2005). Children with congenital hypothyroidsm and their siblings: do they really differ? *Pediatrics*, **115**, e52-e57.

Ruel, J.M. and DeKloet, E.R. (1985). Two receptor systems for corticosterone in rat brain: microdistribution and differential occupation. *Endocrinology*, **117**, 2505–2511.

Ryan, C.M. (1988). Neurobehavioral disturbances: The pancreas. In R.E. Tart, D.H. Van Thiel, and K.L. Edwards, eds.), *Medical neuropsychology: The impact of disease on behavior*. New York: Plenum Press.

Ryan, C.M. and Hendrickson, R. (1998). Evaluating the effects of treatment for medical disorders: Has the value of neuropsychological assessment been fully realized? *Applied Neuropsychology*, 5, 209–219.

Ryan, C.M., and Williams, T.M. (1993). Effects of insulin-dependent diabetes on learning and memory in adults. *Journal of Clinical and Experimental Neuropsychology*, **15**, 685–700.

Salerno, M., Militerni, R., Bravaccio, C., Capalbo, D., Di, M.S., and Tenore, A. (2002). Effect of different starting doses of levothyroxine on growth and intellectual outcome at four years of age in congenital hypothyroidism. *Thyroid*, **12**, 45–52.

Sankar, R., Rai, B., Pulger, T., *et al.* (1994). Intellectual and motor functions in school children from severely iodine deficient region in Sikkim. *Indian Journal of Pediatrics*, **61**, 231–236.

Schlote, B., Nowotny, B., Schaaf, L., *et al.* (1992). Subclinical hyperthyroidism: Physical and mental state of patients. *European Archives of Psychiatry and Clinical Neuroscience*, **241**, 357–364.

Schmidt, P.J., Nieman, L.K., Danaceau, M.A., Adams, L.F., and Rubinow, D.R. (1998). Differential behavioral effects of gonadal steroids in women with and in those without premenstrual syndrome. *New England Journal of Medicine*, **338**, 209–216.

Schucard, P.W., Schucard, J.L., Clopper, R.R., and Schacter, M. (1994). Electrophysiological and neuropsychological indices of cognitive processing deficits in Turner's syndrome. *Developmental Neuropsychology*, 8, 299–323.

Selkoe, D.J. (2000). The origins of Alzheimer disease. *Journal of the American Medical Association*, **283**, 1615–1617.

Shumaker, S.A., Legault, C., Rapp, S.R., Thal, L., Wallace, R.B., Ockene, J.K., Hendrix, S.L., Jones, B.N., Assaf, A.R., Jackson, R.D., Morley Kotchen, J., Wassertheil-Smoller, S., Wactawski-Wende, J., for the Women's Health Initiative Memory Study. (2003). Estrogen plus progestin and the incidence of dementia and mild cognitive impairment in postmenopausal women. *Journal of the American Medical Association*, **20**, 2651–2662.

Singer, C., Tractenberg, R.E., Kaye, J., Schafer, K., Gamst, A., Grundman, M., Thomas, R., Thal, L.J., for the Alzheimer's Disease Cooperative Study. (2003). A multicenter, placebo-controlled trial of melatonin for sleep disturbance in Alzheimer's disease. *Sleep*, **26**, 893–901.

Starkman, M.N., Giordani, B., Gebarski, S.S., Berent, S., Schork, M.A., and Schteingardt, D.E. (1999). Decreases in cortisol reverse human hippocampus storphy following treatent of Cushing's disease. *Biological Psychiatry*, **46**, 1595–1602.

Starkman, M.N., Giordani, B., Gebarski, S.S., and Schteingardt, D.E. (2003). Improvement in learning associated with increase in hippocampal formation volume. *Biological Psychiatry*, **53**, 233–238.

Stern, R.A., Robinson, B., Thorner, A.R., Arruda, J.E., Prohaska, M.L., and Pranges, A.J., Jr. (1996). A survey of neuropsychiatric complaints in patients with Graves' disease. *The Journal of Neuropsychiatry and Clinical Neurosciences*, **8**, 181–185.

Tang, M.X., Jacobs, D., Stern, Y., *et al.* (1996). Effect of oestrogen during menopause on risk and age at onset of Alzheimer's disease. *Lancet*, **348**, 429–432.

Temple, C.M. (2002). Oral fluency and narrative production in children with Turner's syndrome. *Neuropsychologia*, **40**, 1419–1427.

Thoman, M.L. and Weigle, W.O. (1989). The cellular and subcellular bases of immunosenescence. *Advances in Immunology*, **46**, 221–261.

Tremont, G., Stern, R., Westervelt, H.J., Bishop, C.L., and Davis, J.D. (2003). Neurobehavioral functioning in thyroid disorders. *Medicine and Health, Rhode Island*, **86**, 318–322.

Trzepacz, P.T., McCue, M., Klein, I., Levey, G.S., and Greenhouse, J. (1988). A psychiatric and neuropsychological study of patients with untreated Graves' disease. *General Hospital Psychiatry*, **10**, 49–55.

Trivalle, C., Doucet, J., Chassagne, P., Landrin, I., Kadri, N., Menard, J.F., and Bercoff, E. (1996). Differences in the signs and symptoms of hyperthyroidism in older and younger patients. *Journal of the American Geriatrics Society*, **44**, 50–53.

Vander Reijden-Lakeman, I.E., de Sonneville, L.M., Swaab-Barneveld, H.J., Slijper, F.M., and Verhulst, F.C. (1997). Evaluation of attention before and after 2 years of growth hormone treatment in intrauterine growth retarded children. *Journal of Clinical and Experimental Neuropsychology*, **19**, 101–118.

Vitiello, M.V., Moe, K.E., Merriam, G.R., Mazzoni, G., Bucjner, D.H., and Schwartz, R.S. (2006). Growth hormone releasing hormone improves the cognition of healthy older adults. *Neurobiology of Aging*, **27**, 318–323.

Vogel, A., Elberling, T.V., Hording, M., Dock, J., Rasmussen, A.K., Feldt-Rasmussen, U., Perrild, H., and Waldemar, G. (2007). Affective symptoms and cognitive functions in the acute phase of Graves' thyrotoxicosis. *Psychoneuroendocrinology*, **32**, 36–43.

Volpato S., Guralnik J.M., Fried L.P., Remaley, A.T., Cappola, A.R., and Launer, L.J. (2002). Serum thyroxine level and cognitive decline in euthyroid older women. *Neurology*, **58**, 1055–1061.

Watari, K., Letamendi, A., Elderkin-Thompson, V., Haroon, E., Miller, J., Darwin, C., and Kumar, A. (2006). Cognitive function in adults with type 2 diabetes and major depression. *Archives of Clinical Neuropsychology*, **21**, 787–796.

Watt, T., Hegedus, L., Rasmussen, A.K., Groenvold, M., Bonnema, S.J., Bjorner, J.B., and Feldt-Rasmussen, U. (2007). Which domains of thyroid-related quality of life are most relevant? Patients and clinicians provide complementary perspectives. *Thyroid*, **17**, 647–654.

Whybrow, P.C. and Prange, A.J., Jr., Treadway, C.R. (1969). Mental changes accompanying thyroid gland dysfunction. A reappraisal using objective psychological measurement. *Archives of General Psychiatry*, **20**, 48–63.

Williams, C.L., Barnett, A.M., and Meck, W.H. (1990). Organizational effects of early gonadal secretions on sexual differentiation in spatial memory. *Behavioral Neuroscience*, **104**, 84–97.

Williamson, J.D., Miller, M.E., Bryan, N., Lazar, R., Coker, L.H., Johnson, J., Cukierman, T., Horowitz, K.R., Murray, A., Launer, L.J. for the ACCORD Study Group. (2007). The Action to Control Cardiovascular Risk in Diabetes Memory in Diabetes Study (ACCORD-MIND): Rationale, design, and methods. *American Journal of Cardiology*, **99**, 112i-122i.

Winograd, D.L., Sensheima, P., Barrett-Connor, E.L., and McPhillips, T.B. (1990). Community-based study on the prevalence of NIDDM in older adults. *Diabetes Care*, **13** (Suppl 2), 3–8.

Writing Group for the Women's Health Initiative Investigators. 2002. Risks and benefits of estrogen plus progestin in healthy postmenopausal women. Principal results from the Women's Health Initiative Randomized Controlled Trial. *Journal of the American Medical Association*, **288**, 321–333.

Wolkowitz, O.M., Kramer, J.H., Reus, V.I., Costa, M.M., Yaffe, K., Walton, P., Raskind, M., Peskind, E., Newhouse, P., Sack, D., DeSouza, E., Sadowsky, C., Roberts, R., and the DHEA-Alzheimer's Disease Collaborative Research Group. 2003. DHEA treatment of Alzheimer's disease: A randomized, double-blind, placebo-controlled study. *Neurology*, **60**, 1071–1076.

Yaffe, K., Sawaya, G., Lieberburg, I., and Grady, D. (1998). Estrogen therapy in postmenopausal women: Effects on cognitive function and dementia. *Journal of the American Medical Association*, **17**, 1848–1859.

Yeap, B.B., Almeida, O.P., Hydet, Z., Chubb, S.A.P., Hankey, G.J., Jamrozik, K., and Flicker, L. (in press). *Higher serum free testosterone is associated with better cognitive functioning in older men, while total testosterone is not. The health of men study*. Clinical Endocrinology.

Further reading

North, W.G., Moses, A.M., and Share, L. (Eds.). (1993). *The neurohypophysis: A window on brain function*. The New York Academy of Sciences, New York.

Tartar, R.E., Butters, M., and Beers, S.R. (2001). *Medical neuropsychology, Second Edition*. Kluwer Academic/Plenum Publishers, New York.

Snyder, P.J., Nussbaum, P.D., and Robins, D.L. (2006). *Clinical Neuropsychology: A pocket handbook for assessment*. American Psychological Association, Washington, DC.

Chapter 31

The epilepsies

Pamela J. Thompson

1 Introduction

Clinical neuropsychology can make a unique contribution to the management of epilepsy a role identified in the UK National Institute of Clinical Excellence guidelines of 2004 (Stokes *et al.*, 2004).

> *Neuropsychological deficits are commonly associated with epilepsy and its treatment. Awareness of these problems may facilitate education, social integration and employment.*

Neuropsychological deficits are hidden and are often overlooked as most attention is focused on seizures and the need for control. Undetected cognitive deficits will have far reaching negative consequences that extend beyond academic concerns. The longer cognitive problems go unrecognised the worse the outcome and the more difficult to redress the effects. A neuropsychological assessment provides a systematic and standardised record of cognitive strengths and weaknesses and can be vital in the management of the epilepsies.

A verbal learning deficit may present in focal epilepsy arising from left temporal lobe structures. This may cause a child to fall behind at school and fail examinations. Frequent academic knock backs result in loss of confidence. A failing child may also be the butt of jokes at school and a cause of distress within the family. Low self-esteem, social withdrawal and bullying may ensue.

Neuropsychological assessment may assist diagnosis and treatment. It is a major tool in detecting dementia and monitoring its course. It may be important in identifying certain epilepsy syndromes. Neuropsychological test profiles may help differentiate between a focal and a generalised epilepsy and this in turn may result in more effective drug management. Possible adverse drug side effects can be measured with cognitive tests and drug changes can be more promptly implemented if difficulties are demonstrated.

The neuropsychologist has a well-established role in the surgical multidisciplinary team. Cognitive test profiles often yield vital cerebral lateralising and localising information. Pre-operative test scores provide evidence regarding probable post-operative cognitive complications. These can be discussed with the patient and their family and result in better informed surgical decision making.

There is an increasing emphasis on cognitive rehabilitation and this can positively influence epilepsy management. Undetected memory impairments will result in poor compliance. Forgotten tablets will result in an increase in seizures. Teaching and training memory support strategies will improve compliance and may reduce the need for medication increases and in turn improve memory efficiency.

2 Epilepsy - general description

Epilepsy is the most serious, common chronic neurological condition, with a lifetime incidence of 2–5%. The usual prevalence figure given is 5–10 cases per 1000. Rates are higher in those with a learning disability, increasing with the severity of the cognitive impairment (Sander and Shorvon 1996).

Epilepsy refers to a group of conditions that have recurrent seizures as a symptom and consequently *the epilepsies* is the term recommended in the NICE guidelines (Stokes *et al.*, 2004). An epileptic seizure is a transient, abnormal electrical discharge from a set of neurons in the brain; the region involved will shape the behavioural manifestation of the attack. Seizures may involve motor, sensory, psychic or autonomic disturbances, alone or in combination. Epileptic seizures are stereotyped and often have a sudden onset and a brief duration, lasting minutes. Seizure occurrence is generally unpredictable.

There are a number of voluntary organisations that offer information and support to patients, families and health professionals (See Table 31.1 for UK details).

2.1 Classification

The classification of epilepsy is complex and a multi-axial diagnostic system has recently been proposed so that a variety of approaches are possible (Engel, 2001). Seizure type is

Table 31.1 Additional sources of information/support

Organisation	Website	Address	Helpline	Services offered
Epilepsy action	www.epilepsy.org.uk	New Anstey House, Gate Way Drive, Yeadon, Leeds LS19 7XY	0808 800 5050	Local support groups, accredited volunteers, fundraising events, regional conferences for people with epilepsy and their families, epilepsy awareness training, magazines and publications
Epilepsy Scotland	www.epilepsyscotland.org.uk	48 Govan Road, Glasgow G51 IJL	0808 800 2200	Training, fundraising, community support services for one to one service within the community
Epilepsy bereaved	www.sudep.org.uk	PO Box 112, Wantage OX12 8XT	01235 772850	Support services to the bereaved. Free information in relation to epilepsy deaths. Raise awareness of SUDEP. Provide opportunities for bereaved families to meet
National society for epilepsy	www.epilepsy-society.org.uk	Chalfont Centre, Chalfont St Peter, Bucks SL9 ORJ	01494 601400	Helpline, forum, leaflets, books and videos, trained volunteers, membership scheme, epilepsy awareness training, medical, assessment and residential services.

one axis and this is likely to remain the main categorizing tool. The major and long-standing distinction drawn is between partial and generalised seizures. In the newly proposed classification of seizures the term focal is recommended in preference to partial. It is likely this change in terminology will take time to come into common clinical usage and in this chapter partial will continue to be used.

Most seizure types can be classified as partial or generalised although it is recognised some seizures are not adequately encompassed by this dichotomy including multi-focal seizures.

2.1.1 Partial seizures

Partial seizures begin with epileptic activity in a localised brain region. Any area of the cortex can be the epileptogenic zone but the temporal lobes are the most susceptible. 60–70% of partial epilepsies involve onset in the temporal lobes. *Simple partial seizures* are brief in duration and awareness is retained. Common presentations include a strange taste or smell, usually unpleasant in nature; an epigastric rising sensation; flushing and changes in heart rate; memory disturbances such as déjà vu and jamais vu; affective disturbances of which fear is the most common and which can be intense.

Complex partial seizures of temporal lobe origin are relatively long, in the order of 2–3 minutes. Awareness and responsiveness are altered and there is memory loss for the event. Common presentations include automatisms such as lip smacking, chewing, fiddling and rubbing movements. A person may wander around. The attack may be followed by confusion of 5–10 minutes or longer. Post-ictal dysphasia frequently follows seizures arising from the language dominant hemisphere.

The frontal lobes are the next most common site of partial epilepsy. Simple partial seizures include a strange sensation like a 'wave' going through the head, stiffness or jerking on the face or in a limb. *Complex partial seizures* of frontal origin are characteristically short, lasting less than a minute and in contrast to temporal lobe seizures recovery is generally quick. During seizures limbs may raise, there may be tonic or clonic deviation of the head and eyes to one side, unilateral limb jerking or posturing or sudden speech arrest.

Seizures arising in parietal regions may present with tingling, numbness and burning sensations; illusions of size (macropsia, micropsia), shape and sound. Seizures from occipital regions may present with visual perceptual phenomenon (flashing lights, coloured shapes) often restricted to a hemi-field.

Partial seizure activity may spread to involve the whole brain and progress into a generalised seizure.

2.1.2 Generalised seizures

In generalised seizures the epileptogenic activity involves the whole cortex from the outset. Consciousness is lost and accordingly there is no awareness for the event. *Absence seizures* involve only a brief arrest of consciousness in the order of a few seconds. Absences are a common seizure type in children with epilepsy. *Atypical absences* refers to attacks of longer duration that may involve some body jerking.

Generalised *tonic clonic seizures* can last several minutes and are biphasic. The attack begins with muscle contraction and stiffness. The person will fall if standing and muscle tightening around the chest may result in a vocalisation as air is expelled from the lungs (tonic phase). Limb jerking follows (clonic phase). Often breathing is affected with grunting and snorting and the patient may be incontinent. Seizures last a few minutes although exhaustion is common and a period of sleep may be needed.

Tonic seizures are brief. Suddenly all muscles stiffen, the person becomes rigid and will fall if standing. Injuries are common. Recovery of consciousness is rapid. *Atonic* seizures involve a sudden loss of body tone. If standing the person will fall, more usually forwards. As for tonic seizures injuries are common and recovery is quick. *Myoclonic* seizures are the briefest attacks and involve sudden muscle jerks lasting only seconds, most usually affecting the arms.

Most seizures are short-lived and stop spontaneously. Status epilepticus refers to prolonged episodes lasting more than 30 minutes or serial seizures with inadequate recovery between attacks. It can occur for any seizure type but is most dangerous for tonic-clonic seizures and is a medical emergency.

2.1.3 Reflex seizures

Reflex seizures have a specific trigger. Seizures are classified according to the precipitating stimuli. The most common precipitants are visual stimuli (flickering lights and patterns) and the most frequent environmental triggers are watching television, computer games and other computer graphics. Other documented precipitants are hot water, startle and higher mental activity, including reading, writing, arithmetic, memorising, chess and card playing. Seizures can be precipitated by other special circumstances such as fever or alcohol withdrawal but these are not reflex seizures.

2.2 Prognosis

70–80% of people with epilepsy will become seizure free and about 50% will be able to discontinue their antiepileptic medication. The remainder will present with difficult to control epilepsy and it is this group who are at greater risk of cognitive impairments.

At one time epilepsy was considered a benign condition but recent studies have indicated an elevated mortality rate. Death in newly diagnosed epilepsy is invariably due to the underlying aetiology. In more longstanding epilepsy the main cause of death is the seizures and is classified as sudden unexpected death in epilepsy (SUDEP). This accounts for an estimated 500 deaths a year in the UK (Hanna *et al.* 2002; Tomson *et al.* 2005).

Seizure type is of limited utility in assessing prognosis. The underlying cause and any identified syndrome are better indicators.

2.3 Causes

The causes of epilepsy are varied.

◆ Epilepsy may be genetically determined. Idiopathic generalised epilepsies include childhood absence epilepsy. Of these 80% remit by adulthood. The mode of inheritance is unclear and is likely to be multigenetic. There are a large number of rare inherited disorders with seizures as a common feature including tuberous sclerosis and neurofi-bromatosis both autosomal dominant. and Unverricht Lundborgs Disease autosomal recessive.

+ Congenital malformations of the brain may cause epilepsy. Cortical dysgenesis refers to brain abnormalities that have developed as the result of faulty neuronal migration during embryo-genesis. The most severe cases involve gyral abnormalities such as lis-sencephaly, where there is an absence of gyri over the whole brain. Invariably such individuals have severe learning disabilities. Prognosis is usually poor. At the other end of the spectrum there may be more localised small areas of dysgenesis (i.e. dysem-bryoplastic neuroepithemial tumours (DNETs)). Causes of cortical dysgenesis are thought to include intrauterine infection and illness.

+ Hippocampal sclerosis is the most common lesion identified in resected tissue follow-ing temporal lobe resections. It is strongly associated with a prolonged childhood febrile convulsion(s). Habitual epilepsy may not develop for several years. It remains controversial whether hippocampal sclerosis results from epileptic activity or whether it precedes and is the cause of the epilepsy.

+ The incidence of epilepsy is high following cerebral infections and often seizures are difficult to control. Rates for herpes simplex encephalitis are 25%; for bacterial meningitis 10% and for human immune deficiency virus (HIV) related cerebral toxoplasmosis 25%.

+ Epilepsy may be caused by head injuries. The risk is high when the post-traumatic amnesia exceeds 24hrs. Intracranial haematomas and open head injuries increase the risk.

+ Seizures can develop de novo following neurosurgery: The occurrence of seizures will be influenced by the site (increased frontal and temporal), the extent of resection (increased with larger volumes) and the condition for which the craniotomy is performed (e.g. higher for arteriovenous formations than for intracranial aneurysms).

+ Cerebro-vascular disease may cause epilepsy. It depends on the extent and site of the infarction. The rates are low for transient ischaemic attacks and high for haemorra-hagic stroke.

+ Neoplasms increase the risk of epilepsy and the risk varies with type (oligodenroglio-mas 90%; meningiomas and astrocytomas 70%; malignant tumours 35%).

+ Seizures may be a symptom of dementias and neurodegenerative conditions. Approximately 25% of cases with Alzheimer's Disease develop seizures. The response to AED treatment in this group is good.

+ Metabolic disorders may underlie epilepsy. Changes in blood concentrations of sodium, potassium, calcium, magnesium and glucose are implicated.

+ There are reports of epilepsy following drug ingestion. Drugs that have been impli-cated include antibiotics, antimalarials, antidepressants and antipsychotic agents. Illicit drug use and heavy alcohol consumption can cause epilepsy.

3 Investigations for epilepsy

A diagnosis of epilepsy is commonly made on the basis of a behavioural description of the seizure that is generally provided by the family. Rarely do physicians witness an attack.

3.1 Electroencephalography (EEG)

EEG recordings are used to support a diagnosis of epilepsy in patients with a history that suggests an event was epileptic (Stokes *et al.*, 2004). An EEG trace represents the summation of synchronised excitatory or inhibitory postsynaptic potentials. An EEG should never be used in isolation to make a diagnosis of epilepsy. Neither should an EEG be used to exclude a diagnosis of epilepsy. About 10% of patients with epilepsy will have normal EEGs. In about 30% of cases epileptic abnormalities are seen on routine recordings (20–30 minutes). This increases to 95% if a recording captures a seizure; unfortunately the chances of recording a seizure during a routine recording are low.

EEGs may provide useful information about epilepsy type. Generalised spike and wave discharges typically occur during absences and indicate a generalised epilepsy. Evolving temporal slow wave activity may be seen in temporal lobe seizures supporting a diagnosis of a focal seizure disorder.

More prolonged EEG recordings increase the chances of seizure detection. Small portable EEG machines allow longer recordings (ambulatory EEG monitoring). These may be worn for several days in the home environment until an attack occurs. More prolonged EEG recordings can also be undertaken as an inpatient and this also allows for simultaneous video recordings (video-telemetry). During inpatient assessment AEDs can be reduced or withdrawn or the patient can be sleep deprived, conditions that increase the chances of seizures occurring.

3.1.1 Intracranial EEG recordings

These are undertaken on selected surgical candidates usually when epileptic sites are suspected but the precise origin is unclear. Depth electrodes with multi-contact wires are inserted stereotactically under MRI guidance into the region(s) of interest.

Subdural grids and strips consist of larger arrays of electrodes. These are placed directly onto the brain intra-operatively. These are used when the suspected epileptogenic area is extensive and may involve eloquent cortex. Brain stimulation via the electrodes enables mapping of the epileptogenic region. Stimulation when a patient is awake is undertaken to map language and the motor cortex. Intracranial EEG recordings are invasive and carry an increased risk of morbidity.

3.2 Brain imaging

Magnetic Resonance Imaging (MRI) and Computerised Tomography (CT) cannot be used to diagnose epilepsy. Brain imaging plays a vital role in epilepsy in establishing aetiology and in pre-surgical investigations. MRI is the imaging tool of choice and it is recommended best practise to obtain a scan in the majority of patients with epilepsy (Stokes, 2004). The most common abnormalities identified in epilepsy are hippocampal sclerosis, malformations of cortical development vascular malformations, tumours and acquired cortical damage.

Diffusion tensor imaging (DTI) is a method derived from MRI technology that looks at the flow of water within the brain that highlights how different areas of the brain are connected. Trachtography utilises DTI to delineate white matter tracts and demonstrate the connectivity between regions. Recent research has used this technique to delineate language pathways in TLE patients (Powell *et al.* 2007a).

MRI Spectroscopy is an imaging technique that measures neurotransmitter levels and it has been used to explore how the activity of the brain is affected by seizures. This remains largely a research tool.

3.2.1 Functional MRI (fMRI)

fMRI has been a valuable research technique and increasingly is being developed as a clinical tool. In epilepsy, paradigms are being developed to identify the locus of seizure onset. In epilepsy surgery programmes, fMRI paradigms are being developed to assess brain regions involved in critical cognitive functions such as language and memory and to generate data that contributes to surgical decision making. Consensus is growing regarding the utility of such procedures to lateralise language functions but more controversial to date is the use of fMRI data for memory assessment as an alternative to the intracarotid amytal procedure (Powell *et al.* 2004).

3.3 The Intracarotid Amytal Procedure (IAP)

This test used to be carried out prior to all anterior temporal lobe resections and many other surgical procedures. It was originally developed to assess language dominance. Subsequently it was used to screen for the risk of post-operative amnesia in candidates undergoing a temporal lobe resection. Each cerebral hemisphere in turn is temporarily anaesthetised by injecting sodium amobarbital into a single carotid artery via a catheter placed in the femoral artery. The drug effects are variable but last approximately ten minutes. A transient hemiplegia and EEG changes indicate a lateralized effect. The patient is shown stimuli before and after the injection. Speech arrest and dysphasic responses indicate language dominance in the injected hemisphere. Intact memory performance when the 'to be resected' hemisphere is injected indicates no risk of post-operative amnesia. The IAP is an invasive procedure and although complications are rare they can be severe and have included cerebral infarction. The application of this test in many surgical centres has been reduced in recent years due to concerns about such risks together with doubts regarding its reliability and validity (see later).

4 Treatment

4.1 Acute management

Convulsive seizures are usually short-lived and do not require immediate medical treatment. Nothing can be done to influence the course of the seizure.

1 The patient should be made as comfortable as possible, preferably lying down, or eased to the floor if seated.

2 The head should be protected and any tight clothing should be released.

3 Clear a space around the person in order to avoid injury.

4 Do not attempt to open the mouth and do not force anything between the teeth.

5 After the convulsive movements have stopped, roll the person on to their side.

6 Check the airway is not obstructed.

7 Patients may take a variable time to recover and may wish to sleep or rest.

8 Emergency treatment will only be needed if the person sustains an injury, the convulsive stage lasts longer than ten minutes, the patient takes a long time to regain consciousness following the episode, or a second convulsive attack follows on shortly.

Non-convulsive seizures require minimal management.

1 Many attacks are very brief and have little impact on a patient's behaviour.

2 In complex partial seizures the patient may wander and fiddle with items. An attempt should be made to guide the person out of danger if necessary.

3 No attempt should be made to restrain them. Attempts at doing so can make a patient become quite agitated and at times aggressive.

4.2 Medication

Antiepileptic drugs (AEDs) form the mainstay of treatment. The range of drugs available is given in Table 31.2 and the most common side effects in Table 31.3. About 70% of patients developing epilepsy may expect to become seizure free with AED therapy. The majority will achieve control with a single drug and 10–15% with two drugs.

Table 31.2 Antiepileptic drugs

Generic name	Brand name	Abbreviation	Dose range (mgs)
Carbamazepine	Tegretol	CBZ	400–1600
Clobazam	Frisium	CLB	10–30
Clonazepam	Rivotril	CZP	0.5–4
Ethosuximide	Zarontin	ESM	500–1500
Gabapentin	Neurontin	GBP	900–3600
Lamotrigine	Lamictal	LTG	100–400
Levetiracetam	Kepra	LT	750–3000
Phenobarbitone	Luminal	PB	60–180
Phenytoin	Epanutin	DPH	200–400
Pregabalin	Lyrica	PGB	150–600
Oxcarbazepine	Trileptal	OXC	600–2400
Sodium valproate	Epilim	VPA	500–2500
Tiagabine	Gabitril	TGB	30–45
Topiramate	Topamax	TPM	75–400
Zonisimide	Zonegram	ZNS	150–600

Table 31.3 Common AED side effects

Anti-epileptic drug	Common side effects
Carbamazepine	Diplopia, dizziness, headache, nausea
Clobazam	Fatigue, drowsiness
Clonazepam	Fatigue, drowsiness, sedation
Ethosuximide	Nausea
Gabapentin	Somnolence, ataxia, dizziness, diplopia
Lamotrigine	Drowsiness, headache, diplopia, tremor
Levetiracetam	Headache, irritability
Phenobarbitone	Fatigue, depression, insomnia (children), distractibility (children), irritability (children)
Phenytoin	Nystagmus, ataxia
Pregabalin	Dizziness, drowsiness
Oxcarbazepine	Fatigue, diplopia, dizziness
Sodium valproate	Tremor, weight gain, hair loss
Tiagabine	Dizziness, headache, tremor, concentration difficulties
Topiramate	Weight loss, impaired concentration and speech, paraesthesia
Zonisamide	Drowsiness, dizziness

4.3 Surgical treatment

There are two major types of surgery for epilepsy, resective and functional. *Resective surgery* aims to remove the epileptogenic brain region in order to stop seizures (Duncan 2007). Advances in MRI technology have increased the yield of abnormalities that are amenable to this approach. The most commonly performed operation is an anterior temporal lobe resection and the most common pathology hippocampal sclerosis. In such cases up to two thirds can be expected to achieve complete seizure control post-operatively.

A lesionectomy may be performed if there is a small circumscribed area of abnormality. Such lesions include cavernomas, focal cortical dysplasias and indolent tumours such as dysembryoplastic neuroepithelial tumours. A seizure free outcome is highest for extratemporal lesions and is lower when the lesion is within the temporal lobe.

A hemispherectomy represents the most radical procedure; resection of the temporal lobe and central cortex is followed by disconnection of frontal and occipital neocortices from the subcortical structures and corpus callosum. It is most commonly carried out with children when there is evidence of major structural abnormalities and limited functional capacity in the epileptogenic hemisphere.

The aim of *functional surgery* is palliative. It is only considered when resective surgery has been ruled out. The surgical plan is to disconnect the epileptogenic region or to prevent the spread of epileptic discharges to other regions.

Corpus callosotomy involves disconnecting the callosal fibres between the cerebral hemispheres; most operations involve a partial disconnection of the anterior fibres. The procedure is most commonly used in patients with disabling drop attacks.

Multiple subpial transection, also known as Morrel's Procedure, involves multiple cuts being made vertically in the assessed epileptogenic cortical region in an effort to reduce seizure generation while maintaining anatomical function. It is undertaken when seizures arise from language areas or motor cortex.

Vagal nerve stimulation (VNS) is a recently developed procedure. A small device, akin to a cardiac pacemaker, is placed subcutaneously and connected surgically to the left vagus nerve. This generator sends regular mild electrical impulses via this nerve to the brain. The rate of pulse generation is programmed at outpatient hospital visits beginning a few weeks after implantation. The patient also has a magnet which can be used to produce extra impulses following seizure warnings. There are reports of reduced seizure frequency and also reductions in seizure duration and recovery time. A VNS may take several months to have an effect. Side effects include discomfort in the throat, a cough and a hoarse voice. Once implanted, VNS is a contra-indication to higher resolution MRI scanning (even if the VNS has for some reason been disabled).

4.4 Psychological treatment

A number of treatments have been proposed as seizure reducing techniques (Whitmarsh, 2004). From a behavioural viewpoint, a seizure is part of a sequence of events and by interrupting the behavioural chain at some stage, the likelihood of seizure is reduced. Avoidance is a behavioural technique that has been successfully employed in reflex epilepsies. Individuals with photosensitive epilepsy can reduce the likelihood of a seizure by viewing the television at a distance, covering one eye, viewing in good, ambient lighting and by using polarised glasses. Anxiety reduction techniques have been employed with varying success. Recent studies have shown substantial seizure reduction using biofeedback although such approaches require intense input and high levels of motivation. Studies of the efficacy of CBT are few and the support for improving seizure control is limited (Goldstein *et al.* 2003).

4.5 Diet and lifestyle changes

The Ketogenic Diet is the most established dietary control for epilepsy. It is high in fat but low in carbohydrate and protein. It is used almost invariably with children. The diet can be continued for months, or even years, if necessary but many children find it unpalatable and accordingly compliance can be a problem.

In some generalised epilepsies, changes in lifestyle have been associated with improved seizure control and complete seizure freedom. Routines including regularising sleep together with abstinence from alcohol are the most commonly advocated.

5 Neuropsychological deficits

5.1 Intelligence

In the past epilepsy has been associated with limited intelligence. This misperception was a consequence of biased sampling with over-representation of institutionalised and intractable cases. More representative sampling indicates people with epilepsy span the spectrum of intellectual ability.

A few epilepsy syndromes are characterised by failed or arrested cognitive and intellectual development.

- Early infantile epileptic encephalopathy has an onset in early infancy. The MRI shows extensive abnormalities and atrophy. Many infants die and survivors have severe and profound learning disabilities, often with sensory and motor abnormalities.

- In West's Syndrome and Lennox Gastaut Syndrome: There is developmental delay but with plateauing. Sufferers invariably have lifelong, frequent and severe seizures.

- In some other conditions there is co-morbidity and the onset of seizures may not develop until later childhood, adolescence or in adulthood. The estimated risk of epilepsy in Down's Syndrome is 10%; in Autism 30% in Cerebral Palsy 50%, in Tuberous Sclerosis 60%, and in Angelman's Syndrome 80%.

The likelihood of epilepsy increases with the severity of a learning disability. Both the seizures and the cognitive impairment are a consequence of extensive brain damage and immature cerebral development.

5.2 Intellectual deterioration

Longitudinal studies over substantial time periods are few but indicate that intellectual level can remain stable even when seizures are poorly controlled (Thompson and Duncan 2005). Intellectual decline however is a symptom of some rarer syndromes.

Rasmussen's Encephalitis presents with constant partial motor seizures, usually in one limb, with gradual progression to involve the ipsilateral limb, causing a hemiplegia. It is associated with progressive focal brain atrophy. In left hemisphere cases there is a fall in VIQ and language skills and in right hemisphere cases a fall in PIQ and visuo-spatial abilities.

Electrical status epilepticus during slow-wave sleep (ESES) develops in childhood often following several years of normal development. Cognitive decline can be dramatic. EEG studies demonstrate almost continuous periods of abnormal EEG patterns of generalised spike and wave predominant during sleep. EEG abnormalities and seizures remit in the majority in adolescence, but intellectual gains thereafter are small. Landau Kleffner Syndrome involves ESES but in addition with left hemisphere temporo-parietal spike wave discharges while awake and aphasia (see later).

There are a few progressive myoclonic syndromes. Unverricht Lundborg's Syndrome (Baltic myoclonous) is one. The onset is usually between the ages of 5–15. Progressive motor and cognitive deterioration can be dramatic.

5.3 Ictally related cognitive disturbance

Transient cognitive deficits may be temporally related to the seizures. Deficits will vary in severity and type depending on the duration and site of the epileptic discharge. Transient cognitive impairment is a term used to describe fleeting cognitive lapses associated with brief epileptic discharges. These may only become apparent during continuous cognitive activity. When such discharges are frequent cognitive disturbance is marked. Any cognitive activity may be disrupted but cases have been reported of localised discharges having a selective effect (e.g. left temporal discharges impairing verbal but not spatial memory tasks) (Holmes and Lenck-Santini, 2006).

Overt seizures may present as more obvious intermittent cognitive disturbances. For example, word finding difficulties may be the manifestation of partial seizures arising from dominant lateral temporal regions or brief episodes of topographical disorientation may reflect seizures in the non-dominant temporal lobe.

Non-convulsive absence and partial status epilepticus can present as severe cognitive impairment that mimics dementia. Misdiagnosis can occur, most frequently in the elderly and individuals with learning disabilities. EEG recordings confirm this diagnosis and AED treatment can bring about rapid control and reversal of the cognitive disturbance.

There may be post-ictal cognitive changes which persist. For instance verbal memory deficits can persist several days following a cluster of left temporal lobe seizures when other cognitive functions have recovered.

6 Chronic cognitive disturbance

There is no cognitive deficit or neuropsychological test profile that characterises epilepsy. The majority of individuals who are well controlled by drug treatment will not experience problems and accordingly do not come to the attention of a clinical neuropsychologist. Those with intractable epilepsy, however, will be at risk of persisting cognitive difficulties. The most potent factor influencing the nature and severity of a deficit is the presence and location of brain pathology and the epileptic focus. Given the increased risk of epilepsy with temporal and frontal pathology, cognitive deficits associated with these regions are the most frequently encountered in clinical practice.

6.1 Memory

Deficits of new learning have been the subject of most investigations and are the most common cognitive impairment in temporal lobe epilepsy (Thompson, 1997). Memory impairment is most extensive in cases with known bilateral temporal lobe damage, with the amnesic syndrome being the most severe case scenario. Amnesia is most often encountered in adult onset post-encephalitic cases.

Unilateral temporal lobe epilepsy has been associated with material specific memory disorders. Assuming left hemisphere language dominance, left temporal lobe disturbance is reported to be associated with verbal memory difficulties and right temporal lobe disturbance with spatial and other non-verbal memory deficits (Baxendale *et al.* 1998; Baxendale *et al.*, 1998b). Such material specific memory disorders are more likely to be encountered post surgically. In unilateral temporal lobe cases, material specific memory problems may not be found and are less likely in early onset epilepsy, particularly where the underlying pathology is a cortical dysplasia.

Patients' accounts suggest that memory decline may occur several hours or days following successful registration. Research studies have provided some support for this demonstrating that patients with temporal lobe epilepsy can perform adequately when recall is tested with delays up to one hour, but that abnormally accelerated forgetting can occur at longer delays (Blake *et al.* 2000). Routine clinical assessments will miss such memory disturbance.

6.2 Language

Language problems arise most frequently in partial epilepsy emanating from the language dominant hemisphere particularly in the presence of a structural lesion. A seizure focus in fronto-temporal regions will interfere with expressive functions and more posterior temporal lesions with receptive functions. Dominant parietal foci may underlie reading and spelling problems.

6.2.1 Language dominance

Atypical language dominance (i.e. language functions predominantly lateralised to the right hemisphere or bilaterally represented), is not uncommon in epilepsy. Predisposing factors include early cerebral insult to the left hemisphere, early onset of recurrent seizures, left (pathological) handedness or weak right handedness. Language laterality in epilepsy is a clinically relevant variable in individuals being considered for surgery and may influence the decision to proceed to surgery, the extent of a resection, the need for an awake craniotomy and the content of pre-operative counselling outlining post-operative cognitive risks.

6.2.2 Landau Kleffner's syndrome

This is also known as acquired epileptic aphasia and is a rare disorder. Linguistic regression develops in association with severe focal EEG abnormalities. It usually presents between the ages of four to eleven with generally normal language development prior to the onset. Receptive language difficulties may be the first symptom. The majority of cases go on to develop generalised and partial seizures. Language deterioration occurs over time and total mutism can result. EEG recordings show multi-focal spike and wave discharges predominately in temporal and parietal regions. Language functions may improve as seizures become less frequent or stop although many individuals are left with significant language problems (Holmes and Lenck-Santini 2006).

6.3 Executive Functions

Partial epilepsy of frontal lobe origin is associated with an increased risk of executive skills deficits (Upton and Thompson, 1996; Upton and Thompson, 1999; Risse, 2006) Research studies have reported impaired programming and co-ordination of motor sequences, impaired working memory and reduced attention and response inhibition. Executive function deficits are more evident in individuals with bilateral and more extensive pathology. For some, the cognitive burden is very handicapping. A characteristic of frontal lobe epilepsy is rapid seizure propagation, especially to the contralateral lobe and to mesial temporal regions. As a consequence, frontal lateralising and localising cognitive deficits may not be found and, when seizure activity spreads to temporal regions, patients may present with memory deficits more characteristic of temporal lobe epilepsy cases.

Juvenile Myoclonic Epilepsy is a generalised epilepsy syndrome. Neuropsychological studies are few but subgroups with this diagnosis do exhibit working memory and decision making deficits (Pascalicchio *et al.* 2007). Negative social behaviours attributed to dysexecutive syndromes have been described by some authors. Recent imaging studies have raised the possibility of abnormalities in frontal brain regions.

Executive skills deficits have also been described in patients with temporal lobe epilepsy. There are rich connections between frontal and temporal regions, and executive dysfunction in TLE may arise as a result of the propagation of epileptic activity to frontal regions. Executive skills impairments have been reported as more likely when seizures have secondary generalisation (Martin *et al.* 2000).

7 Neuropsychological impact of treatment

7.1 AEDs

There is no evidence that AEDs have any independent cognitive-enhancing properties. Improvements in cognition can occur as a consequence of better seizure control. For individuals with multiple daily absences effective drug treatment will result in improved attention and information processing. For those at risk of status epilepticus effective drug treatment may prevent damage in hippocampal structures and subsequent memory decline. Where seizures take the form of transient cognitive deficits, effective treatment will improve cognition by eliminating such episodes. Control of seizures does not always result in cognitive improvement. AEDs are developed to suppress the symptoms of epilepsy and not the underlying cause. Patients with epilepsy arising from structural brain pathology will tend to experience persisting cognitive problems despite good seizure control.

AEDs should always be considered a possible factor in patients referred with cognitive complaints. AEDs are given to suppress neuronal over-excitability in the brain and they are not selective in their action. Drugs will also affect normally behaving neurons. When a single drug controls seizures at small doses, adverse cognitive effects may be negligible. Where seizures are more difficult to control, the risk of adverse cognitive effects is higher. The aim of drug treatment is to achieve the best seizure control with minimal side effects. This balance can be difficult to achieve. Any drug can exert an effect when blood concentrations are too high. Cognitive disturbance usually presents with other symptoms of intoxication such as ataxia and diplopia. Cognitive blunting however may be the only sign.

Conflicting results predominate in the research literature. Randomized controlled trials tend to report minimal cognitive side effects. Such studies may miss adverse drug effects if the response is not uniform across patients. The pharmaceutical industry sponsors most research which can influence the reporting of results. Case studies and less rigorously designed studies tend to report more negative drug effects. These designs however have their own biases (Ortinski and Meador 2004).

The cognitive profile of individual drugs is far from clear and accordingly, generalisations are difficult. A drug can have an adverse effect in one patient but not another. Genetic factors may underlie side effect susceptibility. A drug effect may manifest as reduced efficiency on a range of tests. Mental slowness and impairments of working memory are more common indicators of a drug effect. However, some patients do experience an exacerbation of pre-existing cognitive problems.

Among the more established AEDs phenobarbitone has been most frequently associated with adverse cognitive effects. Phenytoin is a drug with peculiar pharmacokinetics. A minimal increase in dose can result in a dramatic increase in blood concentrations and in turn impaired concentration and information processing deficits. There have been reports of pseudodementia on this drug. Cases of sodium valproate induced dementia have also been documented often associated with raised ammonia levels (hyperammonaemia). Marked cognitive slowing can arise when phenobarbitone is co-prescribed. Carbamazepine has been associated with fewer cognitive side effects.

The evidence is limited for most of the more recently introduced AEDs with the exception of topiramate. Patients' complaints on this drug highlight effortful thinking and reduced verbal fluency, and this has been confirmed by research studies (Thompson *et al.* 2000). For some, the cognitive loss is marked with VIQ falls of more than ten points recorded, and accompanied by poor academic and work performance. Reports of cognitive decline in young people with epilepsy on TPM should be taken seriously and thoroughly investigated as examination failure can have major social and psychological ramifications.

The risk of cognitive impairment increases with polypharmacy. Unfortunately those with poorly controlled seizures will invariably be prescribed two or more different agents. The cognitive impact of AED combinations has received scant attention and no study has looked at the cognitive risks of co-medications such as antidepressants and antipsychotic agents.

The lack of clear research findings means that objective cognitive monitoring is all the more important. In all patients reporting cognitive decline or deficits, drug treatment should be considered a possible factor. Questions should be asked regarding the onset of cognitive difficulties and changes in drug type or dosage. To assess for drug effects requires assessment before and following changes. Several months should elapse between assessments.

7.2 Surgery

7.2.1 Temporal lobe resections

Neuropsychological assessment has a long established role in the pre-surgical evaluation of candidates for temporal lobe surgery. In the 1950s, the profound amnesia recorded following bilateral hippocampal ablation was instrumental in the discontinuation of this surgical approach. A few cases of post-operative amnesia were recorded following unilateral temporal lobe resections however retrospective analysis in all cases indicated pathological changes in the unresected temporal lobe (Baxendale *et al.* 2003). Impaired memory function in the hemisphere contra-lateral to the proposed surgery highlights the possibility of structural abnormalities and underscores the vital role of pre-operative memory assessment. A good surgical candidate will have a material specific memory deficit which is concordant with MRI identified pathology and with lateralised EEG disturbance (e.g. a verbal memory deficit in a person with left hippocampal sclerosis and ictal epileptic discharges from the left mesial temporal region). However, as described earlier, material specific memory deficits are more likely to be encountered post-operatively. In pre-operative cases, the presence and severity of material specific disorders will be influenced by the underlying pathology, the age of onset and other characteristics of the seizure disorder.

The development of post-operative memory deficits will depend upon the functional adequacy of the tissue removed and the cognitive reserve of the remaining structures. Some plasticity and the development of compensatory strategies post-operatively may also influence the nature and extent of post-operative neuropsychological deficits. Pre-operative neuropsychological scores in conjunction with MRI and other clinical data can be utilised to predict post-operative neuropsychological change. Patients at risk of significant memory decline are older (>40) with higher pre-operative memory scores, and have neuropsychological signs of impaired processing in the contralateral temporal lobe (Baxendale *et al.* 2006). Left temporal lobe resections are associated with memory decline that is more readily apparent to the patient and their family.

Left hemisphere resections are associated with an increased risk of language problems post-operatively. Such deficits are most prominent in the early post-operative period and tend to resolve over time. About one third of cases are left with a mild, persisting nominal dysphasia. A small subgroup of patients, in the order of 10%, do well cognitively view post-operatively and such individuals warrant earlier identification as such cognitive improvements are likely to have a lasting impact on academic, occupational and social functioning.

Intra-carotid Amytal Procedure (IAP) In recent years the reliability and validity of the IAP as a screen for amnesia have been questioned. A systematic review of the literature on post-operative amnesia revealed that all reported cases to date would have had MRI evidence of contra-lateral temporal lobe pathology, had the technology been available. Currently there is an active debate between surgical centres around the world concerning its use and a recent survey indicates several centres have stopped using the procedure or have reduced the number of procedures undertaken (Baxendale *et al.*, 2008). Other centres no longer use the test to screen for amnesic risk but now employ the measure to predict post-operative memory decline and to provide additional data regarding the laterality of the seizure focus. The added value of using the IAP for these reasons, above data derived from other sources remains unproven.

At the National Hospital for Neurology and Neurosurgery in London, the use of the IAP has decreased over time, and we have not undertaken an IAP for four years. Our follow up data in almost 300 cases provides no evidence that this decision has adversely affected surgical outcome, resulted in any unforeseen debilitating cognitive sequelae or has had an adverse impact on patient care. Noteworthy, several patients who had previously had surgery deferred due to a previous IAP 'failure', have since undergone surgery, become seizure free, and are leading fulfilling lives. Currently our assessment of amnesic risk is based primarily on MRI and baseline neuropsychological test findings. Our ongoing research studies are exploring the value of fMRI memory paradigms to predict post-operative memory outcome (Powell *et al.* 2007b).

Reducing the IAP has enabled patients to proceed to surgery more quickly; an important consequence, as this group has an increased risk for epilepsy related death. In addition, the physical and psychological risks accompanying this procedure are avoided and the financial savings are not insignificant (as a 2–3 day hospital admission, and the attendant professional time is no longer required). As important, it has freed up neuropsychology time for patient counselling, follow up and memory rehabilitation work.

7.2.2 Frontal lobe surgery

There are few post-operative cognitive outcome studies. Some cases show exacerbation of existing deficits. Cognitive outcome is poorest in those with continuing seizures who were cognitively intact pre-operatively. Resection involving the pre-motor and sensory motor area increases risk of impaired response inhibition. Marked language disturbance has been reported with dominant hemisphere operations (Helmstaedter *et al.* 1998).

7.2.3 Hemispherectomy

This procedure is most often performed in paediatric cases with evidence of significant hemi-atrophy. Children often have a hemiparesis and cognitive and adaptive abilities are often limited with further decline anticipated (e.g. Rasmussens encephalitis, Sturge-Weber Syndrome). In a recent study with follow up data on 71 children at least five years after surgery, seizure outcome was good with 50% rendered seizure free and half of these off medication (Pulsifer *et al.* 2004). Intelligence and other cognitive functions including language abilities were impaired but had generally not worsened as a consequence of the operation. This must be considered a positive outcome for the cases with Rasmussens Encephalitis as progressive cognitive decline is a feature of this syndrome. Cognitive outcome was poorer in children with hemimegalencephaly and other larger dysplasias particularly in those who continued to have frequent seizures.

7.2.4 Corpus callosotomy

The group undergoing this procedure tend to have severe life threatening seizures including drop attacks. Cognitive data on corpus callosotomy cases indicates a trend towards improved functioning with anterior resections. Outcome is generally less favourable for complete resections. Better cognitive outcome is reported with an early age of surgery. Transient deficits such as alien hand syndrome and mutism are rare and tend to occur earlier in the post-operative period and following total resections (Jenssen *et al.* 2006; Lassonde and Sauerwein 1997).

8 Psychological disorders associated with epilepsy

8.1 Mood disturbance

Mood disturbance can be a direct manifestation of a seizure or it may present as a pre-ictal or post-ictal phenomenon. Pre-ictal mood disturbance may last hours and sometimes days but will resolve following a seizure. Post-ictal mood disturbance often follows seizure clusters and can persist for days. Depression is most commonly encountered and may be severe and involve suicidal ideation. Improving seizure control will reduce ictally related mood disturbance. Helping patients recognise the seizure related cause can help manage these psychologically disturbing episodes.

AEDs can cause mood disturbance. Phenobarbitone, primidone, tiagabine and topiramate have been associated with depression. In such cases the onset of mood disturbance will coincide with the introduction of the drug.

Transient mood disturbance develops following temporal lobe resections in up to 1 in 4 cases, typically 2 to 3 months post-operatively and in a few patients may persist and require treatment.

Research studies have demonstrated high rates of inter-ictal depression in epilepsy. Anxiety has been less frequently studied although it is commonly encountered in clinical neuropsychological practice. Many factors exist which contribute to adverse mood change in epilepsy:

- unpredictability of ongoing seizures.
- intrusive and embarrassing aspects of seizures, such as bizarre behaviours and incontinence.
- risk of injury, particularly for those with drop attacks. Others may be placed in danger, such as small children if a parent has epilepsy.
- fear of death; 20–40 year olds have an eight-fold increased risk of death.
- need to adhere to a restrictive drug regime (especially with side effects such as weight gain, facial hair, acne and cognitive difficulties).
- experience of successive treatment failures in intractable epilepsy. Hopes are raised following the introduction of a new drug, only to be dashed when seizures recur.
- failure of surgical treatment which may occur in approximately a third of cases, particularly when this follows years of freedom from seizures.
- teasing and bullying at school
- employment and financial difficulties
- for potential parents, anxieties may be raised regarding the pregnancy, the birth and subsequent development of the child.
- epilepsy still carries a sizeable social stigma or prejudice and imbues varying degrees of fear and suspicion.

Professionals working in the field need to be aware of possible negative emotional reactions and the potential causes. Allowing time to talk about the experience of having epilepsy and to raise ongoing concerns can be beneficial. Mood rating scales are useful clinical screening tools.

8.2 Psychosis

Post-ictal psychosis is a well recognised phenomenon that generally occurs after seizure clusters but which may develop after several hours or days of recovery. Symptoms include delusions, hallucinations, thought disorder and mania that can last several weeks. Short-term use of benzodiazepines or antipsychotic medication may be helpful and may curtail the episode. Controlling seizures will lessen the occurrence. Psychosis can develop between seizures and become a chronic problem. The onset is usually after several years of seizures and it is more commonly encountered in early onset temporal lobe epilepsy. Psychosis is a rare complication of AED treatment (topiramate, ethosuximide) and temporal lobe surgery.

8.3 Aggression

Aggression is an infrequent complication of epilepsy. Ictal aggressive episodes are rare but will be stereotyped in nature and will occur in the absence of environmental precipitants and be undirected. Aggressive behaviour more commonly occurs in the post-ictal phase often as a result of attempts to restrain before a person has sufficiently recovered. Interictal aggression in epilepsy is more likely to arise in the presence of widespread underlying cerebral damage particularly involving the frontal lobes. Drug treatment may have a role. Irritability has been identified as a side effect of levetiracetam in adults and of phenobarbitone in children.

8.4 Non-epileptic attack disorder (NEAD)

NEAD is a term used to describe transient episodes of altered movement, sensation or experience resembling epilepsy but caused by a psychological process, and not associated with any abnormal activity in the brain (Reuber and Elger 2003). NEAD was previously known as pseudoseizures, a term discouraged due to pejorative connotations. NEAD is recognised as a heterogeneous grouping that may be a manifestation of an anxiety disorder or a dissociative disorder. In the latter group there may be a history of past emotional trauma including physical violence and/or sexual abuse and ongoing psychosocial stressors. Occasionally NEAD may reflect a more conscious process with some obvious secondary financial gain (malingering) or a pathological need (as in Munchausens Disorder). In tertiary referral centres NEAD is diagnosed in up to 25% of cases with a previous diagnosis of epilepsy, and in up to 50% of patients presenting with status epilepticus at A&E departments.

Differentiating between epileptic and non-epileptic seizures is difficult. No characteristics are exclusive to epilepsy and no features occur only in non-epileptic attacks. Incontinence and injury do not reliably distinguish epileptic from non-epileptic seizures. Features suggestive of NEAD include gradual onset, long duration (>5 mins), asynchronous limb flailing, directed actions especially aggression, reactivity to external stimulation and identifiable environmental/psychological triggers.

Treatment begins with a positive presentation of the diagnosis which should be extended to the immediate family. The diagnosis does not mean attacks are consciously put on, but may be the brain's way of dealing with past and/or ongoing stresses. The attacks will not respond to AED drugs and these can be withdrawn, which is likely to have cognitively beneficial effects. CBT is the treatment of choice advocated although the evidence base is limited (Goldstein *et al.* 2004).

Follow up studies of NEAD indicate that in about a third of cases seizures stop, following a change of diagnosis and minimal psychological input. For others, more long-term psychotherapy is beneficial. A favourable prognosis is associated with a shorter duration of seizures and acceptance of a psychological mechanism (Carton *et al.*, 2003).

9 Neuropsychological assessment

9.1 General

- Have a description of seizure(s): In partial epilepsy this may provide pointers to area of cerebral disturbance (e.g. if patient described to have post-ictal dysphasia, suggests language areas implicated and assessment may need to focus on this). Will enable prompt recognition of an attack occurring during the assessment.

- Measurement of mood is recommended; high rates of anxiety and depression will influence the interpretation of the test results.

- Test selection usually influenced by the referral question (although some centres have a standard battery of tests).

- Test selection may also be shaped by the results of investigations (e.g. EEG and MRI findings may indicate localised cerebral disturbance).

- Documentation of drugs taken including dosages.

9.2 Patient complains of memory impairment and/or decline

The most common referral for neuropsychological assessment in patients with epilepsy are:

- Memory tests should include measures of recall, learning, and recognition of both verbal and non-verbal material.

- Immediate and delayed retention: The time available and test standardisation does not permit retention at intervals greater than forty-five minutes, but a longer interval may be helpful for some individuals.

- Measures of general intellectual capacity: WAIS-R, WAIS-III provide an indication of ability level (which provide context for interpretation of memory test scores).

- Measures of other skills, especially language and executive function, as memory declines, may reflect problems in these areas rather than memory per se.

- Subjective rating of memory by patient and ideally an observer provide valuable information as to the nature of memory problems encountered in everyday situations.

- Where negative findings, may need a broader and/or more experimental approach (e.g. remote and autobiographical memory measures; delayed recall > one hour).

9.3 Assessing negative impact of drugs

- Unlikely a single assessment will provide the answer. Ideally, testing should be undertaken before and after a drug change. Recommend two to three months between assessments.

- Require tests available in parallel forms or minimally sensitive to practice effects.

- Include some speeded tests, as drugs seem to impact on speed of processing more than accuracy. Computerised tests enable accurate measure of speed.

- Useful tests include digit span, timed cancellation tasks, verbal fluency and verbal learning.

9.4 Evaluation of candidate for resective surgery

- Assess for cognitive disturbance concordant with known lesion and electrophysiological disturbance. With temporal cases, attention will be on memory skills; with frontal cases, attention to executive functioning.

- Assess for cognitive competency in other areas; a good surgical candidate will be the individual who functions well on other tests.

- Pre-operative counselling: High pre-operative functioning, older age at operation, and discordant neuropsychological deficits, place individuals at risk of cognitive decline post-operatively and this needs to be discussed with patient.

- Arrange post-operative re-assessments to monitor change and to provide rehabilitation if necessary.

10 Neuropsychological rehabilitation

Research evidence of effectiveness is limited, although clinical experience suggests memory training can be useful and have a significant impact on the management of the condition. Patients have to remember appointments, to take tablets, to document seizure frequency. An unreliable memory will result in the physician being presented with a less than accurate picture of seizure control. In a recent unpublished survey of people with epilepsy, 18% indicated that they forget their medication at least on a weekly basis.

People with epilepsy are a good target for memory training. Memory problems are usually less devastating than for other neurological cases and insight is generally retained. Many people with epilepsy live independently and are less likely to have a "carer" on hand to act as an external support for a weak memory.

- Feedback the test results. Individuals may be relieved by the confirmation that a memory difficulty exists and in many cases it is possible to reassure that it is not going to get progressively worse. This would be the case for an individual with well controlled seizures but with known left hippocampal sclerosis.

- If a young person is struggling to achieve academic standards comparable to siblings or parents expectations, confirmation of a memory deficit may result in a reappraisal and redirection to courses with less reliance on written examinations.

- Sessions can be offered to focus on memory support strategies; use techniques employed with other neurological groups. Clinical experience indicates that external memory aids are generally the most valuable (e.g. box organisers, wall planners). Computerised diaries and personal organisers are also useful.

- One of the most valuable external memory aids is the drug wallet. Many people find this device helps them to remember to take their tablets, and also not to take too many. Drug wallets usually consist of seven small containers, one for each day of the week. Compartments can be filled once a week at set times. The seven individual containers are removable. Drug wallets can be obtained from local chemists and are generally not very expensive (less than £10).

- Internal memory aids involving mental strategies may have a use, although generally for small amounts of information which is a, less easily committed to diary or other external memory aids.

Selective references

Baxendale S, Thompson PJ, and Duncan JS 2008, "The role of the Wada test in the surgical treatment of epilepsy:an international perspective", *Epilepsia*, vol. 49, no. 4, pp. 715–720.

Baxendale, S., Thompson, P., Duncan, J., and Richardson, M. 2003, "Is it time to replace the Wada test?", *Neurology*, vol. **60**, no. 2, pp. 354–355.

Baxendale, S., Thompson, P., Harkness, W., and Duncan, J. 2006, "Predicting memory decline following epilepsy surgery: a multivariate approach", *Epilepsia*, vol. **47**, no. 11, pp. 1887–1894.

Baxendale, S. A., Thompson, P. J., and Van, P. W. 1998, "A test of spatial memory and its clinical utility in the pre-surgical investigation of temporal lobe epilepsy patients", *Neuropsychologia*, vol. **36**, no. 7, pp. 591–602.

Baxendale, S. A., Van, P. W., Thompson, P. J., Connelly, A., Duncan, J. S., Harkness, W. F., and Shorvon, S. D. 1998, "The relationship between quantitative MRI and neuropsychological functioning in temporal lobe epilepsy", *Epilepsia*, vol. **39**, no. 2, pp. 158–166.

Blake, R. V., Wroe, S. J., Breen, E. K., and McCarthy, R. A. 2000, "Accelerated forgetting in patients with epilepsy: evidence for an impairment in memory consolidation", *Brain*, vol. **123** Pt 3, pp. 472–483.

Carton, S., Thompson, P. J., and Duncan, J. S. 2003, "Non-epileptic seizures: patients' understanding and reaction to the diagnosis and impact on outcome", *Seizure.*, vol. **12**, no. 5, pp. 287–294.

Duncan, J. S. 2007, "Epilepsy surgery", *Clin.Med.*, vol. **7**, no. 2, pp. 137–142.

Engel, J., Jr. 2001, "A proposed diagnostic scheme for people with epileptic seizures and with epilepsy: report of the ILAE Task Force on Classification and Terminology", *Epilepsia*, vol. **42**, no. 6, pp. 796–803.

Goldstein, L. H., Deale, A. C., Mitchell-O'Malley, S. J., Toone, B. K., and Mellers, J. D. 2004, "An evaluation of cognitive behavioral therapy as a treatment for dissociative seizures: a pilot study", *Cogn Behav.Neurol.*, vol. **17**, no. 1, pp. 41–49.

Goldstein, L. H., McAlpine, M., Deale, A., Toone, B. K., and Mellers, J. D. 2003, "Cognitive behaviour therapy with adults with intractable epilepsy and psychiatric co-morbidity: preliminary observations on changes in psychological state and seizure frequency", *Behav.Res.Ther.*, vol. **41**, no. 4, pp. 447–460.

Hanna NJ, Black M, Sander JE, Smithson WH, Appleton R, Brown S, and Fish DR 2002, *Epilepsy-Death in the Shadows* The Stationery Office, London.

Helmstaedter, C., Gleibner, U., Zentner, J., and Elger, C. E. 1998, "Neuropsychological consequences of epilepsy surgery in frontal lobe epilepsy", *Neuropsychologia*, vol. **36**, no. 4, pp. 333–341.

Holmes, G. L. and Lenck-Santini, P. P. 2006, "Role of interictal epileptiform abnormalities in cognitive impairment", *Epilepsy Behav.*, vol. **8**, no. 3, pp. 504–515.

Jenssen, S., Sperling, M. R., Tracy, J. I., Nei, M., Joyce, L., David, G., and O'Connor, M. 2006, "Corpus callosotomy in refractory idiopathic generalized epilepsy", *Seizure.*, vol. **15**, no. 8, pp. 621–629.

Lassonde, M. and Sauerwein, C. 1997, "Neuropsychological outcome of corpus callosotomy in children and adolescents", *J.Neurosurg.Sci.*, vol. **41**, no. 1, pp. 67–73.

Martin, R. C., Sawrie, S. M., Gilliam, F. G., Palmer, C. A., Faught, E., Morawetz, R. B., and Kuzniecky, R. I. 2000, "Wisconsin Card Sorting performance in patients with temporal lobe epilepsy: clinical and neuroanatomical correlates", *Epilepsia*, vol. 41, no. 12, pp. 1626–1632.

Ortinski, P. and Meador, K. J. 2004, "Cognitive side effects of antiepileptic drugs", *Epilepsy Behav.*, vol. 5 Suppl 1, p. S60–S65.

Pascalicchio, T. F., de Araujo Filho, G. M., da Silva Noffs, M. H., Lin, K., Caboclo, L. O., Vidal-Dourado, M., Ferreira Guilhoto, L. M., and Yacubian, E. M. 2007, "Neuropsychological profile of patients with juvenile myoclonic epilepsy: a controlled study of 50 patients", *Epilepsy Behav.*, vol. 10, no. 2, pp. 263–267.

Powell, H. W., Koepp, M. J., Richardson, M. P., Symms, M. R., Thompson, P. J., and Duncan, J. S. 2004, "The application of functional MRI of memory in temporal lobe epilepsy: a clinical review", *Epilepsia*, vol. 45, no. 7, pp. 855–863.

Powell, H. W., Parker, G. J., Alexander, D. C., Symms, M. R., Boulby, P. A., Wheeler-Kingshott, C. A., Barker, G. J., Koepp, M. J., and Duncan, J. S. 2007a, "Abnormalities of language networks in temporal lobe epilepsy", *Neuroimage.*, vol. 36, no. 1, pp. 209–221.

Powell, H. W., Richardson, M. P., Symms, M. R., Boulby, P. A., Thompson, P. J., Duncan, J. S., and Koepp, M. J. 2007b, "Preoperative fMRI predicts memory decline following anterior temporal lobe resection", *J.Neurol.Neurosurg.Psychiatry.*

Pulsifer, M. B., Brandt, J., Salorio, C. F., Vining, E. P., Carson, B. S., and Freeman, J. M. 2004, "The cognitive outcome of hemispherectomy in 71 children", *Epilepsia*, vol. 45, no. 3, pp. 243–254.

Reuber, M. and Elger, C. E. 2003, "Psychogenic nonepileptic seizures: review and update", *Epilepsy Behav.*, vol. 4, no. 3, pp. 205–216.

Sander, J. W. and Shorvon, S. D. 1996, "Epidemiology of the epilepsies", *J.Neurol.Neurosurg.Psychiatry*, vol. 61, no. 5, pp. 433–443.

Stokes T, Shaw EJ, Juarez A, Camosso-Stefinovic J, and Baker R 2004, "Clinical Guidelines and Evidence Review for the Epilepsies: Diagnosis and management in adults and children in primary and secondary care.," Royal College of General Practitioners, London.

Thompson PJ 1997, "Memory and Epilepsy," in *Clinical Pschologists Handbook of Epilepsy: Assessment and Management*, C.Cull and L.Goldstein, eds., Routledge, London, pp. 35–53.

Thompson, P. J., Baxendale, S. A., Duncan, J. S., and Sander, J. W. 2000, "Effects of topiramate on cognitive function", *J.Neurol.Neurosurg.Psychiatry*, vol. 69, no. 5, pp. 636–641.

Thompson, P. J. and Duncan, J. S. 2005, "Cognitive decline in severe intractable epilepsy", *Epilepsia*, vol. 46, no. 11, pp. 1780–1787.

Tomson, T., Walczak, T., Sillanpaa, M., and Sander, J. W. 2005, "Sudden unexpected death in epilepsy: a review of incidence and risk factors", *Epilepsia*, vol. 46 Suppl 11, pp. 54–61.

Upton, D. and Thompson, P. J. 1996, "General neuropsychological characteristics of frontal lobe epilepsy", *Epilepsy Res.*, vol. 23, no. 2, pp. 169–177.

Upton, D. and Thompson, P. J. 1999, "Twenty questions task and frontal lobe dysfunction", *Arch.Clin.Neuropsychol.*, vol. 14, no. 2, pp. 203–216.

Whitmarsh TE 2004, "Complementary and alternative treatments in epilepsy," in *The Treatment of Epilepsy*, second edn, Shorvon SD, ed., Blackwell Science Ltd, Oxford, pp. 269–276.

Part 7

Neuropsychiatric conditions

Chapter 32

Clinical presentation of neuropsychiatric disorders

Ronan O'Carroll

1 Introduction

Neuropsychology is the study of brain-behaviour relationships, and has traditionally utilised the classical lesion-based approach; relating focal brain damage to patterns of preserved and impaired cognitive functioning. In the majority of psychiatric disorders however, focal brain lesions are rare, and the challenge of the discipline of cognitive neuropsychiatry is to try to understand abnormal behaviour in terms of dysfunctional processing of information (Halligan and David, 2001; Frith, 2008). This is more likely to be related to cognitive processes reflecting abnormalities of brain systems than localised brain damage.

The determination of brain-cognition relationships represents a formidable undertaking in psychopathalogical states. Many neuropsychological studies in major psychiatric disorder are conducted on patients who are taking psychotropic medication, and such drugs may well have confounding effects on measures of cognitive functioning. Most psychiatric disorders disturb affective status, and mood and motivation critically impact on neuropsychological test performance. How does one distinguish between a 'core deficit' and a lack of motivation or effort due to the effects of depression? To take a specific example, imagine you were invited to participate in a neuropsychological research project on PTSD. You fulfilled DSM-IV criteria for PTSD and comorbid major depressive disorder. If your sleep had been disrupted for the previous month, if you were exhausted, felt worthless, a total failure, hopeless and useless and totally lacking in motivation, how well do you think you would perform on a two-hour neuropsychological test battery? Would the test results be a valid representation of your true abilities? One must also address the issue of diagnosis (i.e. how psychiatric disorders are traditionally classified).

The conventional approach is to adopt the medical model and describe 'illness' states that allegedly share common features. However, many critics have challenged the validity and reliability of standard psychiatric diagnoses, such as schizophrenia, arguing that they represent such heterogeneous groupings that effectively 'apples are being mixed with oranges', and classified as the same fruit (Bentall, 1992). In recent years greater attention has been placed on exploring specific syndromes or symptoms rather than 'illnesses'. For example, rather than trying to explain schizophrenia, attempts have been made to explain specific features (e.g. paranoid delusions) in neuropsychological terms (e.g. tendencies to jump to conclusions on limited evidence). Recent work suggests that many people with delusions accept the most salient current hypothesis. They do not reflect on past learning to consider whether the information fits with previous knowledge, with the result that the possibility that one might be mistaken is not considered (Garety *et al.* 2005). Studies are ongoing to test whether these information processing styles are amenable to change.

Clinical neuropsychology also has a crucial role to play in the assessment of cognitive impairment in clinical practice and in research in psychiatry. Recent advances in knowledge have allowed for more fine-grained cognitive analysis of specific impairments. This in turn can lead to a greater understanding of the neural basis of abnormal behaviour. The development of neuropsychological measures allows for the valid and reliable assessment of treatment efficacy. This is particularly important as 'negative features' (including cognitive impairment) have become increasingly recognised as key targets for pharmacological treatment in psychiatry (Kraus and Keefe, 2007; O'Halloran *et al.* 2007). Furthermore, ecologically valid neuropsychological outcome measures are essential in the rapidly developing field of cognitive rehabilitation.

In the following sections, the clinical presentation and common neuropsychological features of some of the major psychiatric disorders will be briefly reviewed.

2 Anorexia nervosa

2.1 Clinical presentation

The essential features of anorexia nervosa are: body weight 15% below the standard weight (i.e. a body mass index below 17.5) and an intense fear of gaining weight or becoming fat, even though the individual is clearly under weight. There is an associated perceptual disturbance in the way the person's body shape is seen (e.g. in the mirror), and in women, the presence of amenorrhea (i.e. the absence of at least three consecutive menstrual cycles). Patients generally eat very little and set themselves very restrictive daily calorie limits (e.g. 500 calories per day). Additional strategies to achieve weight loss include laxative abuse, vomiting and excessive exercise. Anorexia nervosa is approximately ten to twenty times more frequent in women than in men and occurs in approximately 1% of young women. Six to 10% of female siblings of patients with anorexia suffer from the condition, compared to 1–2% found in the general population of the same age. This increase may be due to family environment or to genetic influences.

2.2 Neuropsychological features

A variety of biological, psychological and environmental factors have been implicated in the aetiology of anorexia nervosa. Hypothalamic dysfunction has been proposed in anorexia as there is a profound disturbance of weight regulation. However, the endocrine and metabolic abnormalities may be a *consequence* of low weight and disturbed eating habits, rather than the cause. Brain imaging abnormalities have also been reported (e.g. enlarged ventricles and decreased hippocampal volume in anorexia nervosa). However, these brain changes are often reversed by weight gain, suggesting again that they may represent a consequence rather than a cause. Connan *et al.* (2006) recently reported that after adjustment for total cerebral volume, there was significant bilateral reduction in hippocampal volume in anorexic patients. However there was no evidence of impaired hippocampus-dependent cognitive function and no evidence of a relationship between hippocampal volume and clinical features of anorexia or with changes in cognitive function. They propose that it is important to integrate endocrine, neuropsychological and neuroimaging studies in order to understand the cause and consequence of hippocampal size and function in anorexia nervosa.

Several studies have documented neuropsychological impairments in anorexia, affecting a variety of cognitive domains (memory, attention, set shifting and problem solving).

Fowler *et al.* (2006) recently reported that patients with anorexia nervosa demonstrate subtle neuropsychological impairments, however in those patients with more severe degrees of impairment, these may have important adverse effects on more complex tasks of social and occupational functioning. The authors caution that further work is required to determine the nature of relevant causal mechanisms, including the effects of potential confounders. Cognitive improvements following weight gain suggest again that these impairments are reversible, not primary, and may be related to nutritional status. A recent systematic review and meta-analysis in eating disorders concluded that problems in set shifting as measured by a variety of neuropsychological tasks are common in people with eating disorders (Roberts *et al.* 2007).

3 Asperger's syndrome

3.1 Clinical presentation

Asperger's syndrome is a pervasive developmental disorder, first described by Asperger in 1944. The condition is characterised by marked impairment in social interaction (e.g. avoidance of eye-to-eye gaze and failure to develop relationships, restricted, repetitive and stereotyped patterns of behaviour, with clinically significant impairment in social functioning). Asperger's syndrome differs from autism because in the former there is no general delay or retardation of cognitive development or language. Non-verbal communication problems and clumsiness are common. Asperger's syndrome is well reviewed by Frith (1991).

3.2 Neuropsychological features

There is relatively little known about neuropsychological functioning in Asperger's syndrome, though theory of mind deficits are commonly observed (see section on Autism, below). It has been suggested that right hemisphere impairments may contribute to the behavioural abnormalities seen in Asperger's syndrome (e.g. face processing problems and poor gaze perception (Ellis and Leafhead, 1996)). Autism and Asperger's syndrome have been considered as part of the same spectrum of disorders. Miller and Ozonoff

(2000) proposed that Asperger's may simply reflect high-IQ autism, and that separate categories for the disorders may not be warranted. Thede and Coolidge (2007) recently conducted a comparison of Aspergers children versus high functioning autistic children. Both groups demonstrated marked executive deficits and evidence of Attention Deficit Hyperactivity Disorder compared to healthy controls. The authors concluded that there were more similarities than differences between the Asperger and high functioning autistic children, however the Asperger's children exhibited significantly greater anxiety.

4 Autism

4.1 Clinical Presentation

Autistic children show deficits in social interaction; in particular they fail to show the usual intimate relationship with people close to them, including parents and sibs. Many autistic individuals lack a social smile and do not display an anticipatory posture for being picked up (e.g. when a parent approaches), and abnormal eye contact is frequently observed. Disturbances of communication and language delay are also common. When autistic individuals do learn to converse, they often lack social competence and their conversations do not exhibit the normal reciprocal responsive interchanges. Autistic children often demonstrate abnormalities in play (e.g. engaging in rituals and frequently insisting on 'sameness' and being resistant to change). Autistic children may also be over-responsive or under-responsive to sensory stimuli. Hyperkinesis is also a common behaviour problem in young autistic children.

4.2 Neuropsychological features

Autism is often associated with developmental conditions that have associated neurological lesions (e.g. rubella and in untreated or uncontrolled phenyl ketonuria). EEG abnormalities are common, although no EEG findings are specific to autism. Approximately 40% of children with infantile autism have IQ scores below 50-55. Some autistic children however, demonstrate precocious talents (e.g. in cognitive and visuo-motor abilities). Examples include 'idiots savants', individuals who have exceptional memory, artistic, musical or calculating abilities. Some previous studies have reported working memory deficits in autism, but findings have been inconsistent. Steele *et al.* (2007) claimed that deficits in this domain are present only when working memory load exceeds some limited capacity.

A major current theory proposes that autistic children lack a 'theory of mind' (i.e. the ability to see the world from the perspective of another). This is commonly assessed using tests such as the 'Sally-Anne problem', where two dolls, Sally and Anne, act out a scene: Sally puts a marble in a basket before leaving the room and Anne then moves it to a box. The question is where will Sally look for it when she returns? Autistic children commonly respond 'In the box' (Frith, 1991). Happe and Frith (1996) proposed that it is useful to consider three main neuropsychological areas when attempting to understand autism; mentalizing impairment, executive dysfunction and weak central coherence (a characteristic of normal information-processing, the tendency to draw together diverse information to construct higher-level meaning in context). It is notable that in autism, weak central coherence can result in superior performance to healthy controls on tasks such as the embedded figures test, where one has to try and detect a target hidden in a complex background.

In a recent review, Tonn and Obrzut (2005) concluded that there is overwhelming evidence that individuals with autism have neuropsychological impairments across a number of domains. They conclude that while central coherence, executive function and theory of mind hypotheses are helpful in conceptualising the disorder, it is unlikely that any of them represent 'mutually exclusive' abnormalities. Baron-Cohen (2005) has recently proposed a provocative "extreme male brain" theory to explain autistic behaviour. An important assumption of the model is that all individuals fall on a continuum as regards male and female brain types. His model proposes that autism (and Asperger Syndrome) represents an extreme form of the male brain. Further work is needed to test this model. The interested reader is also referred to a recent special issue of the Quarterly Journal of Experimental Psychology, Vol. 61, January 2008, entitled "Neurocognitive approaches to developmental disorders: a Festschrift for Uta Frith.

5 Bulimia nervosa

5.1 Clinical presentation

Bulimia nervosa is characterised by recurrent episodes of binge eating associated with a lack of control over eating during the binge episode. The binge is usually followed by recurrent eliminatory behaviours aimed at preventing weight gain (e.g. vomiting and laxative abuse). The binge eating and eliminatory behaviours occur, on average, at least twice a week for three months. As in anorexia nervosa, bulimia is much more common in women than in men. Bingeing tends to precede vomiting by about one year in the development of the disorder. Sticking fingers down the throat commonly produces vomiting, though some bulimic patients can vomit at will. Vomiting acts to decrease the abdominal pain and feeling of being bloated. Depressed mood often follows the episode and has been called "post binge anguish".

5.2 Neuropsychological features

Attempts have been made in the past to associate cycles of bingeing and purging with various neurotransmitter abnormalities. Treatment with antidepressants, particularly selective serotonin re-uptake inhibitors have achieved some success, leading to the hypothesis that serotonin is implicated in the aetiology of the disorder. Marked impulsivity, problem-solving and decision making deficits are commonly observed in patients with bulimia (Ferraro et al. 1997). Brand et al. (2007) reported that, in bulimic patients, decision making abnormalities and executive reductions can be demonstrated and may represent neuropsychological correlates of the patent's dysfunctional everyday life decision making behaviour. They proposed that these neurocognitive functions must be taken into consideration in the treatment of bulimia nervosa. A recent systematic review and meta-analysis of neuropsychological studies in eating disorders is provided by Roberts *et al.* (2007), who identified set shifting as a common problem in eating disorders.

6 Capgras Syndrome

6.1 Clinical presentation

The Capgras syndrome involves the belief that impostors have replaced people who the sufferer is emotionally close to (e.g. loved ones or relative). It is believed that the impostors have assumed the roles of the persons they impersonate and behave like them. Some patients who suffer from Capgras syndrome may threaten, harm or even kill the supposed impostor.

6.2 Neuropsychological features

Up to 40% of cases are associated with organic disorders, e.g. head injury and dementia. Right cerebral hemisphere dysfunction has also frequently been reported in patients suffering from Capgras syndrome. Ellis and Young (1990) presented a cognitive account of Capgras syndrome. They proposed two distinct routes to facial recognition, one for the actual identification of the face, and the other to give it emotional significance. They proposed that prosopagnosia results from a disruption of the first route, whereas Capgras syndrome is "a mirror image" of prosopagnosia. Thus, Ellis and Young (1990) propose that Capgras patients have an intact primary route to face recognition but have a disconnection or damage within the route that gives the face its emotional significance. Ellis *et al.* (1997) demonstrated that people with the Capgras delusion fail to show autonomic discrimination between familiar and unfamiliar faces. Their model proposes that to the person with Capgras syndrome, the impostor's face looks identical but the emotional feelings associated with their face are abnormal. Put another way, they receive a veridical image of the person they are looking at, which stimulates the appropriate semantic data about the person, but the patient lacks another set of confirmatory information which may carry the appropriate affective tone for a loved one. The patient then adopts a rationalisation strategy (i.e. the person looks the same but somehow does not feel the same, and therefore the person must be an impostor). The Capgras patient mistakes a change in themselves, for a change in others (i.e. 'they must be impostors'). This area is well reviewed by Ellis and Lewis (2001).

Coltheart (2007) proposes a general two deficit cognitive-neuropsychiatric account of delusional belief that attempts to account for delusions such as Capgras, Fregoli, Cotard etc. He proposes that (a) the patient has a neuropsychological deficit of a kind that could plausibly be related to the content of a patient's delusion, that is a deficit that could plausibly be viewed as having prompted the initial thought that turned into a delusional belief and (b) the patient has right-hemisphere damage (i.e. damage to the putative belief evaluation system located in that hemisphere). He concludes that further studies should focus on the right hemisphere (particularly right frontal lobe) for the brain circuits underlying the fixation and mutation of human beliefs (Coltheart, 2007).

7 Conversion disorder (hysteria)

7.1 Clinical presentation

Hysteria was described by the ancient Greeks to account for a condition where physical and mental symptoms occurred in the absence of the organic pathology which was thought to cause the clinical features. Hysteria has been largely replaced by the terms conversion and dissociative disorders, which distinguish conditions with physical and mental symptoms respectively. Freud proposed that hysteria was caused by emotionally charged ideas that have become lodged in the unconscious of the patient. Classic examples include paralysis of the arm or 'glove anaesthesia' in the absence of organic pathology to account for the paralysis or anaesthesia. Diagnostic features include: (a) symptoms that suggest a neurological or medical condition, (b) psychological features are judged to be associated with the symptom, (c) the symptom is not intentionally produced or feigned, (d) the symptom or deficit cannot be fully explained by a medical condition, (e) the symptom or deficit causes clinically significant distress or impairment, and (f) the symptom is not limited to pain or sexual dysfunction.

Classically, these disorders are said to produce secondary gain (e.g. arm paralysis leading to the sufferer not having to go to work). In addition, patients are said to display 'la belle indifference' (i.e. that the patients show less distress than would be expected of someone with these symptoms). It is often difficult to distinguish between hysteria and malingering.

7.2 Neuropsychological features

It is important to note that diagnostic criteria for conversion disorder state that the symptom or deficit, after appropriate investigation, cannot be fully explained by a general medical condition. However, in a significant study Slater and Glithero (1965) followed up a series of patients who had been referred to a neurological hospital after having been diagnosed as having hysteria. Approximately one third of those patients developed a definite organic illness within 10 years of the original diagnosis and a further third developed depression or schizophrenia. This study has proved very influential, leading to the fear that the diagnosis of hysteria was a fertile source of clinical error, with significant neurological or psychiatric disease often being missed.

However, Crimlisk et al. (1998) followed up 64 patients who had medically unexplained motor symptoms for 6 years. Only three patients were subsequently diagnosed with a neurological disorder that could explain their initial presentation, leading to the conclusion that following up to date thorough evaluation, the chance of a missing a neurological condition that could account for the initial complaint is small.

It has also been proposed that conversion disorders have a neuropsychological basis in that it is possible that excess cortical arousal results in inhibition of afferent sensory motor impulses, thus diminishing the awareness of bodily sensations that in some conversion disorders could explain the observed sensory deficits (e.g. glove anaesthesia). Spence (1999) proposed an interesting avenue to pursue in the study of hysterical paralysis, using functional neuroimaging to test the extent that the pathophysiology of hysteria resembles either (a) the normal functional anatomy of willed action (exercising an intent to deceive) or (b) a failure of the will (through a demonstrable dysfunction of 'higher' centres).

Recent work in this area is reviewed by Vuilleumier (2005), who concludes that the data do not support previous proposals that hysteria might involve an exclusion of sensorimotor representations from awareness through attentional processes. Rather, the data seem to point to a modulation of such representations by primary affective or stress related factors. Vuilleumier (2005) proposes that this may involve primitive reflexive mechanisms of protection and alertness that are partly independent of conscious control, and mediated by dynamic modulatory interactions between limbic and sensorimotor networks. A useful overview of anatomical/neuropsychological mechanisms in hysteria is provided by Halligan *et al.* (2001).

8 Cotard syndrome

8.1 Clinical presentation

Cotard syndrome is essentially the delusion of nihilism. This condition was described by the 19th Century French psychiatrist, Jules Cotard who gave an account of several patients who suffered from a syndrome he referred to as 'délire de négation'. Patients exhibiting this syndrome may complain of having lost possessions, status and strength, and also internal organs such as the heart and lungs. Patients may not only claim that they are dead, but that corpses have replaced their bodies. They may state that they have no feelings, and it is important to note that many are severely depressed.

8.2 Neuropsychological features

Non-specific neurological lesions have been reported in many patients with Cotard's syndrome (e.g. neoplastic, vascular, and encephalopathic lesions). Young and Leafhead (1996) proposed a right hemisphere dysfunction, as evidenced by the observation of face processing impairments in patients with Cotard delusions. In this model, the delusion of being dead is viewed as a misinterpretation of abnormal perceptual experiences in which things seem strange and unfamiliar. There is a lack of emotional responsiveness, together with feelings of emptiness and derealisation. The depressed mood of the patient leads them to exaggerate the negative effects of the perceptual changes while correctly attributing the changes to themselves. In sum, this model proposes that the Cotard delusion represents a depressed person's attempt to account for abnormal perceptual experience.

Recent experimental support for this model is provided by McKay and Cipolotti (2007). Berrios and Luque (1995) have suggested that it is useful to distinguish between patients presenting with Cotard's syndrome in the presence or absence of clinical depression, arguing that the former may be best understood in terms of affective disorder, the latter in terms of delusional disorder. Kudlur *et al.* (2007), provide an overview of the neurological correlates of Cotard syndrome. In a review of over 100 papers on the Cotard syndrome, they report that the most commonly reported neurological abnormalities in these patients include structural brain changes (bilateral cerebral atrophy, dilated lateral ventricles), funcional brain changes (hypoperfusion in the frontal and parietal cortices) and neuropsychological abnormalities, (particularly impaired face recognition). They conclude that, from a clinical perspective, it is important to maintain a low threshold for suspicion for neurological cause in cases of Cotard's and to therefore consider appropriate neurological investigations. A recent review of Cotard's delusion is provided by Edelstyn and Oyebode (2006).

9 De Clerambault's syndrome

9.1 Clinical presentation

De Clerambault's syndrome is one of erotomania. It is currently classified in DSM-IV as a delusional disorder of the erotomanic type. It is exceedingly rare and more commonly a disorder of women. The subject, usually a single woman, believes that a 'higher status' person is in love with her. The target is usually inaccessible as he may be married, or be a famous personality or public figure. The sufferer is convinced that the object of her affection cannot be a happy or complete person without her. People suffering from this syndrome can become extremely difficult for the target of the affection to deal with, and in many cases, police and court involvement may be required in order to protect the target from the sufferer. A proportion of 'stalkers' who threaten celebrities suffer from delusional erotomania (Kamphuis and Emmelkamp, 2000). Many patients suffering from De Clerambault syndrome also suffer from paranoid schizophrenia (Litman, 2004), and it has been suggested that the syndrome may not exist as a separate nosological entity, but rather is a variant of schizophrenia or affective disorder (Ellis and Mellsop, 1985).

9.2 Neuropsychological features

Little is known about neurological or neuropsychological abnormalities in this condition, although the emergence of erotomania has been reported following brain injury. As stated above, the syndrome often presents in the context of schizophrenia, with associated impairments in memory and executive functioning. Kopelman et al. (1995) utilised the case-study approach, and tested the hypothesis that executive dysfunction may underlie delusional memories in erotomania. However, they found executive functioning to be intact, but reported an impairment in retrograde memory for the period around the onset of the patient's psychosis. Kopelman et al. (1995) propose that delusional memories may result from slippage in the relationship between memory schemata, leading to a predisposition to interpret the world in particular ways, contingent upon underlying affective or cognitive factors.

10 Depression

10.1 Clinical presentation

Depression has been recorded since ancient times. Episodes of major depression are characterised by a period of at last two weeks, which represents a change from previous functioning associated with either depressed mood or loss of interest or pleasure.

DSM-IV criteria for a major depressive episode requires five out of the following nine features:

1. Depressed mood most of the day, nearly every day.

2. Markedly diminished interest or pleasure in activities.

3. Significant weight loss or weight gain.

4. Insomnia or hypersomnia nearly every day.

5. Psychomotor agitation and retardation nearly every day.

6. Fatigue or loss of energy nearly every day.

7. Feelings of worthlessness or excessive or inappropriate guilt.

8. Diminished ability to think or concentrate or indecisiveness nearly every day.

9. Recurrent thoughts of death.

Importantly, in addition, the symptoms must not meet criteria for a Mixed Episode, they must cause clinically significant distress and/or impairment, are not attributable to a medical condition or drug effects and the symptoms are not better accounted for by bereavement.

Unipolar depression (i.e. depression with no episodes of mania) is among the most common of psychiatric disorders of adults. In many countries surveyed, at any given moment one person in twenty is significantly depressed, with a life-time prevalence rate of approximately 15%, (twice as prevalent in women as in men). There appears to be a genetic loading for depression in that children of severely depressed patients have a morbid risk of 20% for mood disorder as against about 7% in the relatives of controls. Major depression can be a fatal disorder, approximately two thirds of depressed patients contemplate suicide and 10–15% go on to commit suicide. An excellent overview of depression is provided by Hammen and Watkins (2007).

10.2 Neuropsychological features

Noradrenaline and serotonin abnormalities have been implicated in the pathophysiology of depression. In addition, abnormalities of the limbic hypothalamic pituitary adrenal axis have been the most consistent reported neuroendocrine abnormalities. The dexamethasone suppression test (DST) has been extensively researched in depression. Dexamethasone is a steroid that suppresses the blood level of cortisol and the DST is abnormal in approximately half the depressed patients. However, the DST has been shown not to be specific for depression and may be abnormal in patients with other disorders such as OCD, eating disorders etc. Brain imaging studies have used CT, MRI and PET to investigate possible brain abnormalities in major depression. The results of these studies have not been consistent. However, several have reported decreased blood flow and metabolism in the dorso-lateral prefrontal cortex, the cingulate cortex and in some cases, the basal ganglia. A recent consensus paper on biological markers in depression concluded that no biological markers for major depression are currently available for inclusion in the next set of diagnostic criteria, namely DSM-V and ICD-11 (Moner et al. 2007).

Neuropsychological studies have consistently found psychomotor slowing and impairments in memory and executive functioning (Veiel, 1997). Many studies using affectively-toned stimuli have shown that depressed patients have a memory bias towards negative material, which is thought to help maintain or exacerbate the depressed mood (e.g. Ridout *et al.* 2003).

In bipolar disorder (episodes of depression and mania), the evidence suggests that while neuropsychological functioning is clearly impaired during illness episodes, some residual impairments can be observed in the euthymic state (Ferrier *et al.* 1999). In a recent meta-analysis of neuropsychological functioning in euthymic bipolar disorder, medium to large performance effect size differences were consistently observed between patients and controls, particularly in the domains of attention/processing speed, episodic memory and executive functioning (Torres *et al.* 2007). There is therefore evidence of a trait related neuropsychological deficit in bipolar disorder.

A more severe course of illness and a greater number of illness episodes are often associated with more impaired neuropsychological functioning, suggesting that repeated manic episodes may be neurotoxic. The pathophysiological mechanisms are not fully understood, though hypercortisolaemia may be implicated and may result in impaired neuropsychological functioning (McAllister-Williams *et al.* 1998). Relatively few neuropsychological studies have been conducted on manic patients. Preliminary work suggests that both manic and depressed patients are impaired on tests of memory and planning, but differences have been noted in attentional shifting, with manic patients having difficulty with inhibition of behavioural response and attentional focus, with depressed patients impaired in their ability to shift the focus of their attentional bias (Murphy *et al.* 1999). The same authors confirmed the affective bias for negative material in depression, but also demonstrated the opposite affective bias for positive stimuli in mania.

Taylor Tavares *et al.* (2007) reported a comparison of unmedicated, depressed patients with major depressive disorder and bipolar depression. Both groups were depressed at the time of assessment. The major depression group were impaired on tests of spatial working memory and attentional shifting and were over-sensitive to loss trials on a decision making task, and these deficits were not attributable to current medication status. In contrast, the bipolar depressed group were generally cognitively intact and did not differ significantly from control subjects on the test. Steele *et al.* (2007) also found a blunted response to feedback information in depression. Stoddart *et al.* (2007) recently claim to have described a dissociation between unipolar and bipolar affective illness. They reported that bipolar individuals demonstrate a specific executive deficit that is independent of attention impairment on the Hayling Sentence Completion Test (HSCT).

11 Dissociative Fugue (formally Psychogenic Fugue)

11.1 Clinical Presentation

Fugue state is one of the dissociative disorders. DSM-IV diagnostic criteria include:

1. The predominant disturbance is sudden, unexpected travel away from home or one's customary place of work, with an inability to recall one's past.

2. Confusion about personal identity or assumption of a new identity (partial or complete).

3. The disturbance does not occur exclusively during the course of dissociative identity disorder and is not due to the direct physiological affects of a substance (e.g. drug of abuse) or a general medical condition (e.g. temporal lobe epilepsy).

4. The symptoms cause:

— clinically significant distress

— impairment in social, occupational or other important areas of functioning.

Dissociative Fugue can be mistaken for Malingering, because both conditions occur under circumstances that a person might understandably wish to evade. Critically however, Dissociative Fugue occurs spontaneously and is not faked whereas in Malingering the person feigns illness because it removes them from accountability for their actions. The focus of treatment is helping the person restore lost memories as soon as possible.

11.2 **Neuropsychological Features**

Fugue state seems to appear more often in Hollywood movies than in the scientific literature, however there are a number of notable case-studies where neuropsychological examination has attempted to explain the mechanisms underlying fugue state. Kapur (1991) reported the case of an individual who had memory loss for five days during which he wandered extensively. However, he did not have selective amnesia for the public events which had occurred during the five days for which he claimed memory loss. Kapur (1991) argued that this finding was incompatible with the case having a neurologically based global memory disorder during the fugue state and that this data supports a distinction between personal and public episodic memory. In a later paper, Kapur (1996) argued that most cases of functional retrograde amnesia may represent a combination of conscious simulation and unconscious processes.

Kopelman *et al.* (1994) reported the case-study of a patient who experienced a seven day fugue episode. The patient was assessed soon after admission to hospital and at regular intervals thereafter. Intervention with a sodium amytal abreaction produced substantial recovery of memory. Kopelman *et al.* (1994) proposed a hierarchical model of awareness in memory suggesting that patients with psychogenic amnesia manifest different levels of awareness for differing memories.

Glisky *et al.* (2004), described a case study of psychogenic fugue where the individual lost access, not only to his autobiographical memories, but also to his native German language. A series of laboratory tasks were conducted and led to the conclusion that the individual suffered an episode of psychogenic fugue during which he lost explicit knowledge of his personal past and his native language. However, at the same time, he appeared to retain implicit knowledge of autobiographical facts and semantic or associative structure of the German language. Stracciari *et al.* (2005) proposed that, in Fugue state, the episodes appear as examples of 'functional' memory inhibition, possibly triggered by different conditions, including psychological trauma. The memory profile in fugue state may therefore be explained by a lost access to abstract autobiographical knowledge.

A useful recent review of the dissociative disorders including fugue states is provided Kihlstrom (2005), who concludes that while these disorders have been attributed to trauma and other psychological stress, the existing evidence favouring this hypothesis is plagued by poor methodology. Prospective studies of traumatized individuals reveal no convincing cases of genuine amnesia that could not be attributed to brain insult, injury, or disease.

12 Factitious Disorder

12.1 Clinical Presentation

Factitious disorder is a condition where the person acts as if he or she has an illness by deliberately feigning or exaggerating symptoms. The DSM-IV essential diagnostic criteria are:

1. Intentional production or feigning of physical or psychological signs or symptoms.
2. The motivation for the behaviour is to assume the sick role.
3. External incentives for the behaviour (such as economic gain, avoiding legal responsibility or improved physical wellbeing (as in malingering) are absent.

Factitious disorder differs from malingering in that the motivation for the symptom production in malingering is an external incentive, whereas in factitious disorder, external incentives are absent. Evidence of an internal need to maintain the sick role suggests Factitious disorder. Motivation for the behaviour in factitious disorder must be to assume the 'sick role' and the individual does not 'act sick' for personal gain, as in the case of malingering. When the individual applies the pretended sickness to a dependent (e.g. a child) this is referred to as 'Factitious disorder by proxy'. Munchausen syndrome is a Factitious disorder (see separate entry for Munchausen syndrome).

12.2 Neuropsychological Features

As with Munchausen syndrome, Factitious disorders are poorly understood with no consistent neuropsychological features or widely accepted explanatory neuropsychological models.

13 Frégoli delusion

13.1 Clinical presentation

The essence of the Frégoli delusion is that the patient believes that other people are able to disguise themselves to look like anyone they wish in order to achieve some influence - usually, a sinister one. The patient will identify a familiar person (usually someone who is believed to be his or her persecutor), and insist that this person takes the form of a variety of others he or she comes into contact with. The patient will maintain that although there is no physical resemblance between the familiar person and the others, nevertheless they are the same person. The syndrome is often associated with schizophrenia.

13.2 **Neuropsychological features**

Neurological abnormalities are common in Frégoli delusion (e.g. brain atrophy is often reported (Joseph and O'Leary 1987)). However, transient forms of the delusion have also been described (e.g. following toxic psychoses induced by cannabis). Ellis and Young (1990) offered a cognitive neuropsychiatric explanation for the Frégoli delusion. They employed an information processing model of face recognition which deconstructs into three essential stages: (a) an initial structural encoding (b) the excitation of units sensitive to the unique characteristic of each known phase and (c) the link to other multi-modal nodes that access biographical/episodic information about people.

Ellis and Young (1990) proposed that it is a malfunction in stage (c) that results in the Frégoli delusion. This area is well reviewed by Ellis (2004).

14 **Ganser's syndrome**

14.1 **Clinical presentation**

This syndrome was first reported by Ganser in 1898, in which three prisoners showed an unusual clinical picture. The condition has four main features: (a) giving approximate answers; (b) psychogenic physical symptoms; (c) hallucinations; and (d) apparent clouding of consciousness.

The term 'approximate answers' indicates that although the answer is plainly wrong, it is clearly related to the correct answer in a way which suggests that the correct response is known (e.g. when asked to multiply four times four, the patient answers 'seventeen'). A distinction has been made between the Ganser symptom (approximate answers) and the Ganser syndrome, with the symptom common and the syndrome extremely rare. Ganser's syndrome has variously been regarded as akin to hysterical conversion reactions, malingering, organic confusion and psychotic thought disorder. Ganser's syndrome is often thought to represent the voluntary production of psychiatric symptoms (e.g. in an attempt to avoid imprisonment, and in fact, has been termed 'prison psychosis'). It may be difficult to distinguish whether the condition is genuine or whether the patient is malingering. However, it should be noted that a number of cases have been reported following head injury, indeed of Ganser's original three cases, two had suffered head injury and the third was recovering from typhus fever (Lishman 1998). The syndrome may also occur in people with other disorders such as schizophrenia and depression.

14.2 **Neuropsychological features**

Ganser's syndrome is a poorly understood phenomenon. Originally, Ganser proposed that the condition represented an unusual hysterical confusional state.

Merckelbach *et al.* (2006) described a case study of detecting malingering in an individual who presented with Ganser-like symptoms. The middle aged man had been involved in a car crash and was seeking disability insurance benefits. Malingering tests revealed that he performed below chance on simple memory tests. The authors then collected collateral information which showed the patient was involved in high level sports activities that were difficult to reconcile with the severe cognitive impairment that he claimed to suffer from. The authors conclude that their case highlights that Ganser like symptoms deserve close scrutiny, preferably with tests of malingering.

There are no clear and consistent neuropsychological features that provide an adequate explanation for this disorder. As Lishman (1998) concluded, exactly one hundred years after the syndrome was first described, "Uncertainty surrounds its nosological status and the mechanisms behind its appearance" (p.480).

15 Kluver-Bucy Syndrome

15.1 Clinical Presentation

Kluver-Bucy syndrome is a behavioural disorder that occurs following damage to right and left medial temporal lobes of the brain. The amygdala has been particularly implicated in the pathogenesis of this syndrome. This syndrome is a rare neurological disorder that causes individuals to engage in a number of inappropriate behaviours (e.g. putting objects in their mouth and engaging in inappropriate sexual behaviour). Other symptoms can include visual agnosia, loss or normal fear and anger responses, memory loss, distractibility, seizures and dementia. The syndrome is named after Kluver and Bucy, who removed the temporal lobe bi-laterally in a Rhesus monkey in an attempt to determine its function. The operated monkey developed marked problems including emotional changes, altered sexual behaviour, visual agnosia and oral tendencies. It became notably less fearful of things that would have previously caused marked anxiety (e.g. humans or snakes).

15.2 Neuropsychological Features

There is a relatively limited neuropsychological literature on the Kluver-Bucy syndrome. In a historical review of the Kluver-Bucy syndrome, Nahm (1997) proposed that Kluver's work helped to unify both neuropsychological and neuroanotomical theories regarding the visual and emotive functions of the non-human primate temporal lobe. Approximately 20% of individuals presenting with neuropsychiatric features, characteristic of frontal temporal dementia, went on to develop the Kluver-Bucy syndrome on two year follow-up (Mendez and Perryman 2002). Pestana and Gupta (2007) recently described an interesting case of an 11 year old boy with epilepsy who has fluctuating Kluver-Bucy symptoms. He had three or four daily complex partial seizures over two to three days per month followed by a seizure free interval of approximately three to four weeks. During the seizure free period, he exhibited marked hyper orality, sniffing, irritability, unsolicited sexual gestures etc. The Kluver-Bucy features escalated up to the onset of the seizure cluster and then remitted after the seizures. The authors claim this is the first reported case of Kluver-Bucy syndrome due to congenital bi-temporal malformations.

16 Malingering

16.1 Clinical Presentation

According to DSM-IV, the essential feature of Malingering is the intentional production of false or grossly exaggerated physical or psychological symptoms, motivated by external incentives such as avoiding military duty, avoiding work, obtaining financial compensation, evading criminal prosecution or obtaining drugs. Malingering should be strongly suspected in the following situations:

1. Medical legal context of presentation.
2. Marked discrepancy between the person's claimed stress or disability and objective findings.
3. Lack of co-operation during diagnostic evaluation and in complying with prescribed treatment.
4. The presence of anti-social personality disorder.

As stated previously, Malingering differs from Factitious disorder in that the motivation for the symptom production in Malingering is an *external incentive*. Malingering differs also from Conversion disorder, and other somatoform disorders, by the intentional production of symptoms and the obvious external incentives associated with it.

16.2 Neuropsychological Features

There is a vast literature on attempts to detect Malingering using neuropsychological measures and a detailed review of this area is clearly beyond the scope of this brief section. Many authorities now propose that it is good practice to include both a measure of mood and a measure of malingering in all medico-legal neuropsychological assessments (e.g. The National Academy of Neuropsychology Policy and Planning Committee recently proposed that "the assessment of response validity as a component of medically necessary evaluation is medically necessary" (Bush *et al.* 2005)).

Currently, the Test of Memory Malingering (TOMM) appears to be the most frequently used symptom validity test and appears to be relatively robust. The TOMM is a very simple forced choice visual recognition memory test where even patients with significant cognitive impairment perform well. A low score therefore is suspicious. Both clinical participants and community dwelling adults have been shown to achieve exceptionally high scores.

TOMM scores do not appear to be significantly influenced by self reported symptoms of depression and anxiety (Rees *et al.* 2001; O'Bryant *et al.* 2007). Similarly, Iverson *et al.* (2007) reported that TOMM scores were not affected by chronic pain or depression. A very useful overview of Malingering in relation to illness deception is provided by Halligan *et al.* (2003).

17 **Munchhausen's syndrome**

17.1 **Clinical presentation**

Munchhausen's syndrome is a factitious disorder (i.e. a condition characterised by physical or psychological symptoms that are intentionally produced or feigned). Physical or mental illness is simulated with the objective of assuming the 'sick role' of a patient. Essential features include intentional production of symptoms, the motivation for the behaviour to assume a sick role and external incentives for the behaviour such as financial gain. Munchhausen patients are often admitted to hospital with an apparently serious and acute illness that is often supported by a plausible or dramatic history. However, the history is not true and the patient is often found to have attended hospital and deceived doctors on many previous occasions. Discharge often occurs after hospital staff confront the patient with evidence regarding similar fraudulent presentations. The condition is most often seen in young men. Patients are often resistant to contact with psychologists or psychiatrists and treatment is often refused. Munchhausen syndrome by proxy describes a condition where parents give a false history to explain their child's signs and symptoms (e.g. history suggestive of appendicitis, when in reality, the parent has been poisoning the child). This is clearly child abuse.

17.2 **Neuropsychological features**

Munchhausen is a poorly understood phenomenon, with no consistent neuropsychological features or widely accepted explanatory neuropsychological models.

18 **Obsessive Compulsive Disorder (OCD)**

18.2 **Clinical presentation**

Obsessive/Compulsive Disorder (OCD) is characterised by the presence of obsessions or compulsions. Obsessions are persistent and recurrent thoughts and impulses that cause anxiety and distress that the person tries to suppress, neutralise or ignore and that the person recognises as being the product of his or her own mind. Compulsions are repetitive behaviours or mental acts that the person feels driven to perform, and the behaviour or mental acts are aimed at preventing or reducing distress, or preventing a dreaded event or situation. Common examples include obsessional cleaning and checking. However, the compulsive behaviours or acts are not connected in a realistic way with what they are designed to neutralise or prevent (e.g. removing all hairs from clothing and carpets in the house in order to prevent a loved one dying in a road traffic accident). The obsessions or compulsions are recognised by the individual as being unreasonable and frequently cause marked distress. While OCD is classified as an anxiety disorder, obsessional patients are often depressed.

18.2 Neuropsychological features

Brain imaging findings have suggested that abnormalities in the orbito-frontal cortex and caudate nucleus may be common in OCD (Insel and Winslow, 1992). Cognitive abnormalities often include executive, non-verbal and praxic deficits in OCD, consistent with theories of fronto-striatal functioning which may represent the cognitive substrate of doubt-related phenomena such as checking (Tallis *et al.* 1999).

OCD is a heterogeneous condition. Lawrence *et al.* (2006) showed that OCD patients with prominent hoarding symptoms showed impaired decision making as well as reduced skin conductance responses. Symmetry/ordering symptoms were negatively associated with set shifting. Lawrence *et al.* (2006) claim that this result helps explain previously inconsistent neuropsychological research on OCD and that dissociable neural mechanisms are involved in mediating the different OCD symptom dimensions. On a related theme, Mataix-Cols *et al.* (2004) reported distinct fMRI correlates of washing, checking, and hoarding symptom dimensions in obsessive-compulsive disorder. They concluded that that different obsessive-compulsive symptom dimensions are mediated by relatively distinct components of fronto-striato-thalamic circuits implicated in cognitive and emotion processing. OCD may therefore better be conceptualized as a spectrum of multiple, potentially overlapping syndromes rather than a unitary diagnostic category.

Menzies *et al.* (2007) studied neurocognitive endophenotypes of OCD. They assessed OCD patients, unaffected first degree relatives and matched controls. Interestingly both patients *and relatives* had delayed response inhibition on a stop-signal task compared to healthy controls. They then used magnetic resonance imaging and identified that behavioural impairment on the stop-signal task was significantly associated with the reduced grey matter in orbitofrontal and right inferior frontal regions, and increased grey matter in cingulate, parietal and striatal regions. A structural variation in large scale brain systems related to motor inhibitory control may thus mediate the genetic risk for OCD.

In a recent selective review of memory and executive functioning in obsessive compulsive disorder, Olley *et al.* (2007) concluded that the neuropsychological profile of OCD appeared to be primarily one of executive dysfunction. While memory function is often compromised, they argue that these memory deficits are secondary to a primary executive failure of organisational strategies during encoding. They also note that, given the prominence of chronic doubt and indecision in clinical settings, it is surprising that decision making as related to OCD has not received greater attention in the neuropsychological literature.

19 Othello syndrome

19.1 Clinical presentation

The Othello syndrome is one of delusional jealousy where the person is convinced (without due cause) that his or her spouse or partner is unfaithful. Pathological jealousy is not an uncommon presentation in psychiatric practice, and is more common in men than in women and in some cases, the individual may be highly dangerous. The syndrome often is associated, or may be part of other conditions such as paranoid schizophrenia, depression or alcoholism.

19.2 Neuropsychological features

Organic disorders (e.g. head injury) have been suggested as being present in up to 20% of such cases, often involving right hemisphere damage. In addition, drug abuse (e.g. amphetamine and cocaine) can often precipitate delusional jealousy, as can a wide range of brain disorders, including metabolic and endocrine disorders, degenerative conditions e.g., dementia, infections and neoplasms.

Malloy and Richardson (1994), in a review of the frontal lobes and content specific delusions, concluded that a high proportion of such delusions have a neurological basis and the lesions of the frontal lobes and right hemisphere are often critical to the development and persistence of many content specific delusions. We await convincing and testable neuropsychological models of delusional jealousy.

20 Post-traumatic Stress Disorder (PTSD)

20.1 Clinical presentation

PTSD is a condition where exposure to an intense frightening emotional experience leads to lasting changes in behaviour, affect and cognition. Typically after a life threatening incident (e.g. a violent assault, rape or wartime experience), the individual displays re-experiencing of the event(s) (e.g. via intrusive, distressing thoughts, images, 'flashbacks' or nightmares). The individual may exhibit phobic avoidance and/or physiological reactivity to reminders of the trauma. Increased arousal in terms of sleep disturbance, irritability, and exaggerated startle response are common. In addition, the individual may exhibit a restricted range of affect, sense of a foreshortened future, and may lose interest in previously rewarding hobbies or activities.

20.2 Neuropsychological features

As stated above, PTSD is characterised by intrusive distressing memories of the traumatic event. Paradoxically, it is also often associated with marked impairments in learning and memory for new material. Patients often complain that they remember what they do not want to, yet cannot remember what they now wish to. Heightened arousal at the time of encoding may result in modulation (strengthening) of the memory trace, possibly via noradrenaline release in the amygdala (Cahill 2000). Subsequent anterograde memory impairment may be due to the deleterious effects of stress hormones (e.g. long term hypercortisolaemia) on hippocampal function. Several MRI studies have now shown that PTSD is associated with reduction in volume of the hippocampus, a brain area critically involved in new learning and memory (Bremner 1999). However, this finding was not replicated in Nazi holocaust survivors who had PTSD (Golier *et al.* 2005).

Brewin *et al.* (1996) developed a dual representation theory of PTSD. They propose that two memory systems are implicated in the disorder, one that is verbally accessible and one that is automatically accessed via situational cues. They also propose that clinical features may correspond to chronic or premature inhibition of emotional processing of trauma. Recent neuropsychological studies have suggested that some of the differences in cognitive performance observed between PTSD patients and controls may reflect pre-existing individual differences (Crowell *et al.* 2002). The neuropsychology of PTSD has been well reviewed recently in a book edited by Vasterling and Brewin (2005).

21 Reduplicative paramnesia

21.1 Clinical presentation

Reduplicative paramnesia is a clinical condition where a patient states that there are two or more places with almost identical attributes, although only one exists in reality. Luzzatti and Verga (1996) describe the clinical presentation of several patients presenting with reduplicative paramnesia. For example, a man who had suffered a head injury, stated that he was in Grimsby, when in fact he was in hospital outside Edinburgh and accounted for this state of affairs by saying "I call it Grimsby, you call it Scotland".

21.2 Neuropsychological features

The majority of cases described in the literature suffer from a bilateral frontal lesion associated with lesions in other brain areas. The condition has been proposed as being an orientation problem, a memory problem, a perceptual problem or a mixture of all three. Luzzatti and Verga (1996) proposed that the disorder might be considered as an adaptive rather than a reduplicative phenomenon. In particular, they suggest a difficulty in integrating the actual perceived reality with one's own internal belief. They propose that this is an exaggeration of normal experience, for example waking up in a strange room where the internal belief is compared to the information acquired sensorially from the external world and thus the internal belief adapts to the perceived reality. This integration may be reduced or lost in patients with reduplicative paramnesia and the incapacity to shift from a believed to the perceived reality might be considered a set-shifting or perseverative behaviour. Moser *et al.* (1998) proposed that reduplicative paramnesia is secondary to temporal-limbic-frontal dysfunction giving rise to a distorted sense of familiarity and impaired ability to resolve the delusion via logical reasoning. A recent case report of an elderly patient with Alzheimer's disease who had reduplicative paramnesia confirmed the presence of high neurofibrillary tangle densities in frontal and temporal association cortex (von Gunten *et al.* 2005).

23 Schizophrenia

23.1 Clinical presentation

Schizophrenia has been described as perhaps the most devastating illness known to man, because it appears in early adolescence and can drastically impair the subsequent life of the sufferer and his or her family. A variety of diagnostic systems have been used over the past 100 years, leading to much confusion. Currently, the DSM-IV system requires two or more of the following symptoms: delusions, hallucinations, disorganised speech, disorganised or catatonic behaviour or negative symptoms. These must be accompanied by social/occupational dysfunction, continuous signs of disturbance which persists for at least six months and also that other disorders have been excluded. The life-time risk of developing schizophrenia is about 1%, a figure which varies very little around the world. There appears to be a strong genetic component to schizophrenia. For example, if there is a 1% prevalence of schizophrenia in the general population, the probability of developing schizophrenia in a monozygotic twin of a schizophrenic patient is 47% versus 12% in a dizygotic twin of a schizophrenic patient. Many of the syndromes reviewed in this chapter (De Clerambault, Capgras, Othello etc.) are considered by many to fall within the broad spectrum of schizophrenia.

23.2 Neuropsychological features

A key finding in schizophrenia research was the report by Eve Johnstone and colleagues in 1976 that confirmed ventricular enlargement in CT scans in patients with schizophrenia versus controls (Johnstone *et al.* 1976). In the 1960s, there was a wide spread view that schizophrenia was a socially created disorder and family dynamics, and in particular the 'schizophrenogenic mother' was often blamed. The finding of CT abnormalities shifted the balance back to viewing schizophrenia as a brain/neuropsychological disorder. However, while several studies have found ventricular enlargement in schizophrenia, only about 30% of patients have an increase of one standard deviation greater than the healthy control mean. Furthermore, MRI studies have also confirmed reductions in temporal lobe volume (Nelson *et al.* 1998). Functional brain imaging studies using PET and fMRI have tended to report decreases in frontal lobe blood flow (hypofrontality). This is most readily demonstrated during cognitive challenge tasks where patients have to perform a task, such as the Wisconsin Card Sort Test, and patients typically fail to show the same level of frontal lobe metabolic activity as healthy controls. However, it should be borne in mind that the patients often have difficulty performing the cognitive task, so the finding may tell us more about neural substrate of the cognitive task performance rather than schizophrenia.

Gur *et al.* (2007) recently reviewed brain imaging studies in schizophrenia. They concluded that replicated findings include reduced whole brain and hippocampal volume as potential vulnerability markers with further progression at onset and that these are not attributable to medication effects.

The dopamine hypothesis has been central in attempting to explain schizophrenia, mainly supported by the fact that virtually all effective antipsychotic drugs are dopamine receptor antagonists, particularly D2 receptors. There are at least two problems with the dopamine hypothesis. First, dopamine antagonists are effective in treating virtually all psychotic and agitated patients *regardless of diagnosis* (i.e. response is not unique to schizophrenia and secondly, there is evidence that dopaminergic neurones may, in fact, *increase* their firing rate in response to chronic exposure to antipsychotic drugs, rather than reduce them). Second, many patients who have been resistant to treatment with dopamine antagonists have responded to the atypical antipsychotics such as clozapine and resperidone which target other neurotransmitter systems.

There is a huge neuropsychological literature on schizophrenia. However, as stated in the introduction, this may not have been a particularly fruitful research endeavour given that it may be more profitable from a neuropsychological perspective to try and explain particular signs or symptoms (e.g. auditory hallucinations, passivity or paranoid delusions). Neuropsychological abnormalities are, however, consistently reported in patients diagnosed with schizophrenia. Cognitive deficits are now being increasingly recognised as core features of schizophrenia. These deficits are not secondary to medication or symptoms and have a huge negative impact on everyday functioning (Kraus and Keefe, 2007). The most consistent findings are of impairments in learning, memory and executive functioning (Heinrichs and Zakzanis, 1998). Importantly, these abnormalities can be observed in patients who are drug-free.

The natural history of cognitive impairment in schizophrenia has been much debated. Low intelligence and poor educational achievement precede early onset schizophrenic psychosis (Jones *et al.* 1994). These findings support the view of schizophrenia as a *neurodevelopmental disorder*. Well designed longitudinal studies have produced some conflicting results with some supporting the notion of progressive decline and other refuting it. Morrison *et al.* (2006) published a long term follow-up study where patients with schizophrenia were assessed 33 years after baseline assessment on admission to hospital. At follow-up there was a significant decline in non-verbal intelligence over time (Raven's Progressive Matrices) in patients with schizophrenia but this was not observed in matched controls. No decline was observed in verbal intelligence. Thus there appears to be convincing evidence that some patients with a diagnosis of schizophrenia have detectable cognitive impairments which precede illness onset, and following development of the disorder, continued cognitive decline occurs in some patients.

Attempts to explain schizophrenia *per se* in neuropsychological terms have had limited success, possibly because of the heterogeneity of the disorder. However, certain features (e.g. specific delusions have been explained via recent testable neuropsychological models; see entries for Capgras, Cotard and Frégoli). Frith (1992) has been particularly influential in this area, by developing a model where internal stimuli (e.g. thoughts or intentions) are thought to be misclassified and misattributed to an external source. For example, Frith (1992) proposed that auditory hallucinations in schizophrenia arise from a failure in the self-monitoring of speech processing. In this model, hallucinations are experienced as a result of a failure of the internal registration of the intention to generate inner speech (i.e. the hallucinating person's inner speech is perceived as alien, attributable to an external source). Frith has extended his model to account for a variety of features of schizophrenia including thought broadcasting, insertion and withdrawal. Frith's model has been subjected to several empirical tests with generally supportive results (e.g. Mlakar *et al.* 1994; Stirling *et al.* 1998; Torres *et al.* 2004). A pivotal feature of Frith's theory is that some key features of schizophrenia are due to an inability to monitor the beliefs and intentions of others.

This is similar to the theory of mind deficit in autism, with one key difference: "The autistic person has never known that other people have minds. The schizophrenic knows that other people have minds, but has lost the ability to infer the contents of these minds: their beliefs and intentions. They may even lose the ability to reflect on the contents of their own mind. However, they will still have available ritual and behavioural routines for interacting with people, which do not require inferences about mental states." (Frith, 1992, p.121). Pickup and Frith (2001) reported that TOM impairments in schizophrenia are less severe than in autism, but are specific and not a reflection of general cognitive deficits.

In recent years there has been increasing research on relatives of affected individuals aimed at determining if similar cognitive deficits and brain abnormalities are also found in those with increased genetic vulnerability to schizophrenia. Young adult relatives who are at high genetic risk of developing schizophrenia exhibit memory and executive impairments (Byrne *et al.* 1999) together with reductions in hippocampal/amygdala complex volume (Lawrie *et al.* 1999). In general, findings suggest that deficits are apparent in unaffected relatives and are similar to those observed in schizophrenia (eg memory and executive impairments) but are less marked (Whalley *et al.* 2007).

In a recent review, Reichenberg and Harvey (2007) concluded that the most severe impairments in schizophrenia are apparent in episodic memory and executive control processes, over a background of generalised cognitive deficit. They go on to propose that these neuropsychological impairments may represent genetic liability to the disorder, as similar, milder impairments are evident in schizophrenia patients even before the onset of psychotic symptoms as well as in the non-psychotic relative is schizophrenia patients. The cognitive neuroimaging literature during executive function, episodic memory and working memory tasks in schizophrenia generally report abnormalities in frontal and medial temporal lobe systems (Reichenberg and Harvey, 2007).

24 Somatoform disorders

24.1 Clinical presentation

Somatoform disorders share the common feature of the presence of a physical symptom that suggests an underlying general medical condition, but the symptom is not fully explained by a general medical condition, and the symptoms cause clinically significant distress or impairment. Unlike factitious disorders and malingering, the physical symptoms are **not** thought to be intentional. Gelder (1996) pointed out that there are several problems with the whole concept of somatoform disorder; (a) the lack of clear operational definitions for the overall category and unsatisfactory description of sub-categories, (b) some of the disorders such as hypochondriasis are so enduring that they could be classified as personality disorders rather than mental disorders, and (c) many patients have clinical features which fit the criteria for more than one diagnostic category. Somatoform disorders include somatisation disorder (historically referred to as hysteria or Briquette's syndrome), undifferentiated somatoform disorder, conversion disorder, pain disorder, hypochondriasis, body dysmorphic disorder or somatoform disorder not otherwise specified. It is important to note that patients with chronic somatoform disorder can become grossly disabled, e.g. wheelchair bound (Bass *et al.* 2001).

24.2 Neuropsychological features

Some recent studies have investigated processing of emotional material in somatoform disorder. Lim and Kim (2005) utilised the emotional Stroop paradigm and demonstrated that somatoform patients showed supraliminal interference for physical threat words and showed bias for physical threat words on an explicit memory task. This profile differentiates them from patients with major depression, panic disorder and healthy participants.

There is little consistent evidence regarding neuropsychological abnormalities in the somatoform disorders and, in fact, as indicated above, this may reflect the lack of clear operational definitions for the overall category and the unsatisfactory descriptions of some of the sub-categories (see section on conversion disorder). Recent debates have focused on whether functional somatic syndromes should be defined as separate entities or as one overall syndrome (Moss-Morris and Spence 2006).

25 Tourette syndrome

25.1 Clinical presentation

Tourette syndrome involves multiple motor and one or more vocal tics e.g. shouting profanities, and was first described by Gilles de la Tourette in 1885. The tics can occur many times a day and the disturbance causes marked distress or significant impairment in social and/or occupational functioning. The onset is before age 18 and the condition is not due to drugs or a general medical condition such as Huntingdon's disease. The prevalence of Tourette syndrome is approximately 1 per 2000 and the condition has a high genetic loading with a concordance rate of approximately 50% in monozygotic twins versus 8% in dizygotic twins. Obsessive, compulsive symptoms occur frequently in patients with Tourette's syndrome.

25.2 Neuropsychological features

Visuo-motor difficulties are common in Tourette's disorder and abnormal, non-specific EEG findings are also common (Robertson 1989). CT brain scan studies suggest that approximately 10% of those with Tourette's have non-specific abnormality, with the cingulate gyrus and basal ganglia often suggested as possible candidate sites for the disorder. The central dopaminergic system is thought to malfunction in Tourette's as dopaminergic stimulants exacerbate the disorder and dopamine blockers such as chlorpromazine often improve the condition.

Attentional dysfunction may be central to the disorder as attention difficulties and poor frustration tolerance often pre-date the tics. Indeed, approximately 25% of people with Tourette's have been prescribed stimulants for a diagnosis of attention deficit hyperactivity disorder (ADHD) *before* receiving a diagnosis of Tourette's disorder. Recent work has suggested the presence of executive dysfunction, particularly problems with inhibitory control in patients with the Tourette syndrome (Margolis *et al.* 2006). However, Channon *et al.* (2006) reported that uncomplicated TS is associated with only mild, circumscribed cognitive impairment.

Research has also shown that individuals with Tourettes can suppress their ticks for brief periods of time, and suppression is enhanced when programmed reinforcement is provided for tick free intervals and short periods of suppression do not result in a paradoxical rebound in tick frequency when active suppression has ceased. The ability to suppress tics appears to be correlated with omission but not commission errors on the Continuous Performance Task (Woods *et al.* 2008). Recent neuroimaging research has shown robust activation of cerebellum, insula, thalamus and putamen during tick release. The involvement of cerebellum and insula suggests their involvement in tick initiation and execution (Lerner *et al.* 2007).

26 **Conclusion**

The neuropsychological study of psychiatric disorders is still in its infancy, but the infant appears to be thriving. As Frith stated in a commentary on a paper on a neuropsychological model of schizophrenia: "A few years ago articles of this sort would have been unthinkable. For most psychologists, schizophrenia either did not exist or was a social disorder of no interest to hard-headed experimental psychologists. Today, schizophrenia is unquestionably a disorder of the brain (however caused) and, as such, it provides one of the most exciting challenges for linking brain and cognition" (Frith 1991).

Exciting novel attempts to explain abnormal behaviour in terms of dysfunctional information processing are rapidly being developed. However, it is critical that such models are explicitly amenable to experimental testing and refutation. Only then will significant advances be made in our scientific understanding of abnormal experience. We must be wary of replacing neurotransmitter or structural lesion based explanations of psychopathology with seductive, glossy PET or fMRI illustrations, or simplistic 'black-box' cognitive models. Demonstrating that a particular patient or patient group has abnormal regional brain metabolism, or a specific cognitive deficit is of interest, but it does not provide a causal explanation of abnormal behaviour or experience.

Bentall *et al.* (2007) have recently commented that while there is an increasing recognition of a neuro-developmental approach to psychiatric disorder, this has generally failed to take into account recent advances in the understanding of the psychology of unusual experiences such as hallucinations and delusions. They propose that developmental psychology offers important clues about cognitive and socio-cognitive abnormalities that might be involved in hallucinations and delusions and that an integration of these findings with existing knowledge on the neuro-development of psychosis could offer profitable new avenues of research for investigators working at both biological and psychological levels of explanation.

Furthermore, Garety *et al.* (2007) propose a series of implications for neurobiological research of cognitive models of psychosis. They argue that the evidence increasingly supports hypotheses proposed by cognitive models (i.e. that psychosis is on a continuum;

specific cognitive processes are risk factors for the transition from sub-clinical experiences to clinical disorder, social adversity and trauma are associated with psychosis and with negative emotional processes, and these emotional processes contribute to the occurrence and persistence of psychotic symptoms). They also argue that reasoning biases contribute to the occurrence of delusions. They argue convincingly that the benefits for incorporating cognitive processes into neurobiological research include more sophisticated, bi-directional and interactive causal models. They conclude that cognitive models and their derived phenotypes constitute the missing link in the chain between genetic or acquired biological vulnerability, the social environment and the expression of individual positive symptoms.

I ended the previous edition of this chapter with the following conclusion, which I believe still largely holds true. While significant progress has been made, in most instances we still await truly convincing neuropsychological explanations of many psychopathological states.

Selective references

Baron-Cohen, S. (2005). "Testing the extreme male brain (EMB) theory of autism: let the data speak for themselves." *Cognit Neuropsychiatry* **10**(1): 77–81.

Bass, C., R. Peveler, *et al.* (2001). "Somatoform disorders: severe psychiatric illnesses neglected by psychiatrists." *Br J Psychiatry* **179**: 11–4.

Bentall, R. P. (1992). *The classification of schizophrenia. Schizophrenia: An overview and practical handbook.* D. J. Kavanagh. London, Chapman Hall: 23–44.

Bentall, R. P., C. Fernyhough, *et al.* (2007). "Prospects for a cognitive-developmental account of psychotic experiences." *Br J Clin Psychol* **46**(Pt 2): 155–73.

Berrios, G. E. and R. Luque (1995). "Cotards delusion or syndrome? A conceptual history." *Comprehensive Psychiatry* **36**: 218–223.

Brand, M., C. Franke-Sievert, *et al.* (2007). "Neuropsychological correlates of decision making in patients with bulimia nervosa." *Neuropsychology* **21**(6): 742–50.

Bremner, J. D. (1999). "Alterations in brain structure and function associated with post- traumatic stress disorder." *Seminars in Clinical Neuropsychiatry* **4**(4): 249–55.

Brewin, C. R., T. Dalgleish, *et al.* (1996). "A dual representation theory of posttraumatic stress disorder." *Psychological Review* **103**(4): 670–86.

Bush, S. S., R. M. Ruff, *et al.* (2005). "Symptom validity assessment: practice issues and medical necessity NAN policy & planning committee." *Arch Clin Neuropsychol* **20**(4): 419–26.

Byrne, M., A. Hodges, *et al.* (1999). "Neuropsychological assessment of young people at high genetic risk for developing schizophrenia compared to controls: Preliminary findings of the Edinburgh High Risk Study (EHRS)." *Psychological Medicine* **29**: 1161–1173.

Cahill, L. (2000). Emotional modulation of long-term memory storage in humans: Adrenergic activation and the amygdala. *The Amygdala: A Functional Analysis.* J. Aggleton, Oxford University Press: 425–444.

Channon, S., A. Gunning, *et al.* (2006). "Tourette's syndrome (TS): cognitive performance in adults with uncomplicated TS." *Neuropsychology* **20**(1): 58–65.

Coltheart, M. (2007). "The 33rd Sir Frederick Bartlett Lecture - Cognitive neuropsychiatry and delusional belief." *Quarterly Journal of Experimental Psychology* **60**(8): 1041–1062.

Connan, F., F. Murphy, *et al.* (2006). "Hippocampal volume and cognitive function in anorexia nervosa." *Psychiatry Res* **146**(2): 117–25.

Crimlisk, H. L., K. Bhatia, *et al.* (1998). "Slater revisited: 6 year follow up study of patients with medically unexplained motor symptoms." *British Medical Journal* **316**: 582–586.

Crowell, T. A., K. M. Kieffer, *et al.* (2002). "Neuropsychological findings in combat-related posttraumatic stress disorders." *Clinical Neuropsychologist* **16**(3): 310–321.

Edelstyn, N. M. J. and F. Oyebode (2006). "A review of the phenomenology and cognitive neuropsychological origins of the cotard delusion." *Neurology Psychiatry and Brain Research* **13**(1): 9–14.

Ellis, H. D. (2004). "Cognitive neuropsychology and delusional misidentification of persons." *Annales Medico-Psychologiques* **162**(1): 50–54.

Ellis, H. D. and K. M. Leafhead (1996). Raymond: a study of an adult with Asperger syndrome. *Method in Madness - Case Studies in Cognitive Neuropsychiatry*. P. W. Halligan and J. C. Marshall, Hove Psychology Press.

Ellis, H. D. and M. B. Lewis (2001). "Capgras delusion: a window on face recognition." *Trends in Cognitive Sciences* **5**: 149–156.

Ellis, H. D. and A. W. Young (1990). "Accounting for delusional misidentifications." *British Journal of Psychiatry* **157**: 239–248.

Ellis, H. D., A. W. Young, *et al.* (1997). "Reduced autonomic responses to faces and Capgras delusion." *Proceedings of the Royal Society: Biological Sciences* **B264**: 1085–1082.

Ellis, P. and G. Mellsop (1985). "De Clerambault's syndrome–a nosological entity?" *Br J Psychiatry* **146**: 90–3.

Ferraro, F. R., S. Wonderlich, *et al.* (1997). "Performance variability as a new theoretical mechanism regarding eating disorders and cognitive processing." *Journal of Clinical Psychology* **53**: 117–121.

Ferrier, I. N., B. R. Stanton, *et al.* (1999). "Neuropsychological function in euthymic patients with bipolar disorder." *British Journal of Psychiatry* **175**: 246–251.

Fowler, L., A. Blackwell, *et al.* (2006). "Profile of neurocognitive impairments associated with female in-patients with anorexia nervosa." *Psychol Med* **36**(4): 517–27.

Frith, C. D. (1991). "In what context is latent inhibition relevant to the symptoms of schizophrenia?" *Behavioural and Brain Sciences* **14**: 28–29.

Frith, C. D. (1992). *The Cognitive Neuropsychology of Schizophrenia*. Hove, Lawrence Erlbaum Associates.

Frith, C. D. (2008). "In praise of cognitive neuropsychiatry." *Cognitive Neuropsychiatry* **13**: 1–7.

Frith, U. (1991). *Autism and Asberger's syndrome*. Cambridge, Cambridge University Press.

Garety, P. A., P. Bebbington, *et al.* (2007). "Implications for neurobiological research of cognitive models of psychosis: a theoretical paper." *Psychol Med* **37**(10): 1377–91.

Garety, P. A., D. Freeman, *et al.* (2005). "Reasoning, emotions, and delusional conviction in psychosis." *Journal of Abnormal Psychology* **114**(3): 373–384.

Gelder, M. *et al.* (1996). *Oxford Textbook of Psychiatry*. Oxford, Oxford University Press.

Glisky, E. L., L. Ryan, *et al.* (2004). "A case of psychogenic fugue: I understand, aber ich verstehe nichts." *Neuropsychologia* **42**(8): 1132–47.

Golier, J. A., R. Yehuda, *et al.* (2005). "Absence of hippocampal volume differences in survivors of the Nazi Holocaust with and without posttraumatic stress disorder." *Psychiatry Res* **139**(1): 53–64.

Gur, R. E., M. S. Keshavan, *et al.* (2007). "Deconstructing psychosis with human brain imaging." *Schizophr Bull* **33**(4): 921–31.

Halligan, P., C. Bass, *et al.* (2001). *Contemporary Approaches to the Study of Hysteria*. Oxford, Oxford University Press.

Halligan, P. H., C. Bass, *et al.* (2003). *Malingering and Illness Deception*. Oxford, Oxford University Press.

Halligan, P. W. and A. S. David (2001). "Cognitive neuropsychiatry: towards a scientific psychopathology." *Nature Neuroscience* **2**: 290–215.

Hammen, C. and E. Watkins (2007). *Depression*. Hove, East Sussex, Psychology Press Ltd.

Happe, F. and U. Frith (1996). "The neuropsychology of autism." *Brain* **119**: 1377–1400.

Heinrichs, R. W. and K. K. Zakzanis (1998). "Neurocognitive deficit in schizophrenia: A quantitative review of the evidence." *Neuropsychology* **12**: 426–445.

Insel, T. R. and J. T. Winslow (1992). "Neurobiology of obsessive compulsive disorder." *Psychiatric Clinics of North America* **15**: 813–824.

Iverson, G. L., J. Le Page, *et al.* (2007). "Test of Memory Malingering (TOMM) scores are not affected by chronic pain or depression in patients with fibromyalgia." *Clin Neuropsychol* **21**(3): 532–46.

Johnstone, E. C., T. J. Crow, *et al.* (1976). "Cerebral ventricular size and cognitive impairment in chronic schizophrenia." *Lancet* **2**(7992): 924–6.

Jones, P., B. Rodgers, *et al.* (1994). "Child development risk factors for adult schizophrenia in the British 1946 birth cohort." *Lancet* **344**: 1398–1402.

Joseph, A. B. and D. H. O'Leary (1987). "Anterior cortical atrophy in Fregoli's syndrome." *Journal of Clinical Psychiatry* **48**: 409–411.

Kamphuis, J. H. and P. M. Emmelkamp (2000). "Stalking–a contemporary challenge for forensic and clinical psychiatry." *Br J Psychiatry* **176**: 206–9.

Kapur, N. (1991). "Amnesia in relation to fugue states–distinguishing a neurological from a psychogenic basis." *Br J Psychiatry* **159**: 872–7.

Kapur, N. (1996). "A study of recovery of memory function in a case of witnessed functional retrograde amnesia." *Cognit Neuropsychiatry* **1**(3): 247–58.

Kihlstrom, J. F. (2005). "Dissociative disorders." *Annu Rev Clin Psychol* **1**: 227–53.

Kopelman, M., E. M. Guinan, *et al.* (1995). "Delusional memory, confabulation, and frontal lobe dysfunction: A case in De Clerambault's syndrome." *Neurocase* **1**: 71–77.

Kopelman, M. D., H. Christensen, *et al.* (1994). "The great escape: a neuropsychological study of psychogenic amnesia." *Neuropsychologia* **32**(6): 675–91.

Kraus, M. S. and R. S. Keefe (2007). "Cognition as an outcome measure in schizophrenia." *Br J Psychiatry Suppl* **50**: s46–51.

Kudlur, S. N. C., S. George, *et al.* (2007). "An overview of the neurological correlates of Cotard syndrome." *European Journal of Psychiatry* **21**(2): 99–116.

Lawrence, N. S., S. Wooderson, *et al.* (2006). "Decision making and set shifting impairments are associated with distinct symptom dimensions in obsessive-compulsive disorder." *Neuropsychology* **20**(4): 409–19.

Lawrie, S. M., H. Whalley, *et al.* (1999). "Magnetic resonance imaging of brain in people at high risk of developing schizophrenia." *Lancet* **353**: 30–33.

Lerner, A., A. Bagic, *et al.* (2007). "Neuroimaging of neuronal circuits involved in tic generation in patients with Tourette syndrome." *Neurology* **68**(23): 1979–87.

Lim, S. L. and J. H. Kim (2005). "Cognitive processing of emotional information in depression, panic, and somatoform disorder." *J Abnorm Psychol* **114**(1): 50–61.

Lishman, W. A. (1998). Organic Psychiatry. *The psychological consequences of cerebral disorder* (3rd Edition). Oxford, Blackwell Scientific Publications.

Litman, L. (2004). "A case of de Clerambault syndrome in a male stalker with paranoid schizophrenia." *Can J Psychiatry* **49**(7): 498.

Luzzatti, C. and R. Verga (1996). Reduplicative paramnesia for places with preserved memory. *Method in Madness - Case Studies in Cognitive Neuropsychiatry*. P. W. Halligan and J. C. Marshall, Hove Psychology Press.

Malloy, P. F. and E. D. Richardson (1994). "The frontal lobes and content-specific delusions." *J Neuropsychiatry Clin Neurosci* **6**(4): 455–66.

Margolis, A., M. Donkervoort, *et al.* (2006). "Interhemispheric connectivity and executive functioning in adults with Tourette syndrome." *Neuropsychology* **20**(1): 66–76.

Mataix-Cols, D., S. Wooderson, *et al.* (2004). "Distinct neural correlates of washing, checking, and hoarding symptom dimensions in obsessive-compulsive disorder." *Arch Gen Psychiatry* **61**(6): 564–76.

McAllister-Williams, R. H., I. N. Ferrier, *et al.* (1998). "Mood and neuropsychological function in depression: the role of corticosteroids and serotonin." *Psychological Medicine* **28**: 573–584.

McKay, R. and L. Cipolotti (2007). "Attributional style in a case of Cotard delusion." *Conscious Cogn* **16**(2): 349–59.

Mendez, M. F. and K. M. Perryman (2002). "Neuropsychiatric features of frontotemporal dementia: evaluation of consensus criteria and review." *J Neuropsychiatry Clin Neurosci* **14**(4): 424–9.

Menzies, L., S. Achard, *et al.* (2007). "Neurocognitive endophenotypes of obsessive-compulsive disorder." *Brain* **130**(Pt 12): 3223–36.

Merckelbach, H., M. Peters, *et al.* (2006). "Detecting malingering of Ganser-like symptoms with tests: a case study." *Psychiatry Clin Neurosci* **60**(5): 636–8.

Miller, J. N. and S. Ozonoff (2000). "The external validity of Asberger's disorder: lack of evidence from the domain of neuropsychology." *Journal of Abnormal Psychology* **109**: 227–238.

Mlakar, J., J. Jensterle, *et al.* (1994). "Central monitoring deficiency and schizophrenic symptoms." *Psychological Medicine* **24**: 557–564.

Moner, R., O. Mikova, *et al.* (2007). "Consensus paper of the WFSBP task force on biological markers: Biological markers in depression." *World Journal of Biological Psychiatry* **8**(3): 141–174.

Morrison, G., R. O'Carroll, *et al.* (2006). "Long-term course of cognitive impairment in schizophrenia." *Br J Psychiatry* **189**: 556–7.

Moser, D. J., R. A. Cohen, *et al.* (1998). "Reduplicative paramnesia: longitudinal neurobehavioural and neuroimaging analysis." *Journal of Geriatric Psychiatry and Neurology* **11**: 174–180.

Moss-Morris, R. and M. Spence (2006). "To "lump" or to "split" the functional somatic syndromes: can infectious and emotional risk factors differentiate between the onset of chronic fatigue syndrome and irritable bowel syndrome?" *Psychosom Med* **68**(3): 463–9.

Murphy, F. C., B. J. Sahakian, *et al.* (1999). "Emotional bias and inhibitory control processes in mania and depression." *Psychological Medicine* **29**: 1307–1321.

Nahm, F. K. (1997). "Heinrich Kluver and the temporal lobe syndrome." *J Hist Neurosci* **6**(2): 193–208.

Nelson, M. D., A. J. Saykin, *et al.* (1998). "Hippocampal volume reduction in schizophrenia as assessed by magnetic resonance imaging - A meta-analytic study." *Archives of General Psychiatry* **55**(5): 433–440.

O'Bryant, S. E., L. R. Engel, *et al.* (2007). "Test of memory malingering (TOMM) trial 1 as a screening measure for insufficient effort." *Clin Neuropsychol* **21**(3): 511–21.

O'Halloran, J. P., A. S. Kemp, *et al.* (2007). "*Psychometric comparison of computerized and standard administration of the neurocognitive assessment instruments selected by the CATIE and MATRICS consortia among patients with schizophrenia.*" Schizophr Res.

Olley, A., G. Malhi, *et al.* (2007). "Memory and executive functioning in obsessive-compulsive disorder: a selective review." *J Affect Disord* **104**(1-3): 15–23.

Pestana, E. M. and A. Gupta (2007). "Fluctuating Kluver-Bucy syndrome in a child with epilepsy due to bilateral anterior temporal congenital malformations." *Epilepsy Behav* **10**(2): 340–3.

Pickup, G. J. and C. D. Frith (2001). "Theory of mind impairments in schizophrenia: symptomatology, severity and specificity." *Psychol Med* **31**(2): 207–20.

Rees, L. M., T. N. Tombaugh, *et al.* (2001). "Depression and the Test of Memory Malingering." *Arch Clin Neuropsychol* **16**(5): 501–6.

Reichenberg, A. and P. D. Harvey (2007). "Neuropsychological impairments in schizophrenia: Integration of performance-based and brain imaging findings." *Psychol Bull* **133**(5): 833–58.

Ridout, N., Astell, A.J., Reid, L.C., Glen, T., and O'Carroll, R.E. (2003). Memory bias for emotional facial expressions in major depression. *Cognition & Emotion* **17**, 101–122.

Roberts, M. E., K. Tchanturia, *et al.* (2007). "A systematic review and meta-analysis of set-shifting ability in eating disorders." *Psychol Med* **37**(8): 1075–84.

Robertson, M. M. (1989). "The Gilles de la Tourette Syndrome: The current status." *British Journal of Psychiatry* **154**: 147–169.

Slater, E. T. and E. Glithero (1965). "A follow-up of patients diagnosed as suffering from "hysteria"." *Journal of Psychosomatic Research* **9**: 9–13.

Spence, S. A. (1999). "Hysterical paralyses as disorders of action." *Cognitive Neuropsychiatry* **4**(3): 203–226.

Steele, J. D., P. Kumar, *et al.* (2007). "Blunted response to feedback information in depressive illness." *Brain* **130**(Pt 9): 2367–74.

Steele, S. D., N. J. Minshew, *et al.* (2007). "Spatial working memory deficits in autism." *J Autism Dev Disord* **37**(4): 605–12.

Stirling, J. D., J. S. Hellewell, *et al.* (1998). "Self-monitoring dysfunction and the schizophrenic symptoms of alien control." *Psychol Med* **28**(3): 675–83.

Stoddart, S. D. R., N. J. Craddock, *et al.* (2007). "Differentiation of executive and attention impairments in affective illness." *Psychological Medicine* **37**(11): 1613–1623.

Stracciari, A., K. Mattarozzi, *et al.* (2005). "Functional focal retrograde amnesia: lost access to abstract autobiographical knowledge?" *Memory* **13**(7): 690–9.

Tallis, F., P. Pratt, *et al.* (1999). "Obsessive compulsive disorder, checking, and non-verbal memory: a neuropsychological investigation." *Behav Res Ther* **37**(2): 161–6.

Taylor Tavares, J. V., L. Clark, *et al.* (2007). "Distinct profiles of neurocognitive function in unmedicated unipolar depression and bipolar II depression." *Biol Psychiatry* **62**(8): 917–24.

Thede, L. L. and F. L. Coolidge (2007). "Psychological and neurobehavioral comparisons of children with Asperger's Disorder versus High-Functioning Autism." *J Autism Dev Disord* **37**(5): 847–54.

Tonn, R. T. and J. E. Obrzut (2005). "The Neuropsychological Perspective on Autism." *Journal of Developmental and Physical Disabilities* **17**: 409–419.

Torres, I. J., V. G. Boudreau, *et al.* (2007). "Neuropsychological functioning in euthymic bipolar disorder: a meta-analysis." *Acta Psychiatrica Scandinavica* **116**: 17–26.

Torres, I. J., D. S. O'Leary, *et al.* (2004). "Symptoms and interference from memory in schizophrenia: evaluation of Frith's model of willed action." *Schizophr Res* **69**(1): 35–43.

Vasterling, J. J. and C. R. Brewin (2005). *Neuropsychology of PTSD: Biological, Cognitive, and Clinical Perspectives.* New York, Guilford Press.

Veiel, H. O. (1997). "A preliminary profile of neuropsychological deficits associated with major depression." *J Clin Exp Neuropsychol* **19**(4): 587–603.

von Gunten, A., J. Miklossy, *et al.* (2005). "Environmental reduplicative paramnesia in a case of atypical Alzheimer's disease." *Neurocase* **11**(3): 216–26.

Vuilleumier, P. (2005). "Hysterical conversion and brain function." *Prog Brain Res* **150**: 309–29.

Whalley, H. C., J. C. Harris, *et al.* (2007). "The neurobiological underpinnings of risk and conversion in relatives of patients with schizophrenia." *Int Rev Psychiatry* **19**(4): 383–97.

Woods, D. W., M. B. Himle, *et al.* (2008). "Durability, negative impact, and neuropsychological predictors of tic suppression in children with chronic tic disorder." *J Abnorm Child Psychol* **36**(2): 237–45.

Chapter 33

The clinical assessment of neuropsychiatric disorders

Mervi Pitkanen, Eli J. Jaldow, and
Michael D. Kopelman

1 Introduction

The primary objective of the neuropsychiatric clinical assessment is to make a comprehensive and accurate diagnosis and to set up a plan of management or care. It may be necessary to identify what additional information, if any, is required to substantiate the diagnosis (see Chapter 32). This unambiguous objective is nevertheless difficult to achieve and misdiagnoses are common (e.g. Taggard *et al.* 2006; Kishi *et al.* 2007; Voon *et al.* 2007). It can be intellectually unsatisfying to have to depend upon a range of tests and investigations to determine the correct diagnosis. In general in neuropsychiatry, the greater the care taken in the clinical assessment, the greater the probability of obtaining the correct diagnosis. However, over-investigating can be expensive and stressful for the patient. This chapter will focus on the principles of what a neuropsychiatrist attempts to do, and the particular contributions of the neuropsychologist in assessment and management of neuropsychiatric conditions (see Chapter 32).

2 The clinical interview

Neuropsychiatrists should be self-aware and realize that his or her own general appearance, body language, eye contact and posture will elicit a reaction from the patient and may critically affect the patient's responses. He or she should know how to listen, to be generally perceptive, to take notes and think simultaneously, to deal inconspicuously with interruptions and to give the impression that there is no hurry even when time may be very limited. At the very least, the patient will receive respect and begin to build a therapeutic relationship. It is usually necessary to have at least one follow-up appointment, to review the results of tests and investigations and/or to assess progress after the initial therapeutic intervention. Findings should be reviewed if follow-up appointments are not attended.

Many patients who are referred to a neuropsychiatrist have complex medical histories. It is important that all collected background information is considered carefully before the initial interview. Referral letters often contain essential information. It is often helpful, particularly in complex cases, to begin by clarifying with the patient the reasons for the referral; by reviewing the referral letter with the patient and identifying variations, if there are any, between the referrer's appraisal at the time of writing and the patient's current version of his problems. This should be done carefully and avoid confrontation. In this context, the referrer may be functioning as a collateral historian (see Section 2.1) and in some cases, this may be the only collateral history available. A review of the reason for referral at the beginning of the clinical interview will focus the neuropsychiatrist and the patient on the objectives of the consultation and identify the major topics to be covered in the interview. Also one shouldn't forget that a careful medication review, including prescription and over the counter medication, is required. Discontinuation of all unnecessary medications is important, as medications are an under-appreciated cause of cognitive complaints.

Neurologists and neuropsychiatrists deal with different aspects of both acute and chronic organic reactions. Ideally their approaches are complementary and neurological input may be useful during the neuropsychiatric assessment. Generally the neurologist is primarily concerned with the diagnosis and treatment of specific lesions and diseases. The neuropsychiatrist is concerned with the psychiatric manifestations and complications of known neurological disorders, as well as with the diagnosis and management of disorders evidenced by psychological/psychiatric signs and symptoms. These include delirium and dementia, the management of secondary disorders (e.g. depression after head injury or stroke, psychosis in epilepsy or dementia), the prevention of secondary complications and support for relatives and carers. He/she has responsibility for the coordination of care in the hospital and transfer of care at the time of discharge. Sometimes the neuropsychiatrist will assess an organic contribution to functional disorders, consider detention under the Mental Health Act (if in the UK), or assess issues of compensation or competence. Effective communication skills and the exercise of tact are essential.

In many branches of medicine it is considered good practice to strive to make a single diagnosis that best accounts for all the symptoms (Occam's razor). However, in neuropsychiatric practice there are often several concomitant problems that tend to cluster in familiar patterns. This has an impact on the scope of the neuropsychiatric assessment and will be considered further in Section 6.

The patient's complaints should be asked about early in the interview and should be considered thoroughly. Throughout the clinical interview, the neuropsychiatrist will be collecting information that will either support or reject certain possible diagnoses. He/she will systematically ask questions to help confirm or eliminate the differential diagnosis. Table 33.1 shows the common causes of dementia that a neuropsychiatrist may consider. Patients presenting with amnesia are most likely to have Wernicke-Korsakoff Syndrome, but herpes encephalitis, vascular episode(s), anoxia, head injury, subarachnoid haemorrhage, space-occupying lesion, pituitary excision, radiotherapy, and transient global amnesia are also possible diagnoses. Mild/moderate memory impairment is frequently the result of a vascular episode, epilepsy, alcohol, hypoxia or head injury; whilst non-progressive generalized cognitive impairment is most often due to anoxia or head injury (Kopelman and Crawford, 1996). Tables 33.2 and 33.3 give some examples of aspects of the presenting complaint and the past psychiatric history that may be diagnostically

Table 33.1 Prevalence of different causes of dementia in adults referred for evaluation of progressive intellectual deterioration*

Cause	Prevalence (%)
Alzheimer's disease (presumed)	39
Multi-infarct dementia	13
Dementia associated with psychiatric disorder (pseudodementia)	9
Alcoholic	8
Metabolic disorders	4
Hydrocephalus	4
Cerebral neoplasms	3
Huntington's disease	2
Not demented	2
Miscellaneous	15

* Data based on 708 patients from eight world-wide series (Marsden 1985). Note that Lewy body dementia has subsequently been shown to account for up to 20% of patients with dementia at autopsy. AIDS dementia is not included in this series.

helpful and should be enquired about. If there are a number of complaints or symptoms, it is useful to list them numerically at the outset, and then investigate them one by one.

2.1 Collateral clinical history

A detailed history from close relatives or friends is required to establish the mode of onset of the disorder, the nature and duration of symptoms and their subsequent course. The patient's own account may be distorted by confusion, memory lapses, denial or lack of insight. If possible, it is often advisable to have the collateral history taken by a second interviewer in a separate room, or at least conduct a telephone interview.

Table 33.2 The initial complaint and its diagnostic significance

	Examples and comments
Description	Diagnostically this is the most useful aspect of the history and great care should be taken to obtain detailed and precise information about each complaint or symptom
Mode of onset	
Sudden	Vascular episode, psychiatric disorder
Progressive	Alzheimer's disease, psychiatric disorder
Stepwise	Multi-infarct dementia, multiple sclerosis
Circumstances of onset	Injury/accident (Did the illness cause the accident? Compensation?)
Course	An episodic course is characteristic of epilepsy, Kleine–Levin syndrome, and mental illness

Table 33.3 The past psychiatric history and its diagnostic significance

Type of history	Examples and comments
Family history	**Genetic predisposition?**
Personal history	
Childhood	Brain damage, febrile convulsions, and head injuries all increase the risk of epilepsy
Occupations	Educational attainment and peak occupational level are better indicators of premorbid IQ than end-of-bed evaluations. Periods of unemployment may identify past episodes of illness
Habits	The impact of alcohol and other drugs is related to doses consumed and precise daily intake should be determined if possible. Have there been epileptic seizures, amnesic episodes, and/or withdrawal phenomena? Drug injection exposes the body to infections, emboli, and thromboses
Forensic	There may be genetic predisposition to criminal behaviour, e.g. XYY syndrome, Tourette's syndrome
Psychosexual	Unusual behaviour may be diagnostically helpful, e.g. increased libido and sexual disinhibition in mania and Kleine–Levin syndrome. Having multiple partners increases the risk of sexually transmitted diseases. Pregnancy and breastfeeding may effect some investigations and treatments
Sleep	The timing of insomnia may help distinguish between the type and severity of mood disorder. Insomnia is also a feature of delirium. Excessive daytime sleepiness may be primary or secondary (e.g. drugs/toxins, head injury, sleep apnoea)
Past psychiatric history	Previous symptoms, diagnoses, course of illness, and responses to previous treatments are characteristic of some illnesses and this information is often helpful diagnostically. Old brain scans may be very useful for identifying new pathology
Past medical history	Neurological (e.g. head injuries, epilepsy, meningitis/encephalitis, stroke) and endocrinological (e.g. diabetes, thyroid disease) histories are most often relevant
Personality and social history	A collateral history is important if a personality change is suspected

2.2 Mental state examination

The mental state examination begins with appearance and general behaviour.

◆ Pallor, weight loss, disorders of facial expression, posture and movement and standards of self-care draw attention to the possibility of an organic disorder.

◆ Is the patient impulsive, disinhibited, or insensitive?

◆ Or are they slow, hesitant or unable to understand?

◆ Speech may be impaired in production, perception or comprehension. The patient may be dysarthric, dysphonic, wander off the point or be incoherent. Thought may be impoverished, restricted to certain themes, concrete or impaired in reasoning (Weismer, 2006).

- Mood may be severely disturbed in neuropsychiatric patients (i.e. delirious patient's mood may rapidly change between periods of mild disinhibition or euphoria and hostile agitation whereas in early dementia anxiety or depression may characteristically prevail).

- An empty, shallow quality to emotional expression is quite common, as well as a catastrophic reaction, in which failure at a previously accomplished task elicits an intense emotional reaction with crying, negativity, withdrawal and hostility.

Intelligence has a major modifying effect on the presentation of thought content. A highly intelligent patient may appear less severely impaired by virtue of cognitive compensations for his or her deficits. Doctors should avoid making a glib assessment of IQ based on a conversation - this is a common trap that the medical profession falls into. It is quite possible to have a "normal" conversation with a person who has considerable intellectual impairment. Far more information can be derived from a few 'bedside' clinical screening such as having to copy a few simple shapes (Kopelman, 1986, 1994; Mioshi *et al.* 2006). The tendency to report the experience of unfamiliar abstract phenomena in simple, concrete terms may be due to an inability to appreciate the different modalities of perception and/or a lack of the vocabulary required to accurately describe them. A result may be that delusions or auditory hallucinations are reported as if they were visual phenomena. Ideas of reference and delusions of persecution are common, but often poorly elaborated, vague, shallow, transient or inconsistently related. Anxious, depressive or hypochondriacal ideas may co-occur with perceptual distortions, illusions and hallucinations.

2.3 Assessment of cognitive state

The neuropsychiatrist's assessment of cognitive state is essentially a screening procedure. If abnormalities are found they, combined with the clinical history, should help to focus the referral for neuropsychological assessment by a psychologist (see Section 4). However, it is paramount to remember that when there is a significant psychiatric presentation such as depression, anxiety or psychosis, the importance of cognitive assessment becomes less and one should take extreme caution prior to interpreting anything significant from these tests.

- In acute psychotic or neurotic patients without apparent organic pathology, it may be of importance to assess orientation in time, place and person, as well as recent events (e.g. how they came to the clinic, how long they have been an inpatient).

- In patients with suspected organic disorders, a brief assessment of orientation, attention/concentration, memory (including general information, remote and recent personal memories and current learning), language (including naming, comprehension, expression, repetition, reading and writing, disorders of form and content), mental calculation, drawing and copying, other agnosic or apraxic deficits and frontal function is likely to provide relevant insights and direct further assessments.

The scope for this type of assessment is described in Kopelman (1994).

3 **Physical examination**

A thorough physical examination is required. Twelve per cent of admissions to psychiatric hospitals have physical signs of illness directly contributing to their mental disorders (Lishman 1998). The elderly are particularly vulnerable, with over one third of hospitalised elderly having features of delirium (Marcantonio *et al.* 2003; Kishi *et al.* 2007). Also it should be noted that systemic infections and inflammation can cause acute exacerbation of symptoms and drive the progression of the neurodegenerative disease (Perry *et al.* 2007).

- It is important to examine the patient's face as 'there's no art to find the mind's construction in the face'. A great deal of information can be obtained about mood, perplexity, trust and an impression of character from the face, although beware not to over-interpret. Is there a suspicion that the patient is experiencing hallucinations? This may be obvious or quite subtle. There may be signs of liver disease: spider naevi, jaundice and parotid enlargement in an alcoholic.
- The head should be examined for signs: scars, unusual head shape, size or asymmetry, hair distribution and texture.
- The eyes, windows of the mind, should be examined carefully. Abnormal pupil size may be affected by drugs. Pupillary accommodation and reaction to a light must be checked if there is a suspicion of syphilis; the Argyll-Robinson 'prostitutes' pupil accommodates but does not react.
- The hands may also reveal useful information about the patient's health and lifestyle. Is there a tremor, palmar erythema and leuconychia, nicotine staining, clubbing or calluses? Are the nails long, broken, bitten or unclean?
- The blood pressure must always be measured and the pulse should be taken. Is there an arrhythmia? Is the pulse fast because the patient is anxious or for some other reason (e.g. thyroid disease)?

The traditional neurological examination is often not that abnormal in patients with brain disease. If abnormalities are present they may only be witnessed as 'subtle signs', for example clumsiness, minor Parkinsonism or gait abnormalities. Also "neurological soft signs" should not be ignored (Cuesta *et al.* 2002).

4 **Neuropsychological assessment**

Within the context of a neuropsychiatric clinic, neuropsychological assessment has three main purposes.

- The first is to help with diagnosis in the context of other observations and findings from the background history, clinical and mental state examination and the results of physical investigations. Where all the indexes point in the same direction, the assessment is easy. Where they differ, it is more challenging, but particularly important to find an explanation for the discrepancy. A patient may be found, on formal testing, to be either more or less severely impaired than expected. If more severely impaired, it could be that the clinician had under-estimated the degree of decrement or that the patient is exaggerating or simulating his/her handicap.

* The second main purpose is to identify and quantify the pattern and severity of cognitive impairments. The details of how this is done are discussed elsewhere in this volume.

* The third main purpose of assessment is to plan strategies of cognitive rehabilitation and/or cognitive behaviour therapy: mood disorders and post-traumatic stress disorder being common correlates of cognitive deficits (Kopelman and Crawford, 1996; Jacova *et al.* 2007). Cognitive rehabilitation is carried out according to principles developed elsewhere (Wilson, 1999; Stuss *et al.* 1999).

The actual tests employed in neuropsychiatric settings vary somewhat from clinic to clinic, but do not differ in essence from those considered in relation to specific disorders elsewhere in this volume. Within our own clinic, we commonly employ as initial procedures the National Adult Reading Test–revised (NART-R; Nelson and Willison 1991), or the Wechsler Test of Adult Reading (WTAR; Wechsler, 2001a) for estimating premorbid IQ, the Wechsler Abbreviated Scale of Intelligence (WASI; Wechsler, 1999) as a brief assessment of current intelligence, and the Wechsler Adult Intelligence Scale–III (WAIS–III; Wechsler, 2001b) for more detailed assessment. Measures of anterograde memory, employed in accordance with clinical need and time availability, include the Wechsler Memory Scale-III (WMS–III; Wechsler, 2001c), Wechsler Memory Scale–revised (WMS–R; Wechsler, 1987), the Doors and People test (Baddeley *et al.* 1994), the Recognition Memory Test (Warrington, 1984), the Camden Memory Tests (Warrington, 1996) and the Kendrick Object Learning test (Kendrick, 1985). For naming, we commonly employ the Graded Naming test (McKenna and Warrington, 1983), and for executive function, tests such as verbal fluency (Benton, 1968), Modified Card Sorting (Nelson, 1976), Trail Making (Reitan, 1958), and the Brixton-Hayling tests (Burgess and Shallice, 1996). Autobiographical memory is assessed using the Autobiographical Memory Interview (Kopelman *et al.* 1990). All patients are given the Beck Depression Scale-II (BDI-II; Beck *et al.* 1996) and subjective evaluations of memory are also used occasionally (Sunderland *et al.* 1983).

5 Investigations

Investigations are primarily directed towards excluding or establishing and quantifying organic pathology.

5.1 Blood Tests

A biochemical screen is justified in all cases, even if the diagnosis is known, as any problems in these can often easily be corrected and electrolyte imbalances may complicate and exacerbate other conditions (Rockwood, 2008). Biochemical tests are essential to confirm many suspected diagnosis, for example thyroid disease, parathyroid disease, Cushing's disease, diabetes, uraemia, liver failure and syphilis.

5.2 Electroencephalogram (EEG)

The electroencephalogram is still widely used when organic disorders are suspected, confirming abnormalities of brain structure and function in about 60% of cases. In normal subjects the EEG is symmetrical and classified into four characteristic waveforms depending on frequency: delta, theta, alpha and beta. There are rather specific findings in EEG in certain neuropsychiatric disorders, however the findings always need to be interpreted in the clinical context and they are hardly ever diagnostic. Do note though that the EEG is becoming an increasingly popular tool when combined with advanced imaging techniques (cf. Jeong 2004; Oishi *et al.* 2007; Pomonavera *et al.* in press).

5.3 Structural imaging

Brain structural imaging is considered a crucial component when evaluating neuropsychiatric patients. Magnetic Resonance Imaging (MRI) has a number of advantages over Computerized Tomography (CT) and currently is the examination of choice. However, a CT scan can still be very informative and useful in acute situations.

In a setting of an acute cognitive decline or other acute neuropsychiatric symptoms a CT scan is generally enough to rule out surgically treatable disorders. However, problems easily emerge when interpreting a CT scan due to its poor ability to show subtle lesions particularly in the areas that are difficult to image, but it does remain useful for patients with claustrophobia, pacemaker or other metallic implants (van Straaten *et al.* 2004).

The MRI shows high sensitivity in detecting macroscopic abnormalities occurring in several neuropsychiatric conditions (i.e. Neuropsychiatric SLE related cerebrovascular disease), thus providing a substantial contribution in both diagnosis and management. However, in clinical practice the conventional MRI is typically obtained mainly to exclude the presence of a potentially reversible cause (i.e. brain tumors, subdural hematoma, normal-pressure hydrocephalus) but does not provide any specific support to discriminate among different forms of neurodegenerative disease. In clinical research and more commonly in practice, interest is increasing to measure regional or global brain atrophy and voxel-based morphometry (VBM) is becoming popular (Bozzali *et al.* 2006). However, the information that VBM provides is again related to brain atrophy, which represents the final stage of the pathophysiological processes occurring in neurodegenerative disorders. Recently, more advanced MR techniques (i.e., ^{1}H-MR spectroscopy; diffusion-weighted MRI (DW-MRI), magnetization transfer imaging) have been introduced with the ability to detect subtle changes in brain tissue. Typically these techniques are able to reflect more microscopic aspects of the tissue damage (demyelination, microtubule breakdown, axonal loss), which are supposed to precede the final stage of tissue loss. Even though these techniques are not as yet in common clinical use they do show promising results, improving insight of the brain's microstructural characteristics in neuropsychiatric disorders (Bozzali and Cherubini, 2007; cf. Geuze *et al.* 2005; Farias and Jagust, 2004).

5.4 Functional imaging

Functional imaging, such as Single Photon Emission Computerized (SPECT) and Positron Emission Tomography (PET), provides the means for detecting in vivo metabolic and neurochemical changes in neuropsychiatric disorders. PET and SPECT are nuclear medicine techniques in which temporal changes in the concentrations of radioactive tracers are recorded in brain and other target organs. SPECT assesses brain function by measuring the photon emission from radiotracers which cross the blood brain barrier and distribute in proportion to regional cerebral blood flow shortly after intravenous injection. This provides an indirect measure of cerebral metabolic function. The radioactivity involved is a limiting factor and is an ethical issue. SPECT is cheaper and more widely available than PET, which also permits evaluation of brain metabolism. Transmitter and receptor studies can be done with both SPECT and PET. Overall, PET has become more prevalent in clinical practise but SPECT is being reinvented with new applications (Janssen and Vanderheyden, 2007; cf. Minoshima, 2002; Thobois *et al.* 2001).

6 Concluding the neuropsychiatric assessment

Ideally the clinical history and examination as well as the psychometric testing and the investigations all point to the same diagnosis. However, they often do not, and in those cases all the information should be reappraised carefully.

+ Was part of the history missed?
+ Is there any reason to suspect that the patient may be malingering or embellishing symptoms?
+ Is the patient depressed or suffering from excessive daytime sleepiness (pseudodementia)?

A neuropsychiatrist, having made one probable diagnosis, should then consider other disorders that sometimes cluster with that diagnosis.

+ Head injury may result in neurological signs, cognitive deficits, personality change and/or emotional problems (i.e. depression and PTSD).
+ Alcohol causes a range of problems including withdrawal syndrome, acute hallucinosis or paranoia, hepatic encephalopathy, the Wernicke-Korsakoff syndrome, or more global cognitive deficits as well as a range of psychological problems (i.e. depression, anxiety, and mood lability).

Finding evidence for the presence of the familiar clustering disorders may increase the likelihood that the primary diagnosis was accurate. Using a structured approach to organizing the clinical material, and relying on overall clinical judgement at both the initial and concluding stages will usually furnish the neuropsychiatrist with sufficient information to make a reliable diagnosis and to proceed to set up a plan of management (cf. Cummings and Zhong, 2006).

Selective references

Baddeley, A.D., Emslie, H., and Nimmo-Smith, I. (1994). *Doors and People: a test of visual and verbal recall and recognition.* Thames Valley Test Company, Bury St Edmunds.

Beck, A.T., Steer, R.A. and Brown, G.K. (1996). *Beck Depression Inventory–II.* Psychological Corporation, San Antonio, Texas.

Benton, A.L. (1968). Differential behavioural effects in frontal lobe disease. *Neuropsychologia* **6**, 53–60.

Bozzali, M., Filippi, M., Magnani, G., *et al.* (2006). The contribution of voxel based morphometry in staging patients with mild cognitive impairment. *Neurology* **67**, 453–460.

Bozzali, M. and Cherubini, R. (2007). Diffusion tensor MRI to investigate dementias: a brief review. *Magnetic Res Imaging* **25**, 969–77.

Burgess, P.W. and Shallice, T. (1996). Response suppression, initiation and strategy use following frontal lobe lesions. *Neuropsychologia* **34**, 263–72.

Cuesta, M.J., Peralta, V., Zarzuela, A., *et al.* (2002). Neurological soft-signs in psychosis: threshold criteria for discriminating normal controls and for predicting cognitive impairment. *Schizoph Res* **58**, 263–271.

Cummings, J.L. and Zhong, K. (2006). Treatments for behavioural disorders in neurodegenerative diseases: Drug development strategies. *Nature Rev Drug Discovery* **5**, 64–74.

Farias, S.T. and Jagust, W.J. (2004). Neuroimaging in non-Alzheimer dementias. *Clin Neurosci Res* **3**, 383–95.

Geuze, E., Vermetten, E., and Bremner, J.D. (2005). MR-based *in vivo* hippocampal volumetrics: 2. Findings in neuropsychiatric disorders – Feature Review. *Molecular Psychiatry* **10**, 160–84.

Jacova, C., Kertesz, A., Blair, M., Fisk, J.D., and Feldman, H.H. (2007). Neuropsychological testing and assessment for dementia - Review article. *Alzheimer's and Dementia* **3** 299–317.

Janssen, P.F. and Vanderheyden, J.-L. (2007). The future of SPECT in a time of PET. *Nuclear Medicine and Biology* **34**, 733–5.

Jeong, J. (2004). EEG dynamics in patients with Alzheimer's disease – Invited Review. *Clin Neurophysiology* **115**, 1490–1505.

Kendrick, D. (1985). *Cognitive tests for the elderly.* Windsor: NFER-Nelson.

Kishi, Y., Kato, M., Okuyama, T., *et al.* (2007). Delirium: patient characteristics that predict a missed diagnosis at psychiatric consultation. *Gen. Hospital Psych.* **29** 442–5.

Kopelman, M. D. (1986). Clinical tests of memory. *Br. J. Psychiatry* **148**, 517–25.

Kopelman, M. D. (1994). Structured psychiatric interview: assessment of the cognitive state. *Br. J. Hosp. Med.* **52**, 277–281.

Kopelman, M.D. and Crawford, S. (1996). Not all Memory Clinics are Dementia Clinics. *Neuropsychological Rehabil.* **6**, 187–202.

Kopelman, M.D., Wilson, B.A. and Baddeley A.D. (1990). *The Autobiographical Memory Interview.* Thames Valley Test Company, Bury St Edmunds.

Lishman W.A. (1998). *Organic Psychiatry: The Psychological Consequences of Cerebral Disorder* (3rd ed.). Oxford: Blackwell Scientific Publications.

Marcantonio, E.R., Simon, S.E., Bergmann, M.A., *et al.* (2003). Delirium symptoms in post-acute care: Prevalent, persistent, and associated with poor functional recovery, *J Am Geriatr Soc* **51**, 4–9.

Marsden C.D. (1985). Assessment of dementia. In *Handbook of Clinical Neurology, Vol.2: Neurobehavioural Disorders* (ed. J. A. M. Fredericks) pp. 221–232. Oxford: Elsevier Science.

McKenna, P. and Warrington, E.K. (1983). *The Graded Naming Test.* Windsor: NFER-Nelson.

Minoshima, S. (2002). PET and SPECT imaging of dementia—past, present, and future. *Int. Congress Series* **1228**, 55–61.

Mioshi, E., Dawson, K., Mitchell, J., Arnold, R., and Hodges J.R. (2006). The Addenbrooke's Cognitive Examination Revised (ACE-R): a brief cognitive test battery for dementia screening. *Int J Geriatr Psychiatry*, **21**, 1078–1085.

Morris, R.G. and Kopelman, M. (1992). The neuropsychological assessment of dementia. In *Handbook of neuropsychological assessment* (ed. Crawford, J.R., Parker, D.M. and McKinlay, W.W.) Hove, East Sussex: Lawrence Erlbaum Associates Ltd.

Nelson, H.E. (1976). A modified card sorting test. *Cortex* **12**, 313–24.

Nelson, H.E. and Willison, J.R. (1991). *The National Adult Reading Test*-Revised. Windsor: NFER-Nelson.

Oishi, N., Mima, T., Ishii, K., *et al.* (2007). Neural correlates of regional EEG power change. *Neuroimage* **36** 1301–12.

Perry, V.H., Cunningham C. and Holmes, C. (2007). Systemic infections and inflammation affect chronic neurodegeneration. *Nature Rev. Immunology* **7**, 161–7.

Ponomareva, N.V., Korovaitseva, G.I. and Rogaev, E.I. (in Press). EEG alterations in non-demented individuals related to apolipoprotein E genotype and to risk of Alzheimer disease. *Neurobiology of Aging*.

Reitan, R.M. (1958). Validity of the Trail Making test as an indicator of organic brain damage. *Percept. Motor Skills* **8**, 271–6.

Rockwood, K. (2008). Causes of Delirium. *Psychiatry* **7**, 39–41.

Stuss, D.T., Winocur, G., and Robertson, I.H. (eds.) (1999). *Cognitive rehabilitation*. Cambridge: Cambridge University Press.

Sunderland, A., Harris, J.E., and Baddeley, A.D. (1983). Do laboratory tests predict everyday memory? A neuropsychological study. *J. Verbal Learning Verbal Behav.* **22**, 341–56.

Taggart, C., O'Grady, J., Stevenson, *et al.* (2006) Accuracy of diagnosis at routine psychiatric assessment in patients presenting to an accident and emergency department. *Gen. Hospital Psychiatry* **28**, 330–5.

Thobois, S., Guillouet, S. and Broussolle, E. (2001). Contributions of PET and SPECT to the understanding of the pathophysiology of Parkinson's disease - Review. *Clin. Neurophysiology* **31**, 321–40.

van Straaten, E.C.W., Scheltens, P. and Barkhof, F. (2004). MRI and CT in the diagnosis of vascular dementia. *J. Neurol Sci.* **226**, 9–12.

Voon, V, Lang, A.E. and Hallett, M. (2007). Diagnosing psychogenic movement disorders — which criteria should be used in clinical practice? *Nature – Clin. Practice Neurology* **3**, 134–5.

Warrington, E.K. (1984). *The Recognition Memory Test*. Windsor: NFER-Nelson.

Warrington, E.K. (1996). *The Camden Memory Tests*. Hove: Psychology Press.

Wechsler, D. (1987). *Wechsler Memory Scale-Revised*. San Antonio: Psychological Corporation.

Wechsler, D. (1999). *Wechsler Abbreviated Scale of Intelligence*. San Antonio: Psychological Corporation.

Wechsler, D. (2001a). *Wechsler Test of Adult Reading*. San Antonio: Psychological Corporation.

Wechsler, D. (2001b). *Wechsler Adult Intelligence Scale-III*. San Antonio: Psychological Corporation.

Wechsler, D. (2001c). *The Wechsler Memory Scale-III*. Psychological Corporation, San Antonio, Texas.

Weismer, G. (2006). Speech Disorders. In Traxler M.J., and Gernsbacker M.A: *Handbook of Psycholinguistics* (2nd Ed) pp. 93–124.

Wilson, B.A. (1999). Case studies in neuropsychological rehabilitation. Oxford: Oxford University Press.

Chapter 34

Neuropsychological rehabilitation of schizophrenia

Bjørn Rishovd Rund

1 Introduction

Schizophrenia is a disturbance, or a spectrum of disorders, that is diagnostically defined (*Diagnostic and statistical manual of mental disorders*, 4th edn (DSM-IV); American Psychiatric Association 1994) by a duration of at least 6 months, with at least 1 month of an active psychotic phase. Two or more of the following symptoms should be present during the active phase:

- delusions;
- hallucinations;
- disorganized speech;
- grossly disorganized or catatonic behaviour;
- negative symptoms (i.e. affective flattening, alogia, or avolition).

Even though modern antipsychotics and psychosocial treatment programmes are effective in moderating symptoms and reducing the rate of relapses, most patients with schizophrenia do not function well outside structured, routine settings, such as hospital wards. Outcomes other than symptom improvement and relapse prevention have not been well documented (Lehman *et al.* 1995; Hogarty and Flesher 1999). A majority of patients with schizophrenia interact in ordinary social settings in a conspicuous way and also do not manage an ordinary work or school situation very well. On average, only 10–30% of patients with schizophrenia are employed at any time, and few of these are able to maintain their vocational gains (Attkisson *et al.* 1992; Hogarty and Flesher 1999). What is the reason for this?

1.1 Cognitive dysfunction and outcome in schizophrenia

Many clinicians now claim that the reason is the serious cognitive disturbances of these patients. Several prominent researchers and clinicians have pointed out that cognitive dysfunction is the enduring core feature of schizophrenia. Some have called schizophrenia a thought disorder. Evidence from neuropsychological, neuropathological, and neuroimaging studies has documented schizophrenia as a neuropsychiatric disease. Most cognitive dysfunctions seem to some degree to remain impaired even when symptoms improve.

Andreasen (1999) argues that the definition of schizophrenia should be based on basic cognitive disturbances rather than on phenomenology.

The fundamental importance of cognitive deficits in schizophrenia is also substantiated by the fact that cognitive functions have proven to be of much greater significance in the prediction of prognosis and outcome than the symptoms of the illness. Patients with the most serious cognitive dysfunctions appear to have the poorest outcome. Different dysfunctions seem to relate to different functional outcomes.

- Verbal memory is related to all types of functional outcomes.
- Vigilance predicts social problem-solving and the acquisition of social skills.
- Executive functioning predicts the ability to function in the community (Sharma 1999).
- Impairment in cognitive processing seems to mediate the acquisition of behavioural competencies in schizophrenia.

We still have limited knowledge however, about the underlying mechanisms through which cognitive dysfunctions operate on behaviour and social functions.

1.2 The importance of cognitive prodromal symptoms for early diagnosis

What Hogarty and Flesher (1999) term social cognition (i.e. the ability to act wisely in social interactions), is an important determinant of social and vocational recovery. Klosterkøtter and Schultze-Lutter (2000) have shown that cognitive prodromal symptoms are the only ones with a high diagnostic efficiency. These symptoms have high specificity and positive predictive powers as well as satisfactory percentages of false-positive predictions and a good classification rate. Klosterkøtter and Schultze-Lutter (2000) claim that because of the high predictive value of these cognitive symptoms, a diagnosis in the initial schizophrenic prodrome seems possible. They conclude that in the future an early intervention related thereto might enable prevention of early psychotic episodes.

1.3 Cognitive dysfunction as a target for treatment and rehabilitation

The fact that deviance in cognitive functions is a core deficit in schizophrenia makes them an appropriate target for treatment and rehabilitation. The obvious area to address is the one that is most impaired and most damaging for the person's psycho-social functioning. However, the targeting of cognitive and neuropsychological deficits in schizophrenia for therapeutic interventions has so far been greatly neglected. Attempts at cognitive remediation have been relatively sparse. Effective techniques for normalizing or neutralizing cognitive impairments would be a decisive addition to the treatment armamentarium for patients with a psychotic illness in general and patients with schizophrenia in particular. Neuropsychologists have contributed strongly to the development of the few cognitive remediation programmes for patients with schizophrenia that exist today, primarily the process-oriented approach (see Section 3). This treatment strategy originated in the areas of experimental psychopathology and the neuropsychology of schizophrenia. In this approach, specific cognitive impairments detected in the laboratory are targeted for change, first in the laboratory and later in increasingly realistic situations (Spaulding *et al.* 1999). As such, this treatment approach has much in common with the models for rehabilitation of head traumas.

There are two distinctly different approaches in cognitive therapy with schizophrenic patients. One focuses on cognitive content, while the other is process-oriented, emphasizing the correction of basic cognitive deficits.

2 The content-oriented approach to therapy

This is carried out according to the principles of cognitive therapy (e.g. as described by Beck *et al.* 1979) for the treatment of depression and other emotional disorders. However, some modifications that are necessary for severely disturbed patients are included. Outstanding advocates for this approach in schizophrenia treatment are Perris (1989), Fowler and Morley (1989), Bentall and collaborators (1994), and Kingdon and Turkington (1994).

- ◆ Perris's metacognitive approach has been developed in small, community-based and family-style treatment centres in Sweden. Most of the treatment takes place in small groups.

- ◆ Bentall *et al.* (1994) have developed a more behaviourally oriented treatment package that directly targets persistent auditory hallucinations. Their therapeutic programme consists of procedures for fostering attribution of hallucinations to the self rather than to external sources, and for diminishing distress provoked by hearing voices.

- ◆ Kingdon and Turkington (1994) contend that people with schizophrenia are not inherently irrational, but instead suffer from a circumscribed set of irrational beliefs. Their therapeutic approach attempts to help patients to alleviate the impact of these beliefs.

- ◆ The treatment programme of Fowler and colleagues (Garety *et al.* 1994) focuses on techniques aimed at modifying psychotic thoughts.

3 The process-oriented approach to cognitive therapy

This approach focuses on remediation of deficits in cognitive processes rather than changing distorted thoughts, attitudes, beliefs, or hallucinations (Adams *et al.* 1981). This chapter will be limited to this approach and the empirical studies examining the effects of such therapeutic programmes.

There were a few clinical studies in the late 1960s and 1970s reporting encouraging results. After this promising beginning, research lay dormant for more than a decade. Interest in cognitive training programmes based on empirical research was to some extent rekindled in the 1990s. Some few comprehensive training programmes have been developed, and the effects of certain of these have been examined (Fowler 1992; Brenner *et al.* 1995; Spaulding *et al.* 1999). In addition to these well-founded treatment programmes, there have also been several attempts to remediate more specific elementary attentional and conceptual functions.

3.1 The integrated psychological therapy (IPT) programme

Brenner *et al.* (1992, 1995) developed the most complete therapeutic programme, the so-called Integrated Psychological Therapy (IPT). This is a multi-element hierarchical programme in which there is an attempt to enhance basic cognitive capacities before problem-solving and motor skills training is implemented. IPT is a step-by-step procedure devised for groups of 5–7 patients. It is comprised of five subprogrammes:

- cognitive differentiation;
- social perception;
- communication skills;
- interpersonal problem-solving;
- social skills training.

The rationale behind the IPT is that remediation of cognitive deficits will facilitate acquisition and maintenance of more complex skills. A series of studies of IPT has demonstrated significant treatment effects on cognitive functions and reduction of symptomatology (Hodel and Brenner 1994). However, it has not been documented that remediation of cognitive functions has a pervasive effect on social behaviour.

In the USA, Will Spaulding has adapted and elaborated Brenner's IPT programme. Spaulding *et al.* (1999) published the results from a study in which 90 subjects with severe and disabling psychiatric conditions, predominantly schizophrenia, participated in a controlled-outcome trial. Patients receiving the cognitive training programme, consisting of the three cognitive modules in Brenner's IPT, were compared to control subjects who received supportive group therapy. Patients receiving cognitive training showed incrementally greater gains compared with controls on the primary outcome measures. There was equivocal evidence for greater improvement in the cognitive training group on a disorganization factor for psychiatric symptoms (the Brief Psychiatric Rating Scale), and strong evidence for greater improvement on a laboratory measure of attention processing. Significant improvement was also found on two measures of attention, memory, and executive functioning.

3.2 A trial of individual neurocognitive therapy

Wykes *et al.* (1998) reported the preliminary results of a controlled trial of individual neurocognitive therapy. The effects of cognitive remediation were compared to those of a control therapy that consisted of intensive occupational therapy to control for non-specific effects of treatment. In a randomized control trial of 33 patients with schizophrenia, results suggested a differential effect in favour of cognitive rehabilitation for tests in the cognitive flexibility and memory subgroups, as well as for self-esteem, but not on symptoms or social functioning. However, generalized improvements in cognitive flexibility were related to improvements in social functioning.

3.3 Remediation of conceptual and attentional skills and memory

The attempts to remediate more specific cognitive dysfunction have mainly concentrated on two areas: conceptual skills and attentional skills.

3.3.1 Remediation of conceptual skills

Conceptual skills have been trained primarily by means of the Wisconsin Card Sorting Test (WCST). These studies all show some positive effects of training. The greatest gains have been attained by providing positive reinforcement for correct solutions. It has not been possible to demonstrate any evidence of generalization for improved executive functions. Bellack and co-workers (1996) showed that schizophrenic patients trained on one of two problem-solving tasks similar to the WCST exhibited a marked improvement on the trained task. However, subjects trained on one test performed no better on the other instrument than subjects who received practice only.

3.3.2 Remediation of attentional skills

Regarding attentional skills (cf. Silverstein *et al.* 2001; Suslow *et al.* 2001), two of the most common measures are the Continuous Performance Test (CPT) and the Span Task. Benedict and associates (1994) used six training tasks that all required sustained vigilance and a high degree of mental effort. Results showed improved performance on the training tasks for the experimental group. However, no significant changes on the outcome measures were observed. Benedict and associates (1994) therefore conclude that the rather substantial practice effect demonstrated did not denote an improved fundamental cognitive skill.

The conclusion of Benedict and associates (1994) is in accordance with the view of Bellack *et al.* (1996). They are sceptical as to whether cognitive rehabilitation of schizophrenic patients is an achievable goal. They admit that practice on tasks can improve performance on that specific task, but state that there is little evidence for the generalizability of such training. Thus, they claim that the task for schizophrenia researchers is to develop real-world training programmes.

Several more positive attempts to train attentional deficits in patients with schizophrenia have been carried out recently.

- Kern and associates (1995) compared four groups of schizophrenic patients in regard to improved performance on a Span task. The findings revealed that the combination of monetary reinforcement and instructional cues was superior to other interventions. In the Oslo Cognitive Training Programme that will be outlined in Section 4, we have included an intensive Span training with reinforcement, similar to that used by Kern and associates.

- Hermanutz and Gestrich (1991) showed that it was possible to reduce the distraction of schizophrenic patients on reaction-time tasks.

- Olbrich *et al.* (1993) found clearly positive effects of a training module that addresses a combination of attentional, mnemonic, and conceptual skills.

- Van der Gaag (1992) employed a clinical rehabilitation programme and showed that, although the training programme was effective in some processing domains, it did not affect tasks that rely on fast processing of information.

- Medalia *et al.* (1998) assessed the impact of attention training with chronic schizophrenia patients. They found that it is feasible to use practice and behavioural learning to remediate core attention deficits in this patient group.

3.3.3 Remediation of memory

In addition several attempts have also been made to improve memory in schizophrenic patients. For instance, Koh *et al.* (1976) showed that patients were able to increase recall on a memory task to levels close to that of normal control subjects when their encoding was aided by rating stimuli (words) in terms of pleasantness.

3.4 Other views on cognitive remediation in schizophrenia

In an issue of *Schizophrenia Bulletin* (no. 1, 1999), the theme was interventions for neurocognitive deficits in schizophrenia. Here several outstanding therapists and researchers ask pertinent questions about the results and designs of cognitive remediation research. Bellack *et al.* (1999) point out that the critical question in selecting neurocognitive targets is one of generalizability. They question how far-reaching the effects of training in any basic information-processing domain are. Bellack and collaborators propose an alternative to the cognitive rehabilitation programmes mentioned above. They claim that a compensatory model is much more appropriate. Their emphasis is not on eliminating impairment so much as on minimizing the resulting disability. Bellack and associates are critical of the belief that the neurodevelopmental nature of impairments defies simple solution. Further, they don't find that rehabilitation strategies depending primarily on repeated practice of neuropsychological tasks yield much improvement in the underlying cognitive operations, or have much benefit for community functioning.

Green and Nuechterlein (1999) point out another important issue. Some neurocognitive deficits in schizophrenia are rather stable over time and thus it would be unreasonable to expect longstanding deficits to improve permanently after a short-term treatment. They also point out that the key question is whether changes in neurocognition translate into changes in functional outcome.

Studies using the process-oriented approach are summarized in Table 34.1.

4 The oslo cognitive training programme

The cognitive training programme developed at the Sogn Centre for Child and Adolescent Psychiatry (SCCAP) in Oslo aims to improve cognitive functioning and to develop and strengthen cognitive skills. It takes into account the specific psychopathological characteristics of schizophrenia. The development of the Oslo Cognitive Training Programme is based on research demonstrating that the most significant dysfunctions in schizophrenia can be related to the areas of attention, memory, and executive functions. Using the 'Oslo approach', we have attempted to develop a programme that covers all these areas of dysfunction.

Table 34.1 The process-oriented approach. Characteristics of outcome studies

Study*	Outcome of cognitive training
Koh *et al*. 1976	Increased recall on memory task
Hermanutz and Gastrich 1991	Reduced distraction
Van der Gaag 1992	No sign of improvement
Benedict *et al*. 1994	Improvement on attention task
Hodel and Brenner 1994	Reduction of symptoms
Kern *et al*. 1995	Improved span of apprehension
Bellack *et al*. 1996	Marked improvement on WCST
Medalia *et al*. 1998[†]	Positive effect on attention
Spaulding *et al*. 1999[‡]	Improvement on cognitive function
Wykes *et al*. 1999	Improvement in cognitive flexibility/memory

*The groups studied are schizophrenic patients unless otherwise indicated.
[†]This was a study comprising chronic schizophrenic patients.
[‡]This was a study comprising chronic psychotic patients.

The treatment programme is, however, also based on the presumption that cognitive impairment is a key characteristic in other psychotic disorders. A broad spectrum of psychotic patients is thus included in the study (Rund and Borg 1999).

The controlled treatment study at SCCAP aims to investigate to what extent this cognitive training programme can be a positive clinical supplement to a previously documented psychoeducational training programme that has proven quite effective (Rund *et al*. 1994). The psychoeducational programme was carried out at SCCAP in the late 1980s and early 1990s. The outcome of this programme was compared with that of a standard reference treatment. Clinical outcome was assessed by relapses during the 2-year treatment period and by changes in psychosocial functioning as measured by the Global Assessment Scale (GAS). The results indicated that the most effective programme as measured by relapse was also the cheapest—namely, the psychoeducational programme. Psychosocial functioning improved more, close to significance, in the psychoeducational group. Patients with poor premorbid psychosocial functioning benefit most from this treatment.

In the controlled treatment study now taking place at SCCAP, the question of whether a cognitive training programme can add anything to the effects of a psychoeducational programme alone, will be assessed by comparing two groups at baseline, post-treatment, and at a 1 year follow-up.

- Group A receives a psycho-educational programme alone.
- Group B receives the same psychoeducational treatment package as group A plus the cognitive training programme.

We have chosen a battery of outcome measures for evaluating treatment effects on cognition as well as psychiatric symptoms (Brief Psychiatric Rating Scale (BPRS)) and psychosocial functioning (GAS).

4.1 The training programme

The programme is arranged in four modules: cognitive differentiation; attention; memory; and social perception.

- The *cognitive differentiation module* is based on the supposition of a generalized impairment in verbal intelligence, abstraction–flexibility, and auditory processing that is congruent with a left-hemispheric dysfunction hypothesis. Much of Brenner *et al.*'s (1995) original methodology is adapted for these tasks.

- The *attention module* considers impairment of attention as a central feature of schizophrenia. With the assumption that deficits in attention are part of an underlying mechanism of other cognitive dysfunctions, tasks aim to strengthen sustained attention over time, as well as train selective attention and scanning abilities.

- The *memory module* is based on studies involving both verbal and visual memory. Tasks that primarily involve short-term recall aim to improve the patient's ability to recall an increasing number of items.

- The *social perception module* involves the cognitive processes that allow the patient to respond and adapt appropriately to his or her environment.

Training in verbal communication, attention, memory, and social perception is conducted by administering systematic training procedures.

- During the cognitive differentiation module patients learn to discriminate among stimulus categories by participating in a card-sorting task. After demonstrating competence on this task, patients are introduced to a concept formation task in which they are instructed to match antonyms and synonyms, distinguish concepts with different definitions, and establish a hierarchy of related concepts (Brenner *et al.* 1992).

- Attention and memory modules are presented simultaneously with the concept formation task.

- Following these modules, patients participate in the social perception module where they are trained to encode social stimuli by viewing a series of slides showing actors in different social activities and demonstrating emotions of varied intensity.

In the social perception module the focus is on improving the patient's ability to attend to the statements of others and to understand accurately what was said, as well as to encourage association between the patients' thoughts and the statements of those with whom they interact. This training attempts to address the lack of integration between strategies that target information processing and social learning dysfunction.

4.2 Programme structure

The four modules are systematically introduced to the patient over a period of 8–10 weeks. The training consists of 30–35 hours of individual training with 15-minute work sessions. The programme is designed so that the patient begins with elementary tasks and progresses to more difficult ones. The rate of progression is determined by the individual's functioning, though a standard protocol provides the structure for progression.

In addition to the cognitive training programme outlined in Section 4.1, all patients in Group B participate in an intensive span of apprehension training. Patients are administered the same computerized version of the Span of Apprehension task (Asarnow and Nuechterlein, version 1987) in six different sessions:

- session 1, baseline;
- sessions 2–4, 3 consecutive days of intervention;
- session 5, immediate post-test;
- session 6, at the 10-day follow-up.

The Span task is run on an IBM computer. There are 128 test trials, consisting of 3- and 12-letter arrays. Patients are instructed to identify which of two target letters (T or F) appear on the screen by pressing one of two buttons (marked T or F, respectively) on a control pad as quickly as possible. During interventions 2, 3, and 4, patients receive both monetary reinforcement and enhanced instructions. The reward (50 øre) is given immediately following a correct response by dropping the coin into a metal container placed to the patient's right.

4.3 Initiation of the programme

Following completion of baseline measures of the patient's current level of functioning, he/she is given a standard introduction to the training programme and develops a training schedule together with the therapist. We have chosen to implement our programme individually instead of in a group.

- Early on in the development of the training, it became clear that the patients themselves preferred individual sessions.
- In addition, these allow the therapist to take into consideration patients' tremendous variation in cognitive functioning, and thus progress at an appropriate rate while adhering to the standard protocol.

The cognitive training for the most part takes place in the school at the clinic. A teacher is responsible for this part of the programme. A few tasks, such as the visual scanning task 'Where is Willy', take place in the ward.

4.4 Some preliminary results from the Oslo study

The primary question asked in the present study is whether the Cognitive Training Programme adds anything to the psychosocial (psychoeducative) programme. We have examined two central WCST measures at baseline, at post-test (after 5 months of treatment), and at follow-up 1 year later. The results show an improvement in both groups' performance, but no difference in degree of performance between those who have received cognitive training and those who have not. The same pattern is evident for the Backward Masking task as well as the CPT. (Backward masking is a measure of early information processing.) The conclusion that can be drawn from these preliminary results is that the treatment (or the natural course of the illness) contributes to an improvement in patients' cognitive functioning. However, it is uncertain whether the cognitive training programme contributes specifically to the improvement.

The second question that can be asked at the present stage of the study is, 'Is it possible to improve patients' attentional performance (concentration) by intensive training over a week, and with monetary reinforcement and enhanced instructions added to the intervention?' Results indicate that span of apprehension can be improved by cognitive training (Ueland *et al.* 2003).

5 **Conclusions**

Considering the results from the studies of Hans Brenner, Will Spaulding, and Til Wykes, as well as the preliminary findings in our project, the following answers to the questions asked in this study emerge.

1 **Can basic cognitive functions be remediated?**

Yes, cognitive remediation works in the sense that it is possible to remediate cognitive dysfunctions in psychotic patients. What works is uncertain, however. Our preliminary results provide no basis for assuming that the cognitive training programme is more effective than the psychoeducational programme alone. This stands in a certain contrast to the findings of Will Spaulding and Til Wykes. It might be, however, that our psychoeducational therapy includes elements that are more effective in improving cognitive skills than the treatment given to the comparison groups in the two other studies. It is also possible that the number of training hours in The Oslo Cognitive Training Programme is not sufficient and needs to be increased in order to obtain significant results.

2 **Is it possible to generalize training effects to other functions, and register this by use of appropriate (cognitive and clinical) follow-up instruments?**

There is little evidence in the studies mentioned above for a generalizability of cognitive training.

3 **Is it possible to improve attentional skills by intensive Span training?**

Yes, more intensive training sessions, combined with reinforcement, are effective in improving concentration (continuous focusing of attention). This has been shown in the present study, as well as in several previous studies (Koh *et al.* 1976; Hermanutz and Gestrich 1991; Kern *et al.* 1995). The challenge is to determine how to obtain lasting results which have an impact on the patient's daily functioning.

We have learned that it is difficult to carry out a systematic and consistent cognitive training programme in a clinical setting.

◆ It is difficult to be totally sure that the treatment provided to the two patient groups is in accordance with the therapy manuals.

◆ It is also very difficult to determine the effects of neuroleptics. It would be impossible, for ethical reasons, either to withdraw all patients from antipsychotic medication or to give all patients a standard dosage of medicines.

◆ Further, the researcher cannot require that all patients be on the same drug and the same dosage over a treatment period that lasts for at least 18 months.

Should the 'experiment' of cognitive remediation of psychotic patients continue? In my opinion, the answer is yes. We have sufficient positive results to support this conclusion. We have not received any reports of negative results or negative consequences of cognitive training. More data and new analyses of which variables are related to each other might throw light on which factors are influencing cognitive functions. Most probably, the improvement found in our study cannot be attributed to the inherent process of the illness alone (spontaneous remission), independent of the treatment received. We have sufficient empirical evidence that the typical course of schizophrenia is one with many relapses, in which the level of patients' social and cognitive functioning goes up and down. With a longitudinal design such as ours, with patient assessment at intervals of 5 and 18 months, there is reason to assume that no improvement would have been found on the average for the group if no treatment factors had been influencing cognitive functioning.

It is important to remediate cognitive dysfunctions in patients with schizophrenia. Treatment programmes that do not take cognitive functions into consideration are of limited interest and value. From this point of view, there are no alternatives to cognitive training programmes at the present time. Therefore, it is necessary to further develop useful therapeutic interventions. The only way to do this is to gather empirical evidence for what works in this connection and what does not work. From a clinical perspective, it is warranted to individualize the cognitive training programmes for each patient according to the deficits disclosed through baseline assessments. A related challenge is to find out which patients benefit from cognitive training and which do not.

In order to answer these and related questions it may be necessary to undertake case studies. However, research based on individualized therapeutic interventions continues to be problematic. Thus, a first step in creating evidence-based therapy for patients with schizophrenia—to assess what works and what does not work—seems to be controlled-effect studies in which the effects of therapeutic programmes/manuals are studied at a group level.

Selective references

American Psychiatric Association. (1994). *Diagnostic and statistical manual of mental disorders.* 4th edn. American Psychiatric Association, Washington, DC.

Adams, H.E., Malatesta, W., Brandley, P.J., *et al.* (1981). Modification of cognitive procesesses: a case study of schizophrenia. *J. Consult. Clin. Psychol* **49**, 460–4.

Andreasen, N.C. (1999). A unitary model of schizophrenia. Bleuler's 'Fragmented Phrene' as schizencephaly. *Arch. Gen. Psychiatry.* **56**, 781–6.

Attkisson, C., Crook, J., Karno, M., *et al.* (1992). Clinical services, research. *Schiz. Bull.* **18**, 561–626.

Beck, A.T., Rush, A.J., Shaw, B.J., *et al.* (1979). *Cognitive therapy of depression.* Wiley, Chichester.

Bellack, A.S, Blanchard, J.J., Murphy, P., *et al.* (1996). Generalization effects of training on the Wisconsin Card Sorting Test for schizophrenia patients. *Schizophren. Res.* **19**, 189–94.

Bellack, A.S., Gold, J.M., and Buchanan, R.W. (1999). Cognitive rehabilitation for schizophrenia: problems, prospects, and strategies. *Schizophren. Bull.* **25**, 257–74.

Benedict, R.H.B., Harris, A.E., Markow, T., *et al.* (1994). The effects of attention training on information processing in schizophrenia. *Schizophren. Bull.* **20**, 537–46.

Bentall, R.P., Haddock, G., and Slade, P.D. (1994). Cognitive behaviour therapy for persistent auditory hallucinations: from theory to therapy. *Behav. Ther.* **25**, 51–66.

Brenner, H.D., Hodel, B., Roder, V., *et al.* (1992). Treatment of cognitive dysfunctions and behavioural deficits. *Schizophren. Bull.* **18**, 21–6.

Brenner, H., Roder, W., Hodel, B., *et al.* (1995). *Integrated psychological therapy for schizophrenic patients.* Hogrefe and Huber, Bern.

Fowler, D. (1992). Cognitive behaviour therapy in management of patients with schizophrenia. Preliminary studies. In *Psychotherapy of schizophrenia: facilitating an abstractive factor* (ed. A. Verbart *et al.*), pp. 145–53. Scandinavian University Press, Oslo.

Fowler, D. and Morley, S. (1989). The cognitive behavioural treatment of hallucinations and delusions: a preliminary study. *Behav. Psychother.* **17**, 267–82.

Garety, P.A., Kuipers, L., Fowler, D., *et al.* (1994). Cognitive behavioural therapy for drug resistant psychosis. *Br. J. Med. Psychol.* **67**, 259–71.

Green, M.F. (1998). *Schizophrenia from a neurocognitive perspective.* Probing the impenetrable darkness. Allyn and Bacon, Boston.

Green, M.F. and Nuechterlein, K. (1999). Should schizophrenia be treated as a neurocognitive disorder? *Schizophren. Bull.* **25**, 309–19.

Hermanutz, M. and Gestrich, J. (1991). Computer-assisted attention training in schizophrenics. A comparative study. *Eur. Arch. Psychiatry Clin. Neurosci.* **240**, 282–7.

Hodel, B. and Brenner, H.D. (1994). Cognitive therapy with schizophrenic patients: conceptual basis, present state, future directions. *Acta Psychiatrica Scand.* **90**, (suppl. 384), 108–15.

Hogarty, G.E. and Flesher, S. (1999). Developmental theory for a cognitive enhancement therapy of schizophrenia. *Schizophren. Bull.* **25**, 677–92.

Kern, R.S., Green, M.F., and Goldstein, M.F. (1995). Modification of performance on the span of apprehension, a putative marker of vulnerability to schizophrenia. *J. Abnorm. Psychol.* **104**, 385–409.

Kingdon, D.G. and Turkington, D. (1994). *Cognitive–behavioural therapy of schizophrenia.* Guilford Press, Hillside, New Jersey.

Klosterkøtter, J. and Schultze-Lutter, F. (2000). Diagnosing schizophrenia in the initial prodomal phase [abstract]. *Schiz. Res.* **41**, 10.

Koh, S.D., Kayton, L., and Peterson, R.A. (1976). Affective encoding and consequent remembering in schizophrenic young adults. *J. Abnorm. Psychol.* **85**, 56–166.

Lehman, A.F., Carpenter, W.T., Goldman, H.H., *et al.* (1995). Treatment outcomes in schizophrenia: implication for practice, policy and research. *Schizophren. Bull.* **21**, 669–74.

Medalia, A., Aluma, M., Tryon, W., *et al.* (1998). Effectiveness of attention training in schizophrenia. *Schizophren. Bull.* **24**, 147–52.

Olbrich, R., Voss, E., Mussgay, L., *et al.* (1993). A weighted time budget approach for the assessment of cognitive and social activities. *Soc. Psychiatric Epidemiol.* **28**, 184–8.

Perris, C. (1989). *Cognitive therapy for patients with schizophrenia.* Cassel, New York.

Rund, B.R. and Borg, N.C. (1999). Cognitive deficits and cognitive training in schizophrenic patients: a review. *Acta Psychiatrica Scand.* **99**, 1–12.

Rund, B.R., Moe, L., Sollien, T., *et al.* (1994). The Psychosis Project: outcome and cost-effectiveness of a psychoeducational treatment programme for schizophrenic adolescents. *Acta Psychiatrica Scand.* **89**, 211–18.

Sharma, T. (1999). Cognitive effects of conventional and atypical antipychotics in schizophrenia. *Br. J. Psychiatry.* **174** (suppl. 38), 44–51.

Silverstein, S.M., Menditto, A.A., and Stuve, P. (2001). Shaping attention span: an operant conditioning procedure to improve neurocognition and functioning in schizophrenia. *Schizophren. Bull.* **27**, 247–57.

Spaulding, W.D., Reed, D., Sullivan, M., *et al.* (1999). Effects of cognitive treatment in psychiatric rehabiliation. *Schizophren. Bull.* **25**, 657–76.

Suslow, T., Schonauer, K., and Arolt, V. (2001). Attention training in the cognitive rehabilitation of schizophrenic patients: a review of efficacy studies. *Acta Psychiatrica Scand.* **103**, 15–23.

Ueland, T., Rund, B.R., Borg, N.E., *et al.* (2004). Modification of performance on the span of apprehension task in a group of young people with early onset psychosis. *Scand. J. Psychol.*, **45**(1): 55–60.

Van der Gaag, M. (1992). *The results of cognitive training in schizophrenic patients.* Eburon Publishers, Delft.

Wykes, T., Reeder, C., Corner, J., *et al.* (1999). The effects of neurocognitive remediation on executive processing in patients with schizophrenia. *Schizophren. Bull.* **25**, 291–307.

Chapter 35

Treatment and rehabilitation of neuropsychiatric disorders

Laura H. Goldstein

1 Introduction

This chapter will consider some of the issues and provide a number of guidelines when considering the psychological treatments of neuropsychiatric disorders. Neuropsychiatry itself has been defined in a number of ways (Seli and Shapiro 1997) but for present purposes is best conceptualized as 'an aspect of psychiatry that seeks to advance the understanding of clinical problems through increased knowledge of brain function and structure' (Lishman 1992) and, as indicated by Lishman (1992), neuropsychiatry has greater applicability to some forms of mental illness than others. In practice, neuropsychiatry services tend to see three broad categories of patients:

- those whose psychiatric disorders result from clearly identifiable brain dysfunction;
- patients with psychiatric problems with neurological comorbidity;
- patients who present with neurological symptoms in the absence of underlying neurological disease (Lishman 1992).

It is towards the third of these groups of patients that psychological interventions are most likely to be targeted and therefore most attention will be given to these conditions within this chapter. However, since neurological and psychiatric disorders are clearly not mutually exclusive, issues relevant to the treatment of one class of disorders may be applicable to the other.

2 Assessment

Previous chapters have described some of the neuropsychiatric conditions and investigations necessary to enable the clinician to arrive at a neuropsychiatric diagnosis. However, when commencing treatment, further assessment by the clinical psychologist will inevitably be necessary in order to document the nature of the thought pattern that may be problematic (e.g. in depression, where the patient will be required, in a cognitive behavioural therapy framework, to record negative automatic thoughts as well as activity schedules), the patient's psychophysiological disturbance, or the frequency or pattern of occurrence of the behaviour that is to be changed (e.g. challenging behaviour after head injury or tics in Tourette's syndrome). Even pharmacological treatments of disorders will require good baseline recording of the behaviour or thought pattern to be changed so that clinical psychologists' skills in this area can also contribute to the careful evaluation of treatment efficacy.

2.1 The antecedents–behaviour–consequences (A–B–C) model

In terms of behavioural assessments, the classical approaches to functional analysis remain valuable (cf Goldstein 2003). The simplest of these is the A–B–C model, which assesses the antecedents and setting events of the behaviour, the behaviour itself, and the consequences of the behaviour. This can be applied to challenging behaviour (e.g. aggression following closed head injury) or brief dissociative events such as non-epileptic seizures (see Section 4.2.4), although it would be less commonly applied to the assessment of psychiatric symptoms such as might be present in delusional disorders. However, the A–B link might be worthy of consideration in attempting to examine any potential relationship between psychotic phenomena (the 'behaviour' in this example) and the occurrence of epileptic activity (the 'antecendent' in this example) in individuals being investigated with respect to the possible diagnosis of a post-ictal psychosis.

2.2 Other models of functional analysis

- Other models of functional analysis (e.g. Gardner 1971) extend the area of enquiry to the *interrelationship between problem behaviours*, and the therapist will need to become aware of the broader environment in which the patient exists and identify the resources available to the person to assist in treatment as well as the factors that might exert aversive control over them and their behaviour.

- *Motivational analysis* can also be used to increase the likelihood of treatment success (Kanfer and Saslow 1969), and to identify behavioural strengths as well as weaknesses that can help maximize the opportunities for facilitating progress in therapy (Yule 1987).

- The therapist should also consider *developmental factors* (relevant biological, sociological, and behavioural changes that have occurred in the person's life) since these may also impact on therapy and its likely outcome, as may the interrelationship between the social, cultural, and physical aspects of the person's life.

- It has also become common to consider the *predisposing, precipitating,* and *perpetuating factors* that account for a patient's problems (e.g. Mayou *et al.* 1995; Sharpe *et al.* 1995a).

- Further insight into the nature of the behaviour and the pattern of its occurrence can be gained through the use of *analogue conditions* where the possible A–B–C relationships can be manipulated (e.g. Iwata *et al.* 1982).

- During treatment using cognitive behavioural therapy, the use of *behavioural experiments*, where the validity of patients' automatic thoughts can be challenged, may be used to test out the content of their beliefs and then disconfirm them.

How behaviour is measured will to some extent depend on the behaviour itself and the resources available. For thought patterns, self-report is necessary. Within the context of cognitive-behavioural interventions self-observations and self-monitoring are important for the person to be able to understand the nature of the target behaviour or thought to be changed (Tazaki and Landlaw 2006). More generally for overt behaviours a variety of techniques exists, each with their advantages and disadvantages (Murphy 1987). Wherever possible the clinician should use measures with proven validity and reliability so that the extent of change can be estimated accurately.

3 Applying psychological interventions to neuropsychiatric disorders

3.1 The importance of awareness and insight

As discussed by Manchester and Wood (2000), cognitive behavioural therapy has been applied to a range of psychiatric disorders in which the awareness of, or insight into, the inappropriate behaviour or thoughts might be sufficient to facilitate change in the person's thoughts and behaviour, via therapy. With respect to psychiatric disorders, insight might be conceived as awareness by the person that they are suffering from a mental disturbance that may constitute an illness and acceptance of the resulting medical implications and of the need for treatment (Surguladze and David 1999). As Surguladze and David (1999) indicate, insight is not considered as an 'all-or-none' phenomenon but rather a dimensional one, with individuals having varying levels of awareness of their condition. Understanding cultural variations in insight and belief systems is likely to be important when attempting to facilitate patients' engagement in mental health services (Saravanan et al. 2007).

As Manchester and Wood (2000) note, impaired awareness is an important characteristic of many neuropsychiatric disorders, and as such has implications for the access to and continued contact with services, relapse rates, and morbidity (Kent and Yellowlees 1994; Kemp and David 1995). Husted (1999), defining insight in terms of awareness of having an illness, attributing one's symptoms to the illness, and acknowledging the need for treatment, observes that one of the difficulties in delivering continuous voluntary treatment for people with severe mental illnesses is that these disorders reflect disrupted brain function and in turn affect the person's reasoning ability so that they often do not believe that they are ill or that their illness will respond to pharmacological (or other) treatments.

Impaired insight is frequently found in schizophrenia and is also of importance in bipolar disorder (Husted 1999). It is worth noting that insight in bipolar disorder has been shown to be more severely affected than has insight in affective disorders (Michalakeas et al. 1994; Ghaemi et al. 1995). Importantly, insight may not recover with treatment (Peralta and Cuesta 1998). The clinician should be aware that insight may be impaired in other neuropsychiatric disorders such as obsessive–compulsive disorder (Eisen et al. 1994) and anorexia nervosa (Feighner et al. 1972) and thus the concept is relevant to those undertaking therapy with a wide range of patients. Indeed, data have indicated that patients with Body Dysmorphic Disorder show greater impairment of insight than do patients with Obsessive Compulsive Disorder (Eisen *et al.* 2004).

The clinician should recognize that insight, or lack of it, cannot be simply related to neuropsychological test performance, as the results from a number of studies across different disorders are contradictory (Surguladze and David 1999). Data have suggested that cognitive abilities, whether one is focusing on executive function or more general abilities, may nonetheless be related to measures of insight and to specific activities that require the person to undertake cognitively demanding introspection into particular aspects of their own mental life (Surguladze and David 1999). More recently, Lysaker *et al.* (2006) reported that when considering different domains of insight, awareness of symptoms and treatment need were associated with scores on measures of executive function that particularly involved alternating attention, planning and the ability to derive meaning on the basis of contextual cues. As noted by Surguladze and David (1999), a number of approaches to the assessment of insight in psychiatric disorders have been developed (e.g. McEvoy *et al.* 1989; Amador and Strauss 1990; David 1990; Markova and Berrios 1992; Birchwood *et al.* 1994; Kemp and David 1997) and this may make the elucidation of consistent relationships more difficult. It is widely accepted that lack of awareness or insight is a common feature of people who have sustained brain damage, whether of a traumatic or of a neurodegenerative nature (Migliorelli *et al.* 1995; Zanetti *et al.* 1999). The integrity of insight or awareness has been shown to relate to the success of neurorehabilitation (Ben-Yishay and Gold 1990; Prigatano 1991) although some inconsistencies have been noted, possibly relating to differences in measuring or defining insight and outcome (Malia 1997). Of clinical relevance also are recent observations that individuals may be unaware of some deficits but not others (Dalla Barba *et al.* 1999).

The presence or otherwise of insight may also be relevant to the development of depression in patients with brain damage. Pewter *et al.* (2007) review literature indicating that depression may occur once patients become aware of their impairments and of their inability to function at their premorbid level. They also raise an alternative possibility, (cf. Prigatano 1997, cited Fleminger *et al.* 2003) namely that increased levels of insight permit the brain-damaged individual to deal with their problems more effectively and therefore protect against depression. In a group of encephalitis patients of mixed aetiology, Pewter *et al.* (2007) found that the accuracy of patients' appraisal of their everyday difficulties was important in determining whether or not they were depressed, with more accurate appraisals being associated with lower levels of depression. Their data suggest that once the process involved in changing awareness of deficits has occurred, the development of an accurate appraisal of difficulties may be beneficial in the longer term.

Manchester and Wood (2000) suggest that whilst most therapeutic interventions can be modified to accommodate poor memory, attention, and concentration, it is the need to overcome poor awareness, and also poor motivation that may often be the crucial factor in bringing about treatment success. Issues relating to motivation will be considered next.

3.2 **Motivation to change**

Manchester and Wood (2000) have suggested a pivotal role for the establishment of a good therapeutic relationship as a means of increasing both the awareness of people with brain damage concerning their problems and their motivation to change. They stress the importance of therapist variables such as warmth, support, empathy, non-judgemental attitude, and the expectation that change will occur (Leber and Jenkins 1996). They also emphasize the need for therapists to understand their patients' thinking patterns and to engage in a collaborative rather than confrontational approach to therapy. Although there is no supportive empirical evidence to date, they favour the use of motivational interviewing as a means of raising questions about the viability of the person's thinking and behaviour. They also note that it may be useful, in line with Miller and Rolnick (1991), to consider motivation for change in people with brain damage as something that fluctuates over time and across situations. The potential use of a motivational approach for people with cognitive impairment has also obtained some support from its, albeit limited, application in the field of learning disabilities (Rose and Walker 2000).

3.2.1 A six-stage model of change

Manchester and Wood (2000) outline and recommend the use of Prochaska and DiClemente's (1982) six-stage model of change in providing a useful guide to therapy, both from the point of developing awareness of problems, and increasing motivation to change. These stages are:

- the *pre-contemplation stage* where others are aware that there is a problems but the patient has not yet considered the possibility of changing;
- the *contemplation stage* where the patient is aware of the need to change but may feel ambivalence over this;
- the *determination stage* where the patient decides to take action;
- the *action stage* where the patient undertakes activities to achieve change;
- the *maintenance stage* where additional skills are learned to prevent relapse;
- the *relapse stage* where the patient learns to cope with relapse.

Manchester and Wood (2000) illustrate the use of this model with two patients with very different behavioural problems following acquired brain injury.

With respect to one of these cases, the individual had sustained severe cognitive impairment and therapy was designed to increase his motivation to stop absconding from the treatment unit in response to negative feedback from staff about his sexually inappropriate behaviour.

- The *pre-contemplation* and *contemplation* stages involved first asking the patient why he absconded and what the consequences (positive and negative) of this were, with respect both to the short and longer term. Where negative consequences could not be identified explicitly, the patient was asked to describe how the events following his absconding made him feel.

- The *determination* and *action* stages of treatment involved facilitating the generation of longer-term goals by the patient and his commitment to attempt alternative behaviour in order to achieve these. In this case the longer-term goal was to achieve discharge from the unit and alternative behaviours included more appropriate ways of responding to criticism by unit staff. The process was then reviewed by the therapist and by the patient; the patient was asked to state the behavioural trigger, the old response and its negative consequences, and the new response and its positive consequences. The patient's commitment to change was praised, the difficulty involved in changing behaviour was acknowledged, and the need for practice to achieve the consistent establishment of the new responses was emphasized.

- The *maintenance* stage involved the development of a verbal script for the patient to employ and role-play exercises.

- Finally instances of *relapse* were used to identify difficulties the patient experienced in applying the new behaviours and these were incorporated into role-play exercises.

Other approaches to increasing awareness do exist, however (cf. Malia 1997), and formal evaluation of such approaches will ultimately guide the therapist's choice of techniques. It may also be necessary to bear in mind that it is sometimes difficult to distinguish between the lack of awareness of deficits due to clear evidence of brain damage and the use of denial as a defence mechanism (Malia 1997; Manchester and Wood 2000). Both Malia (1997), and Manchester and Wood (2000) highlight the need for clinicians to consider that both psychological factors and the direct impact of brain damage may interact to produce the level of awareness that is apparent in an individual patient.

4 The application of cognitive behavioural therapy to neuropsychiatric disorders

4.1 Disorders with an identifiable organic basis

Relatively little attention has been paid to the application of cognitive behavioural techniques to neuropsychiatric disorders in which the associated cognitive impairment might itself necessitate modification of the techniques in use, (but see Chapter 34). Manchester and Wood (2000) suggest that where there is cognitive impairment:

- The clinician may need to make therapy sessions more highly structured;

- The sessions may need to occur with greater frequency.

- The sessions might need to deal with more specific behaviours, possibly in a more concrete way.

In addition:

- It may be necessary to adapt therapy techniques and materials to overcome a person's memory or reading impairments (e.g. Newsom-Davis *et al.* 1998), and the clinician should take note of findings from neuropsychological assessments that have been undertaken.

- ◆ Where an assessment of cognitive functions has not been done, such an assessment may be of value in order for therapy to be delivered most effectively.

- ◆ Behavioural experiments may provide concrete feedback to an individual that may lead to balanced appraisals and may also highlight the impact of neuropsychological deficits on everyday function (Dewar and Gracey 2007)

However, in general, there is little to guide the clinician as to when cognitive and neurological signs might predict poor response to treatment. For example, neuropsychological abnormalities and neurological soft signs in adults with obsessive–compulsive disorder did not predict a poor response to behavioural treatment (Bolton *et al.* 2000). Similarly, no data yet exist to indicate whether cerebral activation abnormalities detected in a patient with conversion disorder (Marshall *et al.* 1997) might have any implications for treatment.

In the field of adult mental health, cognitive behaviour therapy (CBT) has been widely applied to people with depression and various anxiety disorders (e.g. Hawton *et al.* 1989) and is also now being applied to disorders such as schizophrenia and bipolar disorder where insight or awareness of difficulties may be an issue (e.g. Kuipers *et al.* 1998; Lam *et al.* 2003).

- ◆ Kuipers *et al.* (1998) reported that 9 months of CBT, directed at medication-resistant symptoms of *psychosis*, led to a reduction in the distress caused by delusions and in the frequency of hallucinations, with the improvement persisting at an 18-month follow-up. They reported clinical improvements in 65% of the CBT group and in only 17% of the standard care group.

- ◆ More generally, family interventions (especially those aimed at a single family) appear effective in preventing psychotic relapses and hospital readmissions, as well as improving medication compliance; CBT has been shown to produce greater 'important improvement' in mental state than other treatments, and appears to be associated with low drop-out rates (Pilling *et al.* 2002).

- ◆ With respect to *bipolar affective disorder*, Lam *et al.* (2003) demonstrated the effectiveness of CBT which incorporated:

  — a psychoeducational model, emphasising the need for combined medical and psychological therapy;

  — using CBT skills to monitor mood and enable people to cope with prodromes and change their behaviour to prevent prodromal symptoms from developing into full-blown episodes;

  — emphasizing the importance of routine and sleep, and

  — the monitoring of behaviours that compensated for lost time due to previous episodes of illness.

In comparison to patients undergoing standard care, patients who were allocated to CBT (undertaken during 12–18 sessions over the first six months and two booster sessions in the second six-month period) had fewer bipolar episodes, days in a bipolar episode and number of admissions for this type of episode. They also had higher social functioning than the standard care group.

- From a broader perspective, successful applications of psychological treatments for bipolar disorder are those that appear to contain psychoeducational components that focus on enhancing compliance and early identification of prodromal signs (Colom and Lam 2005).

However, there are few formal evaluations of the use of CBT to treat affective disorders in patient groups where there is clear evidence of acquired organic pathology such as might be present in disorders more typically presenting with neurological sequelae.

- Davis *et al.* (1984) applied CBT in a group format to a small number of patients with epilepsy, who showed a subsequent reduction in depression scores on various measures.

- Larcombe and Wilson (1984), in an early study, demonstrated the effectiveness of brief, group-based, weekly CBT sessions in reducing depression in a sample of patients with multiple sclerosis (MS) for whom depression was the major problem, and at least of moderate severity.

- While not focusing specifically on depression, Benedict *et al.* (2000) demonstrated that 12 weeks of 'Neuropsychological Compensatory Training' (which set out to use psychoeducational and cognitive-behavioural methods to increase MS patients' and carers' understanding of cognitive, behavioural and personality change) was superior to 12 weeks of non-specific supportive psychotherapy in reducing scores on a measure of social aggression (and in particular excessive egocentric speech); a non-significant reduction in depression scores was found.

- In their Cochrane review, Thomas *et al.* (2006) concluded that existing evidence supports the potential benefit of cognitive-behavioural interventions in the treatment of depression or to generally facilitate coping in people with MS, despite a lack of good randomized controlled trials and manualised treatments.

In neither Davies *et al.*'s (1984) nor Larcome and Wilson's (1984) studies was it reported that the CBT required modification in response to any cognitive difficulties of the participants. When designing cognitive behavioural interventions to treat mood disorders in patients with organic disorders, it will be important however, to consider whether the nature of depressive symptomatology might differ between diseases. Thus, for example, in MS where depression may be under-recognised and under-treated (Ghaffar and Feinstein 2007), irritability, frustration and discouragement are more typical than feelings of guilt and low-self esteem (Minden *et al.* 1987). Similarly, in Parkinson's disease, Cole and Vaughan (2005) have suggested that the presence or otherwise of cognitive symptoms of depression will have implications for the cognitive model of depression applied (in the case of the individual patient), and the focus of therapy.

The mechanisms potentially underlying the development of depression in Parkinson's disease have been summarized by Cole and Vaughan (2005). Using an A-B design with a one-month follow-up, they report a brief, home-based application of CBT with five people with Parkinson's disease; four patients showed a clinically meaningful reduction of depressive symptoms, with the greatest reduction seen in the two people who had been most severely depressed prior to therapy. In their study, in which therapy was based around a structured self-help therapy booklet for people with Parkinson's disease (Beck 2000), they raise a number of issues:

- the slowness of processing speed that is characteristic of Parkinson's disease may affect a person's ability to process information during therapy;
- it is important to hold therapy sessions when anti-Parkinsonian medication is having its maximum effect; so that "off" periods should be avoided;
- it may be necessary to modify therapy to take account of patients' cognitive deficits although there is little evidence on how best to do this;
- medically ill people with less severe depression may show less benefit from CBT in comparison to those who are more severely depressed, and may not maintain therapeutic benefits;
- in conditions such as Parkinson's disease where physical activity may be limited by the severity of the illness, more research is needed to indicate the relevance of physical activity for therapy to achieve a reduction in depressed mood.

Focusing on other neurologically-impaired adults, Lincoln *et al.* (1997) reported a number of A–B single-case designs employing CBT with depressed stroke patients, comparing the results of no more than 10 sessions of treatment within a 3-month period, with baseline. Of the 19 patients treated, only eight were noted to show definite (although modest) improvement. Lincoln *et al.*'s (1997) findings would appear to indicate that:

- stroke patients with intercurrent illness and further stroke might not benefit from treatment;
- patients with impaired memory and reasoning abilities might be less able to understand the concepts underpinning the treatment and therefore might have difficulty applying them independently.

Thus clinicians should bear these difficulties in mind when planning the use of effective CBT for stroke patients. However, clinicians should remember the benefits of facilitating increased leisure activities in improving psychological well-being after stroke if formal CBT proves difficult to implement (Drummond and Walker 1996).

4.2 Medically unexplained disorders

4.2.1 The nature of the problem

Neuropsychiatry services may deal with a range of patients presenting with physical or cognitive disorders for which no medical basis can ultimately be detected, or that are in excess of what is known about the person's medical disorder. These medically unexplained disorders would not include recognized psychiatric symptoms such as delusions and hallucinations.

Within the *Diagnostic and statistical manual of mental disorders*, 4th edition (DSM-IV; American Psychiatric Association 1994) such disorders come within the classifications of somatoform disorders (e.g. somatization disorder, conversion disorder, hypochondriasis), factitious disorders, and dissociative disorders. The clinician should be aware that there is ongoing debate about the extent to which such classifications are adequate (Rief and Hiller 1999). In addition, the terminology itself has been questioned (Sharpe *et al.* 1995*b*). Within ICD-10 (World Health Organisation 1992) disorders of interest here, such as dissociative non-epileptic seizures, are classified within the category of dissociative (conversion) disorders.

It is well recognized that medically unexplained disorders pose a sizeable problem for medical services (e.g. Mayou *et al.* 1995; Bass *et al.* 2001; Nimnuan *et al.* 2001). It is estimated that approximately one third of somatic symptoms seen in primary care, population studies and in neurological clinics are 'medically unexplained' (cf. Kroenke 2003; Stone *et al.* 2005). It is worth remembering that patients referred to specialist tertiary services with somatoform or conversion disorders may experience very severe levels of disability in the absence of any underlying organic disorder (Davison *et al.* 1999) or present with symptoms, only some of which will have a clear medical explanation. Here treatment can be useful in enabling the patient to distinguish between those symptoms that are disease-based and those that have a psychological basis (Sharpe *et al.* 1992). However, it is likely that specialist services will see only a fraction of patients with such presentations (Mayou *et al.* 1995).

4.2.2 Expanatory mechanisms

Tazaki and Landlaw (2006) have outlined how somatoform disorders may be explained in terms of the processes underpinning classical (respondent) and operant conditioning, which may in turn inform the design of therapeutic interventions. Within classical (respondent) conditioning, they suggest that

- in the context of a traumatic experience that gives rise to a negative emotional state such as anger or fear, and which is accompanied by physiological changes, the trauma is an unconditional stimulus (UCS), and the emotional and physiological responses are the unconditional response (UCR);

- repeated presentation of any situation that is similar to the UCS, or that represents part of it, becomes a conditional stimulus (CS), produces a similar emotional state and physiological responses, and gives rise to what become conditional responses (CRs);

- these emotional and physiological responses include a range of symptoms of autonomic arousal.

Within the context of operant conditioning, Tazaki and Landlaw (2006) remind the reader that:

- behaviours are likely to increase in terms of frequency of occurrence if they are followed by what the person views as a positive outcome (i.e. the behaviour is positively reinforced);

- behaviours that allow the person to avoid an undesirable situation will increase in frequency (negative reinforcement);
- this will lead to the occurrence of avoidance behaviour (or, when the fear of the situation is not quite so severe that the person avoids it completely), in the performance of 'safety behaviours'.

Tazaki and Landlaw (2006) indicate how a combination of classical and operant conditioning processes may serve not only to allow a condition to develop, but also to be maintained.

4.2.3 Approaches to treatment

Although not always based on explicit learning theory models (as described above), there is increasing evidence that cognitive behavioural approaches may be of considerable value in treating a number of such disorders (Kroenke and Swindle 2000); however there has been relatively little systematic evaluation of the benefits of psychodynamic psychotherapy (Sharpe *et al.* 1995*a*). Nonetheless, Guthrie (1995) has outlined treatment considerations of relevance to psychodynamic psychotherapists working with patients with functional somatic disorders. Other therapeutic approaches for somatization disorder have included behaviour therapy, exploratory psychotherapy, and group psychotherapy (cf. Wilkinson and Mynors-Wallis 1994). With respect to conversion disorders, where patients present with symptoms that appear to be neurological in nature (e.g. weakness, paralysis, dysphonia, sensory impairment, or memory deficits), the treatment emphasis (within relatively limited studies), appears to be predominantly behavioural (Silver 1996), and the consideration of psychosocial factors also seems crucial. It is likely however, that cognitive behavioural therapy will also be applicable to this group of patients (Halligan *et al.* 2000).

Sharpe *et al.* (1992) described the psychological treatment of what they call functional somatic symptoms, and Speckens *et al.* (1995) described the additional and successful use of CBT in treating what has more recently been termed 'medically unexplained symptoms' (which appear to include somatization disorder).

Cognitive behavioural treatments for these different disorders vary somewhat, but also share common features. It is likely that the aims considered by the clinician will be:

- reducing the patient's stress and disability;
- decreasing the patient's symptoms;
- limiting inappropriate use of medical and other care (Sharpe *et al.* 1992).

4.2.4 Issues to consider when implementing treatment

Prior to treatment by a clinical psychologist or other psychotherapist such patients are likely to have undergone medical investigations for their symptoms. Bass and Benjamin (1993) have suggested that maintenance of symptoms for longer than 6 months would justify describing the person's disorder as chronic, and given the time that many medical investigations may take to organize, clinicians may well find that they are indeed being asked to treat patients whose symptoms appear to fall in this category.

The task facing the clinician embarking on psychological interventions with such patients will depend in part on the prior medical approach the patient has experienced. Bass and Benjamin (1993) suggest that patients require unambiguous information about the results of their medical investigations, and there should be a limit set for the range of investigations which may be appropriate (if possible negotiated and agreed between doctor and patient). They highlight the difficulty posed by doctors worrying about failing to find a treatable medical disorder, but not about missing a treatable psychological problem.

- Patients should come for psychological treatment having been told clearly what illness(es) they do and do not have, and the symptoms and disability that will and will not be attributable to any such illnesses.

- They should come for treatment already knowing that they are to see someone who will be treating their disorder from a psychological perspective, not from a medical one (Bass and Benjamin 1993).

- This should be preceded by a clear account given to the patient to indicate that all necessary investigations have been undertaken. It would be unwise to embark upon a psychological intervention whilst medical investigations are continuing, as it is important that a certainty about diagnosis can be reached, and that the patient can be given an unambiguous account of the aetiology of their disorder, prior to the commencement of treatment.

Despite these recommendations, it is often unclear to the clinician undertaking the psychological intervention exactly what patients have previously been told about the medical basis or otherwise of their condition. Indeed, some patients will perceive that they have been incorrectly referred for psychological treatment, believing that their problems continue to have a physical basis (Salkovskis 1989). They may also be concerned about the stigma attached to having a psychiatric or psychological as opposed to medical diagnosis (House 1995).

- The clinician should seek early clarification from the referring doctor as to what the patient was told prior to referral. It will be important for the treating clinician to understand the basis on which the patient's diagnosis was made so that a consistent explanation can be given to the patient during therapy and any persisting erroneous beliefs can be corrected (Sharpe et al. 1995a).

- It may be appropriate for one person to coordinate all the different aspects of the patient's care (medical and psychological) (Sharpe et al. 1992; Bass and Benjamin 1993) so that throughout the patient receives consistent explanations about their disorder as well as consistent approaches to treatment. This may be particularly relevant for patients with multiple somatic symptoms (e.g. Smith 1995).

- In addition, there ultimately needs to be a clear communication to the patient's general practitioner about the diagnosis and management (Davison et al. 1999) so that treatment is not undermined at this level of care provision.

In all cases, close liaison between the treating and referring teams is extremely important.

Where possible other, parallel treatments for the same symptoms should be terminated or at the very least suspended while the psychological intervention is underway (Sharpe *et al.* 1992). Withdrawal of medication, which in some instances may actually be having a detrimental effect on the person's condition, should be undertaken in consultation with the prescribing doctor (Salkovskis 1989). However, a role remains for antidepressant medication (Bass and Benjamin 1993).

In terms of treatment success, Bass and Benjamin (1993) review evidence which suggests that sociodemographic, pain-related, and psychological factors can predict treatment success. Thus age, employment, pain-related financial compensation, pain nature and history, and the extent of dysfunctional illness beliefs and beliefs about illness aetiology as well as mode of referral may all be relevant. However, it is also of considerable importance that the patient:

◆ engages in treatment;

◆ accepts that psychological/psychosocial factors are important in maintaining the problem;

◆ is willing and able to negotiate treatment goals.

4.2.5 The use of CBT with somatoform, factitious, and dissociative conversion disorders

A CBT approach to the treatment of these disorders will essentially be a collaborative one but, depending on the disorder, may require differing numbers of sessions. The essence will be to formulate the person's problems in psychological terms even when their occurrence is complicated by the presence of an existing medical condition (Salkovskis 1989). The clinician needs to remember that the patient may have been used to a more passive role, undergoing medical tests and taking medication (Sharpe *et al.* 1992), and thus may need time to adjust to playing a more active role in their own treatment. As with any psychotherapeutic intervention it will be important for the clinician to establish a good working relationship with the patient, provide a plausible treatment rationale, offer hope for improvement (as a cure may not be a realistic goal; Salkovskis 1989), and be sympathetic to the patient's worries (Sharpe *et al.* 1992).

In the case of dissociative, somatization, or conversion disorder, it will be important to:

◆ reassure the patient that they are not thought to be 'putting it on' but that their symptoms are real, especially if previous contacts with services have been characterized as dismissive of the patient's symptoms;

◆ determine whether the patient is misinterpreting bodily signs or symptoms as evidence of illness or whether they have misunderstood or misinterpreted what they have been told by doctors or others so that they perceive slight deviations from the norm as representing serious impairment (Salkovskis 1989).

In the case of factitious disorder, where there is deliberate production or feigning of physical or psychological symptoms, this being motivated by the adoption of the sick role, then therapy needs to assist patients to understand why they are acting in that way, in a non-judgemental manner (Kinsella 2001).

An important aspect of treatment will be for the clinician to involve the family members/carers, and to provide them with the same treatment rationale. This will allow for the involvement of a co-therapist, who can facilitate generalization of treatment strategies beyond the treatment session.

Somatization disorders The successful application of a CBT approach to the treatment of somatic symptoms has largely involved the identification and modification of dysfunctional automatic thoughts and the use of behavioural experiments to break the vicious cycle of the symptoms and their consequences (Speckens *et al.* 1995), with this treatment often taking place in specialist services and in-patient units (Bleichhardt *et al.* 2004). Such an approach is often more sophisticated in terms of its components than the previously described, more limited therapeutic approaches designed for use in primary care settings, involving reattribution and problem-solving (Goldberg *et al.* 1989; Wilkinson and Mynors-Wallis 1994). This latter treatment approach seemed to be most beneficial for those people:

- whose somatization had lasted for less than a year;
- who acknowledged prior to treatment that they had psychosocial problems;
- who suffered from anxiety disorders.

In the case of a more traditional CBT approach, clinicians might expect that patients with a high level of illness behaviour might have a relatively poor prognosis (Speckens *et al.* 1997).

Hypochondriasis (i.e. severe and persistent health anxiety) Whereas the clinician treating somatization disorders may be faced with the patient who needs to be reassured that the results of their medical investigations have proved negative, the effective use of CBT with a patient with hypochondriasis will need to enable the patient to identify clear evidence that their problem was health anxiety itself (Warwick *et al.* 1996). This may be important in preventing patients from becoming preoccupied with a new disease once they have successfully overcome their fears about the original illness (Warwick *et al.* 1996). Wattar *et al.* (2005) indicate that treatment requires the patient-specific development of a plausible explanation of how health anxiety and the processes that are maintaining it underpin the patient's problems and the testing out of this less threatening formulation of their disorder, using behavioural experiments. CBT for severe and persistent health anxiety can be effective when implemented in a routine clinical setting and not just in academic research centres (Wattar *et al.* 2005).

Factitious disorder Little guidance is available for the treatment of factitious disorder (used also to describe patients with what has also been termed 'pseudologia fantastica': e.g. Newmark *et al.* 1999, and Munchausen's syndrome, e.g. Fink and Jensen 1989). Certainly it is important to remember that factitious disorder can occur in the context of organic brain damage (e.g. Lawrie *et al.* 1993).

Within DSM-IV, factitious disorder is defined as involving the intentional production or feigning of physical or psychological signs or symptoms, the motivation for which is the assumption of the sick role and there are no external incentives (such as financial gain, avoiding legal responsibility, or improving physical well-being). This is in contrast to *malingering*, where the person again deliberately produces false or exaggerated physical or psychological symptoms but where the motivation is financial (including compensation for injury), evading legal responsibility, avoiding military duty or other forms of work, or obtaining drugs. It is worth pointing out that *factitious disorder* and *malingering* are usually considered to be mutually exclusive. However, there is increasing recognition that the engagement in deceptive behaviour could occur not only for financial benefit but also to maintain the sick role (Bass and Halligan, 2007). Both diagnoses (malingering and factitious disorder) are pejorative and incorrect diagnosis may carry severe financial and social consequences; nonetheless the accurate identification of what is purely conscious deception as opposed to entirely involuntary symptom production (as in conversion disorders) or behaviour that lies somewhere in between these two extremes, may pose a significant challenge for clinicians (Bass and Halligan 2007).

Indeed, a cognitive–behavioural perspective on factitious disorder suggests that, in such patients, the clinician may find the coexistence of symptoms of somatization, factitious disorder, and even malingering (Kinsella 2001). Kinsella (2001) discusses the use of nonpunitive confrontation in cases of factitious disorder. However, nonconfrontational (possibly 'face-saving') approaches may also be of use but require very consistent application by a multidisciplinary team. The clinician should be aware that confrontation may meet with different responses from patients, and Kinsella provides most guidance on the use of CBT with those factitious disorder patients who recognize that they need to stop their pattern of behaviour, are able to admit their need to stop this pattern, and seek help. He suggests that therapy should:

- help the person understand their behaviour;
- address face-saving issues and the benefits and disadvantages of revealing the true picture to family and other professionals;
- identify triggers for the behaviour;
- stress the disadvantages of repeated, often dangerous medical investigations.

In addition, Kinsella recommends that activity scheduling should be used to provide the person with a more pleasurable way of meeting their needs, and the patient's unhelpful cognitive schemas should be addressed. However, as yet there is no formal evaluation of such treatment to guide the clinician as to its effectiveness.

Dissociative conversion disorders In terms of the treatment of dissociative conversion disorders some preliminary evidence, drawn from an open trial of CBT in patients with dissociative non-epileptic seizures (Goldstein *et al.* 2004) indicates that CBT may offer a useful therapeutic model for these patients. Thus approaches similar to those described above for somatization disorders may be effective in reducing the occurrence of events that superficially resemble epileptic seizures but that do not have an organic basis, although at present there is a lack of published adequately-designed randomized controlled trials to demonstrate the use of psychological therapy for dissociative (non-epileptic) seizures (Brooks *et al.* 2007) and the field in general is viewed as one in which treatment development is needed (LaFrance and Barry 2005; LaFrance *et al.* 2006). Mellers (2005) has provided a helpful overview of how to manage such patients, emphasising that these patients can be difficult to engage, having probably had multiple prior contacts with medical services. Inherent in Mellers' (2005) approach are the following points:

- Patients with dissociative seizures will require a clear message that their attacks do not have an epileptic basis, and must have the reasons for this explained to them and to their carers/families. This explanation may require repeating on subsequent occasions.

- It is essential, however, that these patients are not made to feel that are 'mad' or that they have necessarily been fabricating their seizures; it should be acknowledged that they are real events, in that they are significant episodes of disturbed behaviour that are disruptive to the person's life and represent the expression of psychological distress (i.e. one should describe what they *do* have and a description of dissociation may be helpfully provided). At the point at which the diagnosis is presented (or treatment commenced) the underlying psychological triggers may not be/have been apparent, but if these and/or maintaining factors are identified these should be raised with the person.

- If the person has no history of actual epilepsy yet has previously been (incorrectly) prescribed anti-epileptic drugs (AEDs), then they should start a process of medically-supervised AED withdrawal; otherwise persistence with AEDs may, for the patient, represent a 'safety behaviour' in CBT terms and may continue to convey the message that the person has an organic disorder (i.e. epilepsy), as well as exposing them (and in the case of women of childbearing age, their offspring) to unnecessary potentially adverse (including teratogenic) effects from the medication.

While a percentage of patients with dissociative seizures will become seizure-free following diagnosis, engaging those patients who continue to have seizures in psychological treatment may require the therapist to adapt treatments for a range of psychological disorders, given the often complex histories and comorbid problems seen in this patient group. A detailed review of the potential application of different psychological treatment approaches to this patient group is provided by Reuber *et al.* (2005). More generally, however, from a CBT perspective (and see Goldstein *et al.* 2004):

- The treatment of this group of patients is collaborative in nature and will benefit from the involvement of other key people in the person's life to facilitate appropriate changes to behaviour outside of the treatment session, and to assist with exposure to situations and activities that the person had avoided through fear of having a seizure.

- Specific techniques may be used to distract the person from symptoms warning them that they might be about to experience a seizure and to encourage relaxation, thereby reducing symptoms of anxiety that might precede a seizure.

- Treatment would also involve the use of problem-solving techniques and the challenging of negative automatic thoughts.

- Additional problems that might lead to low mood or act as seizure triggers (including reminders of earlier trauma) require attention.
- As with all the other disorders discussed here the therapist needs to consider strategies to enable the patient to prevent relapse of their symptoms.

4.2.6 Treatment of somatic symptoms in older adults

Specific attention has also been paid to the treatment of somatic symptoms in older adults (Pearce and Morris 1995). In this area of work, clinicians will need to consider the many age-related changes that may influence symptoms found in the elderly. Thus, in an older age group, in particular, somatic symptoms may be wholly organic in origin, partially explained by disease, or completely functionally determined. In practice, it is more likely for older adults to present with a mixture of organically and functionally based symptoms than younger adults (Pearce and Morris 1995). Thus there will be an emphasis on determining whether the physical condition is a sufficient explanation for the level of disability experienced. In addition, it will be necessary to remember that physical failings can give rise to emotional distress, and early dementias can be accompanied by mood change and concerns over health. Pearce and Morris (1995) suggest that many of the treatment approaches used for somatoform disorders in younger adults may be appropriately modified for use with older adults.

5 **Conclusions**

Whether treating psychological disorders that have a purely organic basis, that are determined by organic and psychological factors, or that are purely psychological in their aetiology, the clinical psychologist working with a neuropsychiatric population has a number of treatment approaches to employ that require similarly good skills of problem assessment and formulation as well as engagement of what can be very difficult to treat patients. However, the refinement of treatment approaches will be ongoing and the clinician is advised to keep abreast of the rapidly accumulating literature relating to developments that continue to occur in this challenging area of clinical work.

Selective references

Amador, X.F. and Strauss, D.H. (1990). *The Scale to Assess Unawareness of Mental Disorders (SUMD)*. Columbia University and New York State Psychiatric Institute, New York.

American Psychiatric Association (1994). *Diagnostic and statistical manual of mental disorders*, 4th edn. American Psychiatric Association, Washington, DC.

Bass, C. and Benjamin, S. (1993). The management of chronic somatisation. *Br. J. Psychiatry* **162**, 472–80.

Bass, C. and Halligan, P.W. (2007). Illness related deception: Social or psychiatric problem? *J. Roy. Soc. Med.* **100**, 81–84.

Bass, C., Peveler, R., and House, A. (2001). Somatoform disorders: severe psychiatric illnesses neglected by psychiatrists. *Br. J. Psychiatry* **179**, 11–14.

Beck, J.S. (2000). *Coping with depression when you have Parkinson's disease*. Bala Cynwyd, PA: The Beck Institute for Cognitive Therapy and Research.

Benedict, R.H.B., Shapiro, A., Priore, R., Miller, C., Munschauer, F., and Jacobs, L. (2000). Neuropsychological counseling improves social behavior in cognitively-impaired multiple sclerosis patients. *Multiple Sclerosis.* **6**, 391–396.

Ben-Yishay, Y. and Gold, J. (1990). Therapeutic milieu approach to neuropsychological rehabilitation. In *Neurobehavioural sequelae of traumatic brain injury* (ed. R.L. Wood), pp. 194–215. Taylor and Francis Ltd, New York.

Birchwood, M., Smith, J., Drury, V., Healy, J., Macmillan, F., and Slade, M. (1994). A self-report Insight Scale for psychosis: reliability, validity and sensitivity to change. *Acta Psychiatrica Scand.* **89**, 62–7.

Bleichhardt, G., Timmer, B., and Rief, W. (2004). Cognitive-behavioural therapy for patients with multiple somatoform symptoms–a randomised controlled trial in tertiary care. *J. Psychosom. Res.* **56**, 449–54.

Bolton, D., Raven, P., Madronal-Luque, R., and Marks, I.M. (2000). Neurological and neuropsychological signs in obsessive compulsive disorder: interaction with behavioural treatment. *Behav. Res. Ther.* **38**, 695–708.

Brooks, J.L., Baker, G.A., Goodfellow, L., Bodde, N., and Aldenkamp, A. (2007). Behavioural treatments for non-epileptic attack disorder. *Cochrane Database of Systematic Reviews* (**3**). CD006370

Cole, K. and Vaughan, F.L. (2005). Brief cognitive behavioural therapy for depression associated with Parkinson's Disease: A single case series. *Behav. Cogn. Psychotherapy* **33**, 89–102.

Colom, F. and Lam, D. (2005). Psychoeducation: improving outcomes in bipolar disorder. *Eur Psychiatry* **20**, 359-64.

David, A.S. (1990). Insight and psychosis. *Br. J. Psychiatry* **156**, 798–809.

Davis, G.R., Armstrong, H.E., Donovan, D.M., and Temkin, N.R. (1984). Cognitive–behavioural treatment of depressed affect among epileptics: preliminary findings. *J. Clin. Psychol.* **40**, 930–5.

Davison, P., Sharpe, M., Wade, D., and Bass, C. (1999). 'Wheelchair' patients with non-organic disease: a psychological inquiry. *J. Psychosom. Res.* **47**, 93–103.

Dalla Barba, G., Bartolomeo, P., Ergis, A.-M., Boissé, M.-F., and Bachoud-Lévi, A.-C. (1999). Awareness of anosognosia following head trauma. *Neurocase* **5**, 59–67.

Dewar, B-K. and Gracey, F. (2007). "Am not was": Cognitive-behavioural therapy for adjustment and identity change following herpes simplex encephalitis. *Neuropsychol Rehab*, **17**, 602–20.

Drummond, A. and Walker, M. (1996). Generalisation of the effects of leisure rehabilitation for stroke patients. *Br. J. Occup. Ther.* **59**, 330–4.

Eisen, J.L., Phillips, K.A., Coles, M.E., and Rasmussen, S.A. (2004). Insight in Obsessive Compulsive Disorder and Body Dysmorphic Disorder. *Comp. Psychiatry.* **45**, 10–15.

Eisen, S.V., Dill, D.L., and Grob. M.C. (1994). Reliability and validity of a brief patient-report instrument for psychiatric outcome evaluation. *Hosp. Community Psychiatry* **45**, 242–7.

Feighner, J.P., Robins E., Guze, S.B., Woodruff, R.A. Jr, Winokur, G., and Munoz, R. (1972). Diagnostic criteria for use in psychiatric research. *Arch. Gen. Psychiatry* **26**, 57–63.

Fink, P. and Jensen, J. (1989). Clinical characteristics of the Munchausen syndrome. A review and 3 new case histories. *Psychother. Psychosom.* **52**, 164–71.

Fleminger, S., Oliver, D., Williams, W.H., and Evans, J.J. (2003). The neuropsychiatry of depression after brain injury. *Neuropsychol. Rehab.* **13**, 65–87.

Gardner, W.I. (1971). *Behaviour modification in mental retardation*. University of London Press, London.

Ghaemi, S.N., Stoll, A.L., and Pope, H. (1995). Lack of insight in bipolar disorder—the acute manic episode. *J. Nerv. Ment. Dis.* **183**, 464–7.

Ghaffar, O. and Feinstein, A. (2007). The neuropsychiatry of multiple sclerosis: A review of recent developments. *Curr. Op. Psychiatry* **20**, 278–285.

Goldberg, D., Gask, L., and O'Dowd, T. (1989). The treatment of somatization: teaching techniques of reattribution. *J. Psychosom. Res.* **33**, 689–95.

Goldstein, L.H. (2003). Behaviour problems. In *Neurological rehabilitation* (ed. R. Greenwood, M. Barnes, T. McMillan, and C. Ward) pp. 419–32 2nd edn, Erlbaum, Taylor and Francis.

Goldstein, L.H., Deale, A.C., Mitchell-O'Malley, S.J., Toone, B.K., and Mellers, J.D. (2004). An evaluation of cognitive behavioral therapy as a treatment for dissociative seizures: a pilot study. *Cogn. Behav. Neurol.* **17**, 41–9.

Guthrie, E. (1995). Treatment of functional somatic symptoms: psychodynamic treatment. In *Treatment of functional somatic symptoms* (ed. R. Mayou, C. Bass, and M. Sharpe), pp. 144–60. Oxford University Press, Oxford.

Halligan, P.W., Bass, C., and Wade, D.T. (2000). New approaches to conversion hysteria. *Br. Med. J.* **320**, 1488–9.

Halligan, P.W., Bass, C., and Oakley, D. (2001). *Contemporary Approaches to the Study of Hysteria.* Oxford University Press, Oxford.

Hawton, K., Salkovskis, P.M., Kirk, J., and Clark, D.M. (eds.) (1989). *Cognitive behaviour therapy for psychiatric problems.* Oxford University Press, Oxford.

House, A. (1995). The patient with medically unexplained symptoms: making the initial psychiatric contact. In *Treatment of functional somatic symptoms* (ed. R. Mayou, C. Bass, and M. Sharpe), pp. 89–102. Oxford University Press, Oxford.

Husted, J.R. (1999). Insight in severe mental illness: implications for treatment decisions. *J. Am. Acad. Psychiatry Law* **27**, 33–49.

Iwata, B.A., Dorsey, M.F., and Slifer, K.J. (1982). Towards a functional analysis of self injury. *Anal. Intervent. Devel. Disabil.* **2**, 3–20.

Kanfer, F.M. and Saslow, G. (1969). Behavioural diagnosis. In *Behaviour therapy: appraisal and status* (ed. C.M. Franks), pp. 417–44. McGraw Hill, New York.

Kemp, R. and David, A. (1995). Psychosis: insight and compliance. *Curr. Opin. Psychiatry* **8**, 357–61.

Kemp, R. and David, A. (1997). Insight and compliance. In *Treatment compliance and the treatment alliance in serious mental illness* (ed. B. Blackwell), pp. 61–86. Harwood Academic, The Netherlands.

Kent, S. and Yellowlees, P. (1994). Psychiatric and social reasons for frequent rehospitalisation. *Hosp. Community Psychiatry* **45**, 347–50.

Kinsella, P. (2001). Factitious disorder: a cognitive behavioural perspective. *Behav. Cogn. Psychother.* **29**, 195–202.

Kroenke, K. (2003). Patients presenting with somatic complaints: Epidemiology, psychiatric co-morbidity and management. *Int. J. Methods. Psychiatric. Res.* **12**, 34–43.

Kroenke, K. and Swindle, R. (2000). Cognitive–behavioural therapy for somatisation and symptom syndromes: a critical review of controlled clinical trials. *Psychother. Psychosom.* **69**, 205–15.

Kuipers, E., Fowler, D., Garety, P., Chisholm, D., Freeman, D., Dunn, G., Bebbington, P., and Hadley, C. (1998). London East Anglia randomised control trial of cognitive–behavioural therapy for psychosis. III: Follow-up and economic evaluation at 18 months. *Br. J. Psychiatry* **173**, 61–8.

LaFrance, W.C. Jnr., Alper, K., Babcock, D., Barry, J.J., Benbadis, S., Caplan, R., Gates, J., Jacobs, M., Kanner, A., Martin, R., Rundhaugen, L., Stewart, R., and Vert, C. (2006). Nonepileptic seizures treatment workshop summary. *Epilepsy Behav.* **8**, 451-61.

LaFrance, W.C. Jnr. and Barry,J.J. (2005). Update on treatments of psychological nonepileptic seizures. *Epilepsy Behav.* **7**, 364–74.

Lam, D., Watkins, E.R., Hayward, P., Bright, J., Wright, K., Kerr, N., Parr-Davis, G., and Sham, P. (2003). A randomized controlled trial of cognitive therapy for relapse prevention for bipolar affective disorder. Outcome of the first year. *Arch. Gen. Psychiatry.* **60**, 145-152.

Larcombe, N.A. and Wilson, P.H. (1984). An evaluation of cognitive–behaviour therapy for depression in patients with multiple sclerosis. *Br. J. Psychiatry* **145**, 366–71.

Lawrie, S.M., Goodwin, G., and Masterton, G. (1993). Munchausen's syndrome and organic brain disorder. *Br. J. Psychiatry* **162**, 545–9.

Leber, W. and Jenkins, M.R. (1996). Psychotherapy with clients who have brain injuries and their families. In *Neuropsychology for clinical practice* (ed. R.L. Adams, O.A. Parsons, J.L. Cuthbertson, and S.J. Nixon), pp. 489–506. American Psychological Association, Washington, DC.

Lincoln, N.B., Flannaghan, T., Sutcliffe, L., and Rother, L. (1997). Evaluation of cognitive behavioural treatment for depression after stroke: a pilot study. *Clin. Rehabil.* **11**, 114–22.

Lishman, W.A. (1992). What is neuropsychiatry? *J. Neurol. Neurosurg. Psychiatry* **55**, 983–5.

Lysaker, P.H., Whitney, K.A., and Davis, L.W. (2006). Awareness of illness in schizophrenia: Associations with multiple assessments of executive function. *J. Neuropsychiat. Clin. Neurosciences.* **18**, 516–20.

Malia, K. (1997). Insight after brain injury: what does it mean? *J. Cogn. Rehabil.* May/June, 10–16.

Manchester, D. and Wood, R.L. (2000). Applying cognitive therapy to neurobehavioural rehabilitation. In *Neurobehavioural disability and social handicap following traumatic brain injury* (ed. R.L. Wood and T.M. McMillan), pp. 157–74. Psychology Press, Hove, East Sussex.

Markova, I.S. and Berrios, G.E. (1992). The assessment of insight in clinical psychiatry: a new scale. *Act. Psychiatr. Scand.* **86**, 159–64.

Marshall, J.C., Halligan, P.W., Fink, G.R., Wade, D.T., and Frackowiak, R.S.J. (1997). The functional anatomy of a hysterical paralysis. *Cognition* **64**, B1–B8.

Mayou, R., Bass, C., and Sharpe, M. (1995). Overview of epidemiology, classification and aetiology. In *Treatment of functional somatic symptoms* (ed. R. Mayou, C. Bass, and M. Sharpe), pp. 42–65. Oxford University Press, Oxford.

McEvoy, J.P., Apperson, L.J., Appelbaum, P.S., Ortlip, P., Brecosky, J., Hammill, K., Geller, J.L., and Roth, L. (1989). Insight in schizophrenia: its relationship to acute psychopathology. *J. Nerv. Ment. Dis.* **177**, 43–7.

Mellers, J. D. C. (2005). The approach to patients with "non-epileptic seizures" *Postgrad. Med. J* **81**, 498-504.

Michalakeas, A., Skoutas, C., Charalambous, A., Peristeris, A., Marinos, V., Keramari, E., and Theologou, A. (1994). Insight in schizophrenia and mood disorders and its relation to psychopathology. *Acta Psychiatrica Scand.* **90**, 46–9.

Migliorelli, R., Tesón, A., Sabe, L., Petracca, G., Petracchi, M., Leiguarda, R., and Starkstein, S.E. (1995). Anosognosia in Alzheimer's disease: a study of associated factors. *J. Neuropsychiatry Clin. Neurosci.* **7**, 338–44.

Miller, W. and Rolnick, S. (1991). *Motivational interviewing.* Guilford Press, New York.

Minden, S.L., Orav, J., and Reich, P. (1987). Depression in multiple sclerosis. *Gen. Hosp. Psychiatry* **9**, 426–34.

Murphy, G. (1987). Direct observation as an assessment tool in functional analysis and treatment. In *Assessment in mental handicap. A guide to assessment practice, tools and checklists* (ed. J. Hogg and N.V. Raynes), pp. 190–238. Croom Helm, London.

Newmark, N., Adityanjee., and Kay, J. (1999). Pseudologica fantastica and factitious disorder: review of the literature and a case report. *Comprehens. Psychiatry* **40**, 89–95.

Newsom-Davis, I., Goldstein, L.H., and Fitzpatrick, D. (1998). Fear of seizures: an investigation and treatment. *Seizure* **7**, 101–6.

Nimnuan, C., Hotopf, M., and Wessely, S. (2001). Medically unexplained symptoms. An epidemiological study in seven specialities. *J. Psychosom. Res.* **51**, 361–7.

Pearce, J. and Morris, C. (1995). The treatment of somatic symptoms in the elderly. In *Treatment of functional somatic symptoms* (ed. R. Mayou, C. Bass, and M. Sharpe), pp. 371–87. Oxford University Press, Oxford.

Peralta, V. and Cuesta, M.J. (1998). Lack of insight in mood disorders. *J. Affect. Disord.* **49**, 55–8.

Pewter, S.M., Williams, W.H., Haslam, C., and Kay, J.M. (2007). Neuropsychological and psychiatric profiles in acute encephalitis in adults. *Neuropsychol Rehab* **17**, 478–505.

Pilling, S., Bebbington, P., Kuipers, E., Garety, P., Geddes, J., Orbach, G., and Morgan, C. (2002). Psychological treatments in schizophrenia: I. Meta-analysis of family intervention and cognitive behaviour therapy. *Psychol. Med.* **32**, 763–82.

Prigatano, G.P. (1991). Disturbances of self awareness of deficit after traumatic brain injury. In *Awareness of deficit after brain injury: clinical and theoretical issues* (ed. G.P. Prigatano and D.L. Schacter), pp. 111–26. Oxford University Press, New York.

Prochaska, J.O. and DiClemente, C.C. (1982). Transtheoretical therapy: towards a more integrative model of change. *Psychother.: Theory, Res., Practice* **19**, 276–88.

Reuber, M., Howlett, S., and Kemp, S. (2005). Psychologic treatment of patients with psychogenic nonepileptic seizures. *Exp. Rev. Neurother.* **56**, 737–52.

Rief, W. and Hiller, W. (1999). Toward empirically based criteria for the classification of somatoform disorders. *J. Psychosom. Res.* **46**, 507–18.

Rose, J. and Walker, S. (2000). Working with a man who has Prader–Willi syndrome and his support staff using motivational principles. *Behav. Cogn. Psychother.* **28**, 293–302.

Salkovskis, P.M. (1989). Somatic problems. In *Cognitive behaviour therapy for psychiatric problems* (ed. K. Hawton, P.M. Salkovskis, J. Kirk, and D.M. Clark), pp. 235–76. Oxford University Press, Oxford.

Saravanan, B., Jacob, K.S., Johnson, S., Prince, M., Bhugra, D., and David, A.S. (2007). Assessing insight in schizophrenia: East meets West. *Br. J. Psychiatry.* **190**, 243–7.

Seli, T. and Shapiro, C.M. (1997). Neuropsychiatry—the mind embrained? *J. Psychosom. Res.* **43**, 329–33.

Sharpe, M., Peveler, R., and Mayou, R. (1992). The psychological treatment of patients with functional somatic symptoms: a practical guide. *J. Psychosom. Res.* **36**, 515–29.

Sharpe, M., Bass, C., and Mayou, R. (1995a). An overview of the treatment of functional somatic symptoms. In *Treatment of functional somatic symptoms* (ed. R. Mayou, C. Bass, and M. Sharpe), pp. 66–85. Oxford University Press, Oxford.

Sharpe, M., Mayou, R., and Bass, C. (1995b). Concepts, theories and terminology. In *Treatment of functional somatic symptoms* (ed. R. Mayou, C. Bass, and M. Sharpe), pp. 3–16. Oxford University Press, Oxford.

Silver, F.W. (1996). Management of conversion disorder. *Am. J. Phys. Med. Rehabil.* **75**, 134–40.

Smith, G.R. Jr. (1995). Treatment of patients with multiple symptoms. In *Treatment of functional somatic symptoms* (ed. R. Mayou, C. Bass, and M. Sharpe), pp. 175–87. Oxford University Press, Oxford.

Speckens, A.E.M., van Hemert, A.M., Spinhoven, P., Hawton, K.E., Bolk, J.H., and Rooijmans, H.G.M. (1995). Cognitive behavioural therapy for medically unexplained physical symptoms: a randomised controlled trial. *Br. Med. J.* **311**, 1328–32.

Speckens, A.E.M., Spinhoven, P., van Hemert, A.M., and Bolk, J.H. (1997). Cognitive behavioural therapy for unexplained physical symptoms: process and prognostic factors. *Behav. Cogn. Psychother.* **25**, 291–4.

Stone, J., Carson, A, and Sharpe, M. (2005). Functional symptoms and signs in neurology: Assessment and diagnosis. *J Neurol Neurosurg Psychiatry* **76** (Suppl1), i2–i12.

Surguladze, S. and David, A. (1999). Insight and major mental illness: an update for clinicians. *Advan. Psychiatric Treat.* **5**, 163–70.

Tazaki, M. and Landlaw, K. (2006). Behavioural mechanisms and cognitive-behavioural interventions of somatoform disorders. *Int. Rev. Psychiatry.* **18**, 67–73.

Thomas, P.W., Thomas, S., Hillier, C., Galvin, K. and Baker, R. (2006). Psychological interventions for multiple sclerosis. *Cochrane Database Systematic Review* (**1**): CD004431.

Warwick, H., Clark, D.M., Cobb, A.M., and Salkovskis, P.M. (1996). A controlled trial of cognitive–behavioural treatment of hypochondriasis. *Br. J. Psychiatry* **169**, 189–95.

Wattar, U., Sorensen, P., Buemann, I., Birket-Smith, M., Salkovskis, P.M., Albertsen, M., and Strange, S. (2005). Outcome of cognitive-behavioural treatment for health anxiety (hypochondriasis) in a routine clinical setting. *Behav. Cogn. Psychother.* **33**, 165–75.

Wilkinson, P. and Mynors-Wallis, L. (1994). Problem-solving therapy in the treatment of unexplained physical symptoms in primary care: a preliminary study. *J. Psychosom. Res.* **38**, 591–8.

World Health Organisation. (1992). *The ICD-10 classification of mental and behavioural disorders. Clinical descriptions and diagnostic guidelines.* World Health Organisation, Geneva.

Yule, W. (1987). Identifying problems: functional analysis and observation and recording techniques. In *Behaviour modification for people with mental handicaps*, 2nd edn (ed. W. Yule and J. Carr), pp. 8–27. Croom Helm, London.

Zanetti, O., Vallotti, B., Frisoni, G.B., Geroldi, C., Bianchetti, A., Pasqualetti, P., and Trabucchi, M. (1999). Insight in dementia: when does it occur? Evidence for a nonlinear relationship between insight and cognitive status. *J. Gerontol.: Psychol. Sci.* **54B**, 100–6.

Part 8

Forensic neuropsychology

Chapter 36

Forensic issues in neuropsychology

William W. McKinlay, Michaela McGowan
and Jane V. Russell

1 Introduction

Neuropsychologists may be called on to assist in civil cases (e.g. in personal injury claims after traumatic brain injury (TBI)) and other brain injury including medical negligence (e.g. anaesthetic accident). Cases in which there is severe brain injury are amongst the largest personal injury claims coming before the Courts. The large amounts at stake reflect that the costs of providing specialised care to someone with significant disability for the rest of their life are very substantial, together with the fact that there may be substantial loss of earnings.

Neuropsychologists sometimes also assist in criminal cases where issues regarding fitness to plead and fitness to present evidence arise in individuals who may be neuropsychologically impaired. In addition, retrograde amnesia (RA) and post traumatic amnesia (PTA) associated with traumatic brain injury may limit recall of key events, such as an accident or assault, and this can raise important issues so that the Court may require information about the nature and extent of these periods of amnesia.

2 Civil cases

2.1 Why is a neuropsychologist's opinion required?

Serious brain injury typically results in:

- physical/sensory sequelae;
- cognitive sequelae;
- emotional/behavioural sequelae

Psychological factors (cognitive and emotional/behavioural sequelae) are the most important determinants of disability (Jennett *et al.*, 1981) – including reduced ability to work and need for care/supervision. The sequelae of brain injury, especially emotional/behavioural changes, cause stress on family members and sometimes family breakdown, making issues of care more pressing (cf. McKinlay and Watkiss 1999). Loss of earnings and costs of care are often the two main drivers of quantum of damages in these cases. The neuropsychological assessment is often a key assessment in identifying the factors which may impede return to work and give rise to the need for care and supervision.

2.2 **What information do the lawyers and the court need?**

In order to decide what, if any, compensation is due, the court must decide on two broad areas:

- *liability*: did the defending party cause "loss, injury and damage" to the plaintiff (England) or pursuer (Scotland) or claimant/petitioner (some other jurisdictions)?

- *quantum (amount) of damages*, which depends on the extent and implications of the loss, injury and damage suffered.

In cases brought before the courts in the UK damages are awarded under two broad headings. (In America, punitive damages may also arise, and in other jurisdictions the basis of calculation may differ.)

- There is a sum for '*general damages*' (England) or '*solatium*' (Scotland). The extent of pain and suffering is relevant here, as is the extent of the injured person's awareness: the more the injured person is aware of his/her predicament, the greater this element of the damages, other things being equal. At the time of writing this sum is always less than £250,000 in the UK.

- There is a sum for '*special damages*', often by far the larger part of the damages awarded in cases of serious injury. Key factors in calculating quantum of special damages include extent of loss of earnings and extra costs arising from disability. This element of the damages may take the total award to several million pounds after severe disabling brain injury in the UK.

It follows that key information lawyers seek to take from neuropsychologists' reports (and, in their respective fields, from other clinicians) is:

- the nature and extent of any impairment, disorder, or other effect of injury;
- causality: did the injury cause or substantially contribute to the difficulties suffered?
- the prognosis (with and without treatment), including timescale;
- the functional implications, especially for work and care needs.

The neuropsychologist should therefore consider:

- What is the nature/extent of neuropsychological impairment and emotional/ behavioural change? What abilities remain intact? It is important to look for intact as well as impaired abilities as these are relevant to rehabilitation and work prospects, and prognosis.

- Are the impairments/disorders/etc more likely to be due to the injury than to any other cause? Failing this, has the injury made a significant contribution to these impairments/disorders/etc?

- Is further treatment/rehabilitation indicated (and, if so, what kind, with what aims)? What is the prognosis? Is it too soon to estimate long-term outcome? (The likely long-term prognosis will seldom be clear until at least 2-3 years after serious brain injury.)

- What implications – in broad terms – do the impairments and other changes have for functional outcome, including ability to work and lead a social life, and need for care/ supervision?

Civil cases are decided on the *balance of probability*. The question is, for example, whether it is more likely than not that the injury (rather than some other factor) caused – or materially contributed to – the problems found. It is also important to remember that the court will usually make a once-for-all decision, based on the best evidence available at the time. Damages in the UK and many other countries are not punitive, but reflect loss of earnings, care costs, etc. In the UK, an exception to this general rule is that the damages awarded to the victims of criminal assault in the UK via the Criminal Injuries Compensation Authority (CICA) are strictly limited – the maximum total damages for any CICA case in 2008 is £0.5 million, unchanged for several years.

2.3 How should the assessment be conducted?

2.3.1 Stage 1 – Accepting instructions

(i) Before accepting instructions, ensure that you can do what is asked (i.e. can you comment on all of the questions raised?). Amongst the questions there may be some – such as life expectancy and risk of epilepsy – that are matters for other experts. You should point this out at the outset.

(ii) Experts are often asked by potential referring sources about the percentage of instructions they receive from Plaintiff side, Defender side, or on a joint basis. That is information that experts should have to hand, and on which they should reflect if they find that a preponderance of instructions tends to come from one side rather than the other. One has to bear in mind an overriding duty to be fair and impartial.

(iii) A further point about expertise is that there is a good argument that experts should have a current non-litigating practice with the kinds of patients that they are assessing for medico-legal purposes. That this is desirable is generally agreed, at least in public discussion, by both experts and lawyers although it is not a standard which all experts are in fact able to meet.

(iv) There may be strict time requirements, especially in England under the Civil Procedure Rules (CPR) but increasingly also in other jurisdictions. You should only accept instructions if you can meet these time requirements. If you cannot, there may be room for negotiation but you should do this at the outset.

(v) There is no harm in agreeing at the outset, at least broadly, the level of fee and when it will be paid and further comment on this is made below in considering the need to avoid having any financial interest in the outcome.

(vi) It is important to avoid conflict of interest. Obvious conflict of interest may arise where an expert works for, or is affiliated with, a provider of services (e.g. rehabilitation services) and may end up recommending such services. It is important to declare any such conflict or potential conflict of interest. However, it need not be a reason to reject such work so long as conflict of interest is declared. At least those experts who are also rehabilitation providers have current experience in the field – some "experts" commenting on rehabilitation have not practised rehabilitation for many years (or at all). It is always possible for the instructing solicitors/insurers to commission a commentary from a disinterested party if it is felt that a conflict of interest may become active.

(vii) Lawyers will sometimes instruct the treating clinician, will sometimes go to an independent expert, and will sometimes use a mixture of both in an individual case. The advantage of instructing a treating clinician is that he or she is very well acquainted with the case and will have known the injured individual over a period. The potential disadvantages are firstly that they may be (or may be perceived as being) overly sympathetic to the individual because of their personal involvement in the case; and a somewhat contrary concern that they may overstate the degree of recovery without necessarily intending to do so because they are reviewing their own "handiwork". Treating doctors have a place in medico-legal work but very often independent practitioners are preferred and provide the main reports. A potential conflict would arise where a treating clinician was asked by the Defenders to provide a report. In one sense this might not seem to lead to insuperable difficulties, as whatever the source of instructions the report should be impartial. Nevertheless the perception could be that, because of instruction by the Defenders, the treating relationship would be compromised.

(viii) The Civil Procedure Rules in England and Wales which can be found on the website www.dca.gov.uk are particularly helpful in setting out the various matters which an expert should consider before, during and after the assessment. These do not apply in Scotland although the broad principle that experts should be impartial and not partisan certainly does apply. (It would be helpful if the Scottish Courts produced a website setting out what the Courts expect of experts.) An important requirement under the Civil Procedure Rules is that experts should enter the following statement into reports: "I confirm that I have not entered into any arrangement where the amount or payment of my fees is in any way dependent on the outcome of the case". Notwithstanding this requirement the first author has encountered the situation where a legal firm seeks to make arrangements for payment which could run contrary to the CPR requirements. Specifically, a legal firm setting up a panel of experts asked that experts "agree a price structure ... under which, if we are unable to recover your fee from the third party insurers ... you would write your fee off". Legal advice is that this would give the expert a direct financial interest (e.g. where a case was abandoned and the fee not recovered the expert would not be paid). It is important to be sure that arrangements for payment are transparent, with no strings attached which could in effect give the expert a financial interest in the outcome.

2.3.2 Stage 2 – Reviewing records

It is good practice to have all the records you need prior to assessment, so that you are properly briefed, and also so that issues arising can be clarified with patient/ relative. Lack of records can be a reason for assessments being wrong. On the other hand, there is an increasing tendency in UK cases for an extremely large volume of records to be sent to experts and it is worth making plain to those instructing you just which records would be helpful – it will not be helpful for a neuropsychologist to see large volumes of results of blood tests, x-rays films, etc. (Some experts charge an administrative fee for sorting records which arrive poorly ordered.)

The following records are often useful:

- *GP medical records* should make evident any significant pre-injury disorders or handicaps and other factors or conditions (e.g. poorly controlled diabetes, alcohol/drug abuse, previous injuries, etc) which may impact significantly on neuropsychological function.

- *Educational records* (especially for younger people recently in education) or *employment records* (where available) may help confirm test-based estimates of premorbid ability. Sometimes due to young age at injury or acquired language deficits, the usual methods for assessing premorbid ability (e.g. Wechsler Test of Adult Reading – WTAR) cannot be used, and these records will be even more important. It should also be borne in mind that severe brain injury has been found to compromise performance on the WTAR (Mathias *et al.,* 2007), so that exclusive reliance on this test (and probably similar tests) is best avoided, although such tests remain very useful indeed.

- *Acute hospital records* relating to the admission after injury should be reviewed to confirm that there was indeed a significant injury. Information on Glasgow Coma Scale, scan results, and any clinical evidence of focal neurological signs is important. Duration of post traumatic amnesia (PTA) is often not explicitly recorded, but orientation may be. The return of orientation and the ending of PTA cannot be assumed to occur at exactly the same time, but the ending of PTA is seldom long delayed after the return of orientation. Information about orientation is often in the notes – if not in the reports, then in the handwritten clinical notes of the psychologist, speech and language therapist, and other therapists and nurses.

Injury severity is a key consideration if seeming deficits are to be reconciled with the injury. If you do not know from a source independent of the patient/relative how severe the injury was, there is a danger of incorrect assessment/diagnosis. In particular, patients with post-concussion symptoms (PCS) following mild-moderate injury (a condition which is considered to be at least partially maintained by anxiety) may show superficial similarities to patients with more severe brain injury. There is also the risk of malingering: it is not entirely unknown for long coma, long PTA, and great disability to be claimed falsely after what proves from actual records to have been mild or moderate injury.

- *Later hospital/rehabilitation records* should also alert the assessor to behavioural problems. These may not emerge in the calm, contained environment of the neuropsychological examination, but may be a problem in day-to-day interactions with others, and must not be overlooked.

2.3.3 Stage 3 – The examination

It will be apparent from the comments above that the instructing lawyers and the injured party and their family are entitled to expect that expert witnesses will indeed have expertise in the relevant area and that they will be impartial. There are other expectations, however, that may potentially be more problematic.

The instructing solicitors may have 'sold' the expert as a prominent practitioner who will be able to 'help' with the case and there may be a perception on the part of some injured persons and families that you are there to help them win the most damages possible. It is of course not the job of the expert either to maximise damages if instructed by the Plaintiff or to minimise damages if instructed by the Defenders. The expert may explore possible support or rehabilitation, but should be cautious about holding out a firm prospect of such help – the injured person may lose the case or there may be significant contributory negligence (limiting the damages awarded). To the extent that the expert can 'help', it is that a comprehensive and clear report should help to narrow the issues between the parties and help to move the case towards the point of settlement.

A further expectation which has to be treated with caution is to do with confidentiality. There are always limits to confidentiality between psychologists/clinicians and patients. (There are BPS guidelines which set out how to resolve such issues – see www.bps.org.uk.) Injured persons and their families should of course have been made aware by their lawyers that there are further constraints on confidentiality in the medico-legal process. However, one has the impression that they are not always as aware as one might hope of the limitations on confidentiality. It is therefore particularly important to be alert to questions like, "Can I tell you this in confidence?" and to ensure that the limits of confidentiality are explained. A relevant consideration is that when a case is decided it may well enter the public arena. For example, judgements in all cases decided by the Courts in Scotland (as opposed to those settled out of Court) are published on the Internet, and these reports may include considerable detail about the medical and social history of the injured party, the nature and extent of injuries, the effects of injury, and their social circumstances. Further comment on the risk of inadvertent breach of confidentiality is made below.

The assessment should usually include a joint interview between the patient and a significant other; an interview and assessment of the patient; and a separate interview with a significant other. A further possible element in the assessment is a further testing session with a psychological technician or assistant psychologist on which further comment is made below. It is very hard to do a satisfactory assessment without also speaking to a relative or close friend given that the patient may very well have memory gaps and limited insight. In practice it is very rare indeed for patient/relative not to agree to separate interviews (if the need is well explained). It is however not unknown for follow-ups (not neuropsychological follow-ups) to be based on a cursory interview with the patient alone, and therefore to be potentially misleading.

Joint interview Since the patient may well have retrograde amnesia and post traumatic amnesia, information about events around the time of injury is often best collected with a relative also present. Further information which may best be collected with both present – in cases of memory or communication problems – is social and health background.

Separate interviews Due to the problem of lack of insight on the part of the injured person, there is a danger of under-reporting. It is useful to think of insight using the four stages suggested by Fleming et al., (1996):

1 Lack of awareness (or admission) of deficit.

2 Awareness of deficit.

3 Awareness of functional implications of deficit.

4 Ability to set realistic goals.

These stages typically are worked through first in relation to physical limitations, and then cognitive limitations, and lastly emotional/behavioural limitations. However, by no means every injured person completes the process.

It is therefore essential for an interview with a relative or 'significant other' to be carried out – if at all possible, separately. While the relative's view cannot be assumed to be the 'gold standard', there is evidence which suggests it is more likely to be accurate. For example, Sunderland *et al.,* (1983a) found relatives' accounts had greater validity as regards memory failure than those of patients. The separate interviews with patient and relative should *each* cover the main possible sequelae of injury (see McKinlay and Watkiss 1999). Deficits of functional significance may arise in the following areas:

+ The physical/sensory changes (including epilepsy) are of course primarily matters for others, but nevertheless a broad view of them should be kept in mind in considering the psychological picture.

+ There may be symptoms such as headaches, dizziness, poor balance, intolerance of noise, tiredness, changes in sleep/wake pattern, loss of libido. Some of these, especially tiredness, are very common and can be very disabling (Ziino and Ponsford 2005). Tiredness can exacerbate behavioural disturbances, and can 'bring out' otherwise silent residual deficits. It can also impact upon an individual's ability to participate in rehabilitation.

+ The cognitive changes should be reviewed, and an attempt made to identify how they affect daily life.

+ The emotional/behavioural changes should likewise be reviewed. Some patients will deny all such problems while other evidence (relative's account, records) suggests otherwise.

+ Progress in returning to education or employment should of course be considered. Careful questions about how they spend their time ('an average day') should be asked. Family and social life, and maintenance of friendships, should be explored. Social isolation is the major long-term danger for many patients and their families (Morton and Wehman 1995).

The above list is not exhaustive. Questions about other life events and about such factors as alcohol/drug abuse are relevant. Distinctions which are relevant to good clinical practice in any event are even more important in medico-legal reporting, and it is important to be clear about the following points:

+ The distinction between *spontaneous* and *elicited* complaints

+ The *source* of information should be clear (patient, relative, test scores, or records?)

+ The distinction between what is *reported* and *observed* and *inferred* should be made clear.

Neuropsychological examination There are several areas which it is important to assess. It is probably not productive in a chapter such as this to debate the merits and demerits of particular tests. Perfectly sound neuropsychological examinations may be based on varying selections of tests, so long as the tests are suitable for the purpose and the proper range of abilities is sampled. The key areas which should be covered are as follows.

• A language screen should include consideration of spontaneous speech and brief tests of repetition, naming, obeying commands, reading and writing, as Lezak *et al.*, (2004) have described.

• Intellectual level – premorbid and current. A caution should be entered against using an "overall" IQ score in this context. Scores which average subtests vulnerable to the effects of brain injury with subtests which are not vulnerable will mask the nature and extent of impairment. Separate consideration of subtests or indices is therefore better in this context than overall IQ scores.

• Both verbal and visuospatial memory should be assessed. It is worth bearing in mind that verbal memory (especially as assessed by Logical Memory from the Wechsler scale) is one of the tests best related to 'everyday' memory failures (Sunderland *et al.*, 1983b) and failure to return to work (Brooks *et al.*, 1987).

• Another key area to consider is attention/concentration. Difficulties in 'divided attention' are especially common.

• Executive functions, impairment of which is associated with frontal lobe damage, are also common and can be very disabling even where other aspects of cognitive function are not grossly impaired.

• 'Focal' problems (e.g. dyspraxia/agnosia/etc) should not be overlooked, although they are not especially common in marked form after TBI.

• Some clinicians include questionnaire measures of emotional adjustment. However, it should be borne in mind that – in a medico-legal context – these are often essentially a series of leading questions. The manuals of many such measures caution against their use in a medico-legal context. They need to be interpreted with great care.

There has always been a certain divergence between those who adopt a 'battery' approach to neuropsychological assessment and those who use a hypothesis testing approach, with the latter being much more parsimonious in the extent of their testing, and not necessarily using the same set of tests with each patient. There have been developments in testing whereby for example more sophisticated tests of frontal lobe or executive function have become available and where effort tests have become almost *de rigueur* in neuropsychological assessment. Some UK clinicians are increasingly adopting the practice of using a test technician to complete a further session of tests after their initial assessment. The argument can be made that with the improved range of tests and increasingly good norms now available, one should utilise these fully. On the other hand, the argument can also be made that test scores are best interpreted in the context of information from interviews, records, and qualitative observations, and best done by neuropsychologists rather than by test administrators. Moreover there is room for debate about the extent to which the increased demands made of the patient in lengthy testing (which at least some find stressful) is justified by the additional information obtained.

It is increasingly common to incorporate tests of effort. In the American Academy of Clinical Neuropsychology (AACN) Practice Guidelines (2007), it is noted that there is a 'growing literature' which suggests that 'the assessment of motivation and effort is critical when conducting a neuropsychological evaluation'. This document incorporates the following advice: "Clinicians utilize multiple indicators of effort, including tasks and paradigms validated for this purpose, to ensure that decisions regarding adequacy of effort are based on converging evidence from several sources, rather that depending on a single measure or method". I understand that the Division of Clinical Neuropsychology of the British Psychological Society is currently considering the question of offering guidance to neuropsychologists on the need to incorporate measures of effort into their assessments (McMillan, Personal Communication).

The assessment of effort is linked with the issue of malingering although it is a link which has to be made with some caution. Malingering is defined in DSM-IV as the intentional production of false or grossly exaggerated (symptoms or deficits) motivated by external incentives. On the other hand, there has been a view that malingering is more of an accusation than a diagnosis, and that clinical assessments should stop short of reaching the conclusion that there is actual malingering and should be limited to considering whether the symptoms presented are credible. Boone (2007a) notes that non-credible symptoms may be part of somatoform disorders and also conversion disorders and indeed observed that forced-choice methodology (a mainstay of many effort tests) was originally used to help identify conversion.

However, plainly in a personal injury litigation situation there is a potential incentive to 'fake bad'. In some studies subjects, including psychology students, have been asked to simulate ('fake') deficits. Such fakers tend to do badly across the board – as if reluctant to do well even on easy items. TBI patients usually still find some tasks quite easy and typically, although not invariably, show:

- little deficit on measures of personal information, basic language function, verbal IQ, and forwards digit span;
- a degree of difficulty on measures of performance IQ;
- major difficulty on tests of memory and attention/concentration (the latter including backwards digit span, Digit Symbol, and PASAT).
- Some also have great difficulty with 'frontal' (executive function) tests. A 'flat' profile, doing badly across the board, is suspicious. Overall, key areas to look for are:
  - A typical test performance, with seemingly great difficulty on simple tests.
  - Marked inconsistencies in what is expected from the nature of injury and the patient's presentation and self-reports.
- It is also worth bearing in mind:
  - Did the claimant consult a lawyer before seeking full clinical assessment and/or help with 'post-injury' problems?
  - Have symptoms shown typical progression over time?
  - Is the claimant's account at interview consistent with the records?

There is a wide array of effort tests now available and this is a topic which has been receiving increasing attention (e.g. Millis 2008, Boone 2007b; Larrabee 2007). It is important to keep in mind that effort testing is not a straightforward matter of detecting malingerers but a matter of detecting suboptimal effort or non-credible cognitive performance. It is arguable that assessment of effort should become a more prominent part of neuropsychological assessment, not just in forensic (civil or criminal) settings, but also more generally. The simulation of deficit may not only be for external gain (compensation, evading punishment, receiving benefits, or receiving sympathy) but could also relate to internal conflicts – for example Boone (2007a) discusses pseudo-seizures ('several minutes of thrashing and jerking') which are usually accepted as non-conscious behaviour with possibly complex motivations. It is possible that sometimes suboptimal performance could perhaps be analogous to this.

Assessment of effort is in a sense not new. It has always been integral to the neuropsychological assessment (as to a clinical psychological or medical assessment) to form a view about the nature and cause of the symptoms, and that includes forming a view as to whether symptoms/deficits presented are credible or not. The phenomenon of 'answering past the point' (How many legs has a cow? 3; How many weeks in a year? 53) has long been recognised as an indicator of non-credible 'deficit'. Neuropsychologists have long had an array of tests (e.g. the Andre Rey 15-Item test and Dot Counting Test described by Lezak et al., 2004) and also various indices which may be derived from standard IQ/memory tests (Rawling and Brooks 1990; Gudjonnson and Shackleton 1986) to detect simulation. To that extent, the introduction of effort test does not mark a step change in the nature of neuropsychological assessment, but rather an increased level of sophistication in the analysis of the responses that patients give. Boone (2007a) notes some debate about giving 'warning' to patients before using some of these tests but rightly (in the present authors' view) concludes that specific warnings would be inappropriate. They may render the administration of tests non-standard, and not as intended by the test developers. Moreover, as Boone notes, there is an understood social contract that presenting fraudulent data is wrong and indeed may be punishable. In any event the whole neuropsychological assessment, like other medical/psychological assessments, must – if it is to be of any value at all – include the formation of a view about the credibility of the symptoms presented. That said however, it is prudent and reasonable to encourage best efforts on testing.

There are specific tests which have become widely used including the Test of Memory Malingering (TOMM, Tombaugh 1996) and the Word Memory Test (WMT, see Green et al., 1999). Both of these are two-alternative forced-choice tests. Consideration has to be given to the sensitivity of the tests. Green (2007) discusses the relative failure rates on TOMM and WMT effort subtests amongst others, noting that a much higher percentage of the sample studied (32%) failed the effort subtests on the WMT than on the TOMM (11%). An analysis of the evidence is argued to suggest that the difference is mainly due to false negatives on the TOMM. One could debate the relative merits of these tests and that is outside the scope of this chapter but it is important to remember that tests are of varying degrees of sensitivity. It is wise to bear in mind through the whole assessment the need to form a view about the credibility of the symptoms and not to rely only on a single measure.

It is important to remember too that these tests can provide reassurance to the examiner that the deficits being seen are probably real. One case seen by the first author was a young man of 20 with a poor educational record and limited employment history who had sustained a severe head injury. Had he performed poorly on testing, a possible interpretation would have been that this was contributed to by his being unaccustomed to test taking. That concern on the part of the assessor was allayed by a good performance on effort testing, which gave confidence that the poor performance on other aspects of memory testing was likely to represent real deficit. Modern effort tests, however, do have significant advantages over some of the more traditional tests in that they are more likely to detect suboptimal effort in relatively sophisticated test takers. Another case seen by the first author – an academic in middle years – was able to give an intensely detailed account of various aspects of the case, and was running a household including driving a fairly large mileage. On the WMT, performance on the effort tests was close to chance and worse even than the 'hospitalised elderly dements' quoted amongst the norms. This was plainly not credible as a reflection of true memory capacity. Indeed even without the effort test, the very poor memory performance would have been implausible, but the WMT provided detailed evidence and normative comparisons which made that conclusion all the more cogent.

It is important to remember that there may be some rare exceptions, for example Broca's aphasics are routinely misled by aspects of sentence structure and this can lead to below chance performance which is not malingered or representative of a lack of effort (Grodzinsky 1995). There is also a more general caveat that surprising and hard-to-understand behaviour should not too readily be taken to suggest malingering, as there may be an underpinning organic explanation. For example, the first author has come across a case of 'foreign accent syndrome' in which the subject spoke (after a mild stroke allegedly due to medical negligence) with a 'mid-European' sounding accent, despite no connection with that part of the world. The question of malingering had been raised. However, although rare, this condition has been reported to arise sometimes with and sometimes without aphasia and to be related to anterior left (dominant) hemisphere lesions, generally of the frontal and precentral gyri (Kurowski et al., 1996; Moonis et al., 1996; Takayama et al., 1993), as was the case with the subject.

2.3.4 Stage 4 – Reporting and giving evidence

The next stage is to write the neuropsychological report. As the great majority of cases are settled before reaching an actual court hearing, the report will often be the only means by which the neuropsychologist's opinion will be communicated to the court.

What should be included in a medico-legal neuropsychological report? The report (like other medico-legal reports) should set out the instructions given, state where and when the patient and relative were assessed/interviewed, and describe the documentation studied. The nature and severity of injury should be considered, drawing on patient/relative interview and evidence from the records. As always, the social and health background should be described. The information from patient/relative interviews and from the neuropsychological examination should be presented. Neuropsychologists differ in whether they include scores, centiles, etc in their reports or use terms like 'moderate' or 'very severe' impairment. Some argue that actual scores may be misinterpreted by non-psychologists, but without scores one is left only with vague and non-operational terms like 'severe impairment'. Centile scores have the advantage that they can be calculated for most tests and provide a basis for comparison. One solution for those unwilling to include actual scores in the body of the report is to provide a technical summary as an appendix in which scores, test versions used, etc are listed. This facilitates later assessment by other neuropsychologists.

The report should set out conclusions on the key areas of relevance to the court, as set out more fully above (i.e. nature/extent of impairment and change; cause and effect; treatment and prognosis; and functional implications).

What areas should be addressed with caution? There are also areas which it is not appropriate to cover as they are primarily a matter for related reports. To stray into these areas may confuse the issues and give rise to unnecessary contradictions in the evidence. It may be quite appropriate for a neuropsychologist to say that someone has such severe deficits that they are likely to be incapable of open market employment, or would be capable only of restricted/simple work. However, to speculate as to what jobs may be available in more detail may be unwise. Normally such questions are for an employment expert with knowledge of availability of employment in the appropriate travel-to-work area; knowledge of factors which might militate against employment in the relevant field; knowledge of competition for such jobs; and so on.

There will often also be a report on future care which will include costs. It is unhelpful for clinicians to be too specific on care needs: the details are a matter for a care specialist who knows the practicalities of care provision, and can seek to match what is practicable with the patient's needs. It would, however, be appropriate and helpful in a neuropsychological report to offer a view as to the broad level of care/supervision needed.

However, a particular aspect of future care - rehabilitation - may well merit fuller discussion. After brain injury, many patients, at least in the UK, will not receive an adequate (or indeed any) programme of specialised rehabilitation (e.g. Thornhill et al 2000). One cannot consider prognosis without considering what services may be available, and it will often be appropriate to make recommendations for rehabilitation, which may require funding. It is important to remember:

- You should not hold out to patient/family the definite prospect of rehabilitation or other treatment until and unless funding is in place.

- If there is a case for such rehabilitation, you should do no more than discuss it with patient/family as a possibility (to gauge their receptiveness), then raise the matter with your instructing lawyers.

- The lawyers acting for the injured person may be able to obtain funding for this purpose, either by means of an interim award of damages, or through negotiation with the defenders. However, that is a matter for them to pursue where possible and the clinician's role is to provide them with any evidence that such rehabilitation may be of benefit.

- The lawyers acting for the defenders may also be able to arrange funding for this purpose, and the idea of doing so may be attractive to defenders on the grounds that such an investment now may reduce disability (and therefore damages) later. Again the clinician's role is to explain any grounds to believe that such rehabilitation may be of benefit.

- It will sometimes be possible for privately-funded rehabilitation/treatment to be provided by a service with which you (the person who recommended it) have no connection. If the service may be provided by a unit with which you do have a connection, you should declare a possible conflict of interest.

If called to present evidence in court, it is well worth reading some relevant material about the court in advance, or seeking to speak to a colleague with court experience. Carson (1990), a lawyer who describes the methods Barristers or Advocates use to 'test' witnesses, provides a view from the 'other side' which is very helpful for prospective witnesses. Other useful UK publications are: *Psychologists as Expert Witnesses in Scotland* and *Psychologists and the New Rules in Civil Procedure* published by the British Psychological Society.

What happens after an assessment is not always simply a matter of the reports being prepared for negotiations and for Court Hearings, but sometimes rehabilitation decisions follow. In the UK the Association of Personal Injury Lawyers (APIL) and the Forum of Insurance Lawyers (FOIL) have a Rehabilitation Code under which they agree to consider the advantages of rehabilitation, which can produce a potential win-win situation whereby the injured party achieves a better outcome as a result of investment by the insurers and the final cost to the insurers is thereby reduced.

It is clear that some lawyers have a degree of difficulty with this – it is easier to measure one's achievement in winning damages by the size of an award and some more subtlety is required to gauge success in terms of the outcomes achieved by the injured persons. However, it is clear that the leading practitioners in the field do have the welfare of their clients more to the front of their minds than the size of the final award attained.

The use of the Rehabilitation Code should normally lead to an Immediate Needs Assessment prepared by an independent practitioner who is not a compellable witness at Court and to that extent is 'outside' the medico-legal process. It is however important to be careful and disciplined about where instructions come from and who one has permission to report to when this process is in play. The first author has, for example, been instructed to provide a neuropsychological report by an 'independent' rehabilitation provider later to receive a follow-up letter from the defending solicitors asking for further comments. If however, one's report was originally for an independent rehabilitation provider, you cannot assume that you have the consent of the injured party to divulge information in this way – permission should be obtained from their solicitors. It is also sometimes the case that instruction from one party is then followed by agreed joint instruction and it is essential to be clear as to the basis on which one is instructed and to ensure that there is no conflict. Obviously one cannot accept instructions from the defender at one point then (unless the parties agree) go on to accept instructions from the plaintiff/pursuer side or vice versa.

2.4 **Further issues**

2.4.1 Premature ageing

An increased risk of dementia after brain injury has been suggested by some. The idea that the injured brain may be less able to resist the effects of ageing and/or dementia has some plausibility. Bell (1992) was an emphatic proponent of such a link. Lawyers, naturally, may raise the issue: if there was an increased risk of dementia it would have implications for long-term care and therefore costs, and it would only be right that the diligent lawyer pursue the issue. There is a growing literature on this topic.

There are many retrospective studies reporting an association between previous head injury and onset of Alzheimer's Disease. These are of limited interest as the relatives (whose accounts have generally been the basis of these studies) may be making an effort to 'explain' the dementia. Fleminger (2003) provided a systematic review of case control studies and sought to replicate the findings of an earlier meta-analysis by other researchers. He was able to obviate some of the more pressing objections to some of the individual earlier studies. He reported an odds ratio of 2.26 for males (i.e. that males with a head injury were over twice as likely to develop Alzheimer's Disease), although the relative risk for females was slightly below parity. The author comments that, due to the inherent complications in conducting case control studies, other forms of research should be used in the future.

Two other studies which are of particular interest were by Plassman *et al.*, (2000) and Nemetz *et al.*, (1999). The Plassman study was of World War II US Navy or Marine Veterans who were hospitalised during military service with either head injury or with some other condition. Although this was in the era prior to the use of GCS or PTA as markers of injury severity, they nevertheless used satisfactory definitions and a clear and staged procedure to follow up patients to see if they had developed Alzheimer's or other dementias. The hazard ratio for those with moderate head injury was 2.32 and for severe head injury 4.51. This is a study in which the contaminating effects of the expectations of relatives and experimenters are obviated. On the other hand, one has to bear in mind that these patients were injured a long time ago when the nature and extent of rehabilitation, treatment, and support for people with brain injury was significantly different from that which applies nowadays, and so some caution would have to be applied in interpreting these findings.

There is also a study by Nemetz *et al.*, (1999) which is a population-based study of patients injured between 1935 and 1984 in one county in Minnesota. This too provides a good test of the hypothesis insofar as the methodology is not susceptible to expectations or selective recall by relatives. They found no evidence that traumatic brain injury was a significant independent risk factor for Alzheimer's Disease. There were some limitations of the study insofar as the diagnosis of dementia and classification were based on retrospective record review not on current DSM assessments as in the Plassman study. One again would note that some of the patients were injured many years ago, when standards of treatment and care were different. Nevertheless, there was no evidence here of a link.

Two editorials, both of which appeared in the Journal of Neurology, Neurosurgery and Psychiatry in 2003 made comment in this issue. Wilson (2003) provided an editorial which accompanied the Fleminger paper noted above. Wilson hoped that the Fleminger review would stimulate the follow up of cohorts of patients with well-documented head injuries. In the same year, Brooks (2003) commented on a paper by Millar *et al.*, (2003). Brooks noted the possibility of late decline after TBI, although any decline was 'clearly not major'. Brooks also observed that "coming up with good data in this area is going to take dedicated research teams with very long term perspective".

From a medico-legal point of view, therefore, the link between brain injury and increased risk of dementia in later years remains very hard to specify and particularly to specify what it may mean in an individual case. However, it is plainly an area which is potentially relevant in a medico-legal context.

2.4.2 Assessment of capacity

The question of Capacity is one which is often raised with neuropsychologists in civil cases. This is a topic which has been particularly to the fore following the case of Masterman-Lister –v– Brutton & Co in 2002. Lush, Master of the Court of Protection in England and Wales, has provided a summary in which he notes that the decision in this case would be expected to make the assessment of capacity "more arduous for doctors, who have traditionally been gatekeepers of an individual's status as a patient". He notes that they will need to "consider a broader range of social, domestic and economic factors" and he notes the judges' observation that while "the opinions of skilled and experienced medical practitioners are a very important element in the evidence to be considered by the court" that is done in conjunction with other evidence.

The Masterman-Lister judgement (2002, EWCA Civ 1889) included that English law requires a person must have the necessary mental capacity to make legally effective decisions, to make testamentary dispositions, to enter into marriage, consent to divorce and so on. Mental capacity required by law is a capacity "in relation to the transaction which is to be effected" and that what is required therefore is the capacity to understand the nature of "that transaction when it is explained". Capacity is therefore specific and, commonly in personal injury cases, experts are asked to consider whether the individual has capacity to 'compromise' their claim (to reach a settlement of their claim for damages); and whether they have the capacity for 'fund management' (to look after their monies in time to come).

It would not be sufficient to say that someone lacks capacity merely because they might behave unwisely. The Mental Capacity Act of 2005 for England and Wales states that a person is unable to make a decision for him or herself if unable: (a) to understand the information relevant to the decision, (b) to retain that information, (c) to use or weigh that information as part of the process of making the decision, and (d) to communicate the decision (by talking, using sign language, or any other means).

The requirements go on to state that a person is not to be regarded as unable to understand the information relevant to a decision if that person is able to understand an explanation given to him in a way that is appropriate to his circumstances – for example by use of simple language, visual aids or by other means. The fact that the person is able to retain the information for only a short period is considered not to prevent him from being regarded as able to make the decision. The first author has an impression that there is currently a tendency amongst judges to seek to protect individuals who have been injured from what they see as over-zealous professionals wanting to remove capacity.

It is not sufficient to show that memory falls outside a normal range and is grossly defective but it is also relevant to adduce examples of how this affects the ability to make decisions – perhaps by reference to difficulties with decision-making which have arisen already, for example by looking at rehabilitation or case management or social work records. The criteria emphasise communication, retention, and so on. The executive difficulties which are common after head injury do not fall neatly under the rubric in the Act. The fact that making an unwise decision would not mean that one lacked Capacity is something which one has to consider carefully alongside any tendency to be impulsive as a consequence of dysexecutive or frontal lobe problems. It is therefore important to delineate these problems very clearly and to consider whether the extent of these problems means that the person has lost the Capacity to use or weigh information perhaps due to extreme impulsiveness or difficulty in sequencing thoughts. In short it is important to have careful regard to the statements in the Act, to consider the neuropsychological test findings, and also to consider wider examples in order to arrive at a recommendation regarding Capacity. One has to bear in mind too, of course, that the Court will decide at the end of the day, and that lack of Capacity need not be permanent but in some cases is able to be revisited.

There are other very difficult issues, for example, the capacity to consent to sexual relations. There is a judgement (and I am grateful to Helen Dolan of Potter Rees for bringing this to my attention) from a 2007 case (Re: MM [an adult] EWHC 2003 [Fam]). In this judgement it is stated that the law is set out that an adult is presumed to have capacity until the contrary is established, that capacity is issue-specific, and a person may have capacity for one purpose but lack capacity for another. The judgement states: "that is why in cases of this kind it has now become the practice to grant separate declarations (for example) as to a vulnerable adult's capacity: (1) to litigate, (2) to decide where she should reside, (3) to decide who she has contact with, (4) to decide on issues concerning her care, (5) to consent to sexual relations, (6) to consent to marriage and (7) to manage her financial affairs.

The judgement goes on to say that capacity is not merely issue specific in relation to different types of transaction but capacity is also issue specific in relation to different transactions of the same type – "thus a vulnerable adult may have capacity to consent to a simple medical procedure but lack capacity to consent to a more complex medical procedure". It follows therefore that in assessment one has to consider not only the overall findings and level of function, but to apply careful thought to the implications for the specific issues or transactions which are under consideration.

3 Criminal cases

The evidence of a neuropsychologist (as opposed to a forensic psychologist) may also be required in criminal cases. There are certain circumstances in which neuropsychological issues bear on criminal proceedings and it may be that in the future the range of neuropsychological issues arising in this setting will increase, especially given the high reported incidence of neuro-cognitive impairment in criminals (see Denney 2007).

3.1 Peri-traumatic loss of memory in TBI

Possible loss of memory at the time of an accident or assault is a particular issue which sometimes involves neuropsychologists in criminal cases. A period of amnesia (comprising retrograde amnesia – RA; and post-traumatic amnesia – PTA) is the signature of a significant concussional head injury. The individual recalls nothing from sometime before injury until sometime after it. This obviously may lead to difficulty in criminal cases. The victim of an assault may be unable to recall events just prior to assault due to RA, or the immediate aftermath due to PTA, and this can lead to problems in bringing the perpetrators to justice. Another instance is after road traffic accidents when the injured person may have been the victim or may have been a driver suspected of an offence. RA/PTA may mean the injured person has no recall of the event. In all cases where RA/PTA is an issue, study of the contemporaneous records is a key step in trying to clarify how extensive RA and PTA are likely to have been, as the injured person may have a motive for claiming to remember or forget what happened.

It is worth bearing in mind that although RA and PTA are always found with significant concussional head injury, not all assaults are of this sort. In assaults, depressed fractures or penetrating wounds are not uncommon. Where concussion is not the main mechanism of brain injury, the injured person may recall the actual incident, and may have succumbed to unconsciousness later. It should also be borne in mind that many people who commit murder/violent acts claim to have no memory of the act. It is thought that this commonly occurs as a result of emotional shock/psychological trauma (Kopelman 1987). Obviously, this should not be confused with RA/PTA: it is hard to conceive of a concussed person being able to carry out such an act.

3.2 Neuropsychological deficits

The lasting neuropsychological deficits in cognition and emotional adjustment which may follow TBI or other brain insult/disorder are also of potential relevance. Neuropsychologists may be asked to comment on vulnerabilities which affect the competency of a person with brain injury to stand trial, or give evidence as victim or witness. In the context of the police interview and testifying in court, the term 'psychological vulnerabilities' refers to psychological characteristics or mental states which render a witness prone to providing information which is inaccurate, unreliable, or misleading (Gudjonsson 1999).

3.2.1 Cognitive deficits

As well as RA/PTA, people who have had TBI or other brain insult/disorder may have ongoing memory and other cognitive impairments. The issue may arise as to whether such impairments undermine the ability to follow questions and marshal facts in giving evidence. Obviously the bar should not be set too high. In ordinary cases, where there is no neuropsychological deficit, some accused or witnesses may be of well below average ability. It would be wrong and arguably would undermine the aims of justice to say that merely because a witness has some loss of sharpness they could not give evidence, because that might well mean that no charges would be brought and justice would be defeated. However, where there are substantial difficulties (e.g. dysexecutive syndrome, word-finding difficulties, or memory problems) there may be very specific difficulties in giving evidence. Some individuals after severe TBI may be at such a disadvantage in the dock or witness box that attempts at examination and cross-examination would be in serious danger of ending in farce. In this context, the fact that some neuropsychologically com-promised individuals may be subject to extreme emotional responses (e.g. 'catastrophic reaction') is also relevant.

There is, however, a lack of hard indicators (such as test cutting scores), and clinical judgement is required. As regards the defendant, a trial cannot be fair if the individual is unable to understand the court proceedings, instruct their lawyer, and participate in the court proceedings. The exact criteria set down in the law to ensure a fair trial vary to some extent from jurisdiction to jurisdiction.

Where issues of intellectual and related impairment may arise (e.g. due to head injury, neurological disorder, etc), a neuropsychological assessment is necessary to define the nature and extent of the limitations. However, competency cannot be measured by just evaluating mental capacity and there is a need to assess the functional ability of a defend-ant matched to the contextual demands of the case (Grisso 1986).

As regards witnesses, similar considerations apply. A witness may be unable to give evidence if deemed not to have the cognitive capacity to understand questions, articulate answers, and understand the implications of their answers.

3.2.2 Suggestibility

Suggestibility is the tendency to yield to leading questions and submit to interrogative pressure (Gudjonsson 1999). Suggestibility can be assessed by the use of behavioural tests, such as Gudjonsson Suggestibility Scales, which assess an individual's response to 'lead-ing questions' and 'negative feedback'. Many neuropsychologists will have no experience of such measures and may wish to cross-refer to forensic psychologists.

3.2.3 Other variables

A neuropsychologist might also be asked to comment on various further (criminal) forensic issues to the extent that neuropsychological impairments interfere, or may inter-fere, with the ability of the accused, or of a witness, to recall or describe events. The more general factors which may affect the witness' ability to recall details of a crime at later date are primarily of interest to forensic psychologists rather than neuropsychologists. These factors include 'estimator variables' which may affect witness' recall (such witness age, weapon focus, duration of exposure to the crime, effects of stress/arousal), and dura-tion, which occur at the time of the event, and 'system variables' which occur during the investigation process (impact of misleading questions, exposure to 'mug shots'/photographs leading to false memories). Neuropsychological impairments may impact on ability to recall information about crime and perpetrators reliably. However, this is not a mainstream neuropsychological concern and detailed discussion is outwith the scope of this chapter.

3.3 Disposal

An issue which occasionally arises, in the authors' experience, is that of 'disposal', or sentencing. A neuropsychologist may be called upon to comment on whether there is treatment or rehabilitation available which may help, which might be as an alternative to fines or imprisonment.

Acknowledgements

We are grateful to the following for their helpful comments on specific issues:Robert Swanney, Partner, Digby Brown, Solicitors, Glasgow; Hugh Potter and Helen Dolan, Partners, Potter Rees, Serious Injury Solicitors, Manchester; Richard Crabtree, Partner, Pannone, Solicitors, Manchester.

Selective references

American Academy of Clinical Neuropsychology (2007): AACN Practice Guidelines for Neuropsychological Assessment and Consultation, *Clinical Neuropsychologist*, **21**, 209–231.

Bell DS (1992): Late progressive intellectual deterioration in Bell DS: *Medico*-legal *Assessment of Head Injury*.: Charles C Thomas Publisher, Springfield, Illinois.

Boone KB (2007a): A reconsideration of the Slick et al (1999): Criteria for malingered neuro-cognitive dysfunction. In *Assessment of feigned cognitive impairment: a neuropsychological perspective* (Ed: KB Boone) pp 29–49, Guilford Press, New York.

Boone KB (2007b): *Assessment of feigned cognitive impairment: a neuropsychological perspective*. Guilford Press, New York.

Brooks N (2003): Mental deterioration late after head injury – Does it happen? *Journal of Neurology, Neurosurgery and Psychiatry*, **74**, 1014.

Brooks N, McKinlay W, Beattie A and Campsie L (1987): Return to work within the first seven years of severe head injury. *Brain Injury* **1**, 5–19.

Carson D (1990): *Professionals and the Courts: a handbook for expert witnesses*. Birmingham Venture Press.

Denney RL (2007): Assessment of malingering in criminal forensic neuropsychological settings. In: *Assessment of feigned cognitive impairment: a neuropsychological perspective* (Ed: KB Boone) pp 428–52, Guilford Press, New York.

Fleming JM, Strong J, Ashton R (1996): Self-awareness of deficits in adults with traumatic brain injury: How best to measure? *Brain Injury* **10**:1–15.

Fleminger S, Oliver DL, Lovestone S, Rabe-Hesketh S and Giora A (2003): Head injury as a risk factor for Alzheimer's Disease: the evidence ten years on; a partial replication. *Journal of Neurology, Neurosurgery and Psychiatry* **74**, 857–862.

Green P (2007): Spoiled for choice: making comparisons between forced-choice effort tests. In: *Assessment of feigned cognitive impairment: a neuropsychological perspective* (Ed: KB Boone) pp 50–77, Guilford Press, New York.

Green P, Iverson GL, and Allen L (1999): Detecting malingering in head injury litigation with the Word Memory Test. *Brain Injury* **13**, 813–819.

Grodzinsky Y (1995): Trace deletion, Theta roles, and cognitive strategies. *Brain and Language* **51**, 469–497.

Grisso T (1986): *Evaluating Competencies: Forensic Assessment and Instruments*. Plenum Press, New York.

Gudjonsson GH and Shackleton H (1986): The pattern of scores on Raven's Matrices during "faking bad" and "non-faking" performance. *British Journal of Clinical Psychology* **25**, 35–41.

Gudjonsson GH (1999): Testimony from persons with mental disorder. In: *Analysing Witness Testimony: A Guide for Legal Practitioners and Other Professionals*. Blackstone Press.

Jennett B, Snoek J, Bond MR and Brooks N (1981): Disability after severe head injury: observations on the use of the Glasgow Coma Scale. *Journal of Neurology, Neurosurgery and Psychiatry* **44**: 285–293.

Kopelman MD (1987): Amnesia: organic and psychogenic. *British Journal of Psychiatry*, **150**, 428–42.

Kurowski KM, Blumstein SE, Alexander M (1996): The foreign accent syndrome – a reconsideration. *Brain and Language* **54**, 1–25.

Larrabee GJ (2007): *Assessment of malingered neuropsychological deficits*. Oxford University Press, New York.

Lezak MD, Howison DB, Loring DW (2004): *Neuropsychological Assessment*, 4th Edn. Oxford University Press, New York.

McKinlay WW, Watkiss A (1999): Cognitive and behavioural effects of brain injury. In: *Rehabilitation of the Adult and Child with Traumatic Brain Injury*, 3rd Edition (ed M Rosenthal et al), FA Davis Co, Philadelphia.

Mathias JL, Bowden SC, Bigler ED, Rosenfeld JV (2007): Is performance on the Wechsler adult reading test affected by traumatic brain injury? *British Journal of Clinical Psychology*, **46**, 457–466.

Millar K, Nicoll JAR, Thornhill S, Murray GD, Teasdale GM (2003): Long term neuropsychological outcome after head injury: relation to APOE genotype. *Journal of Neurology, Neurosurgery and Psychiatry* **74**, 1047–1052.

Millis SR (2008): Assessment of incomplete effort and malingering in the neuropsychological examination. In *Textbook of Clinical Neuropsychology* (Ed: JE Morgan and JH Ricker) pp 891–904. Taylor & Francis, New York.

Moonis M, Swearer JM, Blumstein SE, Kurowski KM, Licho R, Kramer P, Mitchell A, Osgood DL, Drachman DA (1996): Foreign accent syndrome following a closed head injury – perfusion deficit on Single-Photon Emission Tomography with normal Magnetic-Resonance Imaging. *Neuropsychiatry, Neuropsychology and Behavioral Neurology* **9**, 272–279.

Morton MV, Wehman P (1995): Psychosocial and emotional sequelae of individuals with traumatic brain injury: A literature review and recommendations. *Brain Injury* **9**: 81–92.

Nemetz PN, Leibson C, Naessens JM, Beard JM, Kokmen E, Annegers JF and Kurland LT (1999): Traumatic brain injury and time to onset of Alzheimer's Disease: a population based study. *American Journal of Epidemiology* **149**, 32–40.

Plassman BL, Havlik RJ, Steffens DC, Helms MJ, Newman TN, Drosdick D, Phillips C, Gau BA, Welsh-Bohmer KA, Burke JR, Guralnik JM, Breitner JCS (2000): Documented head injury in early adulthood and risk of Alzheimer's Disease and other dementias. *Neurology* **55**, 1158–1166.

Rawling P and Brooks N (1990): Simulation index: a method for detecting factitious errors on the WAIS-R and the WMS. *Neuropsychology* **4**, 223–238.

Sunderland A, Harris JE, Baddeley AD (1983a): Do laboratory tests predict everyday memory? A neuropsychological study. *Journal of Verbal Learning and Verbal Behaviour* **22**: 341–357, 1983.

Sunderland A, Harris JE, Baddeley AD (1983b): Assessing everyday memory after severe head injury in Harris JE, Morris DE (eds) *Everyday Memory, Actions and Absentmindedness*, London: Academic Press.

Takayama Y, Sugishita M, Kido T, Ogawa M, Akigushi I (1993): A case of foreign accent syndrome without aphasia caused by a lesion of the left precentral gyrus. *Neurology* **43**, 1361–1363.

Thornhill S, Teasdale GM, Murray GD, McEwen J, Roy CW, Penney KI (2000): Disability in young people and adults one year after head injury: prospective cohort study. *British Medical Journal* **320**, 1631–5.

Tombaugh TN (1996): *Test of Memory Malingering.* Western Psychological Services, Los Angeles.

Wilson JTL (2003): Head injury and Alzheimer's Disease. *Journal of Neurology, Neurosurgery and Psychiatry* **74**, 841.

Ziino C and Ponsford J (2005): Measurement and prediction of subjective fatigue following TBI. *Journal of the International Neuropsychological Society* **11**, 1–10.

Part 9

Functional neuroanatomy

Chapter 37

Functional neuroanatomy of spatial perception, spatial processes and attention

Gabriella Bottini, Eraldo Paulesu,
Martina Gandola and Paola Invernizzi

1 Introduction

Functional neuroimaging measures hemodynamic changes (of blood flow in the case of positron emission tomography (PET); Raichle 1987), and blood oxygenation in the case of functional magnetic resonance imaging (fMRI); Turner 1997; Ogawa *et al.* 1998; Logothetis *et al.* 2001). These indices are used as indirect measures of synaptic activity and neural firing. PET and fMRI have rapidly become the major sources of neurophysiological information in humans. Since their early inception, they have been extensively used to characterise the neural bases of spatial cognition. The quantity of empirical information now available is sufficiently large to allow for the formulation of a summary which may prove useful to the clinical and experimental neuropsychologist.

Empirical data from experimental psychology, primate neurophysiology, and neuropsychological observations of brain damaged patients, are the primary generators of experimental hypotheses for functional neuroimaging experiments in spatial neurocognition: the way in which space is mapped from early sensory codes (e.g. retinotopic maps, somatotopic maps) through transformation to higher-order coordinates;

- the multicomponent nature of space representation and the existence of several spatial frames (e.g. far as opposed to near space);
- the distinction between object- and space-based visual cognition;
- the relationship between space and motion cognition;
- the modulation of spatial representation and perception through attentional mechanisms.

In this review we will discuss the above areas of enquiry. These themes will be introduced by a brief summary of the relevant comparative information drawn from the primate physiology literature and neuropsychology. As the reader will notice, there is no complete agreement between lesion data and functional imaging data of spatial processing and attention; this we regard as a source of major interest for further research.

2 Building spatial neural representation from earlier sensory codes

2.1 The higher-order nature of spatial representation

Space, perceived as unitary, is in fact mapped by several systems all of which provide a representation relevant for a given set of actions and for different parts of space itself, including body space (Fig. 37.1) (Andersen *et al.*, 1997; Colby & Goldberg 1999; Rizzolatti *et al.*, 2000).

Evidence for dissociation between spatial representations and individual sensory codes in perception and directional coding of movement is provided by case studies of brain damaged patients:

- with relatively spared elementary perceptual (e.g. visual, tactile) or motor skills and an impaired ability to report, respond to, or orient towards stimuli presented in different portions of space (spatial unilateral neglect: cf. Bisiach & Vallar 2000);

- with altered visuomotor integration in reaching tasks (cf. Jeannerod 1997).

Studies in spatial neglect have allowed us to dissociate elementary somatotopic and retinotopic codes from body-centered coordinate frames (cf. Bisiach & Vallar 2000; Vallar 1998). A third source of evidence for the role of sensory afferents in the building of spatial

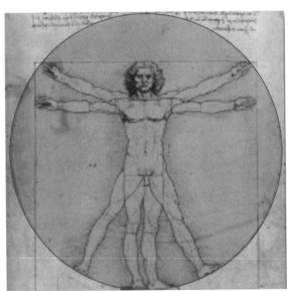

Fig. 37.1 Classification of spatial frames. The body, the space within reaching distance and far space. Neuropsychology and neurophysiology provide evidence that the brain has separate representations for these different spatial frames. Personal space is somatosensory space mapped as a body schema independently from visual space. Extrapersonal space also involves visual space: This can be based on egocentric coordinates (within reaching distance); visual space is organized with reference to head, trunk and limbs. Extrapersonal space can be mapped in allocentric (object-based) coordinates (See also 'Plates' section).

representations comes from the effects of lateralized or direction-specific stimulations of peripheral sensory systems, with methods such as caloric vestibular stimulation (CVS), posterior neck muscle mechanical vibration (NV), and optokinetic stimulation (OKS) (cf. Vallar *et al.*, 1997). In healthy subjects these stimulations can induce a distortion of egocentric coordinates (causing e.g. a deviation of the subjective straight ahead (an index of spatial representation) in pointing tasks (cf. Bottini *et al.*, 2001)). Therefore, the internal representation of space may involve the integration of different sensory inputs - visual, somatosensory-proprioceptive, vestibular, auditory - yielding reference frames that are not based on individual peripheral sensory codes, organised, as they are, in egocentric (e.g., head, trunk, arm), and object- or environment-centered coordinates (Andersen *et al.*, 1997; Rizzolatti *et al.*, 2000; Graziano & Gross 1994). To illustrate the integrative nature of the neural representation of space, we first need to briefly consider the individual sensory modalities. We have constrained our review to visual and somatosensory space. We will discuss how these individual modalities are combined into multimodal representations, and the extent to which functional imaging has contributed to describing the anatomical bases of these representations in humans.

2.2 Visual space

Visual space is mapped primarily by the geniculostriate pathway where magnocellular, parvocellular and koniocellular information arrives segregated to different layers of primary visual cortex (area V1) (Livingstone & Hubel 1988; Zeki 1993; Hendry & Reid 2000). Area V1 information is then conveyed to extrastriate visual cortex through divergent pathways, usually referred to as the ventral (object-centred or 'what') stream and the dorsal (space-related or 'where') stream (Mishkin *et al.*, 1983). Neurons of the visual cortices have receptive fields (RFs) of increasing complexity and size from area V1 to extrastriate visual cortex. The farther from V1, the more complex the receptive fields of the neurons; with neurons having a RF nearly as large as the whole visual field. Cortical visual areas may show retinotopic organization in that a single neuron responds to visual events arising from the same part of the retina. The part of the visual world mapped by these neurons varies with the position of the eyes in the orbit. There is now clear evidence that the brain makes extensive use of both retinotopic and non-retinotopic representations of visual space (cf. Rizzolatti *et al.*, 2000; Graziano & Gross 1994; Andersen 1994; Galletti & Fattori 2002). Even from an intuitive point of view, this appears to be an efficient computational strategy to enable stable phenomenological perception (e.g. when the eyes move, the perceived world remains stable despite the movements of the retinal images). Actions such as reaching and grasping benefit from visual descriptions centred on moving body segments (peripersonal space), or centred on objects in space (allocentric space).

2.2.1 Where are the visual cells with increasingly complex RF properties located?

In the primary visual cortex (area V1), visual space is mapped in purely retinotopic space. Each neuron has a receptive field, a sort of small window which captures a portion of the

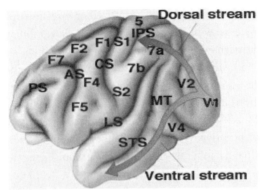

Fig. 37.2 Left cerebral hemisphere of the macaque brain. IPS, intraparietal sulcus; MT, motion temporal area (V5); S1, primary somatosensory area; S2, second somatosensory area; CS, central sulcus; LS, lateral sulcus; STS, superior temporal sulcus; AS, arcuate sulcus; PS, principal sulcus. The nomenclature of motor areas follows Matelli et al. (1985,1991). Some of the visual areas (V3, V6) cannot be seen on the lateral surface of the brain (See also 'Plates' section).

visual field. Suppose we observe a basket full of red apples and fixate on one of the apples. A given single visual cell in V1 will provide the same information when the eyes are fixating on the closest apple at the left end as on the farthest apple at the right end of the basket. That is to say, single neurons in V1 do not discriminate between spatial locations.

A first departure from a purely retinotopic mapping of the visual field is observed in the so-called gaze-dependent cells (Andersen 1994). In these cells the firing frequency depends not only on what strikes their receptive field, but also on the position of the eyes in the orbit or the dynamic component of gaze. Initially found in the posterior parietal cortex (PPC), particularly in area 7a, and in the lateral intraparietal sulcus (LIP), they have been found in extrastriate visual areas V3, V3A, V5/MT, MST, and V6 (see Figs 37.2 and 37.3) (Galletti & Fattori 2002; Galletti *et al.*, 1993). These neurons have retinotopically organized RFs and therefore do not encode visual space in a manner that is independent of eye position.

2.2.2 How does the brain build an eye-position-independent coding of visual space?

There are two competitive hypotheses on this issue.

- One maintains that this further level of visual space representation may arise by the temporal integration of an extensive system of gaze-dependent visual cells (Andersen *et al.*, 1997).

- A second theory postulates the existence of real-position cells, in which visual stimuli given to the same part of space cause similar neuronal responses in spite of the actual direction of gaze and position of the eyes in the orbits. Cells of this kind have been described in the PPC (area V6a or PO; Galletti *et al.*, 1993), in the ventral intra-parietal cortex (Duhamel *et al.*, 1992), and in the pre-motor cortex (area F4)

(Graziano & Gross 1994; Fogassi *et al.*, 1996). Their property may arise from convergent input from a set of gaze-dependent cells. The space coded by such cells, can be called extrapersonal space. Evidence from patients with unilateral neglect and neurophysiological evidence in the monkey show that extrapersonal space can be further divided into peripersonal space (the space within reaching distance) and far space (cf. Rizzolatti *et al.*, 2000).

2.3 Somatosensory and personal space

Cortical somatosensory representation of the body surface, joints, and muscles includes areas of the postcentral gyrus (areas of the S1 complex, Brodmann areas (BAs) 3, 1, 2), areas of the dorsal posterior parietal region (BA 5 of the monkey and human BAs 5 and 7), the secondary somatosensory area (area S2, BA 43) which is located in the ventral bank of the parietal operculum, the granular insula, the retroinsular cortex, and the more rostral part of the inferior parietal lobule (area 7b of the monkey and human area 40) (cf. Kaas 1990; Paulesu *et al.*, 1997). Much as for the visual areas, the RFs of individual neurons of the various somatosensory areas and the overall grain of the resulting maps change from area S1 to area S2, granular insula, retroinsular cortex, and supramarginal gyrus.

- S1 has the finest grained somatotopy with strictly contralateral receptive fields and limited callosal connections.

- S2 has a large proportion of neurons with bilateral or even ipsilateral receptive fields.

  The same applies to the other somatosensory cortices (cf. Paulesu *et al.*, 1997).

- Input to these cortices is purely somatosensory only in area S1 proper (area 3b), and in area 1.

- The retroinsular cortex, part of area 3a, area S2, the cortex at the tip of the intraparietal sulcus, and area 7b receive vestibular input as well.

- Area 7b has approximately 20% of neurons which respond to visual stimuli.

- Signals from the neck muscles reach the retroinsular cortex, the insula, and area S2 (Guldin and Grüsser 1998).

- In keeping with the functional properties of these cortices, the afferent thalamic inputs to these areas are strictly from the specific ventroposterior somatosensory nucleus for area 3b and 1, and from multiple thalamic nuclei for the remaining areas.

  Polymodal neurons with tactile and visual properties have also been found in the lateral premotor cortex (cf. Rizzolatti *et al.*, 2000), which also receives vestibular signals (Guldin & Grüsser 1998).

  The integrative nature of body schema representation goes well beyond a body map of the skin such as that represented in area 3b. The body schema is probably based on a number of body-centred spatial frames, including knowledge of the spatial relationship of body segments. The midsagittal plane of the body appears to be a robust neural/mental construct: its representation is easily tested with tasks involving the appreciation of the straight ahead coordinate on pointing or visual detection tasks, and may arise from the neural operations of the brain regions receiving joint input from tactile, muscle/joint receptors and vestibular receptors. Orientation of the midsagittal plane can be pathologically rotated towards the side of brain damage in patients with spatial neglect, or physiologically rotated in normal subjects by asymmetric input from the vestibular or neck-muscle receptors (Karnath 1994; Karnath *et al.*, 1994). The space coded by this neural system is called personal space.

2.4 Merging visual, somatosensory, and motoric spatial representations

Recently, the important discovery was made of a class of bimodal neurons which respond to visual stimuli and to tactile stimuli. These bimodal neurons have been found in:

- the premotor cortex (area 6 or F4);
- the inferior parietal cortex (area 7b);
- the putamen (Graziano & Gross 1994).

In these regions, a hand bimodal neuron responds to both tactile stimuli (delivered to the hand while the animal's eyes are closed) and to a visual stimulus (delivered in the space surrounding the hand, about 20 to 100 cm away). Interestingly, the visual field of these bimodal neurons moves with the position of the limb and is independent of the position of the eyes. The space coded by these neurons is peripersonal space.

The aforementioned evidence of visual neurons in premotor area 6 contributes to the now overwhelming demonstration that space (visual, somatosensory, and even auditory) is not only represented in posterior sensory regions but also in frontal-lobe regions (including the agranular and dysgranular premotor cortex, which have motor-like functions) (cf. Rizzolatti *et al.*, 2000). The premotor cortex (areas 6 and 8) has neurons which enter in descending motor tracts, or are connected to primary motor cortex. In the same regions, there are visual neurons with clear visual or visuomotor properties, and a recognizable visual receptive field. In the frontal eye-fields (FEFs), the region which triggers saccadic eye movements (to reach spatial location with gaze), there are visual as well as visuomotor neurons whose firing is enhanced by visual stimuli when the stimulus represents a target for an ocular movement (Goldberg & Bushnell 1981). The visual receptive field of these neurons is based on retinotopic coordinates. On the other hand, in the ventral premotor cortex (particularly in area F4), in addition to the motoric neurons involved in reaching and grasping, there are also visual neurons, or bimodal visuotactile neurons (whose visual receptive fields are anchored to body segments and move with them). The response of these neurons does not depend on retinotopic coordinates. Rather, it contributes to egocentric/peripersonal space representation. These premotor cortices are selectively connected to posterior parietal regions of the inferior parietal lobule, of the intraparietal sulcus, and of the superior parietal lobule, sharing some functional properties related to the space mapped. Area F4 is functionally related to the inferior parietal lobule (BA 7b) and to the anterior intraparietal area, which both predominantly encode peripersonal space within reaching distance. The FEFs are functionally connected to the lateral intraparietal cortex and the posterior part of the inferior parietal lobule (BA7a). Their function is concerned with eye movements and visual space, coded in retinotopic and craniocentric coordinates.

Another interesting description of neuronal properties of the premotor and parietal network is based on task-dependent classification of motor behaviour within space which is within reaching distance (Jeannerod *et al.*, 1995; Wise *et al.*, 1997). The dorsal stream is proposed as being a modular visuomotor transformation network.

- There is now abundant evidence that the most dorsal part of the parietofrontal network (superior parietal cortex and dorsal premotor cortex) is primarily concerned with reaching tasks and contributes to computing distance between target and limb, as well as spatial location of targets.
- The more ventral premotor and parietal network is more concerned with grasping, and the relevant dynamic hand-shaping processes.

Objects are therefore represented at multiple levels.

- In the ventral stream, objects are represented in allocentric coordinates related to object semantics (i.e. features such as shape, texture, colour).
- In the dorsal stream objects are coded for their spatial position in an egocentric/peripersonal spatial frame used for the generation of reaching and grasping behaviour.

Dissociation of these spatial frames has been indicated by human neuropsychological evidence: object discrimination can be severely impaired by ventral visual-cortex lesions, while accurate reaching and grasping may still be possible. The opposite anatomo-behavioural dissociation is also on record (Goodale & Milner 1992).

3 Space representation in humans: evidence from lesion studies

A major source of evidence comes from studies of unilateral neglect and from studies of patients with reaching disorders not associated with neglect. The evidence is somewhat limited by the nature of the acquired brain lesions, which are by default, vast and not constrained to discrete cytoarchitectural areas. Acquired lesions also usually involve subcortical white matter, making the interpretation of the anatomoclinical associations more challenging.

3.1 Anatomical basis of spatial neglect (see Chapter 5)

Reviews on the anatomical bases of spatial neglect can be found in Bisiach & Vallar (2000), Mesulam (1990), and Heilman *et al.*, (1994). The distribution of cortical lesions observed in neglect according to Vallar (1998), are presented in Fig. 37.3 (shaded areas). Unilateral neglect, which is characterized by the inability to represent and explore the side of space contralateral to the brain lesion, is usually observed after damage to the inferior parietal lobule: lesions are typically centred on the supramarginal gyrus, with involvement of the neighbouring inferior parietal and superior temporal areas. Lesion of the

Three imaging studies on line bisection

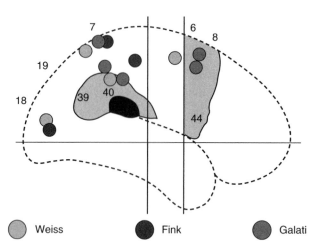

Fig. 37.3 Brain areas associated with spatial neglect (shaded areas) and meta-analysis of three functional neuroimaging experiments in healthy individuals using line bisection. Circles represent the location of activation peaks expressed in stereotactic space from three different imaging studies (Fink *et al.* 2000a; Weiss *et al.* 2000; Galati *et al.* 2000). Only the activations on the lateral surface of the right hemisphere are reported. The horizontal line represents the plane passing through the two commissures. The two vertical lines represent the coronal planes passing through each of the two commissures. Mesial ventral occipital activations are not shown. (See also 'Plates' section).

premotor cortices (BA 6, 44) can bring about neglect dominated by motor symptoms rather than by perceptual symptoms (a dichotomy which remains open to debate, cf. Mattingley *et al.*, 1998).

Neglect has also been observed after thalamic lesions or subcortical white matter lesions. It is much more frequent after right- rather than left-hemisphere lesions. Damage restricted to primary motor or sensory areas does lead to neglect. This supports the higher level nature of the spatial disorder observed in patients with spatial neglect.

It has recently been suggested that parietal neglect may be confounded by visual field deficits. It has been proposed that lesion of the superior temporal cortex (STG) might be a purer anatomical correlate of space exploration deficit (Karnath *et al.*, 2001; Samuelsson *et al.*, 1997). The role of STG (BA 22 and 42) in causing neglect has been further confirmed by Karnath and co-workers (Karnath *et al.*, 2004a) using a large sample of patients (140 right brain damaged patients) which were not selected on the basis of a neurological/symptom based constraint (absence of visual field defects) (Karnath *et al.* 2001).

This evidence is in contrast with the classical literature on neglect anatomy (cf. Heilman *et al.* 1994; Bisiach (Karnath *et al.*, 2001; Karnath *et al.*, 2004a) and Vallar 2000) and the respective role of STG and PPC in the pathogenesis of neglect is unresolved (Karnath *et al.*, 2001; Karnath & Himmelbach 2002; Marshall *et al.*, 2002; Mort *et al.*, 2003; Karnath *et al.*, 2004b; Karnath *et al.*, 2004a). Some authors have suggested that the discrepancies could be due to different tests used to classify patients in the diagnostic phase. In fact, a dissociation between cancellation and bisection tasks has been reported not only in the behavioural domain (Halligan & Marshall 1992; Marshall & Halligan 1995; McGlinchey-Berroth *et al.*, 1996; Ferber & Karnath 2001), but also anatomically (Binder *et al.*, 1992; Rorden *et al.*, 2006). Binder and co-workers observed an association between posterior lesions and impairment in line bisection while more anterior lesions were associated with deficits on cancellation tasks (Binder *et al.* 1992).

More recently, Rorden and colleagues, using modern lesions mapping methods, compared brain lesions of patients with impaired performance in bisection, to those from patients with pathological performance on the cancellation task only. They confirmed an association between deficits in bisection, and temporo-occipital lesions (Rorden *et al.*, 2006). The possibility that the divergences observed in the anatomical-correlation studies of neglect depend on the test used (for the patients' selection) has also been investigated using transcranial magnetic stimulation (TMS) (Ellison *et al.*, 2004). They found that while stimulation of the posterior parietal cortex (PPC) induced a deficit on the landmark task of line bisection judgment, and on hard conjunction visual search, stimulation of the superior temporal cortex, did not impair the landmark performance. Conversely, a stimulation of STG caused a deficit on a hard feature visual task. Furthermore, some authors suggested a correlation between neglect evaluated in the chronic phase, and subcortical white matter lesions connecting the parietal and frontal cortex. In particular, a lesion at different levels of the superior longitudinal fasciculus (SLF) could explain the complex and variegate symptoms associated with hemineglect (Doricchi & Tomaiuolo 2003; Doricchi *et al.*, 2008).

Taken together, the anatomical localization of spatial neglect suggests a distributed neural architecture for spatial representation with a functional specialization in the right hemisphere.

One area in which lesion data have not been informative (as yet) is that of the dissociation between symptoms within the neglect syndrome. Patients may present with neglect symptoms only in one spatial frame (e.g. near space but not far space; Halligan & Marshall 1991) or in the same peripersonal space on one task (e.g. line bisection) but not another (e.g. target cancellation tasks; Halligan & Marshall 1992). These dissociations have not yet been corroborated by clear anatomical differences in lesion locations (cf. Vallar 2001), although different studies have tried to investigate the neural correlates of specific neglect symptoms: the neural correlates of, for example, extinction to double stimulation (Vallar *et al.*, 1994; Karnath *et al.*, 2003), anosognosia (Berti *et al.*, 2005; Karnath *et al.*, 2005), directional hypokinesia (Sapir *et al.*, 2007), perseveration on cancellation tasks (Nys *et al.*, 2006), and personal neglect (Committeri *et al.*, 2007).

3.2 Anatomical basis of deficits in reaching tasks

The other major acquired spatial disorder is characterised by deficits on reaching tasks. Lesions are usually located in the superior parietal lobule, and the disorder typically involves the contralateral limb in reaching to both sides of space (Jeannerod 1997).

3.3 Discrepancies between data from humans and monkeys

How do human and monkey data fit together? While there is substantial agreement for disorders of reaching, there is a clear discrepancy as far as the location of key lesions that underpin neglect.

- In the monkey, neglect is more severe after ventral pre-motor cortical lesions, than lesions in the superior temporal sulcus.

- In humans, the manifestations of neglect are more severe after parietal lesions (cf. Rizzolatti *et al.*, 2000 and Bisiach & Vallar 2000), but not primates.

Another important discrepancy is the hemispheric asymmetry observed in humans and not in primates.

4 Functional anatomical studies of space perception

4.1 Visual and somatosensory space

Functional imaging has the advantage of allowing one to explore the organisation of the healthy, as well as the diseased human brain *in vivo*. Yet, it should be kept in mind that the temporal and spatial resolution of imaging is not equivalent to that of invasive electrophysiology in the primate brain. To give an example of an area where imaging may be difficult to compare to electrophysiology, the progressive making of spatial representation from early sensory visual codes, may prove difficult to demonstrate. With the current techniques it has not been possible to isolate signals of neuronal populations of cells associated with gaze-dependent visual response, nor to isolate responses that can be plausibly interpreted as real-position like. There are obvious reasons why this may remain difficult with imaging. The cells are present in small areas which contain other, simpler cells as well. Even in the primate brain, real-position cells coexist in the same area as gaze-dependent cells.

In spite of these limitations, a substantial portion of the detailed information derived from primate brains is reproducible using functional imaging in humans. Large numbers of retinotopically organized areas have been now identified outside area V1 and area V2. Historically, the existence of separate extrastriate areas which are specialized in colour and motion perception, respectively, were the first to be shown. These are likely homologues of monkey areas V4 and V5 (Zeki *et al.*, 1991). An even more detailed cartography of retinotopically-organized extrastriate areas has now been described through the use of fMRI (see Fig. 37.3) (Sereno *et al.*, 1995). The receptive fields of the neurons within these areas are increasingly complex, with neurons also mapping the ipsilateral visual fields starting from area V3a and area MT/V5 (Tootell *et al.*, 1998). Together with the increasing complexity of the visual receptive fields, an increasing complexity of processing has been observed (e.g. in the ventral stream: while posterior regions are preferentially activated by object attributes such as colours or scrambled objects, more anterior temporal lobe regions are activated by intact objects or faces (cf. Kastner & Ungerleider 2000).

The neural representation of somatosensory space has been explored using a variety of approaches. Simple experiments in which somatosensory stimuli were delivered to the hands or feet have broadly confirmed the well-established notion of somatotopic organization of area S1. A possible somatotopic organization of area S2 has also been reported (Ruben *et al.*, 2001). In keeping with primate data, receptive fields (RF) in S1 appear to be strictly unilateral, while bilateral activation of area S2 is observed for stimuli delivered to either sides of the body, suggesting the presence in the human S2 of cells with at least bilateral, if not ipsilateral RFs (cf. Paulesu *et al.*, 1997).

4.2 The different frames of space as assessed by functional imaging

With respect to higher-order spatial representations, one area of enquiry which was addressed once functional imaging became available, was the demonstration of a broad dichotomy between two visual streams (the 'what' and 'where' pathways). This proved a relatively easy task. Haxby *et al.*, (1991) were the first to compare a face matching task (a ventral 'what' stream task), with a dot location task (a spatial 'where' task). A sensorimotor task with no relevant visual stimuli served as the control task. Compared to baseline, both experimental tasks showed activation of the lateral occipital cortex. Face discrimination alone activated a region of the occipitotemporal cortex, whereas the spatial location alone activated a region of the lateral superior parietal cortex.

This dichotomy was demonstrated and further replicated several times (Haxby *et al.*, 1994), particularly with reference to visual working memory. In keeping with electrophysiological data in the monkey (Goldman-Rakic 1996), when visual processing involves active maintenance of the spatial location of visual stimuli and delayed response, a dorsolateral prefrontal cortex activation is also observed (Courtney *et al.*, 1998). Consistent again with primate data (Wilson *et al.*, 1993; Chelazzi *et al.*, 1993), active maintenance of object-oriented visual information involves the more ventral parts of lateral prefrontal cortex, together with the ventral visual cortex (Courtney *et al.*, 1996). Therefore, the what (ventral) and where (dorsal) dichotomy is also present in frontal cortex (cf. Ungerleider *et al.*, 1998). The experiment of Haxby *et al.*, (1991) involved extra-personal spatial co-ordinates. The systematic exploration of other spatial frames has subsequently become the focus of research in several laboratories.

4.2.1 Object-centred (allocentric) space

Interestingly, a number of tasks have been used in which patients with spatial neglect may fail, showing either an overall impairment or a specific and dissociated impairment, depending on the nature of the task and the spatial frame explored by it. Object-centred (allocentric) spatial judgements have been studied in at least three experiments (Weiss *et al.*, 2000; Fink *et al.*, 2000a; Galati *et al.*, 2000). The stimuli used were computerised variations of Milner's landmark task in which stimuli are pre-bisected segments. The subjects had to judge whether the vertical bar that bisects a longer horizontal segment is placed in the middle of the segment or not. A meta-analysis of the main activations detected in the right hemisphere in these experiments is presented in Fig. 37.3. Baseline tasks were designed to subtract components other than spatial awareness. Activation foci are superimposed on a standard stereotactic view of the right hemisphere. The shaded areas represent the brain regions usually damaged in unilateral neglect (Vallar 1998). The typical involvement of the lateral extrastriate cortex, of the most dorsal part of area 40 in the inferior parietal lobule, and the intraparietal sulcus, the superior parietal lobule, and dorsal premotor cortex are clearly evident. This network closely resembles the visuomotor transformation network involved in reaching tasks in humans and in monkeys (Jeannerod 1997).

In the same experiment, Galati and co-workers (2000) devised an additional task in which subjects had to judge whether the vertical bar was located to the left or right of the subjective (egocentric) midsagittal plane of the body. In comparison with the same baseline, a similar, yet larger, bilateral pattern of activation emerged in the superior posterior parietal cortex (mesial and lateral), in the dorsal premotor cortex (bilaterally), and in left temporoparietal cortex emerged. The premotor cortex, the medial dorsoparietal cortex, and the right intraparietal cortex were more active when compared with the 'allocentric' task. In turn, there was a greater activation in the medial ventral extrastriate cortex when the allocentric task was compared to the egocentric one (not shown in Fig. 37.3). This seems a reproducible result. A similar finding was obtained by Fink et al., 2000b) when comparing a bisection judgement performed on a one-dimensional object (a segment), to a two-dimensional object (a square).

Larger activation of the ventral occipital cortex was also observed by Weiss et al., (2000), when comparing pointing tasks (including bisection) in far, versus near space. On the other hand, they found that the left hemispheric parietal cortex, the dorsal occipital cortex, and the premotor cortices were more active when comparing activations in near versus far space.

4.2.2 Egocentric (personal) space

Representations for egocentric (personal) space have also been explored recently using a different approach (Bottini et al, 2001). As discussed in Section 2, a possible mechanism by which spatial representations could be achieved, is through integration via convergence of different afferent inputs. Within this level of spatial body-centred description tactile, vestibular and proprioceptive stimuli (including those conveyed by the muscle spindles of the neck), play an important role. In the monkey a perisylvian network of cortices including the parietoinsular and retroinsular cortex, the ventral premotor cortex, and the tip of the intraparietal sulcus all receive inputs from the vestibule, the body surface and muscle spindles, including those of the neck muscles. Using this rationale, Bottini et al., (2001) mapped the cortical areas which are activated by either vestibular signals, or by neck muscle spindles; as appropriate stimulations of these systems can induce spatial bias towards the stimulated side in healthy controls, and reduce spatial disorder in unilateral neglect. Specific to the monkey, the perisylvian somatosensory cortex (retroinsular cortex, area S2, supramarginal gyrus) appears to be a site of convergence of these inputs, suggesting that these brain regions contribute to egocentric space representation (Bottini et al., 2001).

4.2.3 Is there dissociation between allocentric and egocentric frames of reference?

The picture which emerges from the experiments detailed above is not yet fully coherent in showing clear-cut dissociations between allocentric and egocentric frames of reference. This may be due to discrepancies between experimental and baseline tasks used in the various experiments (and to the assumption of lack of spatial demands made when choosing such baselines). In addition, subjects responded to the stimuli in different ways in each of the experiments. There was button pressing in three experiments, pointing with a laser light in one, and no response in another. Taken together, however, the results of Fink et al., (2000a), Galati et al., (2000), and Weiss et al., (2000) seem to indicate a weak dissociation within a distributed, partially overlapping system for spatial representation of peripersonal and extrapersonal space.

- The visuomotor transformation network implied in reaching behaviour is activated, with greater emphasis on the dorsal parietal and premotor cortex, when the experimental task implies attending to spatial locations that are within reaching distance.
- Ventral retinotopically organized and object-based visual cortices are more active when the comparisons of blood flow maps isolate the processing of spatial locations (which are either outside reaching distance (far space) or when reaching is (relatively) de-emphasized).

The difference in results between the 'egocentric' task of Galati et al., (2000) and the experiment of Bottini et al., (2001), an experiment which takes into account the convergent afferents which contribute to the representation of egocentric space, remains particularly striking. It is likely that the task, and its reference baseline, dominate the picture of activations which can be observed via imaging; these factors alone may explain the discrepancies. Alternatively, one may speculate on the existence of multiple levels of neural/cognitive representations for the same spatial frame. If this were the case, behavioural dissociations based on lesion data would be required to make this a more convincing possibility. The consistency of each of the above observations with lesion data of neglect will be discussed in Section 6.

5 Spatial attention

The space surrounding us contains far too many items for the brain to simultaneously process efficiently and consciously at once. The mental ability which permits people to deal explicitly with a subset of behaviourally relevant stimuli is usually referred to as attention. In the definition of psychologist William James (1890–1950), "Attention is…the taking possession by the mind…of one out of what seem several simultaneously possible objects or trains of thought.…It implies withdrawal from some things in order to deal effectively with others." This definition emphasizes attention as a process of selection.

The advantage of attention in perceptual/motor task can even be appreciated introspectively. We know that we are more efficient at responding to environmental stimuli when we attend to them. In addition to introspection, there are quantitative behavioural techniques which measure the advantage of attention. Various indices can be used: reaction times are faster for responses to visual stimuli that fall within attended parts of the visual field; discrimination of stimuli is enhanced (cf. Umiltà 2000).

If we consider visual space, the process of orienting attention usually implies fast saccadic eye movements, which are made to bring the visual stimuli into foveal space. Yet there is definitive evidence that spatial attention can also be oriented without eye movements – covert (endogenous) orienting.

- Endogenous orienting of attention is frequently referred to as a top-down or controlled process which is effortful and depends on will. The classic paradigm devised by Posner (1980) taps this form of attention (Umiltà 2000; Posner 1980). This paradigm, with small *ad hoc* adaptations, has been used in a number of functional imaging experiments, as is illustrated in Fig. 37.4.

- Spatial attention can also be attracted automatically by the sudden appearance of a stimulus in the visual field, or by the perceptual salience of a stimulus among others (e.g. a vertical bar among other bars all tilted 30° to the right). These other phenomena are called bottom-up or exogenous processes (Fig. 37.5).

Once attention has been oriented towards a stimulus, it may become necessary to re-orient to a different spatial location, which implies disengagement from the former, to re-orient towards a different one.

5.1 Does spatial attention have a dedicated neural system in the human brain?

The research into spatial attentional processes using functional neuroimaging includes (see also Box 37.1):

- identification of brain regions involved in spatial attention and assessment of the degree of overlap between attentional, perceptual and premotor networks, particularly with reference to the neural systems for eye movement;

- characterization of top-down processes (such as those involved in covert, or endogenous, orienting), as opposed to attentional phenomena based on perceptual salience (bottom-up processes; exogenous orienting);

- assessment of orienting versus disengaging attention;

- space- versus object-based attention;

- global (diffuse) and local attentional processes.

Some of these issues have been investigated using functional imaging.

The contribution of functional imaging to these fundamental issues has been crucial to progress. Lesion data are inconclusive because some disorders of spatial exploration and representation (such as spatial neglect), are not universally interpreted as being due to an attentional deficit (cf. Bisiach & Vallar 2000). Event-related potentials are able to reveal changes of brain response but they cannot tell in which part of the brain these effects are generated. In a very influential paper, Posner and Petersen (1990) summarized the

Covert spatial orientation paradigm of poster

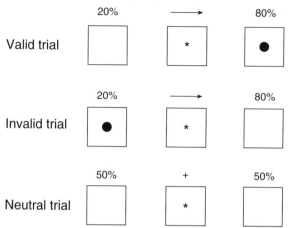

Fig. 37.4 Posner's attentional paradigm. In Posner's paradigm, subjects are instructed by a symbolic central cue (an arrow) that a target stimulus (a filled circle) will occur with 80% of chance in a given spatial location. Subjects are instructed to fixate on a central mark, not to move their eyes, and to press a key as quickly as possible when the filled circle appears. Covert attention is measured as the reaction time benefit in responding to the target which appears in the attended location (valid trials) as opposed to response for targets appearing in unattended locations (invalid trials) or to neutral trials, when another symbol (+) indicates that the filled circle has a 50% chance of appearing in either box (Posner 1980).

Controlled and automatic attention

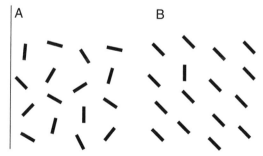

Fig. 37.5 Difference between controlled and automatic attentional processes. In display A, detection of a vertical segment is a demanding attention-seeking (top-down) process that can be oriented endogenously or through verbal instructions. Detection of a vertical segment in display B is stimulus driven and automatic (redrawn from Kastner and Ungerleider 2000).

Box 37.1 Attention from the neurophysiologist's perspective

While psychologists characterize attentional effects in the form of reaction time benefits or costs, the neurophysiologist records the neuronal firing rate associated with the presentation of a stimulus or with the execution of a motoric response. Which response is then interpreted as attentional by the neurophysiologist? The most robust and established effects are 'enhancement effects', increases of baseline activity, and suppression of unwanted information.

◆ *Enhancement effects.* Goldberg and Wurtz (1972) made the important observation that the firing rate of a visual neuron of the superior colliculus can be enhanced when a stimulus is delivered to the receptive field of that neuron if the animal is covertly attending to that spatial location. The enhancement effects in the superior colliculus are present only when the animal is about to generate a saccadic eye movement towards the stimulus. Similar neurons can be found in cortical structures involved in eye-movement control, such as the frontal eye-fields (Goldberg & Bushnell 1981). Importantly, in a given neuron, the 'enhancement effect' is not present if the saccadic eye movement is performed towards a spatial location which lies outside the receptive field of the neuron. Enhancement effects are not necessarily associated with the generation of saccadic eye movements. Such 'purer' enhanced responses have been seen in the pulvinar, but also in parietal cortex (Colby *et al.*, 1996) and temporal cortex (Chelazzi *et al.*, 1993). In the cortex of the parietal lobe, the enhancement is related to spatial location of the stimulus. In the temporal lobe, enhancement effects are related to stimulus attributes, rather than to its spatial location.

◆ *Increase of baseline activity.* While the enhancement effect occurs at the time the stimulus is presented, increase of baseline activity has been observed in neurons of area V2 or V4 even before the presentation of a stimulus (providing that the experimental animal is attending to the spatial location which corresponds to the receptive field of the neuron (Luck *et al.*, 1997)).

◆ *Filtering of unwanted information.* When two objects are present in the receptive field of the same neuron of the temporal lobe (e.g. an object which activates the neuron, and an object which activates it less strongly), a mutual suppression of neural response is observed so that the neural firing is roughly the average of the firing rates induced by each separate object. This suppression can be modulated by attention towards one of the two objects so that the response is similar to that for an object presented in isolation (Reynolds *et al.*, 1999).

All of these general effects have been seen in humans using functional imaging. Enhancement effects have been seen in subjects who were attending to particular visual features of a display, in comparison to when they were passively viewing the same display.

Box 37.1 Attention from the neurophysiologist's perspective *(continued)*

- Attention to colour was associated with enhanced response in modality specific visual cortices such as area V4.

- Attention to shape was associated with enhanced response in area V3.

- Enhancement for speed and motion was associated with area V5/MT (Corbetta *et al.*, 1991).

A shift in baseline activity in specific cortical areas has been described using fMRI. Even in the absence of any actual change in visual stimulus, the baseline activities of the visual motion area V5/MT or of the colour area V4, are enhanced if subjects are expecting to detect a change of motion or colour, in a visual display (Chawla *et al.*, 1999). Conversely, if subjects are distracted by a highly demanding language task while observing a display of moving dots, activation of area V5/MT disappears (contrary to what happens in the same conditions when the distracting task is an easy one (Rees *et al.*, 1997b)). fMRI data which are compatible with the filtering of unwanted visual information by visual cortex have recently been reported (Kastner *et al.*, 1998).

then available evidence, including very early functional imaging data, on the existence of attentional networks. They proposed the following three tenets.

- The attentional system is anatomically separate from the data-processing system, and in this sense it is like other sensory and motor systems.

- The attentional system involves a distributed network:
  - — a posterior attentional system;
  - — an anterior attentional system;
  - — an ascending attentional system.

- Within the network, different components have different specializations that can be described in cognitive terms.

The cognitive operations involved are:

- orienting to sensory events;

- detecting signals for focal processing;

- maintaining vigilance.

In this account of spatial attention, each component has its neural machinery.

- Orienting to sensory events usually implies the foveation of a stimulus (overt orienting). The brain regions involved are: the posterior parietal cortex (Goldberg & Bruce 1985); the pulvinar nucleus of the thalamus (LaBerge & Buchsbaum 1990); and the superior colliculus (Goldberg & Wurtz 1972). These regions represent the posterior attentional system. Based on observation of patients with parietal lesions (Posner *et al.*, 1984), Posner & Petersen (1990) maintain that:

— the posterior parietal cortex is involved in disengagement from an attentional focus towards a target located in the opposite direction to the side of brain lesion;

— the superior colliculus would be also involved in shifting attention, whether or not attention was already focused elsewhere;

— the pulvinar nucleus is thought to contribute to engagement with the new target location of the attentional focus.

◆ Posner & Petersen (1990) also proposed that the anterior (frontal and cingulate) cortical regions might represent an amodal system which primes the posterior system to detect signals for focal processing. The anterior system is postulated to mediate selective attention and cognitive control. Early PET experiments on divided attention and control of response for conflicting stimuli (e.g. Stroop task) support this assumption (Pardo *et al.*, 1990; Corbetta *et al.*, 1991).

◆ Finally, Posner & Petersen (1990) proposed that alerting is a function of the right hemisphere, and of the ascending noradrenergic system (cf. Heilman *et al.*, 1994).

This cognitive-anatomical model for attention is not unanimously accepted. For example, it sharply contrasts with a competing model which postulates that attentional networks are embedded within the same networks involved in perception and action. One such model in fact, postulates that spatial attention is the consequence of the activation (even in the absence of overt motor response), of the neural system that mediates sensory motor transformation (Rizzolatti *et al.*, 1994).

We will next discuss the extent to which assumptions proposed by Petersen and Posner have been supported by the recent imaging literature, together with a short review of other relevant experiments on spatial attention.

5.2 The physiology of eye movements and spatial attention

A crucial test for Posner and Petersen's (1990) model is the assessment of the degree of independence of areas activated by covert orienting of visual attention (as in Posner's paradigm illustrated in Fig. 37.4), and actual performance of saccadic eye movements. Behavioural evidence would suggest that the two systems are somewhat embedded (cf. Umiltà 2000, and Corbetta 1998). On this particular issue there are a number of specific functional imaging experiments (Corbetta *et al.*, 1998; Nobre *et al.*, 2000) and detailed meta-analyses (Corbetta 1998; Nobre *et al.*, 1997).

In short, both covert orienting of attention (as in Posner's paradigm, see Fig. 37.4) and the generation of saccades, share neural resources in:

◆ the parietal regions of the intraparietal sulcus and superior parietal lobule;

◆ the dorsal lateral premotor cortex (human homologue of frontal eye fields);

◆ the mesial dorsal premotor cortex (human supplementary frontal eye-fields) (Fig. 37.6).

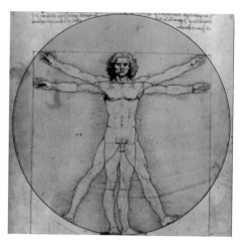

Plate 1 Classification of spatial frames.
The body, the space within reaching distance and far space. Neuropsychology and neurophysiology provide evidence that the brain has separate representations for these different spatial frames. Personal space is somatosensory space mapped as a body schema independently from visual space. Extrapersonal space also involves visual space: This can be based on egocentric coordinates (within reaching distance); visual space is organized with reference to head, trunk and limbs. Extrapersonal space can be mapped in allocentric (object-based) coordinates.

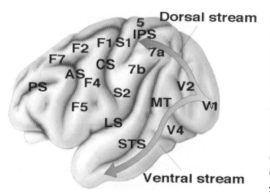

Dorsal stream

Ventral stream

Plate 2 Left cerebral hemisphere of the macaque brain. IPS, intraparietal sulcus; MT, motion temporal area (V5); S1, primary somatosensory area; S2, second somatosensory area; CS, central sulcus; LS, lateral sulcus; STS, superior temporal sulcus; AS, arcuate sulcus; PS, principal sulcus. The nomenclature of motor areas follows Matelli *et al.* (1985,1991). Some of the visual areas (V3, V6) cannot be seen on the lateral surface of the brain.

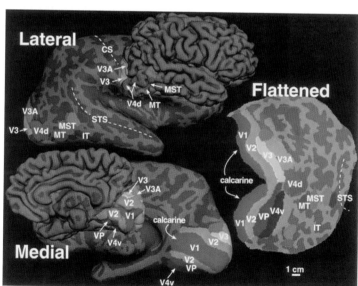

Plate 3 Visual areas with well characterized retinotopic organization identified by fMRI. The brain regions are superimposed on lateral and mesial views of the human cerebral hemispheres and on flattened visual cortex. CS, central sulcus; STS, superior temporal sulcus; MT, motion temporal area; MST, medial superior temporal; IT, inferior temporal; VP, ventral posterior. (Courtesy of Martin Sereno; Copyright (2001), Lippincott, Williams and Wilkins; Sereno *et al.* 1995; Bear *et al.* 2001).

Three imaging studies on line bisection

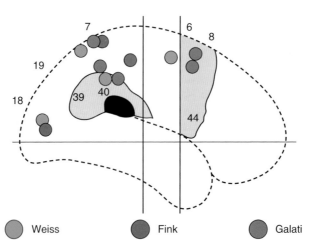

Plate 4 Brain areas associated with spatial neglect (shaded areas) and meta-analysis of three functional neuroimaging experiments in healthy individuals using line bisection. Circles represent the location of activation peaks expressed in stereotactic space from three different imaging studies (Fink *et al.* 2000a; Weiss *et al.* 2000; Galati *et al.* 2000). Only the activations on the lateral surface of the right hemisphere are reported. The horizontal line represents the plane passing through the two commissures. The two vertical lines represent the coronal planes passing through each of the two commissures. Mesial ventral occipital activations are not shown.

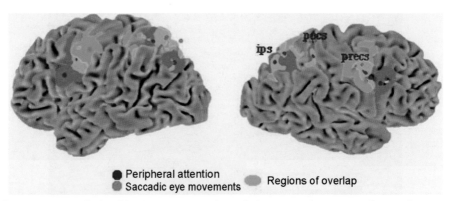

Plate 5 Meta-analysis of brain regions activated during performance of saccadic eye movements and covert orienting of peripheral attention. The picture shows areas for performance of saccadic eye movements, for covert orienting of peripheral attention, and areas shared, at the macroscopic anatomical level, by the two processes. ips, Intraparietal sulcus; pocs, postcentral sulcus; precs, precentral sulcus. (Source: Corbetta 1998; Courtesy of Maurizio Corbetta; Copyright 1998, National Academy of Sciences, USA).

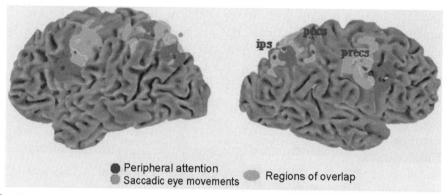

Fig. 37.6 Meta-analysis of brain regions activated during performance of saccadic eye movements and covert orienting of peripheral attention. The picture shows areas for performance of saccadic eye movements, for covert orienting of peripheral attention, and areas shared, at the macroscopic anatomical level, by the two processes. ips, Intraparietal sulcus; pocs, postcentral sulcus; precs, precentral sulcus. (Source: Corbetta 1998; Courtesy of Maurizio Corbetta; Copyright 1998, National Academy of Sciences, USA). (See also 'Plates' section).

Therefore, one can reject the complete independence of regions involved in covert orienting and saccadic eye movements. However in the meta-analysis of Corbetta *et al.*, (1998), the overlap between the two systems (while considerable), is clearly not perfect.

♦ Eye movements are associated with more extensive involvement of regions near the primary motor and somatosensory cortices.

♦ Covert orienting shows a larger involvement of prefrontal, and of lateral occipitoparietal junction regions.

The additional areas seen in the saccadic eye movements can be readily explained by the fact that subjects are actually moving their eyes. The additional areas seen in covert orienting may represent the more cognitive neural counterpart of the task. Indeed, the discrepancy between the motor task (saccadic eye movements), and the more controlled orienting task, is reminiscent of the difference seen in tasks in which one task involves more controlled and cognitive demanding factors. For instance, in the case of articulation of a stereotyped string of digits as opposed to random generation of digits, the latter task also involves more anterior prefrontal regions (Petrides *et al.*, 1993). A meta-analysis performed by Kastner & Ungerleider (2000) also shows that the distribution of the activation during covert orienting of visual attention while maintaining central fixation, is independent of the specific requirements of the visuospatial task (i.e. detecting a stimulus and discriminating or tracking its movement). Interestingly, the pattern of activation resembles that identified in the meta-analysis presented in Fig. 37.3.

What is the impact of eye movements on the firing rate of brain regions outside those directly implicated in the motor commands? There is evidence for a substantial inhibition of occipital visual areas during saccades. This has been seen for reflexive saccades induced by vestibular stimuli, where the lateralization of deactivation (on the side opposite to the areas of major activation by vestibular stimuli), suggests that a specific neurobiological mechanism is involved. It is also interesting that deactivations include, amongst others, the visual motion perception area MT/V5. The modulatory effect of eye movements on visual areas has also been described by Paus *et al.,* (1996). Volunteers lay in the dark and moved their eyes at different rates during a series of scans. Activity in the frontal eye fields was positively correlated with the rate of eye movements. However, in visual cortex and visual association areas, activity was negatively correlated with rate of eye movements.

Fink and colleagues (1997) have explored another important issue, which is the interaction of eye movements in object- as opposed to space-based attention. They found that brain activation during attention is modulated by eye movements, particularly for object-based attention. Greater parietal activations were seen when foveation was not allowed, as if object-based attention in these conditions, becomes 'more spatial' in nature. The stimuli used by Fink and colleagues were devoid of any semantic content (simple lines with a square, and no graspable objects or body segments were used). Further studies are needed to address the same issue using ecologically relevant objects, in two- and three-dimensional presentations.

5.3 Top-down and bottom-up processes in spatial attention: where is 'the top' and where is 'the bottom'?

Whichever model of attention one considers, it is necessary to consider whether there is anatomical distinction between controlled and automatic orienting of attention. While there is general consensus that enhancement effects observed in extrastriate visual cortex (see Box above) may represent the effects of top-down modulations from areas outside visual cortex, the source of the modulation remains elusive.

Kastner and Ungerleider (2000) propose that the source of top-down modulation may be in brain areas involved in covert orienting of attention. The obvious way to test this assumption is to compare Posner's task with another one in which spatial attention is driven exogenously. This was tried by Nobre and collaborators (1997). They compared a task in which a peripheral visual cue indicated that a subsequent stimulus was 80% likely to occur in the same location, with a condition in which the same cue indicated that a subsequent stimulus was 80% likely to occur in the opposite part of the visual field. (The latter task is more closely associated with controlled attentional processes, while the former is an exogenous process.) However, the two tasks did not show any clear-cut dichotomy, either when compared with a reference task, or when the two tasks were compared directly to each other. Both tasks were associated with a system compatible with that described in Fig. 37.6.

Rees *et al.,* (1997a) approached the same problem with an experiment in which top-down factors were assessed with respect to tonic biasing mechanisms versus stimulus-dependent ones. This is not easy to achieve given the temporal resolution of imaging techniques (Rees *et al.,* 1997a). However, by changing the rate of visual stimuli requiring attention, they were able to show that the inferior temporal cortex had rate dependent changes of attention induced activity, while activity in the right dorsal premotor cortex (BA8) was independent of stimulus presentation rate. This data is compatible with the idea that inferior temporal cortex is a site of modulation, while the right premotor region is a source of top-down modulatory effects on visual cortices.

Kastner et al., (1999) used fMRI to investigate patterns of activation in the presence and absence of visual stimuli. Sustained activity was observed, even in the absence of actual stimulation in the dorsal parietal regions and premotor regions usually involved in the covert orienting of attention. This sustained activity was of the same magnitude as the activity observed during stimulus presentation. On the other hand, in ventral extrastriate visual areas, activity in the absence of visual stimuli was comparatively smaller. This evidence supports the notion that dorsal brain areas involved in orienting of attention are the source of modulatory signals directed towards ventral extrastriate visual areas. The role of the superior parietal cortex in orienting attention (rather than stimulus detection), has recently been demonstrated by Corbetta et al., (2000).

Is the source of these modulatory effects unique? We believe that this is unlikely. Although direct imaging evidence remains scanty, there is behavioural evidence which shows that biasing effects in visual stimulus detection can be induced in tasks which are very different from Posner's covert orienting paradigm (or from the other tasks used thus far in imaging experiments). For instance, preparation of a given grasping response, facilitates visual detection of objects which have a shape which is compatible with that grip (Craighero et al., 1999). Grasping and observation of grasping depend on different and more ventral circuits in premotor and parietal cortices than those involved in eye movements (Rizzolatti et al., 2000). As a consequence, it can be speculated that the source of biasing effects will move, according to the nature of the task. This conjecture is supported by recent fMRI evidence. Sustained attention to, and observation of, finger movements modulates ventral premotor and rostral superior parietal regions, involved in both the actual performance of the movements, as well as in their observation. These are regions, particularly the ventral premotor cortex, which are well outside the network for eye movements, which suggests a modular organization of the neural systems for attention (Iacoboni et al., 1999).

6 A discrepancy between imaging data on spatial attention and processing and the anatomy of spatial neglect

As noted by others (Kastner & Ungerleider 2000), the evolving picture of the functional anatomy of spatial attention (and, of spatial processing in general), presents a non trivial discrepancy to the published anatomy of spatial neglect (Vallar 1998, 2001). The distribution of lesions typically observed in neglect are summarized by the shaded areas in Fig. 37.3 (Vallar 1998). It is clear that the pattern of activations reported for line bisection tasks (a sensitive test of spatial neglect; see meta-analysis in Fig. 37.3) involve regions in the parietal lobe; ones which are more dorsal overall. However, the more ventral regions are systematically seen in experiments involving the central projections of the vestibular system, an important finding given the well known ability of vestibular signals to recalibrate spatial misperception (and representation) in neglect patients (cf. Paulesu et al., 1997).

The same point about the topography of parietal and premotor activations applies to the anatomy of the covert orienting of attention circuits (see Fig. 37.6) (Corbetta 1998), which appears to be more dorsal (than the regions associated with spatial neglect). Indeed, given the limited overlap between the two anatomical patterns, the data seem to justify a view that spatial neglect does not merely represent a disorder of attention (cf. Bisiach & Vallar 2000).

Another source of nontrivial discrepancy with respect to the anatomy of neglect pertains to the lateralization of cerebral activations. A predominant activation of the right hemisphere has been found in several studies of spatial attention (e.g. Nobre et al., 1997), and of sustained attention (Pardo et al., 1991). However, meta-analyses of experiments on covert orienting of attention show substantially bilateral and symmetrical patterns of dorsal premotor superior parietal, and intraparietal activity (Kastner & Ungerleider 2000; Corbetta 1998). The functional predominance of the left hemisphere for near space reported in the PET experiment of Weiss et al., (2000), awaits testing in brain-damaged patients.

Recently, Corbetta proposed a model which explains the divergent results emerging from lesion data in neglect patients, and fMRI studies of visuo-spatial orienting. The bilateral dorsal fronto-parietal network, including the intraparietal sulcus (IPS) and frontal eye field (FEF) is involved in voluntary attention and in the selection of stimuli and responses. The ventral network, including the temporo-parietal junction (TPJ) and the inferior frontal gyrus (IFG) (with a strong lateralization to the right hemisphere), is involved in the detection of relevant stimuli (particularly when subjects reorient attention toward a target which appears in an unexpected location). Both these attentional networks interact in normal subjects to permit visual orienting, and both are damaged in patients with visuo-spatial neglect (Corbetta 1998; Corbetta et al., 2002).

Mismatch between functional imaging and lesion data is not new. This has been seen previously for episodic memory, for example (Dolan et al., 1997). Resolution of these discrepancies in spatial neurocognition may contribute to better understanding of spatial neglect, of normal spatial processing and attention, and of the nature of right hemispheric dominance in spatial processing. To achieve this, more studies on the anatomy of neglect are needed as well as on the spatial processing of normal subjects and patients with acquired lesions. The anatomy of neglect needs to be mapped with patients performing a wider range of tasks, to reveal dissociations of behavioural deficit. Indeed, the available data thus far collected, has focused primarily on the cancellation tasks (which cover spatial exploration in peripersonal space alone). If the overall pattern of brain lesion in neglect can be replicated using different tasks, then it becomes important to characterize the spatial properties of those brain areas (in humans); a task which has proved challenging.

Selective references

Andersen, R.A. (1994). Coordinate transformation and motor planning in posterior parietal cortex. In *The Cognitive Neurosciences*. (ed. M. Gazzaniga), pp. 519–33. MIT Press, Boston.

Andersen, R.A., Snyder, L.H., Bradley, D.C., and Xing, J. (1997). Multimodal representation of space in the posterior parietal cortex and its use in planning movements. *Annu Rev Neurosci*. **20**, 303–30.

Bear, M., Connors, B., and Paradiso, M. (2001). *Neuroscience. Exploring the brain*. Lippincott, Williams and Wilkins, Baltimore.

Berti, A., Bottini, G., Gandola, M., *et al.* (2005). Shared cortical anatomy for motor awareness and motor control. *Science*. **309**, 488–91.

Binder, J., Marshall, R., Lazar, R., Benjamin, J., and Mohr, J.P. (1992). Distinct syndromes of hemineglect. *Arch Neurol*. **49**, 1187–94.

Bisiach, E. and Vallar, G. (2000). Unilateral neglect in humans. In *Handbook of Neuropsychology*, 2nd ed. (ed. F. Boller, J. Grafman, and G. Rizzolatti), pp. 1-44. Elsevier, Amsterdam.

Bottini, G., Karnath, H.O., Vallar, G., *et al.* (2001). Cerebral representations for egocentric space: Functional-anatomical evidence from caloric vestibular stimulation and neck vibration. *Brain*. **124**, 1182–96.

Chawla, D., Rees, G., and Friston, K.J. (1999). The physiological basis of attentional modulation in extrastriate visual areas. *Nature Neurosci*. **2**, 671–6.

Chelazzi, L., Miller, E.K., Duncan, J., and Desimone, R. (1993). A neural basis for visual search in inferior temporal cortex. *Nature*. **363**, 345–7.

Colby, C.L., Duhamel, J.R., and Goldberg, M.E. (1996). Visual, presaccadic, and cognitive activation of single neurons in monkey lateral intraparietal area. *J Neurophysiol*. **76**, 2841–52.

Colby, C.L. and Goldberg, M.E. (1999). Space and attention in parietal cortex. *Annu Rev Neurosci*. **22**, 319–49.

Committeri, G., Pitzalis, S., Galati, G., *et al.* (2007). Neural bases of personal and extrapersonal neglect in humans. *Brain*. **130**, 431–41.

Corbetta, M., Miezin, F.M., Dobmeyer, S., Shulman, G.L., and Petersen, S.E. (1991). Selective and divided attention during visual discriminations of shape, color, and speed: functional anatomy by positron emission tomography. *J Neurosci*. **11**, 2383–402.

Corbetta, M. (1998). Frontoparietal cortical networks for directing attention and the eye to visual locations: identical, independent, or overlapping neural systems? *Proc Natl Acad Sci U S A*. **95**, 831–8.

Corbetta, M., Akbudak, E., Conturo, T.E., *et al.* (1998). A common network of functional areas for attention and eye movements. *Neuron*. **21**, 761–73.

Corbetta, M., Kincade, J.M., Ollinger, J.M., McAvoy, M.P., and Shulman, G.L. (2000). Voluntary orienting is dissociated from target detection in human posterior parietal cortex. *Nat Neurosci*. **3**, 292–7.

Corbetta, M., Kincade, M., and Shulman, G.L. (2002). Two neural systems for visual orienting and the pathophysiology of unilateral spatial neglect. In *The Cognitive and Neural Bases of Spatial Neglect*. (ed. H. O. Karnath, A. D. Milner, and G. Vallar), pp. 259–73. Oxford University Press, Oxford.

Courtney, S.M., Ungerleider, L.G., Keil, K., and Haxby, J.V. (1996). Object and spatial visual working memory activate separate neural systems in human cortex. *Cereb Cortex*. **6**, 39–49.

Courtney, S.M., Petit, L., Maisog, J.M., Ungerleider, L.G., and Haxby, J.V. (1998). An area specialized for spatial working memory in human frontal cortex. *Science*. **279**, 1347–51.

Craighero, L., Fadiga, L., Rizzolatti, G., and Umiltà, C. (1999). Action for perception: a motor-visual attentional effect. *J Exp Psychol Hum Percept Perform*. **25**, 1673–92.

Dolan, R., Paulesu, E., and Fletcher, P. (1997). Human Memory Systems. In *Human Brain Function*. (ed. R. Frackowiak), pp. 367–404. Academic Press, San Diego.

Doricchi, F. and Tomaiuolo, F. (2003). The anatomy of neglect without hemianopia: a key role for parietal-frontal disconnection? *Neuroreport*. 14, 2239–43.

Doricchi, F., Thiebaut de Schotten, M., Tomaiuolo, F., and Bartolomeo, P. (2008). White matter (dis) connections and gray matter (dys)functions in visual neglect: gaining insights into the brain networks of spatial awareness. *Cortex*. 44, 983–95.

Duhamel, J.R., Colby, C.L., and Goldberg, M.E. (1992). The updating of the representation of visual space in parietal cortex by intended eye movements. *Science*. 255, 90–2.

Ellison, A., Schindler, I., Pattison, L.L., and Milner, A.D. (2004). An exploration of the role of the superior temporal gyrus in visual search and spatial perception using TMS. *Brain*. 127, 2307–15.

Ferber, S. and Karnath, H.O. (2001). How to assess spatial neglect–line bisection or cancellation tasks? *J Clin Exp Neuropsychol*. 23, 599–607.

Fink, G.R., Dolan, R.J., Halligan, P.W., Marshall, J.C., and Frith, C.D. (1997). Space-based and object-based visual attention: shared and specific neural domains. *Brain*. 120 (pt 11), 2013–28.

Fink, G.R., Marshall, J.C., Shah, N.J., *et al*. (2000a). Line bisection judgments implicate right parietal cortex and cerebellum as assessed by fMRI. *Neurology*. 54, 1324–31.

Fink, G.R., Marshall, J.C., Weiss, P.H., *et al*. (2000b). 'Where' depends on 'what': a differential functional anatomy for position discrimination in one- versus two-dimensions. *Neuropsychologia*. 38, 1741–8.

Fogassi, L., Gallese, V., Fadiga, L., Luppino, G., Matelli, M., and Rizzolatti, G. (1996). Coding of peripersonal space in inferior premotor cortex (area F4). *J Neurophysiol*. 76, 141–57.

Galati, G., Lobel, E., Vallar, G., Berthoz, A., Pizzamiglio, L., and Le Bihan, D. (2000). The neural basis of egocentric and allocentric coding of space in humans: a functional magnetic resonance study. *Exp Brain Res*. 133, 156–64.

Galletti, C., Battaglini, P.P., and Fattori, P. (1993). Parietal neurons encoding spatial locations in craniotopic coordinates. *Exp Brain Res*. 96, 221–9.

Galletti, C. and Fattori, P. (2002). Posterior parietal networks encoding visual space. In *The cognitive and neural bases of spatial neglect*. (ed. H. Karnath, D. Milner, and G. Vallar), pp. 59-69. Oxford University Press, Oxford.

Goldberg, M.E. and Wurtz, R.H. (1972). Activity of superior colliculus in behaving monkey. II. Effect of attention on neuronal responses. *J Neurophysiol*. 35, 560–74.

Goldberg, M.E. and Bushnell, M.C. (1981). Behavioral enhancement of visual responses in monkey cerebral cortex. II. Modulation in frontal eye fields specifically related to saccades. *J Neurophysiol*. 46, 773–87.

Goldberg, M.E. and Bruce, C.J. (1985). Cerebral cortical activity associated with the orientation of visual attention in the rhesus monkey. *Vision Res*. 25, 471–81.

Goldman-Rakic, P.S. (1996). The prefrontal landscape: implications of functional architecture for understanding human mentation and the central executive. *Philos Trans R Soc Lond B Biol Sci*. 351, 1445–53.

Goodale, M.A. and Milner, A.D. (1992). Separate visual pathways for perception and action. *Trends Neurosci*. 15, 20–5.

Graziano, M. and Gross, C. (1994). The representation of extra-personal space: a possible role for bimodal visual-tactile neurons. In *The Cognitive Neurosciences*. (ed. M. Gazzaniga), pp. 1021–34. MIT Press, Boston.

Guldin, W.O. and Grüsser, O.J. (1998). Is there a vestibular cortex? *Trends Neurosci*. 21, 254–9.

Halligan, P.W. and Marshall, J.C. (1991). Left neglect for near but not far space in man. *Nature*. 350, 498–500.

Halligan, P.W. and Marshall, J.C. (1992). Left visuo-spatial neglect: a meaningless entity? *Cortex.* **28**, 525–35.

Haxby, J.V., Grady, C.L., Horwitz, B., *et al.* (1991). Dissociation of object and spatial visual processing pathways in human extrastriate cortex. *Proc Natl Acad Sci U S A.* **88**, 1621–5.

Haxby, J.V., Horwitz, B., Ungerleider, L.G., Maisog, J.M., Pietrini, P., and Grady, C.L. (1994). The functional organization of human extrastriate cortex: a PET-rCBF study of selective attention to faces and locations. *J Neurosci.* **14**, 6336–53.

Heilman, K. M., Watson, R.T., and Valenstein, E. (1994). Localization of lesions in neglect and related disorders. In *Localization and neuroimaging in neuropsychology.* (ed. A. Kertesz), pp. 495–524. Academic Press, San Diego.

Hendry, S.H. and Reid, R.C. (2000). The koniocellular pathway in primate vision. *Annu Rev Neurosci.* **23**, 127–53.

Iacoboni, M., Woods, R. P., Brass, M., Bekkering, H., Mazziotta, J.C., and Rizzolatti, G. (1999). Cortical mechanisms of human imitation. *Science.* **286**, 2526–8.

James, W. (1890/1950). *Principles of Psychology.* Dover, New York.

Jeannerod, M., Arbib, M.A., Rizzolatti, G., and Sakata, H. (1995). Grasping objects: the cortical mechanisms of visuomotor transformation. *Trends Neurosci.* **18**, 314–20.

Jeannerod, M. (1997). *The cognitive neuroscience of action.* Blackwell, Oxford.

Kaas, J.H. (1990). Somatosensory system. In *The Human Nervous System.* (ed. G. Paxinos), pp. 813–44. Academic Press, San Diego.

Karnath, H.O. (1994). Subjective body orientation in neglect and the interactive contribution of neck muscle proprioception and vestibular stimulation. *Brain.* **117**, 1001–12.

Karnath, H.O., Sievering, D., and Fetter, M. (1994). The interactive contribution of neck muscle proprioception and vestibular stimulation to subjective "straight ahead" orientation in man. *Exp Brain Res.* **101**, 140–6.

Karnath, H.O., Ferber, S., and Himmelbach, M. (2001). Spatial awareness is a function of the temporal not the posterior parietal lobe. *Nature.* **411**, 950–3.

Karnath, H.O. and Himmelbach, M. (2002). Science Discussion Topic Strategies of Lesion Localization — Reply to Marshall, Fink, Halligan and Vallar. *Cortex.* **38**, 258–60.

Karnath, H.O., Himmelbach, M., and Kuker, W. (2003). The cortical substrate of visual extinction. *Neuroreport.* **14**, 437–42.

Karnath, H.O., Fruhmann Berger, M., Kuker, W., and Rorden, C. (2004a). The anatomy of spatial neglect based on voxelwise statistical analysis: a study of 140 patients. *Cereb Cortex.* **14**, 1164–72.

Karnath, H.O., Fruhmann Berger, M., Zopf, R., and Kuker, W. (2004b). Using SPM normalization for lesion analysis in spatial neglect. *Brain.* **127**, E10; author reply E11.

Karnath, H.O., Baier, B., and Nagele, T. (2005). Awareness of the functioning of one's own limbs mediated by the insular cortex? *J Neurosci.* **25**, 7134–8.

Kastner, S., De_Weerd, P., Desimone, R., and Ungerleider, L.G. (1998). Mechanisms of directed attention in the human extrastriate cortex as revealed by functional MRI. *Science.* **282**, 108–11.

Kastner, S., Pinsk, M.A., De Weerd, P., Desimone, R., and Ungerleider, L.G. (1999). Increased activity in human visual cortex during directed attention in the absence of visual stimulation. *Neuron.* **22**, 751–61.

Kastner, S. and Ungerleider, L.G. (2000). Mechanisms of visual attention in the human cortex. *Annu Rev Neurosci.* **23**, 315–41.

LaBerge, D. and Buchsbaum, M.S. (1990). Positron emission tomographic measurements of pulvinar activity during an attention task. *J Neurosci.* **10**, 613–9.

Livingstone, M. and Hubel, D. (1988). Segregation of form, color, movement, and depth: anatomy, physiology, and perception. *Science.* **240**, 740–9.

Logothetis, N.K., Pauls, J., Augath, M., Trinath, T., and Oeltermann, A. (2001). Neurophysiological investigation of the basis of the fMRI signal. *Nature.* **412**, 150–7.

Luck, S. J., Chelazzi, L., Hillyard, S. A., and Desimone, R. (1997). Neural mechanisms of spatial selective attention in areas V1, V2, and V4 of macaque visual cortex. *J Neurophysiol.* **77**, 24–42.

Marshall, J. C. and Halligan, P. W. (1995). Within- and between-task dissociations in visuo-spatial neglect: a case study. *Cortex.* **31**, 367–76.

Marshall, J. C., Fink, G. R., Halligan, P. W., and Vallar, G. (2002). Spatial awareness: a function of the posterior parietal lobe? *Cortex.* **38**, 253–7; discussion 258–60.

Matelli, M., Luppino, G., and Rizzolatti, G. (1985). Patterns of cytochrome oxidase activity in the frontal agranular cortex of the macaque monkey. *Behav Brain Res.* **18**, 125–36.

Matelli, M., Luppino, G., and Rizzolatti, G. (1991). Architecture of superior and mesial area 6 and the adjacent cingulate cortex in the macaque monkey. *J Comp Neurol.* **311**, 445–62.

Mattingley, J.B., Husain, M., Rorden, C., Kennard, C., and Driver, J. (1998). Motor role of human inferior parietal lobe revealed in unilateral neglect patients. *Nature.* **392**, 179–82.

McGlinchey-Berroth, R., Bullis, D.P., Milberg, W.P., Verfaellie, M., Alexander, M., and D'Esposito, M. (1996). Assessment of neglect reveals dissociable behavioral but not neuroanatomical subtypes. *J Int Neuropsychol Soc.* **2**, 441–51.

Mesulam, M.M. (1990). Large-scale neurocognitive networks and distributed processing for attention, language, and memory. *Ann Neurol.* **28**, 597–613.

Mishkin, M., Ungerleider, L., and Macko, K. (1983). Object vision and spatial vision: two cortical pathways. *Trends Neurosci.* **6**, 414–17.

Mort, D. J., Malhotra, P., Mannan, S. K., *et al.* (2003). The anatomy of visual neglect. *Brain.* **126**, 1986–97.

Nobre, A.C., Sebestyen, G.N., Gitelman, D.R., Mesulam, M.M., Frackowiak, R.S., and Frith, C.D. (1997). Functional localization of the system for visuospatial attention using positron emission tomography. *Brain.* **120** (pt 3), 515–33.

Nobre, A.C., Gitelman, D.R., Dias, E.C., and Mesulam, M.M. (2000). Covert visual spatial orienting and saccades: overlapping neural systems. *Neuroimage.* **11**, 210–6.

Nys, G. M., van Zandvoort, M.J., van der Worp, H. B., Kappelle, L.J., and de Haan, E. H. (2006). Neuropsychological and neuroanatomical correlates of perseverative responses in subacute stroke. *Brain.* **129**, 2148–57.

Ogawa, S., Menon, R. S., Kim, S. G., and Ugurbil, K. (1998). On the characteristics of functional magnetic resonance imaging of the brain. *Annu Rev Biophys Biomol Struct.* **27**, 447–74.

Pardo, J.V., Pardo, P.J., Janer, K.W., and Raichle, M.E. (1990). The anterior cingulate cortex mediates processing selection in the Stroop attentional conflict paradigm. *Proc Natl Acad Sci U S A.* **87**, 256–9.

Pardo, J.V., Fox, P.T., and Raichle, M.E. (1991). Localization of a human system for sustained attention by positron emission tomography. *Nature.* **349**, 61–4.

Paulesu, E., Frackowiak, R., and Bottini, G. (1997). Maps of Somatosensory Systems. In *Human Brain Function.* (ed. R. Frackowiak), pp. 183–242. Academic Press, San Diego.

Paus, T., Marrett, S., Worsley, K., and Evans, A. (1996). Imaging motor-to-sensory discharges in the human brain: an experimental tool for the assessment of functional connectivity. *Neuroimage.* **4**, 78–86.

Petrides, M., Alivisatos, B., Meyer, E., and Evans, A.C. (1993). Functional activation of the human frontal cortex during the performance of verbal working memory tasks. *Proc Natl Acad Sci U S A.* **90**, 878–82.

Posner, M.I. (1980). Orienting of attention. *Q J Exp Psychol.* **32**, 3–25.

Posner, M.I., Walker, J.A., Friedrich, F.J., and Rafal, R.D. (1984). Effects of parietal injury on covert orienting of attention. *J Neurosci.* **4**, 1863–74.

Posner, M.I. and Petersen, S.E. (1990). The attention system of the human brain. *Annu Rev Neurosci.* 13, 25–42.

Raichle, M.E. (1987). Circulatory and metabolic correlates of brain function in normal humans. In *Handbook of Physiology. The nervous system. Higher functions of the brain.* (ed. V.B. Mouncastle, F. Plum, and S.R. Geiger), pp. 643–74. American Physiological Society, Bethesda, Maryland.

Rees, G., Frackowiak, R., and Frith, C. (1997a). Two modulatory effects of attention that mediate object categorization in human cortex. *Science.* 275, 835–8.

Rees, G., Frith, C.D., and Lavie, N. (1997b). Modulating irrelevant motion perception by varying attentional load in an unrelated task. *Science.* 278, 1616–19.

Reynolds, J. H., Chelazzi, L., and Desimone, R. (1999). Competitive mechanisms subserve attention in macaque areas V2 and V4. *J Neurosci.* 19, 1736–53.

Rizzolatti, G., Riggio, L., and Shaliga, B. (1994). Space and selective attention. In *Attention and Performance, Vol. 15.* (ed. C. Umiltà and M. Moscovitch), pp. 231–65. MIT Press, Cambridge Massachusetts.

Rizzolatti, G., Berti, A., and Gallese, V. (2000). Spatial neglect: neurophysiological bases, cortical circuits and theories. In *Handbook of Neuropsychology*, 2nd ed. (ed. F. Boller, J. Grafman, and G. Rizzolatti), pp. 303–37. Elsevier, Amsterdam.

Rorden, C., Fruhmann Berger, M., and Karnath, H. O. (2006). Disturbed line bisection is associated with posterior brain lesions. *Brain Res.* 1080, 17–25.

Ruben, J., Schwiemann, J., Deuchert, M., *et al.* (2001). Somatotopic organization of human secondary somatosensory cortex. *Cereb Cortex.* 11, 463–73.

Samuelsson, H., Jensen, C., Ekholm, S., Naver, H., and Blomstrand, C. (1997). Anatomical and neurological correlates of acute and chronic visuospatial neglect following right hemisphere stroke. *Cortex.* 33, 271–85.

Sapir, A., Kaplan, J.B., He, B.J., and Corbetta, M. (2007). Anatomical correlates of directional hypokinesia in patients with hemispatial neglect. *J Neurosci.* 27, 4045–51.

Sereno, M.I., Dale, A.M., Reppas, J.B., *et al.* (1995). Borders of multiple visual areas in humans revealed by functional magnetic resonance imaging. *Science.* 268, 889–93.

Tootell, R.B., Mendola, J.D., Hadjikhani, N.K., Liu, A.K., and Dale, A.M. (1998). The representation of the ipsilateral visual field in human cerebral cortex. *Proc Natl Acad Sci U S A.* 95, 818–24.

Turner, R. (1997). Signal sources in bold contrast fMRI. *Adv Exp Med Biol.* 413, 19–25.

Umiltà, C. (2000). Visuospatial attention. In *Handbook of Neuropsychology*, 2nd ed. (ed. F. Boller, J. Grafman, and G. Rizzolatti), pp. 394–425. Elsevier, Amsterdam.

Ungerleider, L.G., Courtney, S.M., and Haxby, J.V. (1998). A neural system for human visual working memory. *Proc Natl Acad Sci U S A.* 95, 883–90.

Vallar, G., Rusconi, M. L., Bignamini, L., Geminiani, G., and Perani, D. (1994). Anatomical correlates of visual and tactile extinction in humans: a clinical CT scan study. *J Neurol Neurosurg Psychiatry.* 57, 464–70.

Vallar, G., Guariglia, C., and Rusconi, M. (1997). Modulation of the neglect syndrome by sensory stimulation. In *Parietal lobe contributions to orientation in 3D space.* (ed. P. Thier and H. O. Karnath), pp. 555–78. Springer-Verlag, Heidelberg.

Vallar, G. (1998). Spatial hemineglect in humans. *Trends in Cognitive Sciences.* 2, 87–97.

Vallar, G. (2001). Extrapersonal visual unilateral spatial neglect and its neuroanatomy. *Neuroimage.* 14, S52–8.

Weiss, P.H., Marshall, J.C., Wunderlich, G., *et al.* (2000). Neural consequences of acting in near versus far space: a physiological basis for clinical dissociations. *Brain.* 123, 2531–41.

Wilson, F. A., Scalaidhe, S. P., and Goldman-Rakic, P. S. (1993). Dissociation of object and spatial processing domains in primate prefrontal cortex. *Science.* 260, 1955–8.

Wise, S. P., Boussaoud, D., Johnson, P. B., and Caminiti, R. (1997). Premotor and parietal cortex: corticocortical connectivity and combinatorial computations. *Annu Rev Neurosci.* **20**, 25–42.

Zeki, S., Watson, J. D., Lueck, C. J., Friston, K. J., Kennard, C., and Frackowiak, R. S. (1991). A direct demonstration of functional specialization in human visual cortex. *J Neurosci.* **11**, 641–9.

Zeki, S. (1993). *A vision of the brain.* Blackwell, Oxford.

Chapter 38

The functional neuroanatomy of learning and memory

Hans J. Markowitsch and Martina Piefke

1 Introduction

This chapter describes the kinds of learning and memory which are relevant for clinical practice and how they are defined and delineated. Two main lines will be followed; one which divides information processing with respect to *time*, and another with respect to *contents*. Questions will be addressed concerning how information is transmitted in the brain (*encoded*, *stored* or represented), and how information is *retrieved*. The anatomical circuits and networks engaged in these processes will be described and reference made to the brain's biochemistry (transmitters, hormones), as far as relevant for learning and memory and disorders thereof.

2 Learning and Memory - the behavioural view

Hering (1870) described the importance of memory by stating that: "Memory connects innumerable single phenomena into a whole, and just as the body would be scattered like dust in countless atoms if the attraction of matter did not hold it together so consciousness – without the connecting power of memory – would fall apart in as many fragments as it contains moments".

Learning is a universal ability of invertebrates and vertebrates. Accordingly, learning abilities range from simple forms of adaptation to the environment, to sophisticated inferential ones. Table **38.1** gives an overview of various forms of learning. Learning and memory can, in general, be conceptualized as defined in the box below.

Memory can be subdivided with respect to *time* and *contents*. Specifications for both dimensions are given in Boxes on page 796 as well as in Figs. **38.1** and **38.2**. The term *anterograde amnesia* is used when the long-term acquisition (i.e., new learning) of information is lost. The term *retrograde amnesia* is applied when a patient is unable to retrieve information which is already stored in long-term memory (see Fig. **38.3**). In most cases of amnesia, the term *global amnesic syndrome*, as applied in early studies of memory loss, is no longer useful: recent research has shown that patients usually have different memory systems affected, and thus suffer from selective deficits of distinct types of memory.

Table 38.1 Taxonomy of learning according to Gagné (1965)

(1) Signal learning or classical conditioning

This form of learning became most well known as Pavlovian conditioning. The dog, who after a few pairings of a bell with a piece of meat soon salivates already to the sound, is an example. In classical conditioning, the unconditioned stimulus occurs independent of the subject's behaviour.

(2) Stimulus-response learning or instrumental conditioning

Instrumental conditioning is dependent on the subject's behaviour. The subject learns the association between a stimulus and a response.

(3) Chaining (including verbal association)

Chaining refers to several consecutive responses where each response determines the next. (E.g., only several responses, which build up on each other may lead to a reward.)

(4) Multiple discrimination

Learning to differentiate between stimuli, which have one or more attributes in common.

(5) Concept learning

Learning to respond in the same way to a variety of objects or attributes of objects, which have something in common.

(6) Principle learning

Acquiring knowledge on how to master a set of problems which have common attributes.

(7) Problem-solving

Making proper use of learned principles and having insight (being able to draw inferences).

Gagné saw this sequence as hierarchical or as proceeding from simple to complex forms of learning.

The hypothetical memory trace is named *engram*. With regard to the retrieval of information from memory, the rather old concept of *ecphory* has regained attention. Ecphory refers to the process wherein retrieval cues interact with stored information such that a representation of the searched information becomes activated. Ecphory furthermore points at the fact that there are different ways in which information can be retrieved.

Box 38.1 Definition of learning and memory

Learning is a relatively permanent change in a behavioural tendency that occurs as a result of reinforced practice (Kimble, 1961).

Memory is the learning dependent storage of ontogenetically acquired information. This information integrates into phylogenetic neuronal structures selectively and with respect to the given species so that it can be retrieved at all times. This means that it can be provided for situation-dependent behaviour. Generally formulated, memory is based on conditioned changes of the transfer properties in neuronal nets so that under specific circumstances those system modifications engrams) which correspond to neuromotoric signals and behavioural tendencies become fully or partially reproducable (Sinz 1979).

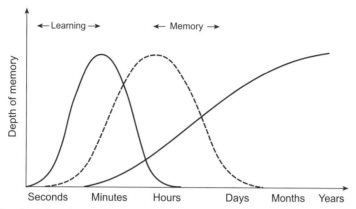

Fig. 38.1 Sketch of the relations between memory strength and duration for the two principal time-related memory systems, short-term and long-term memory.

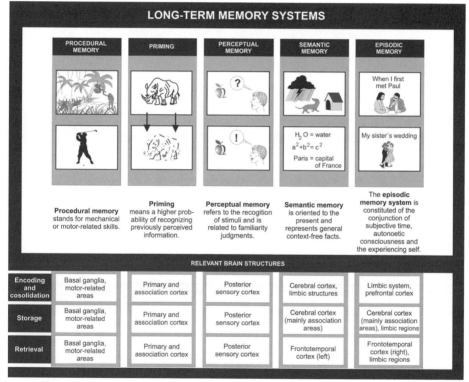

Fig. 38.2 The four principal memory systems important for human information processing. The episodic memory system is context-specific with respect to time and place. It allows a mental time travel. Examples are episodes such as the last vacation or the dinner of the previous night. Declarative memory is context-free and refers to general facts. It is termed semantic memory or the knowledge systems, as well. Procedural memory is largely motor-based, but includes also sensory and cognitive skills ("routines"). Priming refers to a higher likeliness of re-identifying previously perceived stimuli.

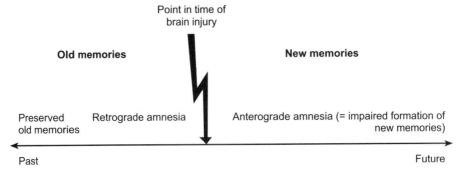

Fig. 38.3 Possible consequences of brain injury on old and new memories.

Box 38.2 The time dimension of memory

Sensory memory ('iconic', 'echoic' memory)	Retaining of information along the sensory channels (duration: ~ 50–500 ms)
Short-term memory (online processing of information)	Storage of memory for seconds to a few minutes (7±2 bits of information)
Long-term memory	Principally life-long retention of information

Box 38.3 The time dimension of memory II (stages)

Registration	Initial perception and transfer to cortical routes
Encoding	Further initial processing of information (binding, associating)
Consolidation	Deep encoding and embedding of information (engram formation)
Storage	Stable representation of information in the nervous system
Retrieval	Reproduction of information (recall)

Box 38.4 The content-dependent dimension of memory

Episodic memory (memory for episodes)	Context-embedded autobiographical memory allowing mental time travelling
Declarative memory (memory for facts) (knowledge system)	Storage of context-free information
Procedural memory	Memory for skills, rules, sequences
Priming	Higher likelihood of re-identifying previously perceived stimuli
Other forms	Lower forms of memory such as classical conditioning or sensitization

The most demanding form is *free recall* which refers to the voluntary *internally cued* recall of learned information without *external help or cueing*. *Cued recall* refers to recall from memory with *the help of external* cues. The most likely least demanding way of retrieving information is its *recognition* by selecting a previously presented stimulus out of a larger number of stimuli.

3 Disorders of learning and memory

Memory disorders represent a complex of symptoms which occur most frequently after brain damage. Moreover, they may arise as a consequence of a number of psychiatric illnesses. The type of memory disorder and the severity of impairments and their course may depend on the locus and extent of damaged brain tissue. In this regard, one has to take into account that in patients with psychiatric diseases, memory disorders are also due to stable or temporary alterations in the nervous system. These are in most cases due to changes in neurotransmitter availability and distribution, or to changes in hormones on the brain level. Indeed, recent neuroimaging data have shown that memory disorders evoked by psychological trauma can lead to lasting changes in brain tissue metabolism (Markowitsch *et al.* 2000), and that there may be considerable similarities to changed neural metabolism found in amnesias occurring after organic brain damage or psychiatric illnesses (Markowitsch 1999a, b, 2003).

Table 38.2 gives an overview of patient groups who usually show memory disturbances.

4 Anatomical bases of learning and memory

Much of current understanding of basic memory-related neuronal changes and modifications stems from the pioneering research of Eric Kandel and co-workers (Martin *et al.* 2000; Kandel 1998) on the invertebrate marine mollusc *Aplysia*. Aplysia contains only a limited number of neurons, many of which are individually identified and labelled. Initially, simple memory mechanisms such as sensitisation and habituation were investigated. It could be demonstrated that there are both short-term and long-term forms thereof. The physiological correlates of short-term forms are facilitated neuronal responses (increases in the magnitude of excitatory postsynaptic potentials formed between sensory and motor neurones). By contrast, the long-term forms (which were elicited by repeated stimulus applications) required new ribonucleic acid (RNA) and protein synthesis, involving the growth of new synaptic connections between sensory and motor neurones.

Kandel's group extended this work to include gene expression and transcription factors; studies which made available new insights into the genetic switch for memory consolidation and storage. Other researchers on invertebrates and vertebrates demonstrated, for example, that adenylyl cyclase is an important enzyme for short-term memory (Zars *et al.* 2000) and long-term potentiation (LTP), as well as long-term depression (LTD); all important mechanisms for memory consolidation (Lynch 2000). Others, however, have questioned the necessity of such mechanisms for memory formation. Zamanillo and

Table 38.2 Overview of patient groups who usually demonstrate memory disorders

Etiology	Common lesion sites
Intra-cranial tumours	Medial and anterior thalamus, medial temporal lobe, posterior cingulate cortex
Cerebral infarcts, ruptured aneurysms	Medial temporal lobe, limbic nuclei of the thalamus (Posterior cerebral artery), orbitofrontal cortex, basal forebrain (anterior communicating artery)
Closed head injury	Temporal pole, orbitofrontal and prefrontal cortex
Viral infections (e.g., herpes simplex encephalitis)	Hippocampal region, limbic and paralimbic cortex
Avitaminoses (e.g., B1 deficiency)	Limbic thalamus, mammillary bodies (e.g., Korsakoff's disease)
Neurotoxin exposure	Hippocampal formation
Temporal lobe epilepsy	Hippocampus and medial temporal lobe
Anoxia or hypoxia (e.g., after a heart attack or drowning)	Hippocampus (CA1 sector)
Degenerative diseases of the CNS (e.g., Alzheimer's or Pick's diseases)	Temporal and other association cortices
Drugs (e.g., anticholinergics, benzodiazepines)	Limbic system
Electroconvulsive therapy	Probably limbic system
Transient global amnesia	Probably medial temporal lobe and/or medial thalamus (when an etiology is found)
Paraneoplastic limbic encephalitis	Limbic structure in medial temporal lobe
Mnestic block syndrome	Massive glucocorticoid release leading to a disruption in the memory processing pathways of the medial temporal lobe
Dissociative disorders	Amnesia possibly due to hormonal changes in the brain

co-workers (1999), for example, provided evidence against LTP as an essential prerequisite for memory formation.

On the vertebrate, and especially the mammalian level, important questions concern not only the issue of how information is processed, but where it is processed, and in what different kinds. From the initial stages of information registration, the brain is, of course involved. However, both the time and the content dimensions of memory interact in the neural processing of information. This complicates the delineation of the neural pathways, circuits, and networks which are implicated in information processing. Firstly, the neural bases of simple forms of memory will be briefly depicted. Thereafter, complex kinds of memory such as semantic and episodic will be described.

Classical conditioning and other simple correlates of memory largely take place within the spinal cord and brain stem; certain other subtypes, however, may engage structures in various other loci of the brain. Fear conditioning, for example, involves the amygdala. Priming (a non-reflected unconscious transmission of information) activates cortical areas - largely, though probably not exclusively, within the particular modality of the stimulus ('unimodal' primary and association cortex). Procedural memory engages the basal ganglia; it may also involve portions of the cerebellum, though the evidence is mixed.

More complex brain circuits are recruited by perceptual, semantic and episodic memory (Tulving & Markowitsch 1998; Tulving 2005; Buckner & Carroll 2007). For these forms, it is necessary to differentiate between the stages of information transfer listed in Box 38.3.

Information of the declarative and episodic memory systems enters the brain via the sensory channels, and is then stored online or short-term (Box 38.1) in cortical association areas, particularly of the lateral parietal cortex (Markowitsch 2000, 2005). From there it is transmitted to the limbic system. Within the various structures and fibre networks involved in this system, the processes of selecting, binding, associating, and assigning occur. The hippocampal formation can be regarded as the core of the limbic system. However, there are several other important components; Table 38.3 lists the most relevant ones.

Most of the case reports on patients who, in former times, were declared globally amnesic, had bilateral damage to either medial temporal lobe or medial diencephalic regions. The most well-known example is patient H.M., who, in 1953, received bilateral resection of the medial temporal lobes due to otherwise intractable epilepsy attacks (Fig. 38.4) (Scoville & Milner 1957). While the attacks were largely reduced after surgery, H.M. suffered from persistent anterograde amnesia.

Medial diencephalic infarcts may also cause bilateral hippocampal damage (Fig. 38.5). This type of amnesia is largely the same as that seen after bilateral medial temporal lesion: However, after medial diencephalic infarct, a patient's capacity for conscious reflection on his memory impairment is, in most cases, also disturbed (Markowitsch 2000, 2008). While H.M. stated *"Every day is alone, whatever enjoyment I've had, and whatever sorrow I've had"*, another patient with bilateral diencephalic damage was unable to acknowledge his severe amnesia, and instead considered his memory to be 'normal' (Markowitsch *et al.* 1993).

These two examples are more or less representative of the two principal groups of patients with major and lasting anterograde amnesia in the episodic and semantic domains – the medial diencephalic, and the medial temporal group. The contribution of distinct parts of nuclei or areas of the medial diencephalon and the medial temporal lobe to memory functions is still a matter of debate (Table 38.2). The issue cannot easily be clarified by lesion studies and neuropsychological testing, since, in amnesic patients, there is rarely damage confined to any single structure. The hippocampal formation may represent an exception; the hippocampus or individual hippocampal sectors are often selectively damaged after hypoxic or toxic states. The high vulnerability of the so-called *Sommer's sector* of the hippocampus to epilepsy or hypoxia was noted by 1880 (Sommer 1880).

The basal forebrain also constitutes a region which is important for unimpaired episodic and semantic memory function. This is, at least in part, due to its intimate connections with other memory-related neural networks (e.g. via the fornix). The basal forebrain is composed of a number of components of divergent evolutionary origin including

Table 38.3 Structures of the limbic system and their principal functional implications

Structure	Functional involvement(s)
Diencephalon	
Anterior nuclear complex	(anterograde) memory, emotion, attention
Mediodorsal nucleus	(anterograde) memory, consciousness, sleep, emotion
Non-specific thalamic nuclei	consciousness?, (anterograde) memory?
Mammillary bodies	(anterograde) memory, emotion?
Telencephalon (subcortical)	
Basal forebrain	emotional evaluation, (anterograde) memory
Amygdaloid body	emotional evaluation of information, motivations, olfaction
Telencephalon (cortical)	
Hippocampal formation	(anterograde) memory, spatial-temporal integration
Entorhinal region	(anterograde) memory
Cingulate gyrus	attention, drive, pain perception
Associated regions	
Medial and orbitofrontal cortex	emotional evaluation, social behaviour, initiative (initiation of retrieval of information)
Insula	sensory-motivational integration?
Temporal pole	memory-related sensory integration, initiation of retrieval, recruitment of engrams
Fiber systems	
Fornix	(anterograde) memory?
Medial internal lamina	(anterograde) memory?
Mammillothalamic tract	(anterograde) memory?
Uncinate fascicle	retrograde memory?

fibre connections. With regard to biochemistry, the cholinergic system (basal nucleus of Meynert, septal nuclei, diagonal band of Broca, the nucleus accumbens, and other parts of the ventral striatum) plays an important role. The cholinergic system has long been implicated in the highest cognitive functions, including memory and consciousness (Perry *et al.* 1999).

5 Brain circuits for encoding and consolidating

A common view of information processing assumes that information enters the brain via the sensory organs and is then stored short-term, most likely in portions of the parietal and also possibly the prefrontal cortices. Information is thereafter transmitted to the limbic system, a phylogenetically old system of structures and fibre connections. It had

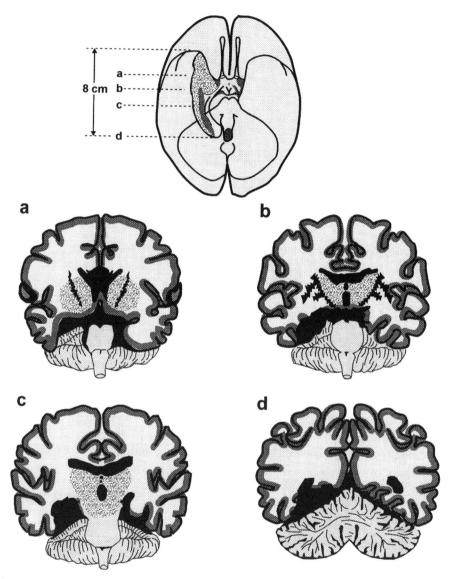

Fig. 38.4 Drawings of the extent of the principal surgical removal within H.M.'s temporal lobe. Part (a) shows a basal view of his brain and part (b) gives coronal sections at the levels A-D indicated in (a). The extent of the surgical resection is blackened on the left side of the brain only, though the removal was bilateral and symmetrical. (After Fig. 2 of Scoville and Milner, 1957.)

originally been associated with olfaction and with emotions in a more general sense. Currently, it is thought to be implicated in the processing of both emotional and cognitive forms of information. In particular, it is assumed that the limbic system is involved in the evaluation of incoming (and short-term stored) information, and in assigning this information to final storage networks. With respect to episodic and semantic memories, these are most likely represented in distributed in cortical circuits.

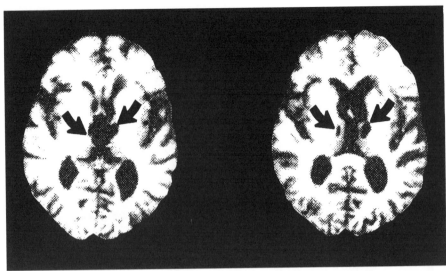

Fig. 38.5 The extent of bilateral diencephalic damage in a patient with preserved intelligence, but severe and persistent anterograde amnesia. (After Figure 2 of Markowitsch *et al.* 1993).

There are several structures within the limbic system which have a closer relation to emotional-affective information processing (e.g., the amygdala and the septum), than others, which are more involved on the cognitive side (e.g., the hippocampal formation). It is thus conceivable that there exist two different circuits for information selection, binding, and transfer (Fig. 38.6). One of them is named the medial circuit (or Papez-circuit), and the other the basolateral limbic circuit. The basolateral limbic circuit is composed of three structures and their interconnecting fibres. The structures are the amygdala, the mediodorsal thalamus, and the subcallosal area within the basal forebrain. The unidirectional ventral amygdalofugal pathway leads from the amygdala to the mediodorsal thalamus. From there, fibres reach the subcallosal area which then projects via the bandeletta diagonalis back into the amygdaloid body. The basolateral limbic circuit evaluates the affective aspects of incoming information. Importantly, it interacts with the medial "cognitive" circuit.

The traditional view includes four structures in the medial circuit: the mammillary bodies, the anterior thalamus, the cingulate cortex, and the hippocampal formation. The cingulate cortex can perhaps be omitted because of both its functional engagement (e.g., Barch *et al.* 2001; Botvinick *et al.* 1999; Piefke *et al.* 2003; Shah *et al.* 2001; Sugiura *et al.* 2005) and the existence of direct projections between the anterior thalamus and parts of the hippocampal formation. The interconnecting fibres are given in Fig. 38.6. The medial circuit is regarded as the circuit which mediates the cognitive evaluation, binding, and assignment of information for long-term storage.

It is evident that both the medial temporal lobe and the medial diencephalic system are embedded in these limbic circuits. Note that there exist most likely more structures which are of relevance for the limbic system (in addition to those directly belonging to the

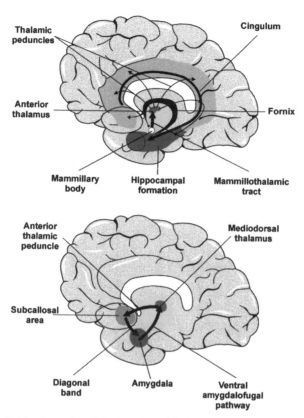

Fig. 38.6 The medial (or Papez-) and the basolateral limbic circuit. The medial circuit is probably more relevant for the cognitive acts of memory processing, the basolateral one for the affective evaluation of information. Both circuits interact with each other. The Papez-circuit interconnects the hippocampal formation via the (postcommissural) fornix to the mammillary bodies, these via the mammillothalamic tract (or tractus Vicq d'Azyr) to the anterior thalamus, the anterior thalamus with its cortical projection targets reaches the cingulate gyrus and the subicular part of the hippocampal formation and the cingulum fibres in addition project back from the cingulate gyrus into the hippocampal formation. (The precommissural fornix in addition provides a bidirectional connection between the hippocampal formation and the basal forebrain.) The basolateral limbic circuit links the amygdala, mediodorsal thalamic nucleus, and area subcallosa with each other by distinct fibre projections, namely the ventral amygdalofugal pathway, the inferior thalamic peduncle and the bandeletta diagonalis.

basolateral and the medial circuits). With regard to the limbic system, there is ongoing discussion as to what is included in it. Structures within the basal forebrain are example candidates. Others are located within the medial temporal lobe system and contain hierarchically organised allocortical structures which converge on subdivisions of the hippocampus (Fig. 38.7).

After the encoding of information and its transfer to the neocortex for long-term storage, the memory engram is not yet fixed. Instead, memories are further consolidated by matching the recently encoded pieces of information with already existing ones, and by

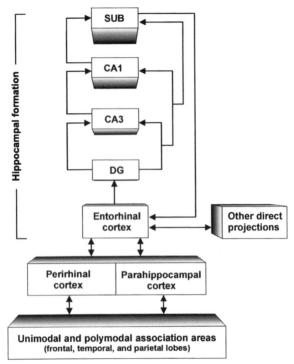

Fig. 38.7 The hierarchical organisation within the medial temporal lobe (according to Squire and Knowlton 2000).

further assimilating, assigning, and embedding recently encoded information within the wealth of already stored engrams. The mind appears to have a tendency to form a congruent and consistent *Gestalt* of its memory repertoire (Markowitsch 2008; Piefke 2007).

5.1 Brain circuits for memory storage

Overall, information is assumed to be stored in widespread neural networks. For episodic and semantic information, these networks are mainly situated within neocortical structures (association cortex, polysensory cortex). However, the storage of these forms of memory may additionally recruit allocortical and subcortical regions. Episodic autobiographical information, which is usually associated with emotions, typically requires input from the amygdala and/or the septal region. As episodic memories are by definition consciously reflected (Tulving & Markowitsch 1998; Tulving 2005), they furthermore depend on a neuronal pathway from the brain stem reticular formation to the neocortex (Markowitsch 2001).

5.2 Brain circuits for memory retrieval

The retrieval of more complex, episodic-autobiographical information is usually reconstructive in nature, that is, retrieved materials need not be identical to the originally encoded information. Interactions of situational cues and a person's mood state at the time of retrieval may, for example, interact with stored memory engrams such that an "updated" representation of the memory may evolve (see the above definition of the process of ecphory). Functional neuroimaging data have shown that portions of the prefrontal and medial temporal cortices are recruited during the recollection of autobiographic episodes (Fink *et al.* 1996; Markowitsch *et al.* 2003; Piefke *et al.* 2003). It is conceivable that the prefrontal cortex provides the impetus or trigger signal to retrieve memories which are largely stored in networks of the posterior association cortices. The regions within the medial temporal lobe may then become active to accomplish the emotional evaluation of retrieved episodes. Moreover, the hippocampal formation may (in particular) mediate the re-encoding of retrieved information. Fig. 38.8 provides an example of the brain regions activated during autobiographical recollection.

6 The brain's biochemistry and psychogenic amnesia

It has long been known that memory and other forms of cognitive processing can not only be impaired after structural brain lesions, but also that psychiatric illnesses may lead to an impaired memory. Neurotransmitter and hormonal alterations, that is, changes in the brains biochemistry, and alcohol or drug abuse may frequently yield psychiatric or neurological disorders. The effects of drugs (as well as hormonal and neurotransmitter alterations) have been the subject of numerous studies in animals and humans (Dujardin & Laurent 2003; Hallam *et al.* 2004; Hasselmo *et al.* 1996). In particular, the process of memory consolidation can be influenced by a wide range of pharmacological substances (Lynch 1998).

Changes in the brain's neurochemistry may lead to well known neurological syndromes such as Parkinson's disease where a lack of dopamine causes motor impairments and occasional procedural memory problems. There is also substantial evidence for an involvement of acetylcholine in memory processing (Hasselmo 1999; Perry *et al.* 1999), and for the view that cholinergic dysfunction may lead to both neurological (Babic 1999) and psychiatric diseases (Sarter & Bruno 1999). Other transmitters such as gamma-amino butyric acid (Kalueff & Nutt 1996), glutamate, serotonin, and noradrenalin have numerous interacting effects especially in the memory related regions such as the hippocampus (Vizi & Kiss 1998). Histamines have been found to enhance memory processing (Passani *et al.* 2000). Vizi and Kiss (1998) suggested that even transmitter release without synaptic contact plays an important role in the fine tuning of communication between neurones within a given circuit.

Kaufer *et al.* (1998) found that changes in cholinergic gene expression may be induced by stress, and Markowitsch *et al.* (1999, 2000) hypothesized that the acute or chronic release of glucocorticoids (i.e., stress hormones) on the brain level may lead to *psychogenic amnesia* (also named '*mnestic block syndrome*'). Psychogenic amnesia may occur in or after stressful phases of life or after traumatic situations such as severe accidents or violent assaults. Posttraumatic stress disorder, which can often be observed in individuals who experience a traumatic event, is also associated with memory impairments. Typically, these are psychogenic amnesias for the trauma and/or intrusive memories

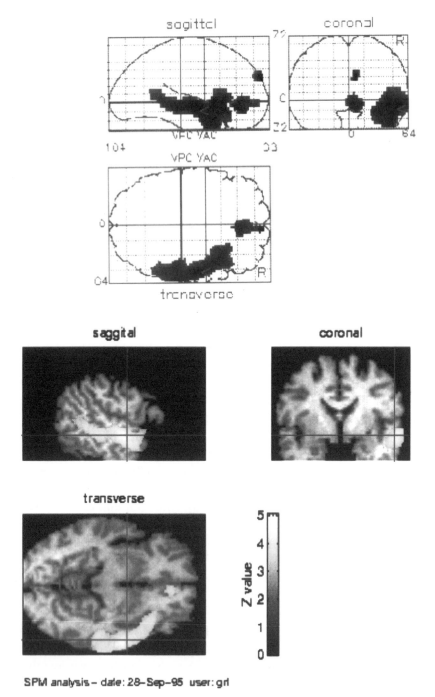

SPM analysis – date: 28–Sep–95 user: grl

Fig. 38.8 Positron emission tomographic results, showing activated brain regions of an individual, imaging episodes of his past.

(Markowitsch *et al.*, 1998; Piefke *et al.* 2008). Psychogenic amnesia may include an inability to retrieve old, or to acquire new information long-term, or both. The syndrome may be transient (Markowitsch *et al.* 2000; Markowitsch 2003), but frequently persists over time. In the latter, slight improvements can sometimes be observed. The occurrence of psychogenic amnesia is an example of the manifold ways in which the environment influences the brain's ability to code and re-code signals (for related aspects of neural plasticity, cf. Piefke 2007; Pascual-Leone *et al.* 2005).

7 Conclusions

The nervous system allows the individual to respond flexibly and to adapt to the demands of the environment. Its functions thus help to improve an organism's possibility of long-term survival. Animals learn to distinguish between edible and poisonous foods and to keep smells in mind in order to distinguish, for example, between dangerous members and putative sexual partners of its own species. Such emotion-related messages are initially processed by the limbic system. The limbic system may thus be referred to as a primary centre for memory control. This is also the case for episodic autobiographical memory in humans where complex interactions between retrieval cues and already stored information during ecphory have to be taken into account. Unconscious forms of memory such as priming and procedural memory are particularly useful in everyday routines, as they increase an organism's adaptability to the environment.

Selective references

Babic, T. (1999). The cholinergic hypothesis of Alzheimer's disease: a review of progress. *Journal of Neurology, Neurosurgery, and Psychiatry*, **67**, 558.

Barch, D.M., Braver, T.S., Akbudak, E., Conturo, T., Ollinger, J., Snyder, A. (2001). Anterior cingulate cortex and response conflict: effects of response modality and processing domain. *Cerebral Cortex*, **11**, 837–848.

Botvinick, M., Nystrom, L.E., Fissell, K., Carter, C.S., Cohen, J.D. (1999). Conflict monitoring versus selection-for-action in anterior cingulate cortex. *Nature*, **402**, 179–181.

Buckner, R.L., Carroll, D.C. (2007). Self-projection and the brain. *Trends in Cognitive Science*, **11**, 49–57.

Dujardin, K., Laurent, B. (2003). Dysfunction of the human memory systems: role of the dopaminergic transmission. *Current Opinion in Neurobiology*, **16**, Suppl 2, S11–S16.

Fink, G.R., Markowitsch, H.J., Reinkemeier, M., Bruckbauer, T., Kessler, J., Heiss, W.-D. (1996). Cerebral representation of one's own past: neural networks involved in autobiographical memory. *Journal of Neuroscience*, **16**, 4275–4282.

Gagné, R.M. (1965). *The conditions of learning*. New York: Holt, Rinehart & Winston.

Hasselmo, M.E. (1999). Neuromodulation: acetylcholine and memory consolidation. *Trends in Cognitive Sciences*, **3**, 351–359.

Hasselmo, M.E., Wyble, B.P., Wallenstein, G.V. (1996). Encoding and retrieval of episodic memories: role of cholinergic and GABAergic modulation in the hippocampus. *Hippocampus*, **6**, 693–708.

Hallam, K.T., Horgan, J.E., McGrath, C., Norman, T.R. (2004). An investigation of the effect of tacrine and physostigmine on spatial working memory deficits in the olfactory bulbectomised rat. *Behavioural Brain Research*, **153**, 481–486.

Hering, E. (1895). *Memory as a general function of organized matter.* Chicago: Open Court.

Kalueff, A., Nutt, D.J. (1996). Role of GABA in memory and anxiety. *Depression and Anxiety,* **4,** 100–110.

Kandel, E.R. (1998). A new intellectual framework for Psychiatry. *American Journal of Psychiatry,* **155,** 457–469.

Kaufer, D., Friedman, A., Seldman, S., Soreq, H. (1998). Acute stress facilitates long-lasting changes in cholinergic gene expression. *Nature,* **393,** 373–377.

Kimble, G.A. (1961). *Hilgard and Marquis' conditioning and learning.* New York: Appleton Century-Crofts.

Lynch, G. (1998). Memory and the brain: Unexpected chemistries and a new pharmacology. *Neurobiology of Learning and Memory,* **70,** 82–100.

Lynch, G. (2000). Memory consolidation and long-term potentiation. In: M.S. Gazzaniga (Ed.), *The new cognitive neurosciences* (pp. 139–158). Cambridge, MA: MIT Press.

Markowitsch, H.J. (1999a). Functional neuroimaging correlates of functional amnesia. *Memory,* **7,** 561–583.

Markowitsch, H.J. (1999b). Neuroimaging and mechanisms of brain function in psychiatric disorders. *Current Opinion in Psychiatry,* **12,** 331–337.

Markowitsch, H.J. (2000). Memory and amnesia. In: M.M. Mesulam (Ed.), *Principles of cognitive and behavioral neurology* (pp. 257–293). New York: Oxford University Press.

Markowitsch, H.J. (2001). Autonoetic consciousness. In: A.S. David, T. Kircher (Eds.), *The self and schizophrenia: A neuropsychological perspective.* Cambridge, MA: Cambridge University Press.

Markowitsch, H.J. (2003). Psychogenic amnesia. *Neuroimage,* **20,** S132–S138.

Markowitsch, H.J. (2005). The neuroanatomy of memory. In: P. Halligan, P. Wade (Eds.). *The effectiveness of rehabilitation for cognitive deficits* (pp. 105–114). Oxford, UK: Oxford University Press.

Markowitsch, H.J. (2008). Anterograde amnesia. In: G. Goldenberg, E. Miller (Eds.), *Handbook of clinical neurology. Vol. 88: Neuropsychology and behavioural neurology.* (pp. 155–184). New York: Elsevier, in press.

Markowitsch, H.J., von Cramon, D.Y., Schuri, U. (1993). Mnestic performance profile of a bilateral diencephalic infarct patient with preserved intelligence and severe amnesic disturbances. *Journal of Clinical and Experimental Neuropsychology,* **15,** 627–652.

Markowitsch, H.J., Kessler, J., Russ, M.O., Frölich, L., Schneider, B., Maurer, K. (1999). Mnestic block syndrome. *Cortex,* **35,** 219–230.

Markowitsch,H.J., Kessler, J., Van der Ven, C., Weber-Luxenburger, G., Heiss, W.-D. (1998). Psychic trauma causing grossly reduced brain metabolism and cognitive deterioration. *Neuropsychologia,* **36,** 77–82.

Markowitsch, H.J., Kessler, J., Weber-Luxenburger, G., Van der Ven, C., Heiss, W.-D. (2000). Neuroimaging and behavioral correlates of recovery from 'mnestic block syndrome' and other cognitive deteriorations. *Neuropsychiatry, Neuropsychology, and Behavioral Neurology,* **13,** 60–66.

Markowitsch, H.J., Vandekerkhove, M.M., Lanfermann, H., Russ, M.O. (2003). Engagement of lateral and medial prefontal areas in the ecphory of sad and happy autobiographical memories. *Cortex,* **3,** 643–665.

Martin, K.C., Bartsch, D., Bailey, C.H., Kandel, E.R. (2000). Molecular mechanisms underlying learning-related long-lasting synaptic plasticity. In M.S. Gazzaniga (Ed.), *The new cognitive neurosciences* (pp. 121-137). Cambridge, MA: MIT Press.

Pascual-Leone, A., Amedi, A., Fregni, F., Merabet, L.B. (2005). The plastic human brain cortex. *Annual Review of Neuroscience,* **28,** 377–401.

Passani, M.B., Bacciottini L., Mannaioni P.F., Blandina, P. (2000). Central histaminergic system and cognition. *Neuroscience and Biobehavioral Reviews,* **24,** 107–113.

Perry, E., Walker, M., Grace, J., Perry, R. (1999). Acetylcholine in mind: a neurotransmitter correlate of consciousness? *Trends in Neurosciences*, **22**, 273–280.

Piefke, M. (2007). Laboratory memory tasks and autobiographical recollection: Cognitive and neuro-functional evidence for differential forms of episodic memory. In: L.N. Bakker (Ed.), *Brain Mapping Research Developments*. (pp. 101–127). New York: Nova Science Publishers 2008.

Piefke, M., Weiss, P.H., Zilles, K., Markowitsch, H.J., Fink, G.R. (2003). Differential remoteness and emotional tone modulate the neural correlates of autobiographical memory. *Brain*, **126**, 650–668.

Piefke, M., Pestinger, M., Arin, T., Kohl, B., Kastrau, F., Schnitker, R., Vohn, R., Weber, J., Ohnhaus, M., Erli, H.J., Perlitz, V., Paar, O., Petzold, E.R., Flatten, G. (2007). The neurofunctional mechanisms of traumatic and non-traumatic memory in patients with acute PTSD following accident trauma. *Neurocase*, **13**, 342–357.

Sarter, M., Bruno, J.P. (1999). Abnormal regulation of corticopetal cholinergic neurons and impaired information processing in neuropsychiatric disorders. *Trends in Neurosciences*, **22**, 67–74.

Scoville, W.B., Milner, B. (1957). Loss of recent memory after bilateral hippocampal lesions. *Journal of Neurology, Neurosurgery, and Psychiatry*, **20**, 11–21.

Shah, N.J., Marshall, J.C., Zafiris, O., Schwab, A., Zilles, K., Markowitsch, H.J., Fink, G.R. (2001). The neural correlates of person familiarity: A functional magnetic resonance imaging study with clinical implications. *Brain*, **124**, 804–815.

Sinz, R. (1979). *Neurobiologie und Gedächtnis*. Stuttgart: Gustav Fischer.

Sommer, W. (1880). Erkrankung des Ammonshorns als aetiologisches Moment der Epilepsie. *Archiv für Psychiatrie*, **10**, 631–675.

Squire, L.R., Knowlton, B.J. (2000). The medial temporal lobe, the hippocampus, and the memory system of the brain. In M.S. Gazzaniga (Ed.), *The new cognitive neurosciences* (pp. 765–779). Cambridge, MA: MIT Press.

Sugiura, M., Shah, N.J., Zilles, K., Fink, G.R. (2005). Cortical representations of personally-familiar objects and places: functional organization of the human posterior cingulate cortex. *Journal of Cognitive Neuroscience*, **17**, 183–198.

Tulving, E. (2005). Episodic memory and autonoesis: Uniquely human"? In: H.S. Terrace, J. Metcalfe (Eds.), *The missing link in cognition: Self-knowing consciousness in man and animals* (pp. 3–56). New York: Oxford University Press.

Tulving, E., Markowitsch, H.J. (1998). Episodic and declarative memory: Role of the hippocampus. *Hippocampus*, **8**, 198–204.

Vizi, E.S., Kiss, J.P. (1998). Neurochemistry and pharmacology of the major hippocampal transmitter systems: synaptic and nonsynaptic interactions. *Hippocampus*, **6**, 566–607.

Zamanillo, D., Sprengel, R., Hvalby, O., Jensen, V., Burnashev, N., Rozov, A., Kaiser, K.M., Koster, H.J., Borchardt, T., Worley, P., Lubke, J., Frotscher, M., Kelly, P.H., Sommer, B., Andersen, P., Seeburg, P.H., Sakmann, B. (1999). Importance of AMPA receptors for hippocampal synaptic plasticity but not for spatial learning. *Science*, **284**, 1805–1811.

Zars, T., Fischer, M., Schulz, R., Heisenberg, M. (2000). Localization of a short-term memory in *Drosophila*. *Science*, **288**, 672–675.

Chapter 39

Functional neuroanatomy of language disorders

Claudius Bartels and Claus-W. Wallesch

Reproduced from *Handbook of Clinical Neuropsychology*, (2003). Oxford University Press.

1 Introduction

This chapter will attempt a synopsis of the representation of language functions in the brain with a focus on disorders based on three sources of information:

- lesion studies (i.e. what is known from the effects of pathology upon language behaviour in patients);

- the anatomical interpretation of normal function based on physiological measurements during language operations in healthy subjects;

- a combination of the two; namely, physiological measurements recorded during language processing in aphasic patients.

Computer-generated three-dimensional brain images into which imaging software places coloured regions of increased or decreased 'function' have great appeal and are well suited for title pages of scientific and other journals. However, the underlying methodology is highly complex and prone to artefacts and misinterpretations. Therefore we shall include a brief discussion of functional imaging methodology.

2 Basic anatomy

The hemispheric surface is divided into the frontal, temporal, parietal, and occipital lobes (Fig. 39.1). The depth of the sylvian fissure, which separates the temporal from the parietal and frontal lobes, harbours a hidden part of cerebral cortex, the insula, which is covered by lips (the opercula) of the adjacent lobes.

The forebrain is walnut-shaped with one strong (the corpus callosum) and two minor (commissura anterior and posterior) interconnections between the hemispheres. The core of the medial surface of the hemispheres does not continue the lobar structure. One single large gyrus, the cingulum, surrounds the corpus callosum.

Cortical processing interacts with the function of subcortical neuronal structures, the basal ganglia and the thalamus, by reciprocal connections with specific nuclei of the latter, and loop systems that include both the basal ganglia and the specific thalamic nuclei (Alexander *et al.* 1986). A similar action upon cortex has been proposed by

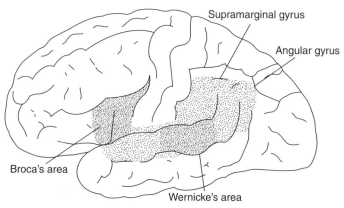

Supramarginal gyrus

Angular gyrus

Broca's area

Wernicke's area

Fig. 39.1 The surface of the left hemisphere. Of special interest for language representations are the following structures of the left hemisphere: the insular cortex and a number of cortical areas that are close to the sylvian fissure, namely, Broca's area in the foot of the second and third frontal convolution, Wernicke's area in the posterior third of the first temporal convolution, and, surrounding the posterior end of the sylvian fissure, the supramarginal and angular gyrus (see the text for a discussion of lateralization of language representations).

Schmahmann and Pandya (1997) for the cerebellum. The basal ganglia consist of the putamen and caudate nucleus, the pallidum, the subthalamic nucleus, and a number of minor nuclei that need not be considered here. The thalamus contains more than 30 nuclei that subserve different relay functions: in cortico–subcortico–cortical loops; in ascending sensory and cerebellar projections; and in non-specific ascending pathways that subserve, e.g. cortical activation and the awake state (Fig. 39.2).

Localization of functions within the brain

The extent to which functions can be localized in the brain is variable. The primary sensory and motor areas are quite circumscribed. The more cognitive a function is, the less well it can be assigned to defined cortical areas. Cerebral maps even of primary areas are not fixed representations but may vary in response to functional demand (Merzenich *et al.* 1983). It has been proposed that neuronal networks are a general feature of cerebral organization with quite distributed networks for cognitive functions (McClelland and Rumelhart 1986; Harley 1996). The extent of such networks has been demonstrated by functional magnetic resonance imaging (fMRI; Carpenter and Just 1999).

In most subjects, almost all right-handers and a majority of left-handers, the left hemisphere dominates language processing, although the degree of cerebral dominance differs interindividually. Anatomically, the planum temporale, which corresponds to the core of Wernicke's area, is larger on the left in about 75 % of normal people (Steinmetz 1996). This asymmetry seems genetically predetermined and can be found in fetuses (Chi *et al.* 1977).

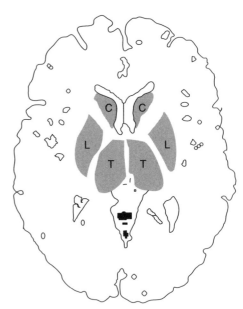

Fig. 39.2 The subcortical nuclei of the cerebral hemispheres.

C = (head of) caudate nucleus
L = lentiform nucleus
T = thalamus

Nevertheless, whether or not the planum temporale is an area that is inherently specialized for language function is currently being debated both on neurobiological and on neurolinguistic grounds (Démonet *et al.*, 2005; Marshall 2000).

The temporal lobe association cortex, of which Wernicke's area is a part, integrates auditory, visual, and even somatosensory information. It is closely interconnected with the temporal limbic cortex and the amygdalohippocampal system that subserve both memory and emotional functions. Broca's area is part of the precentral association cortex, which is located between the cortical motor strip and the prefrontal cortex. The precentral cortex is involved in movement preparation, but the exact function of Broca's area is still under debate. Another frontal lobe cortical area, the left supplementary motor area at the medial aspect of the frontal lobe, is involved in language production, especially in the initiation of speech acts. Functionally, this area is part of the anterior cingulum. (See box below for a discussion of localization of functions in the brain.)

3 **The anatomical foundation of aphasia**

The most common cause of aphasia is stroke in the area of supply of the middle cerebral artery. Stroke results in circumscribed lesions, the anatomical analysis of which is rather unambiguous. Damage to some regions is more likely to cause lasting aphasia than damage to others, and there is some interaction between lesion configuration and chronic aphasia syndromes. Poeck *et al.* (1984) found core lesions for Broca's aphasia in the anterior insula, frontal operculum, and the underlying white matter; for

Wernicke's aphasia in the posterior superior temporal lobe (Wernicke's area); and for global aphasia in the middle and posterior insula and a much larger white matter lesion including the deep white matter. Naeser *et al.* (1987) confirmed the association between Wernicke's area lesion and Wernicke's aphasia, and stressed the role of deep white matter pathways for the pathogenesis of global aphasia (Naeser *et al.* 1989). Whether or not the deep lesion in global aphasia signifies involvement of white matter pathways or rather a lesion of the basal ganglia that combines detrimentally with a cortical lesion is under debate (Wallesch 1997). A recent investigation based on magnetic resonance (MR)-documented lesions came to the following conclusions (Kreisler *et al.* 2000).

- Nonfluent aphasia depends on the presence of frontal or putaminal lesions.
- Repetition disorder depends on insular or external capsule lesions.
- Comprehension disorder depends on posterior lesions of the temporal gyri.
- Verbal paraphasia depends on temporal or caudate lesions.

We will not discuss in detail the anatomy of lesions that may lead to transient aphasia. It may suffice that almost any lesion in the area of supply of the left middle cerebral artery, but also of the left anterior cerebral artery, and lesions of the left thalamus may cause transient speech or language disturbances. Lesions of the left supplementary motor area (SMA) transiently lead to mutism that progresses to transcortical motor aphasia and finally to normal language production with some nonfluency. With bilateral lesions, mustim may persist. There is some agreement that the cingular region, of which the SMA is part, is not involved in linguistic processes, but rather in the initiation of speech (von Stockert 1975).

Kertesz and Wallesch (1993) summarized why the functional neuroanatomy must be different between acute and chronic aphasia: 'The early deficit that may be related to edema, cellular dysfunction, transient ischemia, etc., is followed by a great deal of early spontaneous recovery in trauma or stroke. The chronic deficit is related not only to a loss of function, but to compensatory changes by functionally connected structures such as homologous contralateral areas or neighbouring areas during subsequent stages of recovery'.

Of interest for the issue of lateralization and more widespread, bilateral representations of language functions are cases of aphasia in right-handers with right hemisphere lesions (crossed aphasia). In some well analysed cases an anomalous pattern of lateralization was found, with some linguistic functions lateralized to the right, although for most functions the left hemisphere was dominant (Alexander and Annett 1996). The occurrence of such individual lateralization patterns may explain why the aphasic symptomatology cannot be predicted from imaging data.

There are some language functions that suffer greater impairment from right than from left hemisphere damage (cf. Joanette and Goulet 1993):

- the identification of emotional words and sentences (Borod *et al.* 1992);
- the production of effective prosody in a tonal (Thai) language (Gandour *et al.* 1995).

When analysing the clinical imaging data of large numbers of aphasic patients it becomes apparent that some linguistic functions (e.g. grammaticalization) seem to be focally represented in the left periinsular cortex, whereas others, e.g. the processes that underlie naming and word finding, are more broadly distributed in the brain. It is often argued that the clinical symptomatology should not be attributed to the damaged region but to other undamaged structures that subserve the respective functions after the lesion occurred. This view is based on a localization assumption, namely, that brain regions subserve a function and, if they are destroyed, other brain areas, which originally subserved another function, have to compensate, or that there is redundancy in the system. In recent years, another theory has gained ground, namely, that cognitive functions have a distributed representation in neural networks, which have compensatory facilities of their own. The properties of the network may explain the symptomatology (Plaut 1995).

The role of the basal ganglia and the thalamus in the pathogenesis of aphasic symptoms is still controversial. A central reason is that exact lesion anatomy is difficult to define because of common vascular supply to various structures and anatomical variability. Physiologically, a role for the loop systems, which run from cortex via basal ganglia and thalamus back to executive cortex and which execute an output gating is plausible and can explain the symptoms of so-called subcortical aphasia (Wallesch 1997).

4 The functional neuroanatomy of normal language processing

Literally hundreds of positron emission tomography (PET) and fMRI studies have been published since the landmark investigation of Petersen *et al.* (1988) that described the activation of brain areas in normal subjects during language tasks. With respect to many assumed representations of language functions, the data are conflicting. The studies can be replicated only if the experimental setting is exactly reproduced (for a discussion of methodology, see Section 6). However, certain aspects of language-related activations converge between studies, and some of these are briefly outlined in the box below. Furthermore, PET (Absher *et al.* 2000) and fMRI activations have been found to correlate with electrophysiological event-related potentials, which indicates their validity. In general, fMRI seems more sensitive than PET due to its superior signal-to-noise ratio (Sadato *et al.* 1998). In this review, we shall not separate PET from fMRI studies.

Electrophysiologically, some language processes, especially those that can be analysed by the comparison of two stimuli with identical structure over time and a discrete event that separates them, can be analysed by the method of averaged event-related potentials (ERPs). Of special interest for psycholinguistic analysis is the N400 wave, with which subjects react to semantic or syntactic incompatibility. These phenomena are highly interesting for the physiology of language processing, but give little evidence for its underlying anatomy, even when the method of brain mapping is employed (for further details, see Rugg and Coles 1995).

Some language-related activations of brain areas

PET studies using language comprehension (story listening) and production (covert verb generation to a semantically related noun) paradigms and analysing their covariance in comparison to a resting state were able to identify three areas involved in language processing, roughly the regions of Broca's and Wernicke's area, and the anterior part of the left inferior temporal gyrus (Papathanassiou *et al.* 2000).

Activation of Broca'a area has been found with receptive syntactic processing (Caplan *et al.* 2000). Broca's area was not activated by word repetition, but rather the left anterior insula and lateral premotor cortex were activated (Wise *et al.* 1999).

Lexical–semantic processing of words activates an extensive, mainly left hemisphere network of brain structures (Perani *et al.* 1999*a*, see Fig. 39.3), with a larger left frontal activation for verbs than nouns. A number of studies have found a left fusiform gyrus (a parahippocampal structure of the temporal lobe) activation with semantic access (Murtha *et al*; 1999, Kuperberg *et al.* 2000). With respect to semantic category judgements, Perani *et al.* (1999*b*) found a left fusiform gyrus activation with the processing of living things, and of the left middle temporal gyrus for tools. It can be expected that abundant information on the cerebral basis of semantics will be available from fMRI studies in the near future. It can also be expected that future studies will reveal a great degree of interindividual variability, as subgroups of normal subjects show bilateral temporal activation with semantic retrieval (Warburton *et al.* 1999).

5 The functional neuroanatomy of language processing in aphasics

The lesions underlying aphasia interfere with task-related activation of the affected brain structures. However, functional imaging demonstrated changes in the functional organization of language processing in aphasics. Depending on the language task, aphasic patients seem to activate ipsi- and contralesional cortical areas in addition to spared structures (Ohyama *et al.* 1996). The superior repetition performance in transcortical aphasia seems to be based on right hemisphere mechanisms (Berthier *et al.* 1991). Alterations in language processing in aphasic patients can also be demonstrated by neurophysiological analysis. ERP and MEG (magnetoencephalography) studies have the advantage of superior temporal resolution over fMRI and PET (but inferior spatial resolution). Friederici *et al.* (1998) were able to show that ERP-correlates of the automatic analysis of syntactic structures were absent in Broca's aphasia.

Recovery from aphasia seems to depend mainly upon three functional anatomical mechanisms:

- recruitment of perilesional left cortical areas for language processing (Warburton *et al.* 1999);
- an activation of the left supplementary motor area;
- an activation of contralesional homologues in the right hemisphere.

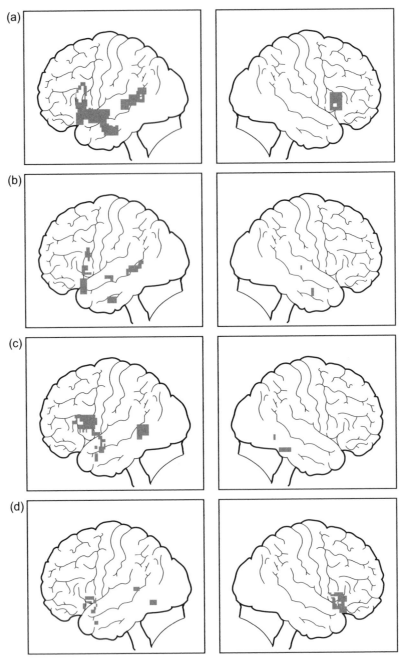

Fig. 39.3 Activation of cortical regions by reading words of different class and concreteness versus pseudowords in a lexical decision task: a) activation by words compared to pseudowords; b) commonalities of activation by all words; c) verbs compared to nouns; d) abstract words compared to concrete words. (Taken with permission from Perani *et al.* 1999*a*, Fig. 1.)

Some studies suggest that early recovery is related to left and long-term improvement to right hemisphere activation (Karbe *et al.* 1998). Patients who were able to recruit dominant language structures exhibited better recovery (Heiss *et al.* 1999). It has been proposed that speech therapy may aid in the activation of the dominant hemisphere and that right hemisphere activation may be dysfunctional (Belin *et al.* 1996). On the other hand, improvement with intensive comprehension training in Wernicke's aphasia was shown to correlate with task-dependent activation in the posterior part of the right superior temporal gyrus (Musso *et al.* 1999).

Pizzamiglio *et al.* (2001) pointed out that the function-related changes in cerebral activation patterns after lesion may have different meanings.

- In some cases, spared neuronal populations involved in a given function may undergo reorganization providing the basis for functional recovery.
- In other cases, different regions of the brain, which process information in a completely different way, are recruited after a lesion to compensate for a functional loss.

6 Methodological problems of functional imaging

Functional images represent spatially and temporally integrated measures of regional cerebral blood flow during the performance of a task in contrast to flow distribution during another task (or a resting state). A detailed discussion of the methodological aspects of functional language studies is given by Grabowski and Damasio (2000). These authors' summary of items to be included in processing the complex data includes:

- modelling and removal of artefacts;
- spatial transformation to a standard anatomical space (usually based upon Talairach and Tournoux 1988);
- spatial filtering to improve signal-to-noise ratio, to overcome anatomical variability, and to meet parametric assumptions of statistical analysis (see end of this section);
- statistical analysis;
- construction of a statistical parametric map;
- significance thresholding of the test statistic images;
- inference;
- representations of the results (Grabowski and Damasio 2000, pp. 430–2).

The method is based on a number of assumptions that are difficult to control.

- It supposes that the experimental task states differ only with respect to the tasks (problems, e.g. effort, demand on working memory, subjective reaction).
- Brains differ anatomically and cannot completely be mapped upon a standard anatomical space (Rajkowska and Goldman-Rakic 1995).
- It is assumed that the experimental tasks isolate a single cognitive function.

◆ It is assumed that task-related activation is insensitive to practice effects.

In fact, practice changes activation patterns. Furthermore, the sheer rate of presentation of stimuli affects activation (Raichle *et al.* 1994).

In many experiments, the crucial experimental task differed in a number of aspects (e.g. difficulty, propositionality, size, and number of activated semantic fields) from those it was compared with. Generally, the so-called subtraction method assumes that cognitive variables that affect different stages of processing are simply added and can be revealed by the subtraction of two states, one that includes the process in question from a similar other that does not. This approach was very fruitful in the analysis of reaction times. The use of this method with language tasks poses many problems, among which the following cause the greatest concern.

◆ Automatic activation of language processing even when subjects are instructed not to pay attention to linguistic content.

◆ Changes in activation may be a characteristic of the control task.

◆ The assumption of addition of a processing state may be inherently false (Friston *et al.* 1996).

Parametric designs are able to overcome some of these problems. Statistical parametric mapping is based upon spatially extended statistical processes that compare spatially distributed events with a probabilistic distribution. Improbable effects within the map are interpreted as regionally specific effects due to the experimental manipulation. 'The fundamental difference between subtractive and parametric approaches lies in treating a cognitive process not as a categorical invariant but as a dimension or attribute that can be expressed to a greater or a lesser extent' (Friston 1997). An important next step is the introduction of nonparametric statistics ('statistical nonparametric mapping'; Poline *et al.* 1997). Functional connectivity between two regions can be statistically established by factorial designs (Friston *et al.* 1997).

7 **Summary**

From the above discussion, it becomes obvious that the methodological problems of functional imaging are not settled. Although experiments can be replicated, if the exact situation is restaged, results are still conflicting, depend upon the strategy of analysis, and cannot be generalized yet (Friston *et al.* 1997; Grabowski and Damasio 2000). However, it is also clear that functional imaging, especially fMRI, has a great potential for the analysis of cerebral processes, particularly those that are involved in cognition and emotion. In our opinion, the analysis of interindividual differences will become increasingly important.

Selective references

Absher, J.R., Hart, L.A., Flowers, D.L., Dagenbach, D., and Wood, F.B. (2000). Event-related potentials correlate with task-dependent glucose metabolism. *NeuroImage.* **11**, 517–31.

Alexander, G., DeLong, M.R., and Strick, P. (1986). Parallel organization of functionally segregated circuits linking basal ganglia and cortex. *Ann. Rev. Neurosci.* **9**, 357–81.

Alexander, M.P. and Annett, M. (1996). Crossed aphasia and related anomalies of cerebral organization: case reports and a genetic hypothesis. *Brain Language.* **55**, 213–39.

Belin, P., van Eeckhout, P., Zilbovicius, M., *et al.* (1996). Recovery from nonfluent aphasia after melodic intonation therapy. *Neurology.* **47**, 1504–11.

Berthier, M.L., Starkstein, S.E., Leiguarda, R., *et al.* (1991). Transcortical aphasia. Importance of the non-speech dominant hemisphere in language repetition. *Brain.* **114**, 1409–27.

Borod, J.C., Andelman, F., Obler, L.K., Tweedy, J.R., and Welkowitz, J. (1992). Right hemisphere specialization for the identification of emotional words and sentences: evidence from stroke patients. *Neuropsychologia.* **30**, 827–44.

Caplan, D., Alpert, N., Waters, G., and Olivieri, A. (2000). Activation of Broca's area by syntactic processing under conditions of concurrent articulation. *Hum. Brain Mapping.* **9**, 65–71.

Carpenter, P.A. and Just, M.A. (1999). Modeling the mind: very-high field functional magnetic resonance imaging activation during cognition. *Topics MRI.* **10**, 16–36.

Chi, J.G., Dooling, E.C., and Gilles, F.H. (1977). Left–right asymmetries of the temporal speech areas of the human fetus. *Arch. Neurol.* **34**, 346–8.

Démonet, J-F., Thierry, G., and Cardebat, D. (2005). Renewal of the neurophysiology of language: Functional neuroimaging. *Physiol. Rev.* **85**, 49–95.

Frackowiak, R.S.J., Friston, K.J., Frith, C.D., Dolan, R.J., and Mazziotta, J.C. (eds.) (1997). *Human Brain Function.* Academic Press, San Diego.

Friederici, A.D., Hahne, A., and von Cramon, D.Y. (1998). First-pass versus second-pass parsing processes in a Wernicke's and a Broca's aphasic: electrophysiological evidence for a double dissociation. *Brain Language.* **62**, 311–41.

Friston, K.J. (1997). Analyzing brain images: principles and overview. In *Human brain function* (ed. R.S.J. Frackowiak, K.J. Friston, C.D. Frith, R.J. Dolan, and J.C. Mazziotta), pp. 25–41. Academic Press, San Diego.

Friston, K.J., Price, C.J., Fletcher, P., Moore, C., Frackowiak, R.S.J., and Dolan, R.J. (1996). The trouble with cognitive subtraction. *NeuroImage.* **4**, 97–104.

Friston, K.J., Price, C.J., Buechel, C., and Frackowiak, R.S.J. (1997). A taxonomy of study designs. In *Human brain function* (ed. R.S.J. Frackowiak, K.J. Friston, C.D. Frith, R.J. Dolan, and J.C. Mazziotta), pp. 141–59. Academic Press, San Diego.

Gandour, J., Larsen, J., Dechongkiet, S., Ponglorpisit, S., and Khunadorn, F. (1995). Speech prosody in affective contexts in Thai patients with right hemisphere lesions. *Brain Language.* **51**, 422–43.

Grabowski, T.J. and Damasio, A.R. (2000). Investigating language with functional neuroimaging. In *Brain mapping: the systems* (ed. A.W. Toga and J.C. Mazziotta), pp. 425–61. Academic Press, San Diego.

Harley, T.A. (1996). Connectionist modelling of the recovery of language functions following brain damage. *Brain Language.* **52**, 7–24.

Heiss, W.D., Kessler, J., Thiel, A., Ghaemi, M., and Karbe, H. (1999). Differential capacity of left and right hemispheric areas for compensation of poststroke aphasia. *Ann. Neurol.* **45**, 430–8.

Joanette, Y. and Goulet, P. (1993). Verbal communication deficits after right-hemisphere damage. In *Linguistic disorders and pathologies* (ed. G. Blanken, J. Dittmann, H. Grimm, J.C. Marshall, and C.W. Wallesch), pp. 383–8. De Gruyter, Berlin.

Karbe, H., Thiel, A., Weber-Luxenburger, G., Herholz, K., Kessler, J., and Heiss, W. (1998). Brain plasticity in poststroke aphasia: what is the contribution of the right hemisphere?. *Brain Language.* **64**, 215–30.

Kertesz, A. and Wallesch, C.W. (1993). Cerebral organization of language. In *Linguistic disorders and pathologies* (ed. G. Blanken, J. Dittmann, H. Grimm, J.C. Marshall, and C.W. Wallesch), pp. 120–37. De Gruyter, Berlin.

Kreisler, A., Godefrey, O., Delmaire, C., *et al.* (2000). The anatomy of aphasia revisited. *Neurology.* **54**, 1117–23.

Kuperberg, G.R., McGuire, P.K., Bullmore, E.T., *et al.* (2000). Common and distinct neural sustrates for pragmatic, semantic and syntactic processing of spoken sentences: an fMRI study. *J. Cogn. Neurosci.* **12**, 321–41.

Marshall, J.C. (2000). Planum of the apes: a case study. *Brain Language.* **71**, 145–8.

McClelland, J.L. and Rumelhart, D.E. (1986). *Parallel distributed processing: explorations in the microstructure of cognition.* Vol. 2: *Psychological and biological models.* MIT Press, London.

Merzenich, M.M., Kaas, J.H., Wall, J., Nelson, R.J., Sur, M., and Felleman, D. (1983). Topographic reorganisation of somatosensory cortical areas 3b and 1 in adult monkeys following restricted deafferentation. *Neuroscience.* **8**, 33–55.

Murtha, S., Chertkow, H., Beauregard, M., and Evans, A. (1999). The neural substrate of picture naming. *J. Cogn. Neurosci.* **11**, 399–423.

Musso, M., Weiller, C., Kiebel, S., Müller, S.P., Bülau, P., and Rijntjes, M. (1999). Training induced brain plasticity in aphasia. *Brain.* **122**, 1781–90.

Naeser, M.A., Helm-Estabrooks, N., Haas, G., Auerbach, S., and Scrinivasan, M. (1987). Relationship between lesion extent in Wernicke's area on computed tomographic scan and predicting recovery of comprehension in Wernicke's aphasia. *Arch. Neurol.* **44**, 73–82.

Naeser, M.A., Palumbo, C.L., Helm-Estabrooks, N., Stiassny-Eder, D., and Albert, M.L. (1989). Severe nonfluency in aphasia. Role of the medial subcallosal fasciculus and other white matter pathways in recovery of spontaneous speech. *Brain.* **112**, 1–38.

Ohyama, M., Senda, M., Kitamura, S., Ishii, K., Mishina, M., and Terashi, A. (1996). Role of the nondominant hemisphere and undamaged area during word repetition in poststroke aphasics. A PET activation study. *Stroke.* **27**, 897–903.

Papathanassiou, D., Etard, O., Mellet, E., Tago, L., Mazoyer, B., and Tzourio-Mazoyer, N. (2000). A common language network for comprehension and production: contribution to the definition of language epicenters with PET. *NeuroImage.* **11**, 347–57.

Perani, D., Cappa, S.F., Schnur, T., *et al.* (1999*a*). The neural correlates of verb and noun processing. A PET study. *Brain.* **122**, 2337–44.

Perani, D., Schnur, T., Tettamanti, M., Gorno-Tempini, M., Cappa, S.F., and Fazio, F. (1999*b*). Word and picture matching: a PET study of semantic category effects. *Neuropsychologia.* **37**, 293–306.

Petersen, S.E., Fox, P.T., Posner, M.I., Mintun, M., and Raichle, M.E. (1988). Positron emission tomographic studies of the cortical anatomy of single word processing. *Nature.* **331**, 585–9.

Pizzamiglio, L., Galati, G., and Committeri, G. (2001). The contribution of functional neuroimaging to recovery after brain damage: a review. *Cortex.* **37**, 11–31.

Plaut, D.C. (1995). Double dissociation without modularity: evidence from connectionist neuropsychology. *J. Clin. Exp. Neuropsychol.* **17**, 291–321.

Poeck, K., de Bleser, R., and von Keyserlingk, D.G. (1984). Computed tomography localization of standard aphasia syndromes. *Advan. Neurol.* **42**, 71–89.

Poline, J.B., Holmes, A., Worsley, K., and Friston, K.J. (1997). Making statistical inferences. In *Human brain function* (ed. R.S.J. Frackowiak, K.J. Friston, C.D. Frith, R.J. Dolan, and J.C. Mazziotta), pp. 85–106. Academic Press, San Diego.

Raichle, M.E., Fiez, J., Videen, T.O., *et al.* (1994). Practice-related changes in human functional anatomy during nonmotor learning. *Cerebral Cortex.* **4**, 8–26.

Rajkowska, G. and Goldman-Rakic, P.S. (1995). Cytoarchitectonic definition of prefrontal areas in the normal human cortex: II: Variability in locations of areas 9 and 46 and relationship to the Talairach coordinate system. *Cerebral Cortex.* **5**, 323–37.

Rugg, M.D. and Coles, M.G.H. (1995). *Electrophysiology of mind. Event-related potentials and cognition.* Oxford University Press, Oxford.

Sadato, N., Yonekura, Y., Yamada, H., Nakamura, S., Waki, A., and Ishii, Y. (1998). Activation patterns of covert word generation detected by fMRI in comparison with 3D PET. *J. Comput. Assisted Tomogr.* **22**, 945–52.

Schmahmann, J.D. and Pandya, D.N. (1997). The cerebrocerebellar system. In 'The cerebellum and cognition' [volume edited by J.D. Schmahmann]. *Int. Rev. Neurobiol.* **41**, 31–60.

Steinmetz, H. (1996). Structure, function and cerebral asymmetry: *in vivo* morphometry of the planum temporale. *Neurosci. Behav. Rev.* **20**, 587–91.

Talairach, J. and Tournoux, P. (1988). *Co-planar stereotaxic atlas of the human brain.* Thieme, New York.

Toga, A.W. and Mazziotta, J.C. (eds.) (2000). *Brain Mapping: the systems.* Academic Press, San Diego.

Von Stockert, T.R. (1975). Aphasia sine aphasia. *Brain Language.* **1**, 277–82.

Wallesch, C.W. (1997). Symptomatology of subcortical aphasia. *J. Neurolinguistics* **10**, 267–75.

Warburton, E., Price, C.J., Swinburn, K., and Wise, R.J. (1999). Mechanisms of recovery from aphasia: evidence from positron emission tomography studies. *J. Neurol, Neurosurg. Psychiatry.* **66**, 155–61.

Wise, R.J., Greene, J., Büchel, C., and Scott, S.K. (1999). Brain regions involved in articulation. *Lancet.* **353**, 1057–61.

Chapter 40

Functional neuroanatomy of executive process

Joaquín M. Fuster

1 Introduction

The cortex of the frontal lobe contains the highest stages of the hierarchy of neural structures dedicated to motor representation and processing. The lowest stage of that hierarchy consists of motor neurons in the anterior horns of the spinal cord. Above, in
ascending order, are the motor nuclei of the brainstem, the cerebellum, and the diencephalon, including nuclei of the hypothalamus, the thalamus, and the basal ganglia. The
cortex of the convexity of the frontal lobe is itself hierarchically organized and devoted to
motor actions. At the bottom of the cortical motor hierarchy lies the primary motor cortex, for the representation and execution of elementary skeletal movements. Above it lies
the premotor cortex, for more complex movements, which are defined by goal and trajectory. Some premotor areas are involved in speech organization. At the top is the cortex
of association of the frontal lobe, commonly called prefrontal cortex. This cortex, especially in its lateral region, contains neuronal networks that represent broad schemas
and plans of sequential action and are crucially involved in their enactment. Thus, the
lateral prefrontal cortex (LPC) has been sometimes identified with the 'central executive'
and also called 'the executive of the brain'. In this chapter, the executive functions of the
LPC are considered (see Chapters 18 and 19). Before dealing with them, the chapter deals
with the anatomy, the connectivity, and the neuropsychology of the prefrontal cortex in
general.

2 Anatomy and connectivity of the prefrontal cortex

The prefrontal cortex is one of latest regions of the neocortex to develop, phylogenetically
as well as ontogenetically. In evolution, it reaches its greatest relative expansion in the
brain of the human, where it constitutes almost one-third of the neocortex. Most of that
expansion takes place in the lateral convexity of the frontal lobe, that is, in the LPC.
In ontogeny, the prefrontal cortex—the LPC in particular—is one of the last regions to
reach full myelination of afferent, efferent, and intrinsic fibres. The LPC is also late in
reaching maturity by other indices, e.g. number and volume of neurons, and size and
number of dendritic spines. In the normal human subject, the prefrontal cortex does not
reach full morphological maturation until late adolescence. The late maturation of the
LPC is probably related to the late maturation of its cognitive functions.

The prefrontal cortex is profusely connected with other brain structures. It receives afferent fibres from the brainstem, the hypothalamus, the limbic system (especially amygdala and hippocampus), the thalamus, the basal ganglia, and other areas of the neocortex, especially the association cortex behind the sylvian fissure (parietal, temporal, and occipital regions).

- The afferents from the brainstem, the hypothalamus, and limbic formations bring the prefrontal cortex information about the internal milieu.

- The inputs from the hippocampus are probably essential for the formation of motor or executive memory.

- The afferents from posterior association cortex appear to be involved in higher-order sensorimotor integrations.

The prefrontal cortex reciprocates afferent inputs from all those cerebral structures with efferent outputs to them.

Several neurotransmitter systems of brainstem origin converge on various areas of the prefrontal cortex. They mediate interactions at the synaptic level between subcortical structures and that cortex. The most prominent among them are the dopamine systems, which vary in terms of the types of receptors by which they mediate the transmission of information between cells.

- Dopamine plays an important role in orbital prefrontal cortex, where it mediates neural transactions related to rewards and emotional behaviour. Furthermore, dopaminergic prefrontal pathways mediate motor behaviour through the basal ganglia.

- Noradrenaline (norepinephrine) and serotonin, with sparser distributions in the prefrontal cortex, are probably involved in cortical arousal and attention mechanisms.

- A powerful cholinergic system, originating in the basal nucleus of Meynert and widely distributed throughout the neocortex, is most probably also involved in those attention mechanisms and in short-term memory.

- In the prefrontal cortex, as in other parts of the cortex, γ-aminobutyric acid (GABA) is the most abundant inhibitory neurotransmitter. It participates in the filtering or exclusionary mechanisms of attention and working memory.

- Glutaminergic neurotransmitters, such as those operating on N-methyl-D-aspartate (NMDA) receptors, most probably play a role in the formation of executive memory in the prefrontal cortex.

Intervening in this process are probably the reciprocal connections between the hippocampus and the LPC, which have been demonstrated in the monkey.

3 Neuropsychology of the prefrontal cortex

For more than a century, the study of the behavioural and cognitive effects of prefrontal damage from disease or trauma has been a major source of knowledge about the functions of the prefrontal cortex. This knowledge is largely inferential, based on the assumption that the deficit from the lesion of a cerebral structure such as the prefrontal cortex results from the interference with the normal function(s) of that structure. This assumption is not always tenable, because the lesion may secondarily and imponderably affect other—neighbouring or connected—structures. Furthermore, the deficit is commonly relative, i.e. only quantitatively different from the dysfunction induced by lesions elsewhere in the brain. In any event, the inferences from clinical lesion are generally confounded by considerable individual variability—in terms of the extent and location of the lesion as well as its effects. Nonetheless, a massive literature is now available on the clinical and psychological manifestations of frontal-lobe injury. This literature allows us to characterize those manifestations with considerable confidence. A particular cluster of symptoms and signs can be reliably observed after damage to each of the three principal regions of the prefrontal cortex (Fig. 40.1):

- medial;
- orbital;
- lateral (LPC).

3.1 Medial/cingulate region

The lesions of the medial region of the prefrontal cortex induce disorders of drive and motivation. Apathy and disinterest are the dominant manifestations of medial prefrontal damage.

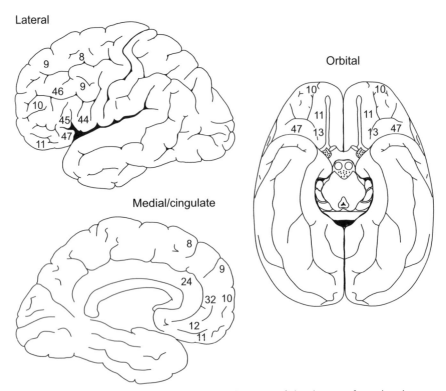

Fig. 40.1 Diagram of the human cerebral cortex. The areas of the three prefrontal regions are numbered in accord with Brodmann's cytoarchitectonic map.

Related to them is the lack of spontaneity in all domains of action, including speech. The patient is generally hypokinetic. In cases with large lesions of medial prefrontal cortex, hypokinesia turns into akinesia (akinetic mutism when speech is involved). Circumscribed lesions of the anterior cingulate cortex (areas 24 and 32) commonly result in deficits of attention. The patient with such a lesion has difficulty focusing on the performance of tasks that require sizeable effort and attention to detail. Thus the patient appears not only neglectful, but also unable to gather the energy to respond to cognitively challenging situations.

In all probability, the lack of interest, the aspontaneity, and the inattentiveness of patients with medial/anterior-cingulate lesion reflect the disruption of a general adaptive function of goal-directed drive that is indispensable for selective attention. The connectivity of medial prefrontal cortex with limbic structures probably plays a role in that general function. Mesulam (1981) has postulated an 'anterior attentional system', of which the anterior cingulate region would be a crucial part. That system also includes gaze-control areas of parietal and lateral prefrontal cortex.

3.2 Orbital region

Lesions of ventral (orbital) prefrontal cortex ordinarily induce a relatively uniform syndrome. An attentional disorder is here again in the foreground, but this one is not so much characterized by absence of drive as by failure of the exclusionary aspect of attention. The patient is abnormally distractable, unable to inhibit the interference from external stimuli that are extraneous to the action in progress, whatever that may be. Together with distractability, and probably related to it, is a general tendency to hyperactivity and hyperreactivity. On formal testing, the patient commonly fails to perform correctly the Stroop task, the Wisconsin Card Sorting Test (WCST), and other tests that require the attentional suppression of interference.

Furthermore, the affect of the orbital patient is labile and unpredictable. Together with a sporadic tendency to euphoria, the patient commonly exhibits inappropriate and coarse humour. In addition, he or she is unable to inhibit instinctive drives, and thus inclined to frequent displays of quarrelsomeness, hypersexuality and hyperphagia. The disinhibition of instinct, accompanied by lack of moral judgement, often leads the patient to unruly behaviour and conflict with the law. Sociopathy is almost the hallmark of the orbital syndrome.

In brief, the patient with damage of the orbital prefrontal cortex commonly exhibits a variety of abnormalities of emotional and social behaviour (Damasio *et al.* 1994; Fuster 1997). At the root of these abnormalities, there appears to be a deficit in the inhibitory control functions of this cortex. In normal attentive processing, inhibitory control is probably exerted through efferent connections of orbital cortex upon the thalamus and upon areas of frontal and posterior association cortex. In normal social behaviour, that control is exerted upon the hypothalamus and other limbic structures. Both kinds of control fail in the patient with orbitofrontal damage.

3.3 Lateral region (LPC)

The most characteristic cognitive deficits from frontal-lobe injury are those that result from damage to the associative cortex of the lateral frontal convexity—the LPC.

In subjects with a large LPC lesion, the most common disorder is the inability to conceptualize and to carry out plans and goal-directed sequences of actions. It is from this disorder that the notion emerged of a critical role of the LPC in the representation and execution of organized behaviour (Luria 1966; Fuster 1997). The planning deficit, which extends to the representation and construction of language (Luria 1970), is now generally considered a consistent manifestation of large lateral LPC lesion. One aspect of this deficit is a difficulty in mentally representing sequences of speech or behaviour. Another is a difficulty in executing them in orderly fashion. The aggregate of these difficulties constitutes what Baddeley (1986) calls the 'dysexecutive syndrome'. This syndrome, like the medial and orbital syndromes, usually includes a severe attentional disorder, though this disorder differs qualitatively from those that result from medial or orbital lesion. Shallice (1988) characterizes the LPC disorder as the failure of 'supervisory attentional control'. By this he means the inability to summon and sustain selective attention on a series of goal-directed actions. This aspect of attention is essential to executive initiative, decision-making, and the temporal organization of novel and complex behaviour.

Any reasonable analysis of the functions of the LPC must distinguish between its *representational* role and its *operational* role. The former can be inferred from the deleterious effects of LPC lesions on the mental representations of plans and schemata of sequential action. The study of these effects has led to the concept of the LPC as the substrate of executive memory, which includes the schemata or plans of past or future action. Plans can be considered 'memory' inasmuch as they consist of fragmentary representations of previous actions—rearranged for future planning. Executive memory is held in wide arrays of interconnected neuronal networks of the LPC (Fuster 1995).

The operational role of the LPC essentially consists of the orderly activation of those networks in the construction of goal-directed sequences or temporal 'gestalts' of executive action. Temporal integration is the most general function of the LPC. This operation is served by at least four cognitive functions that this cortex controls in cooperation with subcortical structures and with other regions of the neocortex. Those functions are:

- attention;
- working memory;
- prospective set;
- response monitoring.

They are closely entwined and cannot be extricated from one another physiologically. None is represented exclusively in any discrete LPC area. Any demonstrable specialization of LPC areas is not so much attributable to the topographical distribution of those cognitive functions as to the kind of executive information they process. Thus some areas are dedicated to motor actions, others to eye movement, and still others to speech. In any given area, all four cognitive functions operate at the service of the temporal integration of the kind of executive information in which the area specializes.

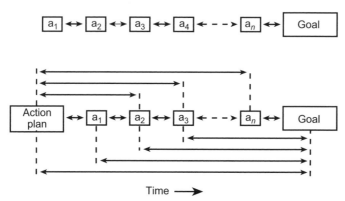

Fig. 40.2 Temporal sequencing of acts (a_1 ... a_n) toward a goal. (Above) Chain of acts in a routine and well-practised sequence. Contingencies (arrows) are present only between successive acts. (Below) A novel and complex sequence of acts that necessitates the mediation of cross-temporal contingencies, a function of the LPC.

4 Temporal integration and its ancillary executive functions

Temporal integration, i.e. the capacity to integrate information across time, is the essence of temporal order. This applies to behaviour, speech, and logical reasoning. The central role of the LPC in the organization of actions in those three domains is crucially based on its ability to mediate contingencies across time ('if now this, then later that; if earlier that, then now this'). Both the choice and the timing of an act in a goal-directed sequence are contingent on the plan of action, on the goal, and on other acts that have preceded that act or are expected to succeed it (Fig. 40.2). Inasmuch as the LPC is needed for the mediation of cross-temporal contingencies, it is needed for the temporal organization of behavioural, linguistic, and cognitive actions.

The most widely used behavioural paradigms for testing the role of LPC in temporal integration are the so-called 'delay tasks', e.g. delayed response, delayed matching- to-sample. In these tasks, the subject is required to retain a discrete item of information in order to execute, a few seconds later, an action that is contingent on that information. For correct performance, therefore, each trial requires the integration of information across time, i.e. across the delay. It has long been known (Jacobsen 1931) that monkeys that have sustained lesions of LPC are rendered incapable of learning and performing delay tasks, especially when the information is complex and the delay long (>10 seconds).

In the past 30 years, electrophysiology and neuroimaging have established the operational role of the LPC in all four of its temporal integrative functions. Many of the studies contributing the supporting evidence have been carried out in monkeys or humans performing delay tasks.

4.1 Sensory attention

Attention is the selective allocation of neural resources to behaviour and cognition. It operates at many levels of sensory and motor systems. It is essential in the cerebral cortex for the efficient processing of information in its vast systems of intersecting networks. For a behavioural sequence to attain its goal, continuous selective attention is required on the sensory stimuli that guide it and on the motor actions that constitute it. This is fundamentally a cortical function. Its mechanisms are still poorly understood and they can be assumed to include excitation as well as inhibition. The results of their operation are:

- selective focusing;
- enhanced contrast;
- suppression of extraneous information.

All forms of attention required for the organization of behavioural and cognitive sequences are under executive prefrontal control. As noted in Section 3, medial and cingulate areas contribute to the motivational aspects of attention and orbital areas to the inhibitory control of interference or distraction. Areas of the LPC, on the other hand, contribute to the aspects of attention more directly related to temporal integration. Sensory attention is one of them. Several LPC areas—notably area 8—are involved in visual attention, as they specialize in the control of gaze and eye movements. Lesions of these areas lead to visual neglect and to the inability to shift attention between locations in the visual field. Functional neuroimaging provides further evidence for the role of LPC in selective sensory attention, as it supports a variety of temporal integrative tasks (Duncan and Owen 2000).

Working memory and prospective set, the two LPC functions that are essential to bridge time (see Sections 4.2 and 4.3), can also be considered forms of selective attention. Both constitute attention that is directed to internal representations. Both appear to depend on the selective activation of cortical and subcortical structures under the control of the LPC (Desimone and Duncan 1995; Fuster 1995).

4.2 Working memory

Working memory (Baddeley 1986) is the temporary retention of information for the performance of an act that is contingent on that information. All forms of cognitive and behavioural performance requiring the mediation of cross-temporal contingencies depend to some degree on working memory. Working memory is the first cognitive function of the LPC to have been substantiated at the neuronal level by microelectrode methods. In delay tasks, during the retention of a sensory cue for a prospective action, neurons in the dorsolateral prefrontal cortex of the monkey exhibit sustained elevated discharge (Fuster 1973). This discharge, which may last anywhere between a few seconds and 2 or 3 minutes, is correlated with accuracy of performance and can be obliterated or attenuated by distraction. Cells with these characteristics have been called 'memory cells'. During the performance of spatial delayed-response tasks, in which the animal must retain the position of a visual cue, some LPC cells are involved in the retention of spatial information. In other kinds of delay tasks, memory cells have been found for colours, auditory cues, and tactile information. In any case, the participation of LPC cells in working memory seems strictly related to the need to retain information for an action that is contingent on that information.

In the human, the use of functional neuroimaging by positron emission tomography (PET) or magnetic resonance (MR) reveals the activation of the LPC in a number of working memory tasks (Grasby *et al.* 1993; Petrides *et al.* 1993; Smith *et al.* 1996). The activation has a different topography depending on the nature of the memorandum or information that the subject must temporarily retain. It is reasonable to assume that the activation reflects the excitation of large assemblies or networks of memory cells that encode that information in working memory. LPC networks have been thus substantiated for visuospatial, visual–nonspatial, and verbal memoranda.

4.3 Prospective set

Prospective or preparatory set is another form of internalized attention under LPC control. Like working memory, it helps the organism to mediate cross-temporal contingencies. Whereas working memory is retrospective memory, prospective set is 'memory of the future'. It is attention focused on the representation of prospective action. Thus, the prospective-set function can be considered a kind of motor, or executive, attention. By this function and mechanisms that are still unknown, the LPC primes executive systems for anticipated action.

A well-known electrical correlate of prospective set is the contingent negative variation (CNV), a slow surface potential that develops over the frontal lobe in the interval between a sensory stimulus and a motor response that depends on it (Brunia *et al.* 1985). Another such correlate is the *Bereitschaftspotential* or 'readiness potential', which develops over motor cortex immediately before the response. In monkeys performing a delay task in which the animal had to remember a colour for a hand movement to the right or to the left, some LPC were found to react specifically to colours and others to direction of manual response (Quintana and Fuster 1999). During the delay or memory period, the cells of the first type (colour-coupled) showed a gradual descent of discharge (Fig. 40.3). Conversely, those of the second type (direction-coupled) showed an acceleration of discharge. Furthermore, the degree of that acceleration varied in proportion to the certainty with which the animal could predict response direction (different colours predicted direction with different degrees of probability).

To sum up, the slow potentials in anticipation of an action, and the presence of cells in LPC that seem to predict the action, indicate that the LPC participates in the preparation of the motor apparatus to act. At lower stages, that apparatus includes structures such as the premotor cortex, the basal ganglia, and the pyramidal system. All may take part in the preparatory modulation of motor systems under LPC control. That kind of preparatory control can also be inferred from the activation of the LPC observed by neuroimaging during planning tasks (Partiot *et al.* 1995; Baker *et al.* 1996).

4.4 Response monitoring

Response monitoring is a fourth integrative function of the LPC. This function is based on both internal and external feedback arriving in this cortex during organized action. The internal feedback consists of signals from internal receptors activated by movement.

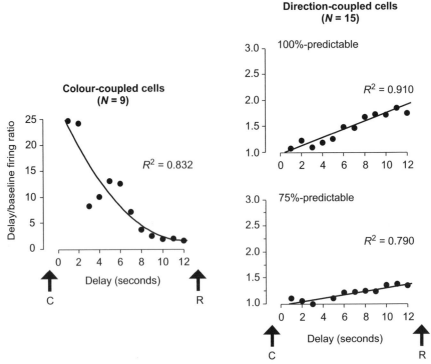

Fig. 40.3 Discharge of LPC cells during the delay between a colour and the manual response associated with it (C, colour; R, response). (Left) Discharge of colour-coupled memory cells. (Right) Discharge of direction-coupled cells. The latter cells anticipate the response with an acceleration of firing that is greatest (top graph) when the animal can predict response direction with certainty.

Such signals include inputs from the motor system in the form of so-called 'efferent copies' of muscular movement and inputs from proprioceptors. The aggregate of these internal signals related to movement generates in the LPC what has been termed *corollary discharge* (Teuber 1972). This consists of neural impulses that flow into sensory systems and prepare them for changes resulting from anticipated movement. Corollary discharge would thus stabilize perception despite changes in the relative position of sensory receptors with respect to the environment.

In addition, various kinds of feedback from sensory receptors carry to the LPC information about the changes that actions in a behavioural sequence induce in the environment. Thus a more or less continuous stream of sensory signals arrive in LPC with information on the consequences of one's successive actions. These signals include indicators of the success or failure of each act with respect to the goal of the sequence. The LPC will integrate that information to prepare the organism for subsequent actions and to induce in them corrective modifications.

Neuroimaging supports the involvement of the LPC in response monitoring (Petrides *et al.* 1993; Fink *et al.* 1999). Further evidence of this involvement comes from electrophysiology in patients with LPC lesions (Gehring and Knight 2000). Both imaging and electrophysiology also indicate a parallel role of the anterior cingulate cortex in the monitoring of response errors.

5 The perception–action cycle

All four integrative functions of the LPC just mentioned operate within the broad physiological framework of the perception–action cycle (Fuster 1997). This physiological cycle constitutes the extension into the cerebral cortex—and thus into the cognitive sphere—of a basic physiological principle of sensorimotor adaptation of the organism to its environment. It may be considered to be part of the 'homeostatic' mechanisms of the organism inasmuch as adaptation to the environment protects stability of the internal milieu. The cycle is made of the circular cybernetic flow of information between the environment, sensory structures, and motor structures. Those neural structures are hierarchically organized along the nerve axis, and so are the levels of the cycle that unites them. The LPC and the posterior association cortex are at the summit of the perception–action cycle (Fig. 40.4).

In the course of a goal-directed sequence of behavioural acts, the sensory information that guides the sequence is processed upward in successive stages of the hierarchy of sensory cortical areas. That processing leads to outputs to motor areas, where actions are integrated.

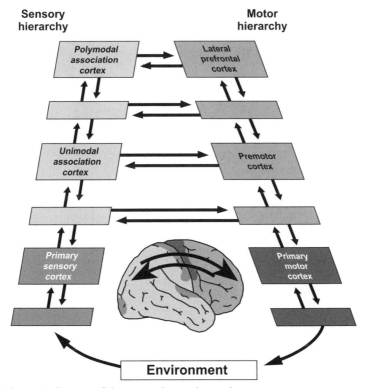

Fig. 40.4 Schematic diagram of the perception–action cycle.

The actions induce changes in the environment, which generate new sensory inputs, which lead to new actions, and so on. Automatic and routine behaviours can be integrated at lower stages of sensory and motor hierarchies, without need for intervention of higher cortices. Novel and complex behaviours, however, require processing at the highest levels of the perception–action cycle and thus involve the prefrontal cortex and the cortex of polymodal sensory association. The LPC intervenes whenever those behaviours necessitate the mediation of cross-temporal contingencies. Temporal integration, and thus the temporal organization of those behaviours, are then made possible by the executive functions of the LPC summarized above.

As can be gleaned from the structure and operations of the perception–action cycle and the position of the LPC in it, the latter performs its executive functions in close cooperation with other cortical regions (Fuster 2001).

- The LPC controls the focus of attention by its modulation of sensory association areas of posterior cortex.
- Working memory is maintained by reverberation of activity in connective loops that link the LPC with those areas.
- Prospective set involves the downflow of priming influences from LPC upon premotor and motor cortices.
- Finally, the monitoring of motor responses and their consequences is in large part mediated by signals that arrive in LPC after being processed in hierarchically lower sensory and motor cortices.

6 Conclusions

The neural substrate for executive processing is organized hierarchically. At every level of the hierarchy, neuronal assemblies serve both the representation and the execution of actions. In the upward progression of executive levels, from the spinal cord to the neocortex, the actions represented and executed increase in complexity, as well as in the spatial and temporal remoteness of their goal. The association cortex of the convexity of the frontal lobes, or lateral prefrontal cortex (LPC), constitutes the highest level of that hierarchy. Its primary function is the temporal organization of goal-directed behaviour, speech, and reasoning. The organization of actions in those domains is essentially based on the capacity of the LPC to integrate temporally discontinuous information. In that process of temporal integration, the LPC mediates contingencies across time by cooperating with other cortical structures in the cognitive functions of the perception–action cycle, which include attention, working memory, prospective set, and response monitoring.

Selective references

Baddeley, A. (1986). *Working memory*. Clarendon Press, Oxford.

Baker, S.C., Rogers, R.D., Owen, A.M., Frith, C.D., Dolan, R.J., Frackowiak, R.S.J., and Robbins, T.W. (1996). Neural systems engaged by planning: a PET study of the Tower of London task. *Neuropsychologia*. **34**, 515–26.

Brunia, C.H.M., Haagh, S.A.V.M., and Scheirs, J.G.M. (1985). Waiting to respond: electrophysiological measurements in man during preparation for a voluntary movement. In *Motor behavior* (ed. H. Heuer, U. Kleinbeck, and K.-H. Schmidt). Springer, New York.

Damasio, H., Grabowski, T., Frank, R., Galaburda, A.M., and Damasio, A.R. (1994). The return of Phineas Gage: clues about the brain from the skull of a famous patient. *Science.* **264**, 1102–5.

Desimone, R. and Duncan, J. (1995). Neural mechanisms of selective visual attention. *Ann. Rev. Neurosci.* **18**, 193–222.

Duncan, J. and Owen, A.M. (2000). Common regions of the human frontal lobe recruited by diverse cognitive demands. *Trends NeuroSci.* **23**, 475–83.

Fink, G.R., Marshall, J.C., Halligan, P.W., Frith, C.D., Driver, J., Frackowiak, R.S., and Dolan, R.J. (1999). The neural consequences of conflict between intention and the senses. *Brain.* **122**, 497–512.

Fuster, J.M. (1973). Unit activity in prefrontal cortex during delayed-response performance: neuronal correlates of transient memory. *J. Neurophysiol.* **36**, 61–78.

Fuster, J.M. (1995). *Memory in the cerebral cortex—an empirical approach to neural networks in the human and nonhuman primate.* MIT Press, Cambridge, Massachusetts.

Fuster, J.M. (1997). *The prefrontal cortex—anatomy, physiology, and neuropsychology of the frontal lobe,* 3rd edn. Lippincott-Raven, Philadelphia.

Fuster, J.M. (2001). The prefrontal cortex—an update: time is of the essence. *Neuron.* **30**, 319–33.

Gehring, W.J. and Knight, R.T. (2000). Prefrontal–cingulate interactions in action monitoring. *Nature Neurosci.* **3**, 516–20.

Grasby, P.M., Frith, C.D., Friston, K.J., Bench, C., Frackowiak, R.S.J., and Dolan, R.J. (1993). Functional mapping of brain areas implicated in auditory-verbal memory function. *Brain.* **116**, 1–20.

Jacobsen, C.F. (1931). A study of cerebral function in learning: the frontal lobes. *J. Comp. Neurol.* **52**, 271–340.

Luria, A.R. (1966). *Higher cortical functions in man.* Basic Books, New York.

Luria, A.R. (1970). *Traumatic aphasia.* Mouton, The Hague.

Mesulam, M.-M. (1981). A cortical network for directed attention and unilateral neglect. *Neurology.* **10**, 309–25.

Partiot, A., Grafman, J., Sadato, N., Wachs, J., and Hallett, M. (1995). Brain activation during the generation of non-emotional and emotional plans. *NeuroReport.* **6**, 1269–72.

Petrides, M., Alivisatos, B., Evans, A.C., and Meyer, E. (1993). Dissociation of human mid-dorsolateral from posterior dorsolateral frontal cortex in memory processing. *Proc. Natl Acad. Sci., USA* **90**, 873–7.

Quintana, J. and Fuster, J.M. (1999). From perception to action: Temporal integrative functions of prefrontal and parietal neurons. *Cerebral Cortex.* **9**, 213–21.

Shallice, T. (1988). *From neuropsychology to mental structure.* Cambridge University Press, New York.

Smith, E.E., Jonides, J., and Koeppe, R.A. (1996). Dissociating verbal and spatial working memory using PET. *Cerebral Cortex.* **6**, 11–20.

Teuber, H.L. (1972). Unity and diversity of frontal lobe function. *Acta Neurobiolagiae Experimentalis.* **32**, 615–56.

Part 10

Clinical context and resources

Chapter 41

Clinical and laboratory examinations relevant to clinical neuropsychology

Udo Kischka

1 Introduction

The methods described in this chapter are used by clinicians to gain insight into the structure and the functions of a patient's nervous system. Computerized tomography (CT) and magnetic resonance imaging (MRI) are the methods of choice to demonstrate the anatomical structure and deviations thereof, such as trauma, stroke, tumour, or inflammation. They help visualize where a lesion is localized. All the other methods mentioned in this chapter are used to examine the extent of functioning of parts of the nervous system. In the context of this handbook, only those methods that deal with the brain rather than the spinal cord and the peripheral nervous system will be considered.

For the neuropsychologist, the outcomes of these examinations are relevant for several different reasons.

◆ The intactness of a patient's sensory and motor functions influences his/her performance in the neuropsychological tests. For instance, a visual field defect renders tests that require reading more difficult, and a weakness (*paresis*) or clumsiness (*ataxia*) in the responding arm will put the patient at a disadvantage in a test demanding motor responses. Thus, the knowledge of a clinical neurological deficit informs the choice of the neuropsychological tests that can be used and can help with the interpretation of their results.

◆ If a patient's cognitive performance fluctuates significantly within a short period of time, he/she might be suffering from *partial complex epileptic seizures*, whereby consciousness is altered for some minutes without being lost completely. In this case, an EEG may provide confirmation of the clinical suspicion of seizures.

◆ The MRI and CT scans make it possible to relate findings of neuropsychological deficits to damaged brain structures.

◆ A patient who displays a slow cognitive decline might suffer from one of a variety of possible neurological conditions, (e.g. tumour, recurring strokes, or progressive brain atrophy in Alzheimer's disease). A CT or MRI scan then demonstrates the nature and extent of the pathological brain process.

Some of the methods described in this chapter (MRI, CT, electroencephalography (EEG), and parts of the clinical neurological examination) therefore, yield results that can be related to neuropsychological findings. In addition, several other methods are briefly described and explained (where such direct links are not possible), which are likely to be encountered by neuropsychologists in their clinical work.

2 The clinical neurological examination

The full clinical neurological assessment includes taking a history, observing the patient's behaviour, and carrying out a formal neurological examination of his/her motor, sensory, and reflex functions. A brief mental status examination also comprises part of this assessment. In about two-thirds of cases, this clinical information alone will enable the neurologist to make a correct anatomical diagnosis regarding the localization of the lesion, and a pathological diagnosis as to the nature of the underlying disease.

2.1 History

Taking the patient's history provides us with important clues about the nature of the disease, and also the patient's ability to cope with it. In addition to listening to the patient's account, the following kinds of questions need to be asked.

- What is the precise description (quality) of the complaints?
- Where are they localized?
- When did they first start?
- How did they start, suddenly or gradually?
- What course have they taken?
- Which situations trigger or relieve them?
- What treatment has been tried?

In conditions that affect the patient's cognitive functions temporarily (such as epilepsy) or continuously (such as dementia), it is necessary to get a relative's or partner's history of the patient.

2.2 Observation of the patient's behaviour

The observation of the patient's spontaneous behaviour comprises the way he/she walks, moves, and talks. Important criteria include the following.

- Level of alertness. Sleepiness is called *somnolence* when it is mild and *stupor* when it is more severe. *Coma* is enduring complete loss of consciousness.
- Speed of movements and speech. Unusual slowness of movement is called *bradykinesia*.
- Involuntary movements. *Tremor* is a rhythmic shaking of the limbs, the head, or, rarely, the whole body. Depending on the underlying disease, it can be most pronounced in rest, in holding the limbs outstretched, or during active movements.
- *Dystonia, dyskinesia, chorea*, and *athetosis* are different types of involuntary movements that are not rhythmic.
- Speech. *Aphasia* is the disturbed production and/or understanding of language; *dysarthria* is a defect in articulation, making the speech slurred.

- ◆ Structuring of the patient's account of his problems.
- ◆ Social appropriateness.

2.3 **Neurological assessment**

The neurological examination usually starts with the head and assessment of the 12 cranial nerves and then proceeds to the motor functions, sensations, and reflexes of the limbs and trunk. It should also include a brief mental status examination.

2.3.1 **The 12 cranial nerves**

The 12 cranial nerves relay motor functions, senses, and reflexes of the head.

- ◆ Motor functions:
  - — facial expression: weakness of facial muscles is called *facial palsy*;
  - — gaze: disturbed control of eye movements can lead to double vision or *nystagmus* (rhythmic movements of the eyes);
  - — speaking (see Section 2.2);
  - — swallowing: disturbed swallowing can cause choking;
  - — turning of the head.

- ◆ Senses:
  - — vision: blindness is called *amaurosis*; a loss of half the visual field within one or both eyes is called *hemianopia*;
  - — smell: loss of smell is called *anosmia*;
  - — taste: loss of taste is called *ageusia*;
  - — hearing: reduced hearing is called *hypacusis*, deafness is called *anacusis*;
  - — feeling: see Section 2.3.3;

- ◆ The vestibular system in the inner ear senses the position and movements of the head and therefore plays an important part in maintaining equilibrium.

- ◆ Reflexes. The most widely used reflex is the light reflex of the pupils.

2.3.2 **Motor functions of the body**

- ◆ Muscle power. The maximum power of each muscle group is described on a scale from 0 (no muscle contraction) to 5 (full power) according to the Medical Research Council. Muscle weakness is called *paresis* or *paralysis*; complete loss of force is called *plegia*. *Hemiparesis* is weakness of one side of the body, *paraparesis* weakness of both legs, and *tetraparesis* or *quadriparesis* weakness of all four limbs.

- ◆ Coordination. The dexterity of both coarse and fine movements is tested by the finger–nose test (touching his/her own nose with his/her index finger) and the shin–heel–test (moving the heel to the opposite knee and along the shin). Clumsiness in these tests is called *ataxia*.

- ◆ Muscle tone. Increased tone can be either *spasticity* or *rigor*; reduced tone is called *flaccid*.

- ◆ Posture and gait. Observe whether the patient stands straight or bent, secure or insecure, and whether the movements seem clumsy (*ataxic*) or asymmetrical.

2.3.3 Sensation

The sensory modalities are:

- touch;
- pain;
- temperature;
- vibration;
- position of limbs.

Reduction of sensation is called *hypaesthesia*, complete loss *anaesthesia*. The feeling of pins and needles is called *paraesthesia*.

2.3.4 Reflexes

The most commonly tested reflexes are the biceps and triceps reflexes in the arms and the knee jerk and the ankle jerk in the legs. Note whether the reflexes are unusually weak or brisk, whether there are side differences, or differences between the reflexes of the arms and those of the legs.

Pathological reflexes indicate a lesion within the central nervous system. The *Babinski reflex* is the most widely used, whereby scratching of the outer side of the foot sole causes a dorsal extension (upward movement) of the big toe.

2.3.5 Cognitive functions

Every patient with known or suspected brain injury or disease should have a brief mental status examination. This detects signs of attentional, memory, or constructional deficits, aphasia, apraxia, agnosia, neglect, or executive dysfunction. This assessment falls under the term *cognitive neurology* (in the UK) or *behavioral neurology* (in the USA). A full neuropsychological examination will then provide a more detailed analysis of the nature and extent of the patient's cognitive deficits.

3 Laboratory examinations

3.1 Computerized tomography (CT)

Computerized tomography uses the extent of absorption of X-rays to demonstrate pathological changes in the body.

In a CT scanner, X-rays are transmitted through the head from different sides, and their strength measured by detectors on the opposite side. The X-rays' weakening (absorption) during the passage through the head depends on the density of the different tissues within and around the brain. The information from these different projections is transformed by a computer into a series of two-dimensional pictures that show air as black, bone as white, and brain tissue in different shades of grey (Fig. 41.1(a)).

The main criteria for analysing CT scans are:

- *Hypodense* areas which are darker than the surrounding tissue. These indicate ischaemic infarctions, oedema, inflammation, or certain tumours.

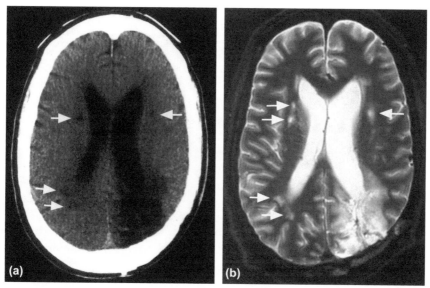

Fig. 41.1 Brain (a) CT and (b) MRI scans of a 57-year-old man 4 months after an ischaemic stroke in the right occipital lobe. He suffered from left hemianopia and hemineglect as well as other visuospatial deficits. There are additional small subcortical infarcts (arrows) that the MRI with its higher resolution shows more clearly than the CT scan.

- *Hyperdense* areas which are lighter than the surrounding tissue. These indicate a fresh bleeding, calcification, or certain tumours.
- Size of the ventricles. An increase in size indicates either hydrocephalus or brain atrophy; a decrease in size indicates brain oedema (swelling of the brain).
- Shape and width of gyri and sulci of the cortical surface. Widened sulci and shrunken gyri indicate brain atrophy; swollen gyri with disappearing sulci indicate brain oedema.

Contrast enhancement can be achieved by intravenous injection of iodide-containing substances. This emphasizes natural and pathological blood vessels, and also areas of disrupted blood–brain barrier, such as infarctions after 2–3 days, abscesses, and some tumours.

The relevance of CT in the context of clinical neuropsychology lies in its ability to depict the anatomical structure of the brain and associated pathologies (Fig. 41.2). These pathologies can be related to findings of neuropsychological deficits. For instance, a patient's expressive aphasia (see Chapter 13) can be explained by the CT finding of a stroke involving Broca's area, and another patient's left hemineglect (see Chapter 5) may correspond to a right parietal tumour. The spatial resolution of CT is approximately 2 mm, which means that anatomical structures or pathological processes have to be at least that big to be detected. CT does not assess the functioning of the brain or its parts.

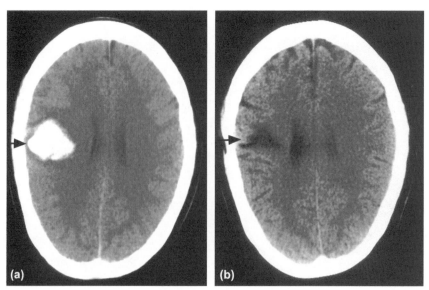

Fig. 41.2 Brain CT scans of a 32-year-old woman who suffered a left hemisphere haemorrhagic stroke (arrows) from an arteriovenous malformation (AVM). She had expressive aphasia and a right hemiparesis. (a) The CT on the day of the stroke shows fresh blood as hyperdense (white) areas. The AVM is not visible here, but was surgically removed after 3 weeks. (b) On the CT scan 8 months later, the blood is completely resorbed, and the resulting brain lesion shows up as hypodense (dark).

3.2 Magnetic resonance imaging (MRI)

MRI uses the magnetic properties of hydrogen protons (H^+) in brain tissue to generate images of the brain. Hydrogen protons constantly rotate ('spin') and therefore act as electrical dipoles. The MRI scanner creates a powerful magnetic field that forces all these protons into a single direction. Their direction is briefly diverted by short electromagnetic impulses and, when they return to their previous state, they emit high-frequency radiation ('echo') that can be measured by the MRI scanner. The characteristic of each proton's echo is influenced by the tissue immediately surrounding it, which allows the computer to generate high-resolution pictures of the different parts of the brain. These images look similar to those of CT, but show in much more detail pathological processes such as ischaemic infarctions (Fig. 41.1(b)), bleedings, inflammation, tumours, pathological blood vessels, hydrocephalus, brain oedema, or atrophy (see Section 3.1). Small lesions that are missed by CT, such as areas of inflammation in multiple sclerosis, can be demonstrated precisely in MRI.

Just as with CT, MRI can be used to examine any part of the body, and the main use of MRI is the depiction of anatomical structures and pathological processes of the brain (Fig. 41.3). The spatial resolution of MRI is better than that of CT, approximately 1 mm. Like CT, MRI does not give us information about the functioning of the brain. Due to the use of a strong magnet, people with pacemakers or with metal implants in their brain or inner ears must not be examined with MRI.

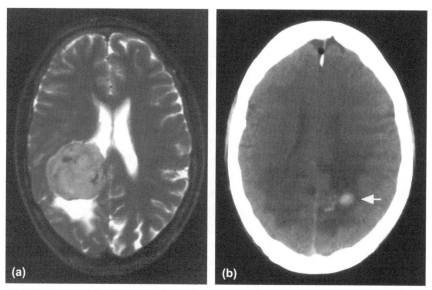

Fig. 41.3 Brain scans of a 46-year-old woman with a meningioma in the left lateral ventricle.
(a) MRI scan before the operation. (b) CT scan 7 days after surgical removal of the tumour. The
right hemisphere was chosen as the surgical access route in order to spare speech-related brain
areas. Note the blood in this region (arrow). After the operation, the patient has moderate
left-sided hemineglect and verbal and nonverbal memory deficits but no disorder of speech.

3.3 Functional MRI (fMRI)

Functional MRI is not a method used in routine clinical practice, but a method of brain
research that shows in which brain areas the blood flow increases while the subject performs a certain activity. It achieves this by making use of the different magnetic properties
of oxygenated haemoglobin and deoxygenated haemoglobin in the bloodstream. An
increased blood flow in a certain brain area is interpreted as a sign of increased activity in
this area. In contrast to MRI itself, fMRI allows us to deduce the functioning of different
brain areas.

3.4 Single-photon emission computer tomography (SPECT) and positron emission tomography (PET)

Both SPECT and PET use radioactive substances ('tracers') that are either injected into
the person's bloodstream or inhaled, and are taken up preferentially into those parts
of the brain which are most active. SPECT and PET therefore provide images of the
blood flow and activity of different brain areas. They are, however, less suited than
MRI and CT to provide a detailed anatomical picture of the brain. Both methods are
increasingly used in clinical routine, e.g. in the evaluation of patients with epilepsy before
surgery, in certain tumours, and in situations where a patient is suspected of having a
mild ischaemia or traumatic brain injury that could not be detected with CT or MRI
scanning.

3.4.1 SPECT

SPECT uses radioactive technetium (^{99m}Tc-HMPAO (hexamethyl propyleneamine oxime)), iodine (^{123}I-IMP (inosine 5'-phosphate)), or ^{133}xenon as its radioactive tracers. During their radioactive decay, they emit photons (γ-quanta), which are measured by one of many γ-cameras which are arranged in a circle around the person's head. From the distribution patterns of the measured γ-quanta, the regional cerebral blood flow (rCBF) in the different parts of the brain can be estimated. The spatial resolution of SPECT is 1–2 cm and the temporal resolution is 30 minutes.

An alternative use of SPECT lies in the use of radioactive tracers that bind specifically to certain receptors. An example of this is the use of ^{123}I-benzamide (IBZM) which binds to D_2 dopamine receptors and therefore provides us with information about the density of these receptors in subjects with (suspected) Parkinson's disease or related conditions.

3.4.2 PET

PET uses radioactive oxygen ($H_2\,^{15}O$), glucose (^{18}F-deoxyglucose), carbon (^{11}C), or nitrogen (^{13}N) as tracers. They are much more unstable than the tracers used in SPECT and emit positrons during their radioactive decay. When one of these positrons collides with a nearby electron, 2 photons (γ-quanta) are released that travel in precisely the opposite direction to each other. Simultaneous measurement of these photons by two γ-cameras on opposite sides of the head ('coincidence measurement') gives information about their source which is more precise than that provided by SPECT. With PET, rCBF and regional cerebral metabolic rate (rCMR) can be estimated. The spatial resolution of PET is 0.5– cm and the temporal resolution approximately 2 minutes.

Like SPECT, PET allows for receptor-binding studies and has been used to examine D_2 dopamine receptors, benzodiazepine receptors, serotonin receptors, and opiate receptors. Because of the fast decay of the tracers used in PET, this method depends on a nearby cyclotron to provide the radioactive substances.

3.5 Angiography

Angiography or arteriography uses conventional X-ray examination after the injection of iodine-containing contrast substance to visualize the arteries and veins. In neurology, one is mostly interested in the arteries and veins of the brain or, sometimes, the spinal cord. Angiography is most useful in showing:

- stenosis (narrowing) of an artery;
- occlusion of an artery or vein;
- aneurysm: a bulging of an artery by a weakness of the artery wall;
- arteriovenous malformation or angioma: a tangle of pathological blood vessels;
- pathological vessels in a brain tumour.

3.6 Electroencephalography (EEG)

This method measures the electrical activity of the cerebral cortex with electrodes that are placed on the scalp (Fig. 41.4(b)).

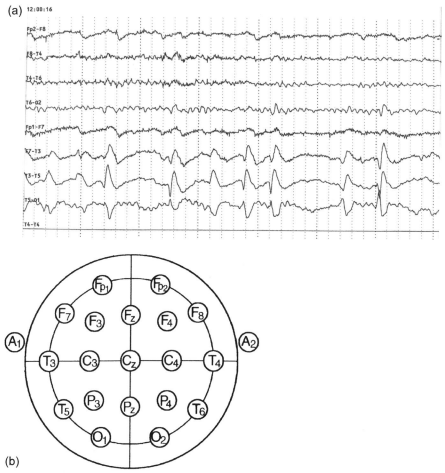

Fig. 41.4 (a) Electroencephalogram (EEG) of a 29-year-old patient with recurring epileptic seizures. The upper four traces demonstrate a normal alpha rhythm over the right hemisphere. The fifth trace is from the frontal part of the left hemisphere and is also normal. The lower three traces are from the posterior part of the left hemisphere and show spike-wave complexes, indicative of an epileptogenic focus in the left temporo-occipital region. (b) The positioning of the EEG electrodes on the skull.

The neurons generate action potentials that spread across the axons and dendrites, and the multitude of action potentials of the cortical neurons adds up to electrical field potentials that can be measured. These field potentials show regular rhythms that are classified as:

- beta, 14–30 Hz;
- alpha, 8–13 Hz;
- theta, 4–7 Hz;
- delta, 1–3 Hz.

These rhythms are probably caused by synchronization of the cortical activity mediated by the thalamus. In rest with the eyes closed, alpha is the predominant rhythm in the healthy adult. During sleep, the slower frequencies become more prominent and sleep-specific wave-forms appear: sleep spindles, vertex sharp transients, and K-complexes.

The EEG gives indications for pathological processes in the brain if the following patterns are found:

- General slowing of the EEG with diffuse theta- and delta-activity occurs in degenerative diseases such as Alzheimer's disease, intoxication, and metabolic encephalopathy (e.g. in liver or kidney dysfunction). In the latter case, the EEG activity can sometimes take the shape of 'triphasic waves' with high amplitude and delta frequency.
- Frontal intermittent rhythmic delta activity (FIRDA) is mainly found in lesions of deep brain structures such as the thalamus.
- Focal changes of rhythm or shape of the EEG waves (e.g. only left parietal) are a sign of an underlying pathological process such as stroke, traumatic brain injury, or brain tumour.
- Epileptic activity is indicated by rhythmic slow waves of unusually high amplitude or by 'sharp waves' that have a pointed rather than sinusoid shape (Fig. 41.4(a)). 'Sharp/slow wave complexes', which show a sharp wave immediately followed by a high-amplitude delta wave, are regarded as proof of epilepsy.

Searching for signs of epileptic activity is by far the most important use of EEG. However, even patients with proven epilepsy can have normal EEG recordings between seizures (inter-ictal EEG). A normal EEG therefore does not exclude epilepsy. If there is sufficient clinical evidence, either a sleep EEG after a wakeful night or a 24-hour EEG recording can then sometimes provide the signs of epileptic activity.

3.7 Evoked responses

Evoked responses are electrical potentials that are recorded from the scalp surface as a response to an external stimulus. They give us information about the functioning of sensory pathways within the nervous system. Visual, auditory, or somatosensory stimuli can be used, and they have in common that hundreds of consecutive stimuli are applied before a reliable evoked response can be measured. The evoked responses consist of a series of waves. The latencies, amplitudes, and shapes of these waves are altered when a sensory system is damaged and therefore allow inferences as to the part of the sensory system that is dysfunctional. A special case is motor-evoked potentials induced by transcranial magnetic stimulation, which are used to examine the functioning of the motor pathways.

- Visual evoked responses (VER) use a flickering draughtboard (checkerboard) for the patient to watch, and they are recorded occipitally over the visual cortical areas.
- Brainstem auditory evoked responses (BAER) are recorded over the mastoid or from the earlobe while the patient listens to click stimuli through headphones.
- Somatosensory evoked responses (SSER) are recorded after stimulation of the median nerve, tibial nerve, peroneal nerve, trigeminal nerve, or pudendal nerve. In addition to

recordings from the scalp over the corresponding somatosensory cortical areas, SSER can also be recorded over the cervical spinal cord.

♦ Motor-evoked potentials (MEP): this method uses electromagnetic impulses to the motor cortex through the scalp (transcranial magnetic stimulation) to elicit electrical potentials in certain target muscles. Their amplitude, shape, and latency give information about the functioning of the motor pathways.

3.8 Event-related potentials (ERPs)

Unlike the evoked responses, which document the reaction of primary cortical areas to an external stimulus, event-related potentials record the responses of secondary cortical areas that occur slightly later. The ERPs are therefore considered to represent cognitive processes such as focusing of attention, detection of a stimulus, and reacting to an unexpected stimulus. The most commonly analysed ERPs are:

♦ P 300: a positive potential with its maximum 300 milliseconds after the stimulus, it can be found during tasks in which the subject is required to watch (or listen to) a series of identical stimuli and recognize occasionally interspersed different stimuli.

♦ N 400: in a task in which the subject reads or listens to sentences, an unexpected word that does not fit into the semantic context and therefore violates expectation is followed by a negative potential 400 milliseconds later.

In spite of intensive research, the precise meaning of the different ERPs is still unclear. They are therefore not commonly used in routine clinical practice.

3.9 Doppler ultrasound

Doppler ultrasound is used to detect a *stenosis* (narrowing) of an artery that leads blood to the brain: the internal carotid artery or the vertebral artery. A probe is pressed on to the skin above one of these arteries in the neck area. It emits ultrasound, which is bounced back from the blood cells and recorded by the same probe. The character of the returning ultrasound signal depends on the speed of the flow of blood cells. This makes it possible to determine where in the underlying artery the speed of the bloodstream is increased, which is an indication of a stenosis in this area. With transcranial Doppler ultrasound, it is even possible to measure the speed of the bloodstream in intracranial arteries, particularly the middle cerebral artery. The finding of a stenosis indicates that the blood supply to a part of the brain may be compromised.

3.10 Cerebrospinal fluid (CSF)

CSF is usually collected by lumbar puncture between the 3rd and 4th or between the 4th and 5th lumbar vertebrae. The analysis of the CSF helps in the diagnosis of the following conditions.

♦ Hydrocephalus: the hydrostatic CSF pressure is increased.
♦ Subarachnoid haemorrhage: the CSF is tainted with blood.

- Inflammation (meningitis or encephalitis): the amount of protein and the number of leukocytes in the CSF are increased. Multiple sclerosis is characterized by oligoclonal bands, with an increase of only a few types of immunoglobulines.
- Tumours: pathological tumour cells can sometimes be found in the CSF.

Selective references

Bradley, W.G., Daroff, R.B., Fenichel, G.M., and Marsden, C.M. (eds.) (2000). *Neurology in clinical practice*. Butterworth Heinemann, Oxford.

Donaghy, M. (ed.) (2001). *Brain's diseases of the nervous system*. Oxford University Press, Oxford.

Gilman, S. (1999). *Clinical examination of the nervous system*. McGraw-Hill, London.

Lee, S.H., Rao, K.C., and Zimmermann, R.A. (1996). *Cranial and spinal MRI and CT*. McGraw-Hill.

Misulis, K.E. (1997). *Essentials of clinical neurophysiology*. Butterworth-Heinemann, Oxford.

Strub, R.L. and Black, W. (1999). *The mental status examination in neurology*. F.A. Davis.

Chapter 42

Neuropsychological deficits within the World Health Organization's model of illness (ICIDH-2)

Derick T. Wade

1 Introduction

Rehabilitation practice needs a conceptual model or framework in which to work. In the past many health professions developed or employed their own model, some explicitly (e.g. Roper's model of nursing), but most less so (e.g. the so-called medical model and the so-called psychosocial model). One advance over the last 20 years has been the growing awareness and acceptance, in research practice at least, of the World Health Organization's (WHO) model of illness embodied in the original International Classification of Impairments, Disabilities, and Handicaps (ICIDH) and more recently revised, expanded, and renamed (as the International Classification of Functioning or ICF) but still referred to as the ICIDH-2 model (Wade and de Jong 2000).

Although widely known in some circles, this model of illness is not always fully understood or used by other health professionals. The WHO's ICIDH is not without controversy and there exist differences of opinion about how certain deficits should be classified. In particular, many clinicians have difficulty placing cognitive difficulties within the WHO's ICIDH-2 model. This appendix provides a possible framework.

The basic ICIDH-2 is shown in Table 42.1 with a revised version in Table 42.2 and Fig. 42.1. This is a slightly revised version that acknowledges that there are subjective (personal to the patient) and objective (observed by outside observers) aspects of most illness (Wade 2001). In addition this version includes pathology (i.e. disease) that is not covered in the ICF, since disease is already covered in the WHO's International Classification of Disease (ICD-10). Finally, the framework includes some acknowledgement of the concept of quality of life (Post *et al.* 1999). Otherwise, the model is essentially the same as the ICIDH-2.

The framework is intended to be used when considering and describing problems faced by patients with brain damage (including cognitive deficits) and provides a common and consistent language between medical and paramedical professionals. Patients seen by clinical neuropsychologists will often (but not necessarily) have an underlying pathology such as frontal lobe infarction (stroke), diffuse axonal injury (after head injury), or degeneration in specific neuronal groups (e.g. Huntington's disease).

Table 42.1 The WHO's ICIDH-2 framework

Level of description	Level of illness	
Term	**Synonym**	**Comment**
Pathology	Disease/diagnosis	Refers to abnormalities or changes in the structure and/or function of an *organ* or *organ system*
Impairment	Symptoms/signs	Refers to abnormalities or changes in the structure and/or function of the *whole body* set in a *personal context*
Activity (was *disability*)	Function/observed behaviour	Refers to abnormalities, changes, or restrictions in the interaction between a person and his/her environment or *physical context* (i.e. changes in the *quality* or *quantity of behaviour*)
Participation (was *handicap*)	Social positions/ roles	Refers to changes, limitation, or abnormalities in the position of the person in their *social context*
Contextual factors		
Domain	**Examples**	**Comment**
Personal	Previous illness	Primarily refers to attitudes, beliefs, and expectations, often arising from previous experience of illness in self or others, but also to personal characteristics
Physical	House, local shops, carers	Primarily refers to local physical structurers but alsoincludes people as carers (not as social partners)
Social	Laws, friends, family	Primarily refers to legal and local cultural setting,including expectations of important others

2 Impairments, disabilities, and handicaps

2.1 Impairments

Abnormal structure or function of the brain (i.e. abnormal neuroanatomy and/or neurophysiology) should be recognized as one cause of impairment to cognitive skills or functions. Emotional disturbance is another potent cause and often a contributing factor. Some patients may have many cognitive impairments such as:

◆ reduced initiation;

◆ reduced ability to recall and/or lay down new memories;

◆ reducing learning;

◆ increased distractability;

◆ inability to shift attention to the left side of space;

◆ inability to use language, etc.

It is difficult to construct a comprehensive framework to encompass all possible cognitive impairments. More importantly, it is crucial to remember that almost all apparent cognitive impairments are extrapolated psychological constructs, largely derived to

Table 42.2 Expanded model of illness

System	Experience/location	
	Subjective/internal	Objective/external
Level of illness		
Person's organ: pathology	Disease: label attached by person, usually on basis of belief	Diagnosis: label attached by others, usually on basis of investigation
Person's body: impairment	Symptoms: somatic sensation, experienced moods, thoughts, etc.	Signs: observable abnormalities (absence or change), explicit or implicit
Person in environment: behaviour	Perceived ability: what person feels they can do, and feeling about quality of performance	Disability/activities: What others note that person does do; quantification of that performance
Person in society: roles	Role satisfaction: person's judgement (valuation) of their own role performance (what and how well)	Handicap/participation: judgement (valuation) of important others (local culture) on role performance (what and how well)
Context of illness		
Internal, personal context	Personality: person's beliefs, attitudes, expectations, goals, etc.	Past history: observed/recorded behaviour prior to and early on in this illness
External, physical context	Salience: person's attitudes towards specific people, locations, etc.	Resources: description of physical (buildings, equipment, etc.) and personal (carers, etc.) resources available
External/social context	Local culture: the people and organizations important to person and their culture; especially family and people in same accommodation	Society: the society lived in and the laws, duties and responsibilities expected from and the rights of members of that society
Totality of illness		
Quality of life: summation of effects	Happiness: person's assessment of and reaction to achievement of or failure to reach important goals *and* sense of being a worthwhile person	Status: society's judgement on success in life; material possessions

explain constrained and naturalistic observed behaviour. As pointed out by Halligan and Marshall (1992), there is, for example, no single brain centre or naturally occurring entity that corresponds to the clinically well established neuropsychological constructs of neglect or aphasia. Both represent constructs employed *post hoc* by clinicians and researchers to refer to specific deficits observed to occur in spatial awareness and language production after right and left brain damage, respectively.

2.2 Disability

Patients may suffer some limitation on or change in the quality of their behaviour (disability or alteration in or limitation of their activities). This can cover anything from maintaining continence through personal activities such as dressing and washing to

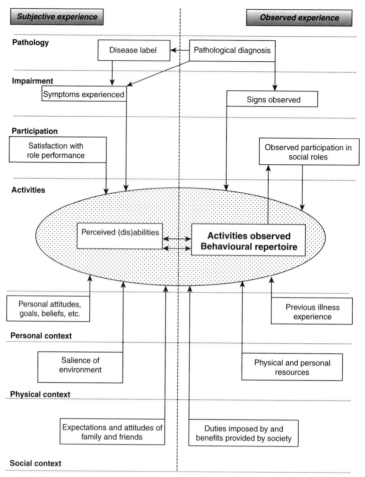

Fig. 42.1 A expanded framework for ICIDH-2.

complex activities such as working, shopping, or participating in conversations. The changes in activities may arise from several different underlying impairments, often in combination. The nature and extent of changes in these activities is greatly influenced by the particular person's physical, personal, and social context (see Section 3).

Some activities of daily living are more likely to be affected by cognitive impairments, but few if any are exclusively and only due to cognitive impairment. Hence it is important to recognize that there are *no* cognitive disabilities, only disabilities that may be attributable to cognitive impairments that are typically demonstrated on clinical or experimental tests.

2.3 Handicap

In illness, patients may experience a change in or limitation on their participation within society, once known as a change at the level of handicap. As for disability, cognitive impairments may be a contributing and, indeed, major factor, but there are no exclusively cognitive handicaps.

3 **The relevance of context**

All patients live within a context that is important for understanding and interpreting the significance of the acquired impairments.

- They have a *personal* context (experiences, beliefs, expectations, attitudes, response styles, etc.). This personal context might be altered by cognitive impairments (but probably less than we expect!). Personal context certainly influences the relationship between cognitive impairment and the resultant disability and handicap.

- Patients also have a *physical* context. The complexity of the environment might well have an influence on how much effect cognitive impairments have and vice versa. For example, an overstimulating environment with complex perceptual demands might lead to aggression in someone with marked cognitive impairments, whereas a well structured environment might help someone.

- Patients have a *social* context. Again this might influence the effect of cognitive impairment. For example, a predictable, stable social context might ameliorate the effects of impaired planning and initiation.

To provide a specific example, a patient might have a subarachnoid haemorrhage (primary pathology) with secondary frontal lobe infarction (secondary pathology) leading to impairment in planning, initiation, and self-awareness (cognitive impairments). In the context of work as a manager in a hospital (social and physical contexts) the person might fail in activities such as chairing meetings or organizing duty rosters, but, at home, in the context of wife and daughter (social and personal contexts), the person might not show any problems and be able to help with such activities as washing dishes. However, if the person's husband fell ill, she might not be able to look after the house.

4 **Implications for treatment**

Treatments can focus on several components and are not mutually exclusive (see Table 42.3), but typically take the form of one of the following four types.

- Some treatments attempt to directly *reduce the impairment*, usually through repetitive practice of the assumed cognitive domain. Usually, this involves a structured set of activities *that are thought to need good function in the impaired domain*. Examples within the area of cognitive deficits are the programmes that are supposed to reduce neglect or improve memory.

- Other treatments focus more on *improving the functional activities* that are affected, again through repeated practice in the specific activities affected. For example, someone with neglect might practise dressing or cooking until able to achieve these activities safely and independently, without the practice being targeted at the assumed impairment.

- Yet other treatments may try to *alter the context*, e.g. through providing external prompts and cues (post-it notes, alarms) or through ensuring a predictable

Table 42.3 Rehabilitation interventions—some examples

Level (term)	Intervention	Comment
Level of illness		
Organ (pathology)	◆ Prevent disease ◆ Reverse or remove pathology ◆ Replace lost physiological function (e.g. insulin) ◆ Give information and advice	Important to know pathology for prognosis and likely impairments; cure often not possible *NB*. Pathology is not always present in an illness
Person (impairment)	◆ Prevent occurrence or worsening of impairment ◆ Reverse or improve impaired skill ◆ Replace lost skill or part with external or internal aid	May use therapy, drugs, orthoses, prostheses, surgery, etc.; may learn technique to overcome loss *NB*. Impairment may improve secondary to functional practice
Person in environment (activities)	◆ Prevent patient learning abnormal behaviours ◆ Teach how to undertake activities in presence of immutable impairments ◆ Practise activities, advising on risks, techniques, etc.	Involves altering behaviour in one way or another. Will often also involve changing the environment. May involve changing patient's goals or goals of others *NB*. This takes time and depends upon learning
Person in society (participation)	◆ Prevent loss of social contacts and roles ◆ Help identify new roles and how to develop them ◆ Ensure patient has opportunities to develop new or maintain old roles	Will almost always involve other people. May involve change in accommodation. For most people work is a central role *NB*. This takes a long time
Context of illness		
Personal context	◆ Prevent development of maladaptive beliefs and expectations ◆ Alter beliefs and expectations if necessary, usually through giving information and psychological therapy	Beliefs and expectations are major determinants of behaviour, but consequences of behaviour may also affect beliefs and expectations
Physical context	◆ Avoid loss of familiar environment if possible ◆ Adjust environment physically, including providing support from other people	Could include environmental control equipment, mobility aids, housing adaptations, etc.
Social context	◆ Adjust or help patient find new social context or help adapt to new social context	Usually strongly linked to accommodation and work
Totality of illness		
Quality of life	◆ Full rehabilitation	

routine through the day. This may involve other people. Many patients with persistent cognitive impairments are best helped in this way.

- Lastly, one may try to *alter expectations and beliefs*, and to find alternative roles and ways of participating in society.

This analysis emphasized that there is no separate cognitive rehabilitation. There is rehabilitation for people with cognitive impairments, rehabilitation that might include trying to reduce the impairment itself but that will include many other interventions. It is also worth noting that much of all rehabilitation involves altering behaviour, a process that depends upon learning, which is a cognitive skill or function. Thus, all rehabilitation is cognitive. It is not surprising, therefore, that patients with neurological disease are perhaps the most difficult to rehabilitate. The very organ and skill needed to succeed in rehabilitation (i.e. the brain and an ability to learn and adapt) are themselves damaged, which often slows the process.

Selective references

Halligan, P.W. and Marshall, J.C. (1992). Left visuo-spatial neglect: a meaningless entity?. *Cortex* **28** (4), 525–35.

Post, M.W.M., de Witte, L.P., and Schrijvers, A.J.P. (1999). Quality of life and the ICIDH: towards an integrated conceptual model for rehabilitation outcomes research. *Clin. Rehabil.* **13**, 5–15.

Wade, D.T. (2001). Disability, rehabilitation and spinal injury. *In Brain's diseases of the nervous system* (ed. M. Donaghy), pp. 185–209. Oxford University Press, Oxford.

Wade, D.T. and de Jong, B. (2000). Recent advances in rehabilitation. *Br. Med. J.* **320**, 1385–8.

Chapter 43

The internet and clinical neuropsychology: privacy, personal safety and effective internet use

Vaughan Bell

1 Introduction

Although only five years have passed since the original version of this chapter was written, it is clear that an update is greatly needed owing to the rapid change in internet technology and culture. This transformation has included the demographics and sophistication of the users, the capabilities of the technology, and the waxing and waning of fashions in both online pursuits and attempts at regulation. To a far greater extent than when the first edition was written, clinical work relies on the internet, and so is increasingly subject to its advantages, problems and dangers. This revised version has a significantly greater focus on personal privacy and safety online, as dangers have become more apparent, and on the diversity and range of internet tools, as the technological possibilities have expanded.

The internet is the single largest and most diverse resource available to clinical neuropsychologists and remains a powerful ally for any patient focused practitioner. It is useful not only because it provides convenient access to a vast array of clinical and scientific information, but also because it allows disparate individuals to widen the informal networks that provide the bedrock of mutual co-operation and education that characterises contemporary clinical science.

This silver lining does not however, come without an accompanying cloud and as with any clinical tool, there are practical and ethical issues that have to be addressed. Increasingly, clinicians need to be aware of the impact of the internet on their privacy and personal safety, as patients, public and other professionals will routinely search for personal information online. Similarly, whilst no clinician would dream of using a novel practice without fully understanding its implications it is not unusual for even the most accomplished of clinical scientists to understand only enough of the internet to facilitate its use without being able to address these issues. This inevitably leads at best to wasted time and frustration, and at worst to serious implications for the welfare of patients (Alejandro et al., 2000).

This chapter aims to provide practical advice so the internet can be used effectively, whilst giving an outline of the additional ethical considerations that internet communication presents.

2 **Personal safety and privacy**

Clinicians have more reasons than most for needing to be competent in managing their online privacy. At the most extreme end, stalking of clinicians has been cited as an 'under-recognised problem' (McIvor and Petch, 2006) and most professionals are unaware of how much personal information can be acquired using the internet. Perhaps less dramatically, clinicians may simply not want their private lives available to anyone who searches for it, and might be concerned that views, opinions or accounts of their participation in informal social events might influence the impression they prefer to portray in their professional lives.

This information comes from two main sources. The first is information that is not intended to be available publicly, but which can be found through unobvious or 'grey' sources; the second is information that is public and appropriate for one audience, but which might be considered inappropriate when found by another.

Many websites or commercial services request personal information and promise to keep it private. Key questions to ask yourself when you enter personal information is 'private from whom?' and 'can I trust the organisation to be honest and competent in their data security?'. It is important to read instructions carefully when entering such information as it may automatically be passed on to other companies (potentially companies who specialise in selling databases of personal information for marketing purposes). Furthermore, the company may be lax in its security, either in terms of its computer facilities (large scale 'personal information theft' from major companies is now a regular occurrence) or its vetting and management of employees. Each individual request should be evaluated in detail, and you may wish to consider using a pseudonym, entering non-identifying details or using a 'throwaway' free webmail account if privacy is of key concern. It is also worth remembering that some online companies specialise in providing access (usually for a fee) to databases of personal information taken from the electoral roll, phone book, or professional registers that would not otherwise be available.

The popularity of online journals, message boards, photo sharing sites, social networking tools and internet dating has meant that people are now revealing much more personal information that was ever possible before. While the majority of this is routine and even banal, the 'ghost of internet past' has come back to haunt certain individuals when circumstances change or unimagined viewers see the material. For example, several high profile cases have been reported where individuals have published fairly unremarkable informal pictures online only to be fired because their employers found them unacceptable. Notably, the law is unclear on the legality of these moves, but if not legally problematic, the unimagined professional or social consequences may be at least uncomfortable.

Clinicians wanting to better control their online privacy need to both be careful of what information they put online, as well as regularly monitor what personal information is available.

Any personal information should be filtered through a consideration of what might be the worst case scenario of the information getting into the wrong hands. While this may seem overly cautious, several projects are now attempting to archive all publicly available internet information, so while the risk now may be minimal, it has to be considered that the information will potentially be available in searchable form indefinitely.

It is also wise to conduct regular internet searches for yourself—searching for your name, email address or titles of personal online resources with popular internet search engines. While some may feel awkward about doing this because of notions about seeming vain, it is an important step in managing your online privacy and will give you an idea of what information can be obtained about you by casual browsers. You may also wish to try with popular 'grey sources' (e.g. online phone directories or registers; 192.com is popular UK service which includes the electoral roll). Notably, many services now have provision for removal of personal information on application.

Importantly, people with uncommon names are at greater risk of being individually identified. A 'Dr Jane Smith' is less at risk of having her privacy breached than a 'Dr Xavier Rubicon', not because she has less personal information online, but because it is less easy to tie specific information with one of the many individuals who share her name.

In terms of patient privacy, patient information is increasingly stored on hospital, service or district-wide databases. While the main responsibility of securing this information from public view and ensuring patient privacy will rest with technical department, choosing secure passwords, not logging in from potentially insecure computers (such as internet cafes) and not printing out unnecessary information will likely to ensure patient confidentiality. One additional concern, however, is that these electronic records are potentially available to a larger number of staff than with paper and file notes. Because records are likely to be stored indefinitely, you may wish to think carefully about what information is entered into these notes, as, for example, details of psychological therapy sessions may contain private details that the person may not want anyone outside their immediate care team to know about.

3 E-mail communication and etiquette

E-mail has always been the *lingua franca* of internet communication by virtue of its ubiquitous nature and flexibility. The utility of a system that allows electronic messages to be delivered to an individual, usually within minutes and regardless of their physical location, would seem to be self evident. As Smith and Senior (2001) have noted, e-mail is becoming the preferred method of communication for the psychologist, and clinical neuropsychologists will undoubtedly find this facility as useful, if not more so, than any other e-mail user. For this reason it is important that clinicians should be fully aware of the facilities, pitfalls and customs that accompany e-mail communication.

Notably, in many countries a 'freedom of information' law may require organisations to make employee emails available to anyone who requests it. Clinicians should therefore be aware that their work emails may become publicly available and are increasingly used as evidence in court. Awareness of this should guide both the style and clarity of writing, as well as decisions about which personal information and communications would be better left to an email system not operated by the employer.

Furthermore, email attachments are a major source of viruses and 'malware': malicious software specifically designed to damage the computer software or steal personal information. Adequate and up-to-date antivirus software should be available and you should be aware that sending non-work material on an employers system is often a dismissible breach of guidelines, regardless of whether anyone takes offence. Similarly, unsolicited email is now a fact of life and much contains innocent looking links to what turns out to be pornographic material or sites designed to fool you into revealing personal information or installing malicious software. Any email from a commercial company (especially a bank) asking you to re-enter login details or payment should be considered highly suspicious. Anything which looks too good to be true probably is. If you are suspicious, searching for the title or text of the email in an internet search engine often reveals the most common (and, only the most common) hoaxes and scams.

3.1 One-to-one email communication

As with any sort of communication, messages must be appropriate to their recipient and so content and style may differ accordingly. However, there are several ways of using the medium to its best advantage for the benefit of both parties.

3.1.1 Write clearly and provide context

Whilst an email may be perfectly understandable in the context of an ongoing dialogue, when read some months or even weeks later it may make little sense. This may not be such an issue for informal communication, but exchanges concerning issues of importance may be referred back to as is frequently the case in clinical settings.

One simple way of doing this is to use context quoting, where the *relevant* section of the received e-mail is quoted with the response added below, like thus:

>I still haven't found the amnesia paper I was after.

Not to worry, I found a copy and will post it to you.

This allows your reply to be concise whilst maintaining context and avoiding the unnecessary bulk of including the whole of the previous email. Quoting or including the whole email may be necessary in some instances (and is becoming increasingly common as fast internet connections are more widely used), but be aware that this can quickly lead to long and confusing emails which may hinder rather than help comprehension of the dialogue.

3.1.2 Use the lowest common denominator

Plain text is preferable to any form of embellishment that an email program may provide such as sending HTML mail (creating and sending email as web pages). Everyone on the internet can read plain text email, not everyone may be able to read any additional features that may be added. Even if you know that the person you are writing to can read your special format of email, this might prevent someone else from reading it if it gets forwarded on as is often the case in the team environments that clinical neuropsychologists commonly work in.

3.1.3 Attachments must be appropriate

Internet connections are becoming faster by the year, and there is no hard and fast rule about what a maximum attachment size should be, but try and be aware of how large attachments are likely to be slower to download and more difficult to manage when retrieved. When sending an attachment state its size and type clearly, as this may not always be obvious to the recipient (e.g. 'the attached paper is a 940k Microsoft Word 2007 file'). If you are technically able and the attachment does not contain private information, it is often better to upload the file to the web and pass on the link to it, so the recipient can download it in their preferred manner.

3.1.4 Remember, email is not written speech

Due to the nature of text based communication many of the subtleties of face to face communication are easily lost, leading to a message being misinterpreted. Particular caution must be taken when using sarcasm, humour or ambiguous statements. Similarly, short functional replies may be interpreted as irritable. Sentences or phrases can be emphasised or softened by the use of punctuation such as asterisks ('I really must *stress* this point') or by using emoticons or 'smileys' to indicate the emotional context of a statement. Excessive use of emoticons is considered a little gauche and most people stick to simplified versions such as :) to indicate positive emotion, for example:

I really enjoyed your talk :)

or :(to indicate a negative emotion, for example:

That's the third time this week :(

3.2 One-to-many email communication

Discussion lists, where email is used to continue an ongoing dialogue with a group of people, can be a source of practical help, support and inspiration as well as a distraction and annoyance. One enquiring email to a group of similarly focused professionals can be worth many hours searching through databases or on the phone, and such lists may also serve as a source of news and announcements and as a way of forming informal associations that can lead to valuable collaborations. Internet discussion lists are however, notorious for bringing out the worst in people, not least because e-mail can so easily be misinterpreted, but also because it is often difficult to fathom the unwritten rules of the group without accidentally violating them.

Simple guidelines (colloquially called 'netiquette') have been formulated to facilitate group interaction in internet discussion groups and include the points covered in our discussion for one to one email communication, with a few additions and alterations.

3.2.1 Attachments should not be sent to a discussion list

Such lists may involve hundreds of subscribers, many of which will not appreciate having to receive a large file that may only be of interest to a minority. If you have a file you wish to disseminate, either ask who wishes to receive it and mail it to them personally, or if possible upload it to a web site and post the location so subscribers can download it at their leisure.

3.2.2 Watch who you are replying to

Additional recipients can be included in an email and by clicking the 'Reply' button you may inadvertently reply to them all. Similarly, if you wish to respond to a public email privately, make sure you are doing so and not accidentally mailing the whole list. Sending a personal email to a public list can be a cause of embarrassment, or in a clinical environment, a potential breach of confidentiality.

3.2.3 Group emails should be of group benefit

Discussion lists are measured by their signal to noise ratio. Lots of irrelevant chatter and 'content-free' contributions encourage an overall decrease in useful interaction and cause genuinely interested people to unsubscribe. That's not to say you necessarily always have to stick exactly to the list topic, but signal heavy content is usually much preferred. In some cases, the discussion list will be moderated so irrelevant messages will not reach the mailing list at all. Furthermore, users often mentally note who sends out useful emails, so sending large numbers of low-relevance messages makes your more important ones less likely to be read.

Recently ethical concerns have been raised about people asking for advice on discussion lists with emails that contain information that may identify the patient (Benkhe, 2007). This is obviously a breach of patient confidentiality and should, of course, be avoided. It is also worth remembering that some comments that will be taken as obviously light-hearted by colleagues may not be similarly appreciated when taken out of context or discovered by later subscribers or people searching the archives.

3.2.4 Don't fan the flames

'Flaming' or the descent into vitriolic argument seems to be a fact of life on internet discussion lists. Clinical practice is, for most practitioners, a passionate interest and is likely to cause heated debate. Whilst it may seem churlish to remind competent professionals that other list members should be treated with respect, I have yet to find a discussion list where this has not happened at least once. Such heated exchanges are usually the result of a perceived but unintended slight, or when the participants do not realise that their exchange has gone beyond an informative debate of general interest into petty pedantry.

4 Using the web

The world wide web has two major advantages for clinical neuropsychologists. Firstly that it allows the targeted retrieval of relevant clinical and scientific information and secondly that it allows information to be easily disseminated with the burden of acquisition placed upon the retriever. Documents, pictures, video or any other sort of digital information need only to be placed on the web, and their existence flagged so interested parties can access them, all without further intervention from the author.

4.1 Targeted searching

It is worth noting that there is more to effective searching than being familiar with the tools. The internet can be thought of as a town. Whilst you may be perfectly competent at buying items in a shop, it is your knowledge of the town that makes this ability useful. Similarly, spending time to overview the general internet resources available to clinical neuropsychologists is often useful for the same reason that general theoretical overviews are useful in any science. Whilst you may not have the information to hand, at least you know the best place to go and find it, saving you valuable time and frustration along the way.

The most useful skill in searching the web for relevant information is not fishing out the gold but filtering out the rubbish. Search engines use entered keywords to identify pages that contain those words somewhere on the page, and hence the best strategy is often not to use words which best describe what you want to find, but to use words which are most likely to appear on pages containing the information you require. For example, searching the web using the keyword 'amnesia' brings up lots of irrelevant information as it is often used as a catchy name for everything from nightclubs to novels. However, a similar search using the keywords 'memory loss' returns lots of highly relevant references.

Humans are inevitably better at evaluating small amounts of information for relevancy than computers, so another useful technique is to use search engines to narrow the field or to give leads. In fields such a clinical neuropsychology where the sources of information may be limited, it is often the case that you may find yourself searching for pages that will then point you to the information you are eventually hoping to find. For example, if I wanted to find information about the notional conference 'Neuropsychology and the Internet' entering these terms may produce a great deal of irrelevant results, either because there may be many pages containing these words which have nothing to do with the conference I wish to find, or because the conference web pages are either non-existent, or have not been catalogued by the search engines' databases. A preferred approach may be to search using the keywords 'Neuropsychology Conferences' to find a page that lists conferences relevant to neuropsychologists (of which there are many) and look for a listing made by an ever reliable human.

Some search engines, and many online databases may allow searches to be made specific by searching for an exact phrase, or by using terms such as AND, OR and NOT. The use of such terms is out of the scope of this particular chapter but almost all facilities that allow such searches have online help and guides in their use. Users of longstanding electronic databases such as PsychINFO/PsychLIT or Medline/PubMed who recognise these terms may find that they can use exactly the same or very similar syntax on many popular internet search engines. These services now typically allow an email alerting service that will regularly run your chosen search and send you any new matching papers added during the week.

One of the key concepts behind the way search engines display their results is an algorithm that works out the popularity of each page that matches the search terms, based on how many other pages link to it. This has now been applied to searches for academic material by using citations rather than links (the most popular being *Google Scholar*; scholar.google.com). This can be a powerful way of quickly getting an overview of an area. For example, if you want to know the key review papers in 'addiction', entering this term will give you a list of which are the most cited (i.e. influential) papers in the field. It is also a useful way of tracking how many citations any particular paper receives over time.

4.2 The power of 'social bookmarking' sites

More recent innovations have included the development of 'social bookmarking' websites. These allow users to maintain an online list of links or references and to add your own keywords to each one. Crucially, it also allows you to search the entire database of all users by a specific keyword. This means when you ask for references tagged 'aphasia', you get all the papers tagged by others as relevant to aphasia. Essentially, you are sampling the distribution of what the user population thinks is relevant and this can often point you towards new conceptual connections or relevant work from other fields. There are now such sites aimed at cataloguing general internet links (e.g. del.icio.us; reddit.com; digg. com) as well as those specifically designed for academic references (e.g. CiteULike.org; Connotea.org). This concept is now standard on many sites that catalogue everything from personal photos to experimental data and can be a powerful way of determining both the depth and breadth of a field or conceptual area.

4.3 Subscribing to 'feeds'

Regularly updated sites often publish 'feeds' or 'RSS feeds', a data format that allows your web browser or dedicated 'feed reader' software to quickly gather and summarise new content (such as new articles, news items or editions of radio programmes) without you having to go to each individual web site to check for updates. These can be integrated into the web browser, work as specific online services (e.g. *Google Reader;* reader.google.com) or as standalone software packages. How to subscribe to each feed varies by method, but an up-to-date list of methods and software is keep on the 'feed reader' page on *Wikipedia* (en.wikipedia.org/wiki/Feed_reader).

4.4 Creating web pages

Internet publishing can, in principal, simplify a great deal of the information distribution problem. Attendees can download notes from your talk, colleagues can retrieve minutes of meetings and important documentation such as ethics forms and other administrative templates, while you can do the same without having to chase after the person with the keys to the right filing cabinet.

In practice, it is a lot more difficult, largely because the easy to use click-and-go tools are not yet available for web publishing as they are for web searching. To publish effectively on the web you either need to put some time and effort into learning the necessary steps, or if working in a suitable institution, have the support of suitably skilled computer or internet technicians.

One of the most important innovations during the last five years has been the widespread use of 'wikis'—websites that use a simplified notation system so users can edit webpage. The most well known is *Wikipedia* (en.wikipedia.org for the English version), an online encyclopaedia where anyone can edit the entries. What sounds like a recipe for disaster actually works remarkably well and demonstrates the power of collective knowledge archiving. Wikis are particularly good for organising information for things like conferences or group projects and work like virtual notice boards that anyone can add useful information to. There are now several services on the net that allow you to set up your own wiki, either for free (e.g. wikia.com) or for a fee (e.g. most commercial internet companies) and often allow you to set the degree of access, so its possible to restrict editing to certain users or administrators if necessary.

To create more complex web sites it is pointless trying to outline all the necessary steps here, both because they will vary wildly depending on the web page hosting arrangements available (institutions own/commercial services/free services) and because high quality easy to understand guides are regularly published in internet magazines and provided by web hosting companies, who often have support lines to aid in technical issues.

As with most technological issues the initial curve is the hardest to climb but once completed, web publishing can be as painless as sending an email.

Some desirable features may or may not be available and it might be worth checking if you feel these might be necessary. Such features may include: password protection for areas or particular documents within your web site, large amounts of storage space, particularly if you wish to disseminate video data, and the ability to run interactive programs, if you wish to make use of certain types of online questionnaires and data collection.

When creating public web pages, you may wish to consider some of the aspects that allow pages to be successfully found via search engines, such as including your own keywords and all the relevant names if a theory, concept or object has alternative naming conventions. Similarly, you may use your own experience of what is pleasant to read and navigate when designing your layout or consult the growing range of books which attempt to explain good web page design to non-computer professionals.

4.5 Making video available online

There are now a multitude of sites (e.g. YouTube.com; video.google.com) which allow video to be uploaded to the web free of charge which can be viewed online, but usually not downloaded to be watched when not connected to the internet. These are often a useful and cheap way of distributing otherwise large video files but bear in mind the quality may be poor in some cases and you may need some assistance with video editing to get optimal results if you are not familiar with the process.

4.6 Blogs and online journals

Blogs are online journals that allow a simple and straightforward way of publishing on the web. There are now a huge number of services that will host your blog for free (with accompanying adverts) and many that will do the same without adverts for only a few dollars a month. Blogs vary in their purpose with some being individual streams of consciousness and others being more journalistic and news-focused. A regular insight into the specialist world of clinical neuropsycholgy can be a powerful way of communicating facts and commentary about recent developments either to a professional or lay audience.

Nevertheless, special care must be taken if you intend to write about your work. A code of ethics has been developed for health care workers who write online (medbloggercode. com) although it is voluntary and has no official status. It is probably worth being aware that while your typical audience may only be a handful of people, anything that is deemed controversial or unwise may have a potential audience of millions so extra care must be taken to ensure that all ethical guidelines are followed. On a more pragmatic level, as blogs can be set up in a matter of minutes with minimal cost they are often a useful way of creating instant news sites for conferences, events, classes or interest groups.

5 **Effective use of internet software**

There are two main problems which may affect a useful internet work session. The first is poor design or broken technology on the remote web site or resource, the second is inefficient use of web browser software.

Frequently, there is little a user can do about remote web site failures or errors, frustrating as they might be. It is however, often worth sending the site administrator a short email pointing out the problem you have encountered. System administrators tend to be somewhat overburdened and are unable to spend vast amounts of time checking every nook and cranny of a complex web site to make sure it still works after every alteration. A polite email pointing out an error in the site is often useful for them, and may mean your required information is fixed within a matter of hours. On a less positive note, technically competent people (especially the overworked ones who are contacted out of the blue), tend to attribute problems to stupidity in the first instance and stop investigating a reported problem (rightly or wrongly) at the first sign that a user might not understand the technology. Less confident users may wish to quickly check with a more experienced colleague that their problem is genuinely with the web site, and not their usage of the software, to increase the chances of a helpful response.

One alternative solution to missing or broken pages is to make use of internet search engines. If you click on a link which leads nowhere, or a web address you have been given does not work, try typing the title of the page into a search engine. If the page has moved, the search engine may have catalogued its new location. Another useful feature, pioneered by the search engine Google (www.google.com) is a system which stores copies of all the pages it knows about. Even if a page has been deleted from its original location, Google may still have a copy in its cache. Simply search for the page as normal, and click the 'Cached' link to see the saved version. A web site called the Way Back Machine (www. archive.org), solely exists for this purpose and has archives of web pages stretching back some years. It is also worth remembering that such archives are kept by third parties if you are considering putting personal or sensitive information on the web. You may be able to remove your own web pages, but will not be able to remove the same information from external archives.

The problem of inefficient web browser use can greatly affect the speed and ease of an internet work session. In the early days of the web, browsers were fairly small and lightweight. They had only limited functionality as web sites were relatively unsophisticated. More recently, due to the demands of newer web site technology, increased multimedia usage and (it has to be said) poor design, browsers have obtained a reputation for being slow, buggy and monolithic. Whilst this situation is gradually improving, a good grasp of how to maximise browser performance may save you a great deal of time and hair-loss.

There are some good practices that apply to almost all computer software you will use. Firstly, it is important to get a good overview of the software, a good habit is to read through all the main menus and familiarise yourself with the options before you start using any new piece of software. This will give you an instant overview of the package's functionality, and will also make any additional documentation (like the electronic help files) much more understandable. Secondly, try and load or enable only the software, features or options that you need. If you feel competent in software configuration, experiment and see which options improve your usage. Often there are many like minded users on the internet, some of which kindly publish their gems of wisdom. A web search using the name of your software package and the word 'hack' or 'optimisation' (or 'optimization' to retrieve pages using the American spelling) as key words will often give you a wealth of information.

An excellent review article by Al-Shahu *et al.* (2002) has lots of useful pointers in this regard, and the table below (Table 43.1) is derived from their paper.

6 Ethics of internet communication

The use of internet communication by clinical neuropsychologists causes some novel ethical dilemmas because of two major considerations. The first is the privacy implications of using the internet and internet software (notorious for their lack of adequate security) for information which you may be legally and ethically bound to keep confidential. The second is the issue of copyright and its use to restrict the dissemination of information which could aid the treatment of patients or education of clinicians, when such dissemination can be conducted for near zero cost when conducted via the internet.

6.1 Internet security and confidentiality

The idea that a patient's medical information should only be available to people directly involved in their medical care, and that it is the carers responsibility to maintain this confidentiality, are core values in the health care system. It will perhaps come as a surprise to many clinicians that sending information over the internet is as confidential as discussing a patient's details on a crowded bus. It may be true that no-one is interested but that does not change the fact that the information is available to many people to whom the patient has not consented access.

With easily available software, any person can intercept and store all of the unencrypted information on your local network without being detected. Government agencies routinely intercept internet traffic, and while this may not be considered a major concern for the majority of patients, it must be noted that in the recent case of General Augusto Pinochet's extradition from the UK, the decision rested on a neuropsychology assessment of his mental fitness. Whilst not all such ethical dilemmas might be as dramatic, each patient should be able to rely on the confidentiality of their clinical records or related information, including when they are communicated via the internet.

Table 43.1 Enhance your use of a browser

Maintain software

- Use the latest version of your browser (determine which version you are using under the 'Help' menu, 'About' in Windows, or Apple menu 'About' on the Macintosh)
- Check for new browser software monthly for the latest security patches.
- Use the latest versions of free software to view multimedia content.
- Install virus protection software and keep it up to date.

Shorten the time you spend on line

- For downloading large amounts of data, use the internet before global use rises (between midnight and noon in Europe).
- If available, use mirror sites (exact copies of web sites) located in, or close to, your own country.
- If the web site allows it, select text-only or low bandwidth options and omit multimedia content if the bandwidth of your connection is low.
- If network response is sluggish, open pages in their own windows and continue working or browsing other pages, and return to them later.

Minimise memory use

- Choose to install only the components of the browser that are essential to you (a full installation can consume many megabytes of disk space)
- Close down browser windows and applications you are no longer using.
- Optimise the size of your cache or "Temporary Internet Files" folder.

Customise your browser

- Set your browser's home page to a blank page (about:blank) or the web site you use the most.
- Organise your 'Favorites' or 'Bookmarks' into folders.
- Set your preferred font type and size (under 'Text Size' on the 'View' menu)
- Maximise the viewable area in your browser by removing the explorer bar and customising toolbars to show only the functions you use (as small icons).

Take short cuts

- When typing web addresses, omit 'http://', as your browser will automatically append it.
- Use copy and paste functions to transfer web addresses between documents and browser.
- Right click (Windows) or click and hold (Macintosh) with your mouse to save images, sounds, or videos from a web site to your hard drive.
- If a web site cannot be found with the web address you have entered use a search engine to see if it available at an alternative location.
- Learn the shortcut keys that allow you to directly type in a web address without having to click on the location bar.

Similarly, much common internet software is susceptible to viruses which can also breach such confidentiality agreements. In the case of one particular virus which exploits vulnerabilities in popular email software, a document is randomly selected and mailed to everyone in the user's address book. This author has personally received a confidential case report which got mailed by this virus to a *public mailing list* which happened to be listed in the infected user's email address book.

One way of assuming responsibility for clinical confidentiality is to ensure that adequate advice is taken on the implications of using particular software and taking precautions to prevent unhappy accidents, such as running up-to-date anti-virus software. In the case of internet communication the use of encryption software to scramble the contents of messages so only the intended recipient can decrypt or unscramble the potentially sensitive information is currently the best method to ensure private communication.

The use of encryption software is, unfortunately, still scarcely used, and not as user friendly as it could be. However, this is rapidly changing, and is becoming accessible to motivated individuals willing to spend a little time learning the ropes. Any clinical neuropsychologists who are provided with their internet access by an employer or institution should push for encryption to be common practice rather than the exception and take good advice from competent computer professionals on suitable software for this purpose.

Clinicians may also wish to consider encryption for storing files on the local disk in case of theft. Luckily, software which creates secure password protected areas is considerably more user-friendly and is readily available. TrueCrypt is a particularly good example of a well-designed, secure and free software package available to do exactly this (truecrypt.org).

6.2 **Electronic publishing**

The debate over the ownership of scientific literature has recently become particularly salient (see Laporte and Hibbitts, 1996, for an excellent analysis), largely because the traditional role of publishers as the cog wheels of journal distribution is becoming increasingly redundant as the internet becomes the preferred method for information dissemination. Since information can be distributed across the internet for near zero cost, questions have been raised about the ethics of using copyright to restrict information which could be used for the benefit of the patient and society at large (Bachrach *et al.*, 1998).

However, whilst no-one would doubt the benefits of peer review in scientific and clinical research, doubts have been raised about the possible decline in quality that may occur if copyright for clinical and scientific journals is abolished (Bloom, 1998).

Clinical neuropsychologists may also face similar dilemmas when producing standardised neuropsychological tests. The question of whether it is ethical to cede copyright to a publisher who may charge large sums of money for a copy of a potentially beneficial clinical test is a thorny issue. For some tests (such as the Block Design subscale of the Wechsler Adult Intelligence Scale) that may require specifically prepared materials that cannot be simply provided as digital templates, it would seem that a third party publisher may be the best method of effective distribution. Many neuropsychological tests are however, produced by publically funded neuropsychologists and can easily be distributed as digital copies to appropriate recipients. Many would argue that to restrict and charge for clinical tests that may be used directly in a patient's care, or in valuable clinical research when a near zero cost distribution method is available, could be considered as unethical, or at the very least, obstructive.

One issue increasingly important issue is the availability of information about neuropsychological tests on the internet which may compromise their validity. Recent surveys of information on medical examinations and tests of malingering found that potentially compromising information was not common, but was available online (Bauer and McCaffrey, 2006; Horwitz and McCaffrey, 2006). Clinicians should be careful not to inadvertently release such information when discussing their work online, and should also attempt to design tests that are not compromised by the material being made available.

References

Alejandro R., Jadad, R., Haynes, B., Hunt, D., Browman, G. P. (2000) The Internet and evidence-based decision-making: a needed synergy for efficient knowledge management in health care. *Canadian Medical Association Journal*, 162 (3), 362–5.

Al-Shahi, R., Sadler, M., Rees, G. & Bateman, D. (2002) Review: The internet. *Journal of Neurology, Neurosurgery and Psychiatry*, 73, 619–628.

Bachrach, S. *et al.* (1998) Intellectual Property: Who Should Own Scientific Papers?. *Science*, 281 (5382), 1459–1460.

Bauer L., McCaffrey R.J. (2006) Coverage of the Test of Memory Malingering, Victoria Symptom Validity Test, and Word Memory Test on the Internet: is test security threatened?. *Archives of Clinical Neuropsychology*, 21 (1), 121–6.

Behnke, S. (2007) Ethics and the Internet: Requesting clinical consultations over listservs. *Monitor on Psychology*, 38 (7), 62. Retrieved from http://www.apa.org/monitor/julaug07/ethicsrounds.html/

Bloom, F. (1998) Editorial: The Rightness of Copyright. *Science*, 281, (5382), 1451.

Horwitz, J.E., McCaffrey, R.J. (2006) A review of internet sites regarding independent medical examinations: implications for clinical neuropsychological practitioners. *Applied Neuropsychology*, 13 (3), 175–9.

Laporte, R. & Hibbitts, B. (1996) Rights, wrongs and journals in the age of cyberspace. *British Medical Journal*, 313, 1609–1612.

McIvor, R.J. & Petch, E. (2006) Stalking of mental health professionals: an underrecognised problem. *British Journal of Psychiatry*, 188, 403–4.

Smith, M.A. & Senior, C. (2001) The internet and clinical psychology: A general review of the implications. *Clinical Psychology Review*, 21 (1), 129–136.

Index